PRIMARY CARE FOR PHYSICIAN ASSISTANTS

PRIMARY CARE FOR PHYSICIAN ASSISTANTS

Editor

Rodney L. Moser, PA-C, PhD

Assistant Professor
Director of Clinical Education
Physician Assistant Program
Central Michigan University
Mount Pleasant, Michigan

Illustrations by Holly R. Fischer, MFA
Ann Arbor, Michigan

McGraw-Hill
Health Professions Division

New York   St. Louis   San Francisco   Auckland   Bogotá   Caracas   Lisbon   London   Madrid   Mexico City
Milan   Montreal   New Delhi   San Juan   Singapore   Sydney   Tokyo   Toronto

McGraw-Hill

A Division of The McGraw·Hill Companies

PRIMARY CARE FOR PHYSICIAN ASSISTANTS

Copyright © 1998 by the McGraw-Hill Companies, Inc. All rights reserved. Printed in the United States of America. Except as permitted under the United States Copyright Act of 1976, no part of this publication may be reproduced or distributed in any form or by any means, or stored in a data base or retrieval system, without the prior written permission of the publisher.

1234567890   QPK QPK   998

ISBN 0-07-043491-3

This book was set in Times Roman by Bi-Comp, Inc.
The editors were John J. Dolan, Lucinda C. Bauer, and Lester A. Sheinis.
The production supervisor was Richard C. Ruzycka.
The cover designer was Joan O'Connor.
The indexer was Kathrin Unger.
Quebecor Printing/Kingsport was printer and binder.

Library of Congress Cataloging-in-Publication Data
Primary care for physician assistants/editor, Rodney L. Moser.
  p. cm.
 Includes bibliographical references and index.
 ISBN 0-07-043491-3
 1. Physicians' assistants—Training of. 2. Physicians'
assistants—Examinations, questions, etc. 3. Primary care
(Medicine)—Examinations, questions, etc. 4. Medical personnel—In-service
training. I. Moser, Rodney L.
 [DNLM: 1. Primary Health Care. 2. Physician Assistants. WB 110
P9524 1998]
R847.P75 1998
616—dc21
DNLM/DLC
for Library of Congress   97-50437
                   CIP

Dedicated to the thousands of
medical professionals
who proudly have "PA" written after their names

CONTENTS

SECTION 6 **Gastroenterology** 187

SECTION 7 **Genetic** 259

SECTION 8 **Hematology** 263

Color plates fall between pages 74 and 75

CONTRIBUTORS

Katherine Adamson, PA-C, MMS
Clinical Coordinator/Instructor
Interservice Physician Assistant Program
Fort Sam Houston, Texas
(Chapters 1–5, 1–12, 9–5)

David P. Asprey, MA, PA-C
Interim Program Director
University of Iowa PA Program
Physican Assistant
Division of Pediatric Cardiology
University of Iowa Hospitals and Clinics
Iowa City, Iowa
(Chapters 1–2, 15–3, 15–8, 15–9)

Laura M. Capozzi, PhD, PA-C
Associate Professor and Program Director
Physican Assistant Program
Central Michigan University
Mount Pleasant, Michigan
(Chapters 10–16, 11–9)

Barry A. Cassidy, PhD, PA-C
Associate Professor and Associate Director
Physician Assistant Program
Midwestern University—Glendale Campus
Glendale, Arizona
(Chapters 17–5, 17–8)

R. Scott Chavez, PA-C, MPA
Physician Assistant Program
Midwestern University
Downers Grove, Illinois
(Chapters 9–31, 11–8)

Stephen M. Cohen, MS, PA-C
Academic Director and Assistant Professor
Physician Assistant Program
Nova Southeastern University
Fort Lauderdale, Florida
(Chapters 10–12, 10–17)

Glen E. Combs, PA-C, MA
Associate Professor
Physician Assistant Program
Bowman Gray School of Medicine
Wake Forest University
Winston-Salem, North Carolina
(Chapters 12–15, 12–16)

Jean M. Covino, PA-C, MPA
Adjunct Associate Professor
Physician Assistant Program
University of Medicine and Dentistry of New Jersey
Piscataway, New Jersey
(Chapters 9–24, 10–9, 12–8, 12–10)

Rick Davis, PA-C
Senior Physician Assistant
Division of Gastroenterology, Hepatology, and Nutrition
University of Florida
Gainesville, Florida
(Chapter 9–30)

Meredith Davison, PhD
Associate Professor and Master's Education Director
Physician Assistant Program
Midwestern University
Downers Grove, Illinois
(Chapter 16–1)

JoAnn Deasy, PA-C, MPH
Director
Physician Assistant Program
Catholic Medical Center of Brooklyn and Queens, Inc.
Jamaica, New York
(Chapters 6–14, 8–1, 8–7, 8–10, 9–4, 9–11, 9–12, 9–15, 17–7)

Richard Dehn, MPA, PA-C
Assistant Director
Physician Assistant Program
University of Iowa
Iowa City, Iowa
(Chapters 3–4, 9–10, 9–16 to 9–18, 9–21, 9–23, 10–5, 15–2, 15–5, 18–3)

Morton A. Diamond, MD, FACP, FACC, FAHA
Professor and Medical Director
Physician Assistant Program
Nova Southeastern University
Fort Lauderdale, Florida
(Chapters 1–1, 1–7, 1–8, 1–11)

Michelle DiBaise, MPAS, PA-C
Physician Assistant and Clinical Research Coordinator
Division of Dermatology
University of Nebraska Medical Center
Omaha, Nebraska
(Chapters 2–5, 2–18, 2–19, 2–23)

Kathleen J. Dobbs, PA-C, MS
Faculty Specialist
College of Osteopathic Medicine
Michigan State University
East Lansing, Michigan
(Chapter 13–3)

John P. Donnelly, PA-C
Director, Cardiac Rehabilitation
Primary Care Clinic
Veterans Affairs Outpatient Clinic
Orlando, Florida
(Chapters 3–10, 17–4)

Timothy C. Evans, MD, PhD
Acting Assistant Professor
School of Medicine
Department of Medicine
University of Washington
Seattle, Washington
(Chapters 5–2 to 5–6, 5–9 to 5–11)

William H. Fenn, PhD, PA-C
Associate Professor
Physician Assistant Department
Western Michigan University
Kalamazoo, Michigan
(Chapters 2–16, 2–17, 2–29, 9–26)

Kathryn Frake, PA-C
Adjunct Instructor
Physician Assistant Program
Central Michigan University
Mount Pleasant, Michigan
(Chapter 9–32)

Dana M. Gallagher, PA-C, MPH
Monterey, California
(Chapters 3–11, 9–25, 12–4, 12–7, 12–9)

Noel J. Genova, MA, PA-C
Staff Physician Assistant
Mercy Family Practice
Portland, Maine
Adjunct Faculty, Research Advisor
Physician Assistant Program
University of New England
Biddeford, Maine
(Chapters 12–12, 12–14)

Anita D. Glicken, MSW
Associate Professor and Psychosocial Coordinator
Child Health Association Physician Assistant Program
University of Colorado Health Science Center
Denver, Colorado
(Chapter 16–4)

Cheryl Gregorio, PA-C
Instructor
Interservice Physician Assistant Program
Army Medical Department Center and School
Fort Sam
Houston, Texas
(Chapters 12–1, 12–6)

Meredith Hansen, MPH, PA-C
Associate Director and Assistant Professor
Physician Assistant Studies Program
The University of Texas Health Science Center–San Antonio
San Antonio, Texas
(Chapters 3–1, 9–6, 9–13, 9–14, 9–22, 9–27)

Anne P. Heinly, PA-C, MMS, MPS
Major, USAF, BSC
Program Supervisor, Phase II, Offutt Air Force Base
Interservice Physician Assistant Program–USAF Branch
Associate Professor of Medicine
University of Nebraska Medical Center
Omaha, Nebraska
(Chapters 6–1, 6–2, 6–4, 6–6 to 6–8, 6–10, 6–11, 6–12, 6–15 to 6–21, 9–3, 13–1)

Janice Herbert-Carter, MD, MGA, FACP
Morehouse School of Medicine
Dept of Medical Education
Atlanta, Georgia
(Chapters 5–1, 5–7, 5–8)

Laura Hess, MSN, ANP
Adult Nurse Practitioner
Sutter Medical Group
Sacramento, California
(Chapter 12–17)

Catherine J. Heymann, RD, CDE, PA-C
Burlingame, California
(Chapters 1–4, 1–6, 17–3)

Katherine D. Hocum, BS, PA-C
Physician Assistant
Federal Medical Center
Rochester, Minnesota
(Chapters 3–5, 3–7)

Pat C. H. Jan, MS, PA-C
Adjunct Faculty
Physician Assistant Program
Midwestern University
Downers Grove, Illinois
Surgical Physician Assistant and PA Educational Coordinator
Thorek Hospital and Medical Center
Chicago, Illinois
(Chapters 6–3, 6–13, 6–22, 6–25, 6–26)

Patricia Kelly, MHS, PA-C
Assistant Professor and Director
Didactic Education
Physician Assistant Program
Central Michigan University
Mount Pleasant, Michigan
(Chapters 13–4 to 13–6, 13–8 to 13–12)

Nadine Kroenke, PA-C
Staff Physician Assistant
Emergency Medicine Specialists
Milwaukee, Wisconsin
(Chapters 3–8, 3–9, 4–5)

Dennis Loudenback, MHS, PA-C
Vascular Surgery
Seattle, Washington
(Chapter 1–3)

David A. Luce, BS, PA-C
Instructor
Physician Assistant Program
Midwestern University
Downers Grove, Illinois
(Chapter 17–1)

Sandra J. Martin, DPM, PA
Department of Orthopaedics
UC David Medical Group
University of California, Davis Medical Center
Sacramento, California
(Chapter 2–10)

Marquitha S. Mayfield, MEd, PA-C
Assistant Professor and Academic Coordinator
Physician Assistant Program
Emory University School of Medicine
Atlanta, Georgia
(Chapters 1–9, 6–5, 6–23)

Joe R. Monroe, PA-C, MPAS
Founder
Society of Dermatology Physician Assistants, Inc.
Vancouver, Washington
(Chapters 2–2 to 2–4, 2–6, 2–8, 2–9, 2–12 to 2–14, 2–20, 2–24
to 2–26)

Rodney L. Moser, PA-C, PhD
Assistant Professor
Director of Clinical Education
Physician Assistant Program
Central Michigan University
Mount Pleasant, Michigan
(Chapters 3–2, 18–6)

William A. Mosier, EdD, PA-C
Director of Research
Center for the Study of Child Development
San Antonio, Texas
(Chapters 7–1, 10–10, 11–1, 11–2, 12–5, 13–2, 16–2, 18–2)

Amelia Naccarto-Coleman, PA-C, MAS
Instructor
Physician Assistant Education
Primary Care Physician Assistant Program
College of Allied Health Professions
Western University of Health Sciences
Pomona, California
(Chapters 12–13, 13–7)

Kelly E. Naylor, PhD
Assistant Professor
Department of Pediatrics
School of Medicine
University of Colorado Health Sciences Center
Denver, Colorado
(Chapter 15–7)

Karen A. Newell, PA-C
Academic Coordinator
Physician Assistant Program
Emory University School of Medicine
Atlanta, Georgia
(Chapters 4–8, 4–9, 6–24, 10–2)

Michaela O'Brien-Norton, PA-C
Emergency Department
Wentworth Douglas Hospital
Dover, New Hampshire
Hahnemann University
Philadelphia, Pennsylvania
(Chapters 4–10, 9–28, 9–29, 18–5)

Claire Babcock O'Connell, MPH, PA-C
Physician Assistant Program
University of Medicine and Dentistry of New Jersey
Piscataway, New Jersey
(Chapters 4–1 to 4–3, 9–1, 9–2, 9–8, 9–9, 17–6)

Maureen MacLeod O'Hara, PA-C
Geriatric Physician Assistant
HealthCare Partners Medical Group
Los Angeles, California
(Chapters 17–2, 17–11)

Wesley T. Ota, OD, FAAO
Staff Optometrist
Sacramento Veterans Administration Outpatient Clinic
Assistant Clinical Professor
UC Berkeley School of Optometry
Clinical Instructor
Department of Ophthalmology
UC Davis School of Medicine
Sacramento, California
(Chapters 14–1 to 14–14, 14–16)

Patti Pagels, PA-C
Instructor
Department of Family Medicine
Health Science Center
University of North Texas
Fort Worth, Texas
(Chapter 10–15)

Kimberly Brown Paterson, MS, RD, PA-C
Emergency Medicine Physician Assistant
Eastern Carolina Emergency Physicians
Wilmington, North Carolina
(Chapters 5–12, 11–7, 15–1)

Daniel P. Radawski, PhD, MD
Associate Professor and Medical Director
Physician Assistant Program
Central Michigan Universigy
Mount Pleasant, Michigan
(Chapter 10–16)

Jill Reichman, MPH, PA-C
Assistant Director and Associate Professor
Rutgers University Physician Assistant Program
University of Medicine and Dentistry of New Jersey
Piscataway, New Jersey
(Chapter 15–6)

Ralph Rice, PA-C
Clinical Assistant Professor
Physician Assistant Program
University of Florida
Gainesville, Florida
(Chapters 4–4, 9–19)

Allan R. Riggs, MS, PA-C
Assistant Professor
Physician Assistant Program
Central Michigan University
Mount Pleasant, Michigan
(Chapter 18–4)

Barbara L. Sauls, MS, PA-C
Clinical Director
Physician Assistant Program
King's College
Wilkes-Barre, Pennsylvania
(Chapters 2–1, 2–7, 2–15, 2–21, 2–22, 2–27, 2–28)

Thomas J. Schymanski, PA-C
Captain
U.S. Army
Physician Assistant

Family Health Center of Fort Belvoir
DeWitt Army Community Hospital
Fort Belvoir, Virginia
(Chapter 15–4)

Pamela Moyers Scott, PA-C
Rainelle Medical Center
Rainelle, West Virginia
(Chapters 3–12, 10–3, 10–4, 10–8, 17–10)

Donald J. Sefcik, DO, MS, RPh
Medical Director
Associate Professor
Physician Assistant Program
Midwestern University
Downers Grove, Illinois
(Chapters 4–7, 18–1)

Freddi Segal-Gidan, PA, PhD
Department of Neurological Sciences and Gerontology
Alzheimer's Disease Diagnostic and Treatment Center
Rancho Los Amigos Medical Center
Downey, California
(Chapters 2–11, 6–9, 11–4, 11–5)

Howell J. Smith III, MMS, PA-C
Associate Director and Assistant Professor
Physician Assistant Program
Nova Southeastern University
Fort Lauderdale, Florida
(Chapters 10–7, 10–14)

Jeffery R. Smith, PA-C
Family Practice and Sports Medicine
Rockwood Clinic, PS
Spokane, Washington
(Chapters 1–10, 4–6)

Francis J. Sousa, MD
Clinical Professor of Ophthalmology, Internal Medicine, and Family Practice
University of California Davis Medical Center
Associate Clinical Professor of Optometry
University of California Berkeley School of Optometry
Sacramento, California
(Chapters 14–1 to 14–14, 14–16)

Don St. John, MA, PA
Physician Assistant
Adult Outpatient Psychiatry
University of Iowa Hospitals and Clinics
Iowa City, Iowa
(Chapters 16–3, 16–5 to 16–7)

Christopher C. Stephanoff, MA, PA-C
Academic Coordinator
Physician Assistant Program
Medical University of South Carolina
Charleston, South Carolina
(Chapter 11–6)

Gloria M. Stewart, EdD, PA-C, ATC
Physician Assistant Studies Program
University of South Dakota School of Medicine
Vermillion, South Dakota
(Chapter 10–1)

Randy Trudeau, PA-C
St. Ignatius, Montana
(Chapter 17–9)

Peggy Valentine, EdD, PA-C
Associate Professor
Physician Assistant Department
Director of National AIDS Minority Information and Education Program
Howard University
Washington, DC
(Chapters 12–2, 12–3, 12–11)

Wayne J. van Deusen, PA-C
Pediatric Provider
Berkeley Primary Care Access Clinic
Berkeley, California
(Chapters 9–20, 10–6)

Suzanne Warnimont, PA-C, MPH
Director and Chairperson
Physician Assistant Program
University of Detroit Mercy
Detroit, Michigan
(Chapters 3–3, 3–6, 14–15)

Andrea G. Weiss, PA-C
Sacramento, California
(Chapter 11–3)

Diane S. Wrigley, PA-C, BS
Blue Hill Hospital
Blue Hill, Maine
(Chapters 8–2 to 8–6, 8–8, 8–9, 8–11, 9–7)

David Zinsmeister, MMS, PA-C
Director
Physician Assistant Program
Assistant Dean
College of Allied Health
Nova Southeastern University
Fort Lauderdale, Florida
(Chapters 10–11, 10–13, 10–14)

PREFACE

Primary Care for Physician Assistants is intended for practicing physician assistants and physician assistant students. Other primary care practitioners, such as nurse practitioners, medical students, and others, will find this thorough, reader-friendly volume beneficial as well.

The book is divided into 18 sections covering the major primary care areas. Within each section are carefully selected presentations that one may encounter in a clinical setting. The consistent chapter structure, index, and cross-references allow easy access to its content. Although quite comprehensive, this book is not intended to replace the encyclopedic works of internal medicine. Rather, the focus is to offer the clinician or student a concise and current overview of a broad spectrum of medical topics, either for rapid clinical reference or as a study guide.

Primary Care for Physician Assistants has a companion question/answer book called *PreTest® Self-Assessment and Review: Primary Care for Physician Assistants.* Containing hundreds of referenced questions, the PreTest will be helpful for self-assessment, as well as preparing for board reviews. Additionally, a concise *Companion Handbook* version of the book will be available as a convenient and portable resource. This "primary care trilogy" should be an invaluable addition to any personal library or curriculum.

ACKNOWLEDGMENTS

The countless hours spent putting this book together has been stressful, exhausting, often overwhelming, but always exhilarating. Without the support of my abused friends, colleagues, and coworkers; my supportive and tolerant PA wife, Lindsey; my five often-neglected children (Kristin, Ryan, Josh, Ben, and Alex); and my aging Macintosh computer, I would not have been able to survive.

There are three overlapping stages of a professional life: *The Learning, the Earning,* and *the Returning.* In the ever-changing science of medicine, learning must be dedicated and lifelong. My *Learning* really began in 1969 when I entered the second class of physician assistants at Alderson-Broaddus College in West Virginia. I entered directly out of high school to join a new and emerging field of medicine—that of the physician assistant. I am grateful to Alderson-Broaddus for taking a chance on this non–banjo-playing Appalachian kid, and to my best friend and brother, Larry, who paved the way.

My *Earning* began in 1973 when I started my first PA job in San Francisco with Bob Haskell, my now-retired lifelong friend and mentor. Those early years in California are now known as my "CAPA years," the years surrounding the founding of the California Academy of Physician Assistants, where friends and colleagues joined together to organize our growing population of physician assistants. To the dinosaurs of CAPA—Juan, Daryl, Harv, Ginny, Frank, and countless others, you have earned my respect and admiration.

My *Returning* started with the thrill of my first publication back in the 70s when I realized that one should educate instead of just medicate. My *Returning* continues now through the editing of the 249 excellent contributions from some of the best writers, clinicians, and educators yet assembled under one cover. Each and every chapter humbled me with the talent that surrounds us. Not to diminish the contributions of all, but some contributors deserve special acknowledgment for agreeing to write a staggering number of topics, for volunteering for extra topics when other contributors dropped out, for tolerating my short deadlines, and for enduring my surgical editing. Those special thanks go to Major Anne Heinly, JoAnn Deasy, Richard Dehn, Timothy Evans, Pat Kelly, Joe Monroe, Will Mosier, Claire Babcock O'Connell, Barbara Sauls, Diane Wrigley, Pamela Moyers Scott, and the ophthalmology team of Francis Sousa and Wesley Ota.

Every contributor helped me share the *Returning* stage of my professional life, and I thank each and every one of them for returning some of their knowledge to this book, and for taking the time to give something back to our profession.

PRIMARY CARE FOR PHYSICIAN ASSISTANTS

Chapter 1–1
CONGESTIVE HEART FAILURE
Morton A. Diamond

DISCUSSION

Heart failure is the only cardiovascular disorder that has increased in frequency in the last decade. Approximately 2 million Americans have this disorder, and it develops in another 400,000 each year. Congestive heart failure (CHF) is best defined in terms of its clinical presentation. The cardinal features include dyspnea, edema, and fatigue. *Congestive heart failure* is a poor diagnostic term, for it does not refer to patients with significant ventricular dysfunction who have no cardiac symptoms, yet those patients can benefit from therapy.

Pathophysiology

CHF patients, regardless of the underlying etiology, can be divided into those with *systolic* failure and those with *diastolic* failure. This classification enables a physician assistant to make an increased correlation between the pathology and the clinical presentation.

Systolic failure is a contractile impairment, a defect in the ability of fibrils to shorten against the load of arterial pressure. An example of pure systolic failure is a patient with CHF secondary to viral myocarditis. Other examples include patients with reduced viable myocardium after infarction and patients with aortic or mitral regurgitation. Patients with systolic failure have a low cardiac output that is manifested as fatigue, weakness, and mental obtundation with the signs of cool skin and reduced blood pressure ("forward failure").

Diastolic heart failure represents an inability of the ventricle to dilate normally during the relaxation phase. The ventricle is abnormally stiff. The problem therefore lies in ventricular filling, not in ventricular ejection. The stiff left ventricle leads to elevated atrial and pulmonary venous pressures without a loss of contractile function. The patient is dyspneic but does not have the symptoms of low cardiac output. Hypertrophy causes a permanent increase in stiffness. In contrast, myocardial ischemia produces a transient increase in stiffness. Examples of pure diastolic failure include hypertrophic cardiomyopathy and infiltrative myocardial diseases such as amyloidosis. It must be recognized that individual patients may manifest concomitant systolic and diastolic impairment.

In CHF, neurohumoral changes occur as a result of the hemodynamic abnormalities in heart failure: increased atrial pressure and reduced cardiac output. These neurohumoral changes relate primarily to the sympathetic nervous system and the renin-angiotensin-aldosterone system. Initially, these compensatory mechanisms are beneficial, since they work to sustain a satisfactory blood pressure and cardiac output. However, the same mechanisms ultimately are destructive and hasten cardiac death.

Risk Factors

Determinants that favor the development of heart failure include increasing age, hypertension, coronary artery disease, diabetes mellitus, obesity, cigarette smoking, and left ventricular hypertrophy of any cause. Both systolic and diastolic forms of hypertension are associated with an increased risk of heart failure. It is noteworthy that these factors have additive risk.

Etiology of Heart Failure

CHF may be caused by coronary artery disease, hypertension, congenital heart disease, cardiomyopathy, rheumatic heart disease, cor pulmonale, and high-cardiac-output states. Regardless of the cause of heart failure, the same underlying pathophysiologic mechanisms—systolic and diastolic dysfunction—are evident.

Precipitating Factors

Many factors may be responsible for the onset of CHF. The primary question a physician assistant must address when caring for a heart failure patient is whether the cardiac disorder is due to myocardial ischemia. If ischemia is the provocation, therapy must increase myocardial perfusion and effect hemodynamic improvement.

A very common precipitating factor is the reduction or cessation of medication intake by a cardiac patient. The medication withdrawal may be due to a sense of well-being or to economic distress. Increased sodium intake, often in the form of snack foods, places an increased burden on the heart and frequently precipitates heart failure. Similarly, medications that increase salt and water retention, for example, nonsteroidal anti-inflammatory drugs, estrogens, and corticosteroids, may initiate clinical heart failure.

Acute hypertension in a previously normotensive patient or a sudden increase in blood pressure in a previously stable hypertensive patient is often responsible for the onset of heart failure.

In caring for a heart failure patient, a physician assistant must consider anemia, infection, and pulmonary embolism as precipitating factors.

Exposure to an uncomfortably high temperature or acute emotional distress in a patient may be responsible for cardiac failure.

Finally, myocardial contractile impairment resulting from acidosis or medications such as beta blockers and doxorubicin may be responsible. Consideration of the precipitating event in heart failure is a primary factor in patient management.

SYMPTOMS AND SIGNS OF LEFT VENTRICULAR FAILURE

The reduced cardiac output in systolic heart failure causes the patient to experience undue fatigue and weakness. As left atrial pressure rises, the patient will note dyspnea and often a nonproductive cough. The breathlessness may initially be present only after effort. As the atrial pressure continues to increase, the patient will note orthopnea, later paroxysmal nocturnal dyspnea, and finally life-threatening pulmonary edema. A pulmonary edema patient coughs up copious quantities of white frothy sputum that may be tinged with blood.

Physical findings in heart failure patients correlate with the degree of hemodynamic compromise. There is generally evidence of increased adrenergic activity manifested as tachycardia, cool skin, and sweating. With mild failure, the patient may be pink and comfortable. With severe failure, the patient is in severe distress and is pale and cyanotic. The blood pressure in a heart failure patient is very variable and is dependent on prior blood pressure, cardiac output, and adrenergic tone. Central venous pressure is normal. Moist pulmonary rales are heard at the lung bases in patients with mild failure. More severe pulmonary congestion causes diffuse rales and pleural effusion. Palpation of the precordium will reflect anatomic and physiologic abnormalities. An apex displaced to the left and downward indicates left ventricular dilatation, while a ventricular lift or heave signifies ventricular hypertrophy. A palpable presystolic (S_4) or protodiastolic (S_3) gallop may be noted. Cardiac auscultation may reveal an S_4 gallop when the atrium contracts more vigorously to fill the stiff left ventricle. A protodiastolic (S_3) gallop and a mitral regurgitant murmur may be heard in a patient with significant ventricular dilatation. Peripheral edema reflects the increased sodium and water retention related to increased aldosterone secretion in heart failure patients. In high-cardiac-output failure, the patient is warm and flushed; this is indicative of peripheral vasodilatation. The pulse pressure is widened, pulses are bounding, and the precordium is active.

SIGNS AND SYMPTOMS OF RIGHT-SIDED HEART FAILURE

Right-sided heart failure most commonly is due to coexistent left-sided CHF. Other important causes include cor pulmonale, pulmonary hypertension caused by congenital disease or another disease, pulmonary valve stenosis, and right ventricular infarction.

Symptoms include weakness and peripheral edema and the symptoms related to hepatic congestion: nausea, anorexia, abdominal discomfort, and increasing abdominal girth resulting from ascites. Physical examination reveals increased central venous pressure, hepatomegaly caused by congestion, hepatojugular reflux, signs of ascites, and peripheral edema. Precordial palpation may reveal the left parasternal lift of right ventricular hypertrophy and the gallop rhythm indicative of systolic or diastolic dysfunction.

HIGH-OUTPUT CARDIAC FAILURE

Cardiac pump function may be supranormal yet inadequate when metabolic demands or requirements for blood flow are excessive. Causes include anemia, arteriovenous fistula (from trauma or arteriovenous shunts), hyperthyroidism, Paget's disease of bone, and beriberi heart disease.

FUNCTIONAL CLASSIFICATION OF FAILURE

The New York Heart Association (NYHA) has defined four categories that assist physician assistants in management and clarify the conclusions reached in clinical heart failure studies:

Class I: no cardiac symptoms with ordinary activity
Class II: cardiac symptoms with marked activity but asymptomatic at rest
Class III: cardiac symptoms with mild activity but asymptomatic at rest
Class IV: cardiac symptoms at rest

LABORATORY TESTS

A complete blood count may reveal anemia that may be a cause of high-output failure or exacerbate underlying cardiac dysfunction. Determination of blood urea nitrogen and serum creatinine may demonstrate prerenal azotemia or chronic renal insufficiency causing hypertensive heart disease. Thyroid and liver function studies and, if recent infarction is suspected, cardiac enzymes should be obtained. Cardiac biopsy and other tests must be considered when an unusual form of cardiomyopathy is suspected.

The electrocardiogram (ECG) will demonstrate arrhythmia, signs of ischemia or infarction, and intraventricular conduction abnormalities.

RADIOLOGIC AND IMAGING STUDIES

A chest x-ray will define the size and shape of the heart, giving information on an underlying heart problem. Examination of the lung fields may demonstrate equalization of blood vessel size at apexes and bases, a sign of early failure, or interstitial (Kerley B lines) or intraalveolar edema. Bilateral or unilateral right effusion is often present. Echocardiography reveals the cardiac chamber size, wall thickness, systolic function (ejection fraction), diastolic (filling) properties of the heart, valvular disease, and pericardial effusion.

TREATMENT

Proper therapy for the patient includes the removal of precipitating factors, education related to diet and activity, medication, and possibly surgery. The severity of the patient's clinical condition will determine whether hospitalization is indicated. Hospitalization generally is recommended for the patient's initial episode of heart failure, for failure related to ischemia or arrhythmia, for those whose symptoms are rapidly accelerating, and for patients who require parenteral therapy.

The patient should be instructed to follow a low-sodium diet, usually 1.5 to 2.0 g daily, engage in moderate activity, and avoid extremes in temperature and humidity. Daily weight measurement can be invaluable in assessing the response to therapy and in early detection of recurrent water retention. Patients with moderate heart failure should receive oxygen and be placed on restricted activity.

Pharmacologic Management

Medication includes diuretics, inotropic agents, vasodilators, and afterload reducing agents such as angiotensin-converting enzyme (ACE) inhibitors. After 200 years of argument, it is now generally accepted that digoxin is valuable in therapy for systolic but not diastolic CHF. The usual dosage is 0.125 to 0.25 mg per day, with adjustment based on concurrent medication, renal function, weight, and any underlying ECG conduction abnormality. Side effects include nausea, vomiting, weakness, and arrhythmias.

Diuretics relieve the breathlessness and edema commonly associated with heart failure. While symptomatic improvement is important, it is noteworthy that these agents do not affect survival favorably. Diuretics lower the cardiac output. Therefore, a heart failure patient taking a diuretic will note lessened dyspnea but increased fatigue. In combination with other agents, diuretics are most efficacious in patients with NYHA class III or class IV failure. Depending on the agent, diuretics have multiple adverse reactions, including hyperglycemia, hyperuricemia, hypercholesterolemia, and hypokalemia. Furosemide and bumetanide producer fewer undesirable metabolic effects. Patients with severe volume overload or significant renal insufficiency should be treated with a loop diuretic.

ACE inhibitors reduce symptoms and lower morbidity and mortality rates in CHF patients. Further, recent studies of patients after a myocardial infarction who had a left ventricular ejection fraction under 40 percent and in whom an ACE inhibitor was started 3 to 16 days after the ischemic event demonstrated a reduction in both recurrent heart failure and mortality rate. All patients receiving diuretics for systolic heart failure should receive an ACE inhibitor. Renal function studies and electrolytes should be checked before the initiation of ACE inhibitor therapy and rechecked at appropriate intervals, since this class of medication may adversely affect blood urea nitrogen (BUN), creatinine, and

Table 1-1-1. Medications Used in the Treatment of
Heart Failure

Drug	Initial Dose mg	Recommended Maximum Dose, mg
Thiazide diuretics		
Hydrochlorothiazide	25 qd	50 qd
Chlorthalidone	25 qd	50 qd
Loop diuretics		
Furosemide	10–40 qd	240 bid
Bumetanide	0.5–1.0 qd	10 qd
Ethacrynic acid	50 qd	200 bid
Thiazide-related diuretic		
Metolazone	2.5*	10 qd
Potassium-sparing diuretics		
Spironolactone	25 qd	100 bid
Triamterene	50 qd	100 bid
Amiloride	5 qd	40 qd
ACE inhibitors		
Enalapril	2.5 bid	20 bid
Captopril	6.25–12.5 tid	100 tid
Lisinopril	5 qd	40 qd
Quinapril	5 bid	20 bid
Digoxin	0.125 qd	As needed
Hydralazine	10–25 tid	100 tid
Isosorbide dinitrate	10 tid	80 tid

* Given as a single test dose initially.

ACE = angiotensin-converting enzyme; bid = twice a day; qd = once
a day; tid = three times a day.

SOURCE: Konstam MA et al (eds): Heart failure: Evaluation and care
of patients with left ventricular systolic dysfunction. Clinical Practice
Guidelines No. 11. Rockville, MD, Department of Health and Human
Services Public Health Service, Agency for Health Care Policy and Research, 1994. AHCPR Publication no. 94-0613.

serum potassium. In certain patients, stable elevations in BUN
and creatinine are acceptable for their symptomatic and clinical
benefit. Potassium supplements should not be ingested, and potassium-sparing diuretics must be used with caution. Other side
effects include cough, which may occur in approximately one-
third of these patients. The medication should be discontinued
only after other causes of cough have been excluded and the
patient finds the cough intolerable. Other potential side effects
include rash, hypotension, and the rare but serious angioneurotic
edema. The initial doses of these agents should be low, with
incremental increases considered at several-day intervals.

Oral vasodilator therapy in the form of hydralazine or nitrates
may be used in addition to or in place of ACE inhibitors. The
vasodilator agents are particularly recommended for heart failure
patients who are unable to tolerate the ACE inhibitors. The
initial doses should be low and should be increased on the basis
of the patient's hemodynamic and symptomatic response.

A patient with acute pulmonary edema should be treated with
oxygen and, if necessary, intubation and assisted ventilation. Intravenous medication generally includes morphine, diuretics, and
nitroprusside or nitroglycerine when blood pressure is preserved.
For a patient in pulmonary edema associated with hypotension
the intravenous inotropic agents dopamine and dobutamine
should be infused. Table 1-1-1 summarizes the medications commonly used to treat heart failure.

OTHER TREATMENT CONSIDERATIONS

Verapamil, nifedipine, and diltiazem should not be used to treat
systolic heart failure. However, in pure diastolic failure these
medications are of value, for they reduce ventricular stiffness. A
diastolic heart failure patient may also receive an ACE inhibitor
to reverse hypertropy and a beta blocker to slow the heart rate.
Beta blocker medication and angiotensin II receptor antagonists
are under investigation as therapy for heart failure. Anticoagulation is indicated in an atrial fibrillation patient who is in CHF.
Heart transplantation should be considered in patients with intractable failure.

BIBLIOGRAPHY

Mair FS: Management of heart failure. *Am Fam Phys* 54:245–254, 1996.
Report to the American College of Cardiology/American Heart Association Task Force on Practice Guidelines; Committee on Evaluation
and Management of Heart Failure: Guidelines for the evaluation and
management of heart failure. *J Am Cell Cardiol* 26:1376–1398, 1995.

Chapter 1–2
CONGENITAL HEART DISEASE
David P. Asprey

DISCUSSION

The incidence of congenital heart disease in the general population is approximately 1 percent (estimates vary from 8 to 12 per
1000 live births). Consequently, most clinicians will provide care
to patients with congenital heart disease during their careers.
Most children with significant congenital heart disease are diagnosed during the first 6 months of life. However, mild forms of
congenital heart disease and occasionally some significant forms
may remain undetected until after 1 year of age.

When a child is diagnosed with congenital heart disease, subsequent siblings have a threefold increase in the likelihood of being
affected. Studies have indicated that the probability of recurrence
is substantially higher when the mother is the affected parent.

There are more than 30 different specific forms of congenital
heart defects. The defects that are most likely to be encountered
by primary care clinicians are

- Ventricular septal defect (VSD): approximately 25 percent of
  all congenital heart defects
- Atrial septal defect (ASD): 6 to 8 percent of all defects
- Patent ductus arteriosus (PDA): 6 to 8 percent of all defects
- Aortic stenosis (AS): approximately 5 percent of all defects
- Pulmonary stenosis (PS): approximately 5 percent of all defects
- Coarctation of the aorta (COA): approximately 5 percent of
  all defects
- Tetralogy of Fallot: approximately 5 percent of all defects

Each of these defects except for tetralogy of Fallot will be discussed in this chapter. The congenital heart defects not included
in this chapter are important but are not covered because of
their infrequent occurrence and the relatively low likelihood that
primary care clinicians will encounter patients with these defects
in their practices.

While many environmental and genetic factors are known to contribute to congenital heart disease, the specific etiology is unknown in approximately 90 percent of cases. Consequently, prevention of congenital heart disease is extremely difficult.

VENTRICULAR SEPTAL DEFECT

Pathology

VSD is the single most common congenital heart defect, accounting for approximately 25 percent of all heart defects. VSD refers to the presence of a communication between the left and right ventricles. This defect occurs as a result of incomplete partitioning of the ventricles during cardiac development. VSDs can occur in numerous places within the ventricular septum. The most common location is the perimembranous region, followed by the muscular or trabecular region of the ventricular septum.

The size of the defect can vary dramatically from a large defect that presents with congestive heart failure and pulmonary hypertension to a very small defect that is hemodynamically insignificant and presents with a murmur but no other signs or symptoms. In VSDs, the pulmonary blood flow is increased above normal. If the increase is significant, it may cause increased pulmonary vascular resistance within the pulmonary arteries, resulting in pulmonary hypertension. When the volume of pulmonary blood flow is twice as great as the systemic blood flow or more, the patient is at significant risk of developing pulmonary hypertension. Pulmonary hypertension develops secondary to the excessive pulmonary blood flow and may become irreversible if it is not corrected by 2 years of age. This pulmonary hypertension can become progressive and ultimately develop into Eisenmenger syndrome, which occurs when the right heart pressures exceed the left heart pressures and the blood begins to shunt from right to left, resulting in systemic cyanosis.

Signs and Symptoms

Often the diagnosis of a VSD is made not during the newborn period but several weeks after birth. This occurs in the newborn because pulmonary vascular resistance remains high as a result of increased smooth muscle mass in the pulmonary arterioles, atelectasis, and alveolar hypoxia. Clinical symptoms are dependent on the degree of shunting, which is determined by the pulmonary vascular resistance and/or the size of the defect. If the VSD is large and the pulmonary vascular resistance is low, the ratio of pulmonary blood flow to systemic blood flow will be high (greater than 2:1). This results in congestive heart failure, which in children is manifested as tachypnea, tachycardia, poor weight gain and growth, diaphoresis with feedings, edema, and decreased exercise tolerance.

Objective Findings

The most characteristic objective finding associated with VSDs is the grade 1 to 5/6 holosystolic murmur that is heard maximally at the middle to lower left sternal border. Often the VSD is small and restrictive (this means that the defect is small enough that it maintains a significant pressure difference between the right and left ventricles), and the characteristic holosystolic murmur is accompanied by a thrill. If the degree of left-to-right shunting is large (the pulmonary blood flow is twice the systemic flow or greater), a diastolic flow rumble will be present at the lower left sternal border. When the pulmonary artery pressure is significantly elevated, P_2 will be increased in intensity.

Diagnostic Considerations

Often a skilled clinician can make the diagnosis of a VSD on the basis of the physical examination and laboratory data alone. While in many instances this diagnosis can be made with a high degree of certainty by examination alone, it is prudent to confirm the diagnosis by echocardiography if it persists beyond 2 years of age.

Laboratory Studies

Electrocardiographic (ECG) findings are useful in grossly quantifying the degree of left-to-right shunting. If the degree of shunting is small, the ECG may be normal. If there is moderate shunting, it may reveal a mild degree of left ventricular hypertrophy (LVH). If the degree of shunting is large, the ECG may demonstrate combined ventricular hypertrophy. In addition, if pulmonary hypertension develops, right ventricular hypertrophy (RVH) will be present.

Radiologic Studies

The chest x-ray finding may vary from normal heart size to cardiomegaly and from normal to increased pulmonary vascular markings, based on the degree of increase in pulmonary blood flow. The echocardiogram is useful in establishing the diagnosis of VSD. In addition, it is instrumental in documenting the location of the VSD and estimating right ventricular pressures and the ratio of pulmonary to systemic blood flow.

Other Diagnostic Studies

In very large VSDs or in children with a VSD in combination with other types of congenital heart defects, cardiac catheterization may be indicated to further delineate the cardiac anatomy and hemodynamics.

Treatment

In the majority of cases, no specific interventions, either medical or surgical, are necessary. However, all individuals who have a confirmed VSD should observe subacute bacterial endocarditis (SBE) prophylaxis.

Medications

In addition to SBE prophylaxis, patients with signs and symptoms of congestive heart failure should be treated with digitalis and/or diuretics.

Surgical Treatment

In patients with a ratio of pulmonary flow to systemic flow greater than 2:1 or pulmonary hypertension, surgical closure of the defect is indicated before age 2. In addition, patients who have congestive heart failure and delayed growth rates are candidates for an elective surgical closure.

Patient Education

Patients with a VSD need to be advised to observe SBE prophylaxis. The parents of newborn infants diagnosed with a VSD should be advised of the signs and symptoms indicating congestive heart failure and should be advised to have the child evaluated by their clinician if those symptoms occur.

Disposition

Approximately one-third of all VSDs undergo spontaneous closure by 2 years of age. One-third remain patent but do not require surgical intervention, and the remaining third require surgical closure.

Complications and Red Flags

Infants who develop congestive heart failure, growth delay, or pulmonary hypertension that is resistant to medical management should be referred for surgical closure of the defect.

Pearls

When a murmur is absent in a newborn and then is detected for the first time at 6 to 8 weeks of life or later, a VSD should be considered. This occurs as a result of the pressure differential that develops as the pulmonary artery pressure decreases after birth.

ATRIAL SEPTAL DEFECT

Pathology

An atrial septal defect refers to any communication or defect in the atrial septum that normally separates the right atrium and left atrium. This communication can occur in one of three different regions of the atrial septum. The most common region for an ASD is the secundum or middle portion of the septum (accounting for approximately 65 percent of all ASDs). This type of defect occurs in the same anatomic location as the foramen ovale, which is the structure that allows the majority of the pulmonary circulation to bypass the lungs in the fetal circulation. In conjunction with the changes that occur in the circulation after birth, the foramen ovale closes and prevents any further right-to-left shunting of the pulmonary blood flow.

The second most common type is the primum ASD, accounting for approximately 30 percent of all ASDs. This defect occurs in the lower portion of the atrial septum and results in a coinciding defect (cleft) in the mitral valve. The primum ASD is typically part of a defect known as an endocardial cushion defect, also referred to as atrioventricular canal defect. The endocardial cushion defect can be partial (primum ASD with cleft mitral valve) or complete (primum ASD, cleft mitral valve, and VSD).

Finally, the ASD can occur at the upper region of the atrial septum near the entrance of the superior vena cava. This defect is known as a sinus venosus ASD and accounts for approximately 5 percent of all ASDs. This particular type of ASD often is associated with a defect known as partial anomalous pulmonary venous return.[1]

In all types of ASDs, left-to-right shunting of blood occurs through the defect. This shunting results in excess blood flow through the right atrium, the right ventricle, and the pulmonary arteries. The degree of shunting can vary dramatically and is dependent on the size and the pressure difference between the right atrium and left atrium. If the degree of excess pulmonary blood flow is significant (ratio of pulmonary blood flow to systemic blood flow greater than 2:1), pulmonary hypertension may develop later in adult life, eventually resulting in Eisenmenger syndrome.

Signs and Symptoms

In the vast majority of cases the patient will be asymptomatic. Occasionally patients report that they fatigue more easily than their peers when the degree of left-to-right shunt is significant.

Objective Findings

In patients with a significant left-to-right shunt, cardiomegaly will result. This may be evident on physical examination by the presence of a slight prominence of the left hemithorax. This finding is most noticeable when one examines the contour of the patient's right and left chest in the supine position, with the examiner standing at the foot of the examining table. Typically, the second heart sound will be widely split and fixed (without variation throughout the respiratory cycle). A systolic ejection murmur, typically grade 2 or 3/6, will be present at the upper left sternal border. If the degree of left-to-right shunt is significant, a diastolic flow rumble will be audible at the lower left sternal border.

Diagnostic Considerations

Patients with an ASD are often asymptomatic, and their physical examination findings are rather subtle; thus, the diagnosis of small ASDs can be very difficult to make. Consequently, it is important that the clinician maintain a high index of suspicion when examining a patient with a systolic ejection murmur in the pulmonary area and/or a fixed, split second heart sound. When these findings are present, an ASD must be ruled out.

Laboratory Studies

The ECG findings may include right axis deviation, right bundle branch block, right ventricular hypertrophy, or an rSr′ pattern in V_1. This pattern in V_1 is indicative of volume overload of the right ventricle.

Radiologic Studies

The chest x-ray findings may include cardiomegaly, prominence of the main pulmonary artery segment, and increased pulmonary vascular markings that are dependent on the degree of left-to-right shunting. The echocardiogram will reveal the presence of the ASD and its specific location. The right atrium, right ventricle, and pulmonary artery may be enlarged.

Other Diagnostic Studies

If the defect is difficult to visualize by echocardiography or if other associated defects are suspected, a cardiac catheterization may be required to further assess the cardiac anatomy and hemodynamics.

Treatment

Medical

Patients with an ASD do not require SBE prophylaxis unless they have other associated abnormalities, such as mitral insufficiency (with primum ASDs) and valvular pulmonary stenosis. Studies are being conducted utilizing nonsurgical closure of ASDs with devices placed into an ASD through a cardiac catheter. When properly placed, these devices can effectively reduce or prevent left-to-right shunting across the ASD.

Surgical

Once the presence of an ASD has been confirmed after the newborn period, surgical closure is indicated. Typically, this repair is recommended before the patient enters school (4 to 5 years of age).

Patient Education

It is important to help the patient and the patient's parents understand that the primary reason for recommending closure of an ASD is preventive. Uncorrected ASDs may result in pulmonary hypertension that will not be detected until well into the adult years. Surgical closure is recommended before school age because the patient is of adequate size to make the procedure safe and it will not interfere with school.

Pearls

Patients with a systolic ejection murmur in the pulmonary region and a fixed split second heart sound should be considered as having an ASD until proved otherwise.

PATENT DUCTUS ARTERIOSUS

Pathology

The ductus arteriosus is an important vascular structure in the fetal circulation that serves to connect the right and left sides of the circulation by allowing a communication between the main pulmonary artery and the descending aorta. In the fetus, this structure allows blood flow to bypass the nonfunctioning lungs. Normally, the ductus arteriosus undergoes closure shortly after birth, thus separating the right and left circulations of the heart. PDAs are more common in infants who are born prematurely.

The amount of left-to-right shunting is dependent on the size of the PDA and the degree of pressure difference between the aorta and the pulmonary artery. In patients with significant left-to-right shunting, pulmonary vascular resistance can become elevated, resulting in the development of pulmonary hypertension.

Signs and Symptoms

The presence or absence of symptoms is dependent on the size of the PDA. If the PDA is small and the amount of left-to-right shunting is insignificant, there will be no symptoms. Conversely, if the PDA is large and the resulting degree of shunting is significant, signs of congestive heart failure may result.

Objective Findings

Typically there is a grade 1 to 3/6 continuous "to-and-fro" murmur at the upper left sternal border. A diastolic rumble may be present at the left lower border in patients who have a moderate to large left-to-right shunt. Accentuated (bounding) peripheral pulses may be noted on examination.

Diagnostic Considerations

PDA typically can be diagnosed by physical examination along with laboratory data. Echocardiography utilizing Doppler color flow mapping is very sensitive in detecting the presence of a PDA.

Laboratory Studies

ECG findings may vary from normal in a small PDA to LVH or even combined ventricular hypertrophy in a large PDA.

Radiologic Studies

The chest x-ray also varies depending on the size of the PDA and its subsequent shunting. In a PDA with a small degree of shunting, the chest x-ray may be normal. In a large PDA, there may be cardiomegaly and increased pulmonary vascular markings. The echocardiogram is very sensitive and can detect PDAs that are not evident by physical examination alone.

Other Diagnostic Studies

Typically there is no need to perform a cardiac catheterization when surgical closure is the chosen treatment. However, some centers are now treating PDAs by closure with a spring or coil device that is placed in a PDA through a catheter. If this treatment is being considered, catheterization also serves as a diagnostic tool in establishing the size of the PDA to help in selecting the correct size of the device.

Treatment

Medical

Patients with a PDA require SBE prophylaxis at times when they are at risk. In children who develop congestive heart failure, digitalis and diuretics may be indicated.

Studies are being conducted utilizing nonsurgical closure of PDAs with devices placed into a PDA through a cardiac catheter. When properly placed, these devices can effectively reduce or prevent left-to-right shunting across a PDA.

Surgical

Once the presence of a PDA has been confirmed beyond the newborn period, surgical ligation and division are indicated. Typically, this repair is recommended after 1 year of age and before the patient enters school (4 to 5 years of age) or at the time of diagnosis in older children.

Patient Education

It is important to help the patient and the patient's parents understand that the primary reason for recommending closure of a PDA is preventive. Closure of the PDA will eliminate the need to observe SBE prophylaxis and reduce the risk of developing SBE. Also, uncorrected PDAs may result in pulmonary hypertension later in life.

Disposition

Once the patient has the PDA closed and has recovered from the surgical procedure, the patient is effectively cured. SBE prophylaxis can be discontinued 6 months after the repair.

Pearls

The continuous number that is characteristic of a PDA can be mimicked by a venous hum (a type of innocent murmur). Be certain you have distinguished between the two murmurs during auscultation.

AORTIC STENOSIS

Pathology

AS results when there is an area of obstruction to blood flow out of the left side of the heart through the aorta. This obstruction most often occurs at the level of the aortic valve but also may occur above the valve (supravalvular) or below the valve (subvalvular). When this obstruction is present, it results in increased left ventricular pressure. This elevated pressure is necessary to create adequate blood flow through the aorta to ensure perfusion of the brain and body. The increased left ventricular pressure results in the development of increased left ventricular muscle mass or LVH.

Valvular AS is the most common form of AS and occurs when the valve is thick and stiffened or is defective, such as a bicuspid aortic valve, which is the most common form of valvular AS. Subvalvular AS can occur as a discrete membrane or can result from more generalized excessive muscle mass, which is the case in idiopathic hypertrophic subaortic stenosis. Supravalvular AS results when the portion of the aorta immediately above the valve has a discrete narrowing.

Signs and Symptoms

At the time of presentation, most patients with mild to moderate AS are asymptomatic. Infants with severe AS may present with the signs and symptoms of congestive heart failure. Children with moderate to severe AS may report decreased exercise tolerance, chest pain, or even syncope.

Objective Findings

Infants with severe AS will have findings consistent with congestive heart failure. Children with AS will have a systolic ejection murmur that is heard maximally at the upper right sternal border. This murmur may be accompanied by a thrill in the suprasternal notch or over the aortic region of the precordium. In addition, if the stenosis is valvular, there typically will be a systolic ejection click that is heard best at the apex. The presence of a high-pitched diastolic murmur is indicative of aortic insufficiency, which may accompany this defect.

Laboratory Studies

ECG findings vary from normal in children with mild AS to LVH in patients with moderate to severe AS.

Radiologic Studies

The chest x-ray findings typically are normal in patients with mild AS. In moderate to severe cases of AS, the ascending aorta may appear enlarged as a result of the poststenotic dilation that results from the turbulent blood flow created by the stenosis. The pulmonary vascular markings will be normal. If cardiomegaly is present, one should also consider aortic insufficiency. The echocardiogram is very useful in establishing the diagnosis along with the location of the obstruction. An estimation of the degree of stenosis can be made by utilizing Doppler measurements of the velocity of the blood flow through the aorta. This test is also useful in screening for the presence of associated aortic insufficiency and for measuring the left ventricle's dimensions.

Other Diagnostic Studies

In infants and children with moderate to severe AS, cardiac catheterization may be indicated to directly measure the degree of obstruction and quantify the degree of associated aortic insufficiency.

Treatment
Medical

Patients with AS should be advised to observe SBE prophylaxis during times of risk. Patients with moderate to severe AS should be advised to avoid strenuous physical exertion. Some centers are attempting to treat valvular AS with balloon dilatation angioplasty during cardiac catheterization, with varying degrees of success.

Surgical

In infants and children with severe AS, surgical treatment may be necessary. There are multiple surgical options available, varying from an aortic valve commissurotomy, to replacing the aortic valve with the patient's pulmonary valve and then placing the aortic valve or a pulmonary homograft in the position of the pulmonary valve (Ross procedure), to artificial valve placement.

Patient Education

AS is a significant and typically progressive form of congenital heart disease. Once a patient has been diagnosed with AS, that patient should be counseled to consider selecting sporting activities and careers that do not require isometric exercise. It is essential that children with AS practice good oral hygiene and observe SBE prophylaxis when indicated.

Disposition

Patients with AS should be monitored frequently during periods of rapid growth. Patients who have significant aortic insufficiency in addition to AS require careful monitoring.

Pearls

AS affects males approximately four times as often as females. In infants and children with confirmed supravalvular AS, consider the diagnosis of William syndrome.

PULMONARY STENOSIS
Pathology

PS results when there is an area of obstruction to the blood flow out of the right side of the heart through the pulmonary artery. This obstruction most often occurs at the level of the pulmonary valve but also may occur above (supravalvular) or below the valve (subvalvular). When the valve is affected, it may be thickened and stiff or dysplastic. When this obstruction is present, it results in increased right ventricular pressure. This elevated pressure is necessary to create adequate blood flow through the pulmonary artery. The increased right ventricular pressure results in the development of increased right ventricular muscle mass or RVH. In addition, the turbulent high-velocity jet of blood that results when the blood is forced through the narrowing causes poststenotic dilation of the pulmonary artery distal to the area of stenosis.

Signs and Symptoms

At the time of presentation, most patients with mild to moderate PS are asymptomatic. Infants with severe PS may present with cyanosis, tachycardia, and tachypnea. Children with moderate to severe PS may report decreased exercise tolerance and dyspnea on exertion.

Objective Findings

A systolic ejection murmur is typically present and is heard maximally at the upper left sternal border. If the stenosis is moderate or severe, the murmur may be accompanied by a thrill that is palpable at the upper left sternal border. The murmur often radiates to the lung fields. When the stenosis is valvular, a systolic ejection click will be present at the upper left sternal border. The presence of a high-pitched diastolic murmur suggests pulmonary insufficiency.

Laboratory Studies

ECG findings vary from normal in mild forms of PS to the presence of RVH in moderate PS and right atrial enlargement and RVH in more severe PS.

Radiologic Studies

Chest x-ray findings are normal in mild PS. The main pulmonary artery segment typically will be dilated in patients with moderate to severe PS as a result of poststenotic dilation. The pulmonary vascular markings are normal; however, in infants who have severe PS, the pulmonary vascular markings may appear diminished. The echocardiogram can be utilized to confirm the specific site of stenosis, assess the pulmonary valve anatomy, and estimate the degree of stenosis through the use of Doppler.

Other Diagnostic Studies

Rarely, a cardiac catheterization is necessary to further define the cardiac anatomy and hemodynamics.

Treatment
Medical

Infants and children with PS should observe SBE prophylaxis. Balloon dilatation angioplasty is a very effective treatment for severe PS. When this treatment is performed at the time of catheterization, it can achieve a significant reduction in the pressure gradient across the pulmonary artery.

Surgical

In infants and children who do not respond to balloon dilatation angioplasty, consideration should be given to surgical treatment. This treatment may consist of pulmonary valvulotomy or the placement of a patch across the right ventricular outflow tract to widen it and thus relieve the obstruction.

Patient Education

It is important for patients with valvular PS to observe SBE prophylaxis. Children with mild PS typically do not progress to severe forms of PS.

Disposition

Children with PS that is not severe should be allowed to participate in all forms of physical activity to their own comfort level.

Pearls

Children with PS and a murmur that is grade 3/6 or less typically have a mild degree of stenosis (less than 30 mmHg gradient across the pulmonary valve).

COARCTATION OF THE AORTA

Pathology

Coarctation of the aorta refers to a narrowing in the descending aorta that occurs during development. When the narrowing is significant, it results in obstruction of blood flow from the heart to the lower half of the body. The degree of narrowing can vary dramatically from trivial to critical in cases where there is a nearly complete interruption of the descending aorta. The body attempts to compensate for the low blood pressure distal to the coarctation (as detected by the renal system) by increasing the systemic blood pressure. This results in systemic hypertension when the blood pressure is measured proximal to the site of the coarctation (i.e., the right arm).

COA affects approximately twice as many males as females. Infants born with severe COA present with the signs and symptoms of congestive heart failure and require immediate medical and surgical management. The discussion in this chapter is limited to children who present with few or no symptoms.

Signs and Symptoms

Most children who do not have critical COA report few or no symptoms. Occasionally these children report a feeling of weakness, fatigue, or even leg pain with vigorous exercise.

Objective Findings

The most consistent finding in children with COA is a differential in the blood pressures obtained in the upper and lower extremities. In association with this finding, the majority of children with COA have a right arm blood pressure that exceeds the ninety-fifth percentile for age. The lower extremity pulses vary depending on the severity of the coarctation and the degree of collateral formation. Collateral arterial blood vessels enlarge and provide a mechanism for blood to bypass the site of the coarctation. If the coarctation is severe and the collaterals are poorly developed, the lower extremity pulses may be absent. If the coarctation is mild to moderate or the collateral formation is extensive, the lower extremity pulses will be decreased but palpable. In addition,

when the pulses are palpable, there will be a delay in the femoral pulse when it is compared in timing to the radial pulse.

A grade 1 to 3/6 systolic murmur is typically audible at the middle left sternal border and in the infrascapular region of the back due to increased blood flow through collateral arteries. Because of the high frequent association of aortic valve disease with this condition, findings of AS or a bicuspid aortic valve also may be present.

Diagnostic Considerations

The findings of the physical examination in patients with a mild COA are often subtle, and therefore a high index of suspicion must be maintained. Patients with mild hypertension or unequal upper and lower extremity pulses must be evaluated carefully for the presence of a COA.

Laboratory Studies

The ECG may range from normal to findings of LVH if the degree of obstruction is severe.

Radiologic Studies

The chest x-ray findings are often subtle but may include mild cardiomegaly. Rib notching may be detectable if a child is of school age or older. Echocardiography is useful in assessing the coarctation site and estimating the degree of narrowing.

Other Diagnostic Studies

Occasionally the coarctation site will be very difficult to visualize by echocardiography, and an MRI may be useful in identifying the anatomy of the aortic arch. In other instances an aortogram may be required to clearly define the arch anatomy.

Treatment

Medical

Children with confirmed systemic hypertension should undergo pharmacologic treatment until the defect is repaired and the blood pressure returns to normal. Some institutions are attempting to treat discrete sites of coarctation with balloon dilatation angioplasty with modest long-term success. SBE prophylaxis should be observed.

Surgical

Asymptomatic patients with confirmed COA and a mild to moderate degree of obstruction can be treated electively at a convenient time. Children with profound hypertension should be considered for repair as soon as possible on a nonemergency basis.

The options for surgical treatment are end-to-end anastomosis and patch repair. An end-to-end anastomosis entails completely dividing the aorta at the site of the coarctation, resecting the defect, and then resuturing the aorta together. A patch repair consists of making a longitudinal slit across the site of the defect and placing a patch in the area of the defect to widen the lumen of the aorta. This patch can be made from a surgical material such as Teflon or from a portion of the left subclavian artery.

Patient Education

Patients with coarctation of the aorta should be advised to monitor their blood pressure closely and should be given guidelines on the indications for notifying their clinicians. Postoperatively, patients may require pharmacologic treatment to control their systemic hypertension.

Disposition

Postoperative patients need routine follow-up for assessment of blood pressure. In addition, if patients are treated surgically before the completion of their growth, they should have the upper and lower extremity blood pressures checked periodically to assess the possibility of a pressure gradient reoccurring. Reoccurrence of a gradient suggests that the coarctation is re-forming. Exercise stress testing including blood pressure monitoring during vigorous exercise is recommended prior to allowing these patients to participate in strenuous exercise such as competitive sports.

Pearls

Most children diagnosed with coarctation of the aorta also have abnormalities of the aortic valve and/or mitral valve. Estimates suggest that as many as 85 percent of patients with coarctation have an associated abnormality of the aortic valve.

REFERENCES

1. Park MK: *The Pediatric Cardiology Handbook,* 2d ed. St. Louis, Mosby, 1997.

BIBLIOGRAPHY

Adams FH, Emmanouilildes GC, Reimenschneider TA, (eds): *Moss' Heart Disease in Infants, Children and Adolescents,* 4th ed. Baltimore, Williams & Wilkins, 1989.

Chapter 1–3
CEREBROVASCULAR ACCIDENT AND TRANSIENT ISCHEMIC ATTACK
Dennis Loudenback

DISCUSSION

Cerebrovascular accident (CVA), or "stroke," is the third leading cause of death in industrialized countries after heart disease and cancer and is a leading cause of long-term disability. More than 500,000 new cases occur each year in the United States, resulting in 150,000 deaths. The most devastating aspect of this disease is the physical and emotional impact on survivors and their families, along with the economic impact on the health care system and the nation in general. The annual cost of stroke in the United States is $30 billion. Roughly 60 percent of this figure involves direct medical costs, while the remainder is due to lost wages and productivity.

Medical and surgical treatments have little or no effect on a completed stroke. These interventions aim only to limit the damage, restore as much function as possible, and reduce the risk of recurrence. Therefore, the most important focus in altering this disease process is prevention. With many recognized modifiable risk factors and predisposing conditions for stroke, it is estimated that 70 percent of all CVAs can be prevented.

A stroke is defined as a neurologic deficit that lasts more than 24 h and is due to infarction of brain tissue. Focal deficits that clear completely within 24 h are called transient ischemic attacks (TIAs); however, they usually last only minutes to a few hours.

Events of intermediate duration—24 h to 1 week—may be called reversible ischemic neurologic deficits (RINDs). This term is seldom used, since a deficit lasting that long is almost certainly due to infarction and such a fine distinction of duration does not change the approach to the patient. These definitions are by convention only, helping to classify a particular event, and not all patients fit precisely into one group. What may be a TIA by the strict definition may actually be a small infarction that is well compensated. Surrounding brain tissues may resume the functions of the infarcted area, resulting in a rapid resolution of symptoms.

A basic knowledge of cerebrovascular anatomy and physiology is crucial in understanding the various mechanisms of stroke. The cerebral blood flow is abundant, receiving 750 ml/min at rest, supplied by four principal vessels: the paired vertebral and carotid arteries. The carotid arteries supply the anterior cerebral circulation, while the vertebrals supply the posterior circulation (Fig. 1-3-1).

Aortic Arch

Three main arteries stem from the aortic arch: the so-called great vessels:

- The innominate artery (or brachiocephalic trunk) divides to become the right subclavian artery and the right common carotid artery (CCA).
- The left common carotid artery.
- The left subclavian artery.

There are well-known congenital anomalies of the great vessels, usually affecting their origins, but they only rarely play a role in stroke.

Carotid Arteries

Each CCA courses upward in the neck, where it branches at the level of the thyroid cartilage to become the external and internal carotid arteries. The external carotid artery (ECA) supplies the face and scalp but also serves as an important source of collateral blood flow around the eye in cases of severe narrowing or occlusion of the internal carotid artery (ICA). Blood flow is capable of reversing direction in the ophthalmic artery, providing an indirect (collateral) source of blood to the brain.

The ICA travels upward behind the angle of the jaw, passes into the base of the skull, and emerges from the temporal bone to take an S-shaped course known as the carotid siphon. This portion of the ICA may occasionally become a source of stenosis, emboli, or occlusion, resulting in cerebral ischemia. The ICA continues to the base of the cerebral hemispheres, where it joins the circle of Willis, but just before this structure it gives rise to the ophthalmic artery, which supplies the eye and the surrounding structures. Impaired flow in this vessel or the terminal branches of the retinal artery may result in the transient visual loss known as amaurosis fugax.

Circle of Willis

A unique vascular structure, the circle of Willis is the most important source of collateral blood flow to the brain when any of the principal feeding vessels become diseased. It lies at the base of the cerebral hemispheres, anterior to the brainstem and encircling the pituitary gland. A single anterior communicating artery (ACOM) and paired posterior communicating arteries (PCOMs) allow for "crossing over" of blood from one hemisphere to the other or from the anterior circulation to the posterior circulation if needed (Fig. 1-3-2). Numerous anatomic variants exist in the circle of Willis, with only 20 percent of the population having the "classic" anatomy described above. Ten to 25 percent of the

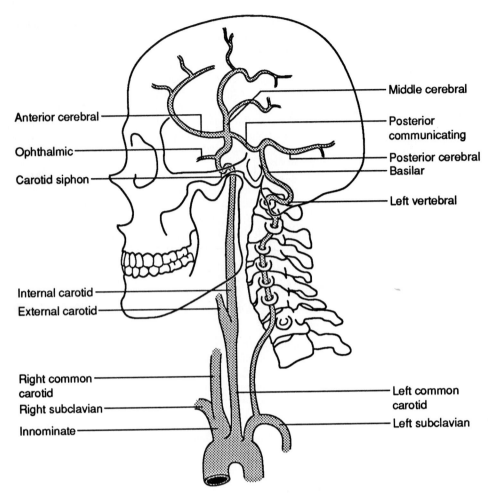

Figure 1-3-1. Cerebrovascular anatomy and aortic arch.

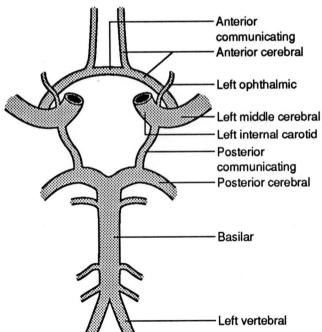

Figure 1-3-2. The circle of Willis as seen from below.

population has a small or functionally absent ACOM or PCOM, severely limiting potential pathways for collateral blood flow.

Vertebrobasilar System

Each vertebral artery originates from its respective subclavian artery, traveling posteriorly and cephalad through the transverse processes of the cervical vertebrae before entering the foramen magnum at the base of the skull. The two arteries then course anterior to the brainstem before joining to become the single basilar artery, which ultimately becomes continuous with the circle of Willis. Ten percent of the population has at least one vertebral artery that is too small to contribute significantly to brainstem blood flow, which is important if the other vertebral artery becomes diseased. Narrowing of the vertebral artery origins is common but rarely causes cerebral ischemia in and of itself.

RISK FACTORS

The major risk factors for stroke are similar to those for heart disease, while others are unique to cerebrovascular disease (Table 1-3-1). Most CVAs occur in the elderly as a result of the increased incidence of atherosclerosis in that group. In the young the etiology is quite different, usually being due to congenital maladies such as aneurysms and arteriovenous malformations (AVMs), trauma, arterial dissection, or drugs such as cocaine and amphetamines. Stroke is slightly more prevalent in males than in females, and whites have more TIAs while black persons have more strokes and therefore deaths.

Table 1-3-1. Risk Factors for Cerebrovascular Disease

Prior stroke or TIA
Hypertension
Diabetes
Smoking
Hyperlipidemia
Obesity
Hypercoagulable states
Alcohol
Drugs (amphetamines, cocaine)
Migraines
Family history
Gender
Ethnicity
Cardiac disease
    atrial fibrillation/flutter
    recent myocardial infarction
    valvular disease
    endocarditis
    ventricular aneurysm
    septal defects
    tumor (atrial myxoma)

The most important modifiable risk factor is hypertension, which plays a crucial role in most causes of stroke and is the primary risk factor in certain types of CVA, such as lacunar infarcts and intracerebral hemorrhage. The important contribution of hypertension was shown in the SHEP study, where lowering the blood pressure of men and women age 60 and older with isolated systolic hypertension (>160 mmHg) resulted in a 36 percent reduction in stroke over 4 years.[1]

Heart disease is also important as it relates to cardiogenic emboli, which cause one-third of all strokes. Every form of cardiac disease carries an increased risk of stroke, but the single most important one is atrial fibrillation, which accounts for roughly 50 percent of all cardiogenic emboli. Recent myocardial infarctions (usually in the first few weeks) cause approximately 20 percent of these emboli as a result of local wall motion abnormalities, where an intramural thrombus may form and enter the arterial circulation. Cardiac valve abnormalities (from rheumatic disease) may result in the valvular vegetations that cause approximately 10 percent of all cardiogenic emboli. The remainder can be attributed to prosthetic cardiac valves and relatively rare causes of stroke such as endocarditis and septal defects.

A stroke risk is associated with female smokers who have a history of migraine headaches and also take oral contraceptive pills (OCPs). This is presumably due to cerebral vasospasm induced by migraines coupled with a hypercoagulable state brought on by OCPs and smoking. The degree of increased risk is not clear, but it is certainly quite small. One group of investigators estimated 19 strokes per 100,000 women with migraines.[2] From a primary care point of view, it is important to recognize that atherosclerosis is the underlying cause of most CVAs, and risk factor modification should be directed at preventing its occurrence.

PATHOPHYSIOLOGY

There are numerous etiologies for stroke, each with its own mechanism, treatment, and prognosis, but they generally may be classified as ischemic or hemorrhagic in nature (Table 1-3-2). The brain maintains an appropriate cerebral blood flow at a given instant through autoregulation, which it can sustain until the mean arterial pressure falls to near 60 mmHg, at which point cerebral perfusion depends on gravity. Isolated episodes of hypotension caused by syncope or orthostasis usually do not result in significant cerebral ischemia or infarction. However, the prolonged hypotension that occurs in cardiac arrest may result in infarction of poorly perfused "watershed" areas between major vascular territories.

Ischemic Stroke

Approximately 85 percent of all strokes are due to ischemia caused by arterial or cardiac pathology. The most common causes of ischemic stroke relate directly or indirectly to atherosclerosis. Atherosclerotic plaques have a predilection for arterial curves, branches, and origins. Severe stenoses may form in the extracranial or intracranial vessels, resulting in ischemia caused by low flow, thrombosis, or embolization. Plaques may rupture, causing embolization by showering debris downstream or by becoming a nidus for platelet and fibrin deposition, which also may embolize.

Atherosclerosis may lead to stroke indirectly through coronary artery disease, resulting in myocardial infarction, arrhythmias, and some forms of valvular disease.

The heart is the most common source of emboli to the brain, with the ICA ("artery-to-artery") emboli being somewhat less common. Roughly 80 percent of cerebral emboli travel to the middle cerebral artery (MCA) distribution, 10 percent go to the posterior cerebral artery (PCA), and the remainder go to the vertebrobasilar system.

Lacunar infarctions cause 20 to 25 percent of all ischemic strokes. They are due to ischemia in small penetrating vessels of the deep white matter that arise from the vertebral and basilar arteries, the circle of Willis, and the MCA. Disease in these very small vessels usually is due to lipohyalinization caused by chronic hypertension. Lacunar infarcts also are found in patients with carotid disease and diabetes.

A TIA is an important clinical entity because it gives the clinician an opportunity to offer treatment before a more devastating CVA can occur. However, fewer than half of all patients with ischemic stroke have premonitory TIAs. Among patients with a TIA, 33 percent will suffer a stroke within 5 years, with no way to predict its severity. The risk of subsequent stroke is highest in the first month after an initial TIA and gradually tapers over the ensuing months. Amaurosis fugax is a monocular visual loss that results from ischemia within the retinal artery caused by low flow, occlusion, or emboli within the ipsilateral (occurring on the same side) ICA. The risk of subsequent CVA is slightly lower in amaurosis fugax than in hemispheric TIA, and permanent visual loss is rare. The mechanisms for TIA and CVA are the same.

Hemorrhagic Stroke

Approximately 15 percent of all strokes are due to intracranial hemorrhage. Nontraumatic subarachnoid hemorrhage (SAH)

Table 1-3-2. Stroke Classifications

Ischemic (85%)

    Embolic
        cardiogenic
        artery-to-artery
        unknown source
    Thrombotic

Hemorrhagic (15%)

    Subarachnoid hemorrhage
        saccular aneurysm
        arteriovenous malformation
        other
    Intracerebral hemorrhage

most often is due to the rupture of an intracranial saccular or "berry" aneurysm, usually presenting between ages 30 and 65. The vast majority (85 percent) of these hemorrhages form in the anterior cerebral circulation, usually at the junction of the anterior cerebral artery and the ACOM. Bleeding into the subarachnoid space may cause vasospasm of nearby cerebral vessels, resulting in further ischemia. Saccular aneurysm rupture has a poor prognosis, with a 10 percent mortality rate in the first 24 h and 25 percent more over 3 months. Twenty percent rebleed within 2 weeks, and at least half the survivors will have severe neurologic deficits.

The majority of the remainder of SAHs are due to AVMs, which refer to an abnormal tangle of vessels between the arteries and veins. They are more common in males, have a heritable component, and primarily affect the young. The highest risk of rupture is at ages 10 to 30, but AVMs may occasionally present as late as 50 years old. SAH caused by an AVM carries a slightly better prognosis than does a saccular aneurysm rupture, as the rate of rebleeding and vasospasm is lower.

An intracerebral hemorrhage (ICH) usually is due to large hypertensive hemorrhages that are not necessarily associated with exertion and most commonly occur during the daytime hours. Other causes of ICH include intracerebral AVMs and aneurysms, blood dyscrasias, trauma, neoplasms, and anticoagulation medications. They may result in mass effects and increased intracranial pressure, with a generally poor prognosis ranging from a 30 to 80 percent mortality rate.

SIGNS AND SYMPTOMS

Perhaps the most common presentation is actually asymptomatic ischemia or infarction. Many so-called silent infarcts are found incidentally on computed tomography (CT) scans, and the patient has no recollection of these infarcts. Similarly, some people are found to have entirely occluded carotid arteries without neurologic sequelae. This is a testament to the rich collateral blood flow to the brain in most individuals. Cerebrovascular disease usually manifests as a focal neurologic deficit affecting motor, sensory, visual, or communication functions. Presenting signs and symptoms reveal which portion of the brain is affected and may suggest a mechanism for the injury. All strokes may vary in severity from nearly asymptomatic to fatal, depending on the location, the extent of injury, and collateral flow (Table 1-3-3).

Hemispheric Stroke

Ischemia and infarction of the cerebral hemispheres constitute the most common presentation for stroke and depend on which cerebral vessel is affected and to what degree. The most common signs and symptoms are contralateral hemiparesis, hemiplegia and hemisensory loss of the face and limbs, homonymous hemianopia, conjugate eye deviations, and ipsilateral monocular visual loss. Aphasia may occur if the dominant hemisphere is affected (the left hemisphere in right-handed individuals and more than 75 percent of left-handed persons). Anosognosia, or hemineglect, is caused by ischemia of the nondominant hemisphere, while dysarthria may result from ischemia of either hemisphere. Strokes resulting from emboli usually have an abrupt onset of symptoms with a maximal deficit, whereas thrombotic or other causes may develop more gradually. Embolic strokes also have a tendency to show fluctuating symptoms as the embolus lyses, migrates, or partially occludes a vessel.

TIAs may present with the symptoms described above but with complete, rapid resolution of the deficit. Amaurosis fugax usually is described as a "shade" coming down or across the visual field or occasionally as a loss of peripheral vision. Patients also may complain of facial or limb numbness (usually the arm).

Table 1-3-3. Common Terms and Definitions in Cerebrovascular Disease

Term	Definition
Hemiparesis	Muscular weakness on one side of the body
Hemiplegia	Paralysis on one side of the body
Ataxia	Lack of muscle coordination
Aphasia	Defect in the expression of language, including speech, reading, and writing, resulting from a central nervous system injury
Dysarthria	Imperfect articulation of speech caused by loss of muscle control in the forming of words
Dysphagia	Difficulty swallowing
Homonymous hemianopia	Defective vision or blindness in half the visual field, occurring in the same location in each eye
Anosognosia	An inability to perceive a defect, especially hemiplegia, on one side of the body
Hemineglect	An impaired response to stimuli from one side of the body

Lacunar infarctions usually have a rapid onset but may present over hours to days. Recovery tends to occur quickly. There are many well-known lacunar syndromes, the most common of which are pure motor hemiparesis, pure sensory hemiparesis, dysarthria and hand weakness, and ataxia and leg weakness. Patients also may present with sensorimotor deficits that are more typical of hemispheric stroke.

Ischemia or infarction in the posterior cerebral (vertebrobasilar) circulation may affect the brainstem, cerebellum, temporal lobes, or occipital lobe. This manifests most commonly as dizziness, vertigo, diplopia, and ataxia (usually without weakness). It also may present with nystagmus, dysarthria, dysphagia, cranial nerve palsies, hemiplegia, eye movement paralysis, pupillary changes, hoarseness, various visual changes, and visual hallucinations. Hemiparesis is rare in patients with posterior infarcts. Since the cranial nerves originate in this region, these infarctions may present with cranial nerve signs contralateral to somatic signs, for instance, left facial numbness and right arm clumsiness.

Cerebellar and brainstem infarctions may rapidly result in respiratory arrest because of brainstem compression, since the posterior fossa of the skull does not allow for much swelling. Edema in this area may cause hydrocephalus, brainstem compression, coma, and death. Early signs and symptoms of this impending disaster may be subtle, consisting only of gait disturbances (inability to stand or walk) or changes in the level of consciousness.

Syncope is usually a manifestation of hypotension or cardiac disease (arrhythmias, aortic stenosis) and usually is not seen in someone presenting with an ischemic stroke or TIA. Similarly, vertigo or dizziness without any other brainstem, cerebellar, or occipital signs is not considered consistent with posterior ischemia. Instead, it usually is due to eighth cranial nerve or labyrinthine disease.

Subclavian steal syndrome is caused by severe narrowing or occlusion of the subclavian artery proximal to the origin of the vertebral artery. When the arm on the ipsilateral side is exercised, the patient may experience symptoms of vertebrobasilar insufficiency (dizziness, diplopia, gait disturbances). This occurs because the vertebral artery undergoes a reversal of flow, becoming a source of blood for the upper extremity, in effect "stealing" blood from the posterior cerebral circulation. Although this phenomenon may be demonstrated in many people by ultrasound examination, it rarely results in ischemia or infarction.

"Stroke in evolution," also known as "stuttering stroke," represents a medical emergency in which a neurologic deficit is found to be progressing in a stepwise fashion over minutes or hours. It frequently is due to a severely stenotic or acutely occluded vessel, and a devastating stroke may be averted if rapid medical or surgical therapy is initiated.

Hemorrhagic Stroke

Hemorrhagic strokes from all causes commonly present with headache but also may show signs of increased intracranial pressure (ICP). Rupture of an intracranial saccular aneurysm usually presents as "the worst headache in my life" and frequently is accompanied by a sudden, temporary loss of consciousness. However, headache may be the only presenting complaint. Patients may have a prodromal phase of headache or cranial nerve signs as the enlarging aneurysm compresses nearby structures.

Intracranial hemorrhage also has a rapid onset and may be accompanied by headache and signs of elevated ICP, including nausea, vomiting, and changes in mental status. Focal neurologic deficits, if present, depend on the site of the bleeding as brain tissues are dissected by an expanding hematoma.

OBJECTIVE FINDINGS

A full history and a physical examination are essential regardless of whether a patient undergoes a routine screening examination or presents with acute stroke. The details and intricacies of this are beyond the scope of this chapter, but a few important points are highlighted below.

A careful patient history may uncover past episodes of minor cerebral ischemia that may have been disregarded by the patient or the patient's family as unimportant or "just due to old age." Direct inquiries should be made about numbness, weakness, or clumsiness of facial and limb movements; changes in vision; "splotches" or "shades" in one eye; clumsiness in writing or handling an object; dizziness and vertigo; and slurring of speech.

Physical examination of the patient should rule out potential cardiac causes of stroke, such as atrial fibrillation and valvular disease. A thorough eye examination should be done, including pupillary responses to light, extraocular movements (to check for nystagmus and gaze paralysis or deviations), visual fields by confrontation (some patients may be unaware of a visual field cut because of hemineglect), and a funduscopic exam to look for small-vessel disease of hypertension and diabetes and rule out papilledema caused by increased ICP.

In both symptomatic and asymptomatic patients a search for arterial bruits should be done. Supraclavicular and carotid bruits are the most frequently encountered, with a high-pitched systolic bruit fading into diastole arousing suspicion of a high-grade stenosis. However, not every bruit is caused by a significant narrowing, and the absence of one does not rule out significant stenosis. The lesion may be so severely stenotic or even occluded that no bruit is generated.

In a symptomatic patient a full neurologic exam should be performed to document any subtle deficits and serve as a baseline if the condition worsens. Elements of the neurologic exam should include mental status (assessment of language, memory, comprehension, etc.), cranial nerves, reflexes, and motor, sensory, and cerebellar functions such as gait and fine movements.

DIAGNOSTIC CONSIDERATIONS

The differential diagnosis for stroke is vast (Table 1-3-4), but if the most common causes are excluded, most of the other etiologies will present in a way that suggests a diagnosis. For example, a patient with stroke symptoms, fever, bacteremia, and intracranial

Table 1-3-4. Differential Diagnosis for Stroke

Cardiac

  arrythmias
  mural thrombus
  septal defects
  valvular disease
  infectious

Vascular

  atherosclerotic
  dissection
  compression
  lipohyalinosis
  inflammatory (granulomatous, arteritides, etc.)
  vasospasm (drugs, migraines, SAH)
  aneurysm/AVM

Hematologic

  hypercoagulable states (SLE, pregnancy, polycythemia, etc.)
  blood dyscrasias, clotting abnormalities (warfarin therapy, etc.)

Other Conditions Causing Focal Neurologic Changes

  intracranial tumor
  hypoglycemia
  subdural hematoma
  migraine headache
  focal seizure
  infectious (tuberculosis, fungal, HIV/AIDS)

abscesses on CT will suggest septic emboli secondary to bacterial endocarditis.

LABORATORY TESTS

Basic laboratory tests required for the initial presentation of stroke include a complete blood count (hematocrit, hemoglobin, platelets, white and red cell indices), electrolytes, blood urea nitrogen, creatinine, serum glucose, prothrombin and partial thromboplastin times, ECG, and chest x-ray. Serum cholesterol should be checked for the purpose of general risk-factor modification. Other tests should be ordered as indicated by each situation, for instance, a toxicology screen if cocaine is suspected, special tests to differentiate hypercoagulable states, and the erythrocyte sedimentation rate (ESR) in vasculitis and other inflammatory conditions.

RADIOLOGIC STUDIES

In the acute CVA presentation, CT examination of the head should be performed to rule out structural problems (such as mass-occupying lesions, dural hematomas, old infarcts, and acute hemorrhages) or if one is considering anticoagulation. CT scans are a good first choice because of their relatively low cost and accessibility in most communities. However, they have deficiencies in some instances. Detection of small hemorrhages (approximately 1 cm) is possible very early, but CT is much less sensitive in finding an early infarction. In acute stroke, CT scans detect infarcts only 5 percent of the time in the first 4 h, 50 percent in the first 24 h, and 95 percent by the eighth day. They also may miss cortical infarcts, lacunar infarcts, and small infarcts in the posterior fossa or brainstem as a result of bony interference.

Magnetic resonance imaging (MRI) is much more sensitive for detecting early infarctions as well as visualizing the entire brain, including the cortex, the lacunae of the deep white matter, and the posterior fossa. However, it is generally more expensive and less commonly found and has contraindications to its use, such as pacemakers, other implanted metal devices, and external equipment such as respirators.

Angiography is considered the gold standard for evaluating the patency of the carotid and the intracranial vessels. It is not an entirely benign procedure, carrying a 2 to 12 percent risk of bleeding, infection, catheter-related trauma, or stroke, and therefore is done only in special clinical situations at the direction of a surgeon, neurologist, or interventional radiologist.

OTHER DIAGNOSTICS

Duplex ultrasonography of the carotid, subclavian, and intracranial vessels is a valuable diagnostic tool. It provides not only physical information such as the locations and severity of stenoses but also physiologic information such as the direction of flow in a given vessel to indicate collateralization. It is also inexpensive and carries none of the risks of an invasive diagnostic procedure. Important potential deficiencies of ultrasound include stenoses in the mild to moderate range (near 60 percent) and very severely narrowed or preocclusive lesions of the carotid artery, which may be misinterpreted as total occlusions.

Echocardiography (transthoracic or transesophageal) is commonly performed to evaluate possible cardiogenic causes of stroke. Valvular vegetations, mural thrombus, and wall motion abnormalities are easily detected by this study.

TREATMENT

Stroke Prevention

The primary care focus should be on altering modifiable risk factors such as hypertension, diabetes, hyperlipidemia, atrial fibrillation, obesity, and smoking. Other treatments are tailored to specific causes of stroke, such as known carotid lesions and structural heart abnormalities.

Anticoagulants

Systemic heparinization is controversial in acute stroke because of the risk of hemorrhage into the infarct zone and probably should be used only under the direction of a neurologist. It is an extremely useful and potent medication for use in recurrent emboli, arterial dissection, and acutely thrombosed vessels and in preparation for surgery as well as for hypercoagulable states in which long-term warfarin (Coumadin) therapy is initiated.

Warfarin has been clearly shown to reduce the risk of stroke in patients with atrial fibrillation. An International Normalized Ratio (INR) of 2 to 3 is recommended for this indication. Warfarin also may be used in situations where antiplatelet agents have failed or are contraindicated (nonsteroidal anti-inflammatory drug sensitivities, gastric irritation, etc.) and in special circumstances such as complete carotid occlusion, in which the uppermost end of the occlusion may serve as an embolic source to the cerebral circulation. Warfarin also may be used in symptomatic patients for whom surgery is contraindicated.

Antiplatelet Agents

Aspirin and ticlopidine (Ticlid) have been shown to decrease the risk of subsequent stroke in patients with a minor completed stroke. Aspirin is the primary antiplatelet agent used in stroke prevention since it is inexpensive and is well tolerated by most people. It is used primarily for asymptomatic carotid stenosis or for symptomatic stenosis in the mild to moderate range. The most effective dose is controversial, ranging from 80 to 325 mg daily. Ticlopidine is as effective as aspirin in stroke reduction but is considerably more expensive and is associated with side effects, including diarrhea and gastrointestinal upset, and it is occasionally associated with neutropenia. Therefore, it requires monitoring of white blood cell counts every 2 weeks for the first 3 months

of therapy. The usual dose is 250 mg twice daily. It generally is reserved for patients who have contraindications to aspirin.

Carotid Endarterectomy

Three randomized studies have shown the superiority of carotid endarterectomy to aspirin alone in preventing subsequent stroke in symptomatic patients with greater than 70 percent carotid stenosis. In asymptomatic patients, the Asymptomatic Carotid Atherosclerosis Study (ACAS) has shown a slightly decreased risk of stroke over 5 years in patients with greater than 60 percent stenosis if the surgical risk is 3 percent or less.[3] The ACAS study determined the degree of stenosis by angiography, which means that the combined risk of angiography and surgery must not exceed 3 percent for a benefit to be seen. Severe asymptomatic stenoses (greater than 80 percent) may be at increased risk of embolizaton and therefore may benefit from surgery coupled with aggressive risk-factor modification if a patient is a good surgical risk and has a life expectancy that is thought to extend beyond 5 years.

ASYMPTOMATIC CAROTID BRUITS

Carotid bruits are commonly found in elderly patients and those with risk factors for atherosclerosis. The first step in their management is to determine the degree of narrowing by duplex ultrasonography. All patients with carotid plaques probably should be instructed to take at least 80 mg of aspirin daily for overall risk reduction. Severe stenoses should be referred to a vascular surgeon for evaluation. Otherwise, periodic examinations and follow-up ultrasound should be performed to determine whether the plaque is stable or progressing. Patients and their family members should be educated about stroke and TIA symptoms and instructed to notify the practitioner immediately if they occur.

MANAGEMENT OF ACUTE STROKE

Management of an acute CVA patient depends on the severity of the presentation. It is recommended to involve a neurologist in all but the most minor CVAs for a thorough evaluation and documentation of the neurologic deficits and to maximize the treatment and rehabilitation potential of the patient. The intricacies of stroke treatment are beyond the scope of this chapter, but some fundamental knowledge is presented here. As always, the initial step is addressing the ABCs of airway, breathing, and circulation. Difficulty handling secretions is common in stroke patients because of dysphagia or impaired gag reflex, and so airways should be protected to prevent aspiration. One should bear in mind that cardiac arrhythmias can be the cause of or can result from a CVA.

Hypertension is commonly seen in acute stroke, with diastolic pressure as high as 115 mmHg. Treatment for this is controversial, but in most cases the blood pressure should not be lowered. This is a protective mechanism induced by the brain to maintain blood flow to the poorly perfused infarct zone. Treatment of hypertension generally should be undertaken only if signs of end organ damage are present, such as angina, congestive heart failure, papilledema, hematuria, and retinal hemorrhages. In large intracranial hemorrhages caused by severe hypertension, the blood pressure may gingerly be lowered by about 25 percent over the first 24 h, but this must be done slowly, as the brain requires high perfusion pressure. It is also important to control pyrexia (occurs in one-third of stroke patients) with acetaminophen because of the increased metabolic demands this places on the brain. Hyperglycemia should be kept to 150 mg/dL or less because excess glucose is converted to lactic acid, which may exacerbate tissue damage.

Stroke in evolution is a medical emergency that should involve a neurologist immediately to determine its cause, which is frequently acute occlusion of an intracranial or extracranial vessel. Anticoagulation, surgery, and thrombolytic therapies are all controversial in acute or evolving stroke patients but may avert a devastating or fatal stroke if applied early and appropriately. These patients should be kept flat in bed to maximize cerebral blood flow.

All subarachnoid hemorrhages require neurosurgical consultation to determine whether cerebral angiography or surgery is required. Patients should be kept in a dark, quiet room with adequate analgesia. These measures are aimed at preventing rebleeding while one is awaiting neurosurgical evaluation.

Large intracranial hemorrhages resulting in increased ICP also may require neurosurgical consultation for decompression if they are anatomically accessible. Patients with infarcts in the posterior fossa can deteriorate rapidly because of brainstem compression. Neurosurgical consultation should be obtained early in these patients if signs of increased ICP are present. All patients with intracerebral hemorrhages should be kept with the head of the bed elevated 30° to prevent cerebral edema.

Future Developments

The latest major advance in the treatment of acute stroke has occurred in the field of thrombolytic therapy. Just as thrombolytics have launched a revolution in the treatment of acute myocardial infarction, tissue plasminogen activator (t-PA) has recently been approved by the U.S. Food and Drug Administration for treatment of acute stroke. However, relatively few clinical trials have been done with this technology, and so the clinical parameters in which it may be used are still narrow. It is expected that as more experience and knowledge are gained, this new treatment may dramatically decrease the severity of stroke and the number of completed strokes if it is initiated early in the course.

REFERENCES

1. SHEP Cooperative Research Group: Prevention of stroke by antihypertensive drug treatment in older persons with isolated systolic hypertension: Final results of the Systolic Hypertension in the Elderly Program (SHEP). *JAMA* 265:3255–3264, 1991.
2. Tzourio C et al: Case-controlled study of migraine and risk of ischaemic stroke in young women. *BMJ* 310(6983):830–833, 1995.
3. Executive Committee for the Asymptomatic Carotid Atherosclerotic Study: Endarterectomy for asymptomatic carotid artery stenosis. *JAMA* 273(18):1421–1459, 1995.

BIBLIOGRAPHY

Bronner LL, Kanter DS, Manson JE: Primary prevention of stroke. *New Engl J Med* 333:1392–1399, 1995.
Dobkin B: The economic impact of stroke. *Neurology* 45(Suppl 1):S6–S9, 1995.
Fauci AS, Braunwald E, Isselbacher KJ, et al, eds: *Harrison's Principles of Internal Medicine,* 14th ed. New York, McGraw-Hill, 1998, pp 2325–2348.
Gorelick P: Stroke prevention. *Arch Neurol* 52:347–355, 1995.
Pryse-Phillips W, Yegappan MC: Management of acute stroke: Ways to minimize damage and maximize recovery. *Postgrad Med* 96(5):75–85, 1994.
Roth GJ, Calverley DC: Aspirin, platelets, and thrombosis: Theory and practice. *Blood* 83(4):885–898, 1994.
Rowland LP, ed: *Merritt's Textbook of Neurology,* 9th ed. Media, PA, Williams & Wilkins, 1995, pp 227–285.
Rutherford RB (ed): *Vascular Surgery*, 4th ed. Philadelphia, Saunders, 1995, pp 1456–1660.
Schwartz GR, Cayten CG, Mangelsen MA, et al, eds: *Principles and Practice of Emergency Medicine,* 3d ed. Malvern, PA, Lea & Febiger, 1992, pp 1523–1533.

Chapter 1–4
ATHEROSCLEROSIS
Catherine J. Heymann

DISCUSSION

Derived from the Greek *athero* ("porridge or gruel") and *sklerosis* ("hardening"), atherosclerosis is one of the leading causes of death in the United States. Atherosclerotic vascular disease (ASVD) affects the intimal layer of the artery, resulting in plaque formation, narrowing of the lumen, decreased elasticity, alterations in contractility, and reduced blood flow.

ASVD begins in early childhood and slowly progresses to symptomatic disease in adults. The disease begins with the formation of a "fatty streak" within the arterial wall. Smooth muscle cells gradually surround the fatty streak, forming a fibrous cap. Through the years, the lesion fills with fibromuscular and/or fibrolipid material. As unhealthy lipid levels and risk factors persist, the lesion continues to grow and eventually encroaches into the arterial lumen. If the lesion ruptures and forms a thrombus, partial or complete occlusion of the artery will occur, producing ischemia, infarction, or sudden death.

A positive correlation between elevated serum lipid levels and atherosclerotic plaque formation is firmly established in the literature. Total cholesterol (TC) is divided into five general lipoprotein subclasses according to the density of each particle. Each lipoprotein subclass has a distinct chemical structure, a specific role in lipid metabolism, and implications for ASVD. It is important to remember that atherosclerotic plaque formation may exist even if the TC is within "normal" ranges. This paradox has focused attention on the role of low-density lipoprotein cholesterol (LDL-C) subclasses in plaque formation.

A strong correlation has been established between several other risk factors and ASVD. If known risk factors are treated, the incidence of ASVD may be reduced and its progression slowed or regressed. Risk factors are classified as modifiable or nonmodifiable (Table 1-4-1); fortunately, a "nonmodifiable" risk factor may be ameliorated by intensive management of treatable risk factors. For example, a family history of premature heart disease is a nonmodifiable risk factor. However, if a low plasma cholesterol and appropriate ratios of lipoprotein subclasses are maintained by optimizing modifiable risk factors, ASVD may be reduced or eliminated.

The preferred treatment modality—prevention—is classified as primary or secondary. In primary prevention, measures to avoid the development of ASVD are initiated. Secondary preven-

Table 1-4-1. Risk Factors for ASVD

Nonreversible	Reversible
Age	Cigarette smoking
Gender	Hypertension
Family history of premature coronary artery disease	Hyperlipidemia
	HDL-C <35 mg/dL
Hyperinsulinemia	Elevated lipoprotein (a)
Genetic factors	LDL-C >160 mg/dL
	Homocysteinemia
	Diabetes mellitus and carbohydrate intolerance
	Abdominal obesity with a waist/hip ratio >0.8 in women and 1.0 in men
	Sedentary life-style

Table 1-4-2. Normal Artery Physiology

Intima
  Inner lining of artery
  Permeable and allows passive transport of LDL-C to subepithelial
    space
  Able to secrete several chemical factors needed for blood flow
Media
  Composed of smooth-muscle cells bound by elastic and fibrous
    tissue
  Secondary site of atherosclerotic plaque formation as disease
    progresses
Adventitia
  Arteries' outermost layer

tion focuses on arresting the progression of ASVD after clinical disease is evident.

PATHOGENESIS

A three-layer permeable pipe, the artery is metabolically active. It maintains and repairs its structural components by secreting fatty acids, cholesterol, phospholipids, triglycerides, growth factors, and enzymes. A free exchange of fluids and solutes in blood takes place through the arterial membrane (Table 1-4-2). Plaque formation has overlapping yet distinct developmental phases: lipid deposition, cellular transport, and plaque thrombosis.

Lipid Deposition

Atherosclerosis begins with the deposition of LDL-C in the subepithelial (intimal) space of the arterial wall. Once inside the subepithelial space, LDL-C is oxidized and taken up by macrophages, producing "foam cells." The foam cells eventually form a fatty streak in the vessel wall and are the earliest manifestation of the atherosclerotic process. A fatty streak has few clinical sequelae and does not encroach into the arterial lumen.

Cellular Transport

Smooth-muscle cells migrate to and proliferate around the fatty streak, eventually forming a fibrous plaque. Ultimately, the lesion protrudes into the arterial lumen, causing stenosis. Vessels with up to 90 percent occlusion may remain patent and relatively asymptomatic and provide an adequate blood supply to distal tissues.

Plaque Thrombosis

A plaque thrombus usually occurs in a soft, unstable lesion of 50 to 60 percent stenosis. These uncalcified plaque formations are more likely to rupture, causing occlusion, ischemia, and infarction of distal tissues. Calcified plaque is more stable and is less likely to rupture. Plaque progression also may result in an arterial wall weakness or aneurysm, especially in the abdominal aorta.

MICROBIOLOGY

No viral or bacterial pathogens have been identified in ASVD. A recent study found *Chlamydia pneumoniae* in 89 percent of the arteries of patients with atherosclerotic plaque and only 4 percent of the arteries of control subjects. Numerous studies will be needed to define this organism's role, if any, in ASVD.[1]

SYMPTOMS

Sudden death may be the first and last symptom of ASVD. Atherosclerotic plaque produces few perceivable symptoms until the stenosis reaches critical levels or ruptures suddenly. Location of the occlusive lesion usually determines any symptomatology. Patients may report a slow onset of angina, dyspnea, intermittent claudication, fatigue, cold extremities, arrhythmias, or transient ischemic attacks (TIAs).

OBJECTIVE FINDINGS

Subtle clues during history taking and physical examination may suggest the presence of ASVD, but a definitive diagnosis must rely on angiography or various radiologic modalities. Disease may be surprisingly localized or widely diffuse. Each major organ system should be evaluated carefully for evidence of atherosclerosis. (Table 1-4-3) Laboratory data, chest radiography, ECG, or exercise stress testing may provide additional evidence of ASVD. Referral to a cardiologist or vascular surgeon may be appropriate.

DIAGNOSTIC CONSIDERATIONS

The diagnosis of ASVD is often presumptive and is based on the functional, physiologic, or metabolic effects of a narrowed arterial lumen. Differential diagnoses of common presenting symptoms—fatigue, dyspnea, chest pain, claudication, and peripheral edema—should be considered (Table 1-4-4).

Etiologies unrelated to atherogenesis also may result in a decreased arterial lumen diameter. Therefore, the course of disease and treatment modalities may be substantially different from those of plaque formation, stenosis, and occlusion.

Table 1-4-3. Clues to ASVD on Physical Examination

Fundoscopic examination
  "Silver wire" veins
  Altered artery/vein ratio
  Arteriovenous "nicking"
  Hollenhorst plaque
Cardiac examination
  New-onset murmurs
  Arrhythmias
  S_3 (atrial gallops) or S_4 (ventricular gallops) heart sounds
  Cardiomegaly
  Shift in cardiac axis
  ECG changes
  Neck vein distention
  Carotid bruits; may indicate atherosclerotic involvement elsewhere
  Paradoxical pulse
Pulmonary examination
  Basilar rales
  Wheezes
Abdominal examination
  Aortic, renal, or iliac bruits
  Pulsating abdominal mass
  Palpable aorta wider than 5 cm
Major artery examination (carotid, aortic, renal, iliac, femoral)
  Bruits
  Palpable thrills
Extremity examination
  Cyanosis or clubbing of nails
  Cool feet or hands
  Decreased or absent pulses in the extremities
  Poor capillary refill (extremities)
  Edema
  Arterial insufficiency
Skin examination
  Cool, dusky, mottled, pale skin
  Abnormally dry, flaking, or thickened skin (extremities)
  Plantar or malleolar ulcerations
  Erythema or rubor of lower extremities
  Shiny hairless skin (extremities)
  Xanthomas of tendon sheaths
  Xanthomas in skin creases of hands, eyelids, or elbows

Table 1-4-4. Differential Diagnosis of ASVD

Edema
   Venous insufficiency or obstruction
   Lymphatic obstruction
   Tumor invasion or compression
   Surgical damage
   Physical trauma
   Lymphedema
   Cor pulmonale
   Malnutrition
   Liver or renal disease
   Myxedema
   Volume overload or alterations in vascular permeability
   Adverse reaction to drugs
Dyspnea
   Pneumothorax
   Pulmonary edema
   Pulmonary emboli
   Trauma
   Sepsis
   Pneumonia
   Tuberculosis
   Emphysema
   Asthma
   Cancer of the lung
   Interstitial lung disease
   Pulmonary hypertension
   Pleural effusions
   Gastric or foreign-body aspiration
   Noxious gas inhalation
   Acute anemia
   Metabolic acidosis
Chest pain
   Skin and subcutaneous lesions
   Breast lesions
   Bruised or fractured rib
   Mitral valve prolapse
   Periosteal hematoma
   Costochondritis
   Intercostal myositis
   Muscular strain
   Shoulder bursitis, strain, tendinitis
   Cervical disk herniation
   Osteoarthritis
   Thoracic outlet syndrome
   Neuralgias
   Pericardial diseases
   Mediastinal disorders
   Pulmonary disease
   Gastroesophageal reflux
   Gastritis
   Peptic ulcer disease
   Cholecystitis
   Pancreatitis
   Psychogenic sources
Arrhthymias
   Hyperthyroidism
   Anxiety
   Hyperventilation
   Anemia
   Fever
   Volume depletion and postural hypotension
   Hypoglycemia
   Adverse drug reaction
   Other cardiac disorder

Mönckeberg's sclerosis is characterized by focal deposits of calcium in the smooth-muscle cells of the medial layer of the artery, causing rigid arteries that are easily visible on radiography, readily palpable, and tortuous. The exact cause is not known,

but long-term use of corticosteroids, smoking, and poorly controlled diabetes may be implicated. Arterial stenosis is seen only if ASVD coexists.

Arteriosclerosis consists of a degeneration and hyalinization of the arteries and/or arterioles of major organs such as the spleen, pancreas, kidney, and adrenal glands. Hypertension is often present. Disease results in arteries that are hyperplastic, elastic, fibrous, or necrosed.

Leriche's syndrome is a chronic obstruction of the aortic bifurcation from arteriosclerosis. Intermittent claudication in the buttocks, impotence, and absent femoral pulses are the usual symptoms.

Age-related thickening of the arterial wall is caused by a diffuse proliferation of smooth-muscle cells and cholesterol esters in the medial layer of the artery. The amount of cholesterol deposition is thought to be directly related to circulating plasma lipid levels. The resulting defects include rigidity, increased arterial wall width, dilation, elongation, tortuous contour, and focal arterial wall weakness that may result in aneurysms. Atherosclerotic plaque formation is a separate process but often coexists.

Small-vessel disease secondary to diabetes, renal insufficiency, autoimmune disorders, hypersensitivity, or congenital structural defects also may result in dysfunctional vasculature.

SPECIAL CONSIDERATIONS

Diabetes mellitus (DM) is associated with an increased risk of atherogenesis and peripheral vascular disease in both insulin-dependent and non-insulin-dependent states. The role of altered carbohydrate metabolism is unclear but is thought to be multifactorial. The increase in circulating insulin observed in type II diabetes mellitus may contribute to atherosclerosis. Whatever the mechanism, there is no histologic difference in atherosclerotic lesions found in diabetic patients and in individuals with normal glucose tolerance. The Diabetes Control and Complications Trial (DCCT) has implied that blood glucose control resulting in a glycosylated hemoglobin within 1 percentage point of the upper end of "normal" may reduce the risk of ASVD.

Obesity alone has not proved to be an independent risk factor for atherosclerosis. However, abdominal adiposity with a waist/hip ratio greater than 0.8 in women and 1.0 in men is strongly correlated with the development of diabetes and/or cardiac disease. Gluteal and femoral obesity are not associated with an increased risk. If obesity is accompanied by carbohydrate intolerance, hypertension, hyperlipidemias, or insulin resistance syndrome, increased rates of ASVD are noted.

Hypertension (HTN) is associated with many forms of cardiovascular disease, including ASVD. Thiazides and beta blockers, which often are used in hypertensive therapy, may potentiate increases in plasma lipid or glucose levels, which both are ASVD risk factors. However, current information is controversial concerning the duration of any metabolic change and the actual long-term risk of utilizing these medications.

A family history of early coronary artery disease or death from myocardial infarction (MI) may indicate a genetic abnormality of lipid metabolism. Although the role of genetic mechanisms is not completely understood, early detection and management of treatable risk factors seem prudent.

Chronic cigarette smoking or exposure to secondhand tobacco smoke is a well-established risk factor for ASVD. The increased risk for the development or progression of ASVD appears to be reversible with smoking cessation.

LABORATORY TESTS

No blood test for atherosclerosis exists. Laboratory testing is directed toward the discovery of accompanying metabolic disorders, evaluation of genetic susceptibility, and evaluation of the efficacy of treatment.

RADIOLOGIC STUDIES

Radiologic visualization by angiography is the gold standard for the diagnosis and evaluation of ASVD. Several less invasive testing methods are available, including Doppler studies, ultrafast CT scans (CINE-CT), magnetic resonance imaging (MRI), positron emission tomography (PET), radionuclide imaging, intravascular ultrasound (IVUS), angioscopy, arterial scans, and echocardiograms. Each technique has its advantages, disadvantages, dangers, costs, availability, and diagnostic value.

A chest radiograph may detect calcification of the aorta or arteries, congestive heart failure, cardiomegaly, aneurysm, or other abnormalities associated with ASVD. However, atherosclerotic plaque is not always calcified, and the extent of calcification noted on x-ray does not always correlate with the severity of disease.

OTHER DIAGNOSTICS

An electrocardiogram (ECG) is the least expensive, least invasive, and most readily available study for the detection of myocardial ischemia. Nonspecific ST changes, Q waves, arrhythmias, and left ventricular hypertrophy may indicate the need for further diagnostic testing. Young women may have a "false-positive" ECG with nonspecific ST-wave changes that may not be indicative of cardiac disease. The decision to perform more intensive testing relies on apparent risk factors, family history, laboratory data, symptomatology, and current medical status. Ambulatory ECG monitoring (Holter monitor) may demonstrate cardiac ischemic changes in an asymptomatic patient. However, a normal ECG does not exclude ASVD or cardiac disease.

TREATMENT

Therapy is directed at reducing lipids and managing the symptoms of vessel stenosis, including angina pectoris, hypertension, claudication, congestive heart failure, and arrhythmias. Additional therapy should focus on the reduction of treatable risk factors, including hyperglycemia, smoking cessation, obesity, physical inactivity, and stress reduction.

Pharmacologic Management

There is no direct pharmacologic treatment for atherosclerotic plaque, although new modalities are under investigation. Partial regression of plaque size has been documented after tight lipid management in several studies.

Aspirin therapy (81 mg/d) has been shown to be an effective tool in lowering the incidence of coronary artery and cerebrovascular events by reducing platelet aggregability. Enteric-coated aspirin may be used in individuals with a history of gastric irritation.

Surgical Treatment

Numerous invasive procedures may be used to reduce or remove vessel stenosis. Percutaneous transluminal angioplasty (PCTA), atherectomy, endarterectomy, laser therapy, intravascular stents, coronary artery bypass surgery (CABS), and arterial graft surgeries are widely available.

PCTA is indicated in patients with angina, ischemia, thrombosis, or acute myocardial infarction. Atherectomy removes rather than stretches the obstructing plaque. Current technology includes directional coronary atherectomy (DCA), rotational ablation, transluminal extraction (TEC), and lasers. Atherectomy often is utilized for difficult lesions or chronic restenosis. Stents

are coiled or interwoven metal "tubes" that provide an internal supporting structure to hold a vessel open against its elastic recoil.

Revascularization also may be achieved through bypass or graft surgery. CABS usually is reserved for severe or multiple-vessel disease. Grafting techniques may be utilized in the repair of aneurysms, major artery stenosis, and cerebral revascularization.

Unfortunately, reocclusion is a common complication. Studies indicate that revascularization procedures are required in approximately 50 percent of these patients within 5 to 10 years. Grafted vessels are three to six times more likely to restenose. Fortunately, medication, diet, and life-style modifications have been shown to prolong the time to restenosis significantly.

Supportive Measures

The treatment and prevention of ASVD involve the triad of medical therapy, pharmacologic management, and life-style modifications.

Life-style modifications include smoking cessation, dietary modification, increased physical activity, and stress reduction. Each component is essential in reducing the risk or limiting the progression of ASVD.

Moderate use of red wine or alcohol may reduce the risk of ASVD. The exact mechanism is not clearly understood but may include increases in protective high-density lipoprotein cholesterol (HDL-C) or the antioxidant properties of the bioflavonoids (phenols) in grapes. Careful counseling on drug-alcohol interactions should be included in any recommendations for alcohol consumption.

Numerous studies have confirmed the benefits of physical activity in the treatment of obesity, stress, hypertension, diabetes, and cardiac disease. Exercise appears to have a favorable impact on serum cholesterol levels (increased HDL-C, decreased TC), improves physical conditioning, and facilitates weight (fat) loss.

Any aerobic activity enjoyed by an individual should be encouraged, with the emphasis placed on frequency and duration rather than intensity. An exercise prescription should include a gradual "conditioning" process and should not be so intense that it discourages compliance. The ultimate goals include a half hour of aerobic exercise three to five times a week within target heart rate ranges (THRs) or target training zone on the Borg scale of perceived exertion. Individuals at risk for ASVD should be carefully evaluated before beginning any exercise program:

- *Target heart rate:* (220 − age) × 0.60 to 0.80. Conditioning should begin at 60 percent and advance to 80 percent.
- *The Borg scale of perceived exertion* is a scale of 0 to 20 on which a patient bases his or her perceived level of exertion. Lower numbers correlate with a minimum exercise level, and higher numbers with a maximum exertion level.

The role of stress is not clearly understood, but stress may be capable of precipitating an acute cardiac episode in a susceptible individual. Knowledge of a patient's personality and life-style is helpful in referring a patient for counseling on stress modification.

Patient Education

Education should describe the disease process and treatment modalities and empower the patient to make life-style modifications. Information is essential if an individual is to understand the expected benefit, methodology, potential adverse effects, and risks of a treatment modality. Compliance usually will increase in direct proportion to effective patient education. The local affiliate of the American Heart Association is one of many organizations that can provide educational materials to the practitioner and patient.

Disposition

Regular follow-up to evaluate for complications, progression of disease, and success of the treatment plan may improve a patient's compliance and quality of life. Referral to a cardiologist or vascular surgeon for evaluation and consultation may be appropriate. Education and medical nutrition therapy provided by a registered dietitian are important for successful dietary modification. Exercise compliance may be enhanced by utilizing an exercise physiologist, physical therapist, or cardiac rehabilitation program.

COMPLICATIONS AND RED FLAGS

A medical practitioner must be alert to the signs and symptoms of disease progression or reocclusion. A patient who is noncompliant with necessary life-style changes or has suboptimal control of a comorbid disease should be monitored closely. Careful questioning and history taking will help elicit information on recurrent symptoms in a timely fashion.

NOTES AND PEARLS

Research on future treatment for atherosclerosis is focused on preventing as well as curing ASVD. Gene therapy, direct intravascular drug delivery systems, advanced pharmacologic agents, new laboratory testing procedures, and innovations in surgical technology are on the horizon. Innovative utilization of "old" drugs such as estrogen, nitric oxide, folate, vitamin B, and vitamin E is promising.

Laboratory tests can now identify and quantitate specific lipoprotein subclasses that are thought to be atherogenic. A lipid panel alone may not be sufficient to diagnose a patient prone to ASVD. The Framingham Study showed that individuals with elevated cholesterol levels are at higher risk for heart disease; however, nearly 80 percent of individuals who developed heart disease maintained TC levels similar to those of individuals who did not.

Although numerous new modalities are on the horizon, individuals will still need to maintain a healthy life-style, utilizing diet, exercise, stress reduction, and smoking cessation, to remain disease-free.

REFERENCES

1. Grundy SM: Relationship of nutritional status and exercise to serum cholesterol levels. Cholesterol and Coronary Disease . . . Reducing the Risk. 3:4–6, 1991.

BIBLIOGRAPHY

Berkow R, ed: *The Merck Manual of Diagnosis and Therapy,* 16th ed. Rahway, NJ, Merck, 1992, pp 409–413.
Bierman EL: Waist-hip ratio and risk of CHD. Cholesterol and Coronary Disease . . . Reducing the Risk. 3:7–8, 1991.
Forrester JS: Efficacy of risk factor management. *J Am Coll Cardiol* 27:964–1047, 1996.
Isselbacher KJ, Braunwald E, Wilson JD, et al (eds). *Harrison's Principles of Medicine,* 13th ed. New York, McGraw-Hill, 1994, pp 1106–1137, 2234–2249.
Muhlestein JB, Hammond EH, Cariquist JF, et al: Increased incidence of Chlamydia species within the coronary arteries of patients with symptomatic atherosclerotic versus other forms of cardiovascular disease. *J Am Coll Cardiol* 27:1555–1561, 1996.
Skillings J, Howes DG: Recertification series hyperlipidemia and atherosclerosis, part I. *Physician Assist* 7:32–68, 1996.
Skillings J, Howes DG: Recertification series hyperlipidemia and atherosclerosis, part II. *Physician Assist* 8:32–62, 1996.
Summary of the Second Report of the National Cholesterol Education Program (NCEP) Expert Panel on Detection, Evaluation and Treatment of High Blood Cholesterol in Adults (Adult Treatment Panel II). *JAMA* 269(23):3015–3023, 1993.
Surperko HR: New aspects of risk factors for the development of atherosclerosis, including small low-density lipoprotein, homocysteine, and lipoprotein (a). *Curr Opin Cardiol* 10:347–354, 1995.
Tierney LM Jr, McPhee SJ, Papadakis MA, eds: *Current Medical Diagnosis and Treatment,* 34th ed. Norwalk, CT, Appleton & Lange, 1995, pp 308–329.
Wood PD: Weight, exercise, and blood lipids. Cholesterol and Coronary Disease . . . Reducing the risk. 3:1–3, 1996.

Chapter 1–5
COR PULMONALE
Katherine Adamson

DISCUSSION

The term *cor pulmonale* refers to enlargement or malfunction of the right ventricle secondary to pulmonary hypertension. The antecedent pulmonary hypertension may result from disease of the lung parenchyma or pulmonary vasculature or from diseases that affect the mechanics of respiration. Cor pulmonale may occur acutely secondary to massive pulmonary emboli. This chapter addresses the more common chronic process.

In the United States, chronic obstructive pulmonary disease (COPD) is by far the most common etiology of cor pulmonale. An estimated 47 million people in this country suffer from COPD;[1] more than half of these individuals have evidence of cor pulmonale.[2]

PATHOGENESIS

To understand the pathophysiology associated with cor pulmonale, it is vital that one appreciate the marked differences in pressure normally found in the pulmonary circulation compared with the systemic circulation. The pulmonary circulation is best thought of as a very compliant reservoir with vascular resistance approximately one-tenth that of the systemic circulation. This relatively easy compliance allows for minute-to-minute changes in flow volume with a minimal increase in pulmonary artery pressure. For pulmonary hypertension to result in cor pulmonale, a significant disturbance in the form of diffuse pulmonary vasoconstriction or occlusion of the pulmonary arterial system has to have occurred. As was stated earlier, COPD leads the list of the etiologies of cor pulmonale. Table 1-5-1 summarizes other common causes.

The pulmonary vessels course through pulmonary parenchymal tissue. With COPD, the alveoli enlarge and place direct pressure on the very thin peripheral vessels. These vessels respond to this external pressure with compression and eventual shunting of blood away from the periphery of the lung toward the more central regions. Added to this abnormal situation is a relative degree of hypoxia-induced vasoconstriction. The result is an increase in pulmonary artery pressure. This pulmonary artery hypertension causes the right ventricle to compensate by increasing its muscle mass, leading to right ventricular hypertrophy (RVH).

Table 1-5-1. Etiologies of Cor Pulmonale

Diseases of the lung parenchyma
  Emphysema
  Chronic bronchitis
  Absence of lung tissue secondary to trauma and/or surgical
    resection
  Cystic fibrosis
Diseases of pulmonary vasculature
  Acute massive pulmonary emboli causing acute cor pulmonale
  Recurrent small emboli resulting in chronic cor pulmonale
Infiltrative processes
  Connective tissue diseases such as sarcoidosis, rheumatoid arthritis,
    systemic lupus erythematosus
  Malignant and/or metastatic disease
Processes that affect the mechanics of respiration
  Morbid obesity
  Thoracic malformations such as kyphoscoliosis
  Sleep apnea syndromes

SYMPTOMS

Chronic cor pulmonale does not exist by itself. These patients present with symptoms of the underlying process that resulted in RVH and eventual failure. The clinician should quantify the type and degree of the pulmonary disease process and then be alert for the development of cor pulmonale. Typically, the patient complains of an increase in chronic respiratory distress in the form of progressive easy fatigability, an increase in dyspnea and sputum production, and the symptoms of right-sided heart failure, particularly peripheral edema.

OBJECTIVE FINDINGS

The patient will be dyspneic and often will show signs of central cyanosis. Examination of the neck veins will demonstrate distention and prominence of the *a* and *v* waves. (Recall that the *a* wave relates to atrial contraction, while the *v* wave relates to atrial filling.) Inspection and palpation of the precordium may reveal a parasternal lift caused by the hypertrophied right ventricle. Upon auscultation, the examiner often notes a systolic murmur along the left lower sternal border that changes with respiration. This is the murmur of tricuspid regurgitation resulting from stretch on the valve annulus by the dilated and hypertrophied right ventricle. When the heart sounds are not too obscured by pulmonary disease, one may appreciate the accentuated closure of the pulmonic valve (loud P_2 of S_2), which is considered diagnostic of pulmonary hypertension. A right-sided S_3 gallop frequently is heard along the left sternal border or in the epigastrium. Abdominal examination may disclose ascites and tenderness in the right upper quadrant from an enlarged liver. Peripheral edema is sure to be found in the sacrum, the pretibial areas, or both.

DIAGNOSTIC CONSIDERATIONS

Chronic cor pulmonale results from any disease process that interferes with adequate ventilation and perfusion from the pulmonary valve to the entry of the pulmonary veins into the left atrium. This chapter has listed several etiologies for cor pulmonale. It is important that the clinician be aware of the relationship between these various processes and the development of RVH and eventual dysfunction.

LABORATORY TESTS

Pulmonary function studies are markedly abnormal with marked airflow obstruction. Arterial blood gases reflect the hypoxia and hypercarbia of the underlying COPD.

RADIOLOGIC STUDIES

Posteroanterior and lateral chest x-rays and Doppler echocardiography may present interpretative challenges because of the hyperinflation that is invariably present. The chest x-ray often shows enlarged central pulmonary vessels and a marked decrease in or even absence of peripheral vessel markings that also is known as pruning. Doppler echocardiography may confirm the enlargement of the right ventricle and the presence of tricuspid valve regurgitation.

OTHER DIAGNOSTICS

A standard 12-lead ECG should demonstrate right ventricular hypertrophy (right axis deviation and reversal of the normal precordial R wave progression in the presence of a QRS of normal duration). Another typical ECG finding is a "P pulmonale," a prominent peaked P wave in leads II, III, and aVF. It is not at all unusual for a patient with cor pulmonale to be in a supraventricular dysrhythmia such as atrial fibrillation. On occasion a patient with cor pulmonale may require cardiac catheterization. The right side of the heart is accessed through the venous system, with blood/oxygen samples and pressure readings taken at various points along the catheter route. Such a procedure is often technically difficult because of the pathology present. Since pulmonary artery wedge pressure is a reflection of left atrial pressure, it is usually normal.

TREATMENT
Medications

The treatment must focus on the underlying disease process. Since this most often involves chronic bronchitis and/or emphysema, the use of bronchodilators, antibiotics, and beta agonists is commonplace. Every effort should be made to decrease the pulmonary arterial hypertension that is at the root of cor pulmonale. Hypoxia-induced vasoconstriction may be improved with chronic oxygen administration. For this reason, oxygen may be the most important medication in the clinician's arsenal against cor pulmonale. Caution must be exercised in the prescription of oxygen therapy, as a large number of patients with cor pulmonale are carbon dioxide retainers. Oxygen can depress the ventilatory drive in this subset of patients, worsening their hypercapnia. There is much discussion in the literature regarding the use of vasodilators, specifically nifedipine (Procardia), in the treatment of cor pulmonale. The consensus seems to be that vasodilator therapy is a useful adjunct acutely but that the resultant decrease in pulmonary vascular resistance and the concomitant increase in right ventricular stroke volume are seen only briefly. The hypotension that often accompanies this therapy places further limitations on its routine use.

Diuretics may be useful in the treatment of cor pulmonale for the relief of systemic edema. The practitioner needs to be alert for resultant electrolyte disturbances, particularly if the patient is taking a cardiac glycoside such as digitalis. Digitalis may be employed in patients with cor pulmonale, especially if a patient presents with uncontrolled atrial fibrillation, but the routine use of digitalis-type medications is controversial at best.[3]

Supportive Measures

Maintaining a clear airway is perhaps the most important supportive measure one can offer a patient with cor pulmonale. The patient and his or her caretakers need to be skilled in the various modalities of pulmonary toilet, including chest physical therapy, breathing exercises, and the employment of airway suction devices.

Patient Education

Prevention of cor pulmonale is centered on prevention of COPD. Patients deserve access to effective smoking cessation programs. Asthma support groups can be helpful in encouraging patients to maintain a difficult but effective medication regimen. One should alert patients to the signs and symptoms of right-sided heart failure so that they can be dealt with on a timely basis.

Disposition

The prognosis in cor pulmonale associated with chronic lung disease is intimately related to the underlying disease process. Emphysema carries a poorer prognosis than does bronchitis. It is clear that the prognosis improves after the administration of long-term oxygen therapy.

COMPLICATIONS AND RED FLAGS

As was noted earlier, patients with pulmonary hypertension and resultant RVH are prone to dysrhythmias. Aberrant rhythms often overtax an already compromised cardiovascular system, leading to dangerous decreases in cardiac output and aggravation of hypoxia. A careful history and physical signs of searching for dysrhythmia should be a part of every clinician-patient encounter. Remember to ask about palpitations, syncope and near syncope, and the telltale discomfort of cardiac ischemia.

NOTES AND PEARLS

Providers learn to focus on the underlying disease, but often at the risk of overlooking the primary problem's sequelae. Chronic cor pulmonale is best viewed as a result of long-standing pulmonary parenchymal or vessel insult. The usually low-pressure right heart cannot deal effectively with these increases in pressure. Long-term compensation in the form of right ventricular dilation, hypertrophy, and eventual dysfunction will follow. Awareness of this pathophysiologic process will enable the physician assistant to anticipate and recognize the symptoms of cor pulmonale when they occur.

REFERENCES

1. Georgiou D, Brundage BH: Pulmonary hypertension, in Kloner RA (ed): *The Guide to Cardiology*, 3d ed. Greenwich, CT, Le Jacq, 1995, p. 620.
2. Butler J, Braunwald E: Cor pulmonale, in Isselbacher KJ, Braunwald E, Wilson JD, et al (eds): *Harrison's Principles of Internal Medicine*, 13th ed. New York, McGraw-Hill, 1994, p. 1085.
3. McFadden E, Braunwald E: Cor pulmonale, in Braunwald E (ed): *Heart Disease: A Textbook of Cardiovascular Medicine*, 4th ed. Philadelphia, Saunders, 1992, pp. 1581–1597.

Chapter 1–6
HYPERLIPIDEMIA

Catherine J. Heymann

DISCUSSION

Cholesterol, triglycerides, and phospholipids are the major lipids in the human body. Hyperlipidemias (or dyslipidemias) result from abnormal transport, accelerated synthesis, and/or retarded degradation of lipid particles in the plasma, vascular endothelial cells, and/or liver. Lipid metabolism varies with gender, age, genetics, and environment. Chemically, cholesterol is not a fat but a molecule from the sterol family with a lipid-like structure. Cholesterol is an essential nutrient that is utilized in cell wall membranes, in the formation of steroid hormones, in the synthesis of vitamin D, as a component of bile acids, and throughout the nervous system. Triglycerides (TGs) represent the body's long-term storage of excess energy in the form of adipose tissue. An integral part of cholesterol metabolism, TGs are composed of three free fatty acids (FFAs) held together by a glycerol molecule. Phospholipids resemble a fat in appearance. They are incorporated into the outer coating of a lipid molecule to increase solubility.

To transport lipids (oil particles) in the bloodstream (an aqueous solution), the body produces a single cell coating called an apoprotein to encompass the particle (Fig. 1-6-1). The body produces many forms of apoproteins, each of which has a unique sequence. During lipid metabolism, apoproteins are readily altered or exchanged to facilitate metabolic, cell synthesis, or transportation requirements.

There are five general lipoprotein subclasses (Table 1-6-1). The three most frequently assayed are high-density lipoprotein (HDL), low-density lipoprotein (LDL), and triglycerides. They are categorized by their lipid composition, weight, size, electrical charge, and apoprotein coating. Abnormal lipid metabolism may result in an increased risk of atherosclerotic vascular disease (ASVD), coronary artery disease (CAD), pancreatitis, and stroke.

PATHOGENESIS

The two metabolic pathways for lipid synthesis are exogenous (dietary sources) and endogenous (within the body). Each pathway may cause hyperlipidemias independently or in synergism with the others.

SYMPTOMS

Mild hyperlipidemias do not produce symptoms until the complications of ASVD become apparent. Angina, dyspnea, claudication, fatigue, transient ischemic attacks (TIAs), or cardiac arrhythmias may be the first indication of vascular damage caused by preexisting abnormal lipid metabolism.

With significant elevations of TGs, patients may report recurrent abdominal pain, nausea, or vomiting related to pancreatitis. As the level of TGs increases, the blood becomes lipemic, thick, and sludgelike. The lipemic blood cannot easily flow through the fine capillaries of the pancreas or liver, resulting in organ damage, inflammation, fibrosis, and pain.

Joint pain resulting from gouty arthritis may be caused by the high uric acid levels associated with elevated TGs. Although the first joint of the great toe is the classic site of gout, any joint may be affected. Migratory polyarthritis may produce warm, erythematous, or swollen joints. The onset is sudden, and the condition lasts a few days to weeks and produces no articular damage.

OBJECTIVE FINDINGS

Extreme elevations of cholesterol or TGs may produce skin eruptions (xanthomas or xanthelasmas), lipemic (pale and creamy) blood samples, pale white retinal vessels (lipemia retinalis), hepatomegaly, splenomegaly, elevated uric acid levels, or foam-cell infiltration of bone marrow. Table 1-6-2 summarizes some of the physical findings in hyperlipidemias.

Skin lesions called xanthomas may bring a patient to a practitioner for cosmetic reasons. Small yellow-white or yellow-

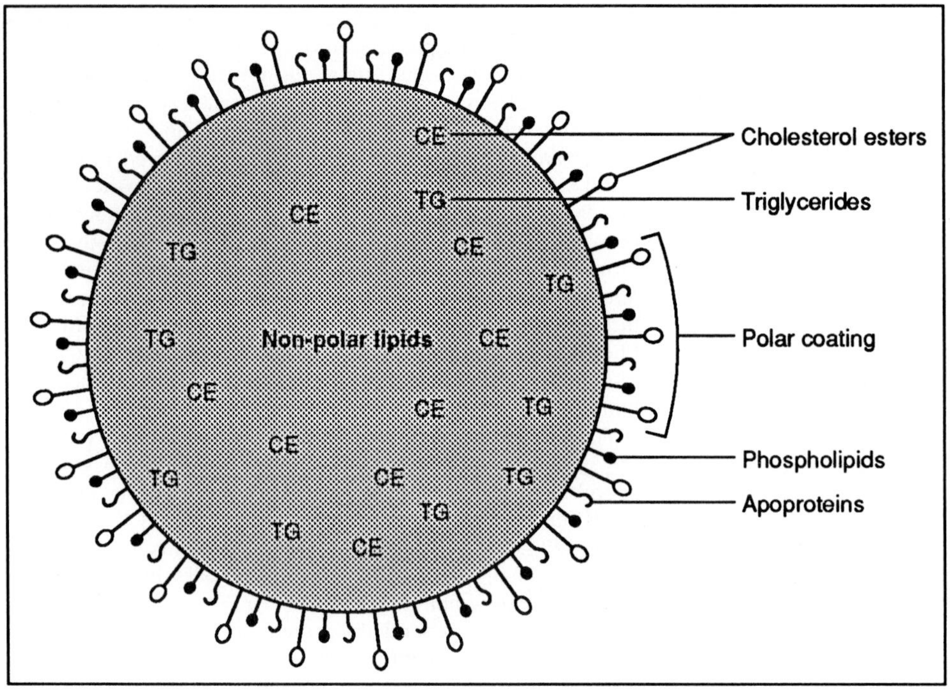

Figure 1-6-1. Lipoprotein molecule.

orange papules with an erythematous "halo" may appear on pressure-sensitive areas such as the buttocks, elbows, and knees. Larger "tuber-like" growths may appear on the Achilles, patellar, elbow, and digital extensor tendons. The lesions usually disappear after the underlying lipid abnormality is corrected.

Yellow-orange discolorations in the creases around the eyelids are called xanthelasmas. Plane xanthomas present as flat yellow-orange patches on the palms of the hands, in the palmar creases, on the face, on the upper trunk, or in scar tissue. More subtle in presentation than large disfiguring tuber xanthomas, they should alert the practitioner to a potentially lethal abnormality of lipid metabolism.

Abdominal examination may reveal an enlarged liver or spleen from chronic inflammation caused by the congested lipemic blood flow observed in hypertriglyceridemia (TGs > 1000 mg/dL).

DIAGNOSTIC CONSIDERATIONS

Abnormal lipid metabolism that is linked to a genetic anomaly is designated as primary. Secondary hyperlipidemias may be associated with several metabolic abnormalities, pharmacologic agents, and excessive alcohol consumption.

Primary hyperlipidemias include several familial hyperlipoproteinemias. Single or multiple variant genes, each with a specific impact on lipids, are often present. Genetically linked abnormalities of lipid metabolism may be associated with inappropriate apoprotein production, various lipid enzyme or receptor site deficiencies, abnormalities of fat metabolism (lipodystrophy), hypopituitarism (dwarfism), and glycogen storage disease. Environmental factors such as obesity, diet, comorbid illnesses, smoking, and physical inactivity play a major role in the expression of genetic disorders of lipid metabolism.

The numerous chronic illnesses that may induce secondary hyperlipidemias include diabetes, hypothyroidism, hepatic diseases, pancreatitis, biliary obstruction, renal disease, nephrotic syndrome, pregnancy, physical and/or emotional stress, anorexia nervosa, acromegaly, autoimmune disorders, porphyria, Cushing's syndrome, and obesity. The underlying disorder must be addressed before the hyperlipidemias can be treated effectively.

Drug-induced hyperlipidemias may result from oral contraceptives, estrogens, androgens, glucocorticoids, thiazides, beta blockers, 13-*cis*-retinoic acid (isotretinoin, Accutane), and alcohol consumption (Table 1-6-3).

Table 1-6-1. Lipoprotein Subclasses

Lipoprotein	Lipid Composition	Role in Metabolism	Role in Disease	Apoprotein Coating
Chylomicrons	Transports dietary TGs and cholesterol esters	Transports dietary TGs	Precursor to TGs	AI, AII, B48, CI, CII, CIII, E
Very-low-density lipoprotein (VLDL-C) or pre-β-lipoproteins	Endogenous TG	Transports endogenous TGs	Precursor to IDL-C and LDL-C	B48, CI, CII, CIII, E
Intermediate-density lipoprotein (IDL-C)	Cholesterol esters, TGs	Precursor to LDL-C	Intermediate step in lipid metabolism	B100, CIII, E
Low-density lipoproteins (LDL-C) or β-lipoproteins	Cholesterol esters	Transports cholesterol to cells	Highly atherogenic LDL-C oxidation is a key step in atherosclerotic plaque formation	B48, B100
High-density lipoprotein (HDL-C) or α-lipoprotein	Cholesterol esters	Transports cholesterol from cells to liver	Protective—returns cholesterol esters to liver, where they are degraded	AI, AII

Table 1-6-2. Physical Findings in Hyperlipidemias

Physical Finding	Hypercholesterolemia	Hypertriglyceridemia
Abdominal pain (recurrent)		X (usually >1000 mg/dL)
Eruptive or planar xanthomas	X	X
Xanthelasma	X	X
Hepatosplenomegaly		X
Lipemia retinalis		X
Atherosclerosis	X	Unknown
Glucose intolerance (associated with certain familial hyperlipidemias)		X

Table 1-6-3. Potential Causes of Abnormal Lipids

Disorder	Resulting Lipid Abnormalities
Hypothyroid	High TC, high LDL
Nephrotic syndrome	High TC, high LDL
Chronic renal failure	High TGs
Diabetes (uncontrolled)	High TGs
Systemic lupus erythematosus	High TGs
Porphyria	High LDL-C
Oral contraceptives	High TGs
Progesterones	Low HDL-C
Alcohol	High TGs
Beta blockers	High TGs, high LDL-C, low HDL-C
Smoking	Low HDL-C

LABORATORY TESTS

The National Cholesterol Education Program II recommends that all adults (20 years or older) be routinely screened for hyperlipidemias by means of a total serum cholesterol level (Table 1-6-4). Since cholesterol levels are not affected by the preceding meal, a random check may be obtained during a routine office visit. If the results are ≤200 mg/dL, the test should be repeated every 5 years. If the total cholesterol is >200 mg/dL, a complete lipid assessment, including a fasting total cholesterol (TC), LDL-cholesterol (LDL-C), HDL-cholesterol, and TGs, should be obtained. Triglyceride and chylomicron levels are affected by the preceding meal; therefore, a fasting sample should be obtained. Further decisions on management and treatment may be based on several indices, including LDL-C, TGs, current disease, comorbid disease, and genetic cardiac risk factors.

LDL-C may be the single laboratory test that is most predictive of future disease. Desirable levels for the general population are <160 mg/dL. If there are significant risk factors but no current evidence of cardiac or vascular disease, acceptable ranges decrease to 100 to 130 mg/dL. An LDL-C level <100 mg/dL has been recommended for all patients with CAD, ASVD, and/or diabetes. LDL-C determinations are commonly made by calculation rather than actual measurement (too expensive).

HDL-C$_2$ is responsible for "reverse cholesterol transport," or removal of excess LDL-C from the blood. Acceptable ranges are >35 mg/dL for males and >50 mg/dL for females. An HDL-C level above 70 mg/dL is considered cardioprotective.

Hypertriglyceridemia is now considered an independent risk factor for ASVD. Newer recommendations advise TG levels <150 mg/dL in all patients.

Ratios of lipid subclasses are often utilized to evaluate a patient's risk of developing ASVD. The most frequently used "cardiac risk ratios" are TC : HDL-C (<4.5, "average risk" or below) and LDL-C : HDL-C (<3.5, "average risk"). The validity of risk ratios is questionable, and they are best utilized if one lipid subclass is unusually high or low. For example, a patient with a total cholesterol of 285 mg/dL may be considered to be at high risk; however, if the HDL-C is 95 mg/dL, the TC : HDL-C is 3 : 1, or

"low risk." The generous HDL-C "counterbalances" the elevation in TC.

There are no "normal" ranges for serum lipids or lipid subclasses, only desirable levels that are thought to prevent or retard atherosclerotic disease (Table 1-6-4). It is important to remember that a "desirable" range in the United States still produces one of the highest rates of coronary artery disease in the world. Epidemiologic studies have documented an increase in ASVD as immigrants come to the United States and adopt its sedentary lifestyle and poor dietary habits.

Tests for additional markers of genetic disorders of lipid metabolism are now available and will soon be the gold standard. Currently utilized laboratory tests are inadequate to diagnose the majority of genetic abnormalities, which are responsible for approximately 80 percent of cardiac and vascular disease. Risk or genetic predisposition to ASVD may be better evaluated with specific assessments of lipid subclasses, apoproteins, homocysteine metabolism, apo E isoforms, and/or enzyme deficiencies. Each of these tests denotes a genetic abnormality of lipid metabolism and is essential in selecting appropriate treatment options.

The laboratory testing described above is new, comparatively expensive, seldom reimbursed, and not an appropriate screening tool for the general population. A family history (genetic map) should alert the practitioner to patients and families that could benefit from specialized testing procedures. Any patient with CAD should have the benefit of advanced testing methods for abnormal lipid metabolism to detect treatable genetic disorders and prevent further ASVD.

RADIOLOGIC STUDIES

Radiologic studies are not done unless CAD, atherosclerosis, peripheral vascular disease, or cerebrovascular disease is suspected.

OTHER DIAGNOSTICS

Classically, the Fredrickenson and Levy phenotyping system has been used to classify specific abnormal patterns of lipid metabolism. Additional genotypes have been identified through the more sophisticated testing methods mentioned above, which may soon

Table 1-6-4. Cholesterol, Triglyceride, and Lipid Subclass Levels

Desirable Ranges	No Risk Factors	No ASVD with Two or More Risk Factors	ASVD and Diabetic Patients
TC	<200 mg/dL	<200 mg/dL	<200 mg/dL
HDL	>35 mg/dL (male)	>35 mg/dL (male)	>35 mg/dL (male)
	>50 mg/dL (female)	>50 mg/dL (female)	>50 mg/dL (female)
LDL	<160 mg/dL	<130 mg/dL	<100 mg/dL
TGs	<200 mg/dL	<150 mg/dL	<100 mg/dL

Table 1-6-5. Genetic Abnormalities of Lipid Metabolism

Lipid Abnormality	Laboratory Tests	Desirable Result	Treatment Options
Small LDL	Gel electrophoresis	Pattern B = majority of LDL <257 Å	Diet minimally effective but may be more effective in pattern A
		Pattern A the majority of LDL >257 Å	Niacin plus fibric acid derivative
Lp(a)	Lp(a)	Upper 10% of normal is >23 mg/dL	Niacin plus estrogen (female) or testosterone (male)
			Vitamin E 400–800 IU/d
Homocysteine	Fasting or postload (methionine) homocysteine levels	Fasting = <0.8 μmol/L	Folate 4–5 mg/d
		Postload = >14 μmol/L	Vitamin B$_6$ 250 mg/day
LDL-C	Gel electrophoresis to determine number of large and small LDL-Cs	LDL-C 100 > LDL-C 48	Resin and niacin
		Smaller particle size is more atherogenic	Statin and niacin
Apo E isoforms	Apo E isoforms	Normal = apo E 3/3	Low-fat diet
			Probucol
			Fibric acid derivatives
Low HDL-C	HDL-C gel electrophoresis to determine distribution of HDL subclasses	Abnormal <25 mg/dL	Resin plus niacin
		Normal	Statins plus niacin
		Female >50 mg/dL	
		Male >35 mg/dL	
		HDL-C should predominate	

render this classification system obsolete. Table 1-6-5 gives a summary of lipid abnormalities, expected lab values, and treatment modalities.

TREATMENT

Before one initiates treatment, other medical conditions or pharmacologic agents that may cause or contribute to hyperlipidemias must be considered (Table 1-6-3).

Medical Nutrition Therapy

Dietary management and life-style modifications should always be the first line of treatment for hyperlipidemias. If therapy fails after an appropriate trial, medications may be added.

Currently, numerous governmental, private, and research organizations recommend a diet that meets the following criteria:

1. Maintenance of a reasonable body weight
2. Fewer calories from fat
3. Reduction of saturated fats to <10 percent of calories
4. Cholesterol intake of <300 mg/d
5. Plenty of fresh fruit and vegetables
6. Increase intake of whole grains, beans, and legumes

The type of fat ingested may be as important as the amount. Fats may be saturated, monounsaturated (MUFA) or polyunsaturated (PUFA). Each type of fat has a distinct impact on lipid metabolism. Saturated fats are implicated in accelerating the production of cholesterol in its most potentially lethal form: LDLs. Always solid at room temperature, saturated fats are found in animal fats, coconut oil, and palm kernel oil. MUFAs are thought to be effective in lowering LDL-C and increasing HDL-C. They are always lipid at room temperature, and their sources are olive, canola, and many nut oils. PUFAs were once thought to be cardioprotective. Although they may produce a reduction of TC, PUFAs increase the amount of LDL-C and may produce a form more prone to oxidation. PUFAs also decrease cardioprotective HDL-C. Again, they are always liquid at room temperature. Solid margarine is made by partially saturating or hydrogenating liquid oils. This transamination of fatty acids has been implicated in an increase in the incidence of ASVD.

The impact of dietary cholesterol on the lipid profile is variable but usually minimal. Chicken, pork, fish, and beef have essentially the same cholesterol content; however, they vary significantly in their saturated fat content. Complex interactions between saturated fats, endogenous and/or exogenous cholesterol metabolism, and genetics influence serum lipid levels. Cholesterol is found only in animal sources, primarily in the flesh of animals, fish, poultry, organ meats, dairy products, and eggs.

Dietary modifications can be implemented successfully only with intensive education, counseling, family support, and realistic goal setting. The American Dietetic Association has a consumer information hot line (800-366-1655) and referral service.

Pharmacologic Management

Medications for hyperlipidemias fall into four basic categories: bile acid–binding resins, HMG-CoA reductase inhibitors, fibric acid derivatives, and nicotinic acid (Table 1-6-6). All these medications have numerous adverse effects that may affect patient compliance. Effectiveness is dependent not only on patient compliance with the medication but on adherence to a healthy diet, regular exercise, smoking cessation, and stress reduction.

Bile acid–binding resins reduce LDL-C by forming an insoluble compound with bile acids in the intestine, restricting their reabsorption, and limiting cholesterol production. These drugs are often used in conjunction with HMG-CoA reductase inhibitors to produce a synergistic effect.

HMG-CoA reductase inhibitors competitively limit LDL-C formation early in cholesterol biosynthesis. The exact mechanism is not completely understood, but a decrease in very-low-density lipoprotein cholesterol (VLDL-C), LDL-C, and TGs and an increase in HDL-C usually is noted. The most effective time to administer the medication appears to be with dinner or at bedtime, as the majority of cholesterol synthesis takes place during the night. This class of drugs is nicknamed the "statins": lovastatin, pravastatin, simvastatin, etc.

Fibric acid derivatives reduce hepatic TG and VLDL-C production while increasing the synthesis of HDL-C. Clofibrate is used infrequently in the United States because of the associated increased incidence of intestinal tumors. Gemfibrozil is the only currently available fibric acid derivative.

Nicotinic acid (niacin) reduces TC, VLDL-C, LDL-C, and TGs and increases HDL-C. The effect appears to be dose-dependent. Niacin often is combined with a bile acid sequestrant to further reduce LDL-C. It is an inexpensive medication, and compliance is dependent on patient tolerance of unpleasant side effects. Slow titration or the addition of aspirin 30 min before the niacin is taken may help reduce the annoying cutaneous flushing and itching. Doses >1000 mg/d may affect glucose tolerance or diabetic control.

Estrogen replacement therapy in postmenopausal women is believed to reduce the incidence of CAD, possibly by maintaining higher HDL-C levels. Progesterone therapy also must be utilized to reduce the risk of uterine cancer if the female has a uterus.

Medications may be combined to increase the lipid-lowering effect. Most CAD patients have more than one genetic abnormality of lipid metabolism, some of which may require separate treatment modalities.

SUPPORTIVE MEASURES

Patient Education

Assessment, education, therapy, and monitoring of life-style modifications require a significant amount of the practitioner's time and unique skills. The use of ancillary professionals such as nurses, dietitians, social workers, psychologists, and physical therapists can facilitate the education and support process. Knowing what to expect, awareness of risks and benefits, and the use of coping mechanisms for any unpleasant side effects of therapy help promote patient compliance.

Exercise

Before beginning an exercise program, patients should be evaluated for ischemic cardiac or atherosclerotic disease. The only effective exercise program is one the patient can comply with on a regular basis. One should utilize nontraditional forms of exercise rather than insisting on something the patient cannot or will not attempt.

Disposition

Patients should be followed with history, physical examination, and laboratory assessments on a regular basis to monitor the efficacy of therapy. Appropriate laboratory surveillance for the complications of pharmacologic therapy should be performed as recommended on the package insert. Close monitoring for evidence of new or progressing cardiac or vascular disease permits early intervention. Referral to a cardiologist or vascular surgeon for consultation and evaluation may be reasonable.

COMPLICATIONS AND RED FLAGS

Pancreatitis, peripheral vascular disease, cardiac disease, cerebrovascular disease, major vessel disease, and death and/or disability are the most frequently seen complications of elevated lipids. A family history combined with appropriate laboratory assessment

Table 1-6-6. Pharmacologic Treatment of Hyperlipidemias

Medication	Effect on Lipids	Adverse Effects	Drug Interactions	Contraindications
Bile acid–binding resins	Lower LDL Lower TC	GI intolerance Constipation Flatulence Bloating Nausea Epigastric pain Elevated TGs Headache	Digoxin Thyroxine Tetracycline Coumadin Thiazides Vitamins A, D, K Folic acid Glipizide Gemfibrozil Iopanoic acid Phosphates Piroxican Propanolol	Peptic ulcers Diverticulitis Allergic reaction Pregnancy Lactation
HMG-CoA reductase inhibitors	Lower LDL-c Raise HDL-c Prevention* Lower VLDL-c Lower TGs Lower TC	Sore muscles High LFTs Rash GI distress Flatuence Constipation	Cyclosporine Fibric acid derivatives Erythromycin Warfarin Gemfibrozil Niacin	Pregnancy Allergic reaction Liver disease Lactation
Fibric acid derivatives	Lower TGs Raises HDL Lower VLDL Lower TC	Flulike illness symptoms Sore muscles (myopathy) Choleliathasis High liver function tests (LFTs) Tumor formation (questionable) Gastrointestinal (GI) distress	Coumadin Cyclosporine "Statins" insulin Sulfonylureas	Liver disease Pregnancy Allergic reaction Gallbladder disease
Nicotinic acid (niacin)	Lowers LDL-c Lowers TGs Lowers VLDL-c Raises HDL-c Lowers TC	Rash Flushing High LFTs Gout (hyperuricemia) Skin discoloration Migraines Decreased vision Glucose intolerance GI intolerance Nausea Vomiting Dyspepsia Peptic ulcers	Aluminum in meds	Liver disease Arrhythmias Peptic ulcers Irritable bowel disease Gout Tartrazines allergy

* New research indicates that HMG-CoA inhibitors may reduce cardiac events in both patients who have had a myocardial infarction and the at-risk population.

of serum lipids may alert a practitioner to patients who are at potential risk. Chapter 1-4 includes information on the detection and evaluation of atherosclerosis.

NOTES AND PEARLS

Abnormal lipid metabolism is now classified as a genetic disorder. Although significant strides in understanding the atherogenic process have been made, it would be premature to think we have all the answers. Certainly, ASVD involves more than hypercholesterolemia and the solution involves considerably more than a "diet." New laboratory tests, lipid management protocols, medications, surgical techniques, gene therapy, and vitamin and mineral supplementation are on the horizon. Numerous well-respected studies have shown that the currently utilized therapies can reduce cardiac events up to 30 percent; inversely, up to 70 percent of coronary events are not prevented. Future technology may well reduce the incidence of ASVD, the number one cause of death and disability in the United States.

BIBLIOGRAPHY

Berkow R (ed): *The Merck Manual of Diagnosis and Therapy*, 16th ed. Rahway, NJ, Merck, 1992, pp 409–413.

Isselbacher KJ, Braunwald E, Wilson JD, et al (eds): *Harrison's Principles of Medicine*, 13th ed. New York, McGraw-Hill, 1994, pp 1106–1116, 2234–2249, 1108–1137.

Skillings J, Howes DG: Recertification series hyperlipidemia and atherosclerosis, part I. *Physician Assist* 7:32–68, 1996.

Skillings J, Howes DG: Recertification series hyperlipidemia and atherosclerosis, part II. *Physician Assist* 8:32–62, 1996.

Summary of the Second Report of the National Cholesterol Education Program (NCEP) Expert Panel on Detection, Evaluation and Treatment of High Blood Cholesterol in Adults (Adult Treatment Panel II). *JAMA* 269(23):3015–3023, 1993.

Surperko HR: New aspects of risk factors for the development of atherosclerosis, including small low-density lipoprotein, homocysteine, and lipoprotein (a). *Curr Opin Cardiol* 10:347–354, 1995.

Chapter 1–7
ISCHEMIC CORONARY ARTERY SYNDROMES
Morton A. Diamond

DISCUSSION

Coronary atherosclerosis is the most common cause of ischemic heart disease. Less frequently, myocardial ischemia may be a result of nonatheromatous coronary disease such as Prinzmetal's variant angina and microvascular angina (syndrome X) or of myocardial hypertrophy, either idiopathic or secondary to aortic valvular disease. This chapter focuses on ischemic coronary syndromes caused by atherosclerosis (see Chap. 1-4).

The atheromatous plaque represents the cardinal substrate of coronary artery disease. The central features of atheroma formation are endothelial injury and low-density lipoprotein (LDL) excess. Increased endothelial permeability to LDL results in subintimal deposition. The LDL is oxidized, attracting macrophages. The macrophages engulf the LDL and become foam cells. In turn, the foam cells elaborate growth factors, free radicals,

Table 1-7-1. Factors Favoring the Development of Coronary Atherosclerosis

Increasing age
Sex (male > female)
Genetics: family history of coronary disease doubles risk
Smoking
Hypertension
Diabetes mellitus
Dyslipidemia
Emotional stress
Obesity
Sedentary life-style

lipases, and proteinases. The growth factors cause smooth muscle cells to multiply and secrete collagen, with resultant atheroma formation.

Superimposed thrombosis is the primary cause of acute coronary syndromes: unstable angina, acute myocardial infarction, and sudden death. Thrombosis is precipitated by endothelial denudation or plaque rupture. Platelets then adhere to the injured endothelium, and this is followed by fibrin deposition, resulting in an occlusive or nonocclusive thrombus. The composition of the atheromatous plaque is the most important determinant of the development of thrombus-mediated unstable angina, myocardial infarction, and sudden death. Thrombosis does not occur until mature plaques are present. Myocardial infarction results from an acute total thrombotic occlusion, while unstable angina usually is due to mural (incomplete) thrombus development.

Since ischemic coronary artery syndromes represent a spectrum of the same pathophysiologic process, they will be considered together rather than as separate disease entities.

Risk Factors

The factors favoring the development of coronary atherosclerosis are listed in Table 1-7-1.

STABLE ("CHRONIC") ANGINA PECTORIS

Chronic angina occurs when myocardial oxygen demand outstrips oxygen delivery by the coronary circulation. Angina typically occurs during physical exertion, emotional upset, fever, and tachyarrhythmias. The frequency of anginal discomfort does not accurately reflect the anatomic or functional severity of the atherosclerotic process. Angina is still a diagnosis made by history.

Signs and Symptoms

The discomfort typically is described as tightness or pressure and is most commonly felt in the chest or arms. Frequently, however, the discomfort may be noted in the neck, jaw, gums, upper back, and even the umbilical area. Sharp or jabbing pain is not suggestive of angina; discomfort affected by breathing, body position, or swallowing is similarly not characteristic of angina. Cardiac patients who describe only exertional dyspnea must have the etiology of the breathlessness clearly defined, for in some patients the dyspnea represents myocardial ischemia ("anginal equivalent"). An anginal patient may experience other cardiac symptoms related to cardiac function, such as peripheral edema, palpitations, and fatigue.

The physical examination in a stable anginal patient is variable. Cardiac examination in a resting asymptomatic patient may be normal or may demonstrate evidence of antecedent myocardial dysfunction. A patient examined during myocardial ischemia often manifests a presystolic (S_4) gallop and/or a transient mitral regurgitant murmur as a result of papillary muscle dysfunction.

Diagnostic Considerations

Esophageal, chest wall, and breast disorders as well as intraabdominal diseases must be considered in a patient who experiences chest discomfort. A careful history and physical examination, complemented by laboratory and imaging studies, will enable a physician assistant to define the correct diagnosis.

Laboratory and Radiologic Studies

There are no laboratory tests that specifically assist in the diagnosis of angina. However, clinical risk factors should be sought, for example, hyperglycemia, anemia, dyslipidemia, hyperthyroidism, and hypoxemia. A chest x-ray may provide information concerning heart size and left ventricular function.

Other Diagnostic Tests

A resting electrocardiogram (ECG) indicates rhythm, the presence of atrioventricular or intraventricular conduction defects, evidence of a previous infarction, and an indication of hypertrophy or ischemia. In the majority of stable anginal patients, the resting ECG is normal when the patient is asymptomatic.

Treatment

General Treatment

Treatment consists of the following:

- *Modify risk factors:* Patients require weight reduction, smoking cessation, dyslipidemia or diabetes treatment, and control of hypertension.
- *Modify activity:* Patients should avoid heavy lifting, sudden bursts of running, and extremes of temperature.
- *Risk assessment:* Since the frequency of anginal attacks does not correlate with anatomic abnormality, patients should undergo exercise or pharmacologic stress testing to define the risk for a cardiac event, that is, an acute myocardial infarction or sudden death. A low-risk patient is treated medically; a high-risk patient is referred for coronary angiography and revascularization.

Pharmacologic Management

Nitroglycerin

Sublingual or inhaled nitroglycerin is used both in the treatment of an acute anginal attack and prophylactically to prevent episodes. For patients having more than four or five attacks per week, long-acting oral or transdermal agents should be added. An 8- to 10-h nitrate-free interval helps prevent nitrate tolerance. The dose of the nitrate is variable, depending on resting blood pressure and concomitant medication intake.

Aspirin

Aspirin 160 mg/d or 325 mg every other day should be prescribed unless a contraindication exists, since this agent reduces cardiac mortality rate.

Beta Blockers and Calcium Channel Blockers

The appropriate choice of a beta or calcium channel blocker depends on the presence of concomitant medical conditions. These disorders, which influence the choice of medication, include resting heart rate, atrioventricular conduction disturbances, arrhythmias, chronic lung disease, congestive heart failure, lipid abnormalities, valvular heart disease, hyper- or hypoglycemia, and peripheral arterial vascular disease. In general, beta blockers are preferred in an anginal patient with resting sinus tachycardia

or a history of ventricular tachycardia. A selected calcium channel blocker is prescribed for patients with sinus bradycardia, hyper- or hypoglycemia, congestive heart failure, peripheral vascular disease, and hypercholesterolemia.

Important side effects of beta blockers include congestive heart failure, unrecognized hypoglycemia, atrioventricular block, and exacerbation of bronchospastic symptoms or peripheral claudication. Calcium channel blockers may precipitate congestive heart failure or orthostatic hypotension. The dose of each agent is variable. One should start low, increasing the medication dose as clinically appropriate.

Clinical Pearls

When talking to a patient with ischemic symptoms, one should use the term *discomfort*, not the term *pain*. A patient with angina will often respond negatively when asked whether he or she has chest pain but affirmatively when asked about discomfort. If a patient with a presumptive diagnosis of angina does not respond to nitroglycerin, one should reexamine the diagnosis. However, an anginal patient may not be receiving the proper dose of the medication.

A simple and effective clinical test is performed by serially measuring blood pressure for 3 min after sublingual nitroglycerin administration. A systolic blood pressure decrease of 10 mmHg is the desired hemodynamic effect. If the patient's systolic pressure does not demonstrate this hypotensive effect, one should increase the tablet dose. Nitroglycerin should be taken while the patient is sitting down. If the patient is unable to sit, leaning against a stationary object may lessen the risk of significant orthostatic hypotension.

Angina lasts continuously for at least 1 min and is experienced in an area at least the size of a silver dollar. One should emphasize to the patient that it is important to take nitroglycerin immediately upon the onset of angina.

Do not allow the patient to "see if I really need it." Further, instruct the patient to notify the physician assistant if there is a change in the pattern of angina, specifically including the appearance of nocturnal angina, angina at rest, or angina with lessened exertion.

UNSTABLE ANGINA PECTORIS

Unstable angina is defined as symptomatic myocardial ischemia occurring at rest or abruptly increasing in frequency in a previously stable anginal patient or new-onset angina.

Signs and Symptoms

Dyspnea, palpitations, and fatigue are the commonly associated symptoms. Single-vessel coronary artery disease is found in 40 to 50 percent of these patients, and multivessel disease in 45 to 50 percent. An acute, nonocclusive thrombus is found in the majority of these patients. The angiogram is normal in the remaining patients.

Physical examination may be normal or may demonstrate transient presystolic (S₄) gallop or mitral regurgitant murmur.

Laboratory and Radiologic Tests

The chest x-ray will define heart size and, if present, evidence of congestive heart failure. An ECG is performed to look for evidence of ischemia, myocardial injury, or infarction. Serial creatine phosphokinase (CPK) and lactate dehydrogenase (LDH) enzyme levels should be obtained three times (every 12 h) to determine whether myocardial necrosis has occurred.

Treatment

Patients experiencing rest angina or worsening angina associated with ECG changes should be urgently hospitalized, placed on bed rest with cardiac monitoring and control of precipitating factors (see "Stable ("Chronic") Angina Pectoris," above), and started on medication. Referral to a physician is indicated.

Pharmacological Management

Treatment of unstable angina includes oral aspirin, intravenous heparin (bolus followed by continuous infusion) to maintain the partial thromboplastin time (PTT) at 1.5 to 2.5 times control, intravenous nitroglycerin, and a beta blocker. Thrombolytic agents are not of clinical value in treating unstable angina. Antithrombotic agents undergoing clinical investigation include hirudin, hirulog, and argatroban. Their efficacy will be defined as clinical studies are reported.

ACUTE MYOCARDIAL INFARCTION

Myocardial infarction is the most frequent cause of death in the United States. Approximately 1.5 million heart attacks occur annually. With modern therapy, hospital mortality rate is 15 percent. Half the deaths occur in the first hour as a result of ventricular fibrillation; the other deaths generally are due to cardiogenic shock or congestive heart failure and occur within 2 days of hospitalization. While atherosclerotic disease is the overwhelming cause of acute myocardial infarction (AMI), it is important to recognize that there are other, nonatherosclerotic etiologies of infarction. In a young adult, cocaine abuse may precipitate an acute, nonthrombotic AMI.

Signs and Symptoms

The patient usually has experienced continuous severe ischemic discomfort for at least 30 min. In some patients, the discomfort may wax and wane ("stutter"). In the elderly, AMI may not be associated with discomfort; instead, the patient will present with left ventricular congestive heart failure or weakness or syncope.

Physical examination often reveals an anguished expression on the patients face. The skin may be moist and cool from adrenergic discharge associated with heart failure. Peripheral cyanosis is noted in AMI patients with cardiogenic shock. The blood pressure and pulse are variable, depending on sympathetic tone and left ventricular function. Precordial palpation may reveal a presystolic impulse correlating with an auscultatory S_4 gallop. Anterior or lateral infarction may be associated with a systolic impulse in the 3d, 4th, or 5th interspace along the left sternal border. A systolic murmur may be heard near the cardiac apex, indicating mitral regurgitation from papillary muscle dysfunction. A pericardial friction rub is heard in approximately 15 percent of AMI patients.

Diagnostic Considerations

The differential diagnosis includes pericardial and pleural pain, pulmonary embolism, aortic dissection, and intraabdominal diseases, including peptic ulcer disease, cholecystitis, and pancreatitis.

Laboratory and Radiologic Tests

Creatine kinase (CK) is abnormal 4 to 8 h after the onset of symptoms and returns to normal in 2 to 3 days. The MB isoenzyme is not entirely specific for myocardium, but an increased MB fraction in the absence of trauma or surgery involving the intestine, uterus, or prostate is indicative of AMI. Troponins T and C are being evaluated as even earlier chemical markers of myocardial infarction.

Table 1-7-2. Patient Selection for Thrombolytic Therapy

Indications
  Ischemic chest pain for more than 30 min
  Electrocardiogram
    ST-segment elevation greater than 1 mm in two contiguous leads
    or new left bundle branch block
  Time window
    Less than 6 h: most beneficial
    6–12 h: less effective but still beneficial
    12–24 h: high risk, continued chest pain
  Special subsets (treat in absence of other contraindications)
    Remote (more than 6 months) history of nonhemorrhagic stroke
    Past history (more than 2 months) of gastrointestinal bleeding
    Hypotension or moderate hypertension
    Cardiopulmonary resuscitation
Contraindications
  Absolute
    Major surgery or trauma in last 2 weeks
    Active internal bleeding (excluding menses)
    Prior intracranial bleed or cerebral neoplasm
    Cerebrovascular events or head trauma (within last 6 months)
    Known allergy to a drug considered for use
  Relative
    Active peptic ulcer
    Pregnancy or within 1 month postpartum
    Severe, persistent hypertension (systolic/diastolic blood pressure
    greater than 200/110 mmHg)
    Current use of anticoagulants

Serial ECGs generally reveal abnormalities in an infarction. It is important, however, to realize that a normal ECG at the patient's initial presentation in the emergency department is not uncommon. Classic ECG changes include the development of Q waves with ST-segment elevation (Q-wave infarction). Frequently, ECGs demonstrate ST-segment depression and/or T-wave inversion (non-Q-wave infarction). In the non-Q-wave group, the diagnosis of AMI rests more on clinical findings and elevation of enzymes than on the ECG.

Treatment

The physician assistant in the emergency department must urgently evaluate patients who experience chest pain to identify those who require perfusion therapy. A history of ischemic discomfort and the standard ECG represent the primary data for patient management.

Patients should be promptly attached to a cardiac monitor, receive nasal oxygen, and have an intravenous 5% dextrose-in-water infusion started.

All patients with an acute coronary syndrome should chew an adult aspirin tablet, and thereafter oral aspirin should be continued indefinitely.

If the ECG shows 1 mm or more ST elevation in contiguous leads, intravenous thrombolytic therapy should be given quickly unless a contraindication is present. Patients whose ECGs demonstrate ST depression and/or T-wave inversion should not be considered for thrombolytic therapy. Thrombolytic agents activate plasminogen, converting it to plasmin, which causes dissolution of a thrombus by digesting the supporting fibrin network. There has been considerable interest in the efficacy of the various thrombolytic agents. Randomized clinical trials suggest that accelerated t-PA is associated with a modestly lower mortality rate but with a slight but definite increase in the risk of bleeding. Table 1-7-2 lists indications for and contraindications to thrombolytic therapy in AMI patients.

Intracranial hemorrhage is the most serious complication of thrombolytic therapy. More common, though relatively minor, is bleeding at vascular puncture sites. Most patients exposed to streptokinase and APSAC will develop antibodies to these agents. Therefore, a patient with AMI should not be treated with streptokinase if he or she has received that agent within the last year.

Analgesia utilizing intravenous morphine or meperidine is effective. Morphine has vagomimetic effects, and meperidine has an atropine-like effect. Oral nitroglycerin should be given as long as the systolic blood pressure is greater than 90 mmHg and there is no evidence of inferior infarction with associated right ventricular infarction. (Right ventricular infarction should be considered when patients with inferior infarction exhibit signs of low cardiac output and elevated central venous pressure.) Intravenous nitroglycerin is most beneficial if the patient is in congestive heart failure or continues to have ischemic discomfort. Close monitoring of blood pressure is essential.

Patients seen within 4 h of the onset of symptoms as well as those with sinus tachycardia or hypertension should receive an intravenous beta blocker as long as no contraindication is present. Such a contraindication would include congestive heart failure, bronchospasm, hypotension, sinus bradycardia, and heart block. At the time of discharge, oral beta blocker therapy should be continued if no contraindication exists. Angiotensin-converting enzyme (ACE) inhibitors also play an important role in AMI therapy. An elderly patient or one with an anterior infarction or a previous infarction and an asymptomatic patient with an ejection fraction of 40 percent or less should receive lifelong ACE inhibitor therapy. The calcium channel blockers verapamil and diltiazem should not be routinely used.

Complications

Major complications of AMI may be arbitrarily divided into two categories: pump failure and electrical instability.

Left ventricular dysfunction continues to be the single most important predictor of death after an AMI. Physiologically, the heart failure may be systolic with a resultant decrease in cardiac output. Alternatively, there may be coexistent systolic and diastolic failure with pulmonary venous congestion and dyspnea.

Heart failure is most effectively treated by a reduction in afterload through the administration of diuretics and nitrates. ACE inhibitors may be added. For severe heart failure not responsive to these agents, beta receptor agonists such as dopamine and dobutamine may be infused. Digitalis is generally reserved for AMI patients with superimposed supraventricular arrhythmia and those whose heart failure is refractory to vasodilator medication, diuretics, and beta agonists.

The most severe manifestation of left ventricular heart failure is cardiogenic shock caused by extensive myocardial damage. These patients exhibit a clouded sensorium, cool skin, and peripheral cyanosis related to a severe reduction in cardiac output. Medical management includes beta agonists, intraaortic balloon counterpulsation, and in selected cases emergency coronary bypass surgery. Despite therapy, the mortality rate remains high at approximately 60 to 70 percent.

AMI is associated with frequent abnormalities in heart rhythm, both supraventricular and ventricular in origin. Sinus tachycardia, sinus bradycardia, atrial fibrillation and flutter, paroxysmal supraventricular tachycardia, ventricular premature beats, ventricular tachycardia, and ventricular fibrillation are common. The hemodynamic consequences of arrhythmia primarily relate to the fact that both tachycardia and bradycardia lower cardiac output. Loss of atrial contraction in atrial fibrillation further reduces cardiac output because of lessened ventricular filling. AMI patients whose course is complicated by arrhythmia require prompt physician consultation.

The treatment of arrhythmia requires careful evaluation of an AMI patient. Therapy may include not only antiarrhythmic drugs and electrical intervention (cardioversion, defibrillation, pacemaker insertion) but also correction of electrolyte and acid-base abnormalities, anemia, and hypoxemia.

Other Complications

Recurrent chest discomfort in a patient with a recent infarction may be due to ischemia (angina or infarct expansion) or nonischemic causes (pericarditis, pulmonary embolism). Careful physical examination, ECG comparison, and the response to nitroglycerin are early measures that may be supplemented with echocardiography or perfusion scans. Pericarditis occurs in transmural infarction, with pain present as early as the first or second day. The pain is typically longer in duration than is that caused by ischemia. The pericardial discomfort is increased during recumbency and deep inspiration and eased when the patient leans forward when sitting.

A transient pericardial friction rub is heard frequently. The echocardiographic presence of a pericardial effusion generally is considered an indication to discontinue anticoagulants. Aspirin in higher doses than are prescribed regularly after an infarction is usually effective and is preferable to corticosteroids and nonsteroidal anti-inflammatory agents.

Mural left ventricular thrombi are common in AMI patients who are not anticoagulated. The incidence of mural thrombi has decreased dramatically in patients receiving thrombolytic agents with heparin or heparin therapy alone. Echocardiography is the most accurate method for diagnosing left ventricular mural thrombi. If they are present, anticoagulation with warfarin for 3 to 6 months generally is recommended.

Predischarge Considerations

A low-level exercise test (5 to 6 Mets) frequently is performed before hospital discharge to identify those at risk for another cardiac event. The provocative test is done to define ventricular arrhythmia and myocardial ischemia. Those who have a normal hemodynamic and ECG response to low-level testing have a 1 to 2 percent annual mortality rate. In contrast, recurrent cardiac events are likely in patients who cannot perform the test or who demonstrate ischemic ST-segment depression or significant ventricular arrhythmia. Patients who demonstrate ischemia may be referred for coronary angiography. Electrophysiologic studies may be indicated for those who exhibit exercise-induced ventricular arrhythmia.

Assessment of left ventricular systolic function, frequently ejection fraction determination by echocardiography, has important therapeutic and prognostic significance. Those whose ejection fraction is 40 percent or less have a significantly higher cardiac mortality rate. However, recent clinical trials have demonstrated the therapeutic benefit of long-term ACE inhibitor therapy in these patients.

At the time of hospital discharge, preventive measures include instruction in diet, activity level, weight control, smoking cessation, treatment of dyslipidemia, and, if no contraindication is present, indefinite aspirin and beta blocker therapy.

SILENT ISCHEMIA

Silent ischemia is myocardial ischemia that occurs in the absence of symptoms. These patients are at increased risk for myocardial infarction and have an increased mortality rate. Silent ischemia is more common in diabetic patients.

The diagnosis is established by defining ischemic ST-segment changes during ambulatory electrocardiography or during treadmill testing in a patient who is not experiencing cardiac symptoms. Silent ischemia may occur in patients who have never had ischemic discomfort. Moreover, silent ischemic episodes are very common in patients who also have anginal discomfort. In fact, the majority of ischemic episodes in this group are asymptomatic.

The presence of ischemic ST-segment depression during an exercise test confers an increased risk of subsequent cardiac events regardless of whether anginal discomfort occurred during the test.

In considering the management of silent ischemia, it is significant that medications that prevent anginal discomfort also prevent silent ischemia. Therefore, aspirin, beta blockers, and nitrates may be prescribed.

SUDDEN CARDIAC DEATH

Sudden cardiac death (SCD) is arguably the primary problem in contemporary cardiology. Approximately 400,000 sudden deaths occur annually in the United States. In one-quarter the sudden death is the initial expression of heart disease. In the majority of cases SCD is due to ventricular fibrillation. Three subsets of patients are at highest risk of sudden cardiac death. The most common substrate of sudden death is myocardial ischemia. In only a small percentage of cases, however, is there associated myocardial infarction. Additionally, patients with left ventricular dysfunction of any etiology and patients with left ventricular hypertrophy are at increased risk. The last subset includes hypertrophic cardiomyopathy, a major cause of sudden death in young adults.

A bifold approach has been taken to this major public health problem. First is the identification of known heart disease patients at greatest risk of sudden death. These patients often demonstrate malignant ventricular arrhythmia. Some of these patients are survivors of sudden cardiac death ("cardiac arrest") who undergo implantation of an automatic defibrillator.

The second approach is the public health measure of placing external defibrillators in public places, for example, sports arenas, with attendant training of nonmedical personnel to be used on those who suddenly collapse and are pulseless. Pilot programs are under way to determine the efficacy of such efforts.

BIBLIOGRAPHY

Falk E, Shah P, Fuster V: Coronary plaque disruption. *Circulation* 92:657–671, 1995.

Chapter 1–8
PERICARDIAL DISEASE
Morton A. Diamond

DISCUSSION

Pericardial disease is increasingly recognized because patients with cancer, renal disease, and connective tissue disease are living longer. Patients with disease of the pericardium may present with acute pericarditis, pericardial effusion, or constrictive pericarditis. When a physician assistant establishes a diagnosis of pericardial

Table 1-8-1. Causes of Acute Pericarditis

Idiopathic
Viral
Purulent
Tuberculosis
Uremia
Myocardial infarction
   Acute pericarditis
   Post–myocardial infarction syndrome
Neoplastic disease
Radiation therapy
Vasculitis–connective tissue disorders
Invasive medical procedures
Medication
Sarcoid
Inflammatory bowel disease

disease, the determination must be made whether a causative systemic illness is present. In the United States, cancer spreading to the pericardium is now the most common cause of disease of the pericardium.

ACUTE PERICARDITIS
Pathophysiology

Pericardial inflammation may be caused by a variety of infectious agents and other disorders (Table 1-8-1). The most common is idiopathic pericarditis that is thought to be due to viruses, usually coxsackievirus and echovirus. Purulent pericarditis is most often due to *Pneumococcus* and *Staphylococcus* from an adjacent intrathoracic infection. Gram-negative organisms and fungi also may produce purulent inflammation. Tuberculous pericarditis is increasing in frequency because of an increase in cases of drug-resistant disease. Tuberculous pericarditis usually occurs in the absence of demonstrable pulmonary disease. AIDS patients may develop acute pericarditis from a wide variety of opportunistic infectious agents. Vasculitis–connective tissue diseases associated with acute pericarditis include systemic lupus erythematosus (SLE), scleroderma, and polyarteritis. SLE must be ruled out in any female patient presenting with acute pericarditis. Uremic pericarditis is common and is dramatic in onset. Its clinical manifestations are similar to those of idiopathic inflammation. Pericardial involvement from neoplasia most frequently is due to lymphoma or contiguous spread from breast or lung cancer. Invasive medical procedures, including heart surgery, pacemaker insertion, and cardiac catheterization, are increasingly common causes of acute pericarditis.

Medications that cause acute inflammation include isoniazid, hydralazine, penicillin, phenylbutazone, procainamide, diphenylhydantoin, and doxorubicin. Aortic root dissection into the pericardium is a rare cause but may quickly cause life-threatening cardiac tamponade.

Symptoms and Signs

The cardinal symptoms and signs of acute pericarditis include chest pain and friction rub. The pain may be precordial or retrosternal and commonly radiates to the neck. The discomfort may be sharp or dull and typically is aggravated by recumbency, inspiration, and body motion. Dyspnea may be noted as the patient is unable to take a full inspiration because of chest pain. The physician assistant must differentiate pericardial pain from that caused by myocardial ischemia. A pericardial friction rub establishes the diagnosis. However, the rub may be transitory, and therefore frequent auscultation is necessary.

Post–myocardial infarction syndrome (Dressler's syndrome), which is manifested by chest pain, malaise, fever, and both pleural and pericardial effusions, is thought to be an autoimmune disorder but is lessening in frequency. Though pericardial effusions may be large, tamponade is rare. Recurrences of Dressler's syndrome are common, but the prognosis of the initial infarction is not altered. Therapy includes nonsteroidal anti-inflammatory drugs (NSAIDs) and, if necessary, corticosteroids.

Laboratory and Radiologic Studies

In idiopathic pericarditis, mild leukocytosis and an elevation of the erythrocyte sedimentation rate are common. Pericarditis associated with SLE frequently reveals leukopenia and a positive antinuclear antibody response. Significant elevation of the white blood cell count, particularly when associated with a leftward shift, suggests bacterial infection. Renal function studies will confirm uremic pericarditis.

The chest x-ray is usually normal unless the pericarditis is associated with significant pericardial effusion or an intrathoracic neoplasm is present. In acute pericarditis, the echocardiogram commonly demonstrates increased pericardial fluid but may be normal.

Electrocardiogram

When not associated with myocardial infarction, the electrocardiogram (ECG) demonstrates ST-segment and T-wave changes without alteration of the QRS complex. The elevated ST segments have a concave upward character and are noted in all leads except V_1 and aVR. There is no reciprocal ST-segment depression as is noted in myocardial injury or infarction. In pericarditis the T wave inverts after the ST segments have returned to baseline, while in myocardial infarction T-wave inversion occurs while ST segments are still elevated. The ECG changes of acute pericarditis also must be differentiated from those of early repolarization. In early repolarization, ST-segment elevation may be diffuse but serial changes are not noted.

PERICARDIAL EFFUSION

Pericardial effusion may be caused by many disorders, including infectious, neoplastic, metabolic, and autoimmune etiologies (Table 1-8-2). The rate of pericardial fluid accumulation determines the clinical state of the patient. Because the pericardium is compliant, a slowly enlarging effusion may contain 2000 mL of fluid without hemodynamic compromise. In contrast, a rapidly developing small effusion may cause life-threatening tamponade related to inadequate cardiac filling. Effusions may be associated with chest pain when they are related to an inflammatory process or may be painless, as may occur in neoplasia.

Clinical Features

Idiopathic pericarditis usually occurs in a young adult who has had an upper respiratory infection during the preceding weeks. The onset of chest pain is often dramatic. The diagnosis is made

Table 1-8-2. Causes of Pericardial Effusion

Neoplasia
Infection
Idiopathic
Myocardial infarction
Congestive heart failure
Trauma
Vasculitis–connective tissue disorders
Medication
Uremia
Nephrotic syndrome
Hypothyroidism

by friction rub, ECG changes, and echocardiographic demonstration of pericardial effusion. No underlying disease is found. NSAIDs commonly suppress the pain within 24 h. Corticosteroids may be given to a patient whose symptoms are resistant to the initial therapy. While effectively suppressing clinical manifestations, corticosteroids may promote exacerbations of inflammation. The illness usually lasts 1 to 3 weeks and is self-limited. In fewer than 5 percent of cases, a recurrence of acute pericarditis will occur. Rarely, tamponade may develop. Bacterial pericarditis should be suspected when a patient has high fever, chills, and night sweats. Suspicion of this disease requires diagnostic pericardiocentesis. If it is present, therapy includes antibiotics and surgical drainage. Mortality rates range from 55 to 75 percent and are particularly high when pericarditis is associated with gram-negative organisms. If pericarditis is mistaken for myocardial infarction, thrombolytic therapy can have life-threatening consequences. Pericarditis is a relative contraindication to both thrombolytic and anticoagulant agents. In transmural myocardial infarction, pericarditis is usually manifest on the second or third day. This pain must be clinically differentiated from myocardial ischemia and infarct extension. Therapy with NSAIDs is generally effective.

Symptoms and Signs

Symptoms and signs are primarily related to the underlying disorder unless tamponade is present. A small effusion may be present in an asymptomatic patient who has a normal cardiac examination. The effusion may be demonstrated only on echocardiographic study. Large effusions may cause cough and dyspnea as a result of compression of adjacent lung tissue and often are associated with muffled heart tones. Tamponade occurs when rapidly developing effusions reduce filling of the heart and subsequently cardiac output. The patient complains of dyspnea, cough, and weakness. Central venous pressure is universally elevated. Tachycardia, tachypnea, paradoxical pulse, and hypotension are very common. Paradoxical pulse—the exaggeration of the normal difference in systolic pressure between inspiration and expiration—can be defined only in a patient in sinus rhythm. The most common cause of a paradoxical pulse is obstructive lung disease.

Radiologic Studies

Radiographic signs in effusion are variable, depending on the size of the fluid accumulation and the presence of an intrathoracic neoplasm. Small effusions are associated with a normal cardiac appearance, while large effusions produce the "water bottle" enlarged cardiac silhouette. The echocardiogram is the best diagnostic tool for the diagnosis of effusion. Tamponade, which is characterized by increased intrapericardial pressure, is diagnosed by demonstration of diastolic collapse of the right atrium and right ventricle.

Management

Therapy is dependent on the presence or absence of hemodynamic compromise. Tamponade requires immediate pericardiocentesis, preferably with catheter drainage. Otherwise, effusion management is related to treatment of the underlying cause. Physician referral is indicated in all cases of pericarditis associated with systemic disease or effusions resulting in hemodynamic impairment.

CONSTRICTIVE PERICARDITIS

Constrictive pericarditis, a tightening vise around the heart, may be due to idiopathic pericarditis, radiation therapy to the chest, neoplasia, cardiac surgery, bacterial and fungal infection, connective tissue disease, uremia, and sarcoid. Constriction may occur quickly, over weeks as in virulent infection or neoplasia, or over years as in tuberculosis. Physiologically, constriction is associated with increased cardiac filling pressure and decreased cardiac output.

Signs and Symptoms

Typical symptoms include fatigue, dyspnea, nausea, and weakness. Physical examination reveals distended neck veins from elevated central venous pressure, congestive hepatomegaly, ascites, and peripheral edema. The lung fields are typically clear. Kussmaul's sign—loss of the inspiratory decrease in jugular venous pressure—is common, but paradoxical pulse is noted in a minority of patients. The physician assistant must differentiate this disorder from right ventricular heart failure and restrictive cardiomyopathy.

Radiologic Studies

The chest x-ray may show pericardial calcification. Echocardiography, as well as CT and MRI, can demonstrate pericardial thickening and small heart chambers.

Electrocardiogram

The ECG generally reveals low-voltage and diffuse T-wave inversion. Atrial fibrillation and atrioventricular and intraventricular conduction defects are common.

Differential Diagnosis

The differentiation of constrictive pericarditis from restrictive cardiomyopathy is still a major diagnostic challenge. Sarcoidosis, hematochromatosis, and amyloid disease of the heart also reduce ventricular filling. Therefore, the clinical appearance of patients in both cardiac disorders is similar. Cardiac catheterization with endomyocardial biopsy is employed to help make the correct diagnosis. Thoracotomy may still be necessary to establish the diagnosis. If constriction is found, pericardiectomy is performed.

BIBLIOGRAPHY

Ameli S, Shah PK: Cardiac tamponade: Pathophysiology, diagnosis and management. *Cardiol Clin North Am* 9:665–674, 1991.

Chapter 1–9
PERIPHERAL VASCULAR DISEASE
Marquitha S. Mayfield

DISCUSSION

Peripheral vascular disease (PVD) is a broad term encompassing a variety of disorders that affect the arteries, veins, and lymphatics. Specifically included in this category of diseases are vessels that provide peripheral circulation to the extracranial cerebral vasculature (carotid and vertebrals), the extremities, and the organs of the thoracic and abdominal cavities. Excluded are disorders caused by pathologic changes involving the coronary and intracranial cerebral vasculature.

Diseases of the peripheral vasculature are common. Ten to twenty percent of the U.S. adult population suffers from varicose veins. Approximately 5 percent of patients over age 70 years have symptomatic arterial disease. Each year, approximately 2 million cases of venous thrombosis and 2000 cases of aortic aneurysms are diagnosed in the United States. Peripheral vascular disease is a leading cause of death and limb loss in the United States. Most of these patients are middle-aged or elderly.

As the patient population continues to age, the prevalence of disorders involving the peripheral vasculature will continue to increase. Many patients with mild to moderate symptoms of chronic vascular disease can be safely managed conservatively in the primary care setting. Others with severe or acute symptoms of vascular disease require intensive diagnostic evaluation and management, often involving the expertise of subspecialty consultants. A primary care provider must be able to differentiate between these two patient population groups to render proper clinical management.

Primary pathologic changes affecting the peripheral vasculature are as follows:

1. *Atherosclerosis:* This is a progressive, systemic disease characterized by the deposition of lipoprotein along the intimal layer of the arterial wall. These deposits become thrombotic and fibrose and calcify, forming an atheroma. Atheromatous plaques build up over time and progressively occlude the lumens of arteries. Atherosclerosis also may cause the medial layer of the vessel wall to degenerate, increasing the risk of developing aneurysms. Because atherosclerosis is a multisystem disease, many patients also have coexisting coronary and/or cerebrovascular disease.
2. *Thrombosis:* This involves the formation of a clot that remains attached to the vessel wall. Clots usually form at sites of previous injury, vessel narrowing, or anastomosis. Clots can occlude the lumens of vessels, diminishing the arterial blood supply or obstructing venous return. Distal tissues become ischemic from arterial occlusion or edematous from venous obstruction.
3. *Thromboembolism:* This involves the detachment or fragmentation of a thrombus (clot) into the bloodstream. This material travels to a distal site, producing vessel occlusion. Both arteries and veins may be affected by the embolic phenomenon. The complications are acute and severe. An embolic event in the arterial tree can precipitate severe ischemia and tissue necrosis (gangrene) from acute arterial insufficiency. In the venous circulation, a pulmonary embolus can result, with catastrophic results.
4. *Aneurysms and varicosities:* When arterial walls weaken and dilate, aneurysms form. These changes in veins produce varicosities. Increased intravascular pressure can distend the vessel lumen, and congenital defects can also weaken vessel walls.
5. *Vasculitis:* Infection or inflammation of the vessel wall can occur. Bacteria introduced into the circulation can seed previously damaged areas of blood vessels. Also, inflammatory disorders of the arteries and veins increase the incidence of thrombosis and vascular obstruction. While these conditions are rare, they should be suspected in patients who are intravenous drug abusers, have a connective tissue disorder, smoke, or have bacterial endocarditis.
6. *Vascular trauma:* The placement of catheters into the lumens of arteries and veins for diagnostic and therapeutic purposes can injure the vessel wall, precipitate the formation of clots that obstruct flow, and/or cause severe vasospasm with vessel occlusion. Vessels also may be transected in a variety of injuries, both major and minor.
7. *Congenital malformations:* Congenital narrowing of the aorta (coarctation), abnormal connections between arteries and veins (arteriovenous fistulas), and the like can form. These

abnormalities produce turbulent blood flow through the vessel lumen, increasing the incidence of thrombosis and embolism.

8. *Vasospasm:* Acute spasm of vessels may produce transient vascular occlusion, sometimes with marked distal tissue ischemia. Small arteries are usually affected. Vasospastic disorders may be primary in origin (Raynaud's disease) or iatrogenic (induced by arterial cannulation procedures).

In thinking about common diseases of the peripheral vasculature, it is useful to divide them into the following major categories:

I. Arterial disease
  A. Arterial insufficiency
    1. Atherosclerotic peripheral vascular disease
    2. Acute arterial insufficiency
    3. Nonatherosclerotic arterial insufficiency
  B. Aortic aneurysms and dissections
II. Venous disease
  A. Varicose veins
  B. Chronic venous insufficiency
    1. Venous stasis and venous ulcers
  C. Venous thrombosis
    1. Deep-venous thrombosis
    2. Superficial thrombophlebitis
III. Lymphatic disease
  A. Lymphedema
  B. Lymphangitis

Arterial Disease (Atherosclerotic Peripheral Vascular Disease)

DISCUSSION

Arterial insufficiency is caused by an occlusive process that reduces or completely obstructs blood flow to the distal tissues. The vascular occlusion may be acute or chronic in origin. Occlusion of 50 percent of the arterial lumen (75 percent of the vessel diameter) produces a clinically significant reduction in blood flow, resulting in tissue hypoxia and ischemia. Severe ischemia can result in tissue necrosis with gangrenous changes and limb loss or distal organ failure.

The most common cause of arterial occlusive disease is atherosclerosis. Atheromatous plaques often develop at points of bifurcation (branching), abrupt curvature, or vascular narrowing because of the shearing forces and turbulent blood flow associated with those areas. Lower extremities are affected more often than are upper extremities because of the higher arterial pressures in the legs.

Common sites for vessel occlusion include aorto-iliac bifurcation, femoral-popliteal bifurcation, popliteal-tibial-peroneal trifurcation, and common carotid bifurcation.

Because atherosclerosis is a chronic, slow process, collateral circulation often develops around areas of chronic occlusion. With adequate collateral flow, patients may be asymptomatic or have minimal symptoms. With time, however, these collateral vessels also become diseased and occlude.

Risk factors for the development of arterial occlusive disease include smoking, hypercholesterolemia, diabetes mellitus, hypertension, a family history, and male sex.

SYMPTOMS AND SIGNS

Pain is the principal symptom of arterial insufficiency. Intermittent claudication is a classic finding in chronic arterial insufficiency. Claudication may be described as a cramping discomfort, weakness, or a tired sensation induced by lower extremity exertion (walking, biking, etc.) and can be relieved with minimal rest. The calf is most commonly affected, although symptoms of claudication can occur in the thigh or buttocks. The area of vascular occlusion is proximal to the site of claudication: Thigh claudication would correlate with aorto-iliac disease, calf claudication with femoropopliteal disease, and foot pain with tibial vessel disease. Most symptoms are unilateral, however occlusive disease at the level of the aortic bifurcation may produce bilateral symptoms and signs. Claudication may become progressive over months or years, and its severity can be monitored by decreasing levels of patient ambulation and activity.

Rest pain is a more ominous sign of severe occlusive disease. This pain is continuous and severe, resulting from constant inadequate tissue perfusion through a severely stenotic artery. It occurs in the foot and is classically described as a burning or aching discomfort in the forefoot or toes that is most intense at night. Dangling the foot on the side of the bed may bring some relief because tissue perfusion is enhanced by gravity. The presence of rest pain is consistent with impending tissue necrosis and is a major indication for surgical intervention.

In males, impotence can be a presenting symptom when aorto-iliac disease is present. Its presence suggests occlusion of the internal iliac artery as is seen in Leriche's syndrome. Thigh and/or buttock claudication also may occur.

Transient ischemic attacks (TIAs) may be manifestations of occlusive disease of the carotid arteries. Amaurosis fugax (transient monocular blindness classically described as a "shade" or "curtain" descending over one eye) is a classic symptom of transient occlusion of the ophthalmic branch of the internal carotid artery. An atheromatous embolus from a diseased carotid artery is commonly the cause. Additional symptoms suggestive of carotid disease include unilateral weakness, numbness or tingling of an extremity, and speech disturbance. TIA symptoms typically develop suddenly and resolve spontaneously within 24 h.

There is a high prevalence of coexisting coronary artery disease, diabetes, cerebrovascular disease, and heart failure, in patients with arterial occlusive disease. Additional symptoms consistent with these disorders also may be present.

OBJECTIVE FINDINGS

Patient examination should be tailored to look specifically for the following clinical features seen in chronic occlusive disease.

1. *Diminished or absent peripheral pulses.* One should compare pulses in both extremities and look for asymmetry. Also, pulses should be compared before and after exercise, as pulses distal to the occlusion may diminish after exercise.
2. *Bruits* heard over the carotid, aortic, renal, iliac, or femoral vasculature. When vessels are severely occluded or stenotic, bruits may be absent.
3. *Ischemic skin changes* such as pallor on leg elevation followed by erythema on dependency (dependent rubor), poor capillary refill, or digital cyanosis.
4. *Trophic changes* such as loss of hair on the extremity (especially the feet and toes), shiny atrophic skin, and thickened toenails.
5. *Collapsed superficial veins* consistent with poor arterial inflow.
6. *Painful ischemic ulcers* that bleed minimally and are located on the distal aspect of digits or the heel of the foot. Gangrenous changes (wet or dry) of the distal extremity may be noted.

DIFFERENTIAL DIAGNOSES

The differential diagnosis for arterial insufficiency includes trauma, arterial embolism, arterial aneurysm or dissection, atherosclerotic vascular disease, and nonatherosclerotic disorders such as Buerger's disease.

A variety of disorders can mimic the pain of claudication, including

- Degenerative disk disease and/or spinal stenosis
- Osteoarthritis of the hip or knee
- Diabetic neuropathy
- Nocturnal leg cramps

Additionally neuropathic ulcers and venous ulcers may be confused with ischemic ulcers of arterial disease.

LABORATORY AND RADIOLOGIC TESTS

In the primary care setting, baseline laboratory studies to detect and evaluate pertinent risk factors (hypertension, diabetes, and hyperlipidemia) should be ordered.

OTHER DIAGNOSTICS

Hand-held Dopplers provide a quick, easy method for detecting nonpalpable pulses in the office. When they are combined with the use of a blood pressure cuff, an ankle/brachial ratio or index (ABI) can be measured and provide more information about the severity of vascular occlusion. Normally, ankle systolic pressures are greater than brachial pressures (ABI > 1.0). ABIs <.90 are hemodynamically significant. ABIs of 0.5 to 0.9 are consistent with arterial claudication. ABIs < 0.4 are seen with rest pain and severe arterial stenosis. Measurements should be recorded before and after exercise (e.g., walking down the hall).

Patients suspected of having significant arterial insufficiency should be referred to a vascular laboratory to have complete segmental arterial Doppler flow studies performed.

Diabetic patients frequently have falsely elevated ABIs as a result of calcification of large vessels as well as small vessel disease. Segmental plethysmography measures changes in pulse volume instead of pressures and provides a better evaluation in diabetic patients. This test should be ordered in these patients.

Arterial duplex scanning combines Doppler with ultrasound imaging to visualize the vessel wall for defects and atheromas as well as to evaluate blood flow. It is extremely useful in evaluating the carotid artery and its branches for stenotic lesions.

Arteriography can be used to determine the precise location and extent of vascular occlusion. However, because of the attendant risk of dye-induced renal failure, anaphylaxis, hematoma, or vascular dissection, it should be reserved for patients in whom surgical intervention is anticipated.

TREATMENT
Medications

Pentoxifylline (Trental 400 mg PO tid) may help some patients with intermittent claudication. Trental improves circulation through stenotic vessels by decreasing blood viscosity and altering the flexibility of red cells. Patients should be warned that it may take as long as 2 to 3 months to achieve significant results and that gastrointestinal side effects are common. Additionally, not all patients may see a significant improvement in their claudication with pentoxifylline therapy.

In patients with thrombotic or embolic events, treatment with aspirin or ticlopidine (Ticlid) may be beneficial. Both medications inhibit platelet aggregation and diminish clot formation. Aspirin is administered in small doses (80 to 325 mg/d). Ticlid is given at 250 mg PO bid.

Pharmacologic measures to control hypertension, diabetes, and hyperlipidemia also should be employed. Anticoagulants (heparin, warfarin, etc.) have no role in the management of chronic arterial occlusive disease.

Supportive Measures

Patients with a history of mild to moderate claudication and ABIs, no rest pain, or ischemic changes may benefit from conservative management. A program of daily walking to the point of claudication followed by 2- to 3-min rest periods repeated throughout the day is the most effective way to enhance the development of collateral vessels and improve circulation. Patients on a progressive exercise program can increase their walking distance by as much as 20 to 30 percent.

Other Treatment Modalities

Vascular reconstruction or angioplasty may be indicated for patients with debilitating claudication, rest pain, or evidence of severe ischemia (cool limbs, digital cyanosis, ischemic ulcers). The best candidates are those with proximal occlusive disease and patent distal vessels. Arterial grafts (prosthetic or saphenous vein) usually are employed to bypass the occluded vessel or vessels.

Thromboendarterectomy is also useful in repairing diseased carotid, iliac, and femoral arteries. Transluminal angioplasty often is utilized in short segmental disease and is a cost-effective alternative to bypass surgery. Amputation of affected limbs may be warranted in patients with gangrenous changes, those who are nonambulatory with severe rest pain, and those who are poor surgical candidates for vascular reconstruction.

Patient Education

The benefits of exercise and smoking cessation should be explained to the patient. Instructions on proper foot care also should be given. Patients placed on an exercise program should be instructed to try to "walk through" periods of claudication a little more each day. They should be instructed to avoid medications that may constrict the arterial vasculature (i.e., ergotamine derivatives and alpha agonists drugs).

Disposition

Follow-up visits for patients with uncomplicated, stable disease may be conducted at 2-, 3-, and 6-month intervals. A consultative evaluation with a vascular surgeon should be obtained for any patient with progressive, refractory, or debilitating symptoms.

COMPLICATIONS AND RED FLAGS

Secondary infections of ischemic ulcers, cellulitis, and tissue necrosis with wet or dry gangrene are complications that may be prevented with appropriate assessment and management. Red flags include new-onset rest pain, painful ulcers, tissue necrosis, and any symptoms suggestive of acute occlusive disease.

OTHER NOTES AND PEARLS

Patients with diabetes mellitus develop atherosclerosis more frequently and earlier. Although large and small vessels may be involved, occlusion of smaller vessels (especially tibial arteries) is more common, making surgical management more difficult. Ischemic ulcers, when present, are more likely to be secondarily infected and are slow to heal. These patients require close supervision and consultative management.

Acute Arterial Insufficiency
DISCUSSION

Arterial insufficiency can occur acutely as a result of thrombosis or embolization. Thrombosis at the site of a previous atheromatous plaque can abruptly obstruct blood flow. Also, thrombi from a proximal aneurysm or atheromatous plaque may fragment, sending embolic material downstream, where it occludes the lumen of smaller vessels, obstructing flow. The most common cause of acute arterial insufficiency, however, is an embolus from the heart. Abnormalities affecting the left side of the heart, such as atrial fibrillation and/or flutter, mitral stenosis, and transmural infarction, can produce clots that embolize. Other causes include trauma, hypercoagulable states, and arterial cannulation procedures. Embolic obstruction of vascular flow is 10 times more likely in the lower extremities than in the upper. The superficial femoral artery is the most common site. When vessel occlusion occurs acutely, severe ischemia develops rapidly because collateral blood vessels have not had time to develop.

Acute arterial occlusion represents a vascular emergency. The final outcome of limb salvage is dependent on the duration of tissue ischemia. There is a 4- to 6-h "golden window" in which limb loss can be minimized by prompt restoration of blood flow.

SYMPTOMS AND SIGNS

Patients present with acute onset of severe pain, loss of pulses, and ischemic changes (cool limbs, possible cyanosis) in an extremity. The symptoms are usually unilateral and may affect only the digits initially. Occlusive disease at the level of the aortic bifurcation may produce bilateral findings. In some patients, the initial manifestation may be that of a stroke, ischemic colitis, or organ failure (renal insufficiency).

In gathering the patient history, one should look for the following:

- Time of onset of the initial symptoms
- Previous history of cardiac disease (cardiac arrhythmias, valvular heart disease, myocardial infarction)
- Previous history of atherosclerotic peripheral vascular disease
- Recent episode of hypotension
- History of recent trauma or vascular procedure

OBJECTIVE FINDINGS

One should look for the classic five Ps:

Pain: constant and aggravated by any movement
Pallor: occurs initially, followed by cyanosis
Pulseless: often associated with a cold limb
Paresthesias: caused by anoxia to peripheral nerves
Paralysis: caused by necrosis of muscular tissue and motor nerves

These clinical findings are distal to the site of vascular occlusion. Both paresthesias and paralysis are relatively late and grave signs seen with tissue necrosis and impending limb loss. Always compare opposite limbs for exam findings.

DIFFERENTIAL DIAGNOSES

The most important diagnostic consideration is whether the acute loss of blood flow is embolic or thrombotic in origin, as the treatment modality is different for each.

Additional diagnostic considerations include:

- Arterial transection from trauma or a vascular procedure
- Aortic dissection with occlusion of peripheral vessels
- Severe arteriospasm
- Acute deep-venous thrombosis with massive swelling obstructing arterial flow
- Severe hypotension

LABORATORY AND RADIOLOGIC TESTS

A standard workup should include the following:

1. *Chest-x-ray* to check for evidence of cardiac disease or thoracic aortic aneurysm
2. *Echocardiogram* to rule out mural thrombus, myxoma, or valvular vegetations that can serve as sources of emboli

3. *Electrocardiogram* to rule out arrhythmias
4. *Serum creative kinase and urine myoglobin* for evidence of muscle necrosis
5. *Prothrombin time (PT) and partial thromboplastin time (PTT)* for baseline monitoring of anticoagulant therapy
6. *Arteriogram* if a noncardiac etiology is suspected and surgical intervention is anticipated

TREATMENT

Time is a critical factor in patient management. Unless contraindicated, immediate anticoagulation with heparin should be started to prevent further propagation of the clot.

Medication

Heparin (5000 to 10,000 units intravenously is given initially as a bolus, followed by 1000 units/h to 1500 units/h titrated to maintain a PTT at 1.5 to 2 times the normal range. The patient remains heparinized until the etiology is clearly established. If a cardiac embolus is the source, often long-term management with oral anticoagulants is needed. Noncardiac thrombi also may be treated with intraluminal clot lysis using urokinase or streptokinase to restore blood flow or an emergent embolectomy-thrombectomy, depending on the duration of tissue ischemia. A surgical consultation is indicated for further patient management.

Supportive Measures

One should provide routine postoperative care for surgical patients. Patients on anticoagulants should be closely monitored for symptoms and signs suggestive of bleeding diathesis (hematuria, rectal bleeding, easy bruising, epistaxis).

Patient Education

Patients with a history of hypertension, diabetes, and hyperlipidemia should be encouraged to follow treatment recommendations for control of their disease. Smokers should be encouraged to quit and provided needed support. Patients placed on long-term anticoagulation should be instructed to report any symptoms of easy bruising or bleeding. Aspirin, nonsteroidal agents, and alcohol should be avoided.

Disposition

Follow-up care should be provided in consultation with a vascular or general surgeon and/or cardiologist. Patients placed on oral anticoagulants should have their PT and/or INR levels monitored weekly until a therapeutic range is achieved. Less frequent monitoring can be instituted for asymptomatic patients under control.

COMPLICATIONS

Limb loss, organ failure, compartment syndrome, and reperfusion syndrome are major complications that increase in incidence the longer affected tissue remains ischemic. Vessels may reocclude, or attempts to remove the offending clot may fail. The overall prognosis for patients with acute occlusive disease is poor. Many of these patients also have significant cardiac disease. Average survival after treatment is 3.1 years.

Nonatherosclerotic Arterial Insufficiency
DISCUSSION

Although less common than acute arterial insufficiency, nonatherosclerotic causes of arterial insufficiency may be encountered.

These patients tend to be much younger at the time of onset (twenties through forties). Most of these patients have symptoms and signs suggestive of chronic arterial occlusive disease; however, acute presentations do occur. The most common disorders in this category are as follows.

Cystic Medial Necrosis

Cystic medial necrosis is a disease that affects primarily young men. Degenerative changes occur in the medial layer of the vessel wall, resulting in aneurysmal formation or aortic dissection.

Buerger's Disease (Thromboangiitis Obliterans)

Buerger's disease is a chronic occlusive inflammatory disease that affects the medium-size and small arteries and veins. Inflammation is followed by healing and thrombosis, resulting in vascular obstruction. Ischemic ulcerations of distal tissue resulting in gangrene may occur. The hands and feet are commonly affected. Smoking is directly related to these changes. Migratory thrombophlebitis is also common.

Raynaud's Disease and Phenomenon

Raynaud's disease is an arteriospastic disorder that produces occlusion of small subcutaneous and cutaneous arteries and arterioles, usually in the hands and occasionally the feet. The disease is characterized by a triphasic color change of the digits (white to blue to red) as well as paresthesias. In Raynaud's disease, arteriospasm may be precipitated by exposure to cold, smoking, or emotional upset. Arteriospasm is paroxysmal and transient and rarely results in significant tissue ischemia. The fingertips and fingers usually are affected bilaterally, with the thumb spared. Rarely are the toes affected. The disease occurs almost exclusively in women between ages 15 and 45. The cause is idiopathic. In Raynaud's phenomenon, an underlying vasculitis produces arteriospasm. Digital cyanosis is prolonged, and gangrenous ulcers are more common. Raynaud's phenomenon is often associated with connective tissue disorders such as systemic sclerosis, lupus erythematosus, and rheumatoid arthritis. Males as well as females are affected.

SYMPTOMS AND SIGNS

Except for the symptoms associated with arterial aneurysm or aortic dissection, patients with cystic medial necrosis are typically asymptomatic. The physical examination findings are the same as those in aneurysmal disease and aortic dissection.

Buerger's Disease

Pain and tenderness of the affected part constitute the chief complaint. On physical examination, one may see rubor or cyanosis. The skin may be thin and shiny, and the nails may be thick and dystrophic. Peripheral pulses are usually palpable and symmetric. In advanced disease, gangrenous changes of the digits may be noted.

Raynaud's Disease and Phenomenon

Patients complain of transient numbness and tingling of digits associated with a classic description of the triphasic color change. Physical examination may be completely normal during symptom-free periods. Peripheral pulses are intact.

In both Raynaud's disease and Buerger's disease, patients may present with clinical manifestations of single or multiple digital involvement.

DIFFERENTIAL DIAGNOSES

The differential diagnosis includes arterial thrombosis, acute arterial insufficiency, thoracic outlet syndrome, and vascular trauma.

LABORATORY AND RADIOLOGIC STUDIES

Arterial Dopplers to obtain digital pressures and evaluate digital blood flow should be ordered. It is important to note that arterial Dopplers may be normal in patients who have transient ischemic events. In some patients, vasospasm may have to be induced in the laboratory by exposing the digits to precipitating factors such as cold to confirm the diagnosis.

Digital plethysmography may be helpful in differentiating Raynaud's disease from Raynaud's phenomenon. Occasionally, an arteriogram is performed if the studies listed above are positive.

TREATMENT

The most important part of treatment for Buerger's disease is cessation of cigarette smoking. For both Buerger's disease and Raynaud's disease and phenomenon, vasodilators (calcium channel blockers, alpha blockers) may be given to relieve vasospasm. In refractory vasospasm, a sympathectomy may be warranted.

Patient Education

Smoking precipitates vasospasm and should be avoided in patients with Buerger's and Raynaud's diseases. Patient's with Raynaud's disease should be advised to avoid exposing their digits to extreme cold. Gloves may prevent ischemic attacks precipitated by exposure to cold.

Disposition

A rheumatology consult may be warranted in patients with Raynaud's disease.

Aortic Aneurysms and Dissections
DISCUSSION

Degeneration of the medial layer of the arterial wall results in the formation of aneurysms. Any artery can be affected, most commonly the aortic (abdominal and thoracic), popliteal, and femoral arteries in order of decreasing frequency. Aneurysms may be fusiform or saccular in shape. Over 95 percent of aortic aneurysms are caused by atherosclerosis. Hypertension is a major risk factor. Men are affected more frequently than are women.

Although aneurysm formation can affect any part of the aorta, most aneurysms are abdominal, with 90 percent originating below the level of the renal arteries. The aorta below the renal arteries averages 2 cm in diameter. An aneurysm is said to be present when the diameter equals or exceeds 4 cm. Other aneurysms in the peripheral arteries often coexist, with the popliteal artery being the most frequently involved.

Aneurysms also may affect any portion of the thoracic aorta from the aortic valve to the descending segment, with the descending aorta being the most frequently affected. In addition to atherosclerosis, deceleration trauma and cystic medial necrosis are common causes of thoracic aneurysms.

Aortic aneurysms have a natural history of expanding in size and rupturing. In fact, the larger the aneurysm, the greater the risk of spontaneous rupture. In arteries 6 cm in diameter, the rate of rupture rapidly increases, with 43 percent of aneurysms this size rupturing within 1 to 2 years. The mortality rate for aortic rupture is extremely high, approaching 90 percent in some populations. Most patients die before they reach the operating room.

Although the term *dissecting aortic aneurysm* is often used, technically, an aortic dissection is not an aneurysm. *Aortic dissection* is caused by extravasation of blood into and along the layers of the arterial wall through an intimal tear that produces a false lumen. The dissection extends not around the circumference of the vessel but along its length. This extension can partially or completely occlude any branch vessel in its path, producing loss of peripheral pulses and multiple organ failure. Dissection may affect any part of the aorta, but the thoracic aorta is the most commonly involved. Sixty percent of intimal tears occur in the proximal ascending aorta, 20 percent in the descending aorta, 10 percent in the aortic arch, and the rest in the abdominal aorta.

In addition to anatomic location, aortic dissections may be classified according to the extension of the dissection. *Type I* dissections originate in the ascending aorta and extend distally to the abdominal aorta. *Type II* dissections are confined to the ascending aorta. *Type III* dissections begin in the descending aorta and may extend distally to the level of the iliac arteries. The most common cause of proximal aortic dissections is cystic medial necrosis. Atherosclerosis is the most common cause of distal aortic dissections. Deceleration trauma, as occurs in motor vehicle accidents, has been implicated in the etiology of some cases of aortic dissection.

SYMPTOMS

Most aneurysms are asymptomatic and are detected as incidental findings on routine physical examination or chest x-ray. The appearance of symptoms is usually an ominous sign indicating aneurysmal expansion, intrathoracic or retroperitoneal bleeding, or an impending rupture. Occasionally, clots formed along the wall of the aneurysm embolize, producing symptoms of acute arterial insufficiency.

When these patients are symptomatic, the most common complaint is abdominal or back pain for abdominal aneurysms and substernal, back, or neck pain for thoracic aneurysms. Pain intensity may vary from mild to severe, and the pain may be constant or intermittent.

In addition to pain, thoracic aortic aneurysms may produce compressive symptoms such as dysphagia, hoarseness, cough, stridor, and dyspnea.

Unlike aneurysms, which may be silent, the clinical manifestations of aortic dissection tend to be sudden and intense. Patients classically present with a sudden onset of severe, tearing pain that is well localized initially but radiates as the dissection extends. Pain beginning in the chest and then radiating to the abdomen or back is described frequently.

Partial or complete occlusion of the branch arteries arising from the aorta may lead to symptoms of syncope, renal failure, bowel obstruction and/or infarction, hemiplegia, and paralysis of the lower extremities.

OBJECTIVE FINDINGS

A pulsatile midabdominal mass in the umbilical region is the most common finding in abdominal aneurysms. A bruit also may be present. With a thoracic aneurysm, distended neck veins and edema in the neck and arms may be seen if the adjacent superior vena cava is obstructed. A murmur of aortic regurgitation may also occur with involvement of the aortic valve. Peripheral pulses may be normal, diminished, or absent. Signs of acute arterial insufficiency may be present if a mural thrombus along the aneurysm wall has embolized.

An aortic dissection rarely presents as a pulsatile mass. Instead, the classic findings on physical examination include clinical signs of shock in the face of frank hypertension, signs of heart failure, a diastolic murmur with retrograde involvement of the aortic valve, and ischemic changes in the lower extremities resulting from occlusion of the iliac artery by extension of the dissection.

DIFFERENTIAL DIAGNOSES

The differential diagnosis includes aortic compression caused by an intrathoracic or abdominal tumor, aortic trauma with partial or complete transection, and pseudoaneurysm.

LABORATORY AND RADIOLOGIC TESTS

CT using contrast media is the gold standard for diagnosing both abdominal and thoracic aortic aneurysms. It is highly sensitive and specific, providing information on the size and exact location of the aneurysm. Abdominal ultrasound is a good noninvasive test for screening and monitoring abdominal aneurysms. Plain film radiography often demonstrates calcifications in the wall of the aneurysm that are denoted as an eggshell pattern. Chest films may demonstrate a thoracic aneurysm as a widened mediastinum. A transesophageal echocardiogram is also a good diagnostic tool for diagnosing thoracic aneurysms. Aortograms may fail to detect an aneurysm if an intraluminal clot exists and should be reserved for preoperative confirmation. Patients with an aneurysm of the ascending aorta should also have studies of the aortic valve and coronary arteries completed, as these structures may require surgical repair.

In aortic dissection, laboratory studies may reveal evidence of end organ failure (abnormal liver function tests (LFTs) and renal insufficiency). Chest x-ray may reveal a widened superior mediastinum. An echocardiogram will reveal a dilated aortic root, pericardial effusion, or a fluctuating intimal flap. Although CT with contrast and MRI are sensitive tests, they are time-consuming and may delay lifesaving emergency surgery. A transesophageal echocardiogram (TEE) of the aorta is the preferred test in hemodynamically unstable patients. An aortogram is indicated preoperatively to determine the precise location and extent of the dissection.

TREATMENT

Asymptomatic aneurysms > 4 cm in diameter may be electively repaired. Control of hypertension may slow the progression of some aneurysms. Symptomatic patients should have surgical repair regardless of aneurysm size. A ruptured aneurysm constitutes a surgical emergency.

Management of aortic dissection is primarily surgical with preoperative control of blood pressure and pain and hemodynamic monitoring. The mortality rate is highest for acute dissections (<2 weeks in duration), with aortic rupture being the most frequent cause of death.

Disposition

Patients with small (approximately 4 cm in diameter), asymptomatic aortic aneurysms are often followed with abdominal ultrasound every 6 to 12 months to monitor the aneurysm for expansion.

All patients with a documented aortic aneurysm or dissection should be managed in consultation with a thoracic surgeon and cardiologist if the thoracic aorta is involved.

COMPLICATIONS

Aneurysms will often continue to expand until they rupture. Digital or leg ischemia secondary to microemboli from an aneurysmal clot is another common complication. Other complications may occur as a result of technical error during surgery and include renal insufficiency from renal artery occlusion, ischemic colitis from inferior mesenteric artery occlusion, paraplegia caused by spinal ischemia, and chylous ascites when the lymphatic vessels are not properly ligated.

OTHER NOTES AND PEARLS

Occasionally, complete disruption of the arterial wall with extravascular accumulation of clotted blood forming a "false aneurysm" may occur. These "pseudoaneurysms" are commonly a consequence of vascular trauma resulting from angiograms, intraarterial thrombolytic therapy, arteriovenous fistulas, infection of vascular grafts, or bleeding at the site of surgical vascular anastomosis. Treatment is primarily surgical.

Venous Disease

DISCUSSION

The venous circulation has three subsystems in the lower extremities.

1. The superficial venous subsystem includes superficial veins that drain blood from the skin, subcutaneous tissue, and feet. Two primary veins and their tributaries constitute this venous network: the greater saphenous vein (GSV), which drains the medial aspect of the thigh and lower leg, and the lesser saphenous vein (LSV), which drains the posterolateral aspect of the calf.
2. The deep-venous subsystem drains most of the venous blood from the leg. Located within intramuscular tissue, these deep veins run parallel with arteries and are named accordingly (femoral vein, iliac vein, etc.).
3. The communicating (perforating) subsystem is a network of vascular channels and smaller veins that connect the deep and superficial subsystem.

Venous blood drains in one direction, from the superficial system to the deep subsystem, via the perforators and then moves toward the inferior vena cava. Veins from the superficial venous subsystem also connect directly to the deep-venous subsystem at the saphenofemoral and saphenopopliteal junctions. Venous valves are present in all three subsystems to prevent retrograde flow of blood from one system to the next.

Veins have thinner and structurally different walls than arteries and are not directly affected by some disorders that damage arteries, such as atherosclerosis and vasospasm. Pathophysiologic changes affecting the venous vasculature commonly involve the development of thrombosis that prevents venous return, destruction or incompetence of the venous valves that allows reflux of blood, or dilatation of the venous lumen as a result of persistent elevation of intraluminal venous pressures.

Venous disorders commonly treated by primary care providers include varicose veins, chronic venous insufficiency (with or without venous stasis ulcers), and thromboembolic disease.

Varicose Veins

DISCUSSION

Varicose veins are caused by incompetence of the saphenous veins, their tributaries, or their connecting perforators. Increased intravascular pressure or defective venous valves cause the greater and/or lesser saphenous veins to stretch, elongate, and become tortuous. The vessel walls may also weaken and thin. Varicosities occur principally in the superficial veins of the medial and anterior thigh, the calf, and occasionally the ankles. Contributing factors include heredity, prolonged standing, pregnancy, obesity, and previous thrombophlebitis. Varicose veins are very common, affecting 10 to 20 percent of the adult population. Varicosities are more common in females, often as a result of pregnancy.

SIGNS AND SYMPTOMS

Aside from the unsightly appearance of varicosities, patients with varicose veins may be asymptomatic. Symptoms, when present, include tiredness or heaviness of the legs, local aching or burning, ankle edema, and easy bruising from minor leg trauma. Standing or sitting for prolonged periods or obesity may aggravate these symptoms.

OBJECTIVE FINDINGS

Inspection for varicose veins in the legs is best performed from behind the patient, with the patient standing. Standing allows any varicosities to fill with blood and dilate. One should look for tortuous vessels that are easily compressed. Mild ankle edema may be noted occasionally. The finding of ulcers is rare and suggests problems in the deep-venous subsystem.

DIFFERENTIAL DIAGNOSES

The differential diagnosis includes thrombophlebitis, venous insufficiency, arterial insufficiency, peripheral neuritis, and arthritis.

LABORATORY AND RADIOLOGIC TESTS

There are no laboratory or radiologic tests for varicose veins.

OTHER DIAGNOSTICS

When varicose veins are present, a manual compression test or Trendelenburg's test may be useful in determining whether valves in the saphenous system or communicating veins are competent. These two modalities help determine whether the patient can benefit from surgical therapy.

Manual Compression Test

One should feel the dilated vein with the patient in a standing position. Using one's fingertips, one should compress the vein at its proximal end with one hand and feel for an impulse transmitted to the fingers of the other hand at the distal end of the vessel. Incompetent valves in the saphenous system allow blood to backflow, creating a palpable thud at the distal end.

Trendelenburg's Test

One elevates the patient's leg to drain venous blood. Next, one occludes the saphenous vein in the upper thigh manually or with a tourniquet and then tells the patient to stand. One should watch for the direction of venous filling with the vein occluded and with the tourniquet removed. Normally, the saphenous vein slowly fills from below. Rapid filling from below is seen with incompetent valves of the perforators. Rapid filling from above once the tourniquet has been removed is seen with incompetence of the saphenofemoral junction.

TREATMENT

Varicose veins may be managed conservatively with custom elastic support stockings. Support stockings sold in department stores do not give a proper fit and are usually too lightweight. Below-the-knee-stockings are preferred. Saphenous vein ligation and stripping constitute the mainstay of surgical therapy. This procedure is warranted in patients with large varicosities. Sclerotherapy uses a sclerosing agent injected into a vessel to scar and shrink it. It is a useful alternative treatment plan for small varicosities.

Patient Education

Patients should be instructed to replace their stockings within 6 months or whenever compression is lost. Tight garments that restrict venous return in the thigh should be avoided. Prolonged standing should be avoided, and the legs should be elevated when the patient is sitting. An exercise routine with daily walking is encouraged. Obese patients should be encouraged to lose weight.

Disposition

Patients who are refractory to conservative management, and have a history of recurrent superficial thrombophlebitis or who are dissatisfied with the cosmetic appearance of their varicosities should be referred for surgical management.

COMPLICATIONS AND RED FLAGS

Long-term varicosities may precipitate valve incompetence secondary to chronic stretching in the vessel wall. This can result in chronic venous insufficiency. Superficial thrombophlebitis may also occur. Additionally, varicosities may enlarge to the point where the overlying skin becomes thin and friable, spontaneously bleeds, or becomes thrombotic or secondarily infected.

OTHER NOTES AND PEARLS

In geriatric patients, conservative management with support hose, exercise, and leg elevation when sitting is preferred to surgical management. Stab evulsion therapy is a newer surgical procedure with a shorter recovery time and may be a viable alternative to sclerotherapy with multiple or small varicosities.

Chronic Venous Insufficiency
DISCUSSION

Previous inflammation or thrombosis can destroy the valves of the deep veins, promoting bidirectional flow of blood and creating incompetent venous perforators. Incompetence of the perforating veins allows blood to backflow from the deep-venous system to the superficial venous system. Chronic elevation of venous pressures develops over time and results in fluid transudation into the surrounding soft tissue. Chronic edema ensues, promoting skin breakdown and the formation of stasis ulcers. Skin ulcers commonly develop along the medial aspect of the leg above the medial malleolus because of the large number of venous perforators in that area. Hemosiderin from stagnant blood accumulates in the subcutaneous tissue and turns the skin dark (stasis dermatitis). Postphlebitic syndrome is the most common cause of chronic venous insufficiency. In some patients, congenital weakness of venous valves may be a precipitating factor.

SIGNS AND SYMPTOMS

The most common complaint in chronic venous insufficiency is edema. Leg edema usually advances above the ankles and may be bilateral. Both of the patient's legs should be measured at the ankle, at the midcalf, and above and below the knees, and a comparison should be made of the results to document edema. Any edema present should be examined for pitting and graded

accordingly. The skin may have a "brawny" discoloration or dermatitis. One should look for evidence of ulceration and any associated signs of cellulitis.

DIFFERENTIAL DIAGNOSES

The differential diagnosis is as follows. For unilateral leg edema it includes deep venous thrombosis, lymphatic obstruction, cellulitis, and trauma. For bilateral leg edema it includes congestive heart failure, nephrotic syndrome, severe malnutrition, liver failure, and lymphedema (rare).

LABORATORY AND RADIOLOGIC TESTS

Venous ultrasound to rule out the presence of deep-venous thrombosis should be performed. In patients with bilateral leg edema, one should order a urinalysis, blood urea nitrogen, and serum creatinine to rule out renal disease; liver function tests, serum albumin, and coagulation profile to rule out liver disease; and chest film for evidence of heart failure.

TREATMENT

Treatment of venous insufficiency is directed primarily at reducing and controlling leg edema and preventing the occurrence of leg ulcers. Bed rest with leg elevation is recommended in the acute presentation. The foot of the bed should be elevated, or the leg should be propped on pillows. When upright, patients should recline rather than sit with the legs elevated higher than the hips. The addition of oral diuretics (hydrochlorothiazide 25 mg qd) may help reduce edema. Once the edema resolves, the mainstay of therapy is the use of custom-fitted vascular elastic support hose (Jobst stockings) to maintain an appropriate venous pressure gradient. Thromboembolic device (TED) hose and many over-the-counter support stockings exert an inappropriate amount of vascular compression (<20 mmHg) to reduce lower extremity edema and should be avoided. Vascular support stockings minimally should be knee-high, avoid constriction at the knee, and should be worn at all times when the patient is erect. Dryness of the skin should be prevented to reduce ulcer formation. The skin should be moisturized daily with lotions or other topical lubricants (Eucerin, Lubriderm, petrolatum).

Management of venous stasis ulcers includes leg elevation and compression dressings. Stasis ulcers that are secondarily infected require treatment with oral antibiotics to cover staphylococcal organisms and gram-negative rods. Normal saline wet-to-dry dressing changes are effective in healing small or shallow ulcers. Dressings should be changed three to four times a day. Occlusive wound care dressings (Duoderm, Tegaderm, Epigard, etc.) in combination with Ace compression bandages are commonly applied to more extensive ulcers. These dressings should be changed every 3 to 7 days or as needed for draining ulcers. A medicated compression boot, the "Unna boot," may be applied to the lower leg. The boot keeps compression on the lower extremity so that edema is minimized. Unna boots are changed weekly or as needed for draining ulcers. Uncomplicated ulcers may take up to 3 to 4 weeks to heal. Deep or extensive ulcers may require local wound debridement with or without skin grafting.

Supportive Measures

Once the ulcer heals, edema of the leg must be controlled throughout life to prevent future ulcers from forming. The mainstay of preventive therapy is the use of custom-fitted elastic vascular support hose.

Patient Education

Patients who use support hose should be instructed to wear them throughout the day, putting them on upon arising and removing them just before retiring. Garments that restrict venous return (girdles, garters) should be avoided.

Disposition

Routine follow-up should be done on a weekly or biweekly basis until uncomplicated edema resolves and then every 3 to 6 months. Patients with stasis ulcers should be seen every 3 to 7 days for dressing changes until the ulcers heal. Refractory edema and recurrent or nonhealing ulcers require consultation with a vascular surgeon. Saphenous vein stripping may be indicated in cases refractory to conservative management.

COMPLICATIONS AND RED FLAGS

Venous stasis ulcers may become secondarily infected if they are not treated promptly. Cellulitis may also develop. Venous stasis ulcers in patients with an associated arterial insufficiency or diabetes may take a long time to heal. Any ulcer that fails to heal after 6 months of therapy should be biopsied to rule out an underlying skin cancer.

OTHER NOTES AND PEARLS

Always do a complete arterial assessment when evaluating venous disease. Venous ulcers will not heal without adequate arterial inflow, and surgery may be indicated to improve the arterial blood supply.

Venous Thrombosis
DISCUSSION

Superficial thrombophlebitis is an inflammation of the superficial veins of the upper or lower extremities caused by thrombus formation. Superficial thrombophlebitis of the arms is a common inpatient problem caused by intravenous catheters. The most common causes of lower extremity involvement are varicose veins and trauma. Other causes include primary hypercoagulable states (antithrombin III deficiency, protein C and S deficiencies), cancer, oral contraceptives, infection, and pregnancy.

Deep-venous thrombosis (DVT) is a thromboembolic disease of the veins of the deep-venous system. Conditions that produce venous stasis (surgery, postoperative immobilization, pregnancy), endothelial injury of the vessel wall (trauma, fractures, central intravenous infusions), and hypercoagulable states (cancer, estrogen use, nephrotic syndrome, thrombocytosis, and the deficiencies noted above) precipitate the formation of clots in the venous vasculature. Within 7 to 10 days, the clots adhere to the vessel wall. They are subsequently dissolved by the fibrinolytic system over the next 3 to 4 months. During the first 3 to 4 days, clots are more likely to embolize and the risk of pulmonary embolism is high. Most clots form in the small veins of the calf, where they are unlikely to embolize. A small percentage may propagate proximally to the deep veins of the knee and thigh, where the risk of pulmonary embolization increases markedly. Patients with clots in the ileofemoral or pelvic veins are at the greatest risk for a pulmonary embolus. Deep-venous thrombosis of the upper extremities rarely occurs unless a central venous catheter is present.

SYMPTOMS AND SIGNS

Patients with *superficial thrombophlebitis* usually complain of dull, aching, or burning pain in the area of the involved vein.

Fever, chills, and malaise may occur if a secondary septic phlebitis is also present.

Patients with deep-venous thrombosis may be asymptomatic. Clinicians must have a high index of suspicion, as the first symptoms may be those associated with a pulmonary embolus. The most reliable symptom, if present, is the acute onset of unilateral persistent swelling of the involved extremity. Additional symptoms include fever and calf or thigh pain.

OBJECTIVE FINDINGS

In superficial thrombophlebitis one should look for tenderness, erythema, increased warmth, and slight swelling along the length of the vein on physical examination. Sometimes the vein is palpable as a subcutaneous "venous cord." Patients with indwelling venous catheters are more likely to be febrile as well. Unless there is an associated deep-venous thrombosis, edema of the extremity rarely occurs.

Physical examination findings in DVT include increased warmth and tenderness of the affected extremity. Homans' sign (calf pain on dorsiflexion of the foot) is considered an unreliable examination clue. The most reliable sign is unilateral edema distal to the site of the clot. Classically, a calf vein DVT produces edema of the ankle and foot, a femoral vein DVT results in edema extending up to the thigh, and a DVT in the iliac vein produces edema of the entire leg. The superficial veins also may be dilated because of collateral flow around the deep venous obstruction. Fever is common. Peripheral pulses are usually palpable, except in the rare case of edema massive enough to compromise arterial flow.

DIFFERENTIAL DIAGNOSES

The differential diagnosis is as follows. For superficial thrombophlebitis it includes cellulitis, erythema nodosum, sarcoidosis, and Kaposi's sarcoma. For deep-venous thrombosis it includes cellulitis, lymphedema, a ruptured Baker's cyst, arthritis, venous compression by tumor, and severe muscle strain or sprain.

LABORATORY TESTS

A white blood cell count to rule out leukocytosis and blood cultures in patients with suspected septic superficial thrombophlebitis should be obtained. Cultures of the intravenous fluids given also may be warranted. Coagulation studies (factor levels, platelet function studies, proteins C and S, antithrombin III) should be performed in patients suspected of having an associated coagulopathy.

RADIOLOGIC TESTS

Color flow or duplex ultrasound with venous Doppler is a noninvasive, highly sensitive test for detecting obstruction of blood flow. It is much more sensitive in detecting DVTs at or above the knee (popliteal and femoral) than below. A venogram is considered the gold standard (high specificity and sensitivity) for confirming the location and extent of a venous thrombosis. It is an invasive test, however, with associated risks and should be reserved for an unequivocal venous Doppler report.

A V/Q scan (ventilation-perfusion scan) is warranted if a pulmonary embolus is suspected. One should look for a ventilation-perfusion mismatch that is "highly suspicious" for pulmonary embolus (PE). The test is not always diagnostic, and a pulmonary arteriogram may be indicated to confirm the diagnosis in symptomatic patients with unequivocal test results.

Venous plethysmography measures changes in venous blood volume from the leg. It is as accurate as duplex ultrasound in detecting popliteal and femoral DVTs and is a widely available and less expensive alternative.

TREATMENT

The clinical course of superficial thrombophlebitis is usually benign, and conservative therapy is recommended. Treatment includes elevation of the extremity, warm compresses, ambulation to prevent the development of deep-venous thrombosis, and the use of support stockings once the initial inflammation resolves. Analgesics (acetaminophen or nonsteroidal anti-inflammatory drugs) may be given for pain relief.

The best treatment for deep venous thrombosis is prevention. Early ambulation in the postoperative period helps prevent venous stasis, a major contributing factor to thrombus formation. Minidose heparin (5000 units subcutaneously bid) may be given 2 h preoperatively and continued during the immediate postoperative period in high-risk patients and those scheduled for lengthy procedures. Low-dose aspirin (<325 mg orally per day) may have prophylactic value.

Patients with DVTs distal to the popliteal vein can be treated conservatively on an outpatient basis. A 1- to 5-day course of bed rest with elevation of the edematous extremity is started. Additionally, anticoagulants are started using intermittent self-injection of subcutaneous heparin or oral warfarin (Coumadin).

Patients with popliteal or ileofemoral DVTs should be hospitalized. Strict bed rest with elevation of the edematous extremity by raising the foot of the bed is initiated. Intravenous anticoagulation is started with heparin (5000 to 10,000 units) given initially as an intravenous bolus followed by 1000 units/h of continuous intravenous infusion. Heparin is then titrated to maintain the PTT at 1.5 to 2 times normal. Patients should remain on heparin and bed rest until the clot matures and pain, tenderness, and leg edema have resolved (usually 3 days). Within 2 to 5 days, patients are switched to warfarin, 5 to 10 mg orally a day for oral maintenance therapy. The warfarin dose is adjusted daily or weekly as needed to maintain the PT at 1.3 to 1.5 times control (approximately 16 to 20 s) or INR at 2.0 to 3.0.

Warfarin therapy should continue for 3 months or until follow-up vascular studies document resolution of the clot. Patients with massive edema obstructing arterial blood flow may require an emergent venous thrombectomy. Patients with a contraindication to anticoagulation (those with a history of gastrointestinal bleeding, bleeding coagulopathy, etc.) and those who have a history of recurrent pulmonary emboli may require the placement of a venous filter in the vena cava to "capture" emboli before they reach the lungs.

Patient Education

All patients with extremity edema should be instructed to elevate the affected part. The upper extremity should be elevated above the heart level by using several pillows. The foot of the bed should be elevated for patients with leg edema. Reclining instead of sitting upright is recommended with the leg elevated higher than the hip. Prolonged sitting or standing is discouraged. Walking is encouraged unless an acute DVT is suspected. Vascular support hose should be worn throughout the day. Patients who have been placed on anticoagulants should be warned about the possible side effects and cautioned to avoid the concurrent use of aspirin, nonsteroidal anti-inflammatory drugs, and alcohol. They also should be encouraged to return for regular monitoring of the coagulation panel.

Disposition

Patients started on warfarin should have the prothrombin time monitored daily until the therapeutic range is achieved, then weekly, and, if stable, monthly until they are taken off the drug.

COMPLICATIONS AND RED FLAGS

The complications of deep-venous thrombosis include the following:

- Pulmonary embolus may occur as late as 1 week postoperatively in a surgical patient.
- Phlegmasia cerulea dolens is a painful acute arterial insufficiency secondary to massive edema. Cyanosis and loss of distal pulse occur, and limb loss is of major concern.
- In postphlebitic syndrome, the accompanying inflammation may destroy the venous valves with the subsequent development of chronic venous insufficiency and secondary varicose veins.

Complications of superficial venous thrombosis are rare. When they occur, the most common is extension of the clot into the deep-venous system with the associated risk of pulmonary embolism.

Complications related to the use of anticoagulants, such as epistaxis, gastrointestinal bleeding, and hematuria, should be observed. Warfarin is a known teratogen and is contraindicated in pregnancy.

Lymphatic Disease
DISCUSSION

Normally, blood flows from the arterial circulation to the venous circulation through the capillary bed. Plasma seeps from the capillary bed into the interstitial tissue, where the exchange of cellular nutrients, wastes, and gases occurs. Most of this "interstitial fluid" is reabsorbed into the bloodstream at the venous end. However, approximately 3 L of fluid each day lags behind in the interstitial tissue and must eventually be returned to the cardiovascular system to maintain adequate blood volume.

The lymphatic system is a special vascular system of lymphatic vessels and lymph nodes that run adjacent to arteries and veins. These vessels drain excess interstitial fluid back to the venous circulation by way of two lymphatic ducts in the chest—the right lymphatic duct and the thoracic duct—that empty into the subclavian veins.

The right lymphatic duct drains lymph from the head, chest, and right arm. The thoracic duct drains lymph from the abdomen, left arm, and both legs. Any pathologic process that obliterates or obstructs the lymphatic vessels will prevent drainage of the affected extremity. Lymphedema, an abnormal accumulation of excess interstitial fluid in the skin and subcutaneous tissue, occurs.

Lymphedema can be primary or secondary. Primary lymphedema is rare and is caused by developmental abnormalities of the lymphatic system (hypoplasia, aplasia, varicose dilation). This condition is more commonly seen in young patients (<35 years). Most cases of lymphedema, however, result from secondary causes such as surgical ligature of lymphatic vessels, radiation therapy for tumors, trauma, and recurrent infections, all of which obliterate lymphatic vessels or nodes.

The most common cause of lymphedema of the lower extremities is a pelvic tumor. Lymphedema is a chronic, progressive condition that frequently is exacerbated by recurrent episodes of secondary infection. In some cases, the extremity may become so edematous that clothing and shoes may be difficult to wear.

Lymphatic vessels also may become inflamed or secondarily infected, producing acute lymphangitis. Extension of staphylococci or beta-hemolytic streptococci from a local infection is the most common cause. In 15 to 20 percent of cases of lymphedema, lymphangitis may occur secondarily.

SYMPTOMS AND SIGNS

Patients with lymphangitis present with pain, malaise, and lassitude of acute onset. Patients with lymphedema classically present with painless, unilateral edema that starts in the feet or hands and progresses proximally. Unlike edema from other causes, elevation of the extremity provides little relief. In some cases, both lower extremities may be involved.

OBJECTIVE FINDINGS

In lymphangitis, one should look for red streaks that follow the course of lymphatic collecting ducts. Multiple, fine erythematous lines are seen streaking up an extremity and may extend from a local wound or an area of cellulitis. Regional lymph nodes are usually enlarged and tender. The skin overlying the area may be indurated and tender as well.

The edema of lymphatic obstruction has a brawny discoloration and is firm, rubbery, and nonpitting. However, unlike the edema of venous insufficiency, ulceration and the hyperpigmentation of stasis dermatitis do not occur. The overlying skin in lymphedema is usually thickened and indurated and may have a *peau d'orange* appearance. Signs of lymphangitis may be present.

DIFFERENTIAL DIAGNOSES

The differential diagnosis is as follows. For lymphangitis it includes cellulitis, superficial thrombophlebitis, and cat-scratch disease. For lymphedema it includes chronic venous insufficiency, lipedema, deep-venous thrombosis, and postphlebitic syndrome.

LABORATORY AND RADIOLOGIC TESTS

Cultures of any exudative wound should be obtained in cases of lymphangitis. If the patient appears acutely ill or is also febrile, blood cultures should be obtained. Lymphoscintigraphy involves the injection of a small amount of radioactive isotope into the lymphatic channels of the interdigital web spaces and the imaging of the extremity for delayed transport of lymph. The test has few adverse side effects, is simple to perform on an outpatient basis, and is the preferred test for diagnosing lymphedema. Lymphangiography is an alternative test that uses radiopaque contrast media to visualize the lymphatic circulation. The test is difficult to perform, and complication rates are high. Nevertheless, it may be useful in differentiating primary from secondary causes of lymphedema.

TREATMENT

Medications

Antibiotic therapy with penicillin G, nafcillin, cephalosporine, or erythromycin is used to treat lymphangitis. A 2-week course of oral antibiotics may be given unless there is an associated cellulitis. Parenteral antibiotics may be indicated in patients who are acutely ill.

Diuretics such as furosemide (Lasix) have limited and temporary effect on edema of lymphatic origin.

Supportive Measures

Heating pads or hot, moist compresses and elevation of the affected extremity may provide some symptomatic relief in patients with lymphangitis. Oral analgesics may help with any discomfort.

Other Treatment Modalities

Any localized abscess associated with lymphangitis should be incised and drained unless there is also an associated cellulitis.

The main objective of treatment for lymphedema is to eliminate as much edema as possible. External compression using a sequential air compression device (lymphedema pump) is very effective in "milking" the edema fluid from the extremity. Lymphedema pumps may be used on an outpatient basis. Bed rest with elevation of the affected extremity in a lymphedema sling on physical therapy in the form of manual lymph massage may also be beneficial. Diuretics such as furosemide (Lasix) have limited and temporary effect on edema of lymphatic origin. Once maximal reduction of edema is achieved, heavy-duty custom-fitted elastic stockings should be worn throughout the day.

Patient Education

Patients with lymphedema should be instructed in proper foot care to minimize trauma and/or acute infections. Dietary restriction of sodium should be encouraged. Any signs of associated lymphangitis or cellulitis should be reported promptly so that proper antibiotic therapy may be initiated.

Disposition

Patients with uncomplicated lymphangitis may be safely managed on an outpatient basis by the primary care provider. Patients with marked lymphedema should be referred to a vascular or general surgeon for a consultative evaluation and management. Referral to an oncologist may be warranted in some patients.

COMPLICATIONS AND RED FLAGS

The most important complication seen in lymphangitis is sepsis resulting from delayed or inadequate treatment. Recurrent cellulitis and lymphangitis are common complications in lymphedema. Lymphangiosarcoma, a rare lymphatic cancer, may occur, particularly in patients with upper extremity postmastectomy lymphedema. Any patient with violaceous, maculopapular skin lesions that coalesce or ulcerate should be referred for biopsy and further evaluation.

BIBLIOGRAPHY

Barker LR, Burton JH, Zieve PD (eds): *Principles of Ambulatory Medicine,* 4th ed. Baltimore, Williams & Wilkins, 1995, pp 1298–1320.

Cohen JR: *Vascular Surgery for the House Officer.* Baltimore, Williams & Wilkins, 1986, pp 1–8, 18–63, 76–84.

Elson JD: Lower extremity ischemia: Interventions to preserve quality of life. *Postgrad Med* 95(1):96–100, 103–108, 1994.

Ernst C, Stanley J: *Current Therapy in Vascular Surgery,* 2d ed. Philadelphia, BC Decker, 1991, pp 1022–1035.

Goroll AH, May LA, Mulley AG Jr (eds): *Primary Care Medicine: Office Evaluation & Management of the Adult Patient,* 3d ed, Philadelphia, Lippincott, 1995, pp 105–110, 201–211.

Griffith W, Dambro MR: *5 Minute Clinical Consult.* Philadelphia, Lea & Febinger, 1996, pp 64–65, 70–71, 1044–1047, 1128–1129, 1189.

Krenzer ME: Peripheral vascular assessment: Finding your way through arteries and veins. *AACN Clin Issues* 6(4):631–644, 1995.

Moore Wesley S: *Vascular Surgery: A Comprehensive Review.* Philadelphia, Saunders, 1991, pp 688–698.

Price SA, Wilson LM: *Pathophysiology: Clinical Concepts of Disease Processes,* 4th ed. St. Louis, Mosby Yearbook, 1992, pp 487–514.

Tierney L, McPhee SJ, Papadakis MA: *Current Medical Diagnosis and Treatment.* Stamford, CT, Appleton & Lange, 1996, pp 806–808.

Young J, Olin J: *Peripheral Vascular Disease,* 2d ed. Philadelphia, Mosby, 1996, pp 3–42.

Chapter 1–10
ACQUIRED VALVULAR HEART DISEASE

Jeffrey R. Smith

DISCUSSION

Valvular heart disease consists of two basic groups of disorders: *congenital* valvular anomalies and *acquired* valvular diseases. Acquired valvular diseases are further defined as *rheumatic* and *nonrheumatic* in origin. Of the four cardiac valves (aortic, mitral, tricuspid, and pulmonic), attention is given in this chapter only to the mitral and aortic valves. The diseases represented by these two valves constitute the most common and significant disorders of acquired valvular disease. Valvular disease can further be defined as *regurgitant* (commonly referred to as "leaky" or "insufficient") and *stenotic* (commonly referred to as "narrowed") or may have components of both types.

RHEUMATIC VALVULAR HEART DISEASE

The frequency and intensity of rheumatic fever caused by group A beta-hemolytic streptococcal bacterial infection has diminished, particularly in developed countries where antibiotics and treatment are readily available. Despite this fact, rheumatic fever continues to play an important role in the development of valvular disease. In fact, there was a resurgence of rheumatic fever in some areas of the United States in the 1980s.[1] If patients with acute rheumatic fever receive appropriate prophylactic antibiotic therapy, about 1 percent subsequently develop severe cardiac disease (class IV rheumatic heart disease) and 4 percent develop debilitating rheumatic heart disease.[2]

The pathogenesis of rheumatic valvular disease involves fibrotic scarring of the valve tissue, leading to thickening, retraction, and fusion of the valve leaflets, after recovery from an episode of rheumatic fever. Actually, valvular stenosis of rheumatic origin progresses gradually through adult life, long after any evidence of rheumatic activity. It may take many years for the valvular disease to develop. The aortic and mitral valves are the most commonly affected.

NONRHEUMATIC VALVULAR HEART DISEASE

Aortic stenosis that occurs as an isolated lesion usually is a result of a congenital bicuspid valve or degenerative thickening and calcification of leaflets that were originally normal.

Pure nonrheumatic aortic regurgitation is usually a result of dilation of the aortic root. Myxomatous changes in the aortic leaflets that are similar to changes seen in the mitral valve are found in many cases as well. These changes may cause severe aortic regurgitation without dilation of the aortic root (floppy aortic valve syndrome).[3] Marfan syndrome, bacterial endocarditis, and in some cases severe trauma are other potential causes of aortic regurgitation.

Mitral regurgitation generally is caused by one of two basic pathogenic sources. The first is coronary artery disease and is related to papillary muscle dysfunction resulting from ischemia or infarction. The second is a prolapsing mitral valve caused by an idiopathic pathologic process typically characterized by loss of fibrous tissue in the chordae tendineae.

Other nonrheumatic causes of valvular disease include damage to valves from radiation therapy.[4] Methysergide, which is used to treat migraine and cluster headaches, has been observed to affect cardiac valves.[5] Rheumatoid arthritis occasionally produces severe valve disease when large rheumatoid nodules involve the leaflets.[6]

SIGNS AND SYMPTOMS

Understanding the anatomy and physiology of stenosis and regurgitation is essential to recognize the signs and symptoms of these disorders. Valvular stenosis obstructs blood flow through the heart. This generally results in elevated pressures in the chamber proximal to the stenosis (in aortic stenosis, left ventricular systolic pressure is elevated; in mitral stenosis, left atrial pressure is elevated above left ventricular diastolic pressure). In aortic stenosis, the increase in pressure load thickens the ventricular wall without affecting the size of the chamber and, combined with a fibrotic myocardium, causes a decrease in diastolic compliance. Over time, the left ventricular chamber dilates and contraction weakens. In mitral stenosis the left atrium becomes hypertrophied because of pressure loads similar to those seen in aortic stenosis. This leads to atrial dilation, decreased atrial contraction, and elevated left atrial pressure. This elevated pressure eventually affects the pulmonary system.

In valvular regurgitation, an amount of blood flows back into the left atrium (mitral regurgitation) each time the ventricle contracts and back into the left ventricle (through an incompetent aortic valve) during diastole. Because the stroke volume of the affected ventricle is increased, systemic flow is kept at nearly normal rates. This produces overwork for the ventricle and eventually dilation of the ventricle (or the atrium in mitral disease) without an increase in wall thickness (differing from stenosis, where there is an increase in wall thickness). Ultimately, ventricular performance decreases, ejection fraction is reduced, and because of long-standing volume overwork the ventricle fails (or the atrium dilates). In combined cases of stenosis and regurgitation, there is an additive affect of strain from overwork and increased pressures.

Most patients with aortic stenosis characteristically present with dyspnea with exertion, angina pectoris, and syncope, any or all of which may be present. Patients with aortic regurgitation may present with symptoms very similar to those of aortic stenosis. Dyspnea, angina pectoris, and palpitations are the most common symptoms.

Angina is seen in both aortic stenosis and aortic regurgitation secondary to a decrease in diastolic perfusion combined with an increase in myocardial oxygen consumption.

In mitral stenosis, the most important symptom is dyspnea, which indicates left atrial pressures high enough to produce transudation of fluid into pulmonary capillaries. Because of this, hemoptysis is also commonly seen. Other signs and symptoms include cough, orthopnea, and paroxysmal nocturnal dyspnea (PND).

Mitral regurgitation often is asymptomatic until the disease becomes very severe. Once that level of severity occurs, the most common presenting symptoms include fatigue, dyspnea with exertion, and palpitations.

OBJECTIVE FINDINGS

Auscultation of the heart is the cornerstone of the detection of valvular heart disease. Knowledge of the location and characteristics of the auscultated murmur is critical to an accurate diagnosis. Understanding how cardiac murmurs should be described is essential in properly communicating physical findings to colleagues.

Aortic stenosis is primarily distinguished from other valvular disorders by its characteristic loud, harsh systolic ejection murmur heard best at the second intercostal space on the right sternal border and radiating into the carotid arteries. Other classic physical findings include narrow pulse pressure, sustained apical pulse, a paradoxically split S_2, a soft S_2, and a present S_4.

In aortic regurgitation, the classic murmur is known as a high-pitched, decrescendo diastolic murmur that begins immediately after the second heart sound and is best heard at the second intercostal space on the right sternal border. Physical findings that are commonly seen include visible bounding and forceful peripheral pulses (Corrigan's pulse), pulsations in the capillary beds of nails (Quincke's pulse), and a systolic ejection murmur resulting from increased flow across the valve area.

Patients with mitral stenosis have a typical murmur that can be recognized by the characteristic opening snap and diastolic rumbling murmur. Patients with long-standing and severe mitral stenosis are often quite thin and frail. Jugular venous distention is seen frequently. Auscultation of the lungs may reveal fine crackles in the bases.

A harsh holosystolic murmur heard best at the apex (left fifth intercostal space, midclavicular line) with radiation into the axilla is the hallmark murmur of mitral regurgitation. Other findings include a laterally displaced and diffuse apical pulse, a widely split S_2, and a present S_3.

DIFFERENTIAL DIAGNOSES

In acquired valvular heart disease, there is no differential diagnosis per se. The challenge during history taking and physical examination lies in differentiating between the different intracardiac possibilities. There may be concurrent processes occurring, such as myocardial infarction, chronic obstructive pulmonary disease, and/or congestive heart failure.

LABORATORY TESTS

No laboratory tests are helpful in securing an accurate diagnosis of valvular heart disease. A discussion of pertinent ECG findings is in the next section.

RADIOLOGIC STUDIES

While the history and physical examination remain the cornerstones for the diagnosis of acquired valvular heart disease, radiographic studies such as echocardiography (using a transesophageal transducer or a standard precordial transducer) and color flow Doppler studies confirm the diagnosis and provide vital information in regard to the severity of disease. Most would agree that the transesophageal electrocardiography (TEE) approach provides more sophisticated images, but it is certainly a more invasive procedure.

In aortic stenosis, echocardiographic studies reveal thickened and calcific valve leaflets with reduced mobility. Pressure gradients and the aortic valve area are calculated by using Doppler studies. These values also can be obtained through invasive procedures such as heart catheterization. Hemodynamically significant stenosis is associated with gradients about 50 mmHg. An aortic valve area less than 1.0 cm^2 is considered significant in most adults. Other studies include chest x-ray, which generally reveals some prominence of the ascending aorta but usually little enlargement of the heart unless significant congestive heart failure is present. Abnormal ECG findings include left ventricular strain patterns such as QRS and T-wave changes that reflect left ventricular hypertrophy.

Echocardiographic findings in aortic regurgitation reveal an incompetent valve during diastole and may include a characteristic flutter-like movement in the anterior mitral leaflet that occurs during diastole. Chest x-ray shows cardiac silhouette enlargement, with the apex being displaced to the left and downward. ECG findings may show signs of left ventricular strain and hypertrophy.

Echocardiographic findings in mitral stenosis generally reveal decreased movement of the mitral leaflets. As in aortic stenosis, the valve area and the diastolic pressure gradient are important in determining the severity of disease and can be calculated with heart catheterization and/or Doppler studies. Gradients of 10 mmHg or more generally suggest the presence of severe stenosis. Chest x-ray almost always reveals left atrial enlargement and also may show pulmonary congestion in the form of "Kerley B lines" (dilated pulmonary lymphatics that become visible as transverse lines in the lower lung fields). ECG findings consistent with left atrial enlargement as well as atrial fibrillation are often present.

Mitral regurgitation is best seen as a regurgitant jet in systole on echocardiography. Quantitative two-dimensional echocardiography can provide a more precise calculation of the severity of regurgitation. A new method—the proximal isovelocity surface area method—measures the size of the regurgitant orifice by quantitating the velocity of regurgitant blood. This technique provides an estimate of the severity of the valvular abnormality that does not depend on hemodynamic variables such as afterload and contractility.[7] Chest x-ray may reveal pulmonary congestion, but this is much less commonly seen than it is in mitral stenosis. Atrial fibrillation may also be seen on ECG.

TREATMENT

Treatment can be divided into nonsurgical and surgical components. General nonsurgical medical management includes treatment of atrial arrhythmias, decreasing the risk of embolism from the left atrium with warfarin therapy, and the use of antibiotics to prevent infective endocarditis. Vasodilator therapy used to treat congestive heart failure also may prove valuable. It may be used in severe but asymptomatic aortic regurgitation with the goal of slowing the development of left ventricular dysfunction and delaying the need for valve replacement.[8]

General surgical treatment involves either repair or replacement. Nonreplacement (repair) procedures play a role in the treatment of valvular disorders, particularly operations such as mitral commissurotomy for the repair of noncalcific forms of aortic valve stenosis.[9] Surgical repair has become the procedure of choice for most patients with floppy-valve syndrome and for many patients with other anatomic types of mitral regurgitation.[10] Valve replacement is the other surgical option, and there are over 30 different models of mechanical and tissue-type valves. The most frequently used prosthetic valves are the Starr-Edwards, CarboMedics, and St. Jude valves.[11,12] Homograft aortic valves and porcine aortic valves are the tissue-type valves used for replacement.

Deciding which patient is a candidate for surgical or nonsurgical treatment remains challenging and must include factors such as severity of disease, age, social and environmental concerns, patient compliance, and patient understanding of the disease process. A delay in surgical treatment may be risky in some patients because of the irreparable damage that may occur to the left ventricle.

DISPOSITION

Meticulous medical management in both nonsurgical and surgical (especially in the postoperative phase) treatment is absolutely crucial to achieving positive outcomes.

Patients who have their cardiac valves replaced are subject to a variety of long-term complications and potential medical problems. Prevention of arterial embolism and monitoring of anticoagulation are probably the most frustrating problems for both the patient and the medical team.

The outcome of valvular replacement surgery is favorable in patients with few comorbid factors and those who are motivated to participate in their own care.

PEARLS

Do not be fooled by the intensity of the murmur in aortic stenosis, either soft or loud. The duration of the murmur and a later peak of intensity suggest more severe aortic obstruction.

Typically, in mitral regurgitation, the murmur radiates into the axilla. An exception is the murmur produced by rupture of the chordae tendineae of the posterior papillary muscle. The murmur produced in this case radiates into the aortic area and neck and mimics the murmur of aortic stenosis.

The single most important predictor of outcome in a patient undergoing cardiac surgery is the ejection fraction.

REFERENCES

1. Bisno AL: Group A streptococcal infections and acute rheumatic fever. *New Engl J Med* 325:783, 1991.
2. Mlandenovic J. (ed): *Primary Care Secrets*, St. Louis, Mosby, 1995, p 121.
3. Agozzino L, de Vivo F, Falco A, et al: Non-inflammatory aortic root disease and floppy aortic valve as cause of isolated regurgitation: A clinico-morphologic study. *Int J Cardiol* 45:129, 1994.
4. Chenu PC, Schroeder E, Buche M, et al: Bilateral coronary ostial stenosis and aortic valvular disease after radiotherapy. *Eur Heart J* 15:1150, 1994.
5. Austin SM, el-Hayek A, Comianos M, et al: Mitral valve disease associated with long-term ergotamine use. *South Med J* 86:1179, 1993.
6. Mullins PA, Grace AA, Stewart SC, et al: Rheumatoid heart disease presenting as acute mitral regurgitation. *Am Heart J* 122:242, 1991.
7. Enriquez-Sarano M, Miller FA Jr, Hayes SN, et al: Effective mitral regurgitant orifice area: Clinical use of the proximal isovelocity surface area method. *J Am Coll Cardiol* 125:703, 1995.
8. Scognamiglio R, Rahimtoola SH, Fasoli G, et al: Nifedipine in asymptomatic patients with severe aortic regurgitation and normal left ventricular function. *New Engl J Med* 331:689, 1994.
9. Shapira N, Lemole GM, Fernandez J, et al: Aortic valve repair for aortic stenosis in adults. *Ann Thorac Surg* 50:110, 1990.
10. Cohn LH, Couper GS, Aranki SF, et al: Long term results of mitral valve reconstruction for regurgitation of the myxomatous mitral valve. *J Thorac Cardiovasc Surg* 107:143, 1994.
11. Copeland JG III, Sethi GK, North American Team of Clinical Investigators for the CarboMedics Prosthetic Heart Valve: Four year experience with the CarboMedics valve: The North American experience. *Ann Thorac Surg* 58:630.
12. Ibrahim M, OiKane H, Cleland J, et al: The St. Jude Medical Prosthesis: A thirteen year experience. *J Thorac Cardiovasc Surg* 108:221, 1994.

Chapter 1–11
CARDIAC ARRHYTHMIAS
Morton A. Diamond

DISCUSSION

Arrhythmias are electrical disturbances in heart rhythm. They may be asymptomatic, or, when the patient is aware of heart action, palpitations may be noted. Palpitations are often described as pounding, thumping, fluttering, or pausing. Moreover, arrhythmias may cause secondary symptoms such as dyspnea, anginal discomfort, faintness, syncope, and congestive heart failure.

Cardiac rhythm disturbances may occur in the absence or presence of underlying structural heart disease. Their varied causes include ingestion of caffeine, alcohol, or over-the-counter medications; electrolyte imbalance; hypoxemia; acid-base disturbances; tobacco use; prescribed medications; and emotional stress as well as organic congenital and acquired heart disease. Finally, in some patients, the etiology of cardiac rhythm disturbance is not defined.

Both the prognosis and the treatment of a patient's arrhythmia depend on the clinical setting in which it occurs. Arrhythmias are more common in older patients and may have more significant hemodynamic effects because of underlying left ventricular dysfunction.

Cardiac rhythm disturbances are classified as supraventricular (SV) and ventricular. SV arrhythmias include sinus bradycardia, sinus tachycardia, atrial premature beats, paroxysmal supraventricular tachycardia, atrial fibrillation, and the Wolff-Parkinson-White syndrome (WPW). A patient with sick sinus syndrome usually manifests a supraventricular bradyarrhythmia intermingled with episodes of atrial flutter or atrial fibrillation. Ventricular rhythm abnormalities include ventricular premature beats, ventricular tachycardia, and ventricular fibrillation. In addition, arrhythmias may be due to atrioventricular conduction disturbances (AV block). First-, second-, or third-degree (complete) heart block may occur.

PHYSIOLOGIC BASIS OF ARRHYTHMIAS

The mechanisms underlying rhythm disturbances include disorders of automaticity, impulse conduction, reentry, and triggered activity. In brief, reentry is the mechanism for many premature beats as well as most paroxysmal tachycardias. Conduction abnormalities are due to prolongation of the refractory periods of cardiac tissue. Triggered activity may be the mechanism responsible for ventricular tachycardia in patients with congenital or acquired long QT intervals.

ARRHYTHMIA EVALUATION

A physician assistant must not only define the presence and character of a rhythm disorder but also establish a causal relationship between the arrhythmia and the patient's symptoms. Patients with life-threatening conditions such as out-of-hospital sudden death, arrhythmia-induced seizures, and congestive heart failure receive inpatient cardiac monitoring. Outpatients who have palpitations have an ECG taken as the initial diagnostic test. Outpatient 24-h ambulatory monitoring, often with an event recorder, is indicated in patients with palpitations or symptoms consistent with arrhythmia. In selected patients, provocative stress testing is indicated to determine the presence of ischemia-induced conduction disturbance or ectopy. Signal-averaged ECG and electrophysiologic testing may be indicated after referral to a cardiologist.

THERAPEUTIC PRINCIPLES

Therapeutic options in the treatment of cardiac rhythm disorders include medication, cardioversion, pacemakers, automatic implantable defibrillators, and cardiac surgery. The physician assistant and the consulting cardiologist determine the appropriate treatment.

Antiarrhythmic medications have been arbitrarily classified into four classes. Class I agents are further subdivided into subsets Ia, Ib, and Ic. Class Ia agents include quinidine, procainamide, disopyramide, and moricizine. Class Ib medications include lidocaine, mexiletine, phenytoin, and tocainide. Class Ic includes flecainide and propafenone. Class II medications consist of the beta sympathetic blockers acebutolol, esmolol, metoprolol, and propranolol. Class III includes amiodarone, sotalol, and bretylium. Amiodarone is gaining increasing importance in therapy for both supraventricular and ventricular arrhythmias.

The calcium channel blockers diltiazem and verapamil are class IV antiarrhythmic agents. A physician assistant must be aware that these agents must be used with caution. They may have side effects superimposed on limited efficacy. For example, flecainide, moricizine, and encainide demonstrated worsening ventricular arrhythmia in post–myocardial infarction patients with asymptomatic ventricular arrhythmia.

SUPRAVENTRICULAR ARRHYTHMIAS

Sinus Bradycardia

In sinus bradycardia, the heart rate is below 60 beats per minute. Each normal P wave is followed by a normal QRS complex unless there is a preexisting intraventricular conduction defect. Sinus bradycardia may be entirely normal in well-conditioned athletes but may occur transiently during periods of increased vagal tone. Other common causes include medication (beta blockers, calcium channel blockers, parasympathomimetic medications, lithium), hypothyroidism, and sinus node disease. This rhythm disturbance should be treated only if it causes symptoms such as weakness and confusion. If necessary, cardiac pacing appears preferable to sympathomimetic agents and atropine-like medication.

Sinus Arrhythmia

A gradual increase in heart rate during inspiration and a gradual decrease during expiration are characteristic of sinus arrhythmia in young patients. In contrast, nonphasic sinus arrhythmia, in which the changing heart rate is not related to respiration, occurs in the elderly and in diabetic patients. Sinus arrhythmia does not require treatment.

Sinus Tachycardia

A heart rate greater than 100 beats per minute in which a normal P wave is followed by a normal QRS complex is characteristic of sinus tachycardia. This arrhythmia may be a normal response to emotional stress, fever, anemia, hypotension, congestive heart failure, hyperthyroidism, myocardial ischemia, cardiogenic or hemorrhagic shock, medication, or foods containing caffeine. Treatment depends on the underlying cause.

Atrial Premature Contractions

Atrial premature contractions (APCs) occur in patients with normal or diseased hearts. APCs commonly are noted in patients with infection, myocardial ischemia, and congestive heart failure (CHF). They also may be found in those who have ingested caffeine products or alcohol and those who smoke tobacco products. In a patient with a history of paroxysmal supraventricular tachycardia, APCs may be a harbinger of recurrent tachyarrhythmia. This patient should be treated with beta blocker, digoxin, or a calcium antagonist. In a cardiac patient who recently has gained weight, APCs may be an important sign of incipient clinical CHF. These patients should receive more vigorous therapy depending on whether systolic or diastolic ventricular dysfunction is present.

Paroxysmal Supraventricular Tachycardia

Paroxysmal supraventricular tachycardia (PSVT) is the most common paroxysmal tachyarrhythmia. It occurs in both normal and diseased hearts. Attacks typically are of abrupt onset and termination. Heart rate is generally in the range of 160 to 220 beats per minute. In PSVT, the P wave may precede, be within, or follow the QRS complex. If the arrhythmia is due to digitalis intoxication, an AV block is also present. Treatment is directed toward termination of the acute episode and prevention of subsequent tachycardia. Carotid sinus massage may be effective in aborting the tachycardia. It should be applied on one carotid artery at a time and never in the presence of carotid bruits. A 6-mg bolus of intravenous adenosine followed if necessary 1 to 2 minutes later by a bolus of 12 mg is often successful in terminating the rhythm disturbance. Adenosine should not be used in asthmatic patients. Theophylline products inhibit the action of adenosine. In contrast, patients receiving dipyridamole are highly sensitive to adenosine. In these patients, one should start with a 1-mg intravenous bolus followed 2 min later, if necessary, by a 3-mg bolus. Intravenous verapamil in incremental doses up to a total of 20 mg in 15 min is also an excellent therapeutic option. Intravenous diltiazem and the short-acting beta blocker esmolol may be appropriate therapeutic options. Cardioversion may be urgently applied in cases of hemodynamic compromise. Further, it may be utilized if medicinal therapy proves ineffective.

A physician assistant has many therapeutic choices in the prevention of recurrent attacks. Oral digoxin (maintenance dose generally 0.125 to 0.5 mg daily) and oral verapamil (maintenance dose generally 120 to 360 mg daily), alone or in combination, are effective. Verapamil increases digoxin blood levels. Additionally, beta blockers are effective. Less frequently, class Ia, class Ic, and class III agents are prescribed. Radiofrequency catheter ablation therapy is considered the treatment of choice in PSVT patients in whom reentry is the underlying mechanism promoting recurrent tachycardia.

Atrial Flutter

In atrial flutter, the atrial rate is generally 250 to 350 per minute with an abnormal contour to the atrial wave (classically a "sawtooth" appearance). The ventricular rate in an untreated patient is generally in the range of 100 to 150 beats per minute. The QRS complex is normal unless there is a preexisting bundle branch block or the ventricular rate is so fast that aberrant intraventricular conduction is evident. Flutter is rarely found in a normal heart and is rarely chronic. This arrhythmia occurs in many congenital and acquired cardiac disorders as well as in constrictive pericarditis, chronic obstructive lung disease, and postoperative cardiac surgery patients. Since pharmacologic control of the ventricular response may be difficult, electrical cardioversion to normal sinus rhythm is usually advisable. The risk of thromboembolism is thought to be low. Nonetheless, anticoagulation is considered advisable in patients with mitral valve disease who are considered for elective cardioversion.

Atrial Fibrillation

Atrial fibrillation (AF) is the most commonly encountered arrhythmia in clinical practice. Its prevalence increases with age; approximately 10 percent of the population over age 80 years has this rhythm disorder. AF may be acute (paroxysmal) or chronic. It may occur in both normal and diseased hearts. AF is common in rheumatic heart disease, coronary atherosclerotic heart disease, pericarditis, hypertension, atrial septal defect, mitral valve prolapse, congestive and hypertrophic cardiomyopathy, and hyperthyroidism. AF is found in 20 percent of patients with acute myocardial infarction. Further, acute attacks may be precipitated by cardiac surgery, alcohol ingestion, and medications.

Atrial activity is very fast, with 400 to 600 impulses per minute reaching the atrioventricular node (AVN). In an untreated patient the ventricular response is approximately 80 to 180 beats per minute. Fast ventricular rates, especially in patients with underlying organic heart disease, may produce ischemic coronary syndromes, hypotension, or CHF.

The principal goals of therapy for AF are control of ventricular rate, restoration of sinus rhythm in patients with paroxysmal arrhythmia, prevention of recurrent episodes, and prevention of stroke and systemic embolism. There is no difference in stroke risk when patients with paroxysmal AF are compared with those with chronic AF.

Control of Ventricular Rate

In the absence of CHF or preexcitation syndrome, verapamil, diltiazem, and beta sympathetic blockers are more effective than digoxin for long-term control. In a patient with an uncontrolled ventricular rate, verapamil may be given intravenously in a dose of 5 to 10 mg over 3 min and repeated in 30 min if necessary. When rate control has been achieved, oral verapamil may be given in a dose range of 40 to 120 mg tid. Intravenous diltiazem 20 mg or 0.25 mg/kg may be administered over 2 min. If necessary, 25 mg or 0.35 mg/kg may be given 15 min later. Oral diltiazem usually is prescribed in a dose of 60 to 120 mg PO tid. Calcium channel blockers are preferred in patients with bronchospasm, diabetes mellitus, and peripheral arterial vascular disease.

When digoxin is the therapeutic option, an intravenous dose of 1.0 to 1.5 mg is given over 24 h in incremental doses of 0.25 to 0.5 mg. The oral maintenance digoxin dose is 0.125 to 0.5 mg daily. One must remember that digoxin blood levels are of little value in assessing an adequate dose. Digoxin must be used cautiously in patients with renal disease. When it is used jointly with verapamil to control the ventricular rate, the verapamil raises serum digoxin levels. Intravenous propranolol is given of 1.0 mg every 2 min until the heart rate is controlled or until a total dose of 7 mg has been injected. The oral maintenance dose is in a wide range of 10 to 120 mg PO bid or tid. Propranolol in low doses may be added to digoxin therapy. In selected patients who do not respond to medicinal therapy, radiofrequency catheter ablation techniques may be necessary to control the ventricular rate.

Restoration of Sinus Rhythm

The physician assistant and the consulting cardiologist must determine which patients will undergo efforts toward the restoration of normal rhythm. There are, however, patients in whom ventricular rate control and anticoagulation are clearly the preferred therapy.

In a patient with acute AF lasting less than 48 h, pharmacologic or electrical cardioversion may be attempted after control of the ventricular rate has been attained. Class Ia or class Ic agents may be used. However, close cardiac monitoring is essential. Electrical cardioversion may be performed urgently in a patient in severe hemodynamic distress. For a patient who has been in atrial fibrillation less than 48 h, electrical cardioversion can be performed without anticoagulant therapy. If fibrillation has been present more than 48 h, the patient should receive, in addition to medication to control heart rate, warfarin therapy for 3 to 4 weeks before cardioversion. The dose of warfarin should maintain the International Normalized Ratio (INR) at 2.0 to 3.0. Those receiving digoxin should have this medication discontinued 24 h before cardioversion. After a successful return to sinus rhythm, warfarin therapy should be continued for a minimum of 4 to 6 weeks. Alternatively, transesophageal echocardiography may be performed to exclude atrial thrombi so that early cardioversion can be accomplished safely. A physician assistant should be cognizant that this clinical approach is not universally accepted.

Prevention of Recurrent Episodes

No available medication has been proved to be clearly superior in maintaining patients in sinus rhythm. All medications, however, have adverse side effects and potential toxicity. Beta blockers, calcium channel blockers, and digoxin have been prescribed frequently. Increasingly, however, low-dose amiodarone (100 to 200 mg daily after the loading dose) is being utilized and may be the medication of choice.

Prevention of Stroke and Systemic Embolism

Cerebral infarction in an AF patient is thought to result from embolization of intracardiac thrombi. Patients with both valvular and nonvalvular heart disease are at risk for this complication. Those with atrial fibrillation and valvular disease, including persons with prosthetic valves, should receive chronic warfarin therapy unless a contraindication exists.

Nonvalvular AF is thought to be the most common cardiac disorder causing cerebral embolism. Studies of patients with paroxysmal and chronic nonvalvular AF have demonstrated six independent predictors of risk for embolism. These high-risk categories include hypertension, diabetes mellitus, previous stroke or transient ischemic attack, history of CHF, left atrial dimension greater than 2.5 cm/m^2, and age above 65 years. In these patients, warfarin reduces ischemic stroke by 70 percent. These patients should receive warfarin to achieve an INR of 2.0 to 3.0. Warfarin should not be discontinued if the patient returns to normal sinus rhythm for a period of time. An adult aspirin should be given daily to noncompliant patients and those who have a contraindication to warfarin. Patients with lone atrial fibrillation, that is, those with atrial fibrillation without underlying structural heart disease or the risk factors listed above, have a very low incidence of stroke. Patients with lone atrial fibrillation under age 60 years do not require anticoagulation or antiplatelet therapy. Those between the ages of 60 and 75 years should take 325 mg aspirin daily. After age 75 years, lone atrial fibrillation patients preferably should receive warfarin therapy.

WOLFF-PARKINSON-WHITE SYNDROME

WPW represents the primary example of preexcitation syndrome, in which atrial impulses may reach the ventricles early via anatomic accessory AV conducting fibers. In preexcitation, the atrial impulse may not traverse the normal AV nodal conducting tissue. Therefore, the heart is prone to the development of AF with an extremely fast ventricular response. This may deteriorate into ventricular fibrillation, accounting for the sudden death observed in these patients.

The typical ECG pattern in WPW includes a PR interval less than 120 ms, a QRS complex greater than 120 ms with slurred upstroke, and secondary ST-T wave changes. Anatomic variants of the preexcitation syndrome manifest different ECG patterns.

The most common tachycardia found in WPW patients is regular at a rate of 150 to 250 beats per minute with a normal QRS complex. More serious is AF with atrial impulses conducted to the ventricles without the normal rate-modulating effect of AV nodal conduction tissue. The ventricular rate in these patients may reach 300 beats per minute. Syncope may result from inadequate cerebral blood flow. Sudden death may occur if the rhythm deteriorates into ventricular fibrillation. The physician assistant and the consulting cardiologist must identify WPW patients who are at risk for AF.

Treatment

In an adult patient with the ECG abnormality of WPW but without a history of tachyarrhythmia, no investigation or therapy is necessary. For a patient with a history of tachyarrhythmia, electrophysiologic testing is indicated. Radiofrequency catheter ablation of an accessory pathway is now considered the treatment of choice in these patients.

For the termination of an acute episode of tachycardia that is regular and has a normal QRS complex, intravenous adenosine or the intravenous calcium channel blockers verapamil and diltiazem may be administered. An external defibrillator must be immediately available if necessary. For the termination of AF with a wide QRS complex, medications that slow conduction in both the accessory pathway and the AV nodal tissues are employed. Procainamide and propranolol may be given intravenously. For a patient exhibiting hemodynamic collapse, electrical cardioversion is the initial treatment.

SICK SINUS SYNDROME

Also known as the brady-tachy syndrome, sick sinus syndrome (SSS) is commonly found in elderly patients. It is characterized by intermittent bradycardia, for example, sinus bradycardia or sinus pauses, interspersed with AF, atrial flutter, or PSVT. The underlying cause is sinus node disease and cardiac conduction abnormalities. However, transient SSS may be caused by digoxin, beta blockers, calcium channel blockers, and other antiarrhythmic agents. Coronary artery disease is an uncommon cause of SSS. The syndrome's initial presentation may be light-headedness, syncope, angina pectoris, or CHF associated with bradycardia or symptoms related to tachycardia with uncontrolled ventricular rates.

Initial therapy consists of the removal of any offending medication. Further treatment includes the insertion of a permanent cardiac pacemaker to prevent bradycardia and an antiarrhythmic agent to prevent paroxysmal tachycardia.

VENTRICULAR ARRHYTHMIAS

Ventricular Premature Beats

Ventricular premature beats (VPBs) are characterized by an early QRS complex that is not preceded by a P wave. They are ubiquitous, found in both normal and diseased hearts. They may be symptomatic or asymptomatic. The importance and treatment of ventricular premature beats depend on the clinical setting in which they occur. In normal hearts, VPBs tend to disappear with exercise. A patient without heart disease who exhibits these premature beats should be treated with reassurance and withdrawal of any offending agents, such as caffeine-containing products. Only a symptomatic patient without heart disease should receive antiarrhythmic medication. Beta blockers are usually efficacious in this setting. VPBs resulting from sinus bradycardia should be treated with medications that increase heart rate, such as parasympatholytic or sympathomimetic agents, or even with cardiac pacing. VPBs in a hypertensive patient without coexistent left ventricular dysfunction would generally benefit from beta blocker therapy. In the setting of acute myocardial infarction, patients who have VPBs that are close to the preceding T wave, occur more frequently than six times per minute, are of multiform contour, or occur in salvos of two or more should be treated with intravenous lidocaine, procainamide, or beta blockers. Consideration must be given to the hemodynamic status of the patient.

Ventricular Tachycardia

Ventricular tachycardia (VT) is defined as three or more VPBs in a row. The VT rate may vary between 70/min (nonparoxysmal) and 250/min (paroxysmal). VT is rarely found in normal hearts. It occurs commonly in patients with ischemic heart disease, rheumatic heart disease, congestive cardiomyopathy, myocarditis, and digitalis toxicity. The physician assistant should seek provocative causes for tachycardia onset, for example, hypoxemia, acute ischemia, and hypokalemia. It may be difficult even for an experienced electrocardiographer to differentiate between VT and SV tachycardia associated with aberrancy.

VT is classified as nonsustained if the arrhythmia lasts less than 30 s and is asymptomatic. VT is sustained when the tachycardia lasts more than 30 s (symptomatic or asymptomatic) or causes hemodynamic collapse within 30 s.

The treatment of nonsustained VT is controversial because the efficacy of antiarrhythmic medication has not been established. It is known that patients with nonsustained VT who have left ventricular dysfunction are at increased risk of sudden death. Electrophysiologic studies of left ventricular dysfunction patients may demonstrate those with inducible VT. This subset of patients should be treated. Class Ia, class II, and class III agents have been prescribed for these patients.

Sustained VT occurs most frequently in patients with an acute or old myocardial infarction. Sustained VT in an acutely infarcted patient is treated with intravenous lidocaine, intravenous procainamide, or, if necessary for a patient in hemodynamic collapse, DC cardioversion. Because of the high risk of sudden death in these patients, electrophysiologic (EPS) studies are frequently performed. The purpose of an EPS study is to determine whether any antiarrhythmic agent can prevent inducible VT in the laboratory. A medication found to be effective on EPS appears to have clinical efficacy. Amiodarone seems to be the most promising medication in this group.

For patients who do not tolerate or benefit from antiarrhythmic medication, consideration is given to the insertion of an implantable cardiac defibrillator, catheter ablation, or surgical aneurysmectomy.

Ventricular Fibrillation

In acute myocardial infarction, ventricular fibrillation (VF) occurs in two clinical settings. Primary VF occurs very early in the illness and typically is not associated with severe left ventricular dysfunction. If it is treated quickly, the patient does not have a negative long-term prognosis. Secondary VF typically occurs on the second or third day and is associated with severe left ventricular mechanical dysfunction. The prognosis is poor in these patients. This arrhythmia is further addressed in the section on sudden death in Chap. 1-7.

Torsade de Pointes

Torsade de pointes is a polymorphic VT in which the QRS complexes change in amplitude around the isoelectric axis. It typically is associated with a long QT interval on ECG. Torsade may be associated with a congenitally long QT interval in which the child frequently collapses during physical exertion. Therapy in the congenital group includes beta blockers, a left stellate ganglion block, or a cervical–high thoracic ganglionectomy. An acquired long QT interval usually is due to class Ia antiarrhythmic agents, but some class Ic and antidepressant agents also may be precipitants. With class Ia medicines, the QT prolongation most frequently occurs within 96 h of the initiation of therapy. It is widely accepted that patients started on class Ia medicines should be under hospital cardiac monitoring during this time period. Torsade occurring at a later time in patients taking these medications frequently is due to complicating hypokalemia or hypomagnesemia. Treatment includes withdrawal of the offending medication and, if necessary, electrolyte replacement, infusion of magnesium, or temporary cardiac pacing.

ATRIOVENTRICULAR BLOCK (HEART BLOCK)

Heart block is classified as first-degree, second-degree, and third-degree. In first-degree block, every atrial impulse is conducted to the ventricles with a PR interval greater than 0.20 s. In second-degree block, some atrial impulses are not conducted to the ventricles when the block is not due to physiologic interference. Second-degree AV block is further subdivided into Mobitz type

I (Wenckebach) and Mobitz type II. Type I is characterized by progressive PR prolongation culminating in a nonconducted P wave. Type I block typically occurs at the level of the AV node so that the QRS complex is narrow. In Mobitz II block, the PR interval is constant before the blocked P wave. The conduction disorder often is in the His-Purkinje system, with a resultant bundle branch QRS complex. Third-degree heart block (complete heart block) may be due to a conduction abnormality at the AV node or in the His-Purkinje system.

First-degree and Mobitz I blocks may occur transiently in normal persons who experience heightened vagal tone. Further, digitalis toxicity, myocardial ischemia or inferior myocardial infarction, acute rheumatic fever, myocarditis, conducting tissue calcification, and degenerative conduction disease may be causative. Medications including digoxin, calcium channel blockers, and beta blockers may cause these rhythm disturbances. Treatment of first-degree block generally consists of the discontinuation of the offending medication. Mobitz I conduction delay is treated by medication withdrawal and, if the ventricular rate is slow enough to cause symptoms, the insertion of a temporary pacemaker.

Mobitz II AV block is not caused by digitalis toxicity. It most commonly is due to acute myocardial infarction, degenerative conduction system disease, or myocarditis. Mobitz II is an unpredictable rhythm, and urgent pacing is required because of its propensity to advance to complete heart block or sudden death. In complete heart block, the ventricular rate is usually 30 to 40 beats per minute. Important causes include digitalis or potassium toxicity, acute infarction, chronic ischemic heart disease, and infiltrative cardiac disease. Complete heart block associated with inferior infarction is associated with a stable junctional (AV nodal) rhythm at a rate of 30 to 60 beats per minute. This conduction defect is typically of short duration, e.g., hours to days, and temporary pacing suffices. In anterior infarction, Mobitz II or complete heart block may occur. Escape rhythm is usually idioventricular and unstable in character. Temporary cardiac pacing is indicated, but the mortality rate remains at approximately 80 percent because of the associated severe myocardial damage. Chronic complete heart block caused by structural disease is treated with permanent cardiac pacing.

BIBLIOGRAPHY

Jung F, DiMarco J: Antiarrhythmic drug therapy in the treatment of atrial fibrillation. *Cardiol Clin North Am* 14:507–520, 1996.

Chapter 1–12
HYPERTENSION
Katherine Adamson

DISCUSSION

Systemic hypertension is one of the most common health problems in this country, affecting as many as 50 million Americans.[1] It is a chronic disease that afflicts more blacks than whites and is found in greater numbers among those in the lower socioeconomic strata. This disease results in more office visits to primary care providers than does any other chronic illness.[2] Hypertension

Table 1-12-1. Classification of Blood Pressure in Adults Age 18 and Older

Category	Systolic, mm Hg	Diastolic, mm Hg
Normal	<130	<85
High normal	130–139	85–89
Hypertension		
Stage 1 (mild)	140–159	90–99
Stage 2 (moderate)	160–179	100–109
Stage 3 (severe)	180–209	110–119
Stage 4 (very severe)	>210	>120

SOURCE: Adapted from the Fifth Report of the Joint National Committee on Detection, Evaluation, and Treatment of High Blood Pressure, National Institutes of Health Publication No. 93-1088.[1]

is a well-established major risk factor for the development of coronary artery disease and is the most important risk factor for cerebrovascular disease. The fifth Joint National Committee on Detection, Evaluation, and Treatment of High Blood Pressure (JNC-V)[1] published guidelines in 1993 that detailed an expanded definition of hypertension and suggested a rational approach to the management of this often complex disease.

For years physicians have been taught that control of diastolic blood pressure is paramount, but it has been confirmed that systolic elevations in blood pressure carry as much significance, if not more, than diastolic elevations. This awareness prompted JNC-V to formulate new parameters for the classification of blood pressure in the adult population (Table 1-12-1).

Those who have been in medicine for a while note that the tolerance level for elevations of blood pressure is changing. It is now recognized that the vast majority of individuals with hypertension fall into the "mild," or stage 1, category. One must not be misled by the assumption that a mild label equals a minimal outcome. Patients with stage 1 hypertension constitute the majority of all hypertensives, and all stages of elevated blood pressure are associated with an increased risk of both fatal and nonfatal cardiovascular events.

It is also important to view hypertension from an etiologic perspective. Over 90 percent of all the patients seen in this country for hypertension fall into the category of primary hypertension. Primary hypertension may be referred to as "essential" or even "idiopathic." This nomenclature underscores the fact that we have not identified the cause of the vast majority of cases of hypertension. The exact causality in essential hypertension may be elusive, but factors involved in the development of essential primary hypertension have been well established: advancing age, ethnicity, gender, family history, sodium intake, excessive alcohol ingestion, socioeconomic status, tobacco abuse, and the presence of high levels of emotional stress.

The term *secondary hypertension* implies that the patient has a clearly identifiable and often treatable cause for the elevation in blood pressure. Secondary hypertension, while rare, usually results from problems in the endocrine or renal system. Approximately 4 percent of cases of hypertension can be related to disease of the kidney and/or the renal vasculature, with another 4 to 5 percent related to an endocrine pathway, such as primary aldosteronism, Cushing's syndrome, pheochromocytoma, hyperthyroidism, hyperparathyroidism, acromegaly, and oral contraceptives.[3] One goal of the clinical evaluation of hypertensive patients is to identify the few individuals who need further investigation to determine the existence of an underlying treatable etiology for hypertension.

Malignant hypertension implies an extreme elevation in blood pressure that is associated with acute end organ damage or failure. This clinical emergency can occur in primary and secondary hypertensive patients.[4]

PATHOGENESIS

Sustained elevated levels of blood pressure result in an acceleration of atherosclerosis. This in turn manifests through coronary artery disease, aortic dissection, peripheral vascular disease, cerebral infarction or hemorrhage, retinopathy, and renal failure. In addition, the heart compensates for the increased workload caused by hypertension by increasing left ventricular wall thickness. If the hypertension is not treated, the hypertrophied heart will eventually cease to compensate and congestive heart failure will ensue. These pathologic presentations are loosely referred to as end organ or target organ manifestations.

There is a direct relationship between the level of blood pressure and the incidence of fatal and nonfatal cardiovascular events and renal disease. As the pressure increases, so does the incidence of end organ damage. From a physiologic point of view, the major factors involved in the maintenance of blood pressure are systemic vascular resistance and cardiac output. These two functions are controlled by a variety of neurohumoral mechanisms (sympathetic outflow) and the kidney (renin-angiotensin and the aldoesterone cascade).

CLINICAL EVALUATION

All health care professionals should measure the blood pressure of every patient at each visit. A diagnosis of hypertension should be made only if the blood pressure readings fall within the parameters reflected in Table 1-12-1 on a minimum of three office visits over a 1-week to several-week period. If a patient's readings fall in the very severe category on a single occasion with no apparent causative event (e.g., acute cocaine intoxication), it is reasonable to make the diagnosis of hypertension on the basis of this single presentation. The goals of clinical evaluation are to evaluate the extent of end organ manifestations and identify patients who require in-depth evaluation or referral for suspected secondary hypertension. All the cardiovascular risk factors should be searched for and properly addressed. This includes evidence of glucose intolerance or diabetes, hyperlipidemia, and life-style considerations.

SIGNS AND SYMPTOMS

Primary hypertension has long been referred to as a silent killer. Symptoms relating to elevated pressure alone are uncommon. Most symptomatology can be tied to long-standing pressure elevations and consequent target organ damage. A minority of patients may be diagnosed with hypertension when they present with occipital headache, dizziness, or epistaxis. In everyday practice, hypertension is uncovered when a patient's pressure is checked routinely as part of a physical examination or health maintenance screening program. Primary hypertension often is first seen in middle-aged individuals with a strong family history of hypertension, whereas secondary hypertension often presents in relatively young patients (<35 years of age).[4] Since hypertension is a major cardiovascular and cerebrovascular risk factor, it is imperative that a thorough cardiac and neurologic review of systems be conducted. It is useful to direct both the history and the physical with the target organ system in mind.

All patients should be historically screened for secondary hypertension by determining the presence of episodic palpitations, headache, and diaphoresis (pheochromocytoma); polyuria, polydipsia, and muscle weakness (from the hypokalemia associated with primary aldosteronism); and mood swings and weight gain (Cushing's syndrome).[4]

PHYSICAL EXAMINATION

A thorough physical examination is mandatory in the evaluation of hypertension. The clinician needs to check the blood pressure readings personally, both supine and upright. The pressures in both upper extremities and one lower extremity are necessary to rule out coarctation of the aorta. While performing a general inspection, one should look for the moon face associated with Cushing's syndrome. A careful funduscopic examination frequently will uncover the earliest physical evidence of uncontrolled hypertension. The Keith-Wagener-Baker classification of retinopathy is a useful reference for the grading of funduscopic changes.[4] Palpation and auscultation of the pulses are of paramount importance. The presence of a bruit will alert the examiner not only to a careful evaluation for accelerated atherosclerosis but also to a consideration of renovascular stenosis as a possible etiology for the hypertension. Examination of the neck must include inspection for venous distention and palpation of the thyroid. A palpable radial femoral pulse delay provides further evidence of aortic coarctation. The suspicion of left ventricular hypertrophy (LVH) on physical examination is significant. LVH is an independent risk factor for cardiovascular disease, and when it is found, aggressive antihypertensive therapy is indicated.[4] One should look for and document the point of maximal impulse (PMI), especially if it is deviated laterally and inferiorly. The presence of an S_4 is not uncommon; however, an S_3, particularly in the setting of pulmonary rates, indicates ventricular dysfunction. Careful auscultation for the presence of cardiac murmurs and extra heart sounds in addition to the rate and rhythm cannot be overemphasized. Auscultation of the abdomen may rarely uncover the bruit of renal artery stenosis. Abdominal palpation should be directed at the discovery of organomegaly or masses, with particular attention paid to the kidneys. Palpation of the abdomen would be incomplete without a gross measurement of the aorta and an assessment of aortic pulsation. The neurologic examination should be thorough and should include a screen for focal deficits in addition to noting the patient's gait and balance.

LABORATORY STUDIES

All hypertensive patients should have the following laboratory diagnostics: complete blood count, urinalysis, serum glucose, potassium, calcium, creatinine, uric acid, lipid profile, and 12-lead ECG.[1,4] This relatively inexpensive battery of tests will assist in the evaluation of target organ status and cardiovascular risk factor analysis and the identification of individuals with secondary hypertension. If ventricular hypertrophy is suspected from the physical examination and/or ECG findings, it is prudent to obtain an echocardiogram. Evidence of heart failure should be further investigated with a chest x-ray. Additional diagnostic studies may be ordered as the situation mandates (Table 1-12-2).

TREATMENT

The goal of treatment of hypertension is to reduce target organ damage while preserving the quality of life. Ideally, the blood pressure should be controlled with life-style modifications and, when necessary, medication. JNC-V has defined hypertension as a blood pressure equal to or greater than 140/90. Therefore, a reasonable goal for blood pressure control is below this level.

Life-Style Modifications

All patients diagnosed with hypertension must be counseled regarding a healthy life-style and strongly encouraged to adopt lifelong healthy habits. Life-style modifications should be viewed as adjunctive therapy for most patients and definitive therapy for some. These modifications are cost-effective and present little or no risk to the patient. Hypertension must be viewed as an independent cardiovascular risk factor, and many of the life-style modifications are aimed at improvement in cardiac risk factor status as well as direct reduction of blood pressure. One should

Table 1-12-2. Considerations in the Evaluation of Secondary Causes of Hypertension

Diagnosis	History	Physical Examination	Diagnostic Tests
Aortic coarctation	Generally young at presentation with long history of hypertension	Diminished or absent lower extremity pulses; decreased lower extremity blood pressure; systolic murmur over precordium	Chest x-ray with rib notching and "3" sign of aortic compression with pre- and poststenotic dilatation; ECG with left ventricular hypertrophy; aortography is definitive test
Parenchymal renal disease	Frequent urinary tract infections		Elevation of blood urea nitrogen (BUN) and creatinine
Renovascular disease	Young women have fibromuscular dysplasia variety	Abdominal bruits; hypertension refractory to treatment	Digital subtraction angiogram or rapid-sequence intravenous pyelography
Polycystic kidneys	Often with family history; flank pain and hematuria may be present	Abdominal or flank masses	Elevated BUN and creatinine; urinalysis with proteinuria and hematuria; cysts identified on renal ultrasound
Hyperthyroidism	Nervousness, tremor, weight loss, heat intolerance, mood swings	Tachycardia and/or atrial fibrillation common, tremor, thyroid enlargement, exophthalmos	Thyroid function studies
Hyperaldosteronism	Weakness, poluria, polydipsia	Nothing specific	Low serum potassium levels, often less than 3.5
Cushing's syndrome	Sexual dysfunction, depression, weight gain	Truncal obesity, hirsutism, striae, ecchymosis	Dexamethasone suppression test, elevated 17-ketosteroids
Pheochromocytoma	Episodic headache, tremor, tachycardia, diaphoresis		24-h urine collection for metanephrines and catecholamines; CT or MRI required to localize tumor preoperatively

encourage patients to attain and maintain ideal body weight, since there is a close correlation between obesity and hypertension. A weight loss program is enhanced by regular aerobic exercise, which of course improves cardiac fitness. The ideal diet is lean in fat and sodium and rich in calcium, magnesium, and potassium. It goes without saying that tobacco must be eliminated from the patient's life. Patients should be instructed to keep alcohol consumption at moderate levels, generally defined as not exceeding 1 oz of ethanol daily (8 oz of wine, 24 oz of beer, or 2 oz of 100-proof whiskey).[3] The role of stress management strategies has not been clearly defined. Nonetheless, it is reasonable to counsel patients about the deleterious effects of sustained high levels of emotional stress.

Medications

Currently, more than 70 different pharmaceutical products are available for the treatment of hypertension, with many more agents on the horizon. With the exception of patients with severe hypertension, a prudent clinician will avoid prescribing medication without allowing a reasonable period of time for life-style modification to have an impact. Generally speaking, if life-style modifications alone are to be effective, this will occur within the first 3 to 6 months. Once it has been determined that medications are necessary, a prudent clinician will use as small a dose as possible to attain control. JNC-V recommends one of six classes of medications for the initial treatment of hypertension: angiotensin-converting enzyme (ACE) inhibitors, alpha$_1$ receptor blockers, alpha-beta blockers, beta blockers, calcium channel blockers, and diuretics. JNC-V goes on to state that "diuretics and beta-blockers have been shown to reduce cardiovascular morbidity and mortality in controlled clinical trials—these two classes of drugs are preferred for initial drug therapy."[1] These recommendations have created significant controversy.[2,5] It is reasonable to follow the treatment algorithm provided in Fig. 1-12-1, which includes allowances for personal preference as well as specific patient situations. The choice of initial therapy needs to be tailored to the patient, with recognition of the increased cost to the patient of many of the newer agents. These cost considerations must be balanced against total cost; i.e., it may be less cost-effective to prescribe a cheaper agent that will require more frequent laboratory follow-up, as may be the case with diuretic therapy and the need for frequent electrolyte measurement.

Because black Americans tend to have low renin levels, this subset of the population is more responsive to diuretics and calcium channel blockers than to ACE inhibitors or beta blockers.[1] ACE inhibitors are known to delay the progression of diabetic nephropathy.[2] This property makes ACE inhibitors ideal agents in the treatment of diabetic hypertensives. There is substantial evidence that ACE inhibitors are effective in preventing congestive heart failure[2] and play a significant role in ameliorating postinfarction ventricular remodeling in patients with evidence of poor ventricular function.[6] In the author's experience, alpha$_1$ blockers have a higher incidence of untoward side effects than do the other suggested antihypertensives. However, the beneficial effect alpha$_1$ blockers have on benign prostatic hypertrophy (BPH) makes them ideal for older male hypertensives with a history of BPH. Experienced clinicians are aware of the synergistic effect of low-dose thiazide diuretics combined with one of several other classes of antihypertensives. The untoward effects of thiazides on glucose, uric acid, and lipids appear to be both dose-related and time-limited.[2,5] Recognition of these metabolic effects leads one away from choosing diuretics as initial therapy in a hypertensive patient with concomitant gout or glucose intolerance.

A pharmaceutical approach that takes the whole patient into account is best. Many of these medications have impotence as a side effect. It is often necessary to question the patient directly about such personal issues so that adjustments in the medication regimen can be made to ensure higher rates of compliance.

COMPLICATIONS AND RED FLAGS

Hypertensive emergencies are situations in which acute organ damage takes place secondary to extreme elevations in blood pressure. Patients in this situation often present with encephalopathy, acute pulmonary edema, dissecting aortic aneurysm, unstable angina, or acute myocardial infarction. Obviously, these patients are cared for in intensive or coronary care units with parenteral medications.

Hypertensive urgency is defined as a diastolic blood pressure in excess of 120 mmHg with no evidence of acute end organ

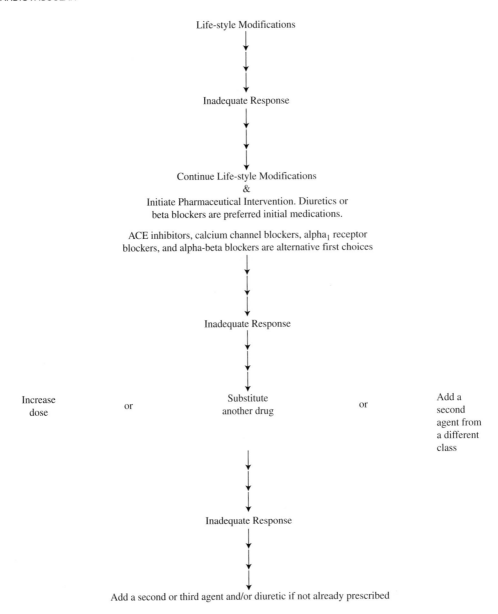

Figure 1-12-1. Treatment algorithm for hypertension. (*Adapted from the Fifth Report of the Joint National Committee on Detection, Evaluation, and Treatment of High Blood Pressure, National Institutes of Health Publication No. 93-1088.*[1])

damage.[1] These patients are often asymptomatic but require blood pressure reduction within 24 h. They can be handled in an outpatient setting using oral medications (Table 1-12-3).

NOTES AND PEARLS

A common practice in emergency rooms and outpatient settings throughout the country is to treat hypertensive urgencies with sublingual nifedipine. This is a practice that should not only be discouraged but abandoned. The sublingual route for nifedipine has never been approved by the U.S. Food and Drug Administration (FDA). This route is fraught with problems because absorption is unpredictable. There have been numerous reports of significant negative sequelae to this treatment approach.[7] Serious hypotensive episodes can result, with the induction of ischemia in the central nervous system or heart.

While ACE inhibitors are generally effective and well tolerated, a few caveats must be remembered. ACE inhibitors carry a boxed warning from the FDA regarding teratogenicity. It is best to avoid this class of drugs in the treatment of hypertension in women of childbearing age. Also, ACE inhibitors in combination with low-dose thiazide diuretics are extremely effective, but one must prescribe the addition of diuretics to ACE inhibitor therapy in the correct sequence. The addition of ACE therapy to a patient on diuretics can result in extreme and dangerous episodes of hypotension. The reverse is not true, and so one must remember that it is acceptable to add a diuretic to an ACE but not to do the reverse. The ACE-diuretic combination is attractive because of the potassium-sparing nature of ACE inhibitors. One must be aware of this effect and avoid using potassium-sparing diuretics in conjunction with ACE inhibitors.

Calcium channel blockers are also very effective antihypertensives. The shorter-acting dihydropyridine nifedipine is very useful in the treatment of hypertensive urgency. However, owing to an unresolved controversy regarding the possibility of increased cardiac mortality rate with the shorter-acting agents, those agents

Table 1-12-3. Management of Hypertensive Urgency:
Outpatient Management with Close Follow-Up

Therapeutic goal is to lower blood pressure by 20% or to a diastolic
  blood pressure <120
    Nifedipine 10–20 mg PO (not SL), repeat q 30–60 min
    Clonidine 0.1–0.2 mg PO, then 0.05 to 0.1 mg q 1 h up to 0.6 mg
    Captopril 25 mg PO, repeated as required
    Labetalol 200–400 mg PO, repeated every 2–3 h as needed
Observe at least 6 h before discharge
Discharge patient on same medication used for initial blood pressure
  reduction

should be used with caution or not at all in the long-term treatment of hypertension.[5]

Hypertension is the most common chronic illness encountered in the primary care provider's office. We now have far more effective and better tolerated forms of therapy, yet only one in five patients is controlled at goal blood pressure levels.[5] These patients may be partially accountable in that noncompliance is a problem. Ultimately, the caregivers need to do a better job in educating patients and being sensitive to the social as well as economic costs of the therapy prescribed.

REFERENCES

1. National High Blood Pressure Education Program: Fifth Report of the Joint National Committee on Detection, Evaluation, and Treatment of High Blood Pressure. Bethesda, MD, 1993. NIH Publication No. 93-1088.
2. Moser M: Management of hypertension, part I. *Am Fam Physician* 53:2295–2302, 1996.
3. Williams G: Hypertensive vascular disease, in Isselbacher KJ, Braunwald E, Wilson JD, et al (eds): *Harrison's Principles of Internal Medicine,* 13th ed. New York, McGraw-Hill, 1994, pp 1116–1131.
4. Griffith C: Hypertension evaluation and management. *Physician Assist* 19:25–42, 1995.
5. Moser M: Management of hypertension, part II. *Am Fam Physician* 53:2553–2559, 1996.
6. Hagar J, Olson H, Kloner R: Acute myocardial infarction, in Kloner RA (ed): *The Guide to Cardiology,* 3d ed. Greenwich, CT, Le Jacq, 1995, pp 299–300.
7. Grossman E, Messerli FH, Grodzieki T, et al: Should a moratorium be placed on sublingual nifedipine capsules given for hypertensive emergencies and pseudoemergencies? *JAMA* 276:1328–1330, 1996.

Chapter 2–1
CONTACT DERMATITIS
Barbara L. Sauls

DESCRIPTION

Contact dermatitis is an inflammatory skin reaction of the dermis and epidermis to an external agent or toxin. When the agent directly damages the skin, it is called *irritant contact dermatitis*. If the reaction is immunologic in nature, it is *allergic contact dermatitis*. Common offending agents are plants, cleaning chemicals, and metals (especially nickel and chromium) in jewelry or clothing. Reactions may range in severity from subacute to acute and chronic, and occur anywhere on the body, possibly even in the nose and mouth. The reaction may occur with the first exposure or may be delayed until the patient has been exposed several times.

The patient's history plays an important role in the diagnosis of contact dermatitis, with occupation, hobbies, changes in household products, and environmental exposures leading the list. Typical jobs at risk for this disease are cleaning personnel, beauticians, chemists, painters, and workers at manufacturing plants using chemicals. Hobbies at risk are model building, arts and crafts (due to the glue and paints), and gardening. Environmental risks are seen in hikers, mountain bikers, campers, and other outdoor enthusiasts. Persons with black skin seem to be less susceptible to contact dermatitis. Changes in soaps and detergents, or the use of ointments and creams, are frequently implicated in contact dermatitis. Even the long-established use of a certain product is not exempt, since manufacturers often change the chemical composition of their products without changing their brand name. Labels such as *new and improved* or *fresher smell* indicate that a chemical change has taken place.

Contact dermatitis (see Fig. 2-1-1) is not contagious to other individuals, a common point of contention between the practitioner and the patient. There is seasonal proclivity only for plant contact dermatitis such as poison ivy, poison oak, and poison sumac during the spring, summer, and fall when the plants are growing. Collectively, these are known as *Rhus dermatitis*. The offending allergen of the *Rhus* species is the urushiol contained in the oleoresin spots found on the undersides the leaves of these plants. The oleoresin is an extremely stable, oily agent and may be carried on inanimate objects such as unwashed clothing or shoes, firewood, and gardening tools and later cause a reaction when a person touches them, even *years* later. Smoke from the burning of *Rhus* is highly allergenic, both from contact and inhalation, commonly causing reactions in firefighters and curious onlookers.

SIGNS AND SYMPTOMS

Patients will complain of burning and itching of the exposed skin areas. Skin may also turn red, become edematous, and form weeping (serous fluid) areas. Patients commonly believe that this serous drainage is "the poison" that is contagious to others.

OBJECTIVE FINDINGS

Physical examination of the subacute reaction reveals areas of mild erythema and fine scales or papules. There may be mild desquamation of the skin. Acute reactions cause areas of erythema that are poorly demarcated and edematous, with vesicular lesions that may have progressed to crusting and drying. These areas of reaction are often linear when caused by direct plant exposure. A random pattern may occur from airborne contact such as burning of plants. Airborne contact may cause a reaction to occur in mucous membranes of the respiratory tract. The vesicles may ooze serous fluid. With chronic contact dermatitis patients develop patches of dry, thickened, mildly red skin. Lichenification is often noted, which includes hyperkeratosis and deepening of skin lines. The pattern of chronic exposure is often in a specific pattern such as a ring or watch band, or a sandal strap. See Fig. 2-1-2 (Plate 1) and Table 2-1-1.

DIAGNOSTIC CONSIDERATIONS

When a patient can relate a history of specific exposure followed by a reaction, it is almost impossible to miss the diagnosis, but identifying the actual offending agent can often be an unrewarding, time-consuming task. Patch testing may be required to make a specific determination, but is not necessary in most cases.

LABORATORY TESTS

It is not necessary to order laboratory tests to make the diagnosis of contact dermatitis. However, if a biopsy of the affected area was ordered, histiocyte and monocyte infiltration of the skin would indicate an allergic origin, whereas vesicles that contain polymorphonuclear leukocytes lead to a diagnosis of primary irritant dermatitis.

TREATMENT

The most important treatment is the recognition and removal of the offending agent. Occupational exposures may be limited by the use of proper protective gear. Hobby enthusiasts should protect their skin as well. Reactions to clothing, shoes, or jewelry are treated the same way. Patients may be able to get jewelry coated to avoid contact with a nickel-based metal. Shoes may be replaced, or a reaction may be prevented by the use of socks. Hikers and campers should be shown photos of *Rhus* species plants so they can try to avoid exposure, or at least they should cover their arms and legs while in the woods.

Topical steroids are used to treat contact dermatitis. Low-potency agents are appropriate for facial and intertriginous areas, middle potency is good for nonfacial and nonintertriginous areas, and high potency is useful on the soles and palms where the skin is thickened. Oral steroids in tapering doses may be needed for a generalized reaction or severe reactions of the face or other areas prone to atrophy from topical steroid use (axillae, groin). The use of steroids in the eyes may precipitate a preexisting fungal or herpetic infection, so extreme care must be taken.

Table 2-1-2, although not meant to be complete, represents some commonly used topical steroids for steroid-sensitive dermatoses.

SUPPORTIVE MEASURES

Cool compresses or tepid baths with Aveeno oatmeal bath or baking soda or starch shakes often helps to relieve the symptoms, albeit temporarily. Calamine lotion is sometimes helpful. Preparations containing topical diphenhydramine (Caladryl) may actually cause a sensitivity reaction and can worsen skin reaction in

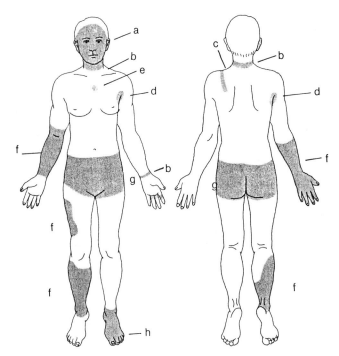

FIGURE 2-1-1. Eczematous dermatitis (contact). a, Airborne allergens, plants, pollens, sprays; b, jewelry, clothing, furs; c, clothing straps; d, deodorant, antiperspirant; e, metal tags; f, plants; g, trunks and panties; h, shoes or hose. (*From Fitzpatrick TB et al.: Color Atlas and Synopsis of Clinical Dermatology: Common and Serious Diseases, 2d ed. New York, McGraw-Hill, 1992, p 18. Used with permission.*)

some cases. Oral diphenhydramine hydrochloride (Benadryl) or other oral antipruritics may be used if the pruritus is severe, but they are not without their well-known side effects, especially sedation. It is important to keep the patient's hands away from the affected area to limit secondary infections. There are no restrictions of activity since this illness is not contagious and rest does not affect disease regression. Since children are often excluded from school or day-care, a note regarding their noncontagiousness may be required.

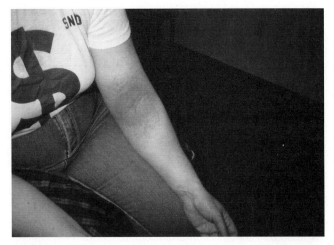

FIGURE 2-1-2 (Plate 1). Acute contact dermatitis of the antecubital area. (*Courtesy of Harold Milstein, MD, The Dermatology Clinic, Hazleton, PA.*)

Table 2-1-1. Various Forms of Contact Dermatitis and Their Manifestations

	Subacute	Acute	Chronic
Color	Mild redness	Erythema	Dark red
Scaling	Yes, small	No	No
Desquamation	Superficial	No	Excoriations
Edema	No	Yes	No
Vesicles	No	Yes	No
Pattern	Exposed area	Linear, random, or specific to exposed area	Shaped like item exposed to
Distribution	Often localized and isolated	Random, isolated, localized, or generalized	Usually localized

PATIENT EDUCATION

Patients must be educated on the avoidance of items causing contact dermatitis reactions. Gloves and long pants and sleeves should be worn to limit contact with *Rhus* plants. *Rhus* dermatitis victims often claim that each subsequent reaction seems worse than the previous. This may be due to an increasing intolerance to the oleoresin with repeated exposure. Those who burn brush should be instructed that the *Rhus* species' oleoresin becomes airborne and remains active. Anyone may be affected by downwind smoke exposure. It is possible to have severe *Rhus* dermatitis in the eyes as well as the entire respiratory tract.

Any inanimate items (boots, garden tools, etc.) that have come in contact with *Rhus* oleoresin as well as any exposure skin should be washed with an effective detergent soap (Fels Naphtha) that deactivates the oleoresin. Carefully wiping the skin, avoiding the face and mucous membranes, with isopropyl (rubbing) alcohol, in a well-ventilated area will also deactivate oleoresin if immediate soap and water washing is not possible. Immediate skin decontamination often prevents any reaction from occurring in a sensitized individual.

Bentoquatam 5% (Ivy Block) is a topical, over-the-counter preparation that is available to protect individuals from *Rhus* dermatitis. It is applied 15 minutes prior to exposure and provides a protective barrier that eliminates or reduces the contact dermatitis reaction to *Rhus* species plants. It must be reapplied every 4 hours.

DISPOSITION

Severe reactions, especially of the face, should be followed at least weekly, or sooner if the reaction worsens. Practitioners must monitor for secondary bacterial infections that may develop in areas that the patient has excoriated. Patients initially treated with topical steroids may need a change to oral steroids if the reaction is not clearing. Full resolution may take up to 3 weeks.

COMPLICATIONS AND RED FLAGS

Severe *Rhus* dermatitis in the eyes typically affects the conjunctiva but may develop on the corneas, though this is a rare occurrence. This condition warrants a referral to an ophthalmologist to monitor for future scarring and vision loss.

Patients who develop respiratory tract lesions from inhalation of a toxin or allergen should be considered for hospital admission. A hand-held nebulizer with a steroid preparation as well as oral or IV steroids may be needed.

In some individuals, future exposures to the same agent may cause more severe reactions with each subsequent contact. This does not occur in every patient.

Chronic contact dermatitis should lessen in severity once the

Table 2-1-2. Topical Steroid Preparations*

Potency Level	Generic	Brand	Dose	Frequency	Cautions
Superhigh	Halobetasol propionate	Ultravate	0.05% cream, ointment	Once or bid	Do not use more than 2 consecutive weeks. Not for use in groin, axilla, or on face. No occlusive dressings.
	Betamethasone dipropionate	Diprolene	0.05% ointment	Once or bid	As above.
High	Clobetasol proprionate	Temovate	0.05% cream, ointment	Bid	As above.
	Diflorasone diacetate	Psorcon	0.05% cream, ointment	Once to tid	As above.
Medium	Amcinonide	Cyclocort	0.1% cream, ointment, lotion	Bid to tid	
	Mometasone furoate	Elocon	0.1% cream, ointment, lotion	Once daily	
	Diflorisone diacetate	Florone	0.05% ointment	Once to qid	
	Halcinonide	Halog	0.1% cream, ointment, lotion	Bid to tid	
	Fluocinonide	Lidex	0.05% cream, ointment, gel, solution	Bid to qid	
	Desoximetasone	Topicort	0.25% cream, ointment; 0.05% gel	Bid	
	Triamcinolone acetonide	Aristocort A	0.1% ointment	Tid to qid	
	Fluticasone propionate	Cutivate	0.005% ointment	Bid	
	Fluocinolone acetonide	Synalar	0.025% cream, ointment 0.01% cream, solution	Bid to qid	
	Hydrocortisone valerate	Westcort	0.2% cream, ointment	Bid to tid	
Low	Hydrocortisone	Hytone	1% cream, ointment, lotion 2.5% cream, ointment, lotion	Bid to qid	

* Although this list of topical steroids is not complete, the level of potency, brand and generic names, dosing, preparation type, frequency, and significant cautions are provided as a starting reference for treatment.

offending agent is removed. Depending on the length of time the reaction has been present, the skin may never completely return to normal. These areas often remain slightly darker and with thickened skin. This does not cause complication, but may be cosmetically disfiguring.

PEARLS

One of the old-time treatments for *Rhus* dermatitis was to take baths with bleach water or to put bleach directly on the affected areas. Some patients may still be doing this. One of the major problems with this treatment is the development of an alkali burn, resulting in a second problem. There is some basis to this treatment, since it has been observed that children with *Rhus* who swim in chlorinated pools seem to heal faster. Tell patients that it is okay to go swimming, and it may even help. The children will love it!

BIBLIOGRAPHY

References

Fauci AS, Braunwald E, Isselbacher KJ, et al (eds): *Harrison's Principles of Internal Medicine,* 14th ed. New York, McGraw-Hill, 1998.
Fitzpatrick TB, Johnson RA, Wolff K, et al: *Color Atlas and Synopsis of Clinical Dermatology: Common and Serious Diseases,* 3d ed. New York, McGraw-Hill, 1997.

Recommended Dermatology Texts to Read

Arndt KA, Robinson JK, LeBoit PE, et al: *Cutaneous Medicine and Surgery.* Philadelphia, Saunders, 1996.
duVivier A: *Dermatology in Practice.* Philadelphia, Lippincott, 1990.
Goldstein BG, Goldstein AO: *Practical Dermatology,* Primary Care Series. St. Louis, Mosby Year Book, 1992.

Weinberg, S, Prose NS, Kristal L: *Color Atlas of Pediatric Dermatology,* 3d ed. New York, McGraw-Hill, 1998.

Advanced Reading

Shelley, WB, Shelley, ED: *Advanced Dermatology Diagnosis.* Philadelphia, Saunders, 1992.

Other Suggestions for Dermatology Education

Internet

For those with access to WWW (World Wide Web), there are numerous dermatology-related URL (Universal Resource Locator) sites of places to go (with a browser such as Netscape, Explorer) that have dermatology information, educational courses, dermatologic drug research, acne and melanoma information, and excellent slide photos (hundreds). A good monitor shows even the skin pores. A highly recommend site is, "You Can Become an Expert at Diagnosing Melanomas" found at the URL site of http://matrix.ucdavis.edu/tumors/new/tutorial-intro.html.

To obtain a list of about 45 of these sites, contact the Society of Dermatology Physician Assistants (SDPA) at the address below or e-mail jomonroe@pacifier.com.

Medline

The easiest access for MEDLINE via WWW is through the National PA home page at http://www.papage.com/papage/.

Two CD ROMS for Basic Dermatology

Reeves JRT: *Clinical Dermatology Illustrated: A Regional Approach.* There is a good review of this CD-ROM product by Jason Chao, MD, in the May 1994 issue of *The Journal of Family Practice.* The CD ROM contains text by John R.T. Reeves (heard frequently on *Audio Digest*) and is written for the primary care practitioner about common skin conditions. There are 340 color photographs, and some of the pictures have a soundtrack recording of Reeves giving some "pearls" from his personal experience. Also included: 15 patient education guides, a formulary section, and 20 hours of Continuing Medical Education credit. Price for individuals: $199. Publisher: Continuing Medical Education Associates, 4015 Hancock St, Suite 120, San Diego, CA 92110.

McLean D, Sober AJ: *Illustrated Dermatology: Synopsis of Diagnosis and Treatment.* Concise description of over 450 prevalent dermatological pathologies, including treatment and differential diagnosis; 2000 high-resolution color images; updated yearly; $195 includes a $50 discount voucher for future editions; phone 1-800-346-0085, ext 477 or fax 218-723-9433.

Dermatology Magazines, Other Methods and Education

To obtain a list of numerous dermatology magazines, contact the Society of Dermatology Physician Assistants, Inc., by fax at 360-253-1446, or write SDPA at: 5705 NE 116th St, Vancouver, WA 98686, or e-mail jomonroe@pacifier.com. Many subscriptions are free.

SDPA is in the process of developing a dermatology home-study course certification for PAs.

Dermatology lectures at American Academy of Physician Assistant and American Academy of Dermatology conferences are another educational source. It is also useful to seek participation in local dermatology grand rounds, morphology conferences, tumor boards, or set up a personal rotation with a local dermatologist.

The distant learning option PA master's program, with concentration in dermatology, is available through the University of Nebraska. Preference is given to University of Nebraska and U.S. Air Force graduates of the PA program there. Contact Jesse Edwards at (fax 402-559-5356) or University of Nebraska PA Program DLO, 600 South 42 St, Omaha, NE 68198-4300.

Research and Patient Support Groups

For a list of addresses or contacts for approximately a dozen skin-disease patient support groups, organized under the Coalition of Patient Advocates for Skin Disease Research (CPA-SDR), write to CPA-SDR at 710 C St, #11, San Rafael, CA 94901, 415-456-4644, fax 415-456-4274.

Chapter 2–2
URTICARIA (HIVES)
Joe R. Monroe

DISCUSSION

Urticaria is a transient, blanchable, wheal-like erythematous dermal swelling of acute onset that is usually highly symptomatic (sting and/or itch). Urticaria is quite common, affecting 20 to 25 percent of all individuals during their lifetimes. The lesions appear suddenly as pale-to-red, well-defined areas of focal, shallow dermal edema that vary from pinpoint to palm size. The individual round lesions frequently coalesce into annular or serpiginous plaques surrounded by an erythematous or pallored rim.

The fact that individual urticarial lesions seldom last more than 24 h is extremely useful in differentiating it from other hive-like conditions. Digital pressure on urticarial lesions produces a brief whitening effect, a phenomenon called blanching, which helps differentiate urticaria from vasculitis, a much more serious condition.

Acute urticaria, traditionally defined as being of less than 6 weeks' duration, is probably more common in children and young adults, whereas recurrent hives, predominately affecting adults, last longer and are termed *chronic*.

On a cellular level, urticaria is caused by the sudden release of histamine from affected mast cells, which leads to increased vascular permeability, and subsequent leakage of serum into the tissues. At least 40 percent of cases are idiopathic, but known causes include food, drink, and medicines (e.g., peanuts, shellfish, wheat and eggs, penicillin, and sulfa drugs) and are more common in atopic (allergy-prone) individuals.

Among non-allergy-related causes of urticaria are the so-called physical urticarias, including those caused by firm stroking of the skin (dermatographism) and exposure to cold, heat, water, sun, exercise, and vibration.

Urticarial lesions can also accompany diseases such as hepatitis A and B, and infectious mononucleosis.

Angioedema is urticaria affecting deeper tissues, presenting with acute focal painless swelling of areas such as lips, nose, eyelids, hands, feet, or genitals. Like urticaria, angioedema may be acute or chronic and may be seen in conjunction with urticaria or by itself.

Hereditary angioedema (HAE) is a potentially life-threatening form of urticaria transmitted in an autosomal dominant mode. Death from laryngeal edema can occur in up to 26 percent of cases of undiagnosed or untreated HAE, so careful history taking is needed to identify a suggestive family history like sudden unexplained deaths of apparent respiratory origin. Eighty-five percent of HAE patients have a deficiency of C_1 esterase, a substance whose level can be measured in most laboratories.

DIFFERENTIAL DIAGNOSIS

Fortunately, the evanescent nature of urticaria is extraordinarily helpful in its diagnosis. No other hive-like lesion goes away so abruptly. This distinguishes it from other hive-like conditions such as urticarial vasculitis and erythema multiforme. Urticarial lesions can be seen in conjunction with other illnesses such as rheumatoid arthritis, lupus erythematosus, viral hepatitis, and infectious mononucleosis, so the clinical context in which the lesions appear needs to be taken into account.

LABORATORY

A diagnosis of urticaria usually requires no laboratory work, but a biopsy may be required to rule out systemic diseases presenting with urticaria, such as the vasculitides. Likewise, blood work may be called for, such as sedimentation rate, antinuclear antibodies (ANA), rheumatoid agglutinin (RA), liver function tests, mononucleosis test, and C_1 esterase levels, as the clinical context dictates.

TREATMENT

Treatment of urticaria involves the following steps:

1. Identify and eliminate the cause, if possible.
2. *Antihistamines* First-generation H_1 blockers such as diphenhy-

dramine hydrochloride (Benadryl and others) or hydroxyzine (Atarax and others), used at bedtime because of their sedative effects, adding second-generation H$_1$ blockers such as cetirizine (Zyrtec) for daytime use, to sidestep problems with sedation. H$_2$ blockers such as ranitidine can be added and may be helpful in some cases, though only in conjunction with the other agents.

3. *Topicals* Other than cool baths or compresses, topical agents are of little use in the treatment of urticaria
4. If these steps fail, the next step should be referral to a dermatologist, not only for confirmation of the diagnosis and possible identification of the trigger, but because the physician will have expertise with a variety of agents that have proved useful in treating urticaria, including calcium channel blockers, systemic corticosteroids, and many others.

PATIENT EDUCATION

Patient education should include the following points:

1. When investigating chronic urticaria, teach patients about the necessity to keep an accurate record of food, drink, and medicine ingested.
2. Educate patients about the early symptoms of anaphylaxis and the necessity for seeking prompt medical attention.
3. Instruct angioedema patients to quiz family members about a possible family history of sudden, unexplained death involving respiratory distress.
4. Educate patients as to the necessity for taking prescribed antihistamines around the clock, and not just "as needed."

PEARLS

Knowledge of the following points can contribute to a satisfactory patient outcome:

- A truly evanescent lesion, that is, one that leaves rapidly, is probably urticaria.
- Viral hepatitis and mononucleosis can present with urticaria.
- OTC medications, especially NSAIDs, can cause urticaria, and are frequently overlooked by patients and providers, as are food additives, such as dyes, or preservatives.
- If the lesions won't blanch (turn white) with pressure, a biopsy is probably indicated to rule out entities such as vasculitis.

PROGNOSIS

Within a year 50 percent are disease-free, but 20 percent will have it 10 years or more. HAE is fatal in up to 26 percent of cases if undetected. The combination of angioedema and urticaria lasts up to 5 years in 50 to 75 percent of cases.

BIBLIOGRAPHY

Arndt, KA, Robinson JK, LeBoit PE, et al: *Cutaneous Medicine and Surgery.* Philadelphia, Saunders, 1996.

duVivier A: *Dermatology in Practice.* Philadelphia, Lippincott, Gower, 1990.

Fitzpatrick TB, Johnson RA, Polano MK, et al: *Color Atlas and Synopsis of Clinical Dermatology: Common and Serious Diseases,* 3d ed. McGraw-Hill, New York, 1997.

Goldstein BG, Goldstein AO: *Practical Dermatology, Primary Care Series.* St Louis, Mosby Year Book, 1992.

Shelley WB, Shelley ED: *Advanced Dermatologic Diagnosis.* Philadelphia, Saunders, 1992.

Weinberg S, Prose NS, Kristal L: *Color Atlas of Pediatric Dermatology,* 3d ed. New York, McGraw-Hill, 1998.

Chapter 2–3
ROSACEA (ACNE ROSACEA)
Joe R. Monroe

DISCUSSION

Rosacea is chronic inflammatory acneiform disorder typically affecting middle-aged or older adults, characterized by intermittent flushing erythema and the recurrent appearance of papules, pustules, and tiny permanent blood vessels called telangiectases, primarily seen on the central cheeks, nose, brow, and chin. Symptoms of burning and itching are common, and there is a tendency toward progression unless treated.

Though the true cause of rosacea is unknown, clearly it is not a type of acne, since there is almost a complete absence of comedones (blackheads and whiteheads), a key diagnostic point. Perhaps the most persistent theory of etiology holds that rosacea is due to the inflammatory response generated by leakage of fluid through dilated vessel walls, in certain individuals with vasomotor instability. After years of vasodilatation, the superficial blood vessels in the affected areas "lock in the open position" giving rise to multiple telangiectases, permanent redness, and, eventually, the formation of papules, pustules, and, on occasion, granulomatous nodules.

Twenty percent of skin biopsies will demonstrate the presence of *Demodex,* a genus of ectoparasitic mites found on all human faces, in the follicles. In rosacea, up to 200 of these organisms are seen in each follicle, compared with only 3 to 5 seen on unaffected individuals. But treatment for *Demodex* (with crotamiton or other pharmaceuticals does not appear to be terribly effective for most cases of rosacea, so researchers are still searching for the true cause of rosacea.

Although the sexes are equally affected by this malady, more women than men request treatment for this condition, which typically begins between the ages of 30 and 50.

It can be complicated by eye involvement (blepharitis, episcleritis, and conjunctival hyperemia) and can progress to rhinophymatous changes, a bulbous appearance of the nose caused by sebaceous hyperplasia, especially in men.

DIFFERENTIAL DIAGNOSIS

Diseases such as acne vulgaris, seborrhea, pityriasis rubra pilaris, lupus erythematosus, syphilis, cutaneous tuberculosis, carcinoid, and sarcoid can all appear like rosacea. Other telangiectatic processes (e.g., scleroderma) may also superficially simulate rosacea, but can usually be readily distinguished on clinical and/or histopathologic grounds.

LABORATORY

Though generally not necessary, biopsy can be helpful, with a histopathologic picture that varies according to the type and stage of the disease process, typically showing a nonspecific lymphohistiocytic perivascular infiltrate and telangiectases. As with all biopsies, it is important to let the pathologist know the differential being considered.

TREATMENT
Oral

Tetracycline 250 mg, one or two capsules bid, for at least 2 months, tapering over a 1- to 2-month period is remarkably effective, but recurrences are common. Side effects include the following: (1)

potentially diminished effectiveness of birth control pills (must use backup like foam, condom, or sponge; (2) potential discoloration to a mottled brown of the permanent teeth of any fetus present during therapy; (3) possible neutralization of the effects of tetracycline by calcium-rich foods like milk products and calcium-containing antacids (which requires avoidance of these foods for 1 h before or after dose), since there is a marked affinity of tetracycline for calcium; (4) potential photosensitivity (sunburn-like rash) in a small but significant number of patients. Other oral antibiotics like erythromycin, amoxicillin, and even trimethoprim sulfamethozole (Septra), have been used but are much less effective.

Topical

Metronidazole (MetroGel) used twice a day has been reported to be effective, but in this author's experience has been a very poor alternative to oral antibiotics, and, at best, takes 6 to 8 weeks to begin working. A less-drying cream form of topical metronidazole is now available.

Anything that is known to exacerbate facial flushing or blushing (e.g., hot foods, alcohol, stress) needs to be eliminated or reduced.

PATIENT EDUCATION

Patients need to know that ocular symptoms of grittiness or irritation may be secondary to the effects of rosacea and may require evaluation by an ophthalmologist. Stress the chronic nature of rosacea and the necessity of staying on medication for extended periods.

PEARLS

Knowledge of the following points can increase positive patient outcome:

- "Acne" primarily affecting the nose is probably rosacea.
- Self-prescribed topical steroids are frequently being used by the patient and are decidedly counterproductive in treating rosacea because of a rebound effect when they are stopped.
- The "typical" patient is perimenopausal with a history of being a blusher.
- Marked sparing of the periorbital area is common in rosacea.

PROGNOSIS

Excellent response to treatment is the rule, but maintenance therapy with as few as two to three capsules of 250-mg tetracycline a week is often a necessity to prevent recurrences. Severe or unresponsive cases require referral to a dermatologist.

BIBLIOGRAPHY

Arndt KA, Robinson JK, LeBoit PE, et al: *Cutaneous Medicine and Surgery.* Philadelphia, Saunders, 1996.

duVivier A: *Dermatology in Practice.* Philadelphia, Lippincott, Gower, 1990.

Fitzpatrick TB, Johnson RA, Polano MK, et al: *Color Atlas and Synopsis of Clinical Dermatology: Common and Serious Diseases,* 3d ed. New York, McGraw-Hill, 1997.

Goldstein BG, Goldstein AO: *Practical Dermatology,* Primary Care Series. St Louis, Mosby Year Book, 1992.

Shelley, WB, Shelley, ED: *Advanced Dermatologic Diagnosis.* Philadelphia, Saunders, 1992.

Weinberg S, Prose NS, Kristal L: *Color Atlas of Pediatric Dermatology,* 3d ed. New York, McGraw-Hill, 1998.

Chapter 2–4
ALOPECIA AREATA
Joe R. Monroe

DISCUSSION

Alopecia areata (AA) is a localized, sharply defined loss of hair in round or oval areas without any visible inflammation or significant skin symptoms. Thought to be an autoimmune disease, this condition may occur on any hair-bearing surface of the body, and may progress to total scalp and brow hair loss (alopecia totalis) or even total body hair loss (alopecia universalis).

Typically affecting younger adults and children, AA is not a sign of multisystem disease, but may be associated with other autoimmune diseases such as vitiligo or Hashimoto's thyroiditis, and can also be brought on by emotional stress.

DIFFERENTIAL DIAGNOSIS

The differential diagnosis includes tinea capitis (will likely demonstrate scaling and inflammation, may be KOH-positive, and may fluoresce) and secondary syphilis (appearance of moth-eaten patches in scalp or beard, with positive VDRL). In AA, the lack of scaling, the redness, and the sharply demarcated loss of hair usually make it easy to distinguish from these other entities.

LABORATORY

Punch biopsy shows infiltrate of mononuclear cells around hair bulbs, a fact often useful in establishing the correct diagnosis. Other laboratory tests can be obtained to rule out coexistent autoimmune diseases such as Hashimoto's thyroiditis (thyroid function tests), lupus erythematosus [antinuclear antibodies (ANA)], pernicious anemia [complete blood count (CBC), iron studies], and syphilis (VDRL).

TREATMENT

Treatment for AA is unsatisfactory. For small, solitary spots, intralesional triamcinolone acetonide, 5 to 10 mg/cm^3, is temporarily very effective. No treatment has been shown to alter the ultimate course of this disease. Avoid systemic corticosteroids since any benefit would inevitably be lost on discontinuing the drug.

PATIENT EDUCATION

Reassure the patient about the usually self-limiting nature of the disease. In severe disease, patients may require counseling to share their feelings about having permanent hair loss.

PEARLS

Knowledge of the following points can contribute to positive patient outcome:

- Sharply demarcated total hair loss in a round configuration without epidermal skin changes (redness, scaling, etc.) is probably alopecia areata.
- There is no good evidence that treatment induces remission or affects the permanent course of the disease.
- Of all indicators for poor prognosis, onset at an early age is the most reliable, with involvement of occipital scalp being the next.

PROGNOSIS

The majority of AA patients recover without any treatment, within 9 months. Predictors of a poor or guarded prognosis are onset at an early age, multiple patches, occipital hair loss, loss of eyebrow and eyelash hair, history of previous attacks, associated atopic disease, and alopecia totalis/universalis.

BIBLIOGRAPHY

Arndt KA, Robinson JK, LeBoit PE, et al: *Cutaneous Medicine and Surgery.* Philadelphia, Saunders, 1996.
duVivier A: *Dermatology in Practice.* Philadelphia, Lippincott, 1990.
Fitzpatrick TB, Johnson RA, Polano MK, et al: *Color Atlas and Synopsis of Clinical Dermatology: Common and Serious Diseases,* 3d ed. New York, McGraw-Hill, 1997.
Goldstein GB, Goldstein AO: *Practical Dermatology,* Primary Care Series. St Louis, Mosby Year Book, 1992.
Shelly WB, Shelly ED: *Advanced Dermatologic Diagnosis.* Philadelphia, Saunders, 1992.
Weinberg S, Prose NS, Kristal L: *Color Atlas of Pediatric Dermatology,* 3d ed. New York, McGraw-Hill, 1998.

Chapter 2–5
ARTHROPOD INFESTATIONS
Michelle DiBaise

DISCUSSION

Pediculosis Capitis (*Pediculus humanus var. capitis*): Head Lice

The head louse infests the scalp and neck of humans most commonly at the occiput and postauricular areas, but rarely in the beard or other hairy sites.[1-4] It deposits eggs, or "nits," on the emerging hair shaft.

Head lice can occur in any age group, but it is most common in school-age children. It is more common in whites and females[1-4] than it is in others. Head lice are not confined to any socioeconomic group and are not related to the patient's hygiene. The head louse can be transmitted via shared brushes, combs, hats, or bedding, in addition to head-to-head contact.

Pediculosis Corporis (*Pediculus humanus var. corporis*): Body Lice

The body louse infests the hair-bearing surfaces of the body, but lives and lays nits predominantly in the seams of clothing. It is relatively uncommon among affluent populations and is also related to poor patient hygiene.[2-4] Unlike other lice, pediculosis corporis is a vector of diseases such as trench fever (*Rickettsia quintana*), typhus (*Rickettsia prowazekii*), and relapsing fever (*Borrelia recurrentis*).[2-4]

Pediculosis Pubis (*Phthirus pubis*): Pubic Lice, or Crabs

The pubic louse is the smallest of the lice species. It is found only on the human host and most commonly infests the hair-bearing areas of the pubic region, but may infest the hair of the chest, axilla, eyebrows, and eyelashes.[1-4] Pubic lice occurs in all age groups, but is most common in young adults, more commonly in males.[1-4] It is spread by close contact, including sexual intercourse, sleeping in the same bed, and possibly by sharing articles of clothing. Pubic lice is one of the most contagious sexually transmitted diseases.[2-4]

Scabies (*Sarcoptes scabiei*): Scabies

Sarcoptes scabiei is a mite that infests the skin. The female mite burrows into the stratum corneum about 2 to 3 mm over a 24-h period, usually at night, and lays eggs during the day.[1,3,4] She deposits fecal pellets, or scybala, in the burrow behind her. Scabies occurs in all age groups, but are more common in children under 5 years, the institutionalized, and young adults who often acquire the mites by sexual contact.[1,3,4] Scabies is transmitted by skin to skin contact, but also by contact with infested bedding or clothing, since the mite can remain alive for more than 2 days after leaving the human host.

SIGNS AND SYMPTOMS

Pediculosis Capitis, Pediculosis Corporis, Pediculosis Pubis

The presenting complaint of the patient is pruritus of the infested area of the body. However, a patient with pubic lice may be asymptomatic. There may also be a complaint of nodularity of the pubic hairs.

Scabies

The patient's first infestation of the scabies mite requires an incubation of 1 month before the onset of pruritus. This is due to the development of a hypersensitivity reaction to the mite. With recurrent infestations, pruritus will begin within 24 h. The pruritus is often described as generalized, intense, and intractable and may be disproportionate to the number of lesions. It often wakes the patient up at night and generally spares the head and neck in adults. Frequently, other family members and close contacts complain of pruritus.

OBJECTIVE FINDINGS
Pediculosis Capitis
Primary Infestation

In a majority of patients there are only about 10 lice present, and they are rarely seen.[1,4] The nits are oval grayish white capsules, approximately 1 mm in length, and are firmly cemented to the hairs [see Fig. 2-5-1 (Plate 2)]. New viable nits have a creamy yellow color, whereas empty nits are white.[1-4]

Secondary Lesions

Excoriations, crusts, and impetiginized lesions are common from scratching and can potentially mask the presence of lice and nits. Secondary lesions may extend onto the neck, forehead, face, and ears. In severe cases, the hair can become matted with lice, nits, crusts, and purulent discharge. With secondary infection, there may also be associated occipital and/or cervical lymphadenopathy.

Pediculosis Corposis
Primary Infestation

The host almost always has poor hygiene. Body lice visit the host only to feed; therefore, nits and lice are observed in the seams of clothing [see Fig. 2-5-2 (Plate 3)]. Sites of feeding may present as red macules or papules.

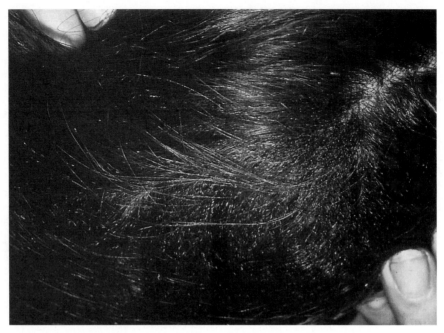

Figure 2-5-1 (Plate 2). Nits. (*From Fitzpatrick, Johnson, Wolff, et al.*)

Secondary Lesions

Primary lesions are commonly excoriated. In atopic individuals, an eczematous dermatitis can develop. These secondary lesions are commonly impetiginized. There may also be associated regional adenopathy present.

Pediculosis Pubis

Primary Infestation

Pubic lice appear as 1- to 2-mm brownish gray specks in the involved hairy areas.[1-4] They are usually few in number. The nits appear as tiny white-gray specks. They can be few to numerous and are initially at the hair-skin junction, predominantly in the pubic area and axilla, but may be present on the perineum, thighs, lower legs, trunk, and periumbilical area. In hairy males, they may be found in the nipple areas and upper arms and rarely the wrists, beard, and mustache area. In children they can appear on the eyelashes and eyebrows and may not have pubic involvement [see Fig. 2-5-3 (Plate 4)].[1-4] Eyelash infestation may be a sign of childhood sexual abuse.

Secondary Lesions

Red macules or papules may be seen at sites of feeding, especially the periumbilical region. Rarely the feeding sites become bullous. With scratching, secondary changes of lichenification and excoriations are common. These lesions can become impetiginized and lead to inguinal lymphadenopathy.

Scabies

Primary Infestation

Burrows are in areas with few or no hair follicles where the stratum corneum is thin, such as the interdigital web spaces, wrists, elbows, buttocks, and axillae. In men the penis and scrotum are usually involved, and in women the breast, especially the areola and nipple, may be infested (see Fig. 2-5-4).

The burrow appears as gray or skin-colored ridges, 0.2 to 10 cm in length either linear, curved, or S-shaped with a pinpoint vesicle, papule and/or halo of erythema at the end of the bur-

row.[1-4] The mite may appear as a black speck at the end of the burrow.

The patient can develop signs of a hypersensitivity reaction including pruritus, generalized, small, urticarial papules predominantly on the anterior trunk, thighs, buttocks, and forearms. In atopic individuals, an eczematous dermatitis can develop at the sites of infestation. With chronic scratching, multiple excoriations are commonly seen. In severe hypersensitivity reactions, the patient can become erythrodermic. Signs of secondary infection include impetiginization, ecthyma, folliculitis, abscess formation, lymphadenitis, and cellulitis.

Nodular scabies is a variant that has been noted to develop in 7 to 10 percent of patients with scabies.[1-4] The nodules range from 5 to 20 mm in diameter and are pink, red, tan, or brown in color.[1-4] An early nodule may have a burrow noted on the surface [see Fig. 2-5-5 (Plate 5)].

Norwegian, or crusted, scabies is another variant seen in the immunocompromised or individuals with neurologic or mental disorders. Crusted scabies appears as well-demarcated markedly hyperkeratotic and/or crusted plaques. Itching may be absent or severe. It can begin as ordinary scabies or present initially with asymptomatic crusting. The distribution can be generalized even involving the head and neck in adults, or it can be localized [see Fig. 2-5-6 (Plate 6)].

Scabies in infants is often misdiagnosed because it can differ from adult infestations. In infants, there is often head and neck involvement. Infants may have multiple vesicles or pustules on the palms and soles. Nodules are seen in the axilla, diaper area, and lateral edge of the foot. Secondary eczematization and impetiginization are common and obscure the primary lesions [see Fig. 2-5-7 (Plate 7)].

Secondary Lesions

Secondary lesions are common and result from scratching. Secondary lesions include pinpoint erosions, excoriations, eczematous dermatitis, and lichen simplex chronicus. With secondary infection, pustules may be seen as well as impetiginization. There may also be associated regional lymphadenopathy.

Figure 2-5-2 (Plate 3). Pediculosis corporis. (*From Fitzpatrick, Johnson, Wolff, et al.*)

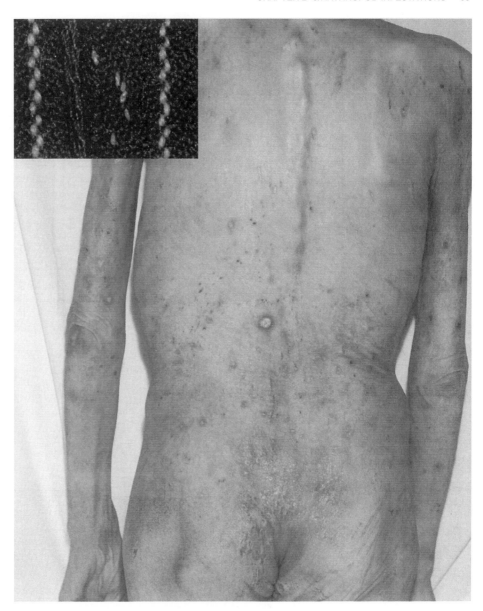

DIAGNOSTIC CONSIDERATIONS

Pediculosis Capitis

The differential diagnosis of head lice includes the use of hair sprays and gels as well as seborrheic dermatitis (dandruff). These however, are easily removed, whereas nits are firmly cemented and are difficult to remove.

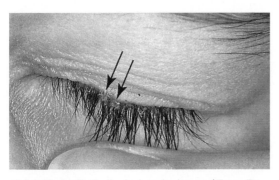

Figure 2-5-3 (Plate 4). Pediculosis palpebrum. (*From Fitzpatrick, Johnson, Wolff, et al.*)

Pediculosis Corporis

The differential diagnosis of body lice includes eczema, folliculitis, and lichen simplex chronicus.

Pediculosis Pubis

The differential diagnosis of pubic lice includes eczema, seborrheic dermatitis, tinea cruris, folliculitis, and molluscum contagiosum.

Scabies

The differential diagnosis of pruritus in scabies includes a cutaneous drug reaction, eczema, contact dermatitis, urticaria, pediculosis corporis or pubis, lichen planus, delusions of parasitosis, and metabolic pruritus. The differential diagnosis for nodular scabies includes urticaria pigmentosa (in young children), papular urticaria, Darier's disease, prurigo nodularis, and secondary syphilis. The differential diagnosis for crusted scabies includes psoriasis, eczematous dermatitis, and seborrheic dermatitis.

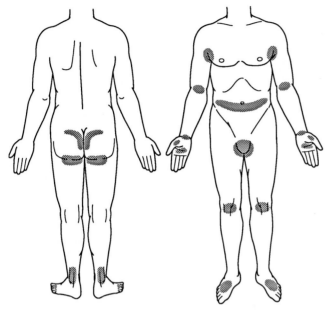

Figure 2-5-4. Distribution of scabies. (*Courtesy of Michel Di-Baise.*)

LABORATORY TESTS

Pediculosis Capitis and Pediculosis Corporis

On microscopy, the nits are oval, whitish eggs. A Wood's lamp examination will fluoresce live nits a pearly color but not dead nits. The louse is a wingless insect with 6 legs, 1 to 4 mm in length with a translucent grayish white body.[1-4] The louse becomes red or rust-colored when engorged with blood (see Fig. 2-5-8).

Pediculosis Pubis

On microscopy, the pubic louse has a short, oval body and prominent claws resembling sea crabs (see Fig. 2-5-9).[1-4] Bacterial cultures should be obtained if lesions appear secondarily infected. Patients should be questioned about risk factors for other sexually transmitted diseases.

Scabies

A healthy adult has 6 to 10 mites infesting the body.[1-4] Therefore, it may be difficult to find a mite on skin scraping. The best yield is from a burrow on the finger web spaces, volar aspect of the wrists, or penis. To identify a burrow, place a drop of blue or black ink on the skin. The burrow will absorb the ink and is highlighted as a dark line. The surface ink is removed with an alcohol pad. A drop of mineral oil is placed over a burrow, and the burrow is scraped with a no. 15 blade. The scraping is placed on a microscope slide with a drop of mineral oil on it. It is diagnostic if the mite, eggs, or fecal pellets (scybala) are seen.

Figure 2-5-5 (Plate 5). Nodular scabies. (*From Fitzpatrick, Johnson, Wolff, et al.*)

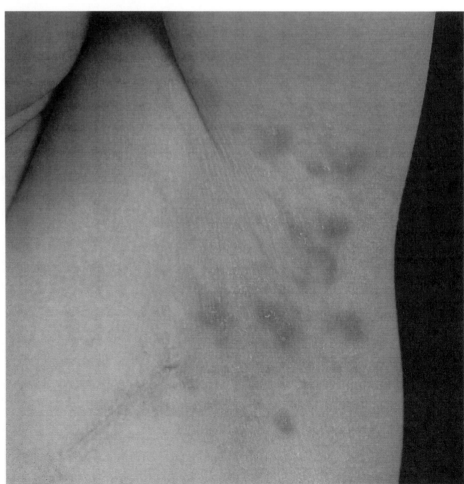

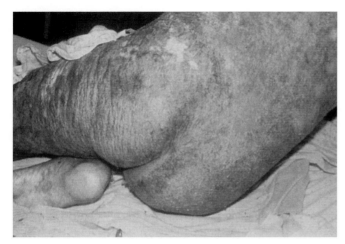

Figure 2-5-6 (Plate 6). Crusted scabies. (*From Fitzpatrick, Johnson, Wolff, et al.*)

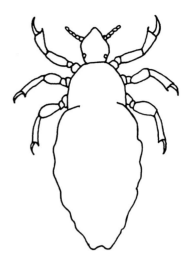

Figure 2-5-8. Body louse. (*Courtesy of Wendy Brunsman.*)

The female mite is 0.3 mm long with a flattened oval body and eight legs, and the eggs are ovoid brown capsules (see Fig. 2-5-10). Scybala are dark masses and are smaller than the eggs [see Fig. 2-5-11 (Plate 8)].

TREATMENT

A hot, soapy bath is contraindicated prior to application of any of these agents, since moisture increases the permeability of the epidermis and increases the chance for systemic absorption.[1–4] Sex partners and close personal or household contacts within the last month should be treated even if asymptomatic.

Pediculosis Capitis, Pediculosis Corporis, and Pediculosis Pubis

Permethrin 1% cream rinse (Nix) is applied to the affected areas and washed off after 10 min. It has less potential for toxicity in the event of inappropriate use. Pyrethrins with piperonyl butoxide are not completely ovicidal. Pyrethrins (RID, A-200, R&C) are applied to the affected areas and washed off after 10 min.

Lindane 1% shampoo, lotion, or cream (Kwell) is applied to the affected area and then thoroughly washed off after 4 min. Seizures and neurotoxicity in infants have occurred with improper

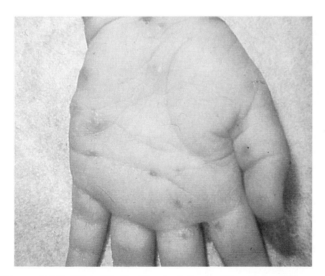

Figure 2-5-7 (Plate 7). Scabies in infants. (*Courtesy of Ramon Fusaro.*)

use of lindane.[1–4] Aplastic anemia has also been reported.[1–4] It is therefore not recommended for pregnant or lactating women, children under 2 years of age, or individuals with extensive dermatitis. Lindane is the least expensive therapy.

Pediculosis palpebrum should be treated by applying petrolatum or other occlusive ophthalmic ointment to the eyelashes bid for 8 to 10 days or tid for 5 days. Alternatives include physostigmine ophthalmic preparations applied bid for 1 to 2 days, baby shampoo applied with a cotton swab tid for 5 days, or fluorescein drops.

Once treatment is complete, the nits must be removed with tweezers or a fine-toothed nit comb. White vinegar on the hair for 15 min may loosen the nits and facilitate removal.

Because the incubation period of louse eggs is 6 to 10 days, the agents should be reapplied in 7 to 14 days.[1–4]

Secondary bacterial infections are generally caused by *Staphylococcus aureus* or group A beta-hemolytic *Streptococcus* and should be treated with appropriate doses of erythromycin, dicloxacillin, topical mupirocin, or other effective antibiotic.

Scabies

For all agents, infants and young children, should be treated on all body areas including the head and neck, and patients with relapse should also be treated head to toe. Reapply any agent to the hands, if hands are washed. The nails should be cut short and medication applied under them vigorously with a toothbrush.

Permethrin cream 5% (Elimite) has low toxicity. It is applied to all areas of the body from the chin down and is washed off after 8 to 14 h.

Lindane 1% lotion, cream, or shampoo is applied thinly to all areas of the body from the chin down and washed off thoroughly, adults after 12 h and infants after 8 h. Resistance to this agent

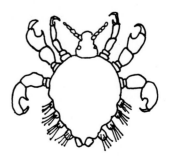

Figure 2-5-9. Pubic louse. (*Courtesy of Wendy Brunsman.*)

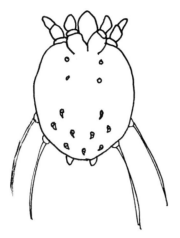

Figure 2-5-10. Scabies mite. (*Courtesy of Wendy Brunsman.*)

has been reported.[1-6] Infants should have lindane applied during the day and be fully clothed and observed to prevent licking of treated sites. If licking cannot be prevented, sulfur or permethrin should be used. With lindane a repeated application should be applied 1 week after first treatment.

Crotamiton cream 10% (Eurax lotion) is applied thinly to the entire body from the chin down nightly for two consecutive nights and is washed off 24 h after the second application. The toxicity of crotamiton is unknown.

Sulfur ointment, 6 to 10% in petrolatum or cold cream, is applied to the entire body from the chin down for 2 to 3 days. The patient bathes 24 h after each application. These preparations are messy, have an unpleasant odor, stain, and cause dryness. The safety of topical sulfur has never been tested.

The pruritus often persists up to several weeks after successful eradication of mite infestation because it is a hypersensitivity reaction to the mite antigens. The pruritus can be treated with antihistamines such as hydroxyzine (Atarax) or diphenhydramine (Benadryl), topical corticosteroid ointments, and in severe cases a tapered course of prednisone for 1 to 2 weeks.

Scabetic nodules may persist for up to a year. Intralesional triamcinolone, 5 to 10 mg/mL into each lesion, is effective.

In crusted scabies, a single application of a scabicide kills 90 to 95 percent of mites.[1,2,4] Multiple applications may be required and in the HIV-infected individual; eradication may be impossible. Ivermectin, 200 μg/kg PO one-time dose, is reported to be effective for crusted scabies in immunocompromised hosts.[1,2,4,7] The associated pruritus was rapidly controlled. Patients with thick, crusted lesions do better with a combination of ivermectin and topical treatment such as permethrin cream.[7]

Secondary infections should be treated with mupirocin ointment or appropriate systemic antimicrobial agents that cover *Staphyloccoccus* and group A *Streptococcus*.

PATIENT EDUCATION

Patients should avoid contact with possibly contaminated items such as hats, headsets, clothing, towels, combs, hairbrushes, bedding, and upholstery. Bedding, linen, clothing, and headgear should be washed and dried on the hot cycle or removed from body contact for 72 h. Combs and brushes should be soaked in rubbing alcohol or Lysol 2% solution for 1 h. The environment should be vacuumed. Otherwise, coats, furniture, rugs, floors, and walls do not need to be cleaned in any special manner.

FOLLOW-UP

Patients should be evaluated after 1 week if symptoms persist. Retreatment may be necessary if lice or nits are observed at the hair-skin junction or if mites and eggs are observed on repeat skin scraping. Patients not responding to one regimen should be retreated with an alternative.

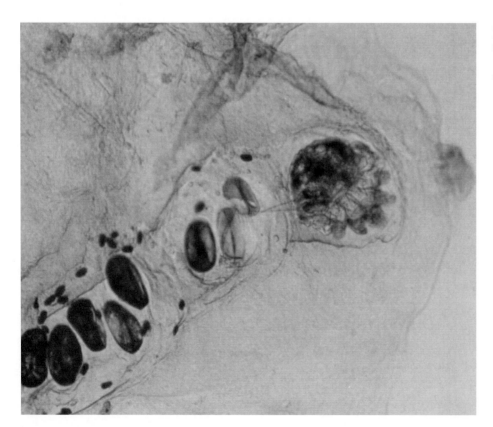

Figure 2-5-11 (Plate 8). Burrow with scabies mite, scybala, and feces. (*From Fitzpatrick, Johnson, Wolff, et al.*)

COMPLICATIONS AND RED FLAGS

Acute streptococcal glomerulonephritis has been reported to follow group A beta-hemolytic *Streptococcus* secondary infections of the skin.[1-4] Bacteremia and death have been reported following secondary *S. aureus* infection of crusted scabies in an HIV-infected individual.[1,4] Therefore, symptoms consistent with glomerulonephritis or bacteremia should be aggressively treated, especially in the presence of immunodeficiency.

REFERENCES

1. Fitzpatrick TB, Johnson RA, Wolff K, et al: *Color Atlas and Synopsis of Clinical Dermatology: Common and Serious Disease.* New York, McGraw-Hill, 1997, pp 836–849.
2. Habif TP: *Clinical Dermatology: A Color Guide to Diagnosis and Treatment,* 3d ed. St Louis, Mosby Year Book, 1996, pp 445–456.
3. Arnold HL, Odom RB, James WD: *Andrew's Diseases of the Skin: Clinical Dermatology,* 8th ed. Philadelphia, Saunders, 1990, pp 512–515, 523–527.
4. Wilson DC, Leyva WH, Kin LE Jr: Arthropod bites and stings, in Fitzpatrick TB, Eisen AZ, Wolff K, et al (eds): *Dermatology in General Medicine,* 4th ed. New York, McGraw-Hill, 1993, pp 2810–2826.
5. Purvis RS, Tyring SK: An outbreak of lindane-resistant scabies treated successfully with permethrin 5% cream. *J Am Acad Dermatol* 25:1015–1016, 1991.
6. Judd LE: Gamma benzene hexachloride resistant scabies. *N Z Med J* 106:61–63, 1993.
7. Meinking TL: The treatment of scabies with ivermectin. *New Engl J Med* 333:26–30, 1995.

Chapter 2–6
ATOPIC DERMATITIS (ATOPIC ECZEMA)
Joe R. Monroe

DEFINITION

Atopic dermatitis is a pruritic inflammation of the dermis and epidermis, frequently in association with a personal or family history of hay fever, asthma, allergic rhinitis, or atopic dermatitis.

CLINICAL DISCUSSION

Atopic dermatitis (AD) is an IgE-mediated papulosquamous process with typical onset in the first 2 months of life, or by the end of the first year in 60 percent of patients, with a highly variable course after that. Sometimes persisting into adulthood, occasionally (fewer than 10 percent) beginning in adulthood, the sine qua non of AD is pruritus, fueling an itch-scratch-itch cycle, and

manifesting as a symmetric papulosquamous patchy rash in flexural locations in adults (antecubital, popliteal, and neck, among others). In contrast, infantile AD tends to be more papulovesicular, and affects facial and extensor skin as well as locations involved in adult AD. Itching in AD is triggered by contact with wool, detergents, soaps, sweating, and stress, but primarily by the act of scratching itself.

Associated clinical findings include xerosis, ichthyosis, vulgaris, pigmentary changes (hypo- and/or hyperpigmentation), eye changes (cataracts, keratoconus), periorbital skin changes (scaling of lid skin, allergic shiners), and hand and foot dermatitis. Complications include increased colonization of affected skin with *Staphylococcus aureus,* which can trigger attacks; increased susceptibility to viral infections of the skin such as warts, molluscum, and herpes; increased susceptibility to fungal infections, especially in hands and feet; generalized exfoliative erythroderma; mental or emotional dysfunction; and growth retardation.

Among complications of AD, especially feared is the development of disseminated herpes (or rarely, vaccinia) infection of AD-involved skin, called eczema herpeticum or Kaposi's varicelliform eruption, which can occur even in patients whose AD is in remission. The virus colonizes eczematous and noneczematous skin, which leads to a widespread eruption of discrete, tense vesicles surrounded by erythema. The patient may therefore be extremely ill and will likely require parenteral acyclovir. Atopic patients should therefore be advised to avoid individuals with an active herpes simplex infection.

DIFFERENTIAL DIAGNOSIS

In infants, seborrheic dermatitis (SD) can resemble AD, but differs significantly in that:

- AD itches, SD is nonpruritic.
- AD is chronic, whereas SD lasts approximately 6 weeks.
- With AD, there is usually a definite family history of atopy, whereas in SD there is none.
- SD involves axillae and diaper area, areas seldom involved in AD.

Other common conditions mimicking AD include contact dermatitis and scabies. Certain rare metabolic disorders can also mimic AD and should be considered. These include gluten enteropathy, acrodermatitis enteropathica, glucagonoma syndrome, and phenylketonuria.

LABORATORY

Biopsy can be helpful in ruling out other conditions, but is not pathognomonic for AD. Serum levels of IgE are often elevated, but not consistently enough to be helpful. Culture for herpes simplex virus (HSV) where indicated.

TREATMENT

The goals of treatment of AD are (1) to hydrate the skin, (2) to identify and eliminate triggers, (3) to decrease pruritus and inflammation, and (4) to educate patients and families about the nature of AD.

For children especially, worsening of AD can be related to stress, so education of parents and patients is crucial. For example, they must understand that no treatment course, however carefully devised, can be effective if the problems of xerosis (dry skin) and scratching are not addressed.

To that end, hydration of the skin is a key element, especially after bathing, while the skin is still moist, using white petrolatum, or products such as Eucerin cream or 12% ammonium lactate lotion (Lac Hydrin), but avoiding common hand lotions, especially those with artificial scent or color. The use of alkaline soaps in bathing should be kept to a minimum because of their drying effects.

AD patients are susceptible to all skin infections, but especially to *S. aureus,* which can colonize or even mildly infect involved skin, producing minimal indications of overt infection, but providing a powerful pruritic trigger. In fact, often the only sign is either a flare of AD or unresponsiveness to the usual AD treatments. A short course of oral antibiotic (erythromycin, dicloxacillin, or cephalosporin) and/or topical application of antibacterial ointment (mupirocin, bacitracin, or Polysporin) can make a dramatic difference.

Other triggers for AD flares include exposure to irritants such as sweat, to environmental irritants, especially on the job (solvents, cleansers, etc.), or to true allergens (airborne or food). Even though AD is not caused by a specific allergen, ongoing exposure to dust mites or seasonal allergens, for example, can be key factors and need to be identified and eliminated if possible.

Topical steroid use in AD has revolutionized its treatment, but there are potential problems with these drugs. Dermal atrophy and striae formation are caused either by prolonged application, and/or by failure to match the concentration of the steroid preparation to the area being treated. The latter is particularly true of thin-skinned areas such as faces (especially lids), and genitals, but also applies to intertriginous skin, that is, skin being rubbed or covered by adjacent skin, such as in the axillae, groin, and intergluteal area. Systemic steroids are seldom indicated in AD because: (1) they can be used for only brief periods (1 to 3 weeks); (2) potential side effects, especially in children, are numerous and potentially severe; (3) withdrawal of the patient from oral corticosteroids can result in dramatic rebound of AD. If the disease is unresponsive to routine therapy, referral to a dermatologist should be seriously considered.

Tar preparations were the mainstay of treatment for AD before the introduction of topical steroids in 1952, and even though tar's mode of action isn't known, it is a potent anti-inflammatory, steroid-sparing topical agent. Commercial preparations such as Estar Gel and PsoriGel are available by presciption or a pharmacist can compound a wide variety of tar-plus-ointment combinations.

The dermatologist to whom a physician assistant may refer more difficult patients has a wide variety of treatment modalities to choose from, including phototherapy, interferon gamma, cyclosporine, and thymopentin, among others, but referral has other values: (1) seeing a dermatologist can be very reassuring to patients and their families; (2) as the primary care provider, a physician assistant can learn more about the management of AD from the dermatologist after following up on the referral; (3) the correct diagnosis can be confirmed or other diagnoses in the differential can be considered, since the diagnosis of AD is not always straightforward, sometimes requiring extraordinary expertise.

PATIENT EDUCATION

The following items can contribute to positive patient outcome:

1. Encourage parents and siblings to discuss any anxiety or feelings of aggression about having a child with AD.
2. Educate parents about increased anxiety in the affected child and how it can manifest itself through increased scratching which will, of course, worsen the disease.
3. Tell parents and siblings that frequent affectionate touching of atopic infants and young children will not only *not* hurt the child, but will help to alleviate anxiety for both the parents and the child.
4. Teach the parents that AD is a chronic, recurring condition that requires daily attention with lubricating lotions; avoidance of wool products, lanolin-containing creams, and other triggers; and adherence to treatment schedules with steroids, tar preparations, and others, with instructions given in writing.
5. Educate as to the necessity for antibiotic therapy with flares or failure to respond to the usual treatments.
6. Explain how and why AD patients should not be exposed to the herpes simplex virus because of the risk of eczema herpeticum.

PROGNOSIS

Spontaneous resolution of AD frequently occurs during childhood, but with occasional, more severe recurrences during adolescence. In most patients, the disease lasts for 15 to 20 years.

BIBLIOGRAPHY

Arndt KA, Robinson JK, LeBoit PE, et al: *Cutaneous Medicine and Surgery.* Philadelphia, Saunders, 1996.
duVivier A: *Dermatology in Practice.* Philadelphia, Lippincott, 1990.
Fitzpatrick TB, Johnson RA, Polano MK, et al: *Color Atlas and Synopsis of Clinical Dermatology: Common and Serious Diseases,* 3d ed. New York, McGraw-Hill, 1997.
Goldstein BG, Goldstein AO: *Practical Dermatology,* Primary Care Series. St Louis, Mosby Year Book, 1992.
Shelley WB, Shelley ED: *Advanced Dermatologic Diagnosis.* Philadelphia, Saunders, 1992.
Weinberg S, Prose NS, Kristal L: *Color Atlas of Pediatric Dermatology,* 3d ed. New York, McGraw-Hill, 1998.

Chapter 2–7
BASAL CELL CARCINOMA
Barbara L. Sauls

DESCRIPTION

Basal cell carcinoma (BCC) is the most common type of skin cancer and arises from the epidermal basal cells. These lesions are slow growing, rarely metastasize, and are relatively easily treated. The incidence of this cancer has risen over the years, particularly in the increasing aged population. Men have a higher incidence of basal cell carcinoma than women, though the difference is decreasing. Risk factors include light-skinned persons, anyone with poor tanning capacity, previous x-ray therapy (such as for acne or cancer), occupations that require extensive exposure to the sun such as road workers and farmers, and increasing age. The most frequently affected skin areas are those exposed to the sun. Brown or black skin is protective.

SIGNS AND SYMPTOMS

The classic presentation of basal cell carcinoma is as a *nonhealing papule, asymptomatic nodule,* or *ulcer.* BCCs can present less often in other forms, such as a scarlike lesion or flat scaly patches,

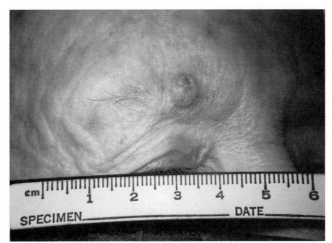

Figure 2-7-1 (Plate 9). Classic presentation of nodular basal cell carcinoma. Note the small area of ulceration in the upper part of the lesion. (*Courtesy of Harold Milstein, MD, The Dermatology Clinic, Hazleton, PA.*)

often misdiagnosed as fungal infection, and even as a deeply pigmented, brown-to-black papule [see Fig. 2-7-1 (Plate 9)].

OBJECTIVE FINDINGS

Physical examination reveals an isolated, elevated, firm, papular or nodular area which often has a central depression. Lesions are round or oval with borders that are described as rolled in appearance. The lesion often looks "pearly" and may be black, red, or pink. Ulcerated lesions may develop, which often have a crusting over them and also have an elevated border. These are referred to as *rodent ulcers*. Close inspection may reveal telangiectasias over the surface of the BCC, which is often a useful diagnostic feature [see Fig. 2-7-2 (Plate 10)].

DIAGNOSTIC CONSIDERATIONS

Nonulcerated nodular lesions look like dermal nevi or cysts, but feel firmer.

LABORATORY TESTS

The diagnosis of basal cell carcinoma is made by shave or punch biopsy, or excision.

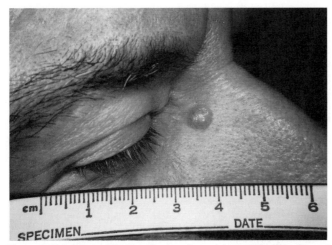

Figure 2-7-2 (Plate 10). Small telangiectasias on left side of basal cell carcinoma. (*Courtesy of Harold Milstein, MD, The Dermatology Clinic, Hazleton, PA.*)

TREATMENT

Eradication of basal cell carcinoma is best produced by surgical excision. Alternative therapies include cryotherapy, laser, radiation therapy, or electrodesiccation. Topical chemotherapy may be used as well as intralesional interferon. The cure rate is high unless the lesions have been neglected and have deeply eroded. Excision in this case often produces a poor cosmetic result.

PATIENT EDUCATION

Patients must be counseled on the use of sunscreens and wide-brimmed hats, covering arms and legs when outside, avoidance of the sun from 10 A.M. until 2 P.M., and avoidance of tanning salons.

DISPOSITION

Routine skin examination by a medical practitioner should be done on a regular basis, paying special attention to the face, ears, and neck. This examination should be performed every 6 months to 1 year for 5 years after a diagnosis of basal cell carcinoma. Patients should be instructed to report any nonhealing or new lesions. These should be examined and possibly biopsied as soon as they are noted.

CONSIDERATIONS

Skin cancers are best treated by dermatologists. The initial biopsy may be done in the family practice office, but it is also appropriate to send the patient to the dermatologist for this initial biopsy. An excisional biopsy can be performed on this initial visit.

BIBLIOGRAPHY

Fauci AS, Braunwald E, Isselbacher KJ, et al (eds): *Harrison's Principles of Internal Medicine,* 14th ed. New York, McGraw-Hill, 1998.
Fitzpatrick TB, Johnson RA, Wolff K, et al: *Color Atlas and Synopsis of Clinical Dermatology: Common and Serious Diseases,* 3d ed. New York, McGraw-Hill, 1997.

Chapter 2–8
BULLOUS BLISTERING DISEASES
Joe R. Monroe

DEFINITION

Bullae are blisters (vesicles) larger than 0.5 cm, most often the result of benign processes such as thermal burns, insect bites, contact dermatitis, impetigo, or part of more serious diseases such as lupus erythematosus or dermatitis herpetiformis. Unfortunately, they can also be one of the first signs of a rather serious group of blistering diseases, which includes some that are potentially fatal, such as pemphigus vulgaris, or bullous pemphigoid.

CLINICAL DISCUSSION

The appearance of bullae is cause for real concern, and should prompt an adequate and timely assessment. Unless that cause is obvious, one key element of such an assessment should be a *punch biopsy* preserved in special fixative (consult the pathology department) for immunofluorescent (IF) studies. Key clinical features of individual diseases are discussed below.

DIFFERENTIAL DIAGNOSES

See discussion and miscellaneous conditions presenting with bullae below.

LABORATORY

Immunofluorescent studies elucidate the precise histologic level at which abnormal antibodies are deposited, separation takes place, and blister formation occurs, and are definitive for each disease entity. They greatly complement the history and physical examination, the latter including Nikolsky's sign, which is said to be positive when the blister margin can be extended by digital pressure. A positive Nikolsky's indicates a shallow level of separation, suggesting a variant of pemphigus, characterized clinically by flaccid, thin-walled bullae, whereas a negative test is consistent with bullous pemphigoid, a less serious disease marked by thick-walled, tense bullae, the roofs of which are composed of the entire epidermis.

TREATMENT

Treatment consists of systemic steroids, often with the addition of azathioprine, usually on long tapering doses (3 months or more) for pemphigus and bullous pemphigoid.

KEY CLINICAL FEATURES OF SELECTED BULLOUS DISEASES

Pemphigus vulgaris has the following features:

- It begins during the fourth or fifth decade.
- Flaccid, easily broken bullae often present with painful erosions.
- Initial areas of involvement often include mucous membranes in mouth and genitals, then face, trunk, and flexures.
- Positive Nikolsky's sign is exhibited.
- It may present as hoarseness.

Bullous pemphigoid has the following features:

- Involvement of elderly patients
- Usually very itchy
- Tense blisters, with surrounding erythema
- Symmetric involvement of limbs and trunk
- Negative Nikolsky's sign

Dermatitis herpetiformis has the following features:

- Symmetric, grouped, excoriated papulovesicular rash
- Involving knees, elbows, buttocks
- Often associated with gluten enteropathy
- Alleviated by gluten-free diet and/or dapsone

Epidermolysis bullosa (*EB*) has the following features:

- 27 different types
- All genodermatoses
- Most common type EB simplex, also known as Weber-Cockayne syndrome, characterized by early onset, no extracutaneous involvement, blistering and hyperhidrosis of palms and soles, and autosomal dominant transmission

Erythema Multiforme's features are listed in Chap. 2-12.

Toxic Epidermal Necrolysis (TEN, Lyell's syndrome) has the following features:

- Cutaneous and mucosal exfoliation, beginning with blisters
- Usually in response to drugs (penicillin, sulfa, etc.), also to infectious agents, but possibly idiopathic

- Potentially life-threatening
- Treated like a burn

Staphylococcal Scalded-Skin Syndrome has the following features:

- Toxin-mediated epidermolytic disease
- Mainly in newborns and infants
- Spectrum of disease ranges from localized bullous impetigo to generalized epidermal sloughing
- Caused by *Staphylococcus aureus* phage group II, type 71
- Treated like a burn

Porphyria Cutanea Tarda has the following features:

- Adults (age 30 to 50) present with complaint of "fragile skin" (bullae) especially on the dorsa of hands
- Major triggers: ethanol and sun
- Periorbital hypertrichosis
- Orange-red fluorescence of urine (plus uroporphyrin)

Pediatric diseases that can present with bullae include varicella, urticaria pigmentosa, and chronic bullous disease of childhood (rare).

Miscellaneous conditions that can present with Bullae include burns (thermal or chemical), contact dermatitis, drug reactions (fixed drug eruptions and others), insect bites (fleas, mosquitoes), lichen planus, lupus erythematosus, and pityriasis rosea.

PEARLS

Knowledge of the following points can contribute to a positive patient outcome:

- The appearance of bullous disease, especially in the very old or very young, should suggest possible referral to a dermatologist.
- Punch biopsies, submitted in special fixative (*not* the usual formalin), can be crucial in the workup of bullous disease.
- Pemphigus can present with hoarseness (eroded laryngeal bullae) as the sole symptom.
- The symmetric distribution of a pruritic papulovesicular/bullous rash on elbows, knees, and buttocks should suggest dermatitis herpetiformis.
- Porphyria cutanea tarda is often induced by alcohol.
- Many common, relatively benign dermatoses (e.g., lichen planus, erythema multiforme, pityriasis rosea) have bullous variants.

PROGNOSIS

Both pemphigus and bullous pemphigoid were quite lethal prior to the advent of steroids in 1952, with death rates of almost 75 percent. The clinical course was inexorably downward, having complications similar to those in burn patients, with fluid loss, overwhelming sepsis, and renal failure ultimately leading to death. Since 1952, the death rate has fallen to about 10 percent, but these disorders are still considered quite serious.

BIBLIOGRAPHY

Arndt KA, Robinson JK, LeBoit PE, et al. *Cutaneous Medicine and Surgery.* Philadelphia, Saunders, 1996.

duVivier A: *Dermatology in Practice.* Philadelphia, Lippincott, 1990.

Fitzpatrick TB, Johnson RA, Wolff K, et al: *Color Atlas and Synopsis of Clinical Dermatology: Common and Serious Diseases,* 3d ed. New York, McGraw-Hill, 1997.

Goldstein BG, Goldstein AO: *Practical Dermatology,* Primary Care Series. St Louis, Mosby Year Book, 1992.

Shelley WB, Shelley ED: *Advanced Dermatologic Diagnosis.* Philadelphia, Saunders, 1992.

Weinberg S, Prose NS, Kristal L: *Color Atlas of Pediatric Dermatology* 3d ed. New York, McGraw-Hill, 1998.

Chapter 2–9
CELLULITIS (INCLUDING ERYSIPELAS)
Joe R. Monroe

DISCUSSION

Cellulitis is an acute infection of the skin and subcutaneous tissue, not involving muscle, most often caused by group A beta-hemolytic streptococci or *Staphylococcus aureus.* True erysipelas denotes cellulitis involving only the face and involves more superficial levels of skin than cellulitis.

Cellulitis can involve any area of skin, but especially those that have been traumatized or which are lymphedematous, particularly legs. A classic presentation of cellulitis is that of the dorsal forefoot starting from a tiny interdigital fissure, itself resulting from tinea pedis. Other risk factors include hematologic malignancies, IV drug use, diabetes mellitus, or immunocompromise. Cellulitis can rapidly produce significant symptomatology with localized tenderness and erythema, as well as fever, chills, and malaise. Recurrences are common in areas of chronic lymphedema such as postmastectomy surgical sites.

Cellulitis is characterized by sharply demarcated, slightly elevated plaques with fiery red-to-bluish purple coloration. Lymphangitic streaking is fairly common, as is tender regional adenopathy.

Other organisms can cause variants of cellulitis, *Haemophilus influenzae* being one of the more common ones seen on the faces of children, as in periorbital cellulitis. Many other examples are seen in severely immunocompromised patients such as cellulitis of cryptococcal origin.

Fortunately, most cases of cellulitis lend themselves well to clinical diagnosis. Exceptions to this would include immunocompromised patients; so-called erysipeloid cellulitis of the hand or fingers, an indolent process typically seen as an occupational condition in those handling fish, poultry, or meat; and necrotizing fasciitis, a rapidly evolving aggressive, centrally necrotic cellulitic process, involving superficial fascia and subcutaneous tissue caused by a rather wide variety of potential pathogens.

DIFFERENTIAL DIAGNOSIS

Contact dermatitis, herpes zoster, stasis dermatitis, deep vein thrombophlebitis, gout, and other diseases can mimic cellulitis.

LABORATORY

Culture (needle aspirate, blister, blood) is only occasionally helpful. Peripheral white count and sedimentation rate may be elevated. Biopsy is only rarely indicated.

TREATMENT

If the organism is not known, treatment should cover both *Streptococcus* and *Staphylococcus,* for example, dicloxacillin, 0.5 to 1.0 g every 6 h PO, or erythromycin, 5 mg every 6 h PO. Predisposing conditions, such as lymphedema or tinea pedis need to be addressed.

PATIENT EDUCATION

Educate patients about the necessity to follow directions for antibiotics and other treatment.

PEARLS

Knowledge of the following points can contribute to a positive patient outcome:

- On feet, think of tinea pedis as a predisposing factor to cellulitis.
- Clearly demarcated, fiery red edematous plaques of skin are clearly suspicious for cellulitis.
- Sequelae of undiagnosed or mistreated cellulitis include hematogenous dissemination of infection, especially to abnormal heart valves.
- Cellulitis can present with sudden onset of fever, chills, vomiting, and confusion, symptoms far worse than the skin findings would suggest.

PROGNOSIS

Dramatic response to antibiotics is typical with staphylococcal and streptococcal infections. In cases where attacks are recurrent (e.g., postmastectomy sites), the patient may have to be placed on prophylactic antibiotics. Lack of response to common antibiotics should prompt a more thorough history (immunocompromised? occupational?) and possible punch or incisional biopsy sent for hematoxylin and eosin (H & E) as well as bacterial, fungal, and acid-fast cultures.

BIBLIOGRAPHY

Arndt KA, Robinson JK, LeBoit PE, et al: *Cutaneous Medicine and Surgery.* Philadelphia, Saunders, 1996.
duVivier A: *Dermatology in Practice.* Philadelphia, Lippincott, 1990.
Fitzpatrick TB, Johnson RA, Wolff K, et al: *Color Atlas and Synopsis of Clinical Dermatology: Common and Serious Diseases,* 3d ed. New York, McGraw-Hill, 1997.
Goldstein BG, Goldstein AO: *Practical Dermatology,* Primary Care Series. St Louis, Mosby Year Book, 1992.
Shelley WB, Shelley ED: *Advanced Dermatologic Diagnosis.* Philadelphia, Saunders, 1992.
Weinberg S, Prose NS, Kristol L: *The Color Atlas of Pediatric Dermatology,* 3d ed. New York, McGraw-Hill, 1998.

Chapter 2–10
COMMON PODIATRIC DISORDERS
Sandra J. Martin

Hyperkeratoses
DISCUSSION

Hyperkeratoses are areas of thickened epidermis that occur as a protective mechanism or reaction of the skin to repeated mechanical and shearing stress. The etiology can be friction from the ground when walking, which creates calluses on the bottom or side of the foot, or from shoes or adjacent toes as the skin is trapped over or between bony prominences. Long-term, chronic hyperkeratoses can cause permanent changes in skin architecture.

The most common plantar hyperkeratoses are caused from friction during weight bearing. They may be diffuse or more concentrated beneath specific pressure points such as metatarsal heads. These become symptomatic when they themselves either become thick enough to cause symptoms or become fissured down to deeper, more sensitive epidermis closer to the dermis.

Diffuse hyperkeratoses on the plantar surface are commonly located beneath the metatarsal heads and around the heel. The calluses around the heel and on the plantar-medial aspect of the first metatarsal head frequently become so thick they fissure and can bleed. They are usually seen in patients who wear open sandals or go barefoot.

TREATMENT

Common plantar hyperkeratoses may be debrided by the clinician, or patients may be taught self-care. Patients can use an emery board or sandpaper to debride a dry, hard callus or a pumice type of stone to debride softened calluses. They should initially debride a little each day until the area has been adequately thinned. Then, they should maintain the area by debriding once or twice a week as needed.

Dry or mildly hyperkeratotic, cracking plantar skin can be softened by placing petrolatum on the area, covering it with plastic wrap and a sock, and leaving this on all night. During the day, emollient creams may be used to maintain hydration of the skin. Lotions and creams containing a large amount of alcohol will dehydrate the skin and should be avoided.

NUCLEATED HYPERKERATOSES

Some hyperkeratoses are nucleated and appear to have firm, hard, tender centers. These may be a diagnostic challenge. When considering the differential diagnosis, it is necessary to consider the location of the lesion, the appearance of the lesion, and the movements that create pain.

Callus with discrete nucleated areas exhibits the following characteristics:

- Usually located in weight-bearing surfaces
- Skin lines through the lesion
- Tenderness with direct pressure
- No pinpoint bleeding with debridement

Plantar verruca (wart) has the following characteristics:

- May be in weight-bearing or non-weight-bearing areas
- Skin lines around the lesion
- Tender to lateral compression
- Pinpoint bleeding at the base with debridement

Foreign body may exhibit the following characteristics:

- Any location on plantar surface
- Skin lines through the lesion
- Frequently a single small puncture
- Tender with direct pressure more than lateral compression

TREATMENT

Nucleated hyperkeratotic lesions may be sharply debrided with a no. 15 blade. Debridement should be gradual, keeping the blade almost parallel to the surface of the skin. Avoid digging out the center, since this can result in cutting the patient. As the lesion is gently debrided parallel to the surface, the central area also becomes thinner. Appropriate padding with an aperture around the area can significantly retard the recurrence of the lesion. Any insole can be used. The area directly under the lesion should be cut out. Padding directly beneath the lesion will cause it to become more painful. The foot can be marked with lipstick or any marking device that will transfer to the insole with pressure. Then, the patient should put the marked foot in a shoe in which the insole

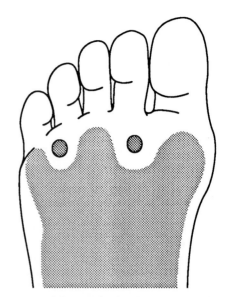

Figure 2-10-1. Padding around calluses or tender metatarsal heads.

has been placed. This delineates where the pressure points hit the insole so that area can be cut out (see Fig. 2-10-1).

Plantar Warts
DISCUSSION

Like other warts, warts on the foot are caused by a virus that invades the skin. The most common is the human papillomavirus, often found on the plantar aspect of the foot. *Verruca plantaris* are plantar warts, and they are often covered with hyperkeratotic tissue, thereby raising them above the surrounding surface. They invade only the epidermis, which is very thick on the plantar aspect of the foot and makes the warts difficult to treat. Warts may present clinically as either singular lesions or multiple (mosaic) verrucae that coalesce with satellite lesions at the periphery. When debriding the hyperkeratotic covering of a plantar verruca, pinpoint bleeding that represents disruption of the small capillaries within the papilla is frequently seen.

TREATMENT

Plantar verrucae are difficult to treat because of the involved thicker epidermis. The lesions do not breach the dermis. Topical keratolytic acids may be used most successfully on solitary lesions, and care should be taken to protect the surrounding healthy tissue from the acid. Debride the hyperkeratotic tissue, then cautiously apply the acid to the lesion. It should be placed under occlusion with adhesive tape for 24 h. Caution patients that they may feel a burning sensation. Debridement and retreatment every few weeks should be continued until the lesion has resolved.

Avoid the use of liquid nitrogen on the plantar aspect of the foot because it does not penetrate to the deeper level of the epidermis and it creates a painful blister that will make walking difficult.

Surgical excision of a verruca that is well demarcated and resistant to topical acids affords the best chance for resolution of the lesion. This involves incision and curettement of the lesion as follows:

1. Use a local anesthetic block with local infiltration or regional block usually with 1% lidocaine plain then infiltrate immediately beneath the lesion with a small amount of 1% lidocaine with epinephrine for hemostasis.

2. Using a no. 15 blade, incise the circumference of the lesion 1 to 2 mm beyond the visual border of the wart and skive it so the wound is wider at the surface. The incision should be down to only the level of the dermal-epidermal junction.
3. Curette the lesion off the dermis. The lesion will shell out, leaving a glistening white dermis intact.
4. Cauterize the base of the lesion with 89% phenol, other chemocautery, or fulguration.
5. Dressing with antibiotic cream such as silver sulfadiazine should be applied. Be aware that this area may bleed liberally when the foot is put in a dependent position.
6. Have the patient remove the dressing in 12 to 24 h and soak in plain warm water for 30 min twice a day. The area should heal without scarring if the dermis has not been violated. Healing time depends on the size and location of the lesion.

Plantar Foreign Bodies

Foreign bodies of all different materials may be found embedded in the plantar aspect of the foot. If they go beneath the epidermis, they can be very painful and become infected. They frequently present with no known history of the patient stepping on something. Diagnosis of a foreign body may be difficult because conventional film x-ray will show only radiopaque objects. Foreign bodies may present like a hyperkeratotic lesion at the site of entry. The area will be tender to direct pressure. Other signs are variable.

Practitioners should not get caught up in a "search and destroy" mission for something they are unsure of even being present. If gentle debridement of the overlying hyperkeratosis does not yield a foreign body, it would be best to refer the patient for further evaluation and treatment.

Corns

Corns are of two general types: *soft* corns (heloma molle) and *hard* corns (heloma durum). The soft corns are present between toes at the base of the digits in an area that is usually moist, thereby creating a macerated hyperkeratotic lesion. They occur from pressure on the skin by adjacent underlying bones. The most common sites for heloma molle are between the fourth and fifth toes or the third and fourth toes when hammertoes are present in such a way as to create underlapping toes.

The best treatment is to separate the toes with some type of interdigital pad, especially when shoes are worn, and use antifungal powder sparingly before stockings are put on. This combination removes the pressure and allows the area to dry out. Acid pads should be avoided because they can create further irritation and encourage infection.

Heloma dura are found on the tops, ends, or sides of toes and are hard because of the lack of moisture such as that seen in the interdigital spaces (see Fig. 2-10-2). They form over pressure points of bony prominences that are present because of either an altered position of the toes (hammertoe, mallet toe, claw toe) or hypertrophy of the bone. Conservative treatment consists of debridement of the hyperkeratosis and appropriate padding or change in shoe gear to alleviate pressure on the area. If this fails to relieve the symptoms, the patient may require referral for surgical intervention.

Ingrown Toenails (Onychocryptosis)
DISCUSSION

Toenails become ingrown most frequently at the distal, lateral, or medial edges. Onychocryptosis on the distal edge of a toenail

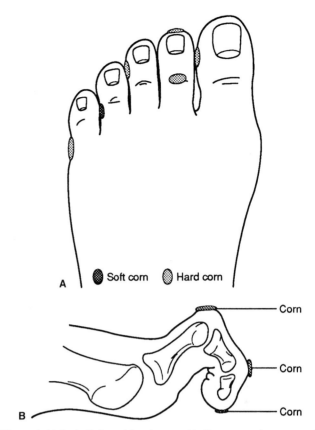

Figure 2-10-2. *A*. Soft and hard corns. *B*. Corns over bony prominences on a mallet toe.

is usually the result of a nail that has previously been removed or lost regrowing into the distal soft tissue. Without the pressure on the nail bed, the distal nail bed becomes bulbous and the new nail must gradually press it down and flatten it out so that the nail can grow over it. Frequently the nail becomes embedded in the distal, bulbous soft tissue. This requires frequent debriding of the nail and pushing the soft tissue down so the nail can grow over it.

Treatment in the office consists of using a very small tissue nipper to debride the distal edge of the nail. Then, the patient should be encouraged to use a cuticle stick to push the skin away from the distal nail edge daily after bathing until the nail makes it over the top of the nail bed.

When the medial or lateral edges of a toenail become ingrown, the cause is usually improper trimming of the nail or pressure on the border from a tight shoe or adjacent toe. Sometimes, there is excessive (hypertrophic) soft tissue in the nail groove secondary to repeated irritation of the area by an ingrown or vertically growing nail border. A less common cause of an incurvated nail is a subungual exostosis that grows up from the distal tuft of the distal phalanx. Therefore, a nail can be simply ingrown, have a hypertrophic ungualabia, or be incurvated. The nail may be ingrown and asymptomatic, ingrown and tender, or ingrown and infected (paronychia).

The simple tender ingrown border that is secondary to improper cutting leaves a small spicule at the edge that will grow distally into the soft tissue and become symptomatic. Figure 2-10-3 illustrates this condition. The spicule acts like a foreign body causing local inflammation, infection, and granuloma.

The initial treatment of an ingrown nail border, infected or not, is to trim the nail border, thereby removing the offending foreign body. This should be trimmed so as not to leave a new spicule proximally. It is not necessary to remove more than the

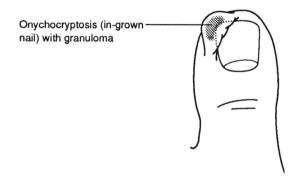

Onychocryptosis (in-grown nail) with granuloma

Figure 2-10-3. Onychocryptosis with granuloma.

distal offending edge as the initial conservative treatment. The patient should be encouraged to soak in warm water a few times a day until the symptoms have resolved.

If the symptoms do not resolve or they return, permanent removal of the offending border is recommended. There is continued controversy regarding the appropriateness of doing a permanent procedure when a paronychia exists. There is always the chance of causing proximal extension of a localized infection when a matrixectomy is performed. It is this author's choice to resolve any gross infection prior to performing chemical matrixectomy. Simply trimming the offending border and placing the patient on soaks twice a day will frequently resolve most of the localized infection. Oral antibiotics may also be used depending on the severity of the infection and the general medical condition of the patient.

Some things to be aware of before performing a permanent removal of a nail border are the following:

1. Chronic paronychia may extend into an osteomyelitis in an immune-compromised patient such as a diabetic. In these patients, it is prudent to take x-rays of the toe to rule out possible bony involvement.
2. Check the vascular status of the patient prior to any minor surgical procedure. Patients who have peripheral vascular disease will experience slow healing and may even progress to more serious ischemic consequences.
3. Patient compliance in the postoperative period is essential to an uneventful postoperative course and a good result. Discuss this with the patient prior to performing any procedure.

The literature describes many different procedures with different approaches and techniques to treat paronychia. One that is technically simple, requires only a few special instruments, and has a favorable success rate is described here. There are many variations of the following procedure. Care should be taken not to remove so much nail that the patient is left with only a small central spicule, to remove as much of the matrix as possible, to not burn surrounding tissues with the phenol, and to provide a mechanism by which the area can drain (see Fig. 2-10-4).

TREATMENT

Phenol and alcohol partial matrixectomy has become the most widely used procedure to permanently remove all or part of a toenail. The procedure is simple, provides for good cosmetic result, has less postoperative discomfort than other procedures, and has a relatively low recurrence rate. The phenol provides antisepsis, and many clinicians perform it when infection is present. If there is a hypertrophied ungualabia, the excessive tissue

can be removed with a tissue nipper and cauterized with the phenol during the procedure.

The following instruments are used:

- 1 Penrose drain, 1/4 in
- 2 straight hemostats
- 1 English anvil nail splitter
- 1 no. 61 miniblade and minihandle
- 1 curette, 2.0 mm
- 1 periosteal elevator or spatula/packer
- 1 tissue nipper

The following supplies are needed:

- Gauze: 2 × 2 and 4 × 4
- Phenol, 89% liquefied
- Cotton-tipped applicators with half the cotton removed or toothpicks with a small amount of cotton on the end
- Nu Gauze 1/4-in plain packing strips
- Silver sulfadiazine or other antibiotic cream (avoid ointments)
- Coban, 3 in

The procedure includes the following steps:

1. Use a local anesthetic block at base of the toe with approximately 3 mL (cc) 1% lidocaine plain (do not use epinephrine).
2. Apply Penrose drain around the base of the toe to obtain hemostasis. Secure this with a hemostat, and use a 2 × 2 between the drain and the skin to protect the skin. Make sure the patient does not have a medical condition that contraindicates the tourniquet.
3. Using the English anvil nail splitter, split the nail (Fig. 2-10-5) longitudinally just where it begins to become incurvated. Split the nail back to the cuticle.
4. Using the no. 61 miniblade, continue the longitudinal split in the nail beneath the cuticle until the tissue is felt to give, which should signify the proximal edge of the nail and matrix.
5. Undermine the portion of the nail to be removed with a packer or periosteal elevator.
6. Grasp the portion of the nail to be removed with a hemostat from distal to beneath the cuticle. Push proximally to loosen the nail border; then roll the hemostat with the border in it toward the center of the nail.
7. Use a curette and tissue nipper to remove any remaining nail matrix (pearly white tissue), granuloma, or fibrous tissue in the nail groove.
8. Apply the phenol. Using the cotton-tipped applicators or toothpicks, dip one in the phenol then blot it to remove excess acid. Apply to the matrix area beneath the cuticle and to the nail bed for 30 sec. Repeat this for a total of three applications.
9. Flush the area with alcohol and remove the tourniquet. Place the silver sulfadiazine or antibiotic cream into the nail groove and loosely pack it with the 1/4-in packing so that the edge of the packing is free. Apply dressing of 2 × 2 and Coban.
10. Prescribe otic solution of neomycin, polymyxin B sulfates, and hydrocortisone or other antibiotic solution.

Postoperative instructions are as follows:

1. A clear, yellowish exudate will drain from the operative area for up to a few weeks. Explain this to the patient.
2. Patient to remove the dressing that evening and soak the toe in warm water for 30 min, leaving the packing in place. Pat the toe dry and apply a few drops of the cortisporin otic

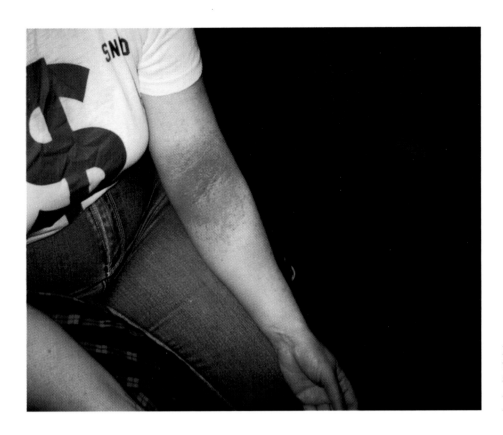

Plate 1 (Figure 2-1-2). Acute contact dermatitis of the antecubital area. *(Courtesy of Harold Milstein, MD, The Dermatology Clinic, Hazleton, PA.)*

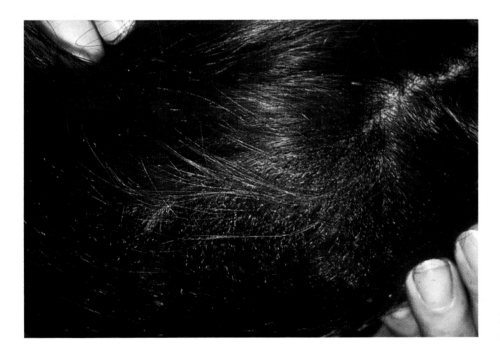

Plate 2 (Figure 2-5-1). Nits. *(From Fitzpatrick, Johnson, Wolff, et al.)*

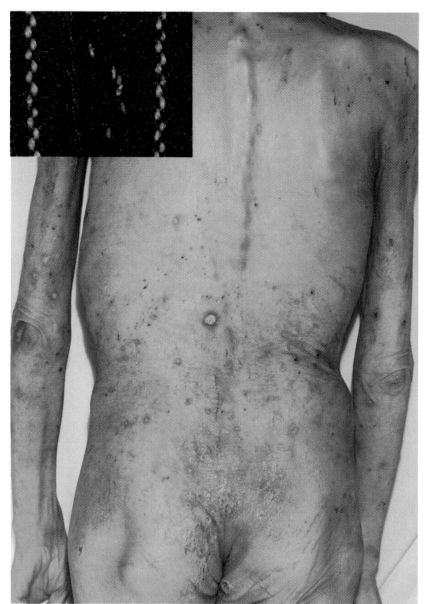

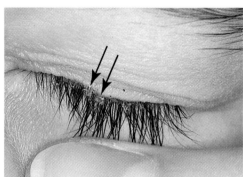

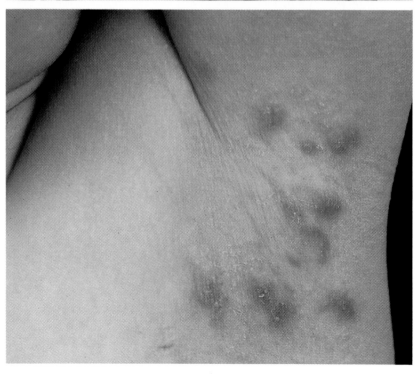

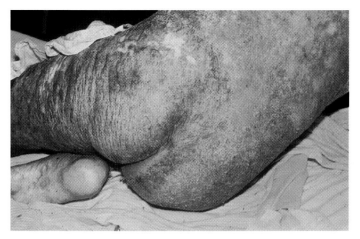

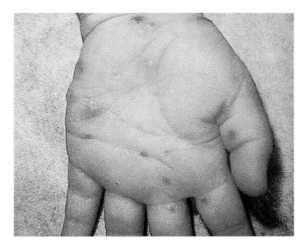

Plate 6 (Figure 2-5-6). Crusted scabies. *(From Fitzpatrick, Johnson, Wolff, et al.)*

Plate 7 (Figure 2-5-7). Scabies in infants. *(Courtesy of Ramon Fusaro.)*

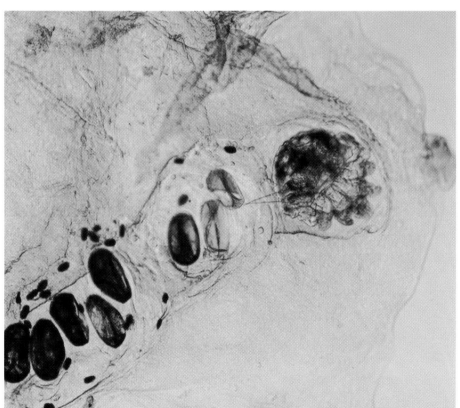

Plate 8 (Figure 2-5-11). Burrow with scabies mite, scybala, and feces. *(From Fitzpatrick, Johnson, Wolff, et al.)*

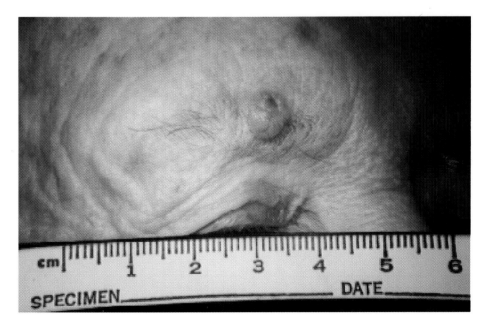

Plate 9 (Figure 2-7-1). Classic presentation of nodular basal cell carcinoma. Note the small area of ulceration in the upper part of the lesion. *(Courtesy of Harold Milstein, MD, The Dermatology Clinic, Hazleton, PA.)*

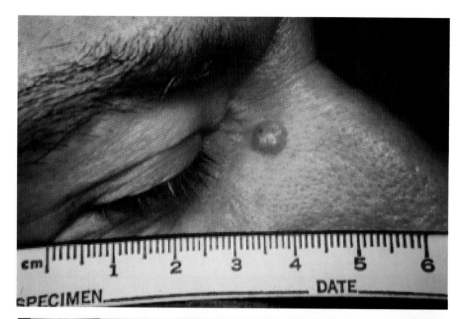

Plate 10 (Figure 2-7-2). Small telangiectasias on left side of basal cell carcinoma. *(Courtesy of Harold Milstein, MD, The Dermatology Clinic, Hazleton, PA.)*

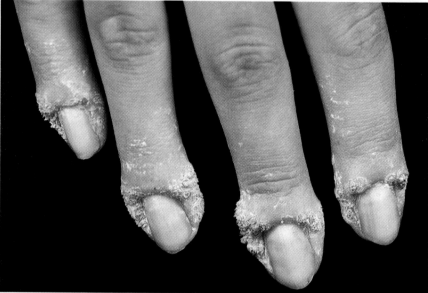

Plate 11 (Figure 2-18-1). Verruca vulgaris. *(From Fitzpatrick, Johnson, Wolff, et al.)*

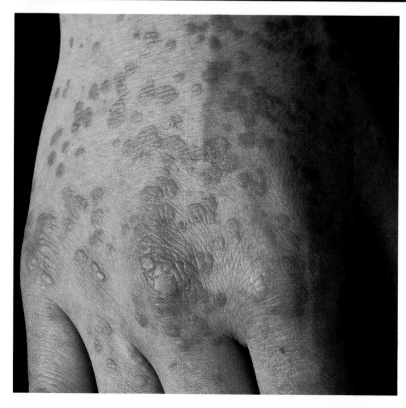

Plate 12 (Figure 2-18-2). *Verruca plana. (From Fitzpatrick, Johnson, Wolff, et al.)*

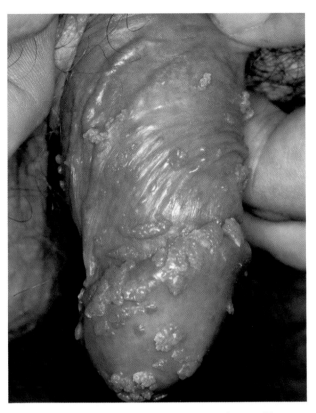

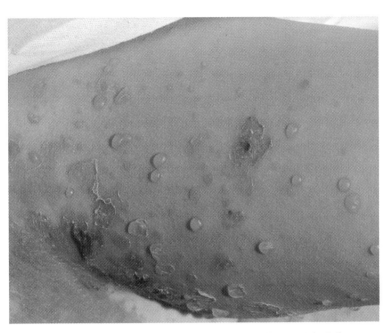

Plate 13 (Figure 2-18-3). Condyloma acuminata. *(From Fitzpatrick, Johnson, Wolff, et al.)*

Plate 14 (Figure 2-19-1). Bullous impetigo. *(From Fitzpatrick, Johnson, Wolff, et al.)*

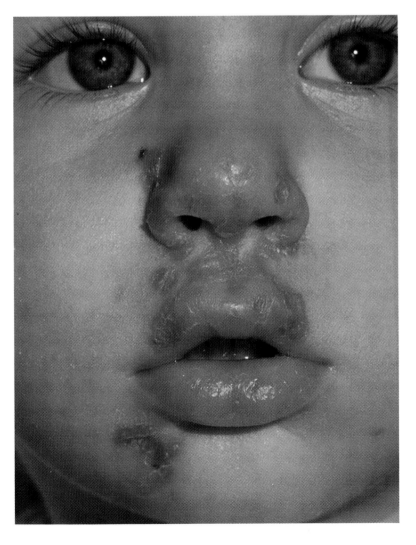

Plate 15 (Figure 2-19-2). Nonbullous impetigo. *(From Fitzpatrick, Johnson, Wolff, et al.)*

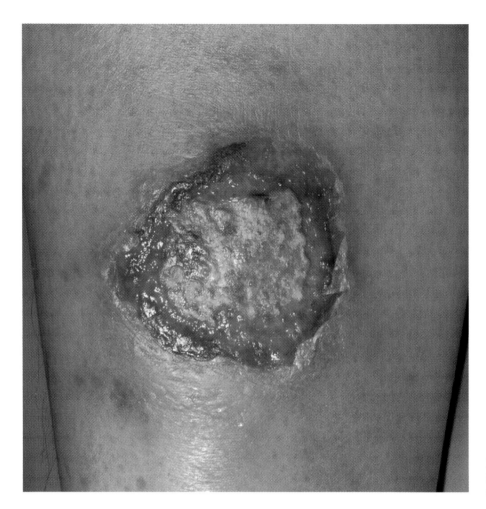

Plate 16 (Figure 2-19-3). Ecthyma. *(From Fitzpatrick, Johnson, Wolff, et al.)*

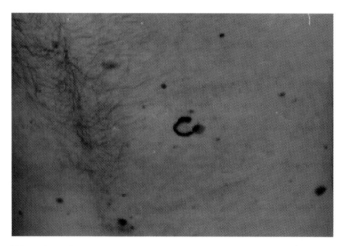

Plate 17 (Figure 2-21-1). A C-shaped malignant melanoma of the abdomen. *(Courtesy of Harold Milstein, MD, The Dermatology Clinic, Hazleton, PA.)*

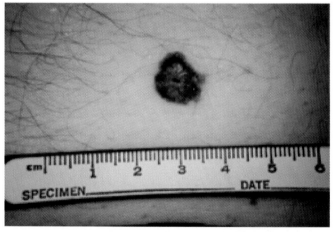

Plate 18 (Figure 2-21-2). A nodular malignant melanoma of the abdomen. *(Courtesy of Harold Milstein, MD, The Dermatology Clinic, Hazleton, PA.)*

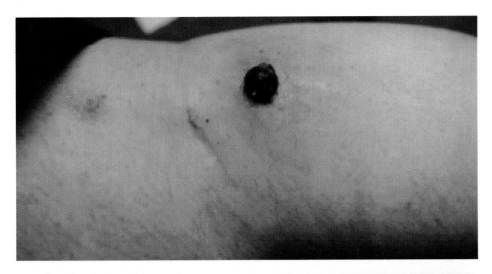

Plate 19 (Figure 2-21-3). Malignant melanoma of the leg. *(Courtesy of Harold Milstein, MD, The Dermatology Clinic, Hazleton, PA.)*

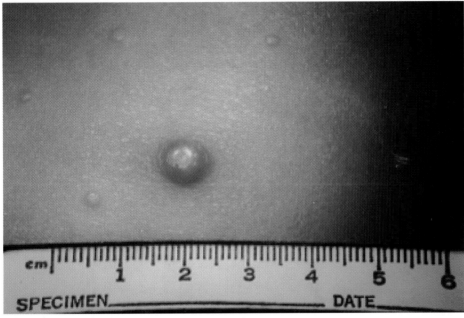

Plate 20 (Figure 2-22-1). Several small molluscum lesions with one giant lesion on the chest. Note the central umbilication and the irritation associated with the larger lesion. In this case, it is appropriate to remove the lesions because of the irritation. *(Courtesy of Harold Milstein, MD, The Dermatology Clinic, Hazleton, PA.)*

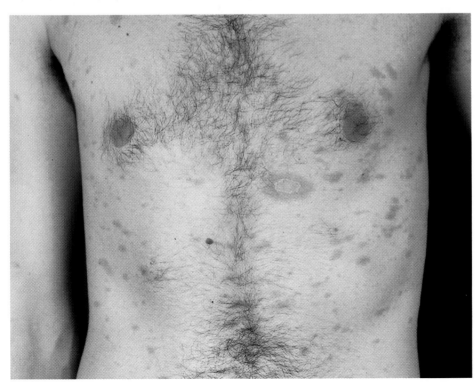

Plate 21 (Figure 2-23-1). Pityriasis rosea. *(From Fitzpatrick, Johnson, Wolff, et al.)*

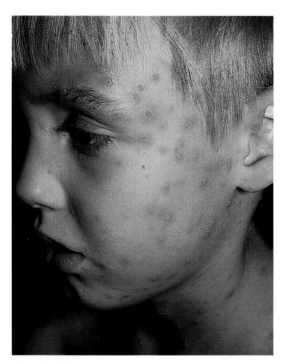

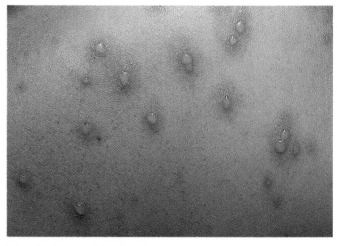

Plate 23 (Figure 9-26-2). Close-up of vesicles showing the characteristic "dewdrop on a rose petal" appearance. *(Photo courtesy of Rodney L. Moser. Used with Permission.)*

Plate 22 (Figure 9-26-1). Pediatric varicella with multiple vesicles and crusting. *(Photo courtesy of Rodney L. Moser. Used with Permission.)*

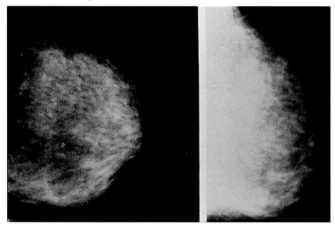

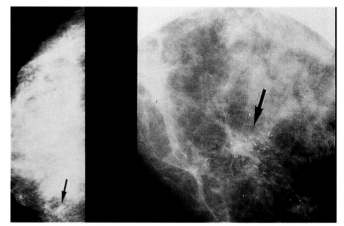

Plate 24 (Figure 12-12-1). Quality assurance for mammography is critical. These images are of the same breast. The image on the left shows a breast that is not properly compressed. It could have mistakenly been read as a dense, glandular breast with no abnormally visualized. The image on the right shows the same breast with proper compression. It is much easier to find a white density indicative of cancer on the right image than on the left image. *(From the American Medical Women's Association for the Breast and Cancer Education Project for Primary Care Providers, under a cooperative agreement with the Centers for Disease Control and Prevention.)*

Plate 25 (Figure 12-12-2). The left side contains a density indicated by the black arrow. The cone compression view on the right reveals a finding even more ominous than the original film, illustrating how useful cone compression mammography can be. This finding represented carcinoma. *(From the American Medical Women's Association for the Breast and Cancer Education Project for Primary Care Providers, under a cooperative agreement with the Centers for Disease Control and Prevention.)*

Plate 26 (Figure 12-12-3). On the left side, the radiologist has noted some white specks. These represent microcalcifications in the breast. Imaging this with a magnification view as shown on the right helps identify the sizes and shapes of the calcifications. These are highly suggestive of carcinoma because they are pleomorphic, that is, of different sizes and shapes. In general, cone compression mammography is used to evalute densities further, and magnification views are done to identify and discern calcifications. *(From the American Medical Women's Association for the Breast and Cancer Education Project for Primary Care Providers, under a cooperative agreement with the Centers for Disease Control and Prevention.)*

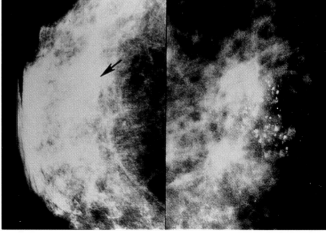

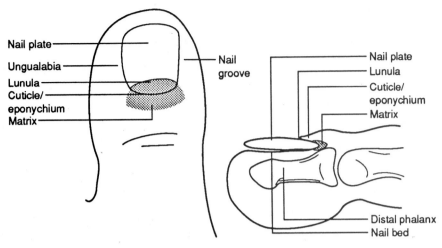

Figure 2-10-4. Nail anatomy.

solution to the area. Redress with *loose* bandage. Letting air into the area is important to aid healing. Therefore, an occlusive dressing should be avoided.

3. Continue soaking and treating as in step 2, twice a day. The packing may be removed after 24 h. After the packing is removed, the patient should begin to debride the area gently with a soft toothbrush or cotton-tipped applicator to tolerance. It is important to keep the nail groove clear of crusted exudate.

4. Soaking, debridement, and medication should continue until there is no more drainage.

The clinician should follow the patient a few days after the procedure, then every few weeks until the area is completely healed. When the nail groove is full of necrotic tissue or crusted exudate, gently debride the area with a curette.

The above phenol and alcohol procedure can also be used for a total matrixectomy. Keep in mind that more phenol should be used, and it may take up to 6 weeks for complete healing.

Subungual Hematoma

Trauma to a nail can cause bleeding of the nail bed beneath the nail. The accumulation of blood in a closed area creates pressure and considerable pain. If the injury is recent and the blood beneath the nail is still liquid, placing a few holes in the nail will release the fluid and alleviate most of the discomfort. If the nail has been broken, it should be removed in total to allow the nail bed to heal. Simple soaks in warm water will provide comfort to the patient and aid healing of the nail bed.

If the trauma has been severe, an x-ray of the toe should be obtained to rule out fracture. If the nail bed is lacerated, depending on the extent of the laceration, it can be sutured or steri-stripped. Counsel the patient that the new nail may have some deformity, depending on the damage to the nail bed and matrix.

Onychomycosis
DISCUSSION

Onychomycosis is an infection of the nail bed and nail by mycotic (fungal) organisms, and may affect more than 20 percent of the adult population. Yeast and bacterial infections can mimic mycotic infections. The pathophysiology is more complicated than commonly thought and usually begins with some type of trauma or disease process that affects the nail bed. This results in compromise of the area's resistance to colonization by microorganisms.

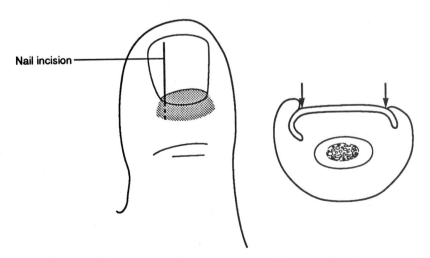

Figure 2-10-5. Area of nail to cut when performing matrixectomy.

A fungal infection of the nail frequently begins as a simple distal subungual onychomycosis in the nail grooves or beneath the nail's distal edge. The infection can then spread proximally involving more and more of the nail bed and, subsequently, the nail. The result may be as severe as complete involvement of the nail plate with discoloration, crumbling, lifting of the nail plate and the accumulation of a lot of malodorous subungual debris.

TREATMENT

Treatment has been a controversial subject for many years. This author believes that minimal nail involvement in the immune-competent patient should be treated either with cosmetic methods or topical treatments. Cosmetically the nail can be improved greatly with filing with an emery-type of file to both thin and shorten the nail plate. Even the most severely involved mycotic nail can be managed by filing it to keep it under control.

However, some patients dislike the appearance of the mycotic nail so much that they insist on treatment. They are willing to take systemic medications or even have the nail permanently removed. However, they may not like the cosmetic result of permanent nail removal, and it is quite tedious to permanently remove multiple mycotic nails.

If only a small distal portion or a portion of one of the sides is involved, some topical medications may control the infection, although cure should not be anticipated. Liquid antifungals designed specifically for nails, such as Mycocide NS or Fungoid Tincture, used as directed, may accomplish significant clearing of the nail plate. However, fungal infections of the nails are usually resistant to topical treatment, and when the medication is discontinued, the onychomycosis will usually recur.

The most effective treatment for onychomycosis with the best possible chance for cure and a resultant normal nail is one of the new oral antifungal agents. As of this writing, there are two, itraconazole (Sporanox), approved by the FDA in October 1995, and terbinafine (Lamisil), approved in May 1996, that have shown significant cure rates for onychomycosis. Fluconazole (Diflucan) is under consideration for approval by the FDA for the treatment of onychomycosis. These new oral antifungals have different side-effect profiles, drug interactions, and dosing schedules. Pretreatment liver function studies should be considered before using these medications. Pulse dosing has been used effectively with all these medications, and patient compliance has been excellent during clinical trials. The effectiveness of treatment is usually first seen in clearing of the new, proximal nail. It may take a few months after the medication has been finished for complete clearing.

These oral antifungals are indicated for the treatment of onychomycosis of the toenail or fingernail due to dermatophytes. A positive culture of the nail should be obtained prior to initiating treatment with these medications. Proper culture technique is important and should be performed by taking the specimen proximal to the distal edge of the infected nail. It is essential that the nail clippings not come from the distal edge but rather be taken from a portion of nail on top of the nail bed and, if possible, some of the subungual debris for submission to the laboratory. Obtaining nail clippings of at least 3 mm will increase the chance for a positive culture. Do not submit specimens if the patient is currently undergoing antifungal therapy because this will often result in a negative culture. If the first culture is negative, a repeat culture is recommended, based on clinical impression.

BIBLIOGRAPHY

Odom RB: New therapies for onychomycosis: *J Am Acad Dermatol* 35:S26–S30, 1996.

Chapter 2–11
DECUBITUS ULCERS
Freddi Segal-Gidan

DISCUSSION

Decubitus ulcers (pressure sores) are the result of prolonged pressure on an area of skin resulting in underlying tissue damage and loss of skin integrity. They usually occur over bony prominences; most commonly the hip, sacrum, lateral malleolus, and heel. With proper patient education pressure sores can usually, but not always, be prevented. The elderly, paralyzed, and those with diabetes, peripheral vascular disease, or peripheral sensory neuropathy are the most likely to develop pressure sores.

PATHOGENESIS

Pressure, shear, and friction are the three primary underlying forces that influence pressure ulcer formation.[1] The presence of moisture increases the deleterious effects of these forces. When external pressure exceeds that of the venous system, total tissue pressure increases. This then causes increased capillary pressure, which results in transudation of fluid from the capillaries, producing tissue edema and autolysis of cells. Pressure also occludes lymphatic drainage, which allows toxic by-products of anaerobic metabolism to accumulate. The duration of pressure is a critical factor; the higher the pressure, the less time is required to cause tissue damage.

Shearing forces are the result of sliding of adjacent surfaces. Such forces are created between body surfaces and that of a bed or chair. They produce stretching and angulation of blood vessels in the subcutaneous tissues, thus causing thrombosis and undermining of the dermis.

Frictional force is the primary factor leading to superficial skin breakdown. Moisture increases the friction between surfaces, thus exacerbating skin breakdown.

SYMPTOMS

Presentation is most typically with a painless open sore over an area of bony prominence or pressure. Detection requires a high index of suspicion for occurrence and frequent, regular complete skin examinations. Those predisposed to pressure sore development must be taught preventive techniques before skin breakdown ever occurs (Table 2-11-1). Prevention of pressure ulcers requires assessment of the individual's overall physical health, medication use, nutritional status, functional problems, psychosocial factors, and pain. Medical conditions that affect peripheral circulation (diabetes, peripheral vascular disease), impair mobility (hip or other lower-extremity fracture, hemiplegia, paraplegia, or quadriplegia), or perception (dementia, neuralgia) increase the probability for pressure ulcer development. Poor nutrition, especially low protein and serum albumin, predisposes to ulcer development and impairs healing. Medications that affect cogni-

Table 2-11-1. Predisposing Conditions for Pressure Ulcer Development

Paraplegia
Quadriplegia
Diabetes mellitus
Peripheral vascular disease
Peripheral neuropathy (sensory)
Immobility

Table 2-11-2. Clinical Staging of Pressure Ulcers

Stage	Description
I	Nonblanchable erythema of intact skin
II	Partial thickness skin loss involving epidermis and dermis
	Presents as abrasion, blister, or shallow ulceration
III	Full thickness skin loss
	Damage or necrosis of subcutaneous tissue
	May extend down, but not through, fascia
IV	Full thickness skin loss with extensive destruction
	Damage through fascia, often involving muscle and/or bone
	Undermining and sinus tracts common

tion and voluntary movements (sedatives) or pain perception (narcotics) may contribute to pressure sores, whereas others (i.e., steroids) impair healing. Knowledge about a patient's level of independent function, and concomitant need for assistance, may point to the need to incorporate others into any prevention or treatment program. Pressure ulcer formation and healing is also influenced by mental status; substance abuse; individual goals, values and life-style; and available resources such as caregivers, money, and equipment.

OBJECTIVE FINDINGS

A complete skin examination, with particular attention to areas prone to skin breakdown, should be routinely performed on all those prone to pressure sore development. This requires the routine removal of socks and shoes, and for wheelchair-bound individuals visual inspection of the sacrum and buttocks. Bed-bound patients in the hospital or nursing home should have skin checks daily.

When a pressure sore is present, note its location and size, including the length, width, and depth. The National Pressure Ulcer Advisory Panel[2] has developed criteria to assess ulcers based on the level of tissue damage (Table 2-11-2). Note the presence of any exudate or necrotic tissue. Examine the surrounding skin for erythema, maceration, and induration. Look for presence of granulation and epithelization. The ulcer should be gently palpated and the edges probed for undermining and/or sinus tract formation. Check the peripheral circulation, noting the presence or absence of pulses and capillary refill, since these will impact on healing.

DIAGNOSTIC CONSIDERATIONS

The differential diagnosis of skin ulcers lies primarily at determining the underlying etiology or predisposing factors.

SPECIAL CONSIDERATIONS

Pressure ulcer formation is much more common in the elderly and among residents of acute- and long-term care settings. Skin changes that accompany aging account for the susceptibility of the elderly to pressure ulcer development. Nearly two-thirds of all pressure ulcers occur in individuals over age 70, and most occur within a few weeks of an acute illness.

LABORATORY TESTS

Laboratory testing is essential for identifying etiologic conditions as well as factors that influence wound healing. Routine blood work, including complete blood cell count (CBC) with differential, erythrocyte sedimentation rate (ESR), serum electrolytes, creatinine, glucose, calcium, protein, and albumin should be performed. Serum glucose is essential for identification of undiagnosed diabetes. In the diabetic a serum hemoglobin A_{1c} provides indirect information about glucose control during the past 3

months. Serum protein and albumin levels are key indicators of current nutritional status.

Blood cultures are important to ascertain for the presence of sepsis. Tissue biopsy or needle aspiration should be performed when an infected ulcer is suspected. Surface swab cultures are inaccurate, may not reveal the true pathogens, and do not differentiate between infecting organisms and commensals.

RADIOLOGIC STUDIES

Routine radiographs are not warranted. If bone is exposed or the pressure ulcer is present for more than a month, suspect underlying osteomyelitis. A radiographic study of the underlying bony skeleton is warranted; this may show lytic lesions, reactive bone formation, and periosteal elevation associated with osteomyelitis.[3] Radionuclide scanning is sensitive, particularly in new lesion development, but has limited usefulness for following the clinical response to the therapy over time. CT scanning is useful for documenting the extent of underlying soft tissue injury.

TREATMENT

Optimal management of pressure ulcers involves prevention, early recognition, and aggressive treatment.[4]

Wound Care

Early pressure ulcer development, stage I or II, is best treated with local measures and pain relief (see below) to avoid further ulcer progression.

Debridement of necrotic tissue is essential for ulcer healing (Table 2-11-3). It may be done mechanically or by instrumentation. Wet-to-dry dressings are the most common form of mechanical debridement. Wound irrigation and hydrotherapy are also forms of mechanical debridement. Sharp debridement involves the use of scalpel, scissors, or other sharp instruments. This is the most rapid form of debridement and is required when there are signs of advancing cellulitis or sepsis. Extensive ulcers require surgical debridement, which may be done at the bedside, but more often require an operating room because of the need for better management of associated pain and bleeding.

Enzymatic debridement uses a topical agent to dissolve necrotic tissue. Agents must be applied according to each manufacturer's instructions. The process may be used alone to break down eschar, after sharp debridement, or in association with mechanical debridement. This is most appropriate when the patient is not a candidate for surgical debridement, such as in a long-term-care resident or homebound patient.

Synthetic dressings allow for autolytic debridement. The wound is covered, and devitalized tissues self-digest from enzymes normally present in the wound fluid. This is a slow and lengthy process that is most appropriate for individuals who cannot tolerate other debridement methods. Autolytic debridement is contraindicated when pressure ulcers are infected.

Optimal healing requires that all necrotic tissue, exudate, and waste be removed from the ulcer. Once the ulcer has been de-

Table 2-11-3. Debridement of Pressure Ulcers

Type	Technique
Sharp	Use of scalpel, scissors, or other sharp instrument
	Often requires operating room and surgeon
Mechanical	Wet-to-dry dressings
	Wound irrigation
	Dextranomers
Enzymatic	Collagenase Santyl Ointment
Autolytic	Wound Dress
	DuoDerm

brided, routine cleansing after each dressing change is necessary to decrease the risk of infection. As with all wounds, pressure ulcers should be cleansed gently and thoroughly. Normal saline is the preferred cleansing agent for most ulcers. Skin cleansers or antiseptics, such as peroxide or povidone iodine, should never be used since these are toxic to healing tissues. The ulcer should be irrigated with enough pressure to be effective (about 4 to 15 lb/in^2) without causing tissue trauma. Use of a large-capacity syringe (>25 mL) with a 17- to 19-gauge angiocatheter is very effective for wound irrigation. Whirlpool cleansings should be considered for pressure ulcers that contain thick exudate, slough, or necrotic tissue and discontinued when the ulcer is considered clean.

Dressings are used to keep the ulcer tissue moist to promote healing and to keep the surrounding skin intact and dry. Dressings do not have to be sterile, but must be clean.

Moist saline or occlusive dressings are optimal for stage I to III ulcers. In stage III or IV ulcers with cavity formation, the cavity needs to be gently filled with moist packing to wick away drainage. Avoid overpacking, which may cause additional damage due to pressure on the wound surface.

Dressings should be monitored regularly and changed at least daily, or more frequently, if necessary, because of drainage or soiling. Those near the anus are especially difficult to keep intact and clean. "Picture framing" the edges of a dressing may help to secure it.

Electrical stimulation is the only adjunctive therapy currently recommended. It involves the application of surface electrodes to the wound site. It may be employed for stage III and IV pressure ulcers that have been unresponsive to conventional therapy or recalcitrant stage II pressure ulcers.

Other adjunctive therapies that have been tried but currently lack sufficient evidence to recommend include hyperbaric oxygen; infrared, ultraviolet, and low-energy laser irradiation; and ultrasound.

Surgical Treatment

Surgical intervention is often required for stage III and IV pressure sores to remove necrotic tissue and scar tissue that may delay healing. Resection of bony prominences that may contribute to recurrent ulceration may also be required. In the operating room surgical closure of the ulcer through a myocutaneous flap or skin homograph may be accomplished. Limb amputation may be required when the ulcer is too large to cover with rotational flats or in the presence of extensive osteomyelitis or severe joint contractures.

Pharmacologic Management

Medication use in the treatment of pressure ulcers should be aimed at pain control and any underlying conditions. Nonsedating analgesics used on a regular, rather than as-needed, basis should be used if pain is an ongoing factor. Chronic pain that is unresponsive to analgesics often responds to an antidepressant such as nortriptyline. Proper treatment of diabetes with either oral hypoglycemic agents or insulin is essential to aid healing. Peripheral circulation may improve with the use of pentoxifylline (Trental). Systemic antimicrobial therapy is required if complications of sepsis or osteomyelitis are suspected.

Supportive Measures

Positioning is the key to prevention of pressure ulcer formation. First, avoid pressure on any existing ulcer; second, reduce pressure on other bony prominences or other areas at risk for pressure ulcer development. Bed-bound and immobile individuals must be turned often, every 2 h, to avoid continuous pressure on any one area. The head of the bed should always be at the lowest elevation consistent with other medical conditions. Avoid positioning immobile individuals on their trochanters, and use devices to relieve pressure on the heels. Foam pads or wedges and pillows should be used to prevent direct contact between an ulcer and the support surface, and between areas at risk for breakdown, particularly bony prominences, and the support surface. Never use rigid doughnut-type ring cushions because these may cause pressure ulcers, not prevent them. When a pressure ulcer is on a sitting surface, avoid the sitting position; place patients on their side or prone.

Proper support surfaces are also essential to preventing pressure ulcer formation and promoting healing of already formed ulcers. Selection should be based primarily on the therapeutic benefit of the product, but the clinical condition of the individual, characteristics of the care setting, and cost must also be considered. The goal is to provide a support surface that provides airflow to dry the skin. Simple mattress overlays include simple foam overlays or water flotation mattresses. These must be monitored for bottoming out. If less than 1 in. of support material remains under the affected ulcer or other bony prominence, the overlay should be replaced. More complex bed support surfaces include alternating-air mattress, low-air-loss bed or an air-fluidized bed. These are indicated primarily for large stage III and IV pressure ulcers on multiple sites.

Surface support is also required for sitting, especially for nonambulatory patients. Wheelchair cushions should be properly fitted to the chair and person. Again, doughnuts should never be used.

Paraplegics and other wheelchair-bound individuals should be taught pressure-relief maneuvers that they can perform regularly to prevent continued pressure on any one surface. Individuals who cannot perform their own pressure-relief maneuvers need to have caregivers properly instructed in these techniques so they are done without producing harm to either the patient or caregiver.

Patient Education

Prevention is the key to pressure sore management. Patients, their families, and caregivers must be engaged both to prevent their development and to promote proper healing. Individuals at risk for pressure sore development should be identified and provided ongoing education about proper skin care, positioning, and overall health. The role of proper nutrition and hygiene to maintain circulatory and skin integrity should be emphasized and assessed routinely by the practitioner. If an ulcer develops, individuals should be educated to contact their provider immediately. Individuals who are able should be instructed in techniques of proper wound care and be active participants in daily dressing changes. Usually, however, it is family or caregivers who must be educated about signs of pressure ulcer development and wound care techniques for the active pressure sore.

Complications and Red Flags

Pressure ulcers that increase in size or fail to heal in the presence of an active wound care program should be referred for surgical evaluation. Surgical debridement is often needlessly delayed and usually required to treat stage III and IV ulcers and sepsis.

Pearls

The time invested in early identification of individuals at risk for pressure ulcer development and education of them and their families is both good medicine and cost-effective. The actual education can be provided by nursing staff either in the office or hospital setting. Videotapes that a patient or family can view and then discuss with the provider or a knowledgeable staff member are a very effective way to teach both prevention (pressure-release maneuvers, transfer techniques, skin assessment) and wound care (irrigation, dressing changes).

REFERENCES

1. Kertesz D, Chow AW: Infected pressure and diabetic ulcers. *Clin Geriatr Med* 8(4):835–852, 1992.
2. National Pressure Ulcer Advisory Panel: Pressure ulcers prevalence, cost, risk assessment: Consensus development conference statement. *Decubitus* 2:24, 1989.
3. Thornhill-Joyness M, Gonzales G, Stewart CA, et al: Osteomyelitis associated with pressure ulcers. *Arch Phys Med Rehab* 67:314, 1986.
4. US Department of Health and Human Services, Agency for Health Care Policy and Research: Treatment of pressure ulcers. Clinical Practice Guidelines, no 15, 1994.

BIBLIOGRAPHY

Linder RM, Morris D: The surgical management of pressure ulcers; A systemic approach based on staging. *Decubitus* 3:32–54, 1990.
Mackelbust A, Sieggreen M: Pressure ulcers: Guidelines for prevention and nursing management. West Dundee, IL, S-N Publications, 1991.
US Department of Health and Human Services, Agency for Health Care Policy and Research: Pressure ulcers in adults: Prediction and prevention. Clinical Practice Guidelines, no 3, 1994.

Chapter 2–12
ERYTHEMA MULTIFORME
Joe R. Monroe

DEFINITION

Erythema multiforme (EM) is a relatively common self-limited inflammatory process of acute onset, often recurrent, manifesting initially as distinctive target-shaped papules, with characteristic histopathology.

CLINICAL DISCUSSION

Most commonly found on the extremities, especially the dorsa of the hands, palms, soles, knees, and dorsal feet, but also on the penis (50 percent) and vulva, EM lesions are frequently tender and can involve mucous membranes as well.

The morphology of EM lesions is somewhat variable, as the name (multiforme) suggests, but the typical picture is striking, and thus readily identifiable. The sudden appearance of iris or target lesions is the hallmark, being a round papule displaying concentric rings of different colors, with darker centers tending to vesiculate (blister), ranging from 1 to 3 cm in size, and distributed symmetrically in characteristic areas (see above).

Atypical lesions frequently resemble hives (urticaria), but, unlike the latter, remain in one location for days.

EM is considered to be a hypersensitivity reaction pattern of an immune response to a variety of potential agents, the best documented of which are recurrent herpes simplex virus (HSV) infection, *Mycoplasma pneumoniae* infection, and drugs. Among the latter, the major offenders include the sulfonamides, anticonvulsant medications (phenytoin and barbiturates), penicillins, allopurinol, and NSAIDs. Lesional HSV antigen can frequently

be demonstrated by polymerase chain reaction, and intradermal injection of HSV antigen has reproduced the condition, facts which some take as proof that most EM, especially the recurrent form, is caused by hypersensitivity to HSV antigen. To proponents of this concept, the other reported triggers for EM, sunlight, infection, foods, and progesterone, do so only because they are well known to trigger overt or clinically inapparent HSV attacks.

EM is traditionally described in two forms, which probably represent opposite extremes of a continuum. EM minor, characterized by the lack of bulla, mucosal lesions, or systemic symptoms, is most often caused by an outbreak of HSV. EM major, usually caused by drugs (see above), by definition involves mucous membranes and demonstrates extensive bullous formation, with fever and prostration. Many authors still use the term, Stevens-Johnson syndrome, as being synonymous with EM major accompanied by erosion of less than 10 percent of the total epidermal surface, whereas the term *toxic epidermal necrolysis* (TEN) is generally reserved for a similar condition in which greater than 10 percent of the epidermis is lost in sloughing of large sheets. Mortality rates from EM major and TEN are 20 to 30 percent, usually from sepsis.

Rare to begin with, EM major is rarely recurrent, and can also be caused by *M. pneumoniae,* most often in children and young adults.

DIFFERENTIAL DIAGNOSIS

Fortunately, the diagnosis is usually easy, with such distinctive lesions. However, it can present with mucosal lesions as the only presenting sign, which should prompt the consideration of bullous disease, or other disease affecting mucosal tissues, such as HSV. In the case of atypical dermal EM, the differential would include urticaria, insect bites, drug eruption, and viral exanthems, among others.

LABORATORY

Punch biopsy for routine hematoxylin and eosin (H & E) pathology can be very helpful, particularly for the bullous form.

TREATMENT

Largely symptomatic with EM minor at least. Topical steroids are of no use in treatment of EM, since the problem is much too deep for these to reach. Suspected herpes triggers are treated with acyclovir. With EM major the following steps are recommended: (1) Give priority to finding the trigger if possible, and eliminating it, as in the case of drugs or treating it as with HSV. (2) Assess and treat potential complications (fluid loss, sepsis, ophthalmic pathology, nutritional deficits). Strong consideration should be given to hospitalization, and in severe cases, transfer to a burn unit.

PATIENT EDUCATION

Reassure the patient about the likely benign, self-limited nature of EM minor. Patients must be made aware of potential triggers in cases where the cause has not yet been found.

PEARLS

Consideration of the following points can contribute to positive patient outcome:

- Target-like (iris) papules of acute onset are pathognomic for EM.
- HSV is the trigger for EM until proved otherwise, though 50 percent of cases are idiopathic.
- EM major is a potentially fatal condition, requiring timely

diagnosis and referral to a dermatologist experienced in treating it.

- Erythematous palmar or plantar lesions that are tender should suggest EM.

PROGNOSIS

The prognosis is self-limited with EM minor lasting up to 4 weeks, whereas EM major can last 6 weeks, with new lesions, especially oral, appearing for weeks after that. Mortality rates from EM major and TEN are 10 to 20 percent, usually from sepsis.

BIBLIOGRAPHY

Arndt KA, Robinson JK, LeBoit PE, et al. *Cutaneous Medicine and Surgery.* Philadelphia, Saunders, 1996.

duVivier A: *Dermatology in Practice.* Philadelphia, Lippincott, 1990.

Fitzpatrick TB, Johnson RA, Wolff K, et al: *Color Atlas and Synopsis of Clinical Dermatology: Common and Serious Diseases,* 3d ed. New York, McGraw-Hill, 1997.

Goldstein BG, Goldstein AO: *Practical Dermatology,* Primary Care Series. St Louis, Mosby Year Book, 1992.

Shelley WB, Shelley ED: *Advanced Dermatologic Diagnosis.* Philadelphia, Saunders, 1992.

Weinberg S, Prose NS, Kristal L: *Color Atlas of Pediatric Dermatology,* 3d ed. New York, McGraw-Hill, 1998.

Chapter 2–13
ERYTHEMA NODOSUM
Joe R. Monroe

Definition

Erythema Nodosum (EN) is an inflammatory reaction pattern, in response to certain drugs, infections, or other disease states, characterized by the bilateral appearance of subcutaneous tender erythematous nodules on extensor surfaces representing an underlying process of septal panniculitis (acute inflammation of fat).

CLINICAL DISCUSSION

Erythema nodosum is the most common of the panniculitides, and, except for certain well-defined causes, is idiopathic (cause unknown) in approximately 40 percent of cases. It presents as an acute process and spontaneously regresses, leaving no surface changes (scarring, ulceration, or atrophy) behind. Most commonly affecting lower extremities, EN can also appear on arms and the neck, and the lesions are quite tender. The lesions themselves are poorly defined, being bright red initially, tending toward more violaceous hues as they mature, sometimes becoming frankly ecchymotic before disappearing after 2 to 6 weeks. They often appear in crops and range in size from 2 to 20 cm. Prior to puberty, the incidence is the same in both sexes, but after that, the female-to-male ratio rises to 3 : 1. Though 40 percent of cases are idiopathic, the rest have discernible causes, the most common of which are streptococcal infections, birth control pills, and sarcoidosis. Less common causes include primary tuberculosis (especially in children), sulfa drugs, coccidioidomycosis, ulcerative colitis, leprosy, and Behçet's syndrome. Most EN patients also complain initially of fever, malaise, and arthralgia, but may have symptoms related to the causative disease, such as cough, sore throat, or gastrointestinal symptoms.

DIFFERENTIAL DIAGNOSES

Diagnosis is usually straightforward with such a striking presentation. Unfortunately, the trigger is often unclear. The most common misdiagnosis is cellulitis or other infectious process, but the latter is not likely to present with multiple subcutaneous lesions showing no break in the skin surface. This lack of epidermal skin change in EN is quite helpful in ruling out a number of other disease processes that might otherwise be considered, such as insect bites or folliculitis.

LABORATORY

For EN itself, a deep skin biopsy (well into the fat) is necessary to demonstrate the characteristic septal panniculitis. For the workup of possible triggering diseases, a basic battery of tests should include complete blood cell count (CBC), erythrocyte sedimentation rate (ESR), chemistry screen, chest films, anti-streptolysin O (ASO) titer, purified protein derivative (PPD), and serum angiotensin converting enzyme level (ACE).

TREATMENT

Find and treat the trigger if possible. NSAIDs, elevation of the affected limbs, and compression with elastic bandages all provide supportive relief while this self-limited disease slowly clears. Unresponsive cases are often treated with potassium iodide 300 to 600 mg tid PO for up to 4 weeks. Recurrent cases are not unusual and should be referred to a dermatologist.

PATIENT EDUCATION

Repeated reassurances are often necessary since the initial presentation of this condition can be fairly impressive, and therefore frightening, in terms of both appearance and symptomatology.

PROGNOSIS

This disease is usually self-limited, lasting 3 to 6 weeks. The underlying trigger may not be as benign, thus a careful search for it is indicated.

PEARLS

Knowledge of the following points can contribute to positive patient outcome:

- EN plus bilateral hilar adenopathy may be the presenting signs of sarcoidosis, but this typically short-lived radiologic finding may be associated with EN in the absence of sarcoidosis.
- When biopsy is needed, a 6-mm punch, or deep incisional biopsy that gets a specimen well into the fat is necessary to diagnose EN, since the actual disease process involves only the fibrotic septa of the subcutaneous adipose (fat) tissue and not the overlying skin.
- Given a choice, never biopsy thin anterior tibial skin, since healing is often a problem here.

- The three most common causes of EN in this country are streptococcal infections (especially in children), birth control pills, and sarcoidosis, but the list of reported triggers is enormous.
- The acute appearance of painful, subcutaneous erythematous nodules on the legs of young women is EN until proved otherwise.
- As EN nodules resolve, they often go through the same color changes as bruises (so-called erythema contusiformis).

BIBLIOGRAPHY

Arndt KA, Robinson JK, LeBoit PE, et al: *Cutaneous Medicine and Surgery.* Philadelphia, Saunders, 1996.
duVivier A: *Dermatology in Practice.* Philadelphia, Lippincott, 1990.
Fitzpatrick TB, Johnson RA, Wolff K, et al: *Color Atlas and Synopsis of Clinical Dermatology: Common and Serious Diseases,* 3d ed. New York, McGraw-Hill, 1997.
Goldstein BG, Goldstein AO: *Practical Dermatology,* Primary Care Series. St Louis, Mosby Year Book, 1992.
Shelley WB, Shelley ED: *Advanced Dermatology Diagnosis.* Philadelphia, Saunders, 1992.
Weinberg S, Prose NS, Kristal L: *Color Atlas of Pediatric Dermatology,* 3d ed. New York, McGraw-Hill, 1998.

Chapter 2–14
FOLLICULITIS
Joe R. Monroe

DISCUSSION

Folliculitis is inflammation of the hair follicle, usually by bacteria, sometimes by other organisms, resulting in the appearance of follicular pustules, that is, tiny pus-filled papules often pierced centrally by a hair. The term *folliculitis* is traditionally used to denote a relatively mild, superficial inflammatory process that heals without scarring. Occlusion of the skin by oils or by impervious dressings seem to be etiologic factors, as does shaving. However, these discrete, superficial pustules can also evolve into furuncles, which involve deeper tissues, and appear acutely as hot, red, tender nodules. Multiple furuncles can then coalesce into larger, even more tender, fluctuant masses called carbuncles ("boils"), caused by *Staphylococcus.*

Apart from this classic presentation, folliculitis can also be caused by a large number of other agents, in an equally wide variety of clinical contexts. A classic example is *Pseudomonas* folliculitis, also known as "hot tub folliculitis," a relatively common self-limited condition promoted by the superhydration inherent in using a hot tub (or sauna), making the follicle susceptible to infection by *Pseudonomas neruginosa,* present in the tub in great numbers because of fecal contamination.

Candida albicans can cause a similar condition, especially common in bed-fast, febrile patients. Folliculitis caused by dermatophytic fungal organisms is common, especially when tinea corporis, cruris, or pedis is mistreated with topical steroids, which, in effect, promote deeper and more vigorous fungal growth.

Even the follicular mite *Demodex* can cause it, usually on the face. So-called pseudofolliculitis is a common condition, especially in black men; it is caused by the sharp end of a shaved, curly hair that, as it grows out, curls back in and actually reenters the follicle from which it came, provoking a chronic folliculitis.

Acne vulgaris (see Chap. 2-29) can evolve into a true folliculitis when it suddenly worsens because of superinfection with gram-negative organisms.

DIFFERENTIAL DIAGNOSIS

Folliculitis can be mistaken for acne, but multiple comedones (blackheads or whiteheads), missing in the former, will be seen in acne. Tiny flat warts, especially common on the face, tiny mollusca, and herpes simplex vesicles can all mimic folliculitis.

Inflamed inclusion cysts can do a good imitation of a carbuncle, with the former being relatively nontender and with modest erythema confined to the immediate perilesional skin, whereas a carbuncles is exquisitely tender ("sore as a boil") and hot to touch, with a relatively large zone of erythematous blush around it.

LABORATORY

Gram stain of pustular material, looking for clusters of gram-positive cocci and polymorphonuclear neutrophil leukocytes (PMNs), bacterial culture and sensitivity, KOH preparation for pustule roof (the need for which should be suggested by failure of antibacterial treatment), and punch biopsies can all be helpful, but are seldom necessary under ordinary circumstances. In chronic furunculosis, consider checking the blood sugar for evidence of diabetes, and doing a complete blood cell count (CBC) for neutropenia.

TREATMENT

For superficial mild folliculitis, use topical antibacterials such as mupirocin (Bactroban) plus warm soaks.

For acute furunculosis, hot packing and incision and drainage (I & D) usually suffice. The same is true for carbuncles if I & D is adequate. Systemic antibiotics are seldom necessary unless systemic symptoms (fever, chills, malaise) are present, suggesting the need for blood cultures prior to antibiotic treatment. Positive blood cultures suggest the need for IV antibiotic therapy.

For chronic furunculosis, long-term (2- to 3-month minimum) treatment with clindamycin 150 mg qid is often used, along with nightly swabbing of nares with mupirocin, and daily use of antibacterial bar soaps.

Pseudomonas folliculitis is usually self-limited and relatively asymptomatic; thus, no treatment is necessary unless pain, fever, or chills are present. Yeast or fungal folliculitis often require treatment with oral antifungals (ketoconazole, fluconazole, itraconazole, or terbinafine), especially if inappropriate steroid treatment has encouraged infection deeper into the dermis.

Demodex folliculitis (diagnosed by KOH preparation) can be treated with crotamiton (Eurax) cream, twice a day.

The best treatment for pseudofolliculitis barbae is to stop shaving. Gram-negative folliculitis, as a complication of acne, is commonly treated with long-term sulfa treatment. However, culture and sensitivity may be necessary to establish the best treatment, as well as the diagnosis.

PATIENT EDUCATION

Stress the importance of home treatment measures such as hot packing and antibiotic ointment application. Educate diabetics and other immunocompromised patients about watching for the development of systemic symptoms. In hot tub folliculitis, after reassuring the patient about the usually benign course, refer patients to the county health department for advice about how to prevent such problems in the future.

PEARLS

Knowledge of the following points can contribute to positive patient outcome:

- Look for the pustule pierced by a hair when folliculitis is suspected.
- Suspect yeast or fungal folliculitis when antibacterial measures fail, when topical steroid application makes things worse, or when the patient is immunosuppressed.
- The morphologic appearance of the lesions of *Pseudomonas* folliculitis are distinctive: a central tiny pustule surrounded by a 0.15- to 0.30-cm circle of bluish red, slightly edematous skin. They are more likely to be found on the skin under the bathing suit, are usually surprisingly asymptomatic, and do not always affect everyone who was in the hot tub.
- Suspect gram-negative folliculitis when acne formerly responsive to tetracycline suddenly gets out of control, and starts to turn cystic.
- When boils begin with menarche, and chronically recur in axillae, groin, and intergluteal skin, it is probably hidradenitis suppurativa.

PROGNOSIS

The prognosis for folliculitis is self-limited in most cases, except as noted.

BIBLIOGRAPHY

Arndt KA, Robinson JK, LeBoit PE, et al: *Cutaneous Medicine and Surgery.* Philadelphia, Saunders, 1996.
duVivier A: *Dermatology in Practice.* Philadelphia, Lippincott, 1990.
Fitzpatrick TB, Johnson JA, Wolff K, et al: *Color Atlas and Synopsis of Clinical Dermatology: Common and Serious Diseases,* 3d ed. New York, McGraw-Hill, 1997.
Goldstein BG, Goldstein AO: *Practical Dermatology,* Primary Care Series. St Louis, Mosby Year Book, 1992.
Shelly WB, Shelley ED: *Advanced Dermatologic Diagnosis.* Philadelphia, Saunders, 1992.
Weinberg S, Prose NS, Kristal L: *Color Atlas of Pediatric Dermatology,* 3d ed. New York, McGraw-Hill, 1998.

Chapter 2–15
HAND-FOOT-AND-MOUTH DISEASE
Barbara L. Sauls

DISCUSSION

Hand-foot-and-mouth disease is a self-limiting viral infection, usually caused by subtype A16 of the coxsackievirus family, but may also result from other enteroviral infection. The most commonly affected individuals are children ages 2 to 8 years. Infectiousness is as a typical virus with a tendency to pass to school or daycare mates and siblings, though many contacts will be spared. This disease occurs most frequently in the spring months.

A variant of this illness is herpangina (subtype A7), which has lesions limited to the pharynx.

SIGNS AND SYMPTOMS

Signs and symptoms of hand-foot-and-mouth disease are fairly classic. Children commonly develop a prodrome of anorexia, nausea, vomiting, and diarrhea with or without mild elevation of temperature. Following this is the development of painful small oral vesicles that ulcerate, commonly found along the soft palate. This results in a sore throat and dysphagia, with children often refusing everything by mouth for several days. A vesicular eruption also develops on the soles of the feet and the palms of the hands. These distal lesions usually do not ulcerate. The development of a rash on the soles and palms is unusual in other viral illnesses since these areas are most often spared.

OBJECTIVE FINDINGS

Physical examination reveals a benign general picture except for the skin and pharynx. Temperature is often normal or with mild elevation. Oral examination shows lesions in various stages beginning as small vesicles whitish to gray in color with a red halo, the lesions often pinpoint in size. The oral lesions are seen along the soft palate, uvula, and tonsillar area, but do not involve the buccal mucosa, lips, or tongue. These areas eventually ulcerate to form a shallow crater with a red base, but do not progress further. Even though there is poor oral intake of fluids, there are usually no signs of dehydration, unless accompanied by a more severe GI illness. Infants and young children are more prone to dehydration.

The lesions on the soles and palms are often discrete. The vesicles are often very small and filled with a minimal amount of fluid. These lesions do not ulcerate and are not usually painful. The patient or parent often does not notice these lesions until the practitioner points them out. It is often difficult to distinguish these lesions clearly in very dark skin individuals.

DIAGNOSTIC CONSIDERATIONS

The differential diagnosis of the oral illness most commonly includes herpesvirus infection (see Chaps. 2-16 and 2-17), although these lesions commonly involve the lips, tongue, gingiva, and buccal mucosa, which are spread in coxsackievirus infection. A rash on the soles and palms may be seen in Rocky Mountain spotted fever, but this has a much more severe onset, is macular in appearance, and occurs on the trunk and extremities as well as the soles and palms. The lesions do not form vesicles in this disease.

LABORATORY TESTS

It is not usually necessary to order any laboratory tests for this illness, although it is possible to order serologic studies for coxsackie if the practitioner believes it is needed. Viral cultures are expensive and of limited value in the treatment of this disease.

TREATMENT

Treatment of hand-foot-and-mouth disease is supportive in nature; there is no specific cure for this illness. If the patient is able to swallow small amounts of fluid, it is usually possible to encourage small sips of fluids every half-hour along with acetaminophen or ibuprofen for pain relief. Over-the-counter sore throat sprays (Chloraseptic) or gargles may offer some relief. Patients who are unable to swallow anything are given either viscous lidocaine to dab on specific areas with a cotton swab or lidocaine solution to swish, gargle, and spit. An alternative is "magic mouthwash" which is mixed by the pharmacist and is a combination of 2 oz Maalox, 1 oz viscous Xylocaine, and 15 mL liquid Benadryl. Some practitioners keep the ingredients on hand and mix it themselves for patients. Patients may swish, gargle, and spit several times daily. Younger infants will not be harmed by swallowing the solution. The numbing effect allows patients to eat and drink adequate amounts. Counsel the parents to watch for signs of dehydration.

SUPPORTIVE MEASURES

Supportive measures include rest and increasing diet as tolerated.

PATIENT EDUCATION

It is important to counsel patients that this illness may take up to 2 weeks to fully resolve. They should not expect their sore throat to go away overnight. Parents often call back in 2 days when their child is still not eating, but proper education helps them overcome their fears. Let them know that fluids are more important than solid food at this point.

DISPOSITION

Follow-up appointments are not necessary unless there is a need to monitor hydration status as in the very young or in longer-lasting illness. Dehydration is an uncommon complication to this illness.

BIBLIOGRAPHY

Fitzpatrick TB, Johnson RA, Wolff K, et al: *Color Atlas and Synopsis of Clinical Dermatology: Common and Serious Diseases,* 3d ed. New York, McGraw-Hill, 1997.
Isselbacher KJ, Braunwald E, Wilson JD, et al (eds): *Harrison's Principles of Internal Medicine,* 13th ed. New York, McGraw-Hill, 1994.

Chapter 2–16
HERPES SIMPLEX
William H. Fenn

DISCUSSION

Herpes simplex viruses types 1 and 2 (HSV-1 and HSV-2) cause superficial mucocutaneous infections in humans. These vesicular eruptions range from the ubiquitous cold sore to the stigmatized genital herpes and together account for well over 100 million outbreaks yearly in the United States alone.

PATHOPHYSIOLOGY

Initial infection with either double-stranded DNA virus occurs after direct transmission from an infected person. Although standing water, such as on the side of a pool, has been shown to harbor the virus for short periods, the virus is incapable of infection via such a route. Inoculation requires direct contact from an infected person to mucous membranes or abraded skin. Most often this dispersion occurs from an active lesion; however, some asymptomatic persons will actively shed the virus also. As the virus penetrates epidermal cells, viral reproduction and host cell destruction occur with resulting intraepidermal vesicles. Symp-

toms occur after a 2- to 20-day incubation period, with 95 percent of patients developing symptoms within 2 weeks. After the initial acute episode, the virus migrates to the sensory or autonomic ganglia and becomes dormant, with reactivation possible following several reported factors, including stress, ultraviolet radiation, and certain foods.

Many conflicting reports attribute differing proportions of HSV-1 and HSV-2 to oropharyngeal versus genital sites. From a clinical point of view, there is no current need to distinguish the two strains, since treatment is based on site and primary versus recurrent eruption. Therefore, it is not useful to get caught up in this issue. However, it is important to avoid drawing conclusions regarding transmission source based solely on viral subtype identification.

SIGNS AND SYMPTOMS

Patients complain of a painful eruption, sometimes accompanied by fever, general malaise, and headaches. In some people, the subjective symptoms precede the eruption, and for some with recurrent disease this prodrome is a reliable predictor of eruption. As a general rule, the discomfort of an initial eruption is more severe than subsequent recurrences, but this is far from universal.

OBJECTIVE FINDINGS

The classic eruption of herpes simplex is one of localized grouped vesicles on an erythematous base. However, these rapidly turn to pustules which rupture, resulting in a weeping erosive lesion that subsequently crusts. Recurrences may consist of a single small vesicle.

The most common location is at or near the vermilion border of the mouth, referred to as herpes labialis. However, it is important to remember that HSV infection can occur anywhere on the skin. When it occurs on the trunk or extremities, it frequently takes on some characteristics of herpes zoster, and is referred to as zosteriform herpes simplex. Herpes genitalis may occur anywhere on the genitals, but in females is most common on the labia. Low-grade fever is common, especially in primary infections. Regional lymphadenopathy is very common in primary and recurrent disease.

DIAGNOSTIC CONSIDERATIONS

As noted, truncal HSV may resemble zoster. Oral HSV may resemble aphthous stomatitis. Contact dermatitis is relatively less likely in the face of pain and systemic signs and symptoms. Impetigo may be ruled out by Gram stain. Genital lesions may suggest chancroid or lymphogranuloma venereum: A syphilitic chancre is relatively less likely in the face of pain.

SPECIAL CONSIDERATIONS

HSV in immunocompromised hosts has a much higher risk for complications, many severe, and therapy must be more aggressive. Although it is beyond the scope of this chapter, neonatal herpes is a dreaded condition. As there is a 50 percent rate of transmission if the virus is present at delivery and the results of infection are devastating, cesarean delivery is indicated. Routine prenatal screening is also recommended owing to the high incidence of clinically inapparent infection. A more diffuse eruption, eczema herpeticum, may occur in patients with atopic dermatitis, especially children. Although the appearance is more dramatic and the course more prolonged, treatment is usually quite successful. Secondary bacterial infection is common.

LABORATORY TESTS

The definitive test remains the viral culture. Polymerase chain reaction (PCR) laboratory studies to identify HSV exist, but are not widely clinically available. A number of antigen detection systems are available, with differing levels of sensitivity and specificity. Serologic testing is of limited value, because of the retrospective nature of the result and the fact that more than 85 percent of adults have antibodies to HSV-1.

Gram stain will help distinguish a bacterial infection, and other serologic tests may be indicated if other disorders are under consideration.

Most protocols call for the routine laboratory screening for other sexually transmitted diseases, including HIV testing with patient consent, any time a diagnosis of primary genital herpes is established.

RADIOLOGIC STUDIES

There are no appropriate radiologic studies for HSV.

OTHER DIAGNOSTIC CONSIDERATIONS

The Tzanck smear is a simple and useful office procedure. The lesion is unroofed (if needed), and the base gently scraped with a blade. The material is placed on a slide, and stained with Wright stain, Giemsa stain or toluidine blue. A positive smear displays multinucleated giant cells. The sensitivity of this test is variable, such that a negative test does not disprove the diagnosis. The test is specific only to herpes viruses in general, and thus will not distinguish simplex from zoster.

TREATMENT
Medications

Therapy is aimed at controlling symptoms, as well as reducing recurrences and sequelae. Although no treatment is available that eradicates infection, prompt institution of therapy has been shown to dramatically reduce healing time and reduce viral shedding.

Primary Infection

Treatment is acyclovir (Zovirax) 200 mg five times daily for 10 days. Therapy should be instituted within 48 h of onset; after this time treatment is of questionable benefit. Valacyclovir (Valtrex) and famciclovir (Famvir) have not been approved for initial infections, but have been used and may presumably offer similar benefits. Acyclovir ointment is much less effective and generally not recommended.

Recurrent Infection

Acyclovir, 200 mg five times daily for 5 days, or valacyclovir, 500 mg twice daily for 5 days, or famciclovir 125 mg twice daily for 5 days.

Since prompt initiation of therapy is essential, patients should be given a single supply of medication to keep at home, with instructions to initiate a course of medication at the first sign of recurrent infection. Patients with predictable prodromal symptoms should begin the medication at the onset of the symptoms.

Suppression of Recurrences

Current recommendations call for suppressive therapy in any patient who experiences six or more recurrent genital infections in a 12-month period. Acyclovir, 400 mg twice daily, administered for up to 1 year, dramatically reduces the frequency and severity of infections, but does not reduce viral shedding. Famciclovir has been shown to be similarly efficacious; however, consensus does not yet exist on dosing protocols.

Special Cases

Immunocompromised patients and other patients with acyclovir-resistant disease may require foscarnet or vidarabine.

Supportive Measures

Cool dressing or soaks may offer short-term relief from discomfort. Prescriptive analgesics may be warranted depending on the site and extent of the eruption. A number of OTC preparations for nongenital lesions are available. Although these preparations have not been subjected to objective clinical trials, sufficient anecdotal reports exist to suggest that they may be of symptomatic benefit.

Patient Education

Preventive measures must be frankly discussed. It is important to assist the patient in dealing with the stigma associated with this disease. Many areas have support groups, and the American Social Health Association maintains a herpes hotline. The myths and realities of the sexual transmission of genital herpes must be explored, including the potential for transmission by asymptomatic patients. Many patients are not aware of this because their knowledge is based on information that is now outdated. In the general population, the risk of contagion is reduced by condom use and increased by contact with multiple sexual partners.

COMPLICATIONS AND RED FLAGS

Autoinoculation to distant sites is possible. Herpetic keratitis, characterized by dendritic fluorescein staining, requires prompt ophthalmic evaluation. HSV-1 is a major etiologic agent for viral encephalitis. Uncommonly, HSV patients may develop erythema multiforme.

OTHER NOTES OR PEARLS

Several new antiviral medications for use in treating HSV infection are currently under development, with release imminent. Additionally, clinical trials of HSV-2 vaccines are underway. A successful vaccine program would dramatically change the approach to this infection.

BIBLIOGRAPHY

Coombs RW: *A Practical Guide to Herpes Infections.* Minneapolis, McGraw-Hill, 1994, pp 7–38.

Fitzpatrick TB, Eisen AZ, Wolff K, et al (eds): *Dermatology in General Medicine,* 4th ed. New York, McGraw-Hill, 1993, pp 2531–2543.

Lookingbill DP, Marks JG: *Principles of Dermatology,* 2d ed. Philadelphia, Saunders, 1993, pp 162–165.

Perry CM, Wagstaff AJ: Famciclovir: A review of its pharmacological and therapeutic efficacy in herpesvirus infections. *Drugs* 50(2): 396–415.

Chapter 2–17
HERPES ZOSTER
William H. Fenn

DISCUSSION

Herpes zoster (shingles) is an acute painful vesicular eruption that occurs along the distribution of a dermatome in patients with a history of varicella. The incidence increases with age, with two-thirds of cases occurring over the age of 50 and less than 10 percent occurring under age 20. The lifetime risk is probably between 10 and 20 percent.

PATHOPHYSIOLOGY

Herpes zoster is the reactivation of latent varicella-zoster virus (VZV) from its latency in sensory ganglia. It occurs after primary VZV infection (varicella), usually many years later. The incidence increases with age, presumably as host immune response declines. Other causes of immune reduction, such as HIV infection, also increase the incidence. When reactivated, the virus migrates down the involved sensory nerve causing prodromal symptoms of pain and pruritus to the skin, where the characteristic eruption ensues.

SIGNS AND SYMPTOMS

Patients complain of pain and altered sensation in the affected area, which may precede the eruption by 3 to 5 days. These symptoms may lessen somewhat with the onset of the eruption, but generally persist throughout the course. A minority of patients may report associated headache, general malaise, and fever.

OBJECTIVE FINDINGS

The principal lesions are groups of vesicles and bullae on an erythematous base, but early presentation will show papules and late presentation will show only confluent crusting and weeping lesions. The defining characteristic of the eruption is its distribution within a unilateral dermatome, although a few discrete lesions across the midline are not uncommon, presumably owing to small nerve fiber crossings. Occasionally infection occurs in adjacent dermatomes, and rarely in bilateral dermatomes. Occasionally zoster occurs without visible lesions. Regional lymphadenopathy is usual, and a low-grade fever may be present.

DIAGNOSTIC CONSIDERATIONS

Herpes simplex can occasionally appear in a dermatome pattern, and multiple recurrences suggest this diagnosis. The prodromal pain may suggest several different diagnoses, depending on location. Involvement of cranial dermatomes may mimic migraine, thoracic dermatomes pleuritis or myocardial infarction, and lumbar dermatome involvement may suggest herniated nucleus pulposus. Onset of the eruption generally makes the diagnosis clear, but appropriate diagnostic measures to rule out underlying pathology should not be delayed pending the eruption.

SPECIAL CONSIDERATIONS

Involvement of the auditory or ophthalmic nerves warrants specialist evaluation. Vesicles on the tip of the nose indicate involvement of the nasociliary branch of the ophthalmic nerve.

Immunocompromised patients may develop disseminated zoster and visceral involvement.

LABORATORY TESTS

Generally testing is not necessary. Viral culture is definitive when needed. Direct immunofluorescence staining is also available. Tzanck smears are easily performed (see Other Diagnostic Considerations, Chap. 2–16), but do not distinguish between zoster and simplex eruptions.

RADIOLOGIC AND OTHER DIAGNOSTIC STUDIES

There are no appropriate radiologic or diagnostic studies for herpes zoster.

TREATMENT
Medications

Treatment is acyclovir (Zovirax), 800 mg five times daily for 7 to 10 days, or valacyclovir (Valtrex), 1 g three times daily for 7 days, or famciclovir (Famvir), 500 mg every 8 h for 7 days.

Prompt institution of therapy reduces acute pain and healing time. Therapy does not appear to affect the incidence of postherpetic neuralgia (PHN), although famciclovir is reported to reduce its duration.

The use of potent analgesics is often warranted. Several recommendations have been made for the use of systemic steroids in older populations to reduce the risk of PHN; however, this benefit has not been confirmed and such treatment is probably not worthwhile. Tricyclic antidepressant therapy, TENS, and topical capsaicin (Zostrix) may be useful in the management of postherpetic neuralgia should it occur.

Supportive Measures

The lesions should be kept clean to avoid secondary bacterial infection. Cool or astringent compresses may reduce weeping, but otherwise topical measures are generally ineffective.

Patient Education

Educate patients as to the cause and course of the disease. Patients should be aware that in at least 30 percent of cases, they can transmit VZV to nonimmune persons, which will cause varicella, not zoster. This is particularly relevant in older patients who may be visiting with grandchildren.

Patients should be aware that recurrence is possible, although the 5 percent rate is less than most patients and health care personnel believe.

Disposition

Patients should be reexamined if the character of drainage changes or if symptoms are progressive. Persistence of pain after the lesions have resolved should prompt evaluation and discussion of PHN.

COMPLICATIONS AND RED FLAGS

PHN is the most likely complication. It is uncommon under the age of 40, but occurs in up to 65 percent of patients over the age of 60. The variation in incidence figures is partly due to the many definitions of PHN. Most commonly it is regarded as pain persisting longer than 1 month.

Treatment reduces symptoms in many patients, and 80 percent of patients with PHN are asymptomatic at 1 year. Radical therapies such as nerve destruction are fortunately seldom indicated.

OTHER NOTES OR PEARLS

The advent of vaccination to prevent varicella offers the possibility of a reduction in the incidence of herpes zoster as well. Proof of this, however, is lacking and it will be some time before results of widespread immunization on zoster incidence are known. As the onset of zoster appears related to reduction in immune status, it is also possible that a booster immunization of the varicella vaccine in aging patients with a history of varicella may reduce the incidence of zoster. The results of ongoing controlled studies are needed before such recommendations can be made.

BIBLIOGRAPHY

Fitzpatrick TB, Eisen AZ, Wolff K, et al (eds): *Dermatology in General Medicine,* 4th ed. New York, McGraw-Hill, 1993, pp 2543–2567.

Levin MJ, Hayward AR: The varicella vaccine: Prevention of herpes zoster. *Infect Dis Clin North Am* 10(3):657–675, 1996.

Lookingbill DP, Marks JG: *Principles of Dermatology,* 2d ed. Philadelphia, Saunders, 1993, pp 165–167.

Chapter 2–18
HUMAN PAPILLOMAVIRUS
Michelle DiBaise

DISCUSSION

The human papillomavirus (HPV) infects keratinized skin and is, therefore, limited to the epidermis. More than 60 HPV subtypes have been identified.[1–5] Some HPV subtypes have been shown to play a role in skin and mucosal oncogenesis, predominantly squamous cell carcinoma. There is an increased incidence of all warts in immunocompromised individuals such as in HIV disease, organ transplantation, and the use of immunosuppressive agents. In these patients, warts tend to be larger, more numerous and are more difficult to eradicate.

Verruca Vulgaris

Known as the common wart, it accounts for approximately 70 percent of all cutaneous warts.[1] As many as 5 to 20 percent of all school-age children develop warts.[1,4,5] It is spread by skin-to-skin contact, especially through minor breaks in the skin from trauma or underlying dermatoses.

Verruca Plantaris

The plantar wart can occur on the palms as well as the soles. It accounts for approximately 30 percent of all warts and is most common in older children and young adults.[1] Like the common wart, it is spread by skin-to-skin contact. A phenomenon called ''kissing warts'' occurs in which two warts develop where skin surfaces touch.

Verruca Plana

This flat wart accounts for only about 4 percent of all cutaneous warts.[1] It is common in children and adults. Like other warts it is spread by skin-to-skin contact. More than other varieties of warts, it is commonly spread by shaving.

Condyloma Acuminata

The most common mucosal form of HPV is condyloma acuminata, or genital wart.[1] It is the most prevalent sexually transmitted disease in all developed countries, including the United States.[1,3,6] It is estimated that between 3 and 28 percent of women have condylomata.[1] Among females with condylomata, nearly 100 percent of their male sex partners are infected and the majority of the lesions are subclinical.

Clinical warts are thought to be more infectious than the subclinical wart. Once infected, it may take weeks to months for an individual to develop lesions. The lesions of condylomata can last for months to years; however, there is some evidence that the infection may last throughout the individual's lifetime.

Condylomata in infants and children can imply sexual abuse. Studies show that up to 50 percent of genital HPV in infants and children actually is related to sexual abuse.[2,4] It may be difficult to prove abuse in that there is a prolonged incubation period before the development of lesions. This hinders pinpointing the exact time of the infection. Also, HPV can be acquired from passage through the birth canal of an infected woman.[1,4,5] Common warts on the hands can occasionally be spread to the genitalia, mouth, or anal area from either the child or a caretaker.[2,4,5]

SIGNS AND SYMPTOMS

Most warts are usually asymptomatic. They may cause cosmetic disfigurement and, therefore, affect the patients self-esteem. They can be painful and interfere with normal daily activity. Plantar warts can be painful enough to interfere with walking. Recurrent trauma such as with shaving can cause the warts to bleed.

OBJECTIVE FINDINGS

Verruca Vulgaris

The common wart is a round, dome-shaped papule, firm to palpation, with thickening of the stratum corneum (hyperkeratosis) and measuring 1 to 10 mm in size.[1,5] The surface has vegetations and is clefted. It is generally flesh-colored and may have black dots that are actually thrombosed capillary loops within the wart. Lesions tend to be discrete, but can at times coalesce into larger plaques [see Fig. 2-18-1 (Plate 11)].

Previously treated warts can form around the area of the old wart in an annular or doughnut shape. The wart is commonly found in areas that are recurrently traumatized, such as the hands, fingers, and knees. When the wart involves paronychia, it can extend underneath the nail plate. A variant of the common wart is the filiform wart. It generally occurs on the head and neck. It has a narrow base and fingerlike projections.

Verruca Plantaris

The plantar wart begins as a small, flesh-colored papule, but eventually enlarges into hyperkeratotic plaques with multiple black dots. Warts on the palms and soles distort the normal skin lines of the finger or footprints and occur over weight-bearing areas such as the metatarsal heads and heel.

Verruca Plana

Flat warts are round or oval, flat, flesh-colored or light-brown papules measuring 1 to 5 mm in diameter and only 1 to 2 mm in thickness.[1–3,6] They are common on the face and dorsum of the hands [see Fig. 2-18-2 (Plate 12)]. In men, they are frequently spread in the beard area from shaving and in women on the legs. When they are spread through autoinoculation from shaving or scratching, they have a linear appearance.

Figure 2-18-1 (Plate 11). Verruca vulgaris. (*From Fitzpatrick, Johnson, Wolff, et al.*)

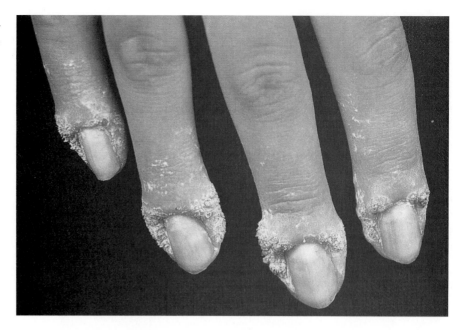

Condyloma Acuminata

Condylomata begin as minute papules and may grow to soft, moist, large cauliflower- or grape-like lesions. If lesions are subclinical, they are best visualized by applying 5 to 7% acetic acid to the skin for 5 min (aceto-whitening), which turns the lesions white. Clinical lesions are flesh-colored in general, but can be pink or red. They usually occur in clusters and tend to occur on the penis and scrotum in men, vagina and cervix in women,

and perineal area, perianal area, urethra, rectum, bladder, and oropharynx in both sexes [see Fig. 2-18-3 (Plate 13)].

DIAGNOSTIC CONSIDERATIONS

Verruca Vulgaris

The differential diagnosis of the common wart includes molluscum contagiosum, seborrheic keratoses, and callus. In a callus,

Figure 2-18-2 (Plate 12). Verruca plana. (*From Fitzpatrick, Johnson, Wolff, et al.*)

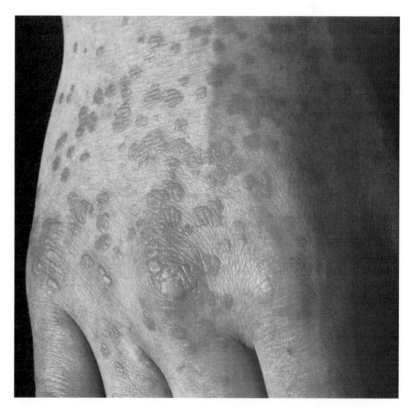

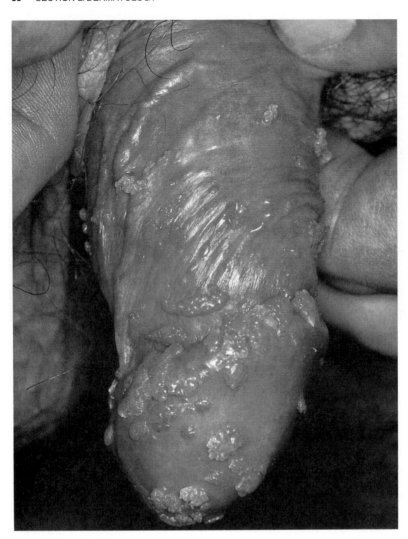

Figure 2-18-3 (Plate 13). Condyloma acuminata. (*From Fitzpatrick, Johnson, Wolff, et al.*)

the normal skin lines are maintained. In older individuals and the immunosuppressed, the differential would also include basal cell carcinoma and squamous cell carcinoma.

Verruca Plantaris

The differential diagnosis for plantar warts includes a callus, corn, and shearing trauma that occurs in sports. Both a callus and corn do not distort the normal skin lines nor do they exhibit black dots.

Verruca Plana

The differential diagnosis for flat warts includes molluscum contagiosum, seborrheic keratoses, syringoma (when present on the face), closed comedones, and lichen planus.

Condyloma Acuminata

The differential diagnosis for condyloma acuminata includes condyloma lata (a manifestation of secondary syphilis), squamous cell carcinoma (invasive or in situ), molluscum contagiosum, bowenoid papulosis (see ''Complications and Red Flags,'' below), lichen planus, seborrheic keratoses, skin tags, pearly penile papules (a benign variant seen on the corona of the penis and occasionally the shaft), nevi, and sebaceous glands.

LABORATORY TESTS

Verruca Vulgaris and Verruca Plantaris

The diagnosis is almost always made on clinical findings. If in doubt, a no. 15 blade can be used to gently pare the wart and confirm the presence of the black dots of the thrombosed capillaries.

Verruca Plana

The diagnosis is usually made by clinical examination. The linear distribution leads away from a diagnosis of seborrheic keratosis and toward that of flat warts.

Condyloma Acuminata

Clinical examination is usually sufficient to make the diagnosis. Subclinical lesions can best be discerned by aceto-whitening. Aceto-whitening is not specific for HPV. Other lesions that whiten with acetic acid include candidiasis, lichen planus, normal sebaceous glands, psoriasis, and areas of healing. Because condylomata is a sexually transmitted disease (STD), the practitioner should consider testing for other STDs such as syphilis and HIV. Women with condylomata or whose partners have condylomata should have annual Pap smears because of the increased risk for cervical dysplasia and squamous cell carcinoma. Anoscopy or proctoscopy should be considered in the presence of perianal warts. The most common HPV types associated with malignant change include 6, 11, 16, 18, 31, and 33.[1-5] HPV subtyping can be performed in cases of sexual abuse.

TREATMENT

In the immunocompetent host, warts are self-limiting. Estimates are that between 35 and 65 percent of warts will spontaneously resolve in 2 years.[3,5] They usually resolve with little or no intervention. It is best, therefore, to avoid overly aggressive treatments that risk scarring. Up to 20 percent of patients will have recalcitrant warts requiring more aggressive therapy.[2] The immunocompromised host may have warts that are very difficult to eradicate. These patients may require monthly visits in which the goal is controlling the bulk of the lesions and not eradication of the warts.

Verruca Vulgaris and Verruca Plantaris

Topical therapy includes over-the-counter medications that contain various strengths of salicylic acid 14 to 17 percent (Occlusal, Duoplant, Compound W, and others). The medicine is painted on and allowed to dry every night. Resolution can be hastened by soaking the area for 10 to 15 min and gently paring the wart with an emery board. Care must be taken to use a new area of the emery board with each wart and disposing of it when finished. The medicine is then applied to the pared wart. Cure rates have been reported at 70 percent for common warts and 84 percent for plantar warts.[6] The topical medications have a plaster variety with salicyclic acid 40% (Mediplast, Duofilm, and others) that is applied directly to the wart and left in place for 24 to 48 h. The plaster is removed, the wart pared down, and a new plaster applied. This is repeated until the wart is gone. The plasters work best on larger warts because normal skin becomes macerated in the process.

Cryosurgery is an alternative for patients for whom topical medications used alone have failed. It can be used in conjunction with the topical medication as well. Liquid nitrogen is applied to the wart using a cryospray or a cotton swab. The wart should be frozen until an ice ball forms on to 1 to 2 mm of surrounding normal skin. The area is allowed to thaw, and the procedure is repeated. The area may blister within 24 h. The patient is instructed not to rupture the blister. If the blister ruptures, it should be covered with antibiotic ointment and a dressing. The blister will eventually crust over in a few days. Once the crust falls off, if there is remaining wart, the topical medicine can be applied until the patient returns to clinic. Repeat freezing usually occurs in 4-week cycles. Cryotherapy does not kill the virus, but rather destroys the normal skin, sloughing the wart off in the process.

Electrocautery is an alternative to freezing. It is more effective than cryotherapy, but has an increased incidence of scarring. The area can be anesthetized prior to the procedure using EMLA (a topical anesthetic cream) or by injecting lidocaine. HPV has been found in the plume of smoke from cautery and can cause infection of the airways.[1] Cure rates range from 60 to 80 percent.[6]

CO_2 *laser surgery* is also effective for recalcitrant warts. The area must be anesthetized. It is expensive and potentially scarring. HPV has been found in the plume of smoke from laser procedures and can infect the airways.[1] Cure rates up to 90 percent have been reported.[6]

Surgical removal can be performed. The least scarring method is curettage. A shave procedure may also be performed. A surgical excision is not necessary because the infection is limited to the epidermis.

Hyperthermia for plantar warts has been advocated.[1] It requires immersion in hot water for 30 to 45 min two to three times a week for up to 16 treatments.

Cimetidine (Tagamet) works as an immune modulator, most likely through the T-cell line although the exact mechanism remains unclear. The doses necessary to show an effect are 400 mg tid in adults or an equivalent based on weight for children. Therapy must be continued for 3 months and be used in conjunction with a destructive method. The literature is mixed about whether the addition of cimetidine is effective when compared with placebo.[4,7-12]

Interferon α (Intron-A, Alferon N) is reserved for warts that do not respond to conventional therapy and when the disease process limits social and physical activity. The patient must be older than 18 years of age. It is given intralesionally three times a week, is extremely painful, and causes influenza-like symptoms. It is quite expensive. Regression has been reported in as high as 60 to 80 percent of lesions.[6]

Bleomycin sulfate is used intralesionally in cases of warts that have failed to respond to all forms of conventional therapy. It cannot be used in pregnant women. It has been shown to have a cure rate of 48 to 92 percent, depending on the location and size of the wart.[2,6] Side effects include pain, necrosis, and the development of Raynaud's phenomenon.

Contact immunotherapy uses agents such as dinitrochlorobenzene (DNCB), diphenylcyclopropenone, and squaric acid dibutyl ester. DNCB may be carcinogenic as well as mutagenic; therefore, its use should be avoided until further safety testing is available. Immunotherapy works by sensitizing the individual to the chemical in a remote site from the wart. The chemical agent is then subsequently applied to the wart causing immune destruction. Reported cure rates for DNCB are 80 percent in one study.[6]

Verruca Plana

Tretinoin (Retin A) has been shown to be effective for the treatment of flat warts. The doses available are 0.025, 0.05, and 0.1% cream and 0.01, 0.025, and 0.1% gel. Treatment may take several months and can produce irritation, excessive erythema, or scaling.

Light cryotherapy is an alternative, but may require treatment over a large surface area.

Topical 5-fluorouracil (Efudex) is applied once or twice a day for approximately 1 month. It should be reserved for recalcitrant warts. It is irritating and may cause hyperpigmentation.

Condyloma Acuminata

Topical treatment can be performed either in the office or at home by the patient. In office treatment is performed with podophyllin, 10 to 25%, in a tincture of benzoin compound. The solution is applied directly to the wart, avoiding normal skin. The amount applied can be no more than 0.5 mL or a surface area of 10 cm² per session. The solution is completely washed off within 1 to 4 h. The treatment can be repeated weekly. Systemic reactions have been noted, including renal effects, paresthesia, ileus, thrombocytopenia, leukopenia, polyneuritis, shock, and death.[2,3] If biopsy is performed after therapy with podophyllin, the pathologist must be informed because the chemical changes may be mistaken for squamous cell carcinoma.[2] After six treatments, if warts persist, an alternative therapy should be considered. Podophyllin cannot be used during pregnancy because of effects on the fetus.[1,3]

The take-home treatment is podophyllin 0.5% (Podofilox, Condylox). The patient applies the solution to the warts twice a day for 3 days and then no treatment for the following 4 days. The cycle is then repeated for up to four times. The volume of solution should not be more than 0.5 mL per day or cover an area greater than 10 cm². Side effects include local pain, burning, inflammation, and erosion of the skin.[2] If the warts are still present after four cycles, an alternative form of therapy should be considered.[1] This treatment should not be used during pregnancy.

Trichloroacetic acid, 25 to 90%, can be used in the office. It is effective but potentially scarring with excessive application. The normal surrounding tissue is protected with petroleum jelly. The solution is applied directly to the wart, which reacts immediately by whitening. The excess acid is then neutralized using sodium bicarbonate. The warts can be treated weekly if necessary, but if they are present after six treatments, an alternative therapy should be considered.[1]

Cryotherapy is an inexpensive alternative, performed in the office. The method is the same as for common warts. It does not result in scarring; however, it is painful. Cryotherapy can be repeated monthly and can also be used in combination with topical at-home therapy.

Electrocautery is an effective method for removal of warts. As in common warts, it requires anesthesia and is potentially scarring; HPV particles are potentially aerosolized in the smoke.

CO_2 laser is best reserved for extensive lesions and in those who have failed other treatment regimens. A "brush" technique has been developed that superficially coagulates normal-appearing skin in an attempt to eradicate subclinical lesions. This technique can be used on the mucosal surfaces.[2]

Interferon α (Intron-A, Alferon N) as in other varieties of warts, should be reserved for cases that have failed conventional therapy. However, it has been shown to clear approximately 36 to 54 percent of recalcitrant lesions.[2,4]

Topical 5-fluorouracil (Efudex) is also reserved for recalcitrant warts. It is applied as a cream to external genital regions and in a suppository form for the vaginal area. The normal skin is protected by the use of petroleum jelly, zinc oxide paste, or hydrocortisone ointment.[2] It cannot be used on pregnant women since it may cause birth defects. Side effects include irritation, inflammation, and ulceration.

FOLLOW-UP

In condyloma acuminata, women with HPV of the genitalia or whose male sex partners are infected with HPV, should have annual Pap smears. The patient should be encouraged to use condoms to prevent transmission of the virus to uninfected partners. Recurrence is more likely due to activation of subclinical infection in the individual rather than reinfection from the patient's sex partner.[1,2]

COMPLICATIONS AND RED FLAGS

Verruca Plana

A rare hereditary disorder, epidermodysplasia verruciformis, mimics verruca plana. The lesions are numerous and large, and they coalesce into larger plaques. Between 30 and 80 percent of cases have been reported to become squamous cell carcinoma, both in situ and invasive, usually in sun-exposed areas.[4–6]

Condyloma Acuminata

Condylomata can undergo malignant change and become squamous cell carcinoma, both in situ or invasive. Any lesion that is not resolving with adequate therapy may warrant a biopsy. Squamous cell carcinoma can arise on any mucosal surface infected with HPV including the oropharynx and the rectum. An uncommon variant is bowenoid papulosis or intraepithelial neoplasia and is caused by HPV subtype 16. It occurs in the genital area of sexually active adults. It is an erythematous or pigmented papule resembling squamous cell carcinoma in situ. It may resolve spontaneously. Females with bowenoid papulosis or female partners of infected men should have annual Pap smears because of the risk of cervical dysplasia.

Laryngeal papillomatosis is a condition that occurs in infants and adults from the nasal passages to the lungs. It presents with stridor, hoarseness and, only rarely, airway obstruction from HPV-associated papillomas.[4,5] It may be acquired in infants born to mothers with active HPV infection. It does not appear that passage through the birth canal is necessary to develop laryngeal papillomatosis since there are reports of affected infants who were delivered by cesarean section.[2] Adult infection has occurred when HPV-infected smoke is inhaled during cautery or laser procedures.

REFERENCES

1. Fitzpatrick TB, Johnson RA, Wolff K, et al: *Color Atlas and Synopsis of Clinical Dermatology: Common and Serious Diseases,* 3d ed. New York, McGraw-Hill, 1997, pp 766–771, 899–909.
2. Habif TP: *Clinical Dermatology, A Color Guide to Diagnosis and Treatment,* 3d ed. St Louis, Mosby Yearbook, 1996, pp 297–303, 325–334.
3. Lookingbill DP, Marks JG Jr: *Principles of Dermatology,* 2d ed. Philadelphia, Saunders, 1993, pp 66–72.
4. Seabury-Stone M, Lynch PJ: Viral warts, in Sams WM, Lynch PJ (eds): *Principles and Practice of Dermatology,* 2d ed. New York, Churchill Livingstone, 1996, pp 127–133.
5. Lowry DR, Androphy EJ: Warts, in Fitzpatrick TB, Eisen AZ, Wolff K, et al (eds): *Dermatology in General Medicine,* 4th ed. New York, McGraw-Hill, 1993, pp 2611–2620.
6. Arnold HL, Odom RB, James WD: *Andrews' Diseases of the Skin, Clinical Dermatology,* 8th ed. Philadelphia, Saunders, 1990, pp 468–476.
7. Wargon O: Cimetidine for mucosal warts in an HIV positive adult. *Australas J Dermatol* 37(3):149–150, 1996.
8. Glass AT, Solomon BA: Cimetidine therapy for recalcitrant warts in adults. *Arch Dermatol* 132(6):680–682, 1996.
9. Yilmaz E, Alpsoy E, Basaran E: Cimetidine therapy for warts: A placebo controlled, double-blind study. *J Am Acad Dermatol* 34(6): 1005–1007, 1996.
10. Ronna T, Lebwohl M: Cimetidine therapy for plantar warts. *J Am Podiatr Med Assoc* 85(11):717–718, 1995.
11. Choi YS, Hann SK, Park YK: The effect of cimetidine on verruca plana juvenilis: Clinical trials in six patients. *J Dermatol* 20(8):497–500, 1993.
12. Orlow SJ, Paller A: Cimetidine therapy for multiple viral warts in children. *J Am Acad Dermatol* 28(5):794–796, 1993.

Chapter 2–19
IMPETIGO AND ECTHYMA
Michelle DiBaise

DISCUSSION

Impetigo and ecthyma are common skin infections caused by *Staphylococcus aureus,* group A beta-hemolytic streptococci, or a combination of both. Impetigo occurs as superficial erosions, whereas ecthyma is a deeper infection. Both diseases can present as a primary or secondary infection. Primary infection requires a minor trauma where breaks in the skin allow bacteria to gain a portal of entry. In *S. aureus* infections, the patient may not remember a traumatic event. However, infection with group A beta-hemolytic streptococci requires more vigorous inoculation, usually from scratching.[1–3] Primary infections occur more often in children.

Primary impetigo can be bullous or nonbullous. Bullous impetigo is due primarily to staphylococci that produce an exotoxin at the site of infection. The exotoxin produces cleavage within the epidermis. Bullous impetigo is seen more commonly in children and young adults.[1-3]

Secondary infection occurs most commonly in inflammatory dermatoses (such as atopic dermatitis), bullous diseases, ulcers, burns, and trauma.[1-3] Lesions secondarily infected are said to be impetiginized. Secondary infections can occur at any age. Both primary and secondary lesions occur more commonly in warm temperatures, high humidity, overcrowded situations, individuals with poor hygiene, and persons with underlying dermatoses.[1-3]

With adequate treatment of impetigo, there is prompt resolution. Untreated lesions may last up to several weeks, but the majority will resolve spontaneously. Some lesions, however, progress to areas of ecthyma usually secondary to poor hygiene and neglect. Recurrence may occur because of failure to eradicate the organism or reinfection from a family member. Recurrent infection may also be an indication that the patient is a carrier of S. aureus. It is estimated that 20 to 40 percent of adult nasal passages are colonized with S. aureus and approximately 20 percent of individuals are colonized on the perineum or axillae.[1,3] In atopic individuals, 90 percent are colonized with S. aureus in areas of active lesions and 70 percent are colonized on apparently normal skin.[1,3]

SIGNS AND SYMPTOMS

Patients with impetigo may experience pruritus, especially in the presence of atopic dermatitis. They may also have mild discomfort in the area of the lesion. Individuals with ecthyma tend to experience more pain or tenderness. Systemic symptoms are not common, although the development of acute streptococcal glomerulonephritis has been reported.[1-4]

OBJECTIVE FINDINGS

Both bullous and nonbullous impetigo begin as vesicles with a very thin roof that is easily ruptured. Lesions can be found anywhere, but most often are located on the face. In bullous impetigo, the vesicles enlarge rapidly to form bullae. The bullous contents become cloudy. The center of the bulla umbilicates, whereas the periphery may retain fluid. A honey-colored crust appears in the center, and if removed, an inflamed base is revealed that exudes serum. As the lesion enlarges, a scaling border replaces the bulla and eventually forms a crust. The lesions have minimal or no surrounding erythema. Individual lesions may increase in size to between 2 and 8 cm^2 [see Fig. 2-19-1 (Plate 14)]. In darker skinned individuals, lesions tend to heal with hyperpigmentation. Regional adenopathy is uncommon with staphylococcal impetigo.

In nonbullous impetigo the small vesicle or pustule is usually not seen. The most commonly encountered finding is the honey-colored crust [see Fig. 2-19-2 (Plate 15)]. The lesions extend radially, and satellite lesions appear beyond the periphery. There is little surrounding erythema. The lesions average 1 to 3 cm in size.[1-3] The skin around the nose, mouth, and the limbs are the sites most commonly affected.[1-4] The palms and soles are not affected. Regional adenopathy is more common with streptococcal impetigo, and it is most common in children 5 to 7 years of age.[2,3]

Ecthyma is caused by group A beta-hemolytic streptococci. It is seen more commonly in excoriations, bites, and areas of trauma, especially in diabetics, the elderly, and alcoholics.[1-3] The presenting lesion is usually a crust, but the more important clinical feature is the depth of infection. In ecthyma, the infection is deep, so when the crust is removed, an ulcer is noted. Because the ulcer of ecthyma extends into the dermis, it more often heals with scarring. The lesion of ecthyma may have a hemorrhagic crust and be indurated or tender. In streptococcal infection, the

erythema surrounding the lesion may be moderate to severe. Ecthyma is usually found on the lower extremities [see Fig. 2-19-3 (Plate 16)].

There may be associated lymphadenopathy.

DIAGNOSTIC CONSIDERATIONS

The differential diagnosis for nonbullous impetigo includes excoriation, perioral dermatitis, seborrheic dermatitis, allergic contact dermatitis, and inflammatory fungal infections.

The differential diagnosis for bullous impetigo includes allergic contact dermatitis such as to poison ivy, herpes simplex, herpes zoster, bacterial folliculitis, burns, bullous pemphigoid, and dermatitis herpetiformis. When the patient presents with crusts, it may be difficult to differentiate impetigo from herpes simplex. A history of a prodrome that includes tingling, burning, or recurrence in the same areas and a history of clear vesicles on an erythematous base will favor a diagnosis of herpes. KOH examination and fungal culture will help differentiate fungal from bacterial infection.

The differential for ecthyma includes chronic herpetic ulcers, excoriated insect bites, neurotic excoriations, porphyria cutanea tarda if limited to the dorsa of the hands, and stasis ulcers if limited to the legs.

LABORATORY TESTS

A Gram stain will reveal gram-positive cocci in chains or clusters. Bacterial culture more commonly will grow S. aureus and less frequently group A beta-hemolytic streptococci. In obtaining material for Gram stain and culture, it is important to first remove the crust so the specimen can be obtained from the base of the lesion.

Further testing in uncomplicated impetigo is costly and may not add information to the clinical picture. In suspected streptococcal impetigo or when symptoms of acute glomerulonephritis are present, serotyping may be necessary. The antistreptolysin O (ASO) titer does not rise to a significant level; however, anti-DNase B rises to high levels and is a sensitive indicator of streptococcal impetigo.[2,4] Antihyaluronidase also increases significantly.[2,4] In acute glomerulonephritis, cultures of the pharynx and skin lesions should be performed and the serotype of the group A streptococci should be determined by typing with M-group and T-type antisera. MT serotypes associated with acute glomerulonephritis are 2, 49, 55, 57, and 60.[2]

TREATMENT

Impetigo may resolve spontaneously, but it can become chronic and widespread. Studies show that 2% mupirocin ointment (Bactroban) is as effective as oral antibiotics and is associated with fewer side effects in the treatment of patients with nonbullous impetigo.[1-3] It is active against staphylococci including methicillin-resistant strains, and group A beta-hemolytic streptococci. In superficial skin infections that are not widespread, mupirocin ointment is the treatment of choice. Mupirocin is applied three times a day until all lesions have cleared. The involved areas should be cleansed once or twice a day with an antibacterial soap. There is a debate about whether the crusts should be removed because they potentially block the penetration of antibacterial creams. It may be sufficient to soften the crusts by soaking the area with a wet cloth compress. Local treatment does not affect evolving lesions in other areas. Infected children should be briefly quarantined until treatment is underway.

A 7- to 10-day course of an oral antibiotic such as cloxacillin, dicloxacillin, cephalexin (Keflex), or the newer macrolide antibiotics such as clarithromycin (Biaxin) or azithromycin (Zithromax) induce rapid healing.[1-3] Erythromycin may not be as effective

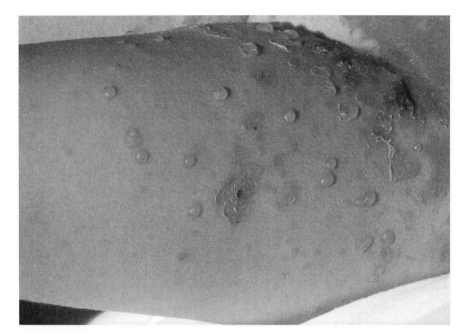

Figure 2-19-1 (Plate 14). Bullous impetigo. (*From Fitzpatrick, Johnson, Wolff, et al.*)

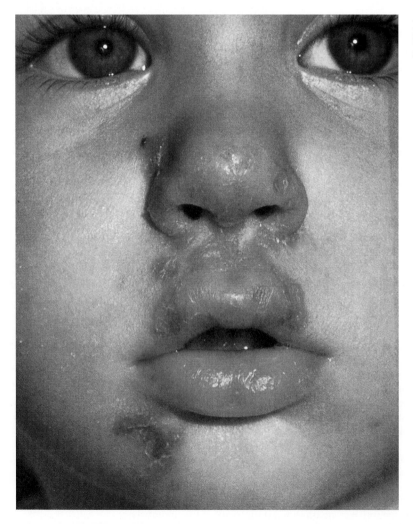

Figure 2-19-2 (Plate 15). Nonbullous impetigo. (*From Fitzpatrick, Johnson, Wolff, et al.*)

Figure 2-19-3 (Plate 16). Ecthyma. (*From Fitzpatrick, Johnson, Wolff, et al.*)

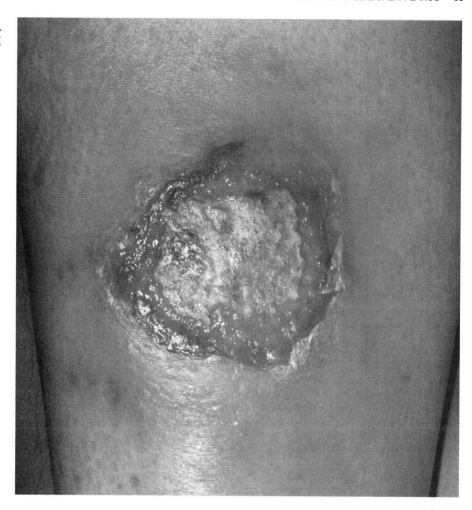

because some strains of staphylococci are resistant.[2,3] Most *S. aureus* strains produce penicillinase, so penicillin is also inappropriate treatment.[2,5]

FOLLOW-UP

Patients with recurrent impetigo should be evaluated for carriage of *S. aureus*. The nares are the most common sites of carriage, but the perineum, axillae, and toe webs may also be colonized.[1–3] Mupirocin ointment applied to the colonized area twice a day for 5 days reduces *S. aureus* carriage. Benzoyl peroxide wash also decreases colonization. Family members should be examined for signs of impetigo.

COMPLICATIONS AND RED FLAGS

Acute glomerulonephritis tends to occur when many individuals in a family have impetigo, mostly in the southern United States, with the highest incidence in children between 2 and 4 years of age.[2] Infants under 1-1/2 years of age are rarely affected by acute glomerulonephritis following impetigo. The overall incidence of acute glomerulonephritis with impetigo ranges from 2 to 5 percent, but when a nephritogenic strain is present, the rate ranges from 10 to 15 percent.[2] The period between formation of the skin lesions and the onset of acute glomerulonephritis ranges from 1 to 5 weeks with an average of 10 days.[2]

The most common clinical features include hematuria with erythrocyte casts, proteinuria, and edema that varies with the amount of dietary sodium.[2] In the morning there may be periorbital and lower extremity edema. Moderate hypertension is also

common. CNS symptoms, congestive heart failure (CHF), and acute renal failure are less common.[2] There is usually marked improvement in most patients within 7 to 10 days. Other complications of superficial skin infections with *S. aureus* and group A beta-hemolytic streptococci have been seen. Group A beta-hemolytic streptococcal impetigo may precipitate or flare an episode of guttate psoriasis. Primary or secondary impetiginous lesions can progress to cellulitis, erysipelas, or bacteremia. Osteomyelitis, septic arthritis, and pneumonia have been reported to occur in infants after episodes of impetigo.[6] Rheumatic fever has not been reported as a complication.[2]

REFERENCES

1. Fitzpatrick TB, Johnson RA, Wolff K, et al: *Color Atlas and Synopsis of Clinical Dermatology: Common and Serious Diseases,* 3d ed. New York, McGraw-Hill, 1997, pp 604–609.
2. Habif TP: *Clinical Dermatology. A Color Guide to Diagnosis and Treatment,* 3d ed. St Louis, Mosby Yearbook, 1996, pp 236–242.
3. Swartz MN, Weinberg AN: Infections due to gram-positive bacteria, in Fitzpatrick TB, Eisen AZ, Wolff K, et al (eds): *Dermatology in General Medicine,* 4th ed. New York, McGraw-Hill, 1993, pp 2310–2313.
4. Rajajee S: Post-streptococcal acute glomerulonephritis: A clinical, bacteriological and serological study. *Indian J Pediatr* 57:775–780, 1990.
5. Demidovich CW, Wittler RR, Ruff ME, Bass JW, Browning WC et al: Impetigo: Current etiology and comparison of penicillin, erythromycin and cephalexin therapies. *Am J Dis Child* 144:1313–1315, 1990.
6. Arnold HL, Odom RB, James WD: *Andrews' Diseases of the Skin, Clinical Dermatology,* 8th ed. Philadelphia, Saunders, 1990, pp 272–273.

Chapter 2–20
LICHEN PLANUS
Joe R. Monroe

DISCUSSION

Lichen planus (LP) is a relatively common inflammatory condition with highly characteristic purple color, distinctive papular morphology, and characteristic histopathologic pattern. It is a curious disorder of unknown etiology, affecting skin, hair, scalp, mucous membranes, and nails. It affects slightly more women than men, ages 30 to 60.

Attacks often begin suddenly, with the appearance of 1- to 3-mm flat-topped (planar) discrete purplish papules, especially on volar wrists, low back skin, legs, and genitals. More likely to itch than not, these papules sometimes coalesce into plaques up to 5 cm. Trauma, especially scratching, can cause arrangement of these papules along lines of trauma, an occurrence known as the Koebner phenomenon. The surfaces of the lesions may also exhibit fine parallel white striations called Wickham's striae, a useful fact identifying LP lesions.

Dermatologic tradition holds that LP can be easily diagnosed in most cases using the "Ps" of LP: papular, pruritic, planar (i.e., flat-topped), polygonal (i.e., multangular), plaque-like, penile, and puzzling.

Several variants of LP have been described, the most common of which is involvement of the buccal mucosa (40 to 60 percent of all LP patients), in which a white, lacy, reticulated papular pattern is seen. This form of LP can become erosive and painful, can affect the lip and tongue as well, and can be very challenging to treat. LP can also affect scalp skin (atrophy and hair loss), and 10 percent of patients will experience destruction of nails. Morphologic variants include bullous and annular forms, whereas on legs, LP tends to present as hypertrophic, hyperpigmented plaques that can resemble psoriasis, especially in people with darker skin.

DIFFERENTIAL DIAGNOSIS

Contact dermatitis, drug eruptions, lupus erythematosus, psoriasis are included in the differential diagnosis. In the mouth, the differential diagnosis includes thrush and oral hairy leukoplakia.

LABORATORY

Biopsy, showing a very characteristic histopathologic picture, can be quite helpful, but the distinctive clinical presentation usually permits an easy diagnosis.

TREATMENT

Steroids (topical, intralesional, systemic) can be very effective in controlling pruritus. PUVA (psoralen, an oral drug, is used in combination with UVA light exposure), especially for widespread eruptions. For oral LP, triamcinolone in Orabase and oral retinoids are used, but often referral to a dermatologist is necessary.

PATIENT EDUCATION

Reassurance about the (usual) self-limited, benign nature of LP is helpful.

PEARLS

Knowledge of the following points can contribute to a positive patient outcome.

- Remember the Ps, especially purple.
- The darker the skin, the darker the purple.
- Genital LP is surprisingly common.
- Pruritus is the rule with LP (80 percent).
- Add LP to the differential diagnosis for "fungal" fingernails.
- The quintessential LP presentation is highly pruritic purple papules on volar wrist skin.

PROGNOSIS

This disease is usually over in weeks, but it may persist for years, especially in the mouth, and on shins with the hypertrophic variety.

BIBLIOGRAPHY

Arndt KA, Robinson JK, LeBoit PE, et al: *Cutaneous Medicine and Surgery.* Philadelphia, Saunders, 1996.
duVivier A: *Dermatology in Practice.* Philadelphia, Lippincott, 1990.
Fitzpatrick TB, Johnson RA, Wolff K, et al: *Color Atlas and Synopsis of Clinical Dermatology: Common and Serious Diseases,* 3d ed. New York, McGraw-Hill, 1997.
Goldstein BG, Goldstein AO: *Practical Dermatology,* Primary Care Series. St Louis, Mosby Year Book, 1992.
Shelley WB, Shelley ED: *Advanced Dermatologic Diagnosis.* Philadelphia, Saunders, 1992.
Weinberg S, Prose NS, Kristal L: *Color Atlas of Pediatric Dermatology,* 3d ed. New York, McGraw-Hill, 1998.

Chapter 2–21
MALIGNANT MELANOMA
Barbara L. Sauls

DISCUSSION

Malignant melanoma is a primary cancer of melanocytes, which are the pigment-producing cells of the epidermis. Melanoma is a life-threatening condition because of the potential for rapid growth and metastases. Most lesions typically begin with a horizontal growth pattern, but all eventually develop a vertical growth phase. One type of melanoma, the nodular form, does not have a horizontal growth phase, growing only vertically into a papule and into the skin. It is during the horizontal growth phase that lesions are detectable and more easily cured. Once deeper growth has occurred, the cure rate and longevity greatly decreases. Sun exposure, light skin, and poor tanning capability predispose an individual to melanoma. Individuals with red and blond hair are especially susceptible. Dark skin is protective. A history of previous, blistering sunburn, especially before age 5, has been statistically correlated to later development of melanoma, as does being immunocompromised. There seems to be a hereditary component, and the presence of a congenital melanocytic nevus or multiple melanocytic nevi is cause for concern. Metastases may occur in any tissue with the brain and liver being favored sites; even the choroid of the eye has been affected.

Figure 2-21-1 (Plate 17). A C-shaped malignant melanoma of the abdomen. (*Courtesy of Harold Milstein, MD, The Dermatology Center, Hazleton, PA.*)

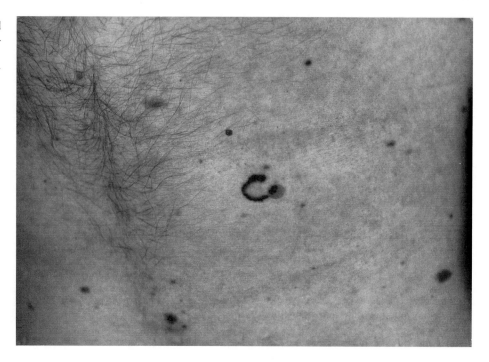

Individuals of all ages are affected, but the average age of 40 is in marked contrast with other types of sun-caused cancer (basal cell carcinoma, and squamous cell carcinoma) whose incidence increases with age. Women frequently develop melanoma on the back or lower legs, while the back is the most common site in men. Melanoma may develop on the palms, soles, and nailbeds of those with dark skin, presumably owing to a lesser amount of pigment in that area. There are three principal types of melanomas that occur in persons with white skin: *lentigo maligna melanoma,* which is the least common; *superficial spreading melanoma,* which is the most common; and *nodular melanoma.* The nodular form has a propensity for rapid vertical growth. *Acral lentiginous melanoma,* which occurs on the soles, palms, and ungual areas, is found most frequently in those with dark skin, whereas whites typically have the superficial spreading form [see Figs. 2-21-1 to 2-21-3 (Plates 17 to 19)].

SIGNS AND SYMPTOMS

Patients present with a lesion that has changed in color, has multiple colors, and exhibits irregular borders. Melanoma may develop in sites of a "mole," or nevus, that becomes larger and irregular, and with colors ranging from black to blue, browns, reds, pink, or tan. There may be itching or bleeding associated with these lesions, but pain is not noted.

OBJECTIVE FINDINGS

Clinicians should be aware of the **ABCDES** of malignant melanoma. Any or all of these conditions warrant further investigation.

A is for **asymmetry** of the lesion. (The right side does not look like the left.)

Figure 2-21-2 (Plate 18). A nodular malignant melanoma of the abdomen. (*Courtesy of Harold Milstein, MD, The Dermatology Center, Hazleton, PA.*)

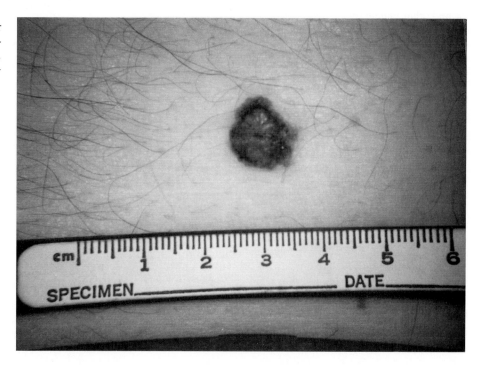

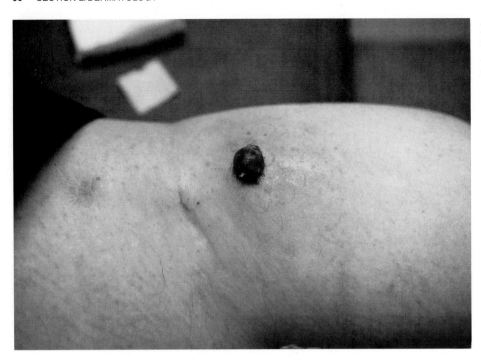

Figure 2-21-3 (Plate 19). Malignant melanoma of the leg. (*Courtesy of Harold Milstein, MD, The Dermatology Center, Hazleton, PA.*)

B is for **border** irregularity. This area can be deeply notched or scalloped, or ill-defined in appearance.

C is for changing or multiple **colors**, or mottling.

D is for a **diameter** of greater than 5 or 6 mm.

E is for **elevation** which is almost always present. It is possible to note this with side lighting, but it may not be palpable.

S is for **shadowing** which is the ''bleeding'' of the border of the lesions into the surrounding tissue. This appears lighter in color.

DIAGNOSTIC CONSIDERATIONS

The differential diagnosis of malignant melanoma includes various benign nevi, basal cell carcinoma, a tattoo from a lead (graphite) pencil, dye, or other procedure or trauma, seborrheic keratosis, and other benign pigmented lesions. More nevi are round or oval and have smooth borders, though this is not always the case. Seborrheic keratoses are dark, waxy, ''stuck-on'' lesions and are usually distinguishable on physical examination. However, if there is any question as to the diagnosis, a biopsy is warranted. The patient may be able to remember a specific incident like having a tattoo or getting a lead pencil stuck in the area.

SPECIAL CONSIDERATIONS

Immunocompromised individuals are at greater risk for the development of skin cancers of any type. Special care for prevention and periodic examination is essential.

Individuals born with a congenital nevomelanocytic or hairy nevus have a high incidence of melanoma developing in that area. The bigger, darker, and more irregular the lesion, the greater the risk of malignant transformation. It is recommended to have all children evaluated by a dermatologist and lesions removed as soon as they are old enough to tolerate the procedure. Extensive lesions of this type often require skin grafting after removal.

LABORATORY TESTS

Prompt referral for excisional biopsy with thin margins is currently recommended to confirm the diagnosis. It is possible to

perform a punch or incisional biopsy initially if an excisional biopsy cannot be performed, such as if the lesion is quite large and would require extensive surgical removal. In this case, it is important to biopsy the darkest, most elevated portion of the lesion.

TREATMENT

Surgical excision is the treatment of choice. Because of the high rate of metastases of this cancer, all patients are staged depending on thickness, extension, node, and organ involvement. Some patients may be candidates for chemotherapy, immunotherapy, or palliative radiation, though metastatic disease is generally considered incurable, so early detection and removal while the lesion is still thin is of utmost importance.

PATIENT EDUCATION

As with all skin cancers the avoidance of sun exposure is essential. Sun screens, long-sleeve shirts and pants, and remaining in the shade from 10 A.M. to 2 P.M. daily is recommended. Patients should perform self-skin examination monthly and report any changing lesion immediately. Their partners should participate in this, since it is difficult to examine all areas of the back and lower extremities completely.

DISPOSITION

After treatment, a fully unclothed skin examination by a medical provider should be performed every 3 months for 1 year, every 6 months for another year, then yearly for the patient's lifetime.

COMPLICATIONS AND RED FLAGS

This condition is most appropriately referred to a dermatologist or plastic surgeon for initial evaluation, follow-up, and treatment. Plastic surgeons often perform excisional surgery for lesions on the face or if skin grafting may be required.

PEARLS

Always maintain an index of suspicion when examining lesions. Give patients the benefit of the doubt and biopsy any lesions that are not definitely and completely benign. In this case, a life may be saved. Be sure to keep the patient in mind during the examination, for instance, a redhead with heavily sun-damaged skin would require careful examination.

BIBLIOGRAPHY

Fauci AS, Braunwald E, Isselbacher KJ, et al (eds): *Harrison's Principles of Internal Medicine,* 14th ed. New York, McGraw-Hill, 1998.

Fitzpatrick TB, Johnson RA, Wolff K, et al: *Color Atlas and Synopsis of Clinical Dermatology: Common and Serious Diseases,* 3d ed. New York, McGraw-Hill, 1997.

Chapter 2–22
MOLLUSCUM CONTAGIOSUM
Barbara L. Sauls

DISCUSSION

Molluscum contagiosum, which is caused by a poxvirus, exhibits discrete, small papular lesions that are scattered and most commonly found on the neck, trunk, and anogenital area. HIV infection may be associated with multiple (often hundreds) facial lesions that often become quite large. The lesions are seen more commonly in males, but are found in both children and adults. Those seen in adults may have been sexually transmitted. Lesions commonly develop over a period of one to several months, and spontaneous resolution over months to years is not uncommon.

SIGNS AND SYMPTOMS

Other than the small, discrete, papular lesions, there are no other associated symptoms such as itching, pain, or burning. These lesions are usually pointed out during a routine visit. If they develop a secondary bacterial infection, they may become pruritic or tender. This may occur in sites of recurrent irritation such as collar areas or areas that are constantly rubbed from sitting or if they are picked at inadvertently by the patient.

OBJECTIVE FINDINGS

Physical examination shows one to many discrete, round or oval papules that are pearly flesh colored and umbilicated. They are usually 1 to 2 mm in diameter and are rarely larger. If seen in an HIV infection, they can be up to five times this size. These lesions are nontender to touch and are usually firm [see Fig. 2-22-1 (Plate 20)].

DIAGNOSTIC CONSIDERATIONS

Differential diagnoses include basal cell carcinoma, which may present as a nodular area with central indentation, and kerato-acanthoma, which is more like a crater with a central plug.

HIV infection should be suspected if an individual presents with a number of large lesions of this type. This may be their initial presentation.

Genital and perianal molluscum lesions in children are suspicious of sexual abuse and require further investigation.

LABORATORY TESTS

It is not necessary to biopsy these lesions, though a Giemsa stain of the core will reveal inclusion bodies called *molluscum bodies.* This sample may be obtained without local anesthesia using the bevel of a needle or a pointed scalpel. With local anesthesia, a punch biopsy or curettage of the lesions may be taken.

TREATMENT

Treatment is often unnecessary, since there is often spontaneous resolution of these lesions. If the lesions are in an area that is

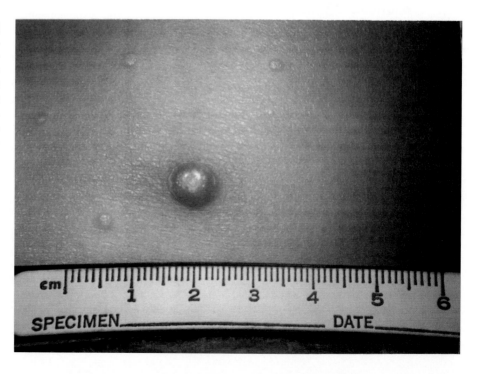

Figure 2-22-1 (Plate 20). Several small molluscum lesions with one giant lesion on the chest. Note the central umbilication and the irritation associated with the larger lesion. In this case, it is appropriate to remove the lesions because of the irritation. (*Courtesy of Harold Milstein, MD, The Dermatology Center, Hazleton, PA.*)

highly visible or frequently irritated, it is possible to lightly freeze or electrocauterize them with complete resolution. Curettage is also possible. It is unnecessary to treat the core completely; a light touch is all that is needed.

Destruction with a topical application of cantherone is occasionally used, particularly in children.

PATIENT EDUCATION

Teach patients to leave the areas alone after treatment and to use a topical antibiotic ointment if they should develop redness. Since this is a poxvirus infection, it is necessary to tell patients that this does not cure the viral infection, and lesions may develop in the future, though not necessarily in the same area. These lesions are not typically infectious, but can be transmitted sexually.

Since children are seen routinely for health maintenance examinations, it is often possible to convince parents to leave the lesions alone for the time being, with reassurance that future treatment will be available should they spread or not resolve spontaneously. This prevents unnecessary stress to children, especially if they are young and uncooperative with the treatments.

BIBLIOGRAPHY

Fauci AS, Braunwald E, Isselbacher KJ, et al (eds): *Harrison's Principles of Internal Medicine*, 14th ed. New York, McGraw-Hill, 1998.

Fitzpatrick TB, Johnson RA, Wolff K, et al: *Color Atlas and Synopsis of Clinical Dermatology: Common and Serious Diseases*, 3d ed. New York, McGraw-Hill, 1997.

Chapter 2–23
PITYRIASIS ROSEA
Michelle DiBaise

DISCUSSION

Pityriasis rosea is an acute, papulosquamous dermatosis of unknown etiology. It is relatively common, usually asymptomatic, and self-limiting. Pityriasis rosea is characterized by the development of a single large lesion, the "herald patch" followed by a generalized eruption with a distinctive pattern, predominantly on the trunk. The majority of patients are between the ages of 10 and 35 years, but pityriasis rosea has been seen in all ages ranging from 4 months to 78 years.[1-4] There is evidence that pityriasis rosea is viral in origin. It demonstrates seasonal variation with a peak in the winter months. As many as 20 percent of patients can relate a recent history of an infectious syndrome including headache, fatigue, sore throat, lymphadenitis, and fever.[2,4] Small epidemics have been noted to occur on military bases and in fraternities.[2] However, despite these findings, pityriasis rosea is seen uncommonly among household contacts. Attempts to isolate an organism have been unsuccessful as have attempts to experimentally transmit the disease. Pityriasis rosea appears to be more common among atopic individuals and slightly more common in women. The entire disease process resolves in approx-imately 6 to 8 weeks. About 2 percent of patients develop a recurrence.[1-4]

SIGNS AND SYMPTOMS

On presentation, the majority of patients are asymptomatic. The patient may relate a history of a recent viral syndrome followed by the development of a single lesion. Within a few days to weeks, the patient develops a generalized eruption. If the patient is symptomatic, the main complaint is pruritus. The pruritus of pityriasis rosea ranges from mild to moderate. Severe itching may accompany extensive eruptions.

OBJECTIVE FINDINGS

The herald patch can usually be identified by the patient as being the first lesion to appear, however, it only occurs in about 80 percent of patients.[1-4] It is the largest of the lesions and ranges in size from 2 to 10 cm. It is an ovoid to round plaque, with a fine scale at the periphery. The scale edge faces toward the center of the lesion and has been described as a trailing or inverse marginal collarette. The generalized eruption follows in a few days to weeks with the average time ranging from 7 to 14 days.[1-4] The early lesions may be papular. In most cases, however, the lesions have the same appearance as the herald patch, but are smaller in size, 1 to 2 cm. The lesions range in color from a pink or salmon color in those with light skin to hyperpigmented in those with darker skin. The multiple lesions are scattered and discrete, reach a peak in 1 to 2 weeks, and number from a few to hundreds. They appear mainly on the trunk and proximal extremities, but can appear on the arms, legs, and face in severe cases [see Fig. 2-23-1 (Plate 21) and Fig. 2-23-2]. The long axis of the lesions follows the lines of cleavage of the skin in a pattern that has been called a Christmas tree. In children, pityriasis rosea can more commonly involve the face. A papular variant is seen more commonly in young children, pregnant women, and those with darker skin. Vesicles, purpura, pustules, and lesions that appear as erythema multiforme but occur in the typical distribution of pityriasis rosea are also seen and develop more commonly in infants and children. Oral lesions, have been reported and have a variety of appearances including erythematous macules, hemorrhagic lesions, and small ulcerations.[1-6] The disease resolves spontaneously in 2 weeks to 2 months with an average of 6 weeks.[1-4] Patients may have residual postinflammatory hyperpigmentation, especially those with darker skin. If pityriasis rosea has an atypical presentation, the practitioner should look for other causes of the eruption. Atypical manifestations include lesions on the face and neck only, the absence of a herald patch or a herald patch that is the only manifestation of the disease, lesions on the palms and soles, and a patient who appears systematically ill. If the eruption persists for more than 6 to 8 weeks, a skin biopsy should be considered to rule out other disorders.

DIAGNOSTIC CONSIDERATIONS

The herald patch can be misdiagnosed as tinea corporis. A KOH preparation will not show the hyphae and spores consistent with a fungal infection.

Erythema chronica migrans is a solitary annular lesion associated with Lyme disease that extends from the periphery. It can be differentiated from the herald patch by a lack of scale. There may also be noted a central punctum where the tick bite occured.

Several disorders can mimic the generalized eruption of pityriasis rosea. Guttate psoriasis has a sudden onset with small, discrete lesions that have a similar distribution to pityriasis rosea. The patient may also have a history of recent streptococcal pharyngitis. For the most part, the scale of psoriasis is thick and silvery

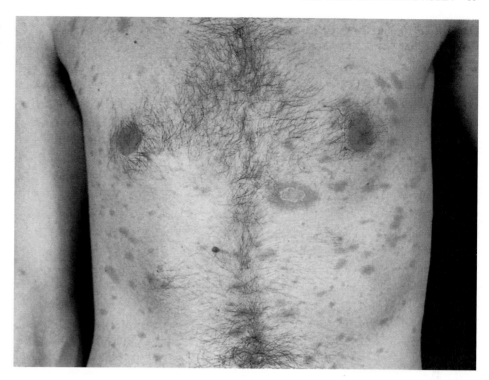

Figure 2-23-1 (Plate 21). Pityriasis rosea. (*From Fitzpatrick, Johnson, Wolff, et al.*)

and distributed throughout the lesion. The course of guttate psoriasis is longer than that of pityriasis rosea.

Generalized lichen planus can also mimic pityriasis rosea in its distribution. The lesions of lichen planus are described as polygonal, purple papules, which can help distinguish it from pityriasis rosea.

Pityriasis lichenoides chronica, also known as chronic or guttate parapsoriasis, is an uncommon disorder in which the lesions may be similar in appearance to those of pityriasis rosea, but is a chronic rather than transient condition.

Drug eruptions should also be considered in the differential diagnosis. Usually, a drug eruption is more confluent and erythematous, there is little or no scaling, and the eruption may be more symptomatic than pityriasis rosea.

Nummular eczema may also mimic pityriasis rosea, but the onset tends to be more insidious and the course more prolonged.

Figure 2-23-2. Distribution of pityriasis rosea.

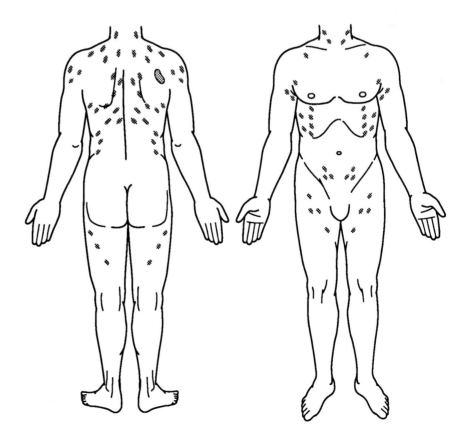

In the presence of atypical pityriasis, the most important differential diagnosis to consider is secondary syphilis. A serologic test for syphilis should be ordered for all sexually active individuals.

AIDS-associated Kaposi's sarcoma demonstrates ovoid, purpuric lesions that follow the lines of cleavage of the skin. It should be considered in the differential of the purpuric variant of pityriasis rosea.

The differential diagnosis of the vesicular variant of pityriasis rosea should include other generalized bullous disorders such as contact dermatitis to the toxicodendrons, generalized bullous impetigo, and in older individuals, pemphigus vulgaris.

LABORATORY TESTS

The diagnosis is made predominantly by the clinical findings. A skin biopsy is nonspecific and rarely indicated. If lesions persist longer than 6 to 8 weeks, a skin biopsy can help in diagnosing other conditions. A KOH test can be performed on the scale of the lesion to rule out tinea corporis. Serologic testing for syphilis should be considered for all sexually active individuals.

TREATMENT

This is a self-limited disease that usually does not require treatment. In instances where pruritus is present, antihistamines, topical corticosteroids and emollients can help alleviate symptoms. A group V topical steroid is usually sufficient to control symptoms. The rare severe case associated with intense pruritus can be treated with a 1- to 2-week course of prednisone. Ultraviolet light therapy (UV-B) has been shown to accelerate the resolution of pityriasis rosea. The treatment is most helpful when started within the first week of the eruption.[1-4]

COMPLICATIONS AND RED FLAGS

There are no complications with the exception of postinflammatory hypopigmentation or hyperpigmentation, which resolves slowly over time, often months. The residual skin changes are more common in darker skinned individuals. In pregnant women, there is no documented risk to the fetus.[2]

REFERENCES

1. Fitzpatrick TB, Johnson RA, Wolff K, et al: *Color Atlas and Synopsis of Clinical Dermatology, Common and Serious Diseases,* 3d ed. New York, McGraw-Hill, 1997, pp 104–106.
2. Habif TP: *Clinical Dermatology, A Color Guide to Diagnosis and Treatment,* 3d ed. St Louis, Mosby Yearbook, 1996, pp 218–220.
3. Arnold HL, Odom RB, James WD: *Andrews' Diseases of the Skin, Clinical Dermatology,* 8th ed. Philadelphia, Saunders, 1990, pp 231–232.
4. Bjornberg A: Pityriasis rosea, in Fitzpatrick TB, Eisen AZ, Wolff K, et al (eds): *Dermatology in General Medicine,* 4th ed. New York, McGraw-Hill, 1993, pp 1117–1123.
5. Vidimos AT, Camisa C: Tongue and cheek: Oral lesions in pityriasis rosea. *Cutis 50:276–280, 1992.*
6. Pierson JC, Dijkstra JW, Elston DM, et al: Purpuric pityriasis rosea. *J Am Acad Dermatol 28:1021, 1993.*

Chapter 2–24
PSORIASIS
Joe R. Monroe

DISCUSSION

Psoriasis is the benign, focal acceleration of the normal production, upward migration, and shedding of epidermal skin, probably of genetic origin, whose course is influenced by a complex interaction of genetic and environmental factors. It is a common skin disease, affecting around 2 percent of the population of Western countries, but a much lower percentage of the population elsewhere. Intensive ongoing research is starting to clarify its pathogenesis, but the exact cause remains elusive. It is fortunate for the patients whose lives are so deeply affected by this disease that treatment has improved tremendously over the last 30 years.

Men and women are affected equally by this disease, which occurs in all age groups. There is probably a multifactorial inheritance mode, the genetic component of which is also influenced by a variety of environmental factors. One-third of affected patients answer in the affirmative when asked about family history of psoriasis.

Exacerbations of psoriasis can be precipitated by drugs such as lithium, beta blockers, oral contraceptives, and NSAIDs; pregnancy; alcohol; any type of skin trauma; stress; and streptococcal infections. Systemic corticosteroids are also considered an exacerbating factor because of a very marked and predictable tendency for psoriasis to rebound as these drugs are withdrawn.

Plaque-type psoriasis is morphologically characterized by the appearance of round-to-oval salmon pink plaques covered by thick adherent silvery scales, tending toward symmetric involvement of extensor surfaces and scalp. Other lesser "stigmata" of psoriasis include umbilical and intergluteal involvement (so-called intergluteal pinking), pitting, and onycholysis of nails. The extent of involvement can vary a great deal and can favor one region (e.g., the scalp) over all others.

The fact that psoriasis also "koebnerizes," that is, forms along lines of trauma such as scratches, surgery, or even sunburns, can be diagnostically useful, but it should be noted that many other dermatologic conditions also koebnerize (warts, mollusca, lichen planus, and others).

CLINICAL PRESENTATION

Psoriasis' appearance can vary considerably, depending on location and type, as follows:

- *Chronic plaque psoriasis (psoriasis vulgaris)* The most common morphologic type, described above.
- *Guttate psoriasis* Characterized by the sudden appearance of multiple guttate, that is, droplike, small psoriatic plaques over widespread areas of the body. Infection [streptococcal pharyngitis or viral upper respiratory infection (URI)] may precede it by 1 to 2 weeks and is suspected as the trigger. An episode of guttate psoriasis, common in those under age 20, may be the first indication of the patient's propensity for the disease.
- *Generalized pustular psoriasis* Also known as Von Zumbusch's psoriasis, this type is characterized by a sudden appearance of widespread tiny pustules on a psoriatic base with progression toward coalescence. It is occasionally fatal, always difficult to treat and, fortunately, unusual.
- *Psoriatic erythroderma* Total involvement ("red man"), mostly in patients with previously diagnosed proriasis, this form may come up with steroid withdrawal. Methotrexate is often needed in these cases.
- *Light-induced psoriasis* This is exaggerated koebnerization to sun damage in a few unfortunate sun-sensitive individuals with preexisting psoriasis.
- *Scalp* The scalp is a favored area for psoriasis. It can be mild, or can present a particular treatment challenge. Often very disturbing to patients because of appearance and itching, it may spill over onto forehead, ears, or neck. Psoriasis itself does not cause hair loss, even with extensive scalp involvement, which may be the only manifestation of the disease. It is often mistaken for tinea capitis.

- *Psoriasis of palms and soles* This may be part of generalized psoriasis but is often the only manifestation. It can look very eczema-like (brownish, maculopapular) or more typically psoriatic (whitish scales on dusky red base). It is also frequently mistaken for fungal infection.
- *Pustular psoriasis of palms and soles.* This is distinguished by painful, tiny pustules along with erythema and scaling.
  Psoriasis of flexural folds Not uncommon, this is also known as inverse psoriasis. Shiny salmon pink to dusky red plaques in axillae, genitals, groin, and intergluteal and inframammary skin probably represents the process of koebnerization. Because of friction and moisture in these areas, scale is notably lacking, producing a confusing clinical picture.
- *Nail psoriasis* This form includes tiny pits in the nail plate, color changes, onycholysis, subungual debris, and dystrophy. Similar changes can been seen in other diseases such as eczema and lichen planus, but the finding of tiny "thimble" pits in nail plates can be very helpful in corroborating the diagnosis of psoriasis. This can be the patient's only manifestation of the disease and presents a particular treatment challenge. It is very commonly mistaken for fungal disease and affects fingernails more than toenails.
- *Psoriatic arthritis* The incidence in the psoriatic population is 7 to 20 percent, with women slightly outnumbering men. The most common pattern is an asymmetric arthritis classically involving a single digit ("sausage finger"). Other types include a seronegative asymmetric polyarthritis resembling rheumatoid arthritis. The most severe form of psoriatic arthritis is called arthritis mutilans, involving osteolysis of the small bones of the hands and feet leading to gross deformity and subluxation, similar to that seen in rheumatoid arthritis. Psoriatic arthritis is common enough that routine history taking from psoriasis patients should always include questions about joint pain.

DIFFERENTIAL DIAGNOSIS

The differential diagnosis varies, depending on the location and type of disease, but includes seborrheic dermatitis, pityriasis rosea, dermatophyte infection, nummular eczema, secondary syphilis, monoarticular arthritis (seronegative), and skin cancers [mycosis fungoides (cutaneous T-cell lymphoma), squamous cell carcinoma, Paget's disease].

LABORATORY

Punch biopsy of skin lesions can be quite helpful showing fusing and elongation of rete ridges, parakeratosis, lymphocytic perivascular infiltrate, or Munro's microabscesses. Biopsy of early psoriatic lesions is notoriously misleading since the above changes are incomplete. Moreover, so-called psoriasiform changes in biopsy reports can be quite nonspecific for psoriasis itself and are commonly found in many other diseases.

TREATMENT

Although no cure is currently available, a number of topical and systemic agents can be quite helpful. However, some attention must first be paid to eliminating possible exacerbators, such as medications (e.g., lithium, beta blockers), alcohol, stress, chronic infection, and scratching.

It is also advisable to determine the patient's expectations for treatment, since patients vary greatly in their tolerance for this disease. Some are very accepting of it and require little treatment, whereas others find it devastating and need ongoing expert treatment.

Other factors to consider before treating include extent and visibility of affected areas, symptoms, type of psoriasis, function of the affected skin (e.g., hands and feet or genitals), patient's age and health, and past treatment history, that is, what worked and what did not.

The primary care provider can safely attempt topical treatment, but should have a very low threshold for referral to a dermatologist as the disease progresses. The dermatologist will not only have a better understanding of the disease and experience with difficult cases but also will have expertise with a wider variety of treatment modalities, particularly UV-A and UV-B phototherapy, and powerful systemic medications. In short, there is no reason for the primary care provider to struggle with an unresponsive psoriasis patient.

Most topical treatments and some systemic medications are subject to the phenomenon called *tachyphylaxis,* in which continued use of the same agent, especially topical steroids, leads to progressive diminution of therapeutic affect and is combatted by rotating treatment with different agents. It should also be noted that combinations of treatment agents and modalities are often used. For example, UV-A and UV-B plus tar and calcipotriene or methotrexate and psoralen plus UV-A light treatment (PUVA) help avoid tachyphylaxis and reduce undesirable side effects such as skin cancer from UV modalities.

TREATMENT AGENTS

Emollients

Safe, effective, and inexpensive, these include petroleum jelly, Eucerin cream, mineral oil, and many other agents that can be very useful to hydrate, soften, and loosen scale.

Topical Corticosteroids

These are the mainstays of psoriasis treatment, especially plaque-type, having anti-inflammatory, antiproliferative, and antimitotic activity. They are much more effective when psoriatic scale has been removed with emollients or after soaking the lesions in warm water. They also work better under occlusion (with plastic wrap or hydrocolloid covering) because of enhanced hydration and decreased trauma.

The thicker the skin, the stronger the steroid preparation to be used. For example, facial (especially eyelids), intertriginous, and genital skin are thinner than elbow, knee, and truncal skin. So, although the latter areas need strong preparations such as betamethasone valerate or clobetasol propionate ointments, the former only require 1 to 2.5% hydrocortisone because they could be adversely affected by the stronger preparations. Even on thicker skin, prolonged application (e.g., more than 2 weeks bid) of the stronger products could not only cause atrophy, but also unsightly striae and telangiectases. The hands and palms, being the thickest skin on the body, can be treated longer and stronger than all other areas.

Tachyphylaxis is a problem, especially with the stronger steroid preparations, and if weekly use exceeds 50 g. Prolonged and widespread use of these agents can even cause adrenal suppression; therefore, steroid-sparing agents like calciprotriene or anthralin are used instead for a time, until they, too, become relatively ineffective.

Intralesional Steroids

For small but persistent psoriatic plaques (up to 3 cm), intralesional injection of triamcinolone acetonide (Kenalog and others) in an aqueous suspension of 5 mg/mL is quite effective. Possible side effects include local atrophy, systemic absorption, and adrenal suppression. *Note:* If the injection does not require a fair amount of force, the medicine is probably being placed too deeply in the tissue.

Other Topical Agents

These include anthralin (Lasan or Anthra-Derm, Drithocreme), calcipotriene ointment (Dovonex), and various tar-containing formulations used in combination with emollients, often under occlusion.

Systemic Corticosteroids

These are very rarely used except in the most extraordinary situations because of the aforementioned tendency for psoriasis to rebound with a vengeance on withdrawal of systemic corticosteroids. For this reason, the presence of psoriasis also constitutes a relative contraindication to the use of such agents for other disease states in a patient.

Other Systemic Agents

Methotrexate, cyclosporine, and sulfasalazine are powerful drugs traditionally reserved for use by dermatologists only in the most difficult cases. Some dermatologists believe that bacterial and/or fungal antigens drive psoriasis in certain difficult cases for which they give drugs such as Duricef and/or Diflucan on a long-term basis, but this is controversial.

Psoralen Plus UV-A Light Treatment

The oral drug psoralen, a potent photosensitizer, is given, followed later by UV-A light exposure on a regular basis as a very effective treatment for recalcitrant psoriasis. This mode requires special equipment and expertise and is therefore used only under the direction of a dermatologist, who will sometimes prescribe UV-B treatment instead. For many patients, natural sunlight is quite beneficial.

TREATMENT OF SCALP PSORIASIS

Scalp psoriasis is particularly difficult to treat because of the hindrance that the hair itself presents, both to local application of medications and in shielding the scalp from phototherapy. Scalp psoriasis quite frequently itches, leading to scratching, which produces even more scale, which must be removed or at least thinned before other medications (e.g., steroids) can reach the actual diseased skin. In that regard, the use of salicyclic acid shampoos (T-Sal shampoo or 20% salicyclic acid in mineral oil) is quite beneficial. Once the scale is removed, tar-based shampoos (Pentrax, T-gel), and topical steroid solutions (betamethasone valerate 0.1%, or clobetasol propionate solution 0.05%) will reduce the itching, redness, and scale formation.

As for long-term maintenance, patients must be convinced that they must shampoo daily with products such as Selsun, Head and Shoulders, or T-gel, rotating these to prevent tachyphylaxis. Patients must then be cautioned to refrain from scratching, since this will negate all treatment efforts.

TREATMENT OF NAIL PSORIASIS

Difficult at best, treatment of nail psoriasis should be left to dermatologists experienced in that area. Some dermatologist–nail specialists inject matrices of involved fingers with triamcinolone. Other treatments used for nail psoriasis include topical agents such as 5-fluorouracil cream, urea paste, calcipotriene, and/or potent topical steroids.

TREATMENT OF OTHER FORMS OF PSORIASIS

Dermatologists have a number of effective agents available for treatment of refractory plaque psoriasis, pustular psoriasis, and erythrodermic psoriasis. These include methotrexate (an anticancer drug), retinoids (vitamin A–derived, such as etretinate), hydroxyurea (an anticancer drug used in combination with UV-A or UV-B therapy), cyclosporine (a powerful immunosuppressant), and others.

Phototherapy, using various combinations of UV-A and UV-B light-wave exposure alone, or in combination with tar, anthralin, and oral drugs like psoralen, is extremely useful in treating difficult cases of psoriasis.

PEARLS

Knowledge of the following points can contribute to positive patient outcome:

- Thinking fungal? Think psoriasis first.
- Ask about family history of psoriasis. Psoriasis patients often assume the practitioner knows about their disease. It's old hat to them.
- Acute exacerbation of psoriasis? Ask about (1) alcohol intake, (2) change in stress level, (3) change in medications, or (4) recent febrile illness.
- Is more than 10 percent of body surface area affected? Strongly consider referral to a dermatologist.
- Psoriasiform changes in skin biopsy do no necessarily mean the patient has psoriasis. Expand the differential diagnoses.
- Intralesional steroid injections (triamcinolone acetonide 5 mg/cm^3) is especially useful for small plaques (smaller than 3 cm), especially in the scalp.
- Never use systemic corticosteroids for psoriasis, and always ask about possible psoriasis before placing patients on it for other conditions.

PATIENT EDUCATION

Especially important for children and adolescents, it can include counseling, sick leave, and vacation (especially to sunny climates). There are special psoriasis camps for kids.

Patients should be encouraged to join the National Psoriasis Foundation: 1-800-723-9166; E-mail: 76135.2746@compuserve.com.

Patients need to know exacerbating factors, so the provider must spend the necessary time with them to make sure they understand their role in treating the disease.

PROGNOSIS

Psoriasis is a lifelong disease with genetic implications for offspring. Exacerbations and remissions characterize the clinical course, and even though treatment has vastly improved, practitioners are still unable to cure it.

BIBLIOGRAPHY

Arndt KA, Robinson JK, LeBoit PE, et al: *Cutaneous Medicine and Surgery,* Philadelphia, Saunders, 1996.

duVivier A: *Dermatology in Practice.* Philadelphia, Lippincott, 1990.

Fitzpatrick TB, Johnson RA, Wolff K, et al: *Color Atlas and Synopsis of Clinical Dermatology: Common and Serious Diseases,* 3d ed. New York, McGraw-Hill, 1997.

Goldstein BG, Goldstein AO. *Practical Dermatology,* Primary Care Series. St Louis, Mosby Year Book, 1992.

Shelley WB, Shelley ED: *Advanced Dermatologic Diagnosis.* Philadelphia, Saunders, 1992.

Weinberg S, Prose NS, Kristal L: *Color Atlas of Pediatric Dermatology,* 3d ed. New York, McGraw-Hill, 1998.

Chapter 2–25
SEBORRHEIC DERMATITIS (SEBORRHEA)

Joe R. Monroe

DISCUSSION

Seborrheic dermatitis (SD) is found in 3 to 5 percent of adults, and is a bit more common in men than in women. It is characterized by scaling and redness in areas of the face, scalp, skin folds, and presternal skin. The percentage of infants affected is unknown, but SD in babies is thought to be common. The cause is controversial.

Since it occurs mostly in areas of skin rich in oil glands also favored by the lipophilic commensal yeast *Pityrosporum ovale,* some practitioners point to the organism as this cause. As further proof, they correctly point out that SD worsens dramatically in HIV disease. However, histologic sections through affected hair follicles show no more of these microorganisms than would be normally expected and SD is often unresponsive to treatment with antifungal agents. Moreover, SD also occurs in oil-poor areas not favored at all by this organism.

Morphologically, SD in adults presents as scaly, pinkish orange patches in highly characteristic symmetric locations, especially alongside the nose, in the brows, behind the ears, and in external auditory meati. Involvement of the scalp (dandruff) is almost universal in SD patients, with diffuse, fine scaling and faint erythema, if any. Patches often crop up in areas of the face covered by a mustache or beard.

As it moves off the face, SD tends to become more weepy and exudative, especially in the umbilicus. On occasion, it can also affect presternal, axillary, genital, upper intergluteal, and even the interscapular skin. Seborrheic blepharoconjunctivitis and styes can accompany SD.

Adult SD often itches, very predictably in the scalp, but variably elsewhere.

This is not the case with infants who have SD; they do not seem to be bothered at all by even moderately severe cases. Infant SD usually presents in the first 6 months of life and is typically gone by 1 year of age, reappearing in late adolescence, if at all. Unlike adult SD, it favors the scalp, where thick, greasy scales develop (so-called cradle cap) but is also seen in the flexural creases and diaper area. Its morphology is a little different from adult SD, being composed mostly of shiny, erythematous plaques with well-defined borders, often with florid intensity.

DIFFERENTIAL DIAGNOSIS

Face

Rosacea (unlike SD, is composed of papules, pustules, and telangiectases) and perioral dermatitis (affects mostly young women, appears acneiform, frequently involves the inappropriate use of exacerbating topical steroids on the face) are part of the differential diagnosis.

Scalp

Psoriasis should be included in the differential diagnosis. SD is characterized by diffuse, fine scaling, with minimal erythema, whereas psoriasis presents with focal heavy scaling on an erythematous base. Pediculosis should be included too. Look for nits and for the tell-tale find red rash on the nape of the neck seen with head lice.

Intertriginous

SD in these areas appears orangish pink and shiny, with little scaling, in contrast to SD look-alikes in these areas, such as fungal infection (KOH-positive), candidiasis (which will exhibit satellites, unlike adult SD), contact dermatitis, and psoriasis, which can sometimes be difficult to distinguish from SD.

LABORATORY

Biopsy is seldom necessary, but it can occasionally be helpful, showing spongiosis (intraepidermal edema), a nonspecific finding, but useful in distinguishing SD from psoriasis.

TREATMENT

Infants

Cradle-cap responds well to a 2% salicyclic acid in olive oil mixture, which breaks up the scale nicely.

Adults

The following steps are recommended:

1. Daily shampooing with OTC dandruff shampoos such as Head and Shoulders, Selsun, or T-gel, leaving it in place for 5 min before rinsing
2. Hydrocortisone 1% cream, up to twice a day application to the face as needed for itching and redness
3. T-sal (OTC) shampoo to thin out heavy scale in the scalp (use carefully, according to directions)
4. For scalp itching: mid-strength steroid solution, such as betamethasone valerate 0.1%, up to twice a day, for no more than 3 days in a row
5. For resistant cases, Nizoral (ketoconazole) shampoo for scalp and face, or an oral antifungal such as fluconazole (Diflucan) 200 mg bid for a week (see package insert for drug interactions)

PATIENT EDUCATION

Teach patients about the following:

1. Daily shampooing is a necessity.
2. Limit hat wearing, which makes SD worse.
3. Make sure the patient understands that a cure is not possible, that control is the goal.
4. Educate as to the noncontagious nature of SD.

PEARLS

Knowledge of the following points can contribute to positive patient outcome:

- Pruritic patchy midsternal scaling and redness is probably SD, which responds well to antifungal creams in this area.
- Sudden appearance or exacerbation of SD suggests two possibilities: HIV disease or Parkinson's.
- SD in infants seems to be asymptomatic, and thus does not require treatment except in the scalp.

PROGNOSIS

No permanent cure exists. SD tends to improve with age in adults. Infant SD associated with diarrhea and failure to thrive suggests an entity called Leiner's disease, which can be life-threatening. These children need prompt evaluation by a dermatologist or pediatrician.

BIBLIOGRAPHY

Arndt KA, Robinson JK, LeBoit PE, et al: *Cutaneous Medicine and Surgery.* Philadelphia, Saunders, 1996.

deVivier A: *Dermatology in Practice.* Philadelphia, Lippincott, 1990.

Fitzpatrick TB, Johnson RA, Wolff K, et al: *Color Atlas and Synopsis of Clinical Dermatology: Common and Serious Diseases,* 3d ed. New York, McGraw-Hill, 1997.

Goldstein BG, Goldstein AO: *Practical Dermatology,* Primary Care Series. St Louis, Mosby Year Book, 1992.

Shelley WB, Shelley ED: *Advanced Dermatologic Diagnosis.* Philadelphia, Saunders, 1992.

Weinberg S, Prose NS, Kristal L: *Color Atlas of Pediatric Dermatology,* 3d ed. New York, McGraw-Hill, 1998.

Chapter 2–26
SEBORRHEIC KERATOSIS ("SENILE KERATOSIS")
Joe R. Monroe

DISCUSSION

Seborrheic keratosis is an extremely common, benign, pigmented epidermal keratotic papular lesion that becomes more common with increasing age. Not a disease at all, but a name for the most common benign lesions found on human beings, seborrheic keratoses are equally common in the sexes, and even though their cause is unknown, a definite familial tendency exists. Although easily confused with precancerous actinic keratoses, they are not related to sun exposure.

These keratoses spare high friction and moist areas such as palms, soles, and genitalia, but can be found on any other area, predominating on trunk and face.

The lesions, which usually appear in multiples, can vary quite a bit in color and configuration, the "norm" being grayish brown, warty, and dry, with a "stuck-on" appearance. However, they can also be yellowish and mostly flat, or even jet black, greasy-looking, and impressively papular, typifying the patient's idea of what skin cancer ought to look like.

In that regard, seborrheic keratoses are benign with almost no potential for malignant degeneration. However, the sudden appearance of multiple lesions has been known to accompany the occult development of internal malignancy, especially that of the gastrointestinal tract. This rare occurrence is called the Leser-Trélat sign.

On blacks, multiple tiny, soft dark-brown-to-black papules develop with age on facial skin, especially around the eyes, and are termed papulosa nigra.

Seborrheic keratoses can be quite dry, tiny, and barely pigmented, especially on legs and dorsal feet, where they are called *stucco keratoses.*

DIFFERENTIAL DIAGNOSES

Usually, the epidermal (stuck-on) appearance makes the diagnosis clear, as does the multiplicity of lesions. Occasionally, though, punch or excisional biopsy is necessary to distinguish these from melanoma, wart, or pigmented basal cell carcinoma.

LABORATORY

None required except biopsy as above.

TREATMENT

Liquid nitrogen or curettement is recomended, and excision is seldom indicated. Of those with darker skin, care needs to be exercised in treating facial seborrheic keratoses (e.g., papulosa nigra) because of a well-documented tendency for residual darkening in treatment locations that can take months to clear, called postinflammatory hyperpigmentation.

PATIENT EDUCATION

Reassure patients about the benign nature of these lesions and the almost total lack of malignant potential. For fair-skinned patients especially, use the opportunity to contrast these to melanomas, which don't often come in multiples, are not epidermal in nature, that is, tend to be more macular, and tend more toward black coloration.

PEARLS

Knowledge of the following points can contribute to positive patient outcome:

- There is no law that says a melanoma cannot occur in the middle of several seborrheic keratoses.
- If it is warty, comes off in pieces, is one of several, and appears on a patient over 35, it is probably a seborrheic keratosis.
- Liquid nitrogen treatment is often diagnostic as well as curative, since it highlights the pseudocysts (appearing as tiny pores) that pock the surfaces of the lesions.
- Seborrheic keratoses are exactly what patients imagine skin cancers look like.

PROGNOSIS

Treatment is very effective, but expect more lesions to appear.

BIBLIOGRAPHY

Arndt KA, Robinson JK, LeBoit PE, et al: *Cutaneous Medicine and Surgery.* Philadelphia, Saunders, 1996.

duVivier A: *Dermatology in Practice.* Philadelphia, Lippincott, 1990.

Fitzpatrick TB, Johnson RA, Wolff K, et al: *Color Atlas and Synopsis of Clinical Dermatology: Common and Serious Diseases,* 3d ed. New York, McGraw-Hill, 1997.

Goldstein BG, Goldstein AO: *Practical Dermatology,* Primary Care Series. St Louis, Mosby Year Book, 1992.

Shelley WB, Shelley ED: *Advanced Dermatologic Diagnosis.* Philadelphia, Saunders, 1992.

Weinberg S, Prose NS, Kristal L: *Color Atlas of Pediatric Dermatology,* 3d ed. New York, McGraw-Hill, 1998.

Chapter 2–27
SQUAMOUS CELL CARCINOMA
Barbara L. Sauls

DISCUSSION

Squamous cell carcinoma is the second most common skin cancer, behind basal cell carcinoma. The lesions arise in the epithelial keratinized cells of the skin. This cancer is able to metastasize and grows rapidly, unlike basal cell carcinoma. The typical patient is older than 50 years, has light skin with poor tanning capacity and a history of frequent sun exposure. Long-term smokers often develop lesions on the lower lip in the area that the cigarette, pipe, or cigar typically rests. These lip lesions have a high rate of metastasis. Exposure to arsenic and coal combustion by-products and chronic heat exposure have also been implicated in the development of squamous cell carcinoma. Dark-skinned individuals may get this disease from toxic agents, rather than sun exposure. Occupations at risk include individuals who work outdoors (e.g., farmers, construction workers, fisherman) and those with industrial exposure to chemical carcinogens. Individuals who travel to foreign countries, either on their own or perhaps with the military, may have been exposed to arsenic in water sources.

Actinic keratosis, cheilitis, and leukoplakia are precursors of squamous cell carcinoma. Squamous cell carcinoma that arises in an actinic keratosis is believed to have less potential for metastases. Bowen's disease is a form of squamous carcinoma that remains superficial, though this form occurs on sun-exposed and protected sites, as well as internally. This lesion is also associated with arsenic exposure.

Patients with a previous diagnosis of certain subtypes of human papilloma virus (HPV) frequently develop squamous cell carcinoma of the anal area, penis, and cervix. Immunosuppression also promotes development of both squamous and basal cell carcinomas.

SIGNS AND SYMPTOMS

Patients typically present with a slowly evolving, nonhealing, ulcerated or scaling lesion, though there is a wide variety of presentation. Presentation may simply be a scaly erythematous patch or a keratotic nodule.

OBJECTIVE FINDINGS

The most common presentation of squamous cell carcinoma is a nonhealing, elevated, ulcerated, nodular lesion, but it may also present as a firm papule or plaque. Erosion may or may not be present. The lesion is usually reddish in color and isolated. Typical areas of occurrence are sun-exposed: tops of ears, nose, cheek, the scalp in bald persons, tops of hands, and forearms.

There may be localized lymphadenopathy.

DIAGNOSTIC CONSIDERATIONS

The differential diagnoses of squamous cell carcinoma are few. Paget's disease, basal cell carcinoma, and eczematous lesions may resemble squamous carcinoma and need to be differentiated through biopsy.

SPECIAL CONSIDERATIONS

Smokers have a predisposition to lip and oropharyngeal lesions, often beginning as leukoplakia. It is common for smokers to develop leukoplakia on the buccal mucosa. Any leukoplakia should be biopsied when first observed, then monitored on a regular basis thereafter if the initial pathology report is benign.

LABORATORY TESTS

Biopsy is required for definitive diagnosis of any suspicious skin lesions.

TREATMENT

Surgery and radiation are used for the treatment of squamous cell carcinoma. The choice depends on the location, size, and shape of the lesion, as well as age and the overall condition of the patient.

Precancerous lesions such as actinic keratoses should be treated with topical chemotherapy such as 5-fluorouracil (5-FU) cream, cryotherapy, or surgical removal.

PATIENT EDUCATION

Since the majority of cases of squamous cell carcinoma are due to sun exposure, patients must be counseled to avoid the sun from 10 A.M. to 2 P.M and to use a sunscreen, hat, long sleeves, and long pants when they are in the sun.

Routine skin examination is required, with close attention paid to developing lesions or areas of leukoplakia. Patients should be instructed to notify the practitioner of any new or changing lesions and not to wait until their next scheduled appointment to have these lesions evaluated.

COMPLICATIONS AND RED FLAGS

These lesions should be treated by a dermatologist. A prompt referral is needed after the initial diagnosis is made.

BIBLIOGRAPHY

Fauci AS, Braunwald E, Isselbacher KJ, et al (eds): *Harrison's Principles of Internal Medicine,* 14th ed. New York, McGraw-Hill, 1998.
Fitzpatrick TB, Johnson RA, Wolff K, et al: *Color Atlas and Synopsis of Clinical Dermatology: Common and Serious Diseases,* 3d ed. New York, McGraw-Hill, 1997.

Chapter 2–28
TINEA INFECTIONS OF THE SKIN (TINEA CORPORIS, TINEA CAPITIS, TINEA CRURIS, TINEA PEDIS, TINEA VERSICOLOR)
Barbara L. Sauls

DISCUSSION

Tinea is a term used to describe superficial dermatophyte infections of keratinized tissue such as the skin, nails, and hair. The most common causative organisms include *Trichophyton, Microsporum,* and *Epidermophyton* species. Tinea versicolor is an exception and is caused by the nondermatophyte fungus *Pityrosporum*. These infections are acquired from other individuals, from the skin of animals, or less commonly from the soil.

Tinea pedis occurs most commonly and often becomes a chronic condition. It is promoted by warm, wet environments and hot and humid weather. Individuals who bathe infrequently, sweat heavily, and do not dry themselves properly, especially between the toes, are at great risk for developing tinea infections of the feet and groin. Tinea capitis is most common in children. Tinea cruris is usually seen in adult male athletes or obese individuals in the warm, moist environment of body folds.

There is an increased incidence of tinea infections in the late spring and summer months when the weather is more hot and humid. Adult blacks seem to have a lower incidence of fungal skin infections, whereas immunosuppressed persons have a higher incidence, and their infections are more difficult to treat.

SIGNS AND SYMPTOMS

Tinea Capitis

Patients most commonly report circular areas of alopecia with little or no pruritus.

Tinea Corporis

This is also referred to as *ringworm*. This infection presents as a reddish, raised, pruritic lesion that grows into a circular (annular) shape. The center of the lesion often clears, and the border tends to be elevated and scaly. There may be more than one lesion present.

Tinea Pedis

This is also known as *athlete's foot*. Patients complain of burning, itching, and peeling of the skin of the feet. This most commonly occurs in the web spaces of the toes. Subacute or chronic conditions may have various stages from dry scaling to edema and maceration.

Tinea Cruris

This condition is also known as *jock itch* and presents as reddened, moist skin in the groin area with itching and burning, notably sparing the scrotum.

Tinea Versicolor

This condition is also known as pityriasis versicolor. Presentation in light-skinned individuals is usually as mildly scaling, well demarcated, hyperpigmented areas. Lesions may occasionally be hypopigmented and confused with vitiligo. Those with dark skin typically have hypopigmented lesions, though they may barely be perceptible. There are no other skin symptoms associated with this infection. Distribution over the shoulders, upper trunk, and arms is called "mantle" distribution and is a common characteristic.

OBJECTIVE FINDINGS

Tinea Capitis

Physical examination of the hair and scalp typically reveals hair shafts that are broken off close to the scalp. This area feels fuzzy when it is rubbed as opposed to alopecia, which does not. *Microsporum* infection usually causes broken hair shafts and is called *gray patch ringworm*. *Trichophyton* infection causes hair to break, and appears as black dots, and is called *black dot ringworm*. *Kerion* has inflammatory pustular areas where hairs fall out when tugged. *Favus* is caused by a *Trichophyton* species. This type of fungal infection develops yellowish crusts and scales called scutula. It has areas of atrophy and scar formation that heal as scarring alopecia. There may also be a secondary bacterial infection of the scalp.

Tinea Corporis

Examination shows one or more lesions that began as red areas and expanded into raised, red borders with central clearing, giving justification to the *ringworm* name. The border is often scaly. These lesions can become quite large and are usually well demarcated.

Tinea Pedis

Examination of the feet shows moist, macerated skin with whitish scales, erosions, vesicles, or bullae. The most common site of infection is the area between the third and fourth toe, which in untreated cases, will often extend to the sole and other interdigital spaces. The sides and soles of the feet may also demonstrate a dry, scaly nonpruritic dermatitis. This is often seen in a "moccasin" pattern.

Tinea Cruris

Physical examination often demonstrates a symmetric, large red plaque with sharp margins that are slightly elevated with light scaling over the intertriginous area and inner thighs. The scrotum is usually not affected by tinea infection, though this is not the case with another fungal infection of the groin, which is caused by *Candida*. Satellite lesions are not seen. Pustules are occasionally seen.

Tinea Versicolor

Physical examination findings include sharply marginated macules that are scattered and discrete. Colors vary from normal skin and range from white to brown, with all shades in between. Caucasians usually have darker patches, whereas those with dark skin have lighter patches. A fine scale may be present. The lesions are most commonly found on the trunk, arms, abdomen, and thighs, and rarely on the face.

DIAGNOSTIC CONSIDERATIONS

The following points should be considered in the diagnosis:

- *Tinea capitis* Alopecia, trichotillomania (hair-pulling), or bacterial folliculitis may resemble the various forms of tinea capitis.
- *Tinea corporis* Psoriasis or cellulitis should be considered.
- *Tinea pedis* In less-severe cases, it is possible to confuse this infection with contact dermatitis.
- *Tinea cruris* Cellulitis or candidiasis may resemble tinea cruris.
- *Tinea versicolor* Hypopigmented lesions may be confused with vitiligo. The presence of scaling is more suggestive of tinea.

SPECIAL CONSIDERATIONS

Fungal infections are often the hallmark of an immunocompromised state, such as diabetes or HIV, and may require further investigation. Fungal infections are notoriously difficult to treat in any immunocompromised patients. The course of treatment is often prolonged and complicated by other medications and therapies.

Care should be taken when prescribing oral antifungal medications since some are potentially hepatotoxic. Intraconazole (Sporanox) and terbinafine (Lamisil) have not been shown to be hepatotoxic.

LABORATORY TESTS

Many tinea skin infections can be diagnosed with a potassium hydroxide (KOH) preparation. This is performed by scraping a small amount of tissue from scales, hair shafts, or pustular areas with the edge of a scalpel onto a microscope slide. A drop or two of 10% KOH solution is placed on the scrapings to lyse the epithelial cells and make the hyphae and buds more easily visible. A glass cover slip is placed over the scrapings, and the slide is gently heated (not boiled). Examine under a microscope at low power. Look for the long filaments of *hyphae*, either straight or coiled together, and multiple *buds*, either alone or attached to the hyphae, like grapes.

A fungal culture will confirm these results and determine the exact organism causing the infection. Since cultures may take several weeks, treatment can be initiated pending results.

A Wood's lamp is sometimes helpful to distinguish tinea infections. Infections will fluoresce different colors depending on the causative organism. Tinea capitis fluoresces bright or grayish green, tinea corporis will appear blue-green, and tinea versicolor tends to be yellow-green. Vitiligo will only show reflected light and not fluoresce.

TREATMENT

The length of treatment varies for both topical and oral antifungal drugs (Table 2-28-1). Package insert materials should be reviewed carefully. Consider the following:

- *Tinea capitis* Oral antifungal medications are required. Baseline liver functions studies are suggested prior to oral therapy.
- *Tinea corporis* Topical antifungals usually are all that is necessary. Persistent or widespread disease may require oral therapy.
- *Tinea pedis* Topical antifungals plus hygiene: frequent washing with complete drying, then use drying powders, and wearing only white cotton socks are beneficial. Resistant cases may require oral antifungal preparations.
- *Tinea cruris* Topical antifungals are required plus hygiene; bathe with complete drying, and use drying powders. Encourage weight loss if obesity is a contributing factor. Resistant cases may require oral antifungal preparations.
- *Tinea versicolor* Depending on the severity, oral or topical antifungal medication may be effective. Selenium sulfide applications are also used with varying success.

SUPPORTIVE MEASURES

Hygiene is a major factor in the management of tinea infections. Bathing followed by complete drying is essential. Reducing humidity is also beneficial but often difficult to accomplish. Powders with cornstarch may help to control moisture. Absorbent cotton socks (white) are important for tinea pedis because the dyes in dark socks can promote fungal growth. Patients should alternate shoes or allow shoes to dry out between use.

PATIENT EDUCATION

Fungal infections are contagious and can spread to close contacts. Other family members should be examined for similar infections, especially if a patient has reoccurent infections. Pets (such as dogs and cats) suspected of having fungal infections should be examined by a veterinarian and treated appropriately. Most cases of tinea corporis in children are from animal vectors. Although obvious to medical practitioners, parents may need to be reminded that "ringworm" infections are not "worms."

DISPOSITION

Patient follow-up depends on the severity and type of infection, and choice of antifungal medications. Usually, patients on oral therapy should be closely monitored for adverse effects. Liver function studies are suggested every 2 months while on oral antifungals. If enzyme levels rise, the medication should be discontinued. Liver enzymes usually return to normal after cessation.

COMPLICATIONS

Secondary bacterial infections are the most common complication of fungal infections and should be treated with an appropriate antibiotic.

PEARLS

Knowledge of the following points can contribute to positive patient outcome:

- Skin scrapings are easy on a compliant patient, but children are often frightened. As an alternative to using a scalpel to scrape the skin, consider using a tongue depressor or the edge of a glass slide for obtaining a specimen.

Table 2-28-1. Summary of the Tinea Infections and Effective Medications.*

Infection	Brand Name	Generic	Frequency	Cautions
Tinea capitis	Grifulvin V, 250- or 500-mg tablets; 125 mg/5 mL suspension	Griseofulvin	500-mg daily in divided doses; children under 50 lbs: 5 mg/ lb daily	Use with care in liver disease. Oral antifungal may adversely react with other medications.
	Fulvicin P/G, 125-, 165-, 250-, and 330-mg tablets	Ultramicrosize Griseofulvin	375 to 750 mg daily in divided dose; children over 2 years: 3.3 mg/lb pound daily, divided	Above
Tinea corporis	Nizoral, 200-mg tablets	Ketoconazole	One tablet daily	Above
	Lotrimin, 1% cream, lotion, solution	Clotrimazole	Twice daily	
	Nizoral, 2% cream	Ketoconazole	Once daily	
	Loprox, 1% cream and lotion	Ciclopirox olamine	Twice daily	
	Spectazole 1 cream	Econazole	Once daily	
	Monistat Derm cream	Miconazole nitrate	Twice daily for 2 weeks	
Tinea pedis	See corporis		For 1 month to 6 weeks	
Tinea cruris	See corporis			
Tinea unguium	See capitis		May require 6 to 12 months of treatment	Above
	Sporanox, 100-mg capsules	Itraconazole	Once daily for 3 months	Above
Tinea versicolor	Selenium sulfide, 2.5% lotion; conjunction with topical antifungals	Selsun	Once daily for 2 weeks; lather, leave on for 10 min, and rinse; repeat after 7 days to 2 weeks	

* Topical therapy that does not give complete response may require a change to oral therapy.

- By putting a drop of KOH immediately on the slide and using a cover slip, it is less likely that the scraping will be lost while being carried to the microscope.

BIBLIOGRAPHY

Fauci AS, Braunwald E, Isselbacher KJ, et al (eds): *Harrison's Principles of Internal Medicine,* 14th ed. New York, McGraw-Hill, 1998.

Fitzpatrick TB, Johnson RA, Wolff K, et al: *Color Atlas and Synopsis of Clinical Dermatology: Common and Serious Diseases,* 3d ed. New York, McGraw-Hill, 1997.

Chapter 2-29
ACNE
William H. Fenn

DISCUSSION

Acne vulgaris is one of the most common skin disorders, affecting as much as 85 to 90 percent of the population at one time or another. Although peak incidence is during the adolescent years, some skin changes of acne are found as early as age 9 in many individuals and lesions may persist or even initially appear between 20 and 40 years of age. So common is the disorder that almost all patients self-diagnose prior to presentation and many have attempted self-treatment.

PATHOPHYSIOLOGY

The lesions of acne are the result of a complex cascade of events. Stimulation of the pilosebaceous unit by androgens results in increased sebum production. It is assumed by many that the increased production of androgens with the onset of puberty accounts for this, but increased sensitivity of the sebaceous glands may be more important. Obstruction of the follicular outlet by adherent keratinized cells, possibly also mediated by androgens, leads to plugging and a cyclical accumulation of keratinaceous debris. In this environment anaerobic bacteria, especially *Propionibacterium acnes*, proliferate and contribute to the inflammatory process along with the release of free fatty acids. The exact mechanism of the bacterial contribution is controversial, with several competing theories being advanced. That *Proprionibacterium acnes* plays a clinically significant role, however, is not in doubt.

As observed in other skin disorders, significant stress (physical, emotional, or psychological) may exacerbate the eruption but is not a causative factor. It is also useful to note that, in general, diet and cleanliness do not play a significant role in the evolution or course of acne.

SIGNS AND SYMPTOMS

Patient complaints are principally related to the cosmetic aspect of the eruption. Some patients also note sensations of burning or pruritus, although these may also be related to attempts at self-therapy.

OBJECTIVE FINDINGS

The initial lesions of acne are the open and closed comedones, often referred to as blackheads and whiteheads, respectively.

These may evolve into papules and pustules, and most patients will have all these lesions simultaneously. In some patients, the disease course involves progression to multiple large scarring cysts and nodules which are often painful. The determinant of which patients suffer from nodulocystic acne is most likely genetic. Lesions predominate on the face in most patients, with the upper back and trunk often involved.

DIAGNOSTIC CONSIDERATIONS

Diagnosis of acne is rarely in doubt. Steroid acne may result from high-strength topical preparations or systemic steroids. The eruption from systemic steroids tends to be more truncal, whereas that of topical steroids is limited to the area of application. Although history is generally revealing in the case of topical steroids and systemic steroids used for legitimate medical purposes, laboratory testing may be required if there is a high degree of suspicion of illicit steroid abuse.

Acne induced by halogenated occupational chemicals tends to have comedones as the predominant lesions. A sudden onset of adult acne may raise the consideration of dysfunction within the hypothalamic-pituitary-adrenal axis. In the older patient, rosacea is a consideration and may be excluded by the absence of telangiectasia.

SPECIAL CONSIDERATIONS

Neonatal acne is generally self-limited and does not require therapy. Comedones occurring in a geriatric population (sometimes referred to as senile acne) generally respond better to mechanical extraction than medication if treatment is desired.

LABORATORY TESTS

There are no relevant laboratory tests, unless secondary causes such as steroid abuse or hormonal disturbances are suggested by other findings.

TREATMENT
Medications

Multiple topical and systemic medications are available for the treatment of acne (see Table 2-29-1). A rational basis for selection focuses on lesion type primarily, along with patient compliance and risk factors. Severity, independent of lesion type, is not a useful basis for medication selection. Topical retinoids are the most effective agents for comedones, whereas topical or systemic antibiotics are more useful against inflammatory and pustular lesions. Providers and patients should expect some changes in medication(s) as the eruption changes. Although more than one preparation is usually beneficial, care should be exercised to ensure the simplest possible regimen.

Supportive Measures

Thoughtful selection of medications used for other reasons may benefit acne. The best example is the informed selection of an oral contraceptive agent in patients desiring such therapy. Rational selection among agents will result in a reduction of acne lesions also. Norgestimate/ethinyl estradiol (Tri-Cyclen) recently became the first oral contraceptive specifically labeled for this situation. Although acne is not perceived as a serious disorder, it is important that the patient hear that the practitioner understands the psychosocial ramifications and takes those seriously. It may be necessary to discuss this with the parents also.

Table 2-29-1. Common Acne Medications

Medication	Dosage Regimen	Comments
Topical Antibiotics		
Erythromycin, clindamycin, tetracycline	Multiple preparations, generally applied twice daily	Little significant difference between meds. Topical tetracycline most efficacious in some studies, but availability limited, higher side-effect profile.
Benzoyl Peroxide Preparations		
Desquam = X, Oxy =5 and =10, Pan Oxyl, etc.	2%, 5%, 10% strengths; lotions, creams, gels, washes	5% most useful strength. Washes of little or no use. Apply qid–bid. When used in combination with other topicals, apply alone daily. The only OTC med of significant benefit.
Topical Retinoids		
Tretinoin (Retin-A, Renova) Adapalene (Differin)	Multiple preparations of tretinoin; most useful, 0.025% gel; twice daily; Differin 0.1% gel; daily application	Wash hands thoroughly after application. Increase in apparent acne prior to improvement. Adapalene more efficacious with fewer side effects.*
Oral Antibiotics		
Tetracycline	Initial: 500 mg bid; tapered to lowest controlling dose (250–500 mg daily)	Need for empty-stomach absorption limits adolescent compliance. Dental staining precludes use during pregnancy or prior to permanent teeth.
Minocycline	Initial: 100 mg daily–bid; tapered to 50 mg daily	If intolerant of or unresponsive to tetracycline.
Erythromycin	Initial: 500 mg bid; tapered to lowest controlling dose (250–500 mg daily)	If intolerant of or unresponsive to tetracyclines. Newer macrolides have little advantage in acne, much higher cost.
Other Agents		
Azelaic acid (Azelex)	20% cream applied bid	May be used daily if skin irritation (common) occurs. Relatively new in U.S., but longer worldwide use. Mechanism uncertain, but may be antimicrobial against *P. acnes.*
Isotretinoin (Accutane)	Multiple slightly differing dosing regimens	Drug of choice for cystic acne. Not indicated for mild to moderate acne vulgaris. High side-effect profile. Pregnancy category X. Use of this medicine by providers without extensive experience is discouraged. Refer likely candidates to qualified provider.

*See Cunliffe et al in Bibliography.

Patient Education

Patient education forms a critical portion of therapy for acne. Because the majority of patients are adolescents, it is very helpful to have both the patient and at least one parent present to boost compliance and avoid conflicting demands on the patient. Patients must be taught proper use of all therapeutic modalities prescribed, as well as proper use of cosmetics, cleansers, and other products. It is critical to tell patients that the medication(s) prescribed will *control,* not *cure,* the acne and that once the lesions have been eliminated, it is important to continue the medication(s) until they are told to discontinue them. Inevitably this leads to questions as to when the acne will go away permanently, and it is important to be honest and acknowledge that this cannot be predicted for each individual.

Teaching the patient how to read and interpret labels on cosmetics and skin and hair care products is not only good general education for patients, but beneficial for relief of the acne as well. Although avoidance of these products would be ideal from a clinical point of view, that is simply not a realistic goal in today's society. The use of any such product should be minimized while acne is present, and all cosmetics used should be labeled as *noncomedogenic.* Other terms, such as *dermatologist-tested* or *hypoallergenic* are not appropriate guides for use.

Incorrect preexisting myths must be debunked; for example, patients must be taught that food products do not play a significant role in acne so long as a generally balanced diet is followed. Scrupulous avoidance of foods such as chocolate or nuts or cheese will not improve acne. Some authors in the field acknowledge this, but believe that patient beliefs are so strong as to make it impractical to discuss. This author believes that it is important to dispense accurate information in a practical fashion and recognize that it is then up to the patient to use or not use the information.

It is also important to note that "dirtiness" is not a factor in the development of acne, and basic good hygiene with twice-daily face washing with a mild soap will suffice. More frequent washing or the use of stronger cleansing preparations may actually aggravate acne. To assist patients (or parents) in understanding this, it may be helpful to remind them that acne is, at its root, a rash and just as with other rashes, such as that of poison ivy, mechanical or chemical irritation is not beneficial.

Disposition

After starting initial therapy, reexamination at 8 to 10 weeks is useful to evaluate efficacy. Once efficacious control is obtained, follow-up every 6 months is reasonable, with instructions to return sooner should an extended period of exacerbation occur. Therapy for control may span many years, and it is necessary to periodically discontinue treatment to determine if remission has occurred. Although there is no right timing for this, a yearly trial off medications is probably warranted.

COMPLICATIONS AND RED FLAGS

With such a good prognosis, complications are limited. While the cystic form of acne is inherently scarring, the more common form is not. The patient must understand that scars may nonetheless result from inappropriate picking, squeezing, or otherwise traumatizing their acne lesions.

OTHER NOTES OR PEARLS

One difficulty often encountered is assessing the degree of improvement from visit to visit. Descriptors such as mild, moderate, and severe are not particularly evocative of the patient's appearance, and although the patient's input is helpful, it is highly subjective. The use of a photographic record is ideal, but is not practical for most general practices for a number of reasons, although progress in digital technology may soon change that. A better method is to record the findings in a manner such as that

Table 2-29-2. Acne Chart with Sample Entries*

	Face	Back
Comedones	1	0
Papules	2	2
Pustules	2	1
Cysts	0	0
Scarring	0	1

* Scale: 0 = none; 4 = extensive, to the point of confluence.

shown in Table 2-29-2, and purchasing a rubber stamp is helpful when treating significant numbers of acne patients. This type of charting allows for rapid recording of findings, and a quick method of assessing interval change—both in severity and lesion type, each of which may have a bearing on potential treatment changes.

BIBLIOGRAPHY

Cunliffe WJ, Caputo R, Dreno B, et al: Clinical efficacy and safety comparison of adapalene gel and tetinoin gel in the treatment of acne vulgaris: Europe and U.S. multicenter trials. *J Am Acad Dermatol* **36:**S126–S134, 1997.

Fitzpatrick TB, Eisen AZ, Wolff K, et al (eds): *Dermatology in General Medicine,* 4th ed. New York, McGraw-Hill, 1993, pp 709–724.

Lookingbill DP, Marks JG: *Principles of Dermatology,* 2d ed. Philadelphia, Saunders, 1993, pp 189–194.

SECTION 3
Ear, Nose, and Throat

Chapter 3–1
SINUSITIS
Meredith Hansen

DISCUSSION

Anatomy and Physiology

The paranasal sinuses are four paired cavities (maxillary, ethmoid, sphenoid, and frontal) within the cranial and facial bones. These sinuses are lined with mucous membranes and cilia that connect with and drain into the nasal cavity. Besides producing mucous, sinuses lighten the skull and serve as resonating chambers for sound.

The maxillary and ethmoid sinuses are present at birth. The sphenoid sinuses develop during adolescence. The frontal sinuses are fully developed by 8 to 10 years of age; however, 10 percent of the population never develops frontal sinuses. Only the maxillary and frontal sinuses are accessible for physical examination.

Pathogenesis

The paranasal sinus ostia are easily obstructed from inflammation of a viral or allergic etiology. The accumulation of mucus then becomes secondarily infected with bacteria.

Microbiology

Sinus pathogens vary with the age of the patient. Most sinusitis pathogens are identical to the agents that produce acute otitis media:

- *Streptococcus pneumoniae:* 40 to 50 percent
- *Haemophilus influenzae:* 20 to 30 percent
- *Staphylococcus aureus:* 2 to 10 percent
- Other streptococci: occasional
- *Moraxella catarrhalis:* 2 to 20 percent
- Gram-negative bacteria: 1 to 15 percent

SIGNS AND SYMPTOMS

Acute Sinusitis

The most common predisposing factor in the development of acute bacterial sinusitis in adults and children is a history of a previous upper respiratory infection (URI) or allergy exacerbation. Purulent nasal discharge, facial pain, congestion, halitosis, headache, cough, and postnasal drainage are commonly present. Many of these patients have a low-grade fever. If a patient presents with a high temperature [>39°C(102°F)], one should suspect a complication of sinusitis.

The maxillary sinuses are by far the most likely paranasal sinuses to become infected. The maxillary sinuses are the largest cavities, and their drainage must defeat gravity. Facial, cheek, or dental pain is a common presentation of maxillary sinusitis. Frontal sinusitis may present with forehead pain and headache.

Chronic Sinusitis

The symptoms of chronic sinusitis are subtle and require an astute index of suspicion. Chronic nasal congestion, cough, and postnasal drainage are the most common symptoms. Fever is uncommon.

OBJECTIVE FINDINGS

Physical evaluation of a patient with a suspected sinusitis consists of ear, nose, and throat (ENT) (including dental), respiratory, and neurologic examinations. In patients with uncomplicated sinusitis, a respiratory and neurologic examination should be unremarkable. The ENT examination may show tenderness on percussion of the forehead (frontal) and cheeks (maxillary). Purulent rhinorrhea and postnasal drainage may be noticed. Sinus x-rays in an uncomplicated sinus infection are not obligatory but may provide a definitive diagnosis.

DIAGNOSTIC CONSIDERATIONS

A variety of diseases should be considered in a patient with facial pain, headache, or cough. Trigeminal neuralgia, dental disease, temporomandibular joint dysfunction, allergic or viral rhinitis, vestibulitis, otitis media, barotitis, and optic neuritis may produce nasal or facial pain.

Neurologic causes of headache are ruled out by a complete neurologic examination and diagnostic tests.

SPECIAL CONSIDERATIONS

Immunocompromised patients are at greater risk of developing complications of sinusitis. Management is best approached in a hospital setting.

Patients who smoke or have chronic allergies have an increased incidence of sinus infections.

LABORATORY STUDIES

In uncomplicated acute sinusitis, laboratory testing is not indicated.

RADIOLOGIC STUDIES

Sinus films, when warranted, should contain a lateral view (sphenoid), a Caldwell view (frontal), and a Water's view (maxillary). A few facilities include a submental vertex view for better visualization of the ethmoid sinuses. Studies show that plain x-rays have little sensitivity in children and 40 to 80 percent sensitivity in adults. Patients with normal x-rays may have sinusitis, and patients with abnormal x-rays may have transitory changes that resolve without therapy.

Sinus CT provides a far better yield than do plain x-rays. Sensitivity on CT ranges from 36 to 66 percent, depending on the sinus involved and the age of the patient. Indications for sinus CT are recurrent acute sinusitis, complicated acute sinusitis, chronic sinusitis, an atypical presentation, an immunocompromised patient, and preoperative evaluation.

The use of MRI should be limited to tumor evaluation by ENT after referral.

OTHER DIAGNOSTICS

Transillumination of the sinuses has not proved helpful but often is used in clinical assessment. If purulent drainage persists, nasal cultures are indicated.

Table 3-1-1. Antibiotic Therapy for Sinusitis

Amoxicillin 250–500 mg orally tid
Amoxicillin/clavulanate potassium 250–500 mg orally tid
Trimethoprim (80–160 mg)-sulfamethoxazole (400–800 mg) orally tid
Cefuroxime 250 mg orally bid
Cefaclor 250 mg orally tid
Clarithromycin 500 mg bid
Cefixime 400 mg daily, orally, single dose

NOTE: All regimens should be continued for 14 days; longer treatment may be indicated.

TREATMENT

Outpatient management of acute uncomplicated sinusitis is recommended.

Pharmacologic Management

The goal of treatment in bacterial sinusitis is to open the sinus ostia to allow appropriate drainage of the pus accumulation in the sinuses. Table 3-1-1 describes recommended antibiotics for the management of acute bacterial sinusitis in adults.

Oral and nasal decongestants may be used, but some controversy exists about ciliastasis with decongestant usage. Intranasal corticosteroids may facilitate the ostial patency. Parenteral steroids, antihistamines, and combination decongestant-antihistamines have no proven use in sinusitis. Acetaminophen and ibuprofen should manage the facial pain associated with sinusitis. Guaifenesin at high doses (1200 mg twice a day) will thin mucus and facilitate passage.

Surgical Management

Endoscopic surgery may be indicated in patients who have anatomic blockage (mucoceles), recurrent acute sinusitis, acute complicated sinusitis, or chronic sinusitis.

Patient Education

Smoking cessation should be stressed to all patients. Parents with children who have ENT infections should be counseled about the hazards of secondhand smoke. Steam inhalation accelerates mucus passage.

Disposition

Ambulatory management is suggested for patients with uncomplicated acute sinusitis with minimal symptoms. Hospitalization is indicated in patients with pansinusitis (multiple cavities affected), sinus complications (meningitis, osteomyelitis, cavernous sinus thrombosis, mucocele, septicemia), and immunocompromised patients.

Follow-up should occur before the patient stops antibiotics because of a high incidence of longer antibiotic treatment being needed.

COMPLICATIONS AND RED FLAGS

Studies have shown that frontal sinusitis has a 3 to 10 percent change of progressing to a complication: osteomyelitis, intracranial complications, or septicemia. Aggressive outpatient treatment and follow-up or hospitalization are indicated.

Complications of acute sinusitis are rare. The most common complication is chronic sinusitis. The incidence of chronic sinusitis can be minimized by longer antibiotic treatment initially and judicious follow-up.

Mucoceles are a complication of sinusitis from a prolonged ductal obstruction. The treatment for mucoceles is surgical removal.

Osteomyelitis or periorbital cellulitis may result from the spread of infection from the sinus cavity to the surrounding bone or tissue. The frontal sinus is indicated in the majority of complications of osteomyelitis. Osteomyelitis requires prolonged intravenous antibiotics and surgical removal of the diseased bone.

Other complications of sinusitis include intracranial involvement that produces a cavernous sinus thrombosis, meningitis, or brain abscess. Intracranial complications are rare.

Sinus cancer should be considered in the assessment of recurrent or chronic sinusitis.

BIBLIOGRAPHY

Fauci AS, Chester AC: Chronic sinusitis. *Am Fam Phys* 53:877–887, 1996.
Fauci AS, Braunwald E, Isselbacher KJ, et al (eds): *Harrison's Principles of Internal Medicine*, 14th ed. New York, McGraw-Hill, 1998, pp 179–181.
Ferguson, BJ: Acute and chronic sinusitis. *Postgrad Med* 97:45–56, 1995.
Gwaltney JM Jr, Jones JG, Kennedy DW: Medical management of sinusitis: The International Conference on Sinus Disease. *Ann Otol Rhinol Laryngol* 167 (suppl):22–30, 1995.
Tierney LM Jr, McPhee SJ, Papadakis MA (eds): *Current Medical Diagnosis and Treatment*, 36th ed. Norwalk, CT, Appleton & Lange, 1997, pp 182–189.

Chapter 3–2
ACUTE OTITIS MEDIA
Rodney L. Moser

DISCUSSION

Middle-ear infections affect nearly 90 percent of all children before age 6, prompting frequent office visits. Otitis media (OM) and otitis media with effusion (OME) may be associated with conductive hearing loss, deficient verbal abilities, and learning problems. Upper respiratory infection is the most common predisposing factor, followed closely by day-care attendance. Allergies, enlarged adenoids, bottle feeding instead of breast feeding, exposure to secondary smoke (including wood-burning stoves), and low-income families are all considered additional risk factors. Boys and Native American children also have a higher incidence. The incidence of OM peaks between ages 6 months and 6 years and is highest in the winter and spring. OM occurs less often in later childhood and adulthood.

PATHOGENESIS

Most cases of AOM (acute otitis media) occur when nasopharyngeal pathogens enter the warm, moist middle-ear space via the eustachian tube. Eustachian tubes in children under age 6 tend to be short, narrow, and more horizontal, resulting in poor drainage and ventilation, and are easily obstructed by enlarged adenoids, nasopharyngeal irritation and/or infection, and allergies. The presence of pathogens leads to mucosal swelling in the middle ear and inflammatory obstruction of the eustachian tube. The resultant purulence and pressure usually lead to pain and fever. As the child grows, the eustachian tube elongates and angles downward, improving drainage. This change, along with the strengthening of the pediatric immune system, accounts for the reduced incidence of AOM in later childhood.

Table 3-2-1. Microbiologic Causes of Otitis Media

Streptococcus pneumoniae:	35–40% (5% may be resistant strains)
Haemophilus influenzae:	23–25% (up to 50% may be β-lactamase producers)
Moraxella (Branhamella) catarrhalis:	14% (about 90% produce β-lactamase)
Beta-hemolytic Streptococcus group A:	5–8% (most biologically common cause of spontaneous rupture of the tympanic membrane)
Viral:	up to 25 percent

MICROBIOLOGY

Up to 25 percent of middle-ear cultures are sterile and are felt to be viral. Middle-ear pathogens may vary with the population and geographic location. There is empirical evidence that some middle-ear pathogens are becoming more drug-resistant. Penicillin-resistant *Streptococcus pneumoniae* has been reported in middle-ear pathogens at some day-care centers. There has been a steady increase in the incidence of β-lactamase-producing strains of *Haemophilus influenzae* and *Moraxella* (*Branhamella*) *catarrhalis* (Table 3-2-1).

SYMPTOMS

In a young child, nonspecific irritability, crying, malaise, fever, diminished appetite, and ear pulling may be observed. Upper respiratory infection (URI) and allergic symptoms (runny nose, congestion, conjunctival inflammation, etc.) are often present. Less commonly, associated symptoms may include purulent ear discharge (from a perforation), diarrhea, and vomiting. OM also may be relatively asymptomatic. Previous experience with OM leads some parents to believe that virtually any mood change or ear pulling is OM until proved otherwise. In an older child or adult, well-localized otalgia is the most common symptom.

OBJECTIVE FINDINGS

On otoscopic examination, the tympanic membrane (TM) appears red, bulging, or opacified, having decreased motility and poorly visible landmarks. Strategic cerumen removal may be necessary for proper viewing. A pneumatic otoscopic, using the proper soft pneumatic ear specula, should always be performed. Decreased motility of the TM appears to be more predictive than are color changes in diagnosing AOM. As OM develops, pain may precede eardrum redness. Also, many children are examined before strong clinical signs are evident, and so OM often is diagnosed and treated simply on the basis of symptomatology and suspicion, perhaps resulting in an unnecessary overuse of antibiotics. Most providers have their own personal criteria for diagnosing and managing OM, and it is notoriously overdiagnosed.

DIAGNOSTIC CONSIDERATIONS

Otalgia can result from a variety of causes,[1] the most common being

- Otitis externa
- Serous otitis media
- Cerumen impaction/foreign body
- Furunculosis/skin infections
- Dental problems
- Trauma
- Sinusitis
- Lymphadenitis
- Tonsillitis/pharyngitis
- Barotitis/pressure changes

SPECIAL CONSIDERATIONS

Children in grouped-care situations develop OM more than do children cared for at home or in smaller home day-care settings. Children who are immunocompromised and those with cleft palate, hypotonia, and Down syndrome also have a greater risk of OM. Parents who smoke put their children at risk and should be encouraged to stop or never to smoke around children. Mothers should be encouraged to breast feed or to avoid propped bottles with the child in the supine position. Cleaning ears with cotton-tipped applicators should be discouraged to avoid TM and ear canal trauma.

LABORATORY TESTS

Unless the child is toxic-appearing, no laboratory tests are needed in primary care settings. Tympanocentesis with culture may be done by an ear, nose, and throat (ENT) specialist. Concurrent pharyngitis can be screened for group A beta-hemolytic streptococci. Nasopharyngeal cultures may not correlate with middle-ear pathogens and are unnecessary in most cases. Allergy testing is indicated only in carefully selected allergic patients and never is done routinely.

RADIOLOGIC STUDIES

No radiologic studies are necessary unless diagnostic considerations include mastoiditis, sinusitis, neoplastic disease, or other complications requiring special imaging.

OTHER DIAGNOSTICS

A pneumatic otoscopic examination is quick, easy, and rarely uncomfortable for the patient and should be done in most cases. Tympanometry and acoustic reflex testing are important diagnostics. Gross hearing evaluation or whisper tests are commonly used screening tools in the clinical setting but should not replace audiometric studies if hearing loss is suspected. Video otoscopy with magnification may be available in some specialty practices. More specialized studies, such as CT to show images of the middle ear and the surrounding bone structure and MRI to check for soft tissue problems, nerve damage, or tumors, are most often ordered by ENT after referral.

TREATMENT

Pharmacologic Management

Antibiotics remain the mainstay of treatment in clear-cut cases of OM, although there is growing controversial evidence that early antibiotic intervention may be counterproductive in "borderline" cases. Effectiveness, cost, safety, compliance, side effects, and knowledge of community strains are major considerations in choosing antibiotics for treating OM. There are a wide variety of treatment options (Table 3-2-2). Depending on the antibiotic selected, most practitioners use a 10-day course of therapy, although shorter courses may be effective. Amoxicillin and trimethoprim-sulfamethoxazole (Bactrim, Septra) tend to be the initial drugs of choice in uncomplicated OM. If OM fails to resolve with first-line antibiotics, a β-lactamase-producing organism is often involved. Amoxicillin/clavulanate potassium (Augmentin) and a cephalosporin antibiotic are common next-line choices. Cephalosporins should be used with caution in penicillin-allergic individuals. The patient should be basically asymptomatic after 2 to 3 days of antibiotic therapy, or an alternative medication should be considered. The practitioner should be wary of common side effects (nausea, vomiting, diarrhea, rash, etc.) of the selected antibiotics and inform the patient or parent. Antibiotics with once- or twice-daily dosing are the preferred choices for children in school or day care. Medication noncompliance (missed or

Table 3-2-2. Antibiotics for Otitis Media

Antibiotic	Dose	Comments
Amoxicillin (Amoxil)	20–40 mg/kg/d in divided doses tid × 7–10 days; doses as high as 60–80 mg/kg/d have been used in resistant cases	Most frequent, cost-effective first-line choice; well tolerated, available in suspension, chewable tablets, and capsules; few side effects; treatment failure could indicate resistant organism
Trimethoprim-sulfamethoxazole (Septra or Bactrim)	Based on 40 mg/kg/d divided bid × 10 days of sulfamethoxazole	Not for children under 2 months; twice-daily dosage convenient for day care; suspension does not require refrigeration; sulfa rash is common side effect.
Erythromycin-sulfisoxazole (Pediazole)	50 mg/kg/d erythromycin and 150 mg/kg/d sulfisoxazole divided qid × 10 days	Not for children under 2 months; inconvenient qid dosage; gastrointestinal (GI) side effects common with erythromycin, and rash with sulfa
Amoxicillin-clavulanate (Augmentin)	40 mg/kg/d based on amoxicillin in divided doses tid × 10 days (twice-daily dosage form now available)	Available in tablets, chewables, and suspension; very effective but costly; diarrhea is common side effect that may be related to improper dosing
Cefaclor (Ceclor)	40 mg/kg/d in divided doses tid × 10 days; can be divided bid for convenience	Available in liquid suspension or tablets; costly; generally well tolerated and effective
Cefixime (Suprax)	8 mg/kg/d in single doses for 10 days	Available in suspension (100 mg per 5 mL) and 400-mg tablets; good once/day compliance; GI side effects most common
Cefprozil (Cefzil)	30 mg/kg/d in bid dosage	Well-tolerated, with diarrhea and nausea the most common side effects; not used in children under 6 months
Cefuroxime (Ceftin)	30 mg/kg/d divided bid	Available in tablets and suspension; tablets taste terrible if chewed and must be swallowed whole; oral suspension more tolerable; diarrhea and/or vomiting most common side effects; used in children over 3 months.
Loracarbef (Lorabid)	30 mg/kg/d divided bid	Best tasting of all oral suspensions for OM; side effects of diarrhea, vomiting, and nausea less than with other cephalosporines
Cefpodoxime (Vantin)	10 mg/kg/d	Convenient once-a-day dosage; side effects include diarrhea and diaper rash; not studied in infants under 5 months; bitter-tasting but works well
Ceftriaxone (Rocephin)	50 mg/kg in single IM injection	Efficacy, simplicity, and convenience of a single-dose therapy are desirable; cost, pain of injection, and lack of long-term studies are downside; IV for serious infections
Clarithromycin (Biaxin)	15 mg/kg/d divided bid for 10 days	Convenient dosage; GI side effects (diarrhea and vomiting) most common; tolerated well; reasonable price; suspension has objectionable taste to some children
Aziithromycin (Zithromax)	10 mg/kg/d on first d, then 5 mg/kg/d on days 2–5	Once-per-day dosing for only 5 days; no refrigeration; only 1–2% GI side effects; reasonably priced
Ceftibuten (Cedax)	9 mg/kg/d for 10 days (1 tsp per 10 kg once per day)	Once-per-day dosing; GI side effects most common: 4% diarrhea and 2% vomiting

improperly measured doses, stopping prematurely, etc.) is a major factor in treatment failure.

Supportive Measures

One should treat the pain. Ibuprofen or acetaminophen will effectively control most pain related to OM. It is not necessary to treat simple fever. Auralgan (antipyrine and benzocaine) otic solution works well for ear pain. One should fill the ear canal with body-temperature drops, insert a cotton plug, and repeat every 2 h if needed. One should not use Auralgan if the TM is perforated or myringotomy tubes are in place. Controlling ear pain helps limit late-night calls and after-hours care. Oral decongestants usually are not recommended but may be used if there is concurrent congestion. Antihistamines are not recommended because of their drying effects and have limited value in allergy-complicated OM. At present, steroid therapy is not recommended, although its role may change in the future.

Patient Education

Patient education is vital in the comprehensive management of OM. It is necessary to discuss risk factors and modify the ones that can be changed, particularly secondhand smoke exposure and day care. Suggesting a less populated day-care setting (fewer than eight children) or smaller pods will help limit exposures. Medication noncompliance can be limited by selecting antibiotics

with fewer daily doses and fewer side effects. Proper measuring of doses is also important. Properly instructed and encouraged, any parent can learn to use an inexpensive home otoscope.[2] Acoustic reflectometers are also beginning to appear in the consumer market. Patient education may reduce unnecessary visits and allow the parent to participate more in the care of a child with OM. An educated parent may be less likely to solicit unnecessary antibiotics.

Disposition

One must recheck in 2 to 3 weeks or sooner if patient is not responding to treatment and is worse. Earlier rechecks may still reveal postinfection effusion that could be unnecessarily treated as a nonresolving infection. Some effusions can last 3 to 4 months and require careful monitoring.

COMPLICATIONS AND RED FLAGS

Chronicity, recurrent infections, and temporary hearing loss are among the most common complications. If hearing loss is unilateral, it may go undetected for a long period. In preverbal children, middle-ear effusion (OME) can delay speech development. In older children, it can result in behavioral and learning difficulties and lead to a more permanent hearing loss. Mastoiditis (see Chap. 3-12) is a rare and potentially serious complication. Redness, tenderness, and swelling of the mastoid should be diagnostically confirmed by x-ray or CT. Treatment is with aggressive antibiotic therapy and occasionally surgical intervention. Meningitis (see Chap. 9-28), labyrinthitis (see Chap. 3-5), facial paralysis, and other intracranial complications can occur as a result of OM but are rare.

Surgical Intervention and Tubes

A simple myringotomy, or lancing of the TM, is a supportive treatment and a pain-relieving procedure that can be done if the patient is seriously ill or toxic-appearing. It is rarely done in primary care settings anymore. According to the 1994 U.S. Department of Health and Human Services Task Force on Otitis Media,[3] children ages 1 to 3 with uncomplicated OME, especially those with hearing loss, should be evaluated for possible myringotomy tubes only after 4 to 6 months of watchful waiting. Myringotomy tubes should be reserved for children who have failed on antibiotics and those with hearing loss and other complications. The tubes tend to last about a year, although they can extricate or obstruct at any time. Adenoidectomy is not recommended for the surgical management of OME in the absence of specific adenoidal pathology, such as obstruction or encroachment of the eustachian tubes. Tonsillectomy has no proven value in the management of OM.

Suppression Therapy for Chronic/Recurrent Otitis Media

Antimicrobial chemoprophylaxis using daily doses of amoxicillin (20 mg/kg/h) or sulfisoxazole (50 mg/kg/d of Gantrisin) is commonly used in primary care. Prescribing criteria range from daily doses for up to 6 months to 6-week bursts of therapy followed by an antibiotic-free "vacation." Suppression therapy often is timed to occur in the peak OM season. Many primary care providers feel that suppression therapy should be tried before myringotomy is considered.

Other Complications

Chronic ear infections can lead to the formation of cholesteatomas, or pockets of scar tissue and debris on the TM. Cholesteatomas can seriously damage the ossicle chain, leading to permanent hearing loss, pain, or dizziness. If this is suspected, the patient should be referred to ENT for evaluation and management.

NOTES AND PEARLS

Preliminary studies have shown a reduction in the incidence of OM after the administration of flu vaccine and/or Pneumovax, especially in children with asthma or other chronic respiratory problems. Other bacterial or viral vaccines are being investigated. There is a growing trend to reduce the astronomic amounts of antibiotics used in the management of OM. The disturbing emergence of resistant strains of pneumococcal organisms in hospitals and day-care centers is likely to continue. One can expect newer antibiotics and treatment modalities to combat these evolving microorganisms and a trend toward more conservative management.

REFERENCES

1. Moser RL: Ear Infections in children. *Phys Assist* 13:23–45, 1989.
2. Moser RL: *Ears: An Owner's Manual.* Ferndale, CA, Notoco, 1994.
3. US Department of Health and Human Services: *Otitis Media with Effusion in Young Children.* Washington, DC, AHCPR Publication No. 94–0622, 1994.

Chapter 3–3
MONONUCLEOSIS
Suzanne Warnimont

DISCUSSION

Infectious mononucleosis is an acute illness that presents classically with sore throat, fever, and adenopathy. It usually is caused by the Epstein-Barr virus (EBV), which affects people of all ages but mainly teenagers and young adults of middle to upper socioeconomic status.

College students develop mononucleosis at an annual rate of 0.5 to 12 percent. Infectious mononucleosis is known as the "kissing disease." It is transmitted by repeated intimate oral contact with an asymptomatic person who is shedding the virus through saliva.

EBV is rarely transmitted by transfusion of fresh blood or organ transplantation. Uncommon (<10 percent) causes of mononucleosis include cytomegalovirus, human immunodeficiency virus (HIV), *Toxoplasma gondii,* and human herpesvirus type 6.

SIGNS AND SYMPTOMS

After an incubation period of 30 to 50 days (4 to 8 weeks), there is an abrupt onset of fever, malaise, and pharyngitis. The patient also may complain of chills, headache, photophobia, anorexia, dysphagia, myalgia, and distaste for cigarettes. The infection may be asymptomatic or may be manifested by a brief febrile illness in infants and young children.

The acute phase lasts 1 to 3 weeks, with most patients experiencing recovery in 6 to 8 weeks.

OBJECTIVE FINDINGS

Physical findings include periorbital edema, enlarged tonsils with erythema and exudate, palatine petechiae, cervical adenopathy, and splenomegaly. Less common findings include jaundice and hepatomegaly. A maculopapular rash develops in 10 percent of these patients.

Ampicillin causes a generalized rash in 90 percent of patients treated during acute infectious mononucleosis.

DIAGNOSTIC CONSIDERATIONS

Primary infection by the HIV-1 virus causes a monolike illness that lasts 2 to 4 weeks. There is no exudative pharyngitis. One must rule out the following:

- *Bacterial disease:* strep pharyngitis, mycoplasma, bacteremia
- *Viral disease:* cytomegalovirus, toxoplasmosis, respiratory viruses, viral hepatitis, rubella, mumps
- HIV, human herpesvirus type 6
- Drug reaction
- Hematologic malignancies: leukemia or lymphoma

LABORATORY TESTS

In the complete blood count (CBC), the white blood cell (WBC) count is elevated to 12,000 to 50,000/mm^3 with most of the increase in lymphocytes; 8 to 10 percent of the WBCs are atypical. A mild reduction in platelet count is seen in 50 percent of these patients. Serum transaminases are elevated to two to three times normal in more that 80 percent of these patients. Serum heterophile antibodies are found in 75 percent of patients with EBV mononucleosis by the seventh day of illness and in 95 to 97 percent by the twenty-first day. Testing is done with the "Monospot" test.

RADIOLOGIC STUDIES AND OTHER DIAGNOSTICS

No radiologic studies or other diagnostics are necessary.

TREATMENT

Uncomplicated mononucleosis requires only supportive therapy. Warm saline gargles and acetaminophen, 650 to 1000 mg every 4 h are given for fever.

Antibiotic treatment is necessary for bacterial superinfection of the pharynx.

Pharmacologic Management

Corticosteroids (40 to 80 mg daily tapered over 5 to 14 days) are useful in the management of airway obstruction and thrombocytopenia. Otherwise steroids are not useful, since they have no effect on the clinical course.

Acyclovir reduces oropharyngeal shedding but has no effect on the clinical course.

Penicillin and erythromycin can be taken for 10 days to treat bacterial superinfection by group A beta-hemolytic *Streptococcus pyogenes* (ampicillin or amoxicillin should be avoided, as they produce a rash).

Supportive Measures

The patient should avoid strenuous exercise to decrease the risk of splenic rupture. The patient should limit activity during acute illness.

Patient Education

No contact sports are allowed for 4 to 8 weeks or as long as the spleen is palpable or is enlarged on x-ray. Intimate contact during acute illness is restricted to reduce transmission. Isolation is not necessary, as the virus is not likely to be transmitted by aerosol or fomites.

Disposition

Symptoms resolve slowly, with 50 percent of patients symptom-free by 2 weeks, 80 percent by 3 weeks, and 97 percent by 4 weeks. Malaise is the most persistent symptom, and occasional patients remain so fatigued that they have difficulty returning to school or work for months.

COMPLICATIONS AND RED FLAGS

Complications are uncommon and include hemolytic anemia, immune thrombocytopenia, neutropenia, upper airway obstruction, pneumonia, myopericarditis, splenic rupture, severe hepatitis, bacterial superinfection, and CNS infection (encephalitis, aseptic meningitis, transverse myelitis, hearing loss, cranial nerve palsy, and peripheral neuropathy, including Guillain-Barré syndrome). Rarely, symptoms of fever, malaise, pharyngitis, or cervical adenopathy or neuropsychiatric symptoms can reoccur months or years after acute EBV mononucleosis.

BIBLIOGRAPHY

Cohen JI: Epstein-Barr virus infections, including infectious mononucleosis, in Fauci AS, Braunwald E, Iselbacher KJ, et al (eds): *Harrison's Principles of Internal Medicine*, 14th ed. New York, McGraw-Hill, 1998, pp 1089–1091.
Scheible WR: Infectious mononucleosis, in Rakel RE (ed): *Saunder's Manual of Medical Practice*. Philadelphia, Saunders, 1996, pp 872–874.
Stobo JD, Hellman DB, Ladenson PW, et al (eds): *The Principles and Practice of Medicine*, 23d ed. Stamford, CT, Appleton & Lange, 1996, pp 614–615.

Chapter 3–4
ALLERGIC RHINITIS
Richard Dehn

DISCUSSION

Allergic rhinitis is a disease that affects primarily the nasal mucous membranes. Allergic rhinitis is quite common, and it has been estimated that up to one-sixth of the U.S. population is affected. Symptoms usually begin by the fourth decade of life and tend to decrease with age. Most cases of allergic rhinitis are caused by airborne allergenic particles that initiate an IgE-mediated response in the nasal mucosa.

Patients presenting with allergic rhinitis usually can be classified into two subgroups depending on whether the symptoms are seasonal or perennial. The seasonal subgroup is the most common, and patients with this classification present with recurring symptoms that are limited to a certain time of the year every year. Spring and late summer are the most common times of presentation for seasonal allergic rhinitis, which is often called *hay fever*. This type of allergic rhinitis usually is triggered by airborne plant pollens or mold spores; therefore, the symptoms follow the pollination season of the sensitizing plant or mold. Pollen cycles are often unique for each geographic area, and so symptoms present in a consistent annual pattern if the patient stays in the same environment. Allergenic plants often pollinate in the early morning hours, and so symptoms can be worse in the morning. It is not uncommon for a patient to be allergic to more than one pollen, and this complicates the identification of the allergen. The most common allergens are ragweed, grass, and tree pollens.

The perennial subgroup is sensitive to allergens that are present year-round. The allergenic agents are usually present in the home or work environment. The most common allergens are house dust, mites, animal dander, and mold spores. Occasionally chemical allergens from the home or work environment are the causative agent, with the most common being vapors released from construction materials or furniture. On very rare occasions the allergen is contained in the patient's food.

PATHOGENESIS

Allergens in the environment enter the respiratory system through the nose, where they are trapped by the mucosal surfaces of the turbinates. The allergen elicits an IgE-mediated response that causes nearby mast cells to release histamine and other mediators. The effects of this release may occur within a few minutes or may take several hours to develop. Histamine release produces tissue edema and eosinophilic infiltration and indirectly stimulates sensory nerve receptors, resulting in a centrally mediated parasympathetic reflex that produces itching, sneezing, and increased nasal secretions. Histamine also increases mucosal cell permeability, which then allows the allergen access to submucosal regions, where additional IgE-mediated responses are initiated.

SIGNS AND SYMPTOMS

The immune response resulting from the allergen's contact with the nasal mucosa produces the classic symptoms of allergic rhinitis. The most common of these symptoms include sneezing, increased nasal secretions, and nasal congestion. They often are accompanied by itching of the eyes, ears, nose, or throat. Severe cases may present with conjunctival inflammation with excessive tearing and mucoid discharge. Persistent postnasal drainage can result in sore throat and a productive cough. Recurrent or chronic allergic rhinitis also may present with fatigue, headache, irritability, ear pain, decreased hearing, and malaise.

The nasal mucosa appears edematous, boggy, and a pale or bluish color coated with clear secretions, though it is not uncommon for the mucosa to appear erythematous. Nasal polyps, which are hypertrophic areas of mucosa that appear as yellow masses, sometimes are seen on examination. Severe mucosal edema is often present and in severe cases can produce airway obstruction and compromise the visualization of the nasal airway. Commonly the conjunctiva is somewhat injected, and a watery and clear discharge is present. In severe and chronic cases, periorbital edema may be present, with a pooling of venous blood around the eyes producing a characteristic sign called *allergic shiners*. In response to chronic nasal itching, children often use the side of the hand to rub the nose in an upward motion known as the *allergic salute,* and this process over time can produce a horizontal mark across the bridge of the nose. The mucosa of the posterior pharynx can be inflamed in severe cases, and a postnasal drainage can be visualized. Irritation of the eustachian structures can lead to occlusion, which can produce a reduction of tympanic membrane mobility, serous otitis media, or acute otitis media.

SPECIAL CONSIDERATIONS

Allergic rhinitis often is found in individuals with a predisposition to chronic or recurrent sinusitis, atopic dermatologic conditions, otitis media, and asthma. Sometimes these conditions occur secondary to a flare-up of allergic rhinitis so that treatment of the allergic rhinitis will improve the secondary condition. In some cases treatment that prevents the symptoms of allergic rhinitis reduces the number and frequency of occurrences of the secondary condition. Chronic allergic rhinitis can result in the development of nasal polyps, which can contribute to obstruction and the development of sinusitis.

DIAGNOSTIC CONSIDERATIONS

Allergic rhinitis must be distinguished from viral and bacterial infections of the nasal mucosa. This differentiation usually can be made by physical examination, since infections often present with erythematous mucosa. Additional information can be obtained by microscopically examining the nasal secretions, which will contain significant neutrophilia in an infectious process, in contrast to the eosinophilia seen with allergic rhinitis.

Allergic rhinitis also can be confused with vasomotor rhinitis, in which nasal secretions are due to functionally hyperactive mucosa. In vasomotor rhinitis, precipitating factors include sudden temperature change, strong odors, air-conditioning, alcoholic beverages, and even sexual activity. In patients with vasomotor rhinitis, itching and sneezing are usually absent, since the syndrome does not involve the release of histamine.

The chronic use of nasal decongestants (rhinitis medicamentosa) also can produce symptoms of allergic rhinitis. Rebound nasal congestion after overuse of these drugs can precipitate a purulent rhinitis in which the mucosa appears bright red. Obstructions also can contribute to the symptoms of allergic rhinitis. These symptoms can have many primary etiologies, such as septal deviation, tumors, foreign bodies, and adenoidal hypertrophy. Several endocrinologic states also can produce symptoms of allergic rhinitis, including hypothyroidism and pregnancy.

LABORATORY TESTING

Identification of significant eosinophilia from a swabbing of the nasal secretions is highly suggestive of allergic rhinitis. The presence of neutrophils in nasal secretions is more suggestive of sinusitis.

Radioallergosorbent testing (RAST) and skin testing are useful in identifying the specific allergens to which a patient is sensitive. A RAST test measures in vitro specific IgE present in the serum, while skin testing measures the skin's direct response to antigen exposure. Information from a RAST test or skin testing can be useful if the goal of therapy is allergen avoidance or immunotherapy.

TREATMENT

The treatment of allergic rhinitis involves allergen avoidance, pharmacologic therapy, and immunotherapy. Although allergen avoidance is the cheapest and least invasive form of therapy, pharmacologic therapy is the most commonly used first-line treatment since it does not require the identification of the offending allergen or allergens.

Drug therapy is most appropriate for patients with seasonal or mild perennial allergic rhinitis. First-line drugs include antihistamines and decongestants. Antihistamines work by competitively blocking histamine at the H_1 receptor sites. Commonly used antihistamines and the adult doses are chlorpheniramine (Chlor-Trimeton) 4 mg qid, brompheniramine (Dimetane) 4 mg qid, and diphenhydramine (Benadryl) 25 to 50 mg qid. The major advantages of these antihistamines are low cost and nonprescription availability; however, there are major side effects of sedation and anticholinergic effects. Nonsedating antihistamines are available but cost significantly more and are available only by prescription. The most common nonsedating antihistamines and the adult doses are astemizole (Hismanal) 10 mg qd and loratadine (Claritin) 10 mg qd. Astemizole has been known to cause QT-interval prolongation when taken with macrolide antibiotics, or the antifungal agents ketoconazole and itraconazole and in patients with liver failure.

Decongestants also are used as first-line therapy for allergic rhinitis. They work as sympathomimetics, producing vasoconstriction, and are available as both systemic and topical agents. The most common oral preparations and adult dosages are pseudoephedrine (Sudafed) 60 mg every 4 h and phenylpropanolamine 25 mg every 4 h. Systemic decongestants can produce nervousness as a side effect, limiting their usability. Decongestants should be used carefully in patients with hypertension or cardiac disease, since the sympathomimetic effects often raise the blood pressure, increase the heart rate, and cause coronary vasoconstriction. Most of the systemic side effects can be avoided by using topical preparations, since a much smaller quantity of the drug is systematically absorbed. Commonly used topical decongestants include oxymetazoline (Afrin) and phenylephrine (Neo-Synephrine); however, the use of topical decongestants should be limited to 5 days to avoid rhinitis medicamentosa. Often oral over-the-counter and prescription preparations contain a formulation of both antihistamines and decongestants. The side effects of these combination preparations are unpredictable from patient to patient, depending on how well the drowsiness from the antihistamine is balanced against the nervousness from the decongestant.

Corticosteroid preparations are utilized when symptoms are more severe, are more chronic, or do not respond to antihistamines or decongestants and when the side effects of antihistamines or decongestants are intolerable. Corticosteroids work by reducing the release of histamine and other mediators from mast cells; this reduces eosinophilic migration and prevents the centrally mediated parasympathetic reflex. Corticosteroids work best if treatment begins before mast cell exposure to the allergen. Systemic oral or intermuscular corticosteroids are occasionally used; however, topical corticosteroid preparations are equally effective and do not have the side effects of systemic absorption. Several preparations of topical nasal corticosteroids are available.

The usual recommendations are that two puffs be placed in each nostril twice daily, with some improvement expected in 1 to 2 weeks and an optimum effect apparent in 1 or 2 months. Severe cases may require increased dosing, though many patients are able to decrease to a small maintenance dose once the symptoms have been controlled. Since little systemic absorption occurs with the topical preparations, very few systemic side effects are reported; however, local side effects of stinging and epistaxis are not uncommon. A topical corticosteroid is being considered for approval as an over-the-counter product and may be available in the future without a prescription.

Cromolyn is effective in inhibiting mast cell degranulation. Intranasal cromolyn sodium is available as a 4% solution (Nasalcrom), and one spray should be used in each nostril three or four times daily. Similar to topical corticosteroids, cromolyn is most effective if treatment precedes mast cell contact with the antigen, and a maximum effect is noted after 4 to 6 weeks of regular use. Cromolyn is not systematically absorbed, but it can cause local irritation and sneezing. It is not very effective when the nasal mucosa is thickened, and so efficacy can be increased in those cases by using a nasal decongestant before the chromolyn application.

Anticholinergic preparations have been found to be effective in reducing the symptoms of allergic rhinitis. Ipratropium bromide (Atrovent) can be sprayed twice into each nostril bid, using an infant feeding nipple with the hole enlarged and placed over the outlet of the inhaler mechanism. The major side effect is nasal mucosal dryness.

Allergen avoidance is important for the long-term management of allergic rhinitis in patients who are not responsive to or are intolerant to medications. Occasionally a patient is able to identify the offending allergen; however, most of the time skin testing or RAST testing must be performed to identify the allergen or allergens responsible. Identification of the allergens will allow the patient to attempt to remove those substances from the environment. In the case of outdoor seasonal pollens, this may involve avoiding outdoor activity during the peak season or wearing a filtering mask while outside. Indoor allergens can be reduced substantially by frequent cleaning of furniture and bedding, placing mattresses and pillows in plastic cases, removing pets from the household, fixing areas where molds grow, and eliminating carpet in favor of wood floors.

Patients with chronic and severe allergic rhinitis who are unable to avoid allergens are candidates for immunotherapy. With immunotherapy, or hyposensitization therapy, small quantities of allergen are regularly injected subcutaneously in increasing doses. As many as 80 percent of patients undergoing immunotherapy experience improvement after 1 to 2 years of treatment. Successful immunotherapy requires careful identification of the allergen and a compliant patient, since treatment should continue for 4 to 5 years. Primary management of immunotherapy should be done by practitioners capable of interpreting the reactions in order to adjust the doses appropriately.

BIBLIOGRAPHY

Coren J, Rachelefsky GS: *Conn's Current Therapy.* Philadelphia, Saunders, 1995.
Dixon HS, Dixon BJ: *Common Problems of the Head and Neck Region, American Academy of Otolaryngology, Head and Neck Surgery Foundation.* Philadelphia, Saunders, 1992.
Fauci AS, Braunwald E, Isselbacher KJ, et al (eds): *Harrison's Principles of Internal Medicine,* 14th ed. New York, McGraw-Hill, 1998.
Jackler RK, Kaplan MJ: *Current Medical Diagnosis and Treatment,* 35th rev ed. Appleton, WI, Appleton & Lange, 1996.
Salvaggio JE: *Cecil Textbook of Medicine,* 19th ed. Philadelphia, Saunders, 1992.

Chapter 3–5
LABYRINTHITIS
Katherine D. Hocum

DISCUSSION

Acute labyrinthitis (vestibular neuronitis, inner-ear infection) is a benign condition that is more accurately described as a peripheral non-Meniere's vestibular disorder. While labyrinthitis may be caused by various bacteria (suppurative labyrinthitis), most often it is viral in origin and is more commonly known as vestibular neuronitis. Vestibular neuronitis (VN) is an acute unilateral infection or inflammation of the vestibular system. It is a common clinical condition that presents as severe vertigo, nystagmus, nausea, and vomiting. Symptoms such as tinnitus and hearing loss are most often absent. Patients often report a history of recent upper respiratory infection (URI). They also may have recently suffered from otitis media (DM) or sinusitis. Adolescents and young adults appear to be affected most often. There also appears to be a familial and/or seasonal component associated with this condition.

PATHOGENESIS

The pathophysiology of this syndrome appears to be secondary to a sudden unilateral disruption of the normal vestibular neural input to the brainstem and cerebral cortex. The brain erroneously interprets the altered neural input as violent head movement, and that misinterpretation is responsible for the vertigo. The vestibular symptoms are due in part to an isolated infection of the labyrinth or vestibular nerve by a virus after a recent URI. Paralysis of the vestibular nerve, as found in Bell's palsy, or inflammation of the nerve trunk, has been suggested as a cause. After a viral URI, it appears that the virus may distribute itself into the ganglionic nuclei of the cranial nerves, where it remains latent for a short period. Upon replication, there is a sudden autoimmune reaction that causes inflammation and edema. Spontaneous reactivation of the virus is common after periods when inflammation is minimal. Inflammation and edema cause the vertigo.

SIGNS AND SYMPTOMS

The clinical features of vestibular neuronitis are severe rotational vertigo, nystagmus, nausea, and vomiting. There is an absence of tinnitus or hearing loss. Vertigo at first is persistent and then becomes paroxysmal. The patient also may present with ataxia. Nystagmus is horizontal-rotatory away from the affected ear. Central nervous system (CNS) deficits are not present. The condition lasts 7 to 10 days and is usually self-limited. VN may occur as a single episode or, as in the majority of patients, paroxysmal episodes over 12 to 18 months. Generally, each subsequent attack is less severe and of shorter duration than the first.

OBJECTIVE FINDINGS

The evaluation of a patient presenting with a sudden onset of vertigo or dizziness presents a diagnostic challenge. Numerous disease states and conditions may cause vertigo, nystagmus, or ataxia. It is essential that the practitioner elicit an accurate and detailed history when evaluating a patient with dizziness. The diagnosis of vestibular neuronitis is often a presumptive one based on the patient's history of sudden vertigo, nausea, and vomiting after a URI. While hearing loss and tinnitus usually are absent, disorders of the CNS or cardiovascular system and

Table 3-5-1. Differential Diagnosis of Vestibular Neuronitis

Benign paroxysmal positional vertigo
Meniere's disease
Acoustic neuroma
Ototoxic medications
Vertebrobasilar insufficiency
Faintness and syncope
Vertiginous migraine
Hypo- and hypercapnia, hypoxia
Multiple sclerosis
Aortic stenosis
Anemia, hypovolemia
Depression, anxiety, other psychiatric illness
Epilepsy
Cervical spondylosis
Otosclerosis
Orthostatic blood pressure changes
Cerebellar disease
Space-occupying lesions
Trauma
Hyperventilation
Diabetes, hypoglycemia

Table 3-5-2. Differential Diagnosis for Dizziness

Peripheral Causes	Central Causes	Other Causes
Benign paroxysmal positional vertigo	Vertebrobasilar insufficiency	Diabetes mellitus
Labyrinthitis/vestibular neuronitis	Transient ischemic attack/ischemia	Anemia, hypovolemia
Trauma	Multiple sclerosis	Psychiatric illness
Ototoxic medications	Tumors/neuroma	Orthostatic blood pressure changes
Otosclerosis	Vestibular epilepsy	Medications
Neurosyphilis	Cerebellar injury/disease	Aortic stenosis
Herpes zoster oticus	Cerebrovascular accident	Migraine

metabolic and psychiatric disorders should be considered. (Table 3-5-1).

The evaluation of any patient presenting with dizziness must include a complete physical examination of the head, eyes, ears, neck, nose, and throat. Hearing acuity and speech discrimination also should be tested. Examination of the tympanic membranes, unless the patient is suffering from otitis media, often is normal. Nystagmus is generally present and should be described accurately. Nystagmus should be horizontal-rotatory in nature and should move away from the affected side. A complete neurologic examination including mental status should be performed. Ataxia is not an uncommon finding in patients with VN. Evaluation of the endocrine, pulmonary, and cardiovascular systems should be included in any workup of a patient with dizziness.

DIAGNOSTIC CONSIDERATIONS

The initial step in the evaluation of the patient is to obtain an accurate description of "dizziness." The vertigo associated with VN will remain present whether the patient opens or closes the eyes. Precipitating factors and the frequency or timing of vertigo should be elicited. Associated signs suggesting central vertigo (neurologic deficits) should be absent. There may be evidence of URI, OM, or sinusitis.

Benign paroxysmal positional vertigo (BPPV) and Meniere's disease are the diagnoses most likely to mimic VN. Ototoxicity and otosclerosis may present with similar symptoms. Acoustic neuroma should always be considered, although the lack of neurologic deficits should make this disorder unlikely. Metabolic disorders and psychiatric disorders should also be included in the differential diagnosis (Table 3-5-2).

SPECIAL CONSIDERATIONS

VN often follows a viral URI. Adolescents and young adults are the most frequently affected. There is often an occurrence of this disorder in members of the same family or during certain periods of the year. Patients with VN may have a past medical history of similar, more severe episodes.

LABORATORY TESTS

There is no laboratory test to confirm diagnosis of VN.

DIAGNOSTICS

If the presence of neurologic signs associated with vertigo cannot be adequately differentiated, computed tomography (CT) and magnetic resonance imaging (MRI) are essential to rule out central lesions. Electronystagmography (ENG) also helps in the diagnosis of peripheral versus central vertigo.

TREATMENT

While vestibular neuronitis is usually a self-limiting condition, vertigo may be severe enough to require symptomatic treatment during the acute phase. Diazepam (Valium) 5 to 10 mg intramuscularly or orally may initially be helpful. Trimethobenzamide hydrochloride (Tigan) 200 mg intramuscularly every 12 h or 250-mg capsules orally every 8 h may relieve nausea and vomiting. Medications that sedate the vestibular system may be appropriate. Meclizine (Antivert) 25 to 50 mg orally every 6 h or dimenhydrinate (Dramamine) 50 mg orally every 6 h should relieve most patients. Patients who take vestibular sedatives should be advised of the drowsiness associated with these agents and should not operate machinery while under treatment. The use of steroids has also been successful in reducing inflammation of the vestibular nerve in some cases (Table 3-5-3).

RED FLAGS

Isolated acute vertigo in an elderly patient may signify vascular disease (cerebral infarct, transient ischemic attack) in 25 percent of cases. Careful attention should be paid to the presence of neurologic signs and/or confusion. Diagnostic imaging studies (CT, MRI) are warranted in an elderly patient presenting with dizziness.

Table 3-5-3. Pharmacologic Management of Vestibular Neuronitis

Agent	Dose/Route	Comments
Diazepam (Valium)	5–10 mg IM or PO	Used most often for acute attacks
Trimethobenzamide hydrochloride (Tigan)	200 mg IM q12h	For severe nausea and vomiting
	250 mg PO q8h	For nausea and vomiting
Meclizine (Antivert)	25–50 mg PO q6h	Nausea and vomiting: 12.5 mg PO tid in elderly patients
Dimenhydrinate (Dramamine)	50 mg PO q6h	Do not operate machinery

PEARLS

Most patients with VN require only reassurance and symptomatic treatment. Complications and sequelae are uncommon.

BIBLIOGRAPHY

Bates B, Bickley L, Hoekelman R (eds): *A Guide to Physical Examination and History Taking,* 6th ed. Lippincott, Philadelphia, 1995, pp 147–227.
Fauci AS, Braunwald E, Isselbacher KJ, et al (eds): *Harrison's Principles of Internal Medicine,* 14th ed. New York, McGraw-Hill, 1998.
Gorroll AH, May L, Mulley A (eds): *Primary Care Medicine: Office Evaluation and Management of the Adult Patient.* Lippincott, Philadelphia, 1995, pp 985–1010.
Rakel RE: *Conn's Current Therapy,* 1995.
Shea JJ: Classification of Meniere's disease. *Am J Otol* 14(3):224–229, 1993.
Tran Ba Huy P: Physiopathology of peripheral non-Meniere's vestibular disorders. *Acta Otolaryngol* 513(Suppl):5–10, 1994.

Chapter 3–6
LARYNGITIS
Suzanne Warnimont

DISCUSSION

Laryngitis is a viral disease that usually lasts a few days to a week. Adenoviruses and influenza are the most common causes. Laryngitis often is associated with upper respiratory infection (URI) and may persist even after other symptoms of URI have resolved. Bacterial causes include *Moraxella catarrhalis* and *Haemophilus influenzae. Streptococcus pneumoniae, Staphylococcus aureus,* and group A streptococci also may cause laryngitis associated with pharyngitis, sinusitis, or tonsillitis.

History usually determines the cause of laryngitis. It should include a history of vocal abuse, URI, trauma to the throat (including intubation), infectious or toxic exposure (including tobacco smoke, alcohol, fumes, smoke inhalation, and radiation), and gastrointestinal or pulmonary complaints.

SIGNS AND SYMPTOMS

Hoarseness and dysphonia (variation in vocal quality) are the most common symptoms. Occasionally, mild difficulty swallowing and/or an irritating cough are reported. Pain may be present, localized to the larynx or referred to the ear.

OBJECTIVE FINDINGS

Usually there are no objective findings. Fever with infectious causes may be present. There may be vesicles on the soft palate and lymphadenopathy. Indirect laryngoscopy reveals red, swollen true vocal cords.

A thorough head and neck examination should be done. Indirect laryngoscopy should be done to look for inflammation, masses, vocal cord dysfunction, and structural abnormalities.

DIAGNOSTIC CONSIDERATIONS

Other causes of hoarseness should be ruled out. Persistent hoarseness that does not resolve with conservative treatment may include the following:

- *Laryngeal polyps*: caused by voice abuse or direct trauma (intubation). Appear as discrete polypoid growths on the true vocal cords.
- *Vocal nodules*: also known as "singer's nodules" or "preacher's nodules," caused by poor voice use or overuse. Seen as bilateral, discrete, pearly white lesions at the junction of the anterior and middle thirds of the true vocal cords.
- *Contact ulcers*: caused by voice abuse. Occur as bilateral ulcerations at the tips of the vocal processes of the laryngeal cartilages, causing hoarseness and pain on phonation. Biopsy is required to rule out carcinoma.
- *Hyperkeratosis* ("whiskey voice"): associated with smoking and/or alcohol abuse. Vocal cords are thickened, rough, and covered with hyperkeratotic plaques, which are often premalignant. The patient should be referred for biopsy and follow-up.
- *Leukoplakia:* related to voice and alcohol abuse and smoking. Appears as white, raised plaques at the anterior extremity of one vocal cord. It is premalignant, and biopsy with close follow-up is necessary.
- *Carcinoma*: the most serious cause of hoarseness. Any patient with a suspicious laryngeal lesion should be referred for direct laryngoscopy and biopsy.
- *Vocal cord paralysis*: paralysis of one vocal cord can cause hoarseness. The patient should be referred for evaluation.

SPECIAL CONSIDERATIONS

Smoking and alcohol can aggravate simple laryngitis and are risk factors for more serious causes of persistent hoarseness.

LABORATORY TESTS

A white blood cell count with a differential should be done if infection is suspected. A culture from the throat or larynx is taken in certain cases.

RADIOLOGIC STUDIES

No radiologic studies are necessary in most cases.

OTHER DIAGNOSTICS

Indirect or direct laryngoscopy is used to view the vocal cords. Biopsy may be necessary in selected cases.

TREATMENT

The underlying cause should be treated. In most cases, voice rest, elimination of throat clearing, humidified air, and hydration will speed recovery. The condition is self-limiting.

Medications

Cough suppression may be necessary for irritative coughing. Relief of nasal congestion may help humidify air. Other medications are given as indicated for bacterial infection or gastroesophageal reflux.

Patient Education

Patients should be instructed to use the voice as little as possible. Both shouting and whispering strain the vocal cords, and so if speaking is necessary, a normal tone should be used. Patients should avoid breathing extremely cold air. The use of tobacco and alcohol should be discouraged.

Disposition

Laryngitis is a self-limiting condition. Most patients recover their voices within 2 to 3 weeks or sooner. Chronic laryngitis or acute laryngitis that does not respond to treatment should be further investigated. Laryngeal polyps and vocal nodules require surgical removal. Patients with suspicious or premalignant lesions must be referred to an otolaryngologist for direct examination and biopsy.

COMPLICATIONS OR RED FLAGS

Voice abuse will cause repeated hoarseness. Speech therapy may be necessary to eliminate further abuse.

BIBLIOGRAPHY

Curtis LG: Common ear, nose and throat problems. *Phys Assist* 14:17–22, 1990.

Tierney LM Jr, McPhee SJ, Papadakis MA (eds): *Current Medical Diagnosis and Treatment*, 35th ed. Stamford, CT, Appleton & Lange, 1996, p 208.

Wang BM: Laryngitis, in Rakel RE (ed): *Saunders Manual of Medical Practice.* Philadelphia, Saunders, 1996, pp 108–109.

Chapter 3–7
MENIERE'S DISEASE

Katherine D. Hocum

DISCUSSION

Meniere's disease (Meniere's syndrome, endolymphatic hydrops) is a pathologic condition of the inner ear characterized by episodic vertigo, tinnitus, and fluctuant sensorineural hearing loss. It is a poorly understood progressive disorder that affects over 2 million people in the United States. It is four times as prevalent as otosclerosis and more common than all carcinomas and tumors involving the larynx and salivary glands. It is most frequently seen in adults 20 to 60 years of age. The frequency with which Meniere's disease occurs in the right or left ear is equal. Similarly, there is no gender predilection; it occurs in males as often as in females. One in three patients may suffer from bilateral disease. While the triad of vertigo, tinnitus, and hearing loss dominates the clinical presentation, many patients may complain of a sensation of "fullness" in the affected ear. Vegetative symptoms such as nausea and vomiting are also commonly reported.

PATHOGENESIS

It is believed that the symptoms of Meniere's disease result from a malfunction of the endolymphatic sac in the inner ear. Although the etiology is often idiopathic, it is postulated that the condition results from an imbalance in the amount of endolymph produced by the cochlea and the amount absorbed by the endolymphatic sac, leading to a consistent finding of endolymphatic hydrops. The increased hydrostatic pressure produced by the accumulation of endolymph subsequently causes dizziness and the sensation of aural fullness. As the hydrops becomes more extensive, hearing loss ensues. This chronic distention of the endolymphatic system results in a dysfunction of vestibular and cochlear hair cells that is presumed to cause the chronic disequilibrium and irreversible hearing loss reported by these patients. The etiologic basis of Meniere's disease appears to be multifactorial as well as inherited in many patients. Whites appear to be at increased risk for Meniere's disease, along with those with a history of allergy or excessive exposure to noise. While no single mechanism leading to endolymphatic hydrops can be identified, currently most clinical research and therapeutic measures focus on elimination of the hydrops and identification of viral, autoimmune, and metabolic factors (lipid disorders, allergy) that may lead to the formation of endolymphatic hydrops. Clearly, further research into the pathophysiology of Meniere's disease is necessary to develop stricter diagnostic criteria and suitable treatment modalities.

SIGNS AND SYMPTOMS

The clinical features of Meniere's disease have been described as a triad of symptoms: recurrent debilitating vertigo, progressive sensorineural hearing loss, and tinnitus. Patients also may complain of aural pressure or fullness in the affected ear as well as nausea and vomiting associated with vertiginous episodes. Usually these symptoms appear together, although it is not uncommon for tinnitus or diminution of hearing to precede the onset of vertigo. The onset of vertigo is usually sudden and often disabling. The vertigo may last minutes or hours but rarely lasts longer than 24 to 48 h. Persistent vertigo lasting longer than this suggests a diagnosis other than Meniere's disease. Some patients may report loudness recruitment and diplacusis associated with this condition. Vestibular nystagmus may be present during attacks; however, neurologic signs such as loss of consciousness, aphasia, headache, aura, and paraesthesias are clinically absent. Progressive loss of speech discrimination leads to an irreversible hearing loss that does not improve with the use of a hearing aid. Meniere's disease attacks, while unpredictable, are usually short-lived and self-limiting. Patients frequently are well between vertiginous episodes.

OBJECTIVE FINDINGS

A patient presenting with vertigo or dizziness can represent a diagnostic challenge. Numerous disease states and conditions may cause vertigo, deafness, tinnitus, disequilibrium, or a combination of these symptoms. It is essential that the practitioner elicit an accurate and detailed history when evaluating a dizzy patient. The diagnosis of Meniere's disease is often a presumptive one based on patient complaints of fluctuating sensorineural hearing loss, episodic vertigo, and tinnitus. It is also a diagnosis of exclusion, as conditions affecting the central nervous system and the cardiovascular system and metabolic or psychiatric disorders all may present with similar features and must be considered (Table 3-7-1).

Table 3-7-1. Differential Diagnosis of Dizziness

Benign paroxysmal positional vertigo
Labyrinthitis or vestibular neuronitis
Meniere's disease
Acoustic neuroma
Ototoxic medications
Vertebrobasilar insufficiency
Faintness and syncope
Vertebrobasilar migraine
Hypo- and hypercapnia, hypoxia
Multiple sclerosis
Aortic stenosis
Anemia, hypovolemia
Depression, anxiety, other psychiatric illnesses
Epilepsy
Cervical spondylosis
Otosclerosis
Orthostatic blood pressure changes
Cerebellar disease
Space-occupying lesions
Temporal bone trauma, perilymphatic fistula
Hyperventilation
Diabetes, hypoglycemia

Table 3-7-2. Central versus Peripheral Vertigo

Signs or Symptoms	Peripheral Vertigo	Central Vertigo
Severity of vertigo	Marked, spontaneous	Often mild, gradual
Tinnitus/hearing loss	Usually present	Usually absent
Vertical nystagmus	Never	Occasionally
Horizontal nystagmus	Uncommon	Common
Duration	Finite, intermittent	Variable, chronic
Central nervous system signs	None	Common

A complete physical examination of the head, eyes, ears, nose, neck, and throat is a must. Hearing acuity and speech discrimination should be tested. Examination of the tympanic membranes (TMs) often is normal, as no observable anatomic or morphologic changes are associated with the vertigo, hearing loss, tinnitus, and aural fullness of Meniere's disease. Nystagmus, if present, should be described accurately. A thorough neurologic examination, including reflexes, mental status, and gait, should be performed. Care should be taken to adequately assess the cardiovascular, pulmonary, and endocrine systems. Frequently, patients presenting with Meniere's disease have an unremarkable physical examination.

DIAGNOSTIC CONSIDERATIONS

The initial step in evaluating the patient is to obtain an accurate description of "dizziness." True vertigo, as experienced in Meniere's disease, is typically described as a sensation of one's environment "spinning" or "everything moving." Precipitating factors, if any, and the frequency and timing of the vertigo should be elicited. The patient also should be encouraged to relate any other symptoms associated with the episodes. Vestibular vertigo may be central or peripheral in origin, and the practitioner should remain aware of conditions that mimic Meniere's disease but arise from significantly different causes. Typically, isolated vertigo with or without tinnitus and hearing loss arises from a peripheral lesion. In central lesions, vertigo often is accompanied by neurologic deficits (Table 3-7-2).

Benign paroxysmal positional vertigo (BPPV) is sudden isolated vertigo experienced when the head is moved into specific positions. Symptoms are self-limiting but may resume when the patient moves into a "trigger" position. BPPV may last up to 6 months, and recovery is often spontaneous and complete. Labyrinthitis, sometimes called a vestibular neuronitis, develops in the inner ear after a viral upper respiratory infection (URI). Any vertigo, hearing loss, or tinnitus is temporary and usually resolves spontaneously within 3 to 6 weeks. Ototoxicity, otosclerosis, and herpes zoster oticus may have a similar presentation. Acoustic neuroma should always be considered, though the accompanying neurologic signs (decreased corneal reflex, ataxia) often make the diagnosis clear. Central causes of vertigo are often more worrisome. Multiple sclerosis (MS), vertebrobasilar insufficiency, and a decompensated cardiovascular system may present initially as vertigo. Often these conditions, like transient ischemic attacks (TIAs), are accompanied by other signs and symptoms, making the diagnosis of Meniere's disease less likely. Psychiatric illness (depression, anxiety states) and metabolic disorders (hypoxia, drug overdose) should also be considered in evaluating a patient with dizziness (Table 3-7-3).

SPECIAL CONSIDERATIONS

An elderly patient with vertigo is likely to be the most difficult to diagnose. Many geriatric patients complain of dizziness as well as suffer from one or more multisystem disorders (diabetes, TIA) that may make the diagnosis complicated.

LABORATORY TESTS

No single laboratory test or battery of tests can confirm the diagnosis of Meniere's disease. The diagnosis is often presumptive after a thorough history and physical examination.

RADIOLOGIC STUDIES

Computed tomography (CT) and magnetic resonance imaging (MRI) of the internal auditory canal and cerebellopontine angles should always be performed to rule out localized or space-occupying lesions.

OTHER DIAGNOSTICS

Electronystagmography (ENG) with warm and cold calorics will differentiate between central and peripheral causes of vertigo. Audiologic testing to document hearing loss is also indicated. If neuroma of the eighth cranial nerve is suspected, brainstem auditory response testing should be performed. Electroencephalography (EEG) will aid in the diagnosis of epilepsy or migraine. Patients should not be medicated with vestibular sedatives during testing, as these agents may affect the response or invalidate the diagnostic study altogether.

TREATMENT

Treatment of Meniere's disease may be medical or surgical. While it is clear that there is no universally effective treatment for patients with Meniere's disease, most treatment modalities are aimed at reducing endolymphatic hydrops or symptomatically suppressing the vertigo. Until the definitive etiology of Meniere's disease is elucidated, treatment will remain only moderately effective in the majority of patients.

Pharmacologic Treatment

For an acutely disabled patient, diazepam (Valium) 5 mg intramuscularly or 10 mg orally may be helpful. Trimethobenzamide hydrochloride (Tigan) capsules 250 mg every 8 h (adults) or 100 mg every 8 h (children) may be administered to control nausea and vomiting. If the nausea and vomiting are severe, the intramuscular route, 200 mg every 12 h, should be considered. Medications that sedate the vestibular system, such as meclizine (Antivert) and dimenhydrinate (Dramamine), are also effective. Antivert 25 to 50 mg orally every 6 h or Dramamine 50 mg orally every 6 h should relieve most patients. Both agents may cause considerable drowsiness. Patients should be warned against driving or operating machinery while medicated. Lower doses in elderly patients may be less sedating yet equally effective. For a patient with an established diagnosis of Meniere's disease, treatment is aimed at preventing vertiginous episodes through diet modification and diuretics. Hydrochlorothiazide (Hydro-Diuril) 25 to 50

Table 3-7-3. Differential Diagnosis of Meniere's Disease

Peripheral Causes	Central Causes	Other Causes
Benign paroxysmal positional vertigo	Vertebrobasilar insufficiency	Diabetes mellitus
Labyrinthitis/ vestibular neuronitis	Transient ischemic attack/ ischemia	Anemia, hypovolemia
Trauma	Multiple sclerosis	Psychiatric illness
Ototoxic medications	Tumors/neuroma	Orthostatic blood pressure changes
Otosclerosis	Vestibular epilepsy	Medications
Neurosyphilis	Cerebellar injury/ disease	Aortic stenosis
Herpes zoster oticus	Cerebrovascular accident	Migraine

Table 3-7-4. Pharmacologic Management of Meniere's Disease

Agent	Dose/Route	Comments
Diazepam (Valium)	5–10 mg IM or PO	Used most often for acute attacks
Trimethobenzamide hydrochloride (Tigan)	200 mg IM q12h	For severe nausea and vomiting
Meclizine (Antivert)	250 mg PO q8h	For nausea and vomiting
Dimenhydrinate (Dramamine)	25–50 mg PO q6h	Nausea and vomiting: 12.5 mg PO tid in elderly patients
Hydrochlorothiazide (Hydro-Diuril)	50 mg PO tid	Do not operate machinery
Triamterene (Dyrenium)	25–50 mg PO, 50 mg PO	Check serum potassium, Check serum potassium

mg orally or triamterene (Dyrenium) 50 mg once a day is effective as a long-term treatment. Patients are also encouraged to maintain a low-salt diet (1 to 2 g sodium per day). Some clinicians believe that a vasodilating agent such as papaverine hydrochloride (Pavabid) 150 mg orally bid or cyclandelate (Cyclospasmol) 200 mg orally tid may aid endolymph resorption. The majority of patients with Meniere's disease, however, can be adequately controlled on diuretic therapy coupled with diet modification and vestibular sedatives as needed. Patients who are unresponsive to pharmacologic management may be candidates for surgical intervention (Table 3-7-4).

Surgical Management

While medical therapies are the first-line treatment for patients with Meniere's disease, some patients do not respond to these conservative measures. Procedures designed to drain the endolymphatic system or ablate the eighth cranial nerve and/or the labyrinth may be warranted in aggressive cases. Decompression of the endolymphatic sac and internal shunt placement may be achieved by sacculotomy or cochleosacculotomy. The results are highly variable with these procedures, and while they may reduce vertigo, they often precipitate sensorineural hearing loss. Labyrinthectomy is currently the gold standard in surgical treatment of Meniere's disease, relieving episodic vertigo in the majority of cases. Intratympanic instillation of ototoxic antibiotics such as gentamicin and streptomycin has been successful in relieving vertigo while preserving hearing in many patients. Surgical resection of the eighth nerve has also had some success in controlling vertigo but is associated with postsurgical complications such as headache, hearing loss, and an incomplete vestibular response. Patients affected with bilateral disease make the choice of treatment a greater challenge, as preservation of hearing in at least one ear is desirable.

COMPLICATIONS AND RED FLAGS

Irreversible sensorineural hearing loss is the major complication of Meniere's disease. These patients are also at increased risk for falls and accidents secondary to vertigo, disequilibrium, and/or sedation associated with medical therapy. Patients on diuretic therapy should be encouraged to keep well hydrated, and practitioners may want to periodically evaluate their serum potassium levels.

OTHER NOTES AND PEARLS

Current management of Meniere's disease provides most patients with symptomatic relief only. Patients are advised to avoid caffeine, alcohol, and smoking. Stress reduction may help. Newer diagnostic tools such as electrocochleography (ECoG), inner-ear specific immunoassays, and labyrinthine MRIs may be employed. Human genetic studies may one day allow gene manipulation therapy, making symptomatic treatment obsolete. Future diagnostic techniques and treatment modalities will require well-controlled, multicenter research studies.

BIBLIOGRAPHY

Bates B, Bickley L, Hoekelman R (eds): *A Guide to Physical Examination and History Taking,* 6th ed. Lippincott, Philadelphia, 1995, pp 147–227.

Fauci AS, Braunwald E, Isselbacher KJ, et al (eds): *Harrison's Principles of Internal Medicine,* 14th ed. New York, McGraw-Hill, 1998.

Gorroll A, May L, Mulley A (eds): *Primary Care Medicine: Office Evaluation and Management of the Adult Patient.* Lippincott, Philadelphia, 1995, pp 985–1010.

Isenhower WD: The evaluation and diagnosis of the dizzy patient. *J S C Med Assoc* 90(10):517–522, 1994.

Merchant SN: Meniere's disease. *Eur Arch Oto-Rhino-Laryngol* 252:63–75, 1995.

Monsell EM: Therapeutic use of aminoglycosides in Meniere's disease. *Otolaryngol Clin North Am* 26(5):737–746, 1993.

Norrving B: Isolated vertigo in the elderly: Vestibular or vascular disease? *Acta Neurol Scand* 91:43–48, 1995.

Rakel RE: *Conn's Current Therapy 1996.* Saunders, Philadelphia, 1995, pp 858–878.

Rakel RE: *Textbook of Family Practice,* 5th ed. Saunders, Philadelphia, 1995, pp 441–480.

Shea JJ: Classification of Meniere's disease. *Am J Otol* 14(3):224–229, 1993.

Sullivan M: Psychiatric and otologic diagnoses in patients complaining of dizziness. *Arch Intern Med* 153(12):1479–1484, 1993.

Tran Ba Huy P: Physiopathology of peripheral non-Meniere's vestibular disorders. *Acta Otolaryngol* 513(Suppl):5–10, 1994.

Chapter 3–8
PERITONSILLAR ABSCESS
Nadine Kroenke

DISCUSSION

Peritonsillar abscess (PTA) is one of the most commonly seen abscesses of the head and neck area. PTA is a complication of tonsillitis, peritonsillar cellulitis, and mononucleosis. The abscess forms as a result of an infection extending from within the tonsil through its fibrous capsule into the peritonsillar space and then the peritonsillar fascial planes. The peritonsillar space is designated as the area of the neck between the capsule of the palatine tonsil medially and the fascia of the superior constrictor muscle laterally.

The classic onset of PTA symptoms usually begins only 3 or 5 days before patients seek treatment. Many patients are currently on appropriate antibiotics for a preceding tonsillitis.

Peritonsillar cellulitis and abscess formation are fairly common occurrences in young adults, with the average patient's age being less than 30. It is relatively rare in young children and adults. Occurrences in young children and older adults should alert the clinician to an underlying susceptibility to infection from immune deficiency, malnutrition, leukemia, or another systemic disease.

Peritonsillar abscess is most often polymicrobial, with anaerobic bacteria being recovered most often. The most common aerobic isolates are *Streptococcus pyogenes, Streptococcus milleri, Haemophilus influenzae,* and *Streptococcus viridans.*

Generally, the abscess forms in the supratonsillar space of the soft palate immediately above the superior pole of the affected tonsil. The supratonsillar space initially becomes inflamed, and cellulitis begins. This results in pus formation in the supratonsillar space and the surrounding muscles, especially the internal pterygoids, producing spasm of the muscle that produces trismus.

There has been no agreed-on sex distribution. PTA has the highest incidence in the winter months.

No reliable criteria exist for differentiating PTA from peritonsillar cellulitis (PTC) on physical examination. Differentiating the diagnoses of PTA and PTC can be done by means of careful needle aspiration of the affected tissue by a practitioner familiar with the procedure. If aspiration in three loci yields negative findings, the patient is diagnosed as having PTC. Aspiration may be stopped after one positive aspirate. The diagnosis also may be made by an otolaryngologist [ear, nose, and throat (ENT)] after the patients' clinical course has been followed.

SIGNS AND SYMPTOMS

The typical presentation of a patient with PTC or PTA occurs about 2 to 3 days after the onset of a sore throat. Many of these patients are on appropriate antibiotics for pharyngitis. Patients will describe many of the classic symptoms of pharyngitis, such as fever, sore throat, and odynophagia (pain on swallowing). They also may complain that the sore throat pain is much worse on the side of the abscess. Other symptoms include referred ear pain, headache, and malaise. Patients also may complain of trouble handling secretions and be actively drooling.

OBJECTIVE FINDINGS

Physical examination of a patient with PTA/PTC will show a patient in mild to moderate distress secondary to pain. Low-grade fever and mild tachycardia will be present. A distinctive "hot potato" voice is often noted during the history taking. Palpation of the neck will reveal tender ipsilateral anterior chain lymphadenopathy. The patient may be drooling, spitting, or having trouble handling oral secretions. Trismus will be present in attempts to visualize the oral pharynx. Trismus is considered the leading clinical finding that is helpful in differentiating PTA/PTC from severe tonsillitis. Visualization of the oropharynx will show a deviated uvula with unilateral peritonsillar swelling. The posterior pharynx will be diffusely erythematous. Exudate may or may not be present.

DIAGNOSTIC CONSIDERATIONS

Diagnostic considerations include pharyngitis/tonsillitis, PTC, and retropharyngeal abscess.

SPECIAL CONSIDERATIONS

All pediatric patients should be treated with a trial of intravenous hydration and antibiotics when no airway compromise is present and if no improvement is observed within 24 h. If symptoms worsen, surgery should be performed. It is not recommended to attempt a needle aspiration on a child without general anesthesia.

LABORATORY TESTS

Fluid aspirate culture from a PTA may be obtained, depending on the practitioner's preference. It is recommended in every immunosuppressed patient. Cultures often do not change patient management and outcome.

RADIOLOGIC STUDIES

Because the treatments of PTA and PTC are different and since needle aspiration is a painful invasive procedure, neck CT and intraoral ultrasound are being used increasingly by ENT in some institutions to aid in the differential diagnosis.

OTHER DIAGNOSTICS

No other diagnostics are used.

TREATMENT

PTC can be treated with antibiotics alone, whereas a PTA should be drained. Treatment options when the abscess has already formed include incision and drainage, needle aspiration, and immediate tonsillectomy followed by intramuscular or intravenous penicillin.

None of the surgical interventions has been identified as the optimal procedure for the drainage of a PTA. Tonsillectomy is considered the definitive treatment. There have been reports of recurrence with this method, however.

Pharmacologic Management

Currently, penicillin is the recommended drug of choice; with 1.2 million units of Bicillin LA being administered intramuscularly. Other antibiotics, such as clindamycin, Augmentin (amoxicillin/clavulanic acid), and third-generation cephalosporins are appropriate. However, they should be administered only after consultation with ENT.

DISPOSITION

Primary outpatient management of PTA is recommended by present and prior studies. Patients appropriate for outpatient treatment are those who are nontoxic, compliant, without drooling or severe pain, and taking oral fluid well. Follow-up by ENT should be done within 24 h. The patient should be seen midway through the course of treatment and again 1 week after finishing antibiotics.

Patients who should be admitted for general anesthesia incision and drainage are those who are dyspneic, in severe pain, have excessive trismus on physical exam, or are too young to undergo needle aspiration. Inpatient treatment is required in approximately 15 percent of cases, and an individual stay usually does not exceed an average of 2 days. Patients should be seen again promptly for any recurrence of symptoms.

COMPLICATIONS AND RED FLAGS

The most common complications are recurrent tonsillitis and recurrent PTA, which occur in about 10 percent of these patients. The factors related to the recurrence of PTA are unclear. The general time frame for recurrence is 3 months.

An untreated PTA may rupture, leading to aspiration and pneumonia. Spreading infection of the parapharyngeal spaces can lead to mediastinitis and meningitis. Other complications of peritonsillitis and PTA are endocarditis, polyarthritis, cervical abscess, and sepsis. When the patient is treated early with appropriate incision and drainage and antibiotics, these complications can be avoided. Antibiotic treatment has led to rare complications and limited mortality.

BIBLIOGRAPHY

Ahmed K, Jones A, Smethurst A: Radiology in focus: The role of ultrasound in the management of peritonsillar abscess. *J Laryngol Otol* 108:610–612, 1994.

Blokmanis A: Ultrasound in the diagnosis and management of peritonsillar abscesses. *J Otolaryngol* 23:260–262, 1994.

Callahan M (ed): *Current Practice of Emergency Medicine.* Philadelphia, Decker, 1991.

Fauci AS, Braunwald E, Isselbacher KJ, et al (eds): *Harrison's Principles of Internal Medicine,* 14th ed. New York, McGraw-Hill, 1998.

Jousimies-Somer H, Savolainen S, Makitie A, Ylikoski J: Bacteriologic findings in peritonsillar abscesses in young adults. *Clin Infect Dis* 16(suppl 4):S292–S298, 1993.

Parker G, Tami T: The management of peritonsillar abscess in the 90's: An update. 13:284–288, 1992.

Passy V: Pathogenesis of peritonsillar abscess. *Laryngoscope* 104:185–190, 1994.

Patel K, Ahman S, O'Leary G, Michel M: The role of computed tomography in the management of peritonsillar abscess. *Otolaryngol Head Neck Surg* 107:727–732, 1992.

Roberts J: Emergency department considerations in the diagnosis and treatment of peritonsillar abscess. *Emerg Med News* 2:4–7, 1996.

Roberts J, Hedges J (eds): *Clinical Procedures in Emergency Medicine.* Philadelphia, Saunders, 1991.

Sakaguchi M, Sate S, Asawa S, Taguchi K: Radiology in focus: Computed tomographic findings in peritonsillar abscess and cellulitis. *J Laryngol Otol.* 109(5):449–451, 1995.

Saunders C, Ho M (eds): *Current Emergency Diagnosis and Treatment.* Norwalk, CT, Appleton & Lange, 1992.

Savolainen S, Jousimies-Somer H, Makitie A, Ylikoski J: Peritonsillar abscess: Clinical and microbiological aspects and treatment regimens. *Arch Otolaryngol Head Neck Surg* 19:521–524, 1993.

Schwartz G, Cayten C, Mangelson M, et al (eds): *Principles and Practice of Emergency Medicine.* New York, Lea & Febiger, 1992.

Strong E, Woodward P, Johnson L: Intraoral ultrasound evaluation of peritonsillar abscess. *Laryngoscope* 105:779–782, 1995.

Tintinalli J, Ruiz E, Krome R (eds): *Emergency Medicine: A Comprehensive Study Guide.* New York, McGraw-Hill, 1996.

Weinberg E, Brodsky L, Staniewich J, Volk M: Needle aspiration of peritonsillar abscess in children. *Arch Otolaryngol Head Neck Surg* 119:169–172, 1993.

Wolf M, Even-Chen I, Kronenberg J: Peritonsillar abscess: Repeated needle aspiration versus incision and drainage. *Ann Otol Rhinol Laryngol* 103:554–557, 1994.

Chapter 3–9
PHARYNGITIS/TONSILLITIS
Nadine Kroenke

DISCUSSION

Sore throat is one of the most frequently encountered outpatient complaints, accounting for 40 million outpatient visits per year. Pharyngitis/tonsillitis is reported to be anywhere from the third to the seventh most common emergency department diagnosis. These statistics demand a well-structured treatment plan and follow-up.

The disease involves inflammation and infection of the oropharynx and the associated lymphoid tissue. Microbiology reveals that up to 80 percent of adult patients have pharyngitis/tonsillitis that is viral in etiology. Some of the more common viral agents are adenovirus and herpesvirus, which cause more significant symptoms, and rhinovirus and coronavirus, which are more common and typically cause a milder course. Anywhere from 5 to 20 percent of bacterial infections are due to group A beta-hemolytic streptococci (GABHS) in adults. GABHS accounts for up to 50 percent all cases of pediatric pharyngitis/tonsillitis, making this the most common bacterial pathogen in both the pediatric and the adult populations. GABHS has the most serious consequences to health; therefore, treatment is directed at GABHS. Other bacterial etiologic agents in adults are *Mycoplasma, Chlamydia,* and *Corynebacterium.*

Pharyngitis/tonsillitis is most commonly seen in children ages 5 to 15, with no noted sex prevalence. This infection is most common in the winter and spring. Children are at increased risk because of exposure at school. The disease is spread through direct contact via droplet spread.

The course of all types of pharyngitis/tonsillitis is about 1 week. Fever usually resolves in about 3 to 5 days, with improvement of the sore throat and other associated symptoms afterward. Lymphadenopathy and tonsillar hypertrophy may take several weeks to resolve.

SIGNS AND SYMPTOMS

The typical incubation period of streptococcal pharyngitis is 2 to 4 days. Classically, GABHS infection is described as the abrupt onset of sore throat and odynophagia (pain on swallowing). Other associated symptoms include headache, malaise, fever, anorexia, "sandpaper" rash, arthralgias, and myalgias. Nausea, vomiting, and abdominal pain are common complaints in children. It is important to remember that the sore throat complaint may be a minor component in the patient's presentation.

Cough and rhinorrhea suggest a viral etiology. Viral pharyngitis has no distinguishing clinical features to suggest a specific causative agent.

OBJECTIVE FINDINGS

Regardless of the specific etiology, the patient is likely to be moderately ill with tachycardia and fever usually higher than 38.3° C (101° F). Examination of the throat will reveal injection, erythema, and lymphoid hyperplasia of the posterior pharynx. The tonsils, if present, may be enlarged and erythematous and may or may not be exudative. Neck examination will reveal tender and enlarged anterior cervical chain lymphadenopathy. Patients who have had a tonsillectomy tend to experience a milder clinical course.

Fever is considered the most commonly occurring symptom in children with GABHS. The combination of fever, exudate, and tender lymphadenopathy tends to be regarded as the most sensitive indicator of GABHS. Patients with these symptoms have positive throat cultures 30 to 45 percent of the time. Petechiae of the soft palate tend to be found only in streptococcal infection. A scarlatiniform rash or "strawberry" tongue is also considered pathognomonic of streptococcal disease.

Physical examination is considered unreliable in differentiating streptococcal infection from a viral or other bacterial infection. Even the best practitioners have been found to be correct on the basis of physical findings alone only about 50 percent of the time.

DIAGNOSTIC CONSIDERATIONS

While GABHS is the most common bacterial pathogen, other bacterial and viral causes should be considered in the differential diagnosis. *Chlamydia* occurs in adults predisposed by orogenital sexual activity. *Mycoplasma* is associated with lower respiratory tract infections and headache. *Haemophilus influenzae,* which is more commonly found in pediatric patients, is usually found in a syndrome of symptoms including pharyngitis, otitis media, laryngotracheitis, and epiglottitis.

Diphtheria, which is rare in the current immunized population, is characterized by the presence of a gray exudative membrane that bleeds easily.

Mononucleosis should be considered in patients with exudative tonsillitis that is unresponsive to antibiotics, has a lingering course, and features posterior chain neck lymphadenopathy and abdominal pain.

Noninfectious causes should be considered when the patient does not improve as expected. Other diagnoses to consider include agranulocytosis, leukemia, and lymphoma.

SPECIAL CONSIDERATIONS

Patients who are refractory to antibiotic therapy suggest a resistant bacteriologic or viral etiology. Therefore, other laboratory tests may be indicated at that time. In known streptococcal infections, the Infectious Diseases Society of America's guidelines recommend that treatment failure may be considered after no clinical response at 3 to 5 days of therapy and alternative therapy, and diagnostics may be considered at that time.

It is important to remember that lack of compliance accounts for a significant proportion of treatment failures. It is important to ascertain compliance before regarding a patient as a treatment failure.

LABORATORY TESTS

The Rapid Strep Latex Agglutination Test

While 90 percent sensitive, the rapid strep latex agglutination test has a specificity of only about 80 percent. A negative strep screen does not indicate the absence of GABHS. Literature review recommends that all negative rapid strep screens be followed with routine culture. Obtaining this test depends on the individual clinical situation, compliance, and the availability of follow-up. Rapid strep screens are helpful when there are multiple children in the same family. The known presence or absence of GABHS can help determine the treatment of other family members if they become symptomatic. It is important to remember that a routine culture that is positive for GABHS may not always indicate the pathogen. Approximately 5 to 30 percent of all patients are considered chronic carriers of GABHS.

Other Diagnostics

A Monospot test may be obtained to rule out mononucleosis. This test is often negative in the early phase. In a complete blood count with differential, looking for reactive lymphocytes can be helpful. An ASO titer may be obtained but is rarely useful in the acute setting.

RADIOLOGIC STUDIES

No radiology studies are indicated for routine pharyngitis/tonsillitis unless the diagnosis is unclear.

PHARMACOLOGIC MANAGEMENT

The treatment of pharyngitis is directed at preventing complications of GABHS. Penicillin remains the drug of choice.

Treatment Options for Adults

For adults, the following medications can be used:

- Bicillin LA, 1.2 million units intramuscularly
- Penicillin VK 250 mg or 500 mg four times a day for 10 days
- Amoxicillin 250 or 500 mg three times a day for 10 days
- Erythromycin 20 to 40 mg/kg/d divided bid or qid for 7 to 10 days if the patient is allergic to penicillin
- Cephalexin (Keflex) 500 mg PO qid for 7 to 10 days
- Cefadroxil (Duricef) 1 to 2 g divided qd/bid for 7 to 10 days
- Cefaclor (Ceclor) 250 mg PO tid for 7 to 10 days
- Cefuroxime (Ceftin) 250 to 500 mg bid for 7 to 10 days
- Azithromycin (Zithromax) 500 mg daily for 3 days

Treatment Options for Children

For children, the following medications can be used:

- Bicillin LA, 600,000 units intramuscularly for patients 27 kg or less
- Penicillin VK suspension (or tablets) 125 to 250 mg qid for 10 days
- Amoxicillin suspension 40/mg/kg/d divided tid for 10 days
- Erythromycin elixir 30 to 50 mg/kg/d divided tid/qid for 10 days
- Pediazole suspension 50/mg/kg/d divided qid for 10 days
- Azithromycin (Zithromax) suspension 12 mg/kg once daily for days 1 through 5

Steroids have recently become accepted adjuncts to the treatment of both bacterial and viral pharyngitis. Decadron 10 mg intramuscularly has been shown to provide quicker resolution of symptoms with no increased incidence of complications.[1]

SUPPORTIVE MEASURES

Hydration, antipyretics, rest, and pain medication can provide supportive care. Aspirin should be avoided in children and teenagers because of the possibility of Reye's syndrome (see Chap. 15-4). Ibuprofen is an excellent choice for pain and inflammation in both adults and children.

PATIENT EDUCATION

Patients should be encouraged to complete the full course of antibiotics and maintain adequate hydration. A patient should be seen if a rash or arthralgia develops or if it is not progressively improving. Children are no longer considered infectious after 24 h of continuous antibiotic therapy and may return to day care or school without restrictions while on medication.

DISPOSITION

Virtually all these patients can be managed on an outpatient basis. Patients can return to their usual activities when they are improved.

COMPLICATIONS

Streptococcal pharyngitis is associated with two delayed nonsuppurative sequelae: acute rheumatic fever, which can be prevented by treatment up to 2 weeks after onset, and acute glomerulonephritis, which may occur regardless of treatment.

Streptococcal infection of the pharynx may lead to acute otitis media and sinusitis. Other diseases that may develop secondarily to streptococcal infection include cervical lymphadenitis, retropharyngeal and parapharyngeal abscess, peritonsillar cellulitis and/or abscess, toxic shock syndrome, and scarlet fever.

REFERENCE

1. O'Brian J, Meade J, Falk J: Dexamethasone as adjuvant therapy for severe acute pharyngitis. *Ann Emerg Med* 22:212–215, 1993.

BIBLIOGRAPHY

Barken R, Rosen P (eds): *Emergency Pediatrics: A Guide to Ambulatory Care.* St. Louis, Mosby Year Book, 1994.
Bonilla J, Bluestone C: Pharyngitis: When is aggressive treatment warranted? *Postgrad Med* 97:61–69, 1995.
Burke P: Sore throat. *Practitioner* 237:854–856, 1993.
Denny F: Tonsillopharyngitis 1994. *Pediatr Rev* 15:185–191, 1994.
Dippel D, Touw-Otten F, Habbema D: Management of children with acute pharyngitis: A decision analysis. *J Fam Pract* 34:149–159, 1992.

Fauci AS, Braunwald E, Isselbacher KJ, et al (eds): *Harrison's Principles of Internal Medicine,* 14th ed. New York, McGraw-Hill, 1998.

Feldman W: Pharyngitis in children. *Postgrad Med* 93:141–145, 1993.

Joslyn S, Hoekstra G, Sutherland J: Rapid antigen detection testing in diagnosing group A beta-hemolytic streptococcal pharyngitis. *J Am Board Fam Pract* 8:177–182, 1994.

Knudtson M: Differential diagnosis of pharyngitis in children. *J Pediatr Health Care* 8:33–35, 1994.

Markowitz M: Changing epidemiology of group A streptococcal infections. *Pediatr Infect Dis J* 13:557–560, 1994.

Peter G: Streptococcal pharyngitis: Current therapy and criteria for evaluation of new agents. *Clin Infect Dis* 14:S218–S223, 1992.

Pichichero M: Group A streptococcal tonsillopharyngitis: Cost-effective diagnosis and treatment. *Ann Emerg Med* 25:390–403, 1995.

Saunders C, Ho M (eds): *Current Emergency Diagnosis and Treatment.* Norwalk, CT, Appleton & Lange, 1992.

Schwartz G, Cayten C, Mangelsen M, et al (eds): *Principles and Practice of Emergency Medicine.* New York, Lea & Febiger, 1992.

Shulman S: Streptococcal pharyngitis: Diagnostic considerations 1994. *Pediatr Infect Dis J* 13:567–571, 1994.

Stevenson L, Yetman R: Practice guidelines. *J Pediatr Health Care* 8:39–40, 1994.

Stollerman G: Penicillin for streptococcal pharyngitis: Has anything changed? *Hosp Pract* 3:80–83, 1995.

Tintinalli JE, Ruiz E, Krome RL (eds): *Emergency Medicine: A Comprehensive Study Guide,* 4th ed. New York, McGraw-Hill, 1996.

Vukmir R: Adult and pediatric pharyngitis: A review. *Emerg Med Rev* 10:607–616, 1992.

Chapter 3–10
UPPER RESPIRATORY ILLNESS
John P. Donnelly

DISCUSSION

Upper respiratory illness (URI), or the common cold, is one of the most common community illnesses. URI is an acute infection caused by a virus. It generally is self-diagnosed and treated by the patient and is self-limited in its duration. The economic impact of URI is staggering. Estimates of annual expenditures for medications used in therapy for the common cold exceed $2 billion annually.[1]

PATHOGENESIS

The common cold (URI) is caused by viruses, the most common of which are rhinoviruses, followed by coronavirus, adenovirus, parainfluenza virus, respiratory syncytial virus, and influenza virus (Table 3-10-1).

Rhinovirus accounts for more than 30 percent of common colds and has over 100 antigenically different types. Coronavirus accounts for 10 to 20 percent of URIs and is followed by parainfluenza, respiratory syncytial virus, adenovirus, and influenza virus at 5 percent each.[5]

Influenza virus, parainfluenza virus, and adenovirus present with a more severe influenza-like syndrome often involving the lower respiratory tract, whereas rhinovirus and coronavirus present with the more common nasal mucosal irritation and scratchy, irritated sore throat. Seasonal peaks of URIs in the early fall and spring usually are caused by rhinovirus, while winter peaks are attributed to coronavirus.

Table 3-10-1. Etiologic Viruses in the Common Cold

Virus	Frequency, %
Rhinovirus	30
Coronavirus	10–20
Parainfluenza virus	5
Influenza virus	5
Respiratory syncytial virus	5
Adenovirus	5

It is often difficult to distinguish between the various viruses from a clinical examination alone, and often the severity of the illness may be the only clue. Early fall peaks of the common cold often are attributed to the start of school and the spread of virus particles by schoolchildren. Contrary to popular belief, cold temperature (or temperature changes) is not an important factor in the epidemiology of colds, though the crowding associated with colder weather does promote the spread of viruses. Psychological stress has been shown to be a factor in the frequency of colds, probably through compromise of the immune system.

SYMPTOMS

The signs and symptoms of URI can of course vary with the etiologic agent and present with an acute mild to moderate infection lasting about a week. URIs present with the familiar scratchy throat, malaise, headache, and nasal discharge. The nasal discharge is clear at first and may become purulent after a day or so. Sore throat is present in about two-thirds of cases.

Cough may be present and can be prolonged in smokers. A primary differential diagnostic concern in a patient presenting with pharyngitis, especially exudative, is group A streptococcus. Appropriate cultures should be obtained if indicated by the physical examination.

Adenovirus presents with a more severe illness and is the etiologic agent in febrile pharyngoconjunctival illness.

Respiratory syncytila virus (RSV) presents with a more severe illness and can be an important etiologic agent in day-care and nursery outbreaks.

OBJECTIVE FINDINGS

Objective findings on physical examination may be few. Red irritated nasal mucosa, rhinorrhea, and pharyngeal erythema are common physical signs. Mild respiratory wheezing can accompany some viral infections, especially in children, and can be precursors to exacerbations of asthma.

Sinus pain can be elicited in many patients with URIs. CT of sinuses during a recent study in patients with the common cold revealed that 60 percent had abnormalities of the ethmoid or maxillary sinuses and that 30 percent had abnormalities of the frontal sinuses.[2]

Cervical adenopathy and a low-grade fever may be present.

DIAGNOSTIC CONSIDERATIONS

In patients with pharyngitis, the differential diagnosis should include beta-hemolytic streptococcus, though the presence of coryza and cough is generally not consistent with streptococcal pharyngitis (see Chap. 3-9).

Acute infections with mononucleosis (see Chap. 3-3) should be considered when the illness appears to be prolonged. Measles and chickenpox may present with the symptoms of the common cold in the early stages, resulting ultimately in the usual exanthems typical of the disease.

Influenza (see Chap. 9-15) may present in the early stages with typical cold symptoms, but usually other constitutional symptoms are present and the severity of the symptoms is greater.

Allergic rhinitis (see Chap. 3-4) is also a consideration in the differential diagnosis.

SPECIAL CONSIDERATIONS

There are possible complications of the common cold, especially in patients who are prone to asthma. Viruses have been shown to be precursors to exacerbations of acute asthma attacks,[3] especially in children. Acute exacerbations may require corticosteroids to control bronchospasm. New therapies for the treatment or prevention of viral URIs could greatly reduce mortality and morbidity rates in this population (see Chap. 17-1).

Bacterial infections of the middle ear are a consideration, especially in children. Sinusitis may appear at any time during the course of a URI and may require antibiotic therapy. There has been an increase in the frequency of pneumonia and bronchitis after URIs, especially in the debilitated and elderly populations.

LABORATORY TESTS

No specific laboratory tests are recommended for the common cold. Strep screens may be appropriate for patients with pharyngitis and adenopathy. Viral cultures and immunoassays are generally unnecessary; however, in major outbreaks, such tests can indicate which virus is the prevailing type.

RADIOLOGIC STUDIES

There are no specific recommendations for radiologic studies. In patients with severe illness and wheezing, chest x-ray may be helpful in ruling out an underlying pneumonitis.

TREATMENT

Sir William Osler was quoted as saying, "There is just one way to treat a cold . . . with contempt."

Most cases of the common cold are diagnosed and treated by the patient without medical intervention. Though billions are spent for over-the-counter preparations, many of these medications have been shown to be ineffective or to actually prolong symptoms. In a study by Grahm and associates,[4] aspirin and acetaminophen were shown to have a detrimental effect on URI therapy through neutralization of antibodies, which resulted in an increase in symptoms, especially nasal.

Naproxen has been shown to produce a significant reduction in the symptoms of the common cold without altering viral shedding[5] or prolonging the symptoms.

Antihistamines do not appear to be effective in the majority of URIs.[6,7] Symptomatic relief by antihistamines may derive more from the sedative effect than from the actual local effect.[2] The oral sympathomimetics (pseudoephedrine, phenylephrine) help reduce secretions from the nasal mucosa by neutralizing the effects of kinin production. Recently, nasal ipratropium was advocated as a local measure in colds to reduce nasal congestion and secretions. The mechanism of action is again a reduction in kinin production or neutralization. Topical sympathomimetics in nasal sprays should be used for very short periods. Because of the rebound effect and dependence resulting in chronic use, they should be used only a few days.

Antibiotics are not indicated for the common cold. Patients often request antibiotics, and providers sometimes are pressured into prescribing these. As a result of the emergence of numerous strains of antibiotic-resistant bacteria, antibiotic utilization should be confined to cases of documented bacterial infection.

Patient Education

Patients should be instructed in good hand-washing techniques to prevent or reduce spread by surface contact or hand-to-hand contact. There is empirical evidence that increased surface disinfection (especially in day-care centers, schools, etc.) with an effective antiseptic product may reduce the incidence of viral spread. Children should be instructed not to touch the eyes and nose, important portals of entry for respiratory viruses.

Disposition

Patients should follow up if symptoms are prolonged, i.e., last over 5 to 7 days. Fever appearing late in the illness may be a warning of a secondary bacterial infection such as sinusitis or pneumonia, particularly in an immunocompromised host.

REFERENCES

1. Spector SL: The common cold: Current therapy and natural history. *J Allergy Clin Immunol* 95:1133–1138, 1995.
2. Engel JP: Viral upper respiratory infections. *Semin Respir Infect* 10:3–13, 1995.
3. Abramson MJ, Marks GB, Pattermore PK: Are non-allergic environmental factors important in asthma? *Med J Aust* 163:542–545, 1995.
4. Graham NM, Burrell CJ, Douglas RM, et al: Adverse effects of aspirin, acetaminophen and ibuprofen on immune function, viral shedding and clinical status in rhinovirus infected volunteers. *J Infect Dis* 162:1277–1282, 1990.
5. Sperber SJ, Levine PA, Sorrentino JV, et al: Ineffectiveness of recombinant interferon-beta serine nasal drops for prophylaxis of natural colds. *J Infect Dis* 160:700–705, 1989.
6. Hutton N, Wilson MH, Mellits ED, et al: Effectiveness of an antihistamine-decongestant combination for young children with the common cold: A randomized, controlled clinical trial. *J Pediatr* 118:125–130, 1991.
7. Smith MG, Geldman W: Over the counter cold medications: A critical review of clinical trials between 1950 and 1991. *JAMA* 269:2258–2263, 1993.

BIBLIOGRAPHY

Ansari SA, Springthorpe VS, Sattar SA, et al: Potential role of hands in the spread of respiratory viral infections: Studies with human parainfluenza virus 3 and rhinovirus 14. *J Clin Microbiol* 29:2115–2119, 1991.
Gwaltney JM Jr, Phillips CD, Miller RD, et al: Computed tomography study of the common cold. *New Engl J Med* 330:25–30, 1994.
Morrison VA, Pomeroy C: Upper respiratory tract infections in the immunocompromised host. *Semin Respir Infect* 10:37–50, 1995.
Sattar SA, Jacobson H, Springthorp VS, et al: Chemical disinfection interrupts transfer Rhinovirus type 14 from environmental surfaces to hands. *Appl Environ Microbiol* 59:1579–1585, 1993.

Chapter 3–11
ORAL HAIRY LEUKOPLAKIA
Dana M. Gallagher

DISCUSSION

Oral hairy leukoplakia (OHL) is a white striated or corrugated mouth lesion that typically is found on the sides of the tongue, although it also may occur on the soft palate and the floor of the mouth. OHL may affect mere millimeters or cover the dorsum of the tongue entirely.

Although OHL was first observed in 1981 in homosexual males with HIV infection, it is not pathognomonic. Approximately 25 percent of people with HIV develop OHL;[1] it also has been found in people with iatrogenically induced immunosuppression (those with organ transplants or leukemia, asthmatics on steroids) and in three patients with no evidence of immunocompromise.[2] OHL occurs more frequently in smokers.

PATHOGENESIS

OHL is not a malignant or even a premalignant lesion. It is likely that cell turnover, as evidenced by the keratinization of the lesion, is actually reduced.[3] OHL is a signal of advancing HIV infection[4] and is not infectious.

Microbiology

OHL is caused by Epstein-Barr virus (EBV) and also has been associated with human papillomavirus (HPV) infection. The shedding of EBV from saliva to the mucosa maintains the leukoplakia. It has been noted that there are a variety of EBV types, strains, and variants. Coinfection and recombination of EBV are consistently found in those with OHL, regardless of their immune status.

SYMPTOMS

OHL is asymptomatic. Unlike another common HIV-related mouth condition, oral candidiasis, or "thrush," OHL does not cause bad breath, unpleasant tongue sensations, or taste changes.

OBJECTIVE FINDINGS

A white corrugated lesion unilaterally or bilaterally on the tongue is visible on gross examination. In contrast to thrush, OHL cannot be scraped away with a tongue depressor or toothbrush.

DIAGNOSTIC CONSIDERATIONS

The diagnosis of OHL usually is made clinically and therefore is frequently treated presumptively. OHL often is seen in conjunction with oral candidiasis and can be confused with smoker's leukoplakia and oral cancers.

LABORATORY TESTS

Biopsy is the gold standard; however, in primary care settings, it usually is not performed until a treatment trial has failed. Unfortunately, viral cultures cannot be used to make the diagnosis.

RADIOLOGIC STUDIES

No radiologic studies are necessary.

TREATMENT

Pharmacologic Management

The following agents can be used.

1. Acyclovir 800 mg PO five times a day has been shown to be effective. Lesions probably will recur if the medication is stopped.
2. A one-time application of 25% topical podophyllin is efficacious[5] (but this is not currently an FDA-approved use for podophyllin). Patients report minimal transient side effects, including a burning sensation and pain and altered taste. Patient tolerance is high. Considerable short-term resolution of lesions can be expected.

Supportive Measures

Good mouth hygiene (tongue and mouth self-examinations, frequent brushing and flossing) is critical for all HIV-positive people.

Patient Education

Patients should be told the following facts:

1. OHL cannot be spread by kissing, sharing utensils, or drinking from the same cup. People with HIV should not share toothbrushes with others, since bleeding gums can theoretically spread the virus.
2. Treating OHL is not mandatory (but often the patient will want to for cosmetic or psychological reasons). OHL can be treated but probably will recur when the treatment stops.
3. If the patient is a smoker, a smoking cessation program should be recommended and instituted.

DISPOSITION

HIV-positive patients should have a mouth examination at every office visit. The finding of OHL on a routine examination should prompt testing in a patient whose HIV status is unknown.

NOTES AND PEARLS

Ganciclovir (DHPG) used in the treatment of cytomegalovirus infection has simultaneously been used to treat OHL. The newer acyclovir-like drugs (famciclovir, valacyclovir) may prove useful in treatment.

REFERENCES

1. Walling DM, Clark NM, Markovitz DM: Epstein-Barr virus co-infection and recombination in nonhuman immunodeficiency virus-associated oral hairy leukoplakia. *J Infect Dis* 171:1122, 1995.
2. Zakrzewska JM, Aly Z, Speight PM: Oral hairy leukoplakia in a HIV-negative asthmatic patient on systemic steroids. *J Oral Pathol Med* 24:282, 1995.
3. Greenspan JS, Greenspan D: Oral complications of HIV infection, in Sande MA, Volberding PA (eds): *The Medical Management of AIDS,* 5th ed. Vienna, VA, Antimicrobial Therapy, 1997, p 174.
4. Sanford JP, Sande MA, Gilbert DN: *The Sanford Guide to HIV/AIDS Therapy.* Vienna, VA, Antimicrobial Therapy, 1996, p 33.
5. Gowdey G, Lee RK, Carpenter WM: Treatment of HIV-related hairy leukoplakia with podophyllum resin 25% solution. *Oral Surg Oral Med Oral Pathol* 79:64–67, 1995.

Chapter 3–12
MASTOIDITIS
Pamela Moyers Scott

DISCUSSION

Mastoiditis is a bacterial infection that causes coalescence of the mastoid air cells by destroying the bony partitions between them. It is generally a complication of otitis media; hence, the primary pathogens tend to be the same: *Streptococcus pneumoniae, Haemophilus influenzae,* and *Moraxella catarrhalis.* Other pathogens include *Streptococcus pyogenes* and *Staphylococcus aureus.*

In the preantibiotic era, acute mastoiditis complicated up to 20 percent of all cases of acute otitis media. With the advent of appropriate antibiotic therapies and early treatment of acute otitis media, the incidence of acute mastoiditis declined to an estimated 0.2 and 2.0 percent. A chronic, subclinical mastoiditis is probably more prevalent than acute mastoiditis in today's medical practice.

SIGNS AND SYMPTOMS

Acute mastoiditis is characterized by the return of otalgia, fever, and diminished hearing approximately 2 weeks after the initial onset of acute otitis media. Additionally, the patient generally complains of postauricular pain and swelling.

Chronic mastoiditis is asymptomatic, although the individual may experience frequent episodes of acute otitis media. Therefore, symptoms related only to the otitis media will be present.

OBJECTIVE FINDINGS

In acute mastoiditis, the tympanic membrane has the appearance of acute otitis media: erythematous, bulging, and poorly distinguishable landmarks. If a perforation is present, a purulent creamy discharge also is usually present. Additionally, there are varying degrees of postauricular tenderness, erythema, and edema.

In chronic mastoiditis, there are no concomitant physical findings unless otitis media is also present.

DIAGNOSTIC CONSIDERATIONS

If there is marked postauricular edema, erythema, or tenderness, a careful examination is imperative to evaluate the possibility of an associated fluctuant postauricular mass that indicates the presence of an abscess.

Chronic mastoiditis in adults frequently is associated with an underlying allergic condition.

LABORATORY TESTS

Unless a patient with acute mastoiditis appears toxic, no specific laboratory analysis is indicated.

RADIOGRAPHIC STUDIES

Early in the course of acute mastoiditis, the mastoid x-ray can be normal or can show minimal cloudiness of the mastoid air cells. As the disease progresses, the cloudiness increases. As mastoiditis becomes chronic, mastoid films reveal destruction of the bony partitions separating the mastoid air cells (Fig. 3-12-1).

Computed tomography (CT) can reveal the cloudiness of the mastoid air cells and the destruction of the mastoid bony partitions that result in the coalescence of these air cells.

TREATMENT

Pharmacologic Management

If the patient is not toxic, a trial of 24 to 48 h of oral antibiotics on an outpatient basis in a compliant patient is appropriate.

First-line therapy generally consists of a cephalosporin, such as cefixime (Suprax) 400 mg daily for adults and 8 mg/kg/d for children, cefuroxime axetil (Ceftin) 500 mg bid for adults and 30 mg/kg/d for children, or cephalexin (Keflex) 500 mg qid for adults and 50 mg/kg/d for children. Amoxicillin/clavulanic potassium (Augmentin) 500 mg q 8 h for adults or 40 mg/kg/d for children is another acceptable alternative. Another acceptable first-line agent is dicloxacillin.

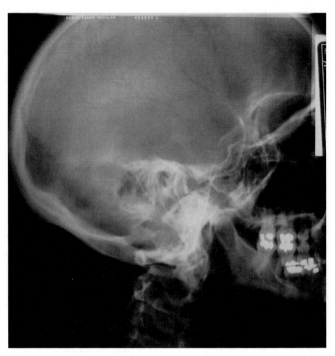

Figure 3-12-1. Cloudiness of the mastoid air cells and frank loss of the air cells as a result of the destruction of the bony partitions between them are common radiographic findings in mastoiditis.

In individuals allergic to or intolerant of these medications, erythromycin and the macrolide antibiotics are acceptable alternatives. All therapy should last for 14 days.

If the patient does not respond or worsens in the first 48 h, he or she should be referred for hospital admission to receive intravenous antibiotics and possible surgery. Some authorities feel that all patients with acute mastoiditis should be hospitalized initially.

Surgical Interventions

If the patient does not respond to empiric antibiotic therapy and the tympanic membrane is intact, a tympanocentesis and myringotomy with or without tympanostomy tubes should be performed. This facilitates drainage of the middle ear and provides a specimen for culture and sensitivity testing. Again, some experts feel that this should be performed immediately after the diagnosis.

If a patient with acute mastoiditis does not respond to treatment or has chronic mastoiditis, he or she needs some form of mastoidectomy, depending on the severity of the disease. The goals of a mastoidectomy include resolving the infection, preventing intracranial complications, improving hearing to preinfection levels, reventilating the middle ear, and allowing healing of the tympanic membrane if perforation was present or myringotomy was performed. The estimated success rate of a simple or modified radical mastoidectomy is approximately 80 percent.

Supportive Measures

Pain relief is essential. Nonsteroidal anti-inflammatory drugs (NSAIDs) such as ibuprofen 800 mg tid to qid are generally effective. Occasionally, narcotic pain medications are required to alleviate the pain. Fever may be controlled with ibuprofen and/or acetaminophen.

Patient Education

If acute mastoiditis is treated on an outpatient basis, it is imperative that the patient understand the potential sequelae resulting from mastoiditis and the importance of frequent, regular follow-up visits as well as compliance with the antibiotic regime to minimize complications.

If a perforated tympanic membrane is present, the patient must be instructed in the proper use of earplugs, the importance of follow-up, and the potential need for surgical repair.

DISPOSITION

If outpatient therapy is chosen for a patient, that patient should be seen again in 24 to 48 h. Follow-up visit frequency depends on the response and whether perforation of the tympanic membrane is present.

COMPLICATIONS AND RED FLAGS

The complications of acute and chronic mastoiditis can be divided into intra- and extracranial conditions. Extracranial complications can consist of hearing loss, labyrinthitis, weakness or complete paralysis of the ipsilateral seventh cranial nerve (facial), and Gradenigo's syndrome, which is characterized by otalgia, otorrhea, and paralysis of the ipsilateral sixth cranial nerve (abducens).

Intracranial complications from acute or chronic mastoiditis are the same as those from otitis media: meningitis, brain abscess, epidural abscess, lateral sinus thrombophlebitis, and otitic hydrocephalus.

The following situations require immediate referral to an otorhinolaryngologist for hospitalization:

• Presence of an abscess

• Paralysis of the sixth or seventh cranial nerve
• Failure to respond by 24 or 48 h

Any patient who has incomplete resolution of all symptoms or develops chronic mastoiditis should be referred to an otorhinolaryngologist.

OTHER NOTES AND PEARLS

In choosing a cephalosporin for the treatment of acute mastoiditis, it is imperative to consider the frequency of methicillin-resistant *S. aureus* and β-lactamase-producing *H. influenzae* and *M. catarrhalis* in your geographic region.

BIBLIOGRAPHY

Bailey J, Struck CL, Smith C: Otolaryngology, in Rakle R (ed): *Textbook of Family Practice,* 5th ed. Philadelphia, Saunders, 1995, pp 455–456.

Giebink GS: Epidemiology and natural history of otitis media, in Lim D, Bluestone C, Klein J, Nelson J (eds): *Recent Advances in Otitis Media with Effusion.* Philadelphia, Decker, 1994, pp 5–9.

Lebovics R: Diseases of the upper respiratory tract, in Wilson JD, Braunwald E, Isselbacher KJ, et al (eds): *Harrison's Principles of Internal Medicine,* 12th ed. New York, McGraw-Hill, 1991, pp 1096–1099.

Niparko J: Hearing loss and associated problems, in Barker LR, Burton J, Zieve P (eds): *Principles of Ambulatory Medicine,* 4th ed. Baltimore, Williams & Wilkins, 1995, pp 1410–1411.

Sanford J, Gilbert D, Sande M: *Guide to Antimicrobial Therapy 1995.* Dallas, Antimicrobial Therapy, 1995, p 6.

Snow J: Surgical disorders of the ears, nose, paranasal sinuses, pharynx, and larynx, in Sabiston D (ed): *Textbook of Surgery,* 14th ed. Philadelphia, Saunders, 1991, pp 1190–1191.

Chapter 4–1
ACID-BASE DISORDERS
Claire Babcock O'Connell

DISCUSSION

The plasma pH is constantly adjusting to changes in hydrogen ion content and the concentration of other substances such as bicarbonate, carbon dioxide, and organic acids that are inherently acidotic or alkalotic in nature. Through the adjustments made mainly by the lungs and the kidneys, the extracellular pH is held relatively constant at 7.35 to 7.45. The intracellular pH is slightly lower because of cellular metabolism; for practical application, the pH of the extracellular fluid is used for clinical assessment and evaluation.

Determination of pH is based on the Henderson-Hasselbalch equation (see Fig. 4-1-1), which describes the relationship between bicarbonate and carbonic acid, the principal players in the acid-base balance of the extracellular fluid. Carbonic acid is very short-lived and readily converts to water and carbon dioxide (see Fig. 4-1-2). The overall pH is determined by the ratio between the concentrations of HCO_3^- to CO_2. The normal ratio is 20 HCO_3^- to 1 CO_2. When the ratio exceeds 22, the condition is alkalotic; below 18 it is acidotic. The ratio changes with variations in the concentration of either substance. An increase in bicarbonate or a decrease in carbon dioxide causes an increase in the ratio (alkalosis); a decrease in bicarbonate or an increase in carbon dioxide causes a decrease in the ratio (acidosis). In general, the pH varies directly with change in HCO_3^- and indirectly with change in CO_2.

Regulation of pH balance is conducted by the lungs and kidneys, which are continually responding to minute changes in ion concentration and bringing the overall condition of the body back to equilibrium. The lungs affect pH by blowing off CO_2, a volatile gas that, through its release, decreases the concentration of hydrogen ions. Through changes in the rate and depth of respirations, the pH is finely adjusted. The blood-brain barrier is freely permeable to CO_2 and reacts rapidly to changes in the CO_2 content in the blood by stimulating or inhibiting respirations. High CO_2 (low pH) stimulates an increase in respiration; low CO_2 (high pH) inhibits respirations. This respiratory response to changes in pH is rapid but can become blunted.

The kidneys are not as fast as the lungs in their role in the maintenance of pH balance. The kidneys respond to changes in hydrogen ion concentration by adjusting the ability to retain HCO_3^- and excrete H^+. The kidneys are responsible for the more chronic adjustments through this alteration in renal excretion. High levels of CO_2 drive the bicarbonate–carbonic acid equation to the left, producing increased H^+. Acidosis (high H^+) stimulates hydrogen ion secretion and, hence, the production of ammonia. H^+ is then excreted as ammonium with new HCO_3^- produced and reabsorbed. Decreased CO_2 has the opposite effect. Alkalosis (low H^+) inhibits hydrogen secretion, reducing HCO_3^- generation. In alkalosis, there is already a high concentration of HCO_3^-, which results in increased HCO_3^- excretion.

Acid-base status is clinically evaluated through measurement of arterial blood gases. Pao_2 (normally >80 mmHg), $Paco_2$ (nor-

mally 35 to 45 mmHg), and pH (7.35 to 7.45) are measured directly; HCO_3^- (normally 22 to 26 mmHg) is determined using a nomogram. Proper technique is necessary to assure accurate blood-gas analysis. Specimens should be put on ice promptly; the CO_2 will rise over time, especially at room temperature, which will also cause a fall in pH. Long delays in analyzing the specimen will cause lysis of cells, which will cause a false acidosis. Body temperature at either extreme will affect the gases: high fevers and hypothermia necessitate correction of the pH (increased in fever, decreased in hypothermia) and the Pao_2 and $Paco_2$ (decreased in fever, increased in hypothermia). Large air bubbles caught in the specimen introduce additional O_2 into the specimen and, therefore, a relative reduction in $Paco_2$ and a falsely higher pH.

In general, metabolic disorders indicate a change in HCO_3^-, and respiratory disorders indicate a change in CO_2. The clinical assessment of acid-base status for the most part can be evaluated using the pH and the $Paco_2$. The suffix, *emia*, denotes the status of hydrogen ion in the blood; the suffix *osis* indicates the condition of the patient. Alkalemia occurs whenever there is a rise in HCO_3^- or a fall in CO_2; acidemia occurs whenever there is a rise in CO_2 or a fall in HCO_3^-. The pH rises in alkalemia and falls in acidemia. Compensation is carried out by the body in reaction to these changes in hydrogen ion concentration and pH. If the primary condition causing the imbalance is metabolic, the lungs will be the principal player in compensation; if the primary condition is respiratory, the kidneys will attempt compensation.

The first step in evaluating acid-base disorders in practice is the history and physical examination. Analysis of arterial blood gases confirms and quantitates the condition and helps to direct and monitor treatment. However, the interpretation of the blood gases should not be complicated.

Simply look at the pH first and determine whether it is normal, elevated, or low. Then look at the $Paco_2$. If the pH is acidotic and the $Paco_2$ is elevated, there is a respiratory acidosis; if the $Paco_2$ is low or normal, there is a metabolic acidosis. In this case, the HCO_3^- will be low; any decrease in $Paco_2$ represents respiratory compensation. Alternatively, if the pH is alkalotic and the $Paco_2$ is decreased, there is a respiratory alkalosis; if the $Paco_2$ is high or normal, there is a metabolic alkalosis. Here the HCO_3^- will be elevated, and any increase in $Paco_2$ represents respiratory compensation. Compensation may bring the pH back into the normal range (7.35 to 7.45) but will never move past the midline (7.4) and "overcompensate." Figure 4-1-3 illustrates the major changes in acidosis and alkalosis.

METABOLIC ACIDOSIS

Bicarbonate loss or consumption underlies all metabolic acidosis. Bicarbonate is consumed whenever there is an increase in acid production (lactic acid, ketoacids, etc.) or a decrease in renal excretion of H^+. Bicarbonate loss results from renal dysfunction. Differentiation among causes of metabolic acidosis is aided by the determination of the anion gap $[Na^+-(Cl^- + HCO_3^-)]$. The major cation in the plasma is sodium; the major "measured" anions are chloride and bicarbonate. The unmeasured anions (mainly albumin, phosphate, sulfate, lactate, and the salts of other weaker acids) are collectively known as the anion gap. An increase in these unmeasured anions increases the anion gap. Conditions of metabolic acidosis that are associated with increased

$$pH = pk + \log \frac{(HCO_3^-)}{(H_2CO_3)}$$

$$pH = pk + \log \frac{(HCO_3^-)}{(H_2O + CO_2)}$$

Figure 4-1-1. The Henderson-Hasselbalch equation.

anion gap are known as high anion gap metabolic acidosis; those that are not are known as normal anion gap metabolic acidosis.

High anion gap metabolic acidosis is usually an acute process and caused by increased production of nonvolatile acids [ketoacidosis (diabetes, starvation, alcohol), lactic acidosis (cardiopulmonary failure), salicylate, methanol, or ethylene glycol poisoning] or by decreased acid excretion by the kidney (uremia, renal failure). Normal anion gap metabolic acidosis is more commonly a chronic process and caused by renal tubular dysfunction or by the loss of bicarbonate (severe or prolonged diarrhea or malabsorption). The pH is low, and the HCO_3^- is low; respiratory compensation may be evident by a reduction in Pa_{CO_2}.

Clinically, metabolic acidosis is manifested by dehydration, thirst, weakness, and restlessness. The patient may complain of fatigue, appear confused, and progress to stupor or coma. The respiratory rate is commonly increased in an effort to blow off CO_2 and raise the pH. Treatment should be directed at the underlying cause and based on the patient condition. Severe acidosis (generally below 7.10) should be treated with administration of intravenous bicarbonate. Dosage is based on body weight and base excess and given in small increments as the pH is monitored. Indiscriminate use of bicarbonate may produce further lactate production and worsen the metabolic acidosis and so should not be used unless the condition is severe. Overzealous administration of bicarbonate may also produce a rebound alkalosis, especially in chronic forms of metabolic acidosis such as renal tubular dysfunction.

METABOLIC ALKALOSIS

Metabolic alkalosis can be associated with volume depletion states (vomiting, gastric drainage, diuretics), hyperadrenocorticoid states which stimulate H^+ secretion (Cushing's disease, Bartter's syndrome, primary hyperaldosteronism), or abundance of alkali (iatrogenic overdose, milk-alkali syndrome, antacid abuse). The condition consists of increased pH and increased HCO_3^-. The bicarbonate level is elevated owing to either the gain of bicarbonate or the loss of hydrogen ion. Severe hypokalemia impairs renal tubular function by producing intracellular acidosis; this acidosis in turn stimulates bicarbonate retention and can lead to metabolic alkalosis. Vomiting causes a loss of H^+ and Cl^- as well as volume depletion; the kidneys respond by generating and retaining bicarbonate and excreting potassium. Mineralocorticoids cause excess Na^+ retention with H^+ loss in exchange; mineralocorticoids also cause hypokalemia, further perpetuating the metabolic alkalosis.

Metabolic alkalosis does not produce many clinical signs. Apathy and confusion may occur. Diagnosis is based on history and laboratory values. A clue to the differential diagnosis of metabolic alkalosis is the measurement of urinary chloride. In volume-depletion causes of metabolic alkalosis, urinary chloride is low; in hyperadrenocorticoid states or hypokalemia, urinary chloride is high. Metabolic alkalosis rarely requires specific treatment.

$$H_2O + CO_2 \leftrightarrows H_2CO_3 \leftrightarrows H^+ + HCO_3^-$$

Figure 4-1-2. The bicarbonate–carbonic acid exchange system.

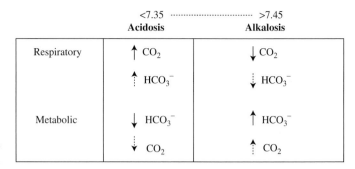

	<7.35 .... >7.45	
	Acidosis	**Alkalosis**
Respiratory	↑ CO_2	↓ CO_2
	⇡ HCO_3^-	⇣ HCO_3^-
Metabolic	↓ HCO_3^-	↑ HCO_3^-
	⇣ CO_2	⇡ CO_2

Figure 4-1-3. The primary (solid lines) and compensatory (dotted lines) mechanisms in common acid-base disorders.

Volume-depleted states should respond to the administration of fluid and chloride salts.

RESPIRATORY ACIDOSIS

Hypoventilation causes retention of CO_2, which drives the bicarbonate-carbonic acid equation to the right, increasing the concentration of H^+—respiratory acidosis. Acute respiratory acidosis can be caused by trauma, drugs, or cerebral dysfunction as in cardiac arrest. The rapid rise in tissue acidosis is buffered somewhat, but because the blood-brain barrier is easily permeated by carbonic acid, confusion, obtundation, asterixis, and papilledema indicating increased intracranial pressure rapidly occur. Chronic states of respiratory acidosis are most commonly seen in patients with chronic alveolar hypoventilation [chronic obstructive pulmonary disease (COPD), Pickwickian syndrome]. In chronic acidotic states, the kidneys increase production of ammonia and enhance the excretion of ammonium; bicarbonate retention increases, and the urine becomes acidotic.

Diagnosis of respiratory acidosis depends on the history, evidence of hypoventilation, and increased Pa_{CO_2} with decreased pH. The bicarbonate level is high in chronic states of respiratory acidosis as renal (metabolic) compensation becomes evident. It is necessary to correlate the changes in blood gases with the patient history to direct treatment. In acute, severe respiratory acidosis, such as in cardiac arrest, administration of bicarbonate, in addition to increasing ventilation, may be justified with careful monitoring. In cases of chronic hypoventilation and chronic respiratory acidosis, treatment of the underlying cause, that is, increasing ventilation, is the sole means of treatment.

RESPIRATORY ALKALOSIS

Hyperventilation causes a reduction in Pa_{CO_2}, which drives the bicarbonate–carbonic acid equation to produce alkalosis. Hyperventilation may be self-induced or in response to hypoxia. The decreased oxygen level in hypoxic states activates the respiratory centers in the brain to stimulate breathing. These centers may also be activated by anemia or severe hypotension in response to reduced oxygen delivery to the cells. Anxiety, sepsis, fever, pregnancy, and toxins may also excite the respiratory centers and lead to respiratory alkalosis.

Clinically, respiratory alkalosis is manifested by irritability, anxiety, vertigo, paresthesia, and numbness of the mouth, hands, and feet. In severe cases, confusion and loss of consciousness may occur. Tetany may develop with normal serum calcium owing to the increased excitability of neuromuscular tissue. ECG recordings may show ST- or T-wave flattening. Arterial blood gases will reveal increased pH and decreased Pa_{CO_2}; renal elimination of bicarbonate indicates compensation. The objective in the treatment of respiratory alkalosis is to remove the underlying cause. Assurance, sedation, and supplemental oxygen is usually sufficient to alleviate symptoms. In the acute hyperventilation syndrome, rebreathing into a paper bag may help by raising the Pa_{CO_2}.

BIBLIOGRAPHY

Bennet JC, Plum F (eds): *Cecil Textbook of Medicine*, 20th ed. Philadelphia, Saunders, 16(3):17–45, 1996.
Bongard FS, Sue DY (eds): *Current Critical Care Diagnosis and Treatment.* Norwalk, CT, Appleton-Lange, 1994.
Guyton AC: *Textbook of Medical Physiology*, 6th ed, Philadelphia, Saunders, 1981.
Hafstad L: Evaluation of acid-base disturbances. *Phys Assist* 16(3):17–45, March 1992.
Isselbacher KJ, Braunwald E, Wilson JD, et al (eds): *Harrison's Principles of Internal Medicine*, 13th ed. New York, McGraw-Hill, 1994.
Kelley WN, DeVita VT Jr, DuPont HL, et al (eds): *Textbook of Internal Medicine*, 2d ed. Philadelphia, Lippincott, 1992.
Kelley WN, Watanabe AM, Yamada T, et al (eds): *Essentials of Internal Medicine.* Philadelphia, Lippincott, 1994.
Marini JJ, Wheeler AP: *Critical Care Medicine—The Essentials.* Baltimore, Williams & Wilkins, 1989.
Marino PL: *The ICU Book.* Philadelphia, Lea & Febiger, 1991.
Williamson JC: Acid-base disorders: Classification and management strategies, *Am Fam Phys* 52(2):584–590 Aug, 1995.

Chapter 4–2
ELECTROLYTE DISORDERS
Claire Babcock O'Connell

SODIUM

Sodium is the major extracellular cation, accounting for 92 percent of the positive charge in the extracellular fluid (ECF). It is exchanged for potassium in cell depolarization and returned to the extravascular space by active transport. The body content of sodium determines the extracellular fluid volume, including the plasma volume. Serum sodium and interstitial sodium are in equilibrium; therefore serum level represents ECF sodium. Normal serum sodium is 136 to 145 meq/L. This amount is kept relatively constant despite variations in intake.

The average American takes in about 3 g of sodium per day in the form of various sodium salts, mainly sodium chloride. About 3 g of sodium is excreted each day. Sodium is filtered at the glomerulus; 70 percent is reabsorbed in the proximal tubule, most of the remaining sodium is reabsorbed in the distal tubule under the influence of aldosterone. Aldosterone accelerates the exchange of sodium and potassium in all cells and promotes the retention of sodium and the excretion of potassium in the kidney. Therefore, a deficiency in aldosterone results in excess loss of sodium and retention of potassium. Conversely, estrogen may cause a cyclic retention of sodium and loss of potassium, leading to menstrual bloating.

Increased concentration of sodium in the circulatory fluid stimulates the thirst mechanism and release of antidiuretic hormone (ADH). This, in turn, causes the body to retain water, increasing the ECF volume and leading to edema. The key to correcting the excess volume state is to treat the underlying cause [congestive heart failure (CHF), hepatic cirrhosis, nephrotic syndrome, etc.]. Sodium deficiency may prompt osmotic water excretion leading to water depletion, decreased ECF, and clinical dehydration. Changes in the ECF volume (water) cause greater clinical effects than changes in the absolute sodium content. Hyponatremia or hypernatremia may exist with normal, high, or low levels of sodium.

Hyponatremia

Hyponatremia exists whenever the ratio of solute to water is reduced (Table 4-2-1). If water intake exceeds water loss or water loss is defective, a relative reduction of sodium to water content occurs. Total body water can be normal, reduced, or increased. Any condition that generates a reduction in effective circulatory volume will stimulate the release of ADH owing to the diminished delivery to the diluting segments of renal tubules. ADH will prompt increased reabsorption of water beyond the amount of sodium reabsorbed, thereby producing hyponatremia. In chronic impaired water excretion states, the excess water is distributed between intracellular fluid (ICF) and ECF; no edema results. Generally, the clinical manifestations are more directly related to the volume state than the sodium level.

Clinical manifestations of hyponatremia depend on the degree and the rapidity of sodium loss. Acute rapid increases in body water relative to sodium concentration will cause rapid influx of water into cells. Swelling of cells in the central nervous system will cause lethargy, confusion, stupor, or coma. Rapid reduction in sodium concentration causes hyperexcitability, which is evident by muscle twitching, irritability, and seizure activity. Chronic slower processes that lead to hyponatremia are handled better. The central nervous system is able to excrete inorganic ions (potassium and other) and produce idiogenic osmoles that assist in maintaining water balance within the central nervous system cells and preserving neurologic function. Moderate hyponatremia will cause increased salivation, lacrimation, and watery diarrhea in an attempt to rid the body of the excess water relative to sodium content.

Diagnosis is made through history, physical examination, and laboratory values. The history should concentrate on water intake and fluid losses. The physical examination will allow categorization into normal volume, excessive volume (fluid overload), or reduced volume (dehydration) states. The blood urea nitrogen (BUN) and creatinine levels are drawn to verify the suspected volume states: high values indicate dehydration or renal losses

Table 4-2-1. Common Causes of Hyponatremia

Volume depletion states (water and sodium depleted)
  Diuretic abuse (loop diuretics, thiazides, other)
  Proportionally greater loss of sodium than water (vomiting, diarrhea, burns, etc.)
Fluid overload states, edema
  Congestive heart failure
  Cirrhosis
  Nephrotic syndrome
  Hepatic cirrhosis
Normal volume states (or moderately increased volume states, no edema)
  Syndrome of inappropriate ADH (SIADH)
  Chronic renal failure
  Endocrine disorders
    Adrenal insufficiency
    Hypothyroidism
  Psychogenic polydipsia
  Essential hyponatremia
Other
  Oncotic losses (glucose, mannitol)
  Artifactual (laboratory error, interference by proteins or lipids in sample)

Table 4-2-2. Common Causes of Hypernatremia

Pure water deficits
  Extrarenal losses
    Fever
    Burns
    Increased respiratory states
  Renal losses
    Diabetes insipidus
    Hypothalamic disorders
Water and sodium loss (hypotonic loss)
  Extra renal losses
    Sweating without adequate intake
  Renal losses
    Osmotic diuresis
      Mannitol
      DKA
    Urea diuresis (high-protein diets)
    Hyperosmolar nonketotic diabetic coma (glucose diuresis)
Excess sodium states
  Iatrogenic sodium overload
  Adrenal hyperfunction (Cushing's syndrome)

(or renal failure); normal or low values support fluid overload causes or normal volume states of hyponatremia.

Treatment of hyponatremia is targeted to the underlying cause. In most situations, the hyponatremia does not require specific treatment and will be corrected promptly with removal of the causative disorder. In the rare case of severe, acute hyponatremia, correction can be assisted by infusion of hypertonic saline with careful monitoring to avoid shrinkage of central nervous system cells in response to the osmotic gradient of the infused solution into the ECF.

Hypernatremia

In hypernatremia, the ratio of solute to water is increased (Table 4-2-2). Excess sodium concentration can be the result of pure water losses, water and sodium loss (proportionally more water than sodium is lost), or states of excess sodium. Assessment of overall fluid is essential because treatment options will differ. Clinical manifestations resulting from the high concentration of sodium reflect the status of dehydration which often coexists with hypernatremia: decreased lacrimation, decreased salivation, dry mucous membranes, flushed skin, decreased skin turgor, restlessness, weakness, tachycardia, and hypotension. The high solute concentration causes an osmotic flow of water from the ICF into the ECF. The central nervous system is affected less, in as much as it can counterbalance the osmotic loss with the production of idiogenic osmoles to help retain water in neurons. Change in mental status, confusion, delirium, muscle twitching, seizures, obtundation, stupor, and coma may result as the sodium concentration rises above this ability to counter the increased osmotic pressure. Acute rapid increases in sodium concentration are more detrimental than slower, more chronic increases because of the production of these idiogenic osmoles occurring over 1 to 3 days.

Overall correction of hypernatremia relies on treatment of the underlying cause. In the acute setting, treatment decisions are based on whether the high sodium concentration is accompanied by volume loss, volume expansion, or normal volume states. Increased solute without expansion of volume necessitates solute diuresis with accompanying replacement of obligate water losses. In states of diminished volume (loss of hypotonic fluid which results in overall hypertonic vascular fluid), both water and sodium must be replaced. Normal (isotonic) saline is hypotonic to the patient and is usually recommended as the first line of replacement fluid. After some expansion of the ECF is evident, switch to half-normal saline or $D_5\frac{1}{2}NS$ to contine water replace-

ment. D_5W may correct the hypernatremia too quickly flooding the brain cells. Glucose may cause hyperglycemia and therefore an osmotic diuresis and worsen the hypertronic state, so it should be used with caution.

POTASSIUM

Potassium is the main cation of the intracellular fluid, accounting for 77 percent of all intracellular cations and providing the bulk of intracellular osmotic pressure. Of total body potassium, 98 percent is found within cells. The ratio of potassium to sodium is essential for cellular metabolism, proper membrane potential, and depolarization. Small changes in concentration can be detrimental to physiologic function. Serum potassium concentration is used as a rough indicator of overall potassium balance.

Obligate daily potassium losses are small. Most of the dietary intake of potassium is excreted by the kidneys. Excretion of potassium is facilitated by high sodium levels and high intracellular concentrations of potassium; it is inhibited by low potassium filtration and low sodium loads in the distal nephron. The shift of potassium from the ECF to the ICF is enhanced by insulin, catecholamines, and metabolic alkalosis. Potassium is shifted out of the cells and into the ECF by metabolic acidosis, such as diabetic ketoacidosis (DKA). In DKA, the initial measurement of serum potassium may be increased, but the actual total body potassium may be normal or low.

Acid-base disorders upset potassium balance. Alkalosis causes hypokalemia by increasing renal secretion of potassium with the excess bicarbonate and also, to some extent, trading extracellular potassium ions for intracellular hydrogen ions. Acidosis, such as in DKA, causes a shift of potassium ions from the intracellular space to the extracellular space in exchange for hydrogen ion. The high potassium load presented to the kidney may cause excess potassium secretion, thereby producing a true low total body potassium in the face of normal or high serum potassium levels. Correction of the acidotic state may therefore uncover a hypokalemia.

Hypokalemia

True potassium deficits can occur through GI losses or excessive renal excretion. False potassium deficit may arise from any condition that causes a shift of potassium ions into cells without true overall body potassium depletion (Table 4-2-3). Clinical manifestations of potassium depletion are influenced by the amount and the rapidity of loss. Severe or abrupt potassium depletion can lead to neuromuscular losses, paralysis, rhabdomyolysis, myoglobinuria, diminished reflexes, and paralytic ileus. Impaired renal tubular function secondary to low potassium concentration in

Table 4-2-3. Common Causes of Hypokalemia

GI losses
  Vomiting (metabolic alkalosis induces potassium wasting)
  Diarrhea (rarely severe enough to produce symptoms)
Renal losses
  Metabolic alkalosis
  Diuretics (thiazides, loops, carbonic anhydrase inhibitors)
  Osmotic diuresis (including DKA and hyperosmolar nonketotic diabetic coma)
  Excess mineralocorticoids
  Renal tubular diseases
  Magnesium depletion
Hypokalemia without total body potassium depletion
  Insulin, hyperalimentation
  Alkalosis
  Catecholamines (bronchodilators)

Table 4-2-4. Common Causes of Hyperkalemia

Inadequate potassium secretion
  Renal disorders
    Renal failure, acute and chronic (oliguria)
    Tubular disorders
      Systemic lupus erythematosus
      Amyloidosis
      Posttransplant rejection
  Decreased effective circulatory volume (enhances reabsorption, in-
    hibiting secretion
  Hypoaldosteronism
    Adrenal disorders
    Hyporeninemia
    Potassium-sparing diuretics
Extracellular potassium addition
  Tissue damage (muscle crush, hemolysis, internal bleeding)
  Drugs that alter K^+ uptake (succinylcholine, arginine, digitalis tox-
    icity)
  Metabolic acidosis
  Hyperosmolality
  Insulin deficiency
  Hyperkalemic period paralysis
Excessive intake
  Iatrogenic overload
Pseudohyperkalemia
  Thrombocytosis
  Leukocytosis
  Hemolysis of sample in vitro
  Poor laboratory technique

tubular fluid causes decreased concentrating ability and may produce polyuria and polydipsia.

Cardiac manifestations of hypokalemia include flattening and inversion of T waves, prominence of U waves, and a sagging ST segment. Severe or rapid loss of potassium may precipitate cardiac arrest. Hypokalemia in the presence of digitalis can increase the likelihood of digitalis toxicity and produce arrhythmias.

Treatment of hypokalemia is potassium replacement. Oral potassium is preferred if it can be tolerated. Parental potassium is indicated in true potassium deficits if there is GI impairment or neuromuscular or cardiac manifestations indicating moderate to severe deficit. False hypokalemia does not necessitate potassium replacment. Treatment of the underlying cause of potassium shift should correct the hypokalemia. In instances where hypokalemia exists despite treatment of the underlying cause, potassium should be replaced.

Hyperkalemia

Excessive dietary intake of potassium should not cause hyperkalemia in persons with normal renal function. Renal excretion should be equal to dietary intake. However, additions of excess potassium directly into the extravascular space by intravenous therapy or a reduced ability of the kidneys to excrete potassium loads may lead to hyperkalemia (Table 4-2-4). Hyperkalemia is often asymptomatic until the potassium level has risen above 7.0 meq/L. Hyponatremia, hypocalcemia, and acidosis will potentiate the effects of increased potassium levels. Correction of these abnormalities will aid in the avoidance of hyperkalemic complications. The most common symptom of a rising potassium level is muscle weakness. Associated features of mild to moderate hyperkalemia include nausea, vomiting, diarrhea, and intestinal colic. As the weakness progresses, flaccid paralysis and respiratory disturbances may occur; cerebral function remains normal.

The most devastating effect of hyperkalemia is cardiac arrhythmias. Mild hyperkalemia (5.0 to 6.0 meq/L) produces peaked T waves. Potassium levels between 6.0 and 8.0 meq/L prolong the PR interval and produce heart block. Severe hyperkalemia

(>8.0 meq/L) causes a loss of P waves, widened QRS, ventricular fibrillation, and cardiac standstill. Patients suspected to be at risk for hyperkalemia should be followed with electrocardiography as well as laboratory measurements of potassium.

Correction of hyperkalemia hinges on the treatment of the underlying cause. Elimination of the cause of hyperkalemia will allow the body's metabolism to bring the potassium back to normal levels. In the acute setting, it is imperative to treat any concurrent volume deficit and acidosis and monitor the patient with serial ECGs and plasma measurements. Calcium can be administered to directly counteract the effects of the potassium on cardiac tissue and avoid fatal arrhythmias. Specific measurements aimed at rapid reduction in serum potassium include promoting potassium transfer from the ECF to the ICF (glucose with insulin, sodium bicarbonate, and beta agonists) and enhancing potassium elimination (non-potassium-sparing diuretics, dialysis, exchange resins).

CALCIUM

Much of the calcium in the human body is locked in bone. The ionized calcium found in the ECF is important, though, for proper function of muscles and neurons. Dietary calcium intake is important to maintain adequate body stores of calcium. Absorption of calcium in the GI tract is dependent on vitamin D. In the normal individual, about 30 percent of the ingested calcium is absorbed. In times of deficient calcium status, the absorption can rise to 90 percent. Children and pregnant women require higher daily intake of calcium to support skeletal growth. Prolonged immobilization precipitates bone loss and calcium efflux to the blood.

About half of the nonbone calcium is bound to protein in the plasma; most of the remaining calcium is unbound, ionized calcium, and a small amount exists as calcium salts (citrates, phosphates). Laboratory analysis of total calcium levels must always be assessed in light of serum protein status. Hypoalbuminemia is associated with a measured hypocalcemia. Specimens for calcium level measurement should be taken with the patient fasting and seated or recumbent to stabilize the albumin.

Ionized calcium is filtered and reabsorbed in the kidney. Conditions that interfere with sodium and potassium reabsorption will also affect absorption of calcium and increase calcium excretion in the urine. Calcium balance is regulated by parathyroid hormone (PTH) and vitamin D—active metabolite {1,25-dihydroxycholecalciferol[1,25-$(OH)_2D_3$]}; increases in PTH can cause release of calcium from the bone, decreased calcium excretion from the kidney, and augmented absorption of calcium in the gut. PTH release is primarily governed by serum calcium level.

Hypercalcemia

The vast majority of cases of hypercalcemia result from one of two causes: a defect in calcium regulation (hyperparathyroidism) or increased release of calcium from bone due to endogenous parathyroid-like substances, commonly produced in malignancy. High levels of calcium on routine blood screening or manifestations of hypercalcemia (renal stones, bone pain) are often the earliest indicators of underlying disease (hyperparathyroidism, Paget's disease, sarcoidosis, malignancy, hyperthyroidism, adrenal insufficiency). Excessive vitamin D intake causes increased absorption of calcium and increased bone resorption leading to hypercalcemia. Lithium therapy is also associated with a hypercalcemia.

Hypercalcemia induces an osmotic diuresis and resultant polydipsia and polyuria. If the patient can maintain adequate fluid intake and functional kidneys, the high calcium levels may go undetected until other symptoms occur. If the high calcium levels and associated interference with ADH action continue for a prolonged period, permanent renal damage may occur, especially if there is a concomitant elevation in phosphate level.

High levels of calcium effect the motility of the gastrointestinal tract producing abdominal pain, nausea, vomiting, anorexia, decreased bowel sounds, and constipation. Acute pancreatitis is not uncommon in hypercalcemia. Lethargy, fatigue, and weakness are encountered in hypercalcemia secondary to neuromuscular dysfunction. The QT interval may be shortened. Severe hypercalcemia (>15 mg/dL) is a medical emergency which can result in coma or cardiac arrest.

Diagnosis of the cause of hypercalcemia can, for the most part, be made through a medical history and PTH level. Asymptomatic individuals with a chronic increase in calcium most likely are exhibiting primary hyperparathyroidism. Decreased parathyroid hormone with an acute presentation of hypercalcemia indicates malignancy. Low or normal levels of parathyroid hormone with chronically elevated calcium warrant investigation for other causes such as sarcoidosis, vitamin D excess, or conditions of high bone turnover.

Mild, asymptomatic hypercalcemia does not need to be treated. Search for and treatment of the underlying cause of the hypercalcemia is warranted. Very high levels of serum calcium (>12 mg/dL) or hypercalcemia associated with symptoms should be treated while searching for the cause. Expansion of extracellular volume with isotonic saline will result in a decreased reabsorption of sodium and calcium thereby lowering the serum calcium level. Addition of furosemide will enhance this process. When hypercalcemia is due to pathologic losses from bone, pharmacologic therapy to enhance bone reuptake can be attempted (mithramycin, diphosphates). Calcitonin has short-lived effects but is used to promote renal excretion of calcium, inhibit bone breakdown, and slow gastrointestinal absorption of calcium. Hemodialysis is effective for patients with inadequate renal function.

Hypocalcemia

Low levels of serum calcium must be assessed in view of the plasma proteins because the calcium that is measured in routine laboratory testing is protein-bound. If the serum albumin is low, the serum calcium level should be corrected by adding 0.75 mg/dL for every 1.0 g/dL below 3.5 g/dL of albumin. Hypocalcemia is a result of lack of efficient parathyroid hormone function. When deficient calcium levels are detected by the body, PTH secretion is increased within seconds; within days there is evidence of increased biosynthesis of PTH followed by parathyroid cell hyperplasia within weeks. This process is known as secondary hyperparathyroidism and causes an increase in renal secretion of $1,25\text{-}(OH)_2D_3$ and increased calcium flow into the blood from the intestinal lumen, bone, and renal tubules. Primary hypoparathyroidism (inherited or acquired) and hypomagnesia result in a severe depletion or absence of hormone. Whenever the responses to low calcium are weakened or blunted (either primarily or secondarily), hypocalcemia results.

Clinically, a low calcium state is associated with increased neuromuscular excitability, which is first manifested as paresthesia in the fingers and toes and around the oral cavity. As the serum level drops lower, muscle cramping, carpopedal spasm, laryngeal stridor, and convulsions may occur. Appearance of symptoms is related to the degree and rate of calcium deficit. Latent tetany associated with calcium deficit may be demonstrated with Chvostek's sign (twitching of the upper lip upon tapping on the facial nerve) and Trousseau's sign (carpal spasm after inflating a cuff above systole for 2 to 3 min).

Low serum calcium is also associated with mental disturbances including irritability, depression, and psychosis. Papilledema may indicate increased intracerebral pressure. Cataracts may occur in long-standing calcium-poor status.

Diagnosis is based on the history and physical examination and confirmed with laboratory results. Hypocalcemia, hyperphosphatemia, and normal renal function supports primary hypoparathyroidism; this is confirmed by low levels of PTH. Low calcium with normal or low phosphate indicates malabsorption of vitamin D; the PTH levels should be elevated, and the patient's GI function should be evaluated.

Treatment of hypocalcemia is based on the underlying cause. In an acute situation, calcium can be administered intravenously. Oral calcium supplementation is recommended for persons at risk of calcium loss or in need of excess calcium—children, pregnant women, patients facing prolonged immobilization, peri- and postmenopausal women, and others.

PHOSPHORUS

Phosphorus is the major anion of the intracellular compartment. It is found in virtually all soft tissue although the majority of it is in bone. Its functions include the building of cell membrane phospholipids and participating in various energy-producing reactions. It is absorbed in the gut under the influence of vitamin D, and filtered and reabsorbed in the kidney. When phosphorus levels exceed a transport maximum (TmP), phosphorus will be excreted in the urine; an increase in PTH will inhibit renal phosphate reabsorption.

Hypophosphatemia

Low phosphate can result from either ion shift or depleted stores. Ingestion of a high carbohydrate load or alkalosis will cause a transient shift of phosphate into cells. More commonly, hypophosphatemia results from depleted stores. Poor intake or poor gastrointestinal absorption (hyperalimentation, prolonged use of phosphate-binding antacids) account for some depletion; more often hypophosphatemia is a result of inadequate renal reabsorption, which is seen in poorly controlled diabetes mellitus, alcoholism, and in the recovery period following severe burns or starvation.

A sustained hypophosphatemia causes widespread cellular enzymatic dysfunction and decline in phosphate-dependent energy sources. Phosphate deficiency causes changes in the cell membrane structure and function, depletes intracellular phosphorylated compounds such as adenosine triphosphate (ATP) and 2,3-diphosphoglycerate, and increases the intracellular calcium levels. The effects are seen throughout several organ systems. There is weakness and possible paralysis, rhabdomyolysis, and cardiomyopathy; altered RBC function including hemolytic anemia, impaired leukocyte function, and poor platelet aggregation; increased bone resorption, osteomalacia, and rickets; or impaired hepatic and renal function, metabolic encephalopathy, and hypoglycemia.

Treatment is aimed at correcting the underlying disorder. In severe or symptomatic hypophosphatemia, the goal is to minimize urinary losses and enhance absorption from the gut. Supplemental phosphates given intravenously are associated with changes in other electrolytes including calcium and magnesium and therefore should be closely monitored. Oral phosphate supplements are associated with diarrhea, metabolic acidosis, hypertension, and loss of calcium from the gut.

Hyperphosphatemia

Increased renal reabsorption or reduced renal excretion of phosphate lead to hyperphosphatemia. With normally functioning kidneys, increased oral intake is only rarely associated with hyperphosphatemia; all excess phosphate will be excreted. Iatrogenic overload via intravenous phosphate can occur. A transient rise in phosphate levels will be seen in any state that causes rapid cell destruction.

High levels of phosphate will bind with calcium and deposit into soft tissue. This will cause a hypocalcemia and possible tetany. Chronic hyperphosphatemia-hypocalcemia will cause a resultant secondary hyperparathyroidism. Phosphate also reduces the action of vitamin D and therefore reduces the amount of calcium absorption in the gut. Clinically, the signs and symptoms of hypocalcemia are more important than the hyperphosphatemia. Correction of the underlying process will prompt a return to balance for both calcium and phosphate.

MAGNESIUM

Magnesium is the second most abundant intracellular cation after potassium. It is vital for proper enzymatic actions, including ATP, and, with calcium, proper neuromuscular functioning. One quarter of serum magnesium is protein-bound; its distribution is not controlled by hormones or acid-base status. Free magnesium is reabsorbed and a steady state is readily established with a normal diet. Excess amounts of magnesium are not protein-bound and are excreted up to a limit imposed by the glomerular filtration rate.

Hypomagnesemia

Decreased intake and/or increased excretion account for most hypomagnesemia. Poor dietary intake is rarely a cause of low magnesium; conditions that affect gastrointestinal absorption will cause hypomagnesemia. Severe diarrhea, steatorrhea, and familial malabsorption syndromes are associated with low body magnesium with a low urinary magnesium. Renal magnesium loss is associated with normal to high urinary magnesium levels. Renal wasting can be divided into intrinsic renal disorders (familial or sporadic renal tubular disorders, Bartter's syndrome, nephrotoxic agents) and extrinsic renal disorders (volume expansion, hypercalciuria, diuretic abuse, diabetic ketoacidosis).

Other disorders associated with magnesium loss include thyrotoxicosis, pancreatitis, lactation, alcoholism, and severe burns. Acute myocardial infarction is often accompanied by hypomagnesemia, and treatment of this magnesium deficit will greatly reduce the risk of ventricular arrhythmias. Forty percent of patients found to be deficient in magnesium will have a coexisting hypocalcemia and a refractory potassium depletion state. Addition of magnesium will rapidly assist in treatment.

Hypomagnesemia is often manifested clinically in association with hypokalemia and hypocalcemia. Weakness, anorexia, apathy, fasciculations, and tremors indicate neuromuscular dysfunction. Chvostek's and Trousseau's signs may progress to overt tetany. Ventricular arrhythmias occur, especially in light of digitalis toxicity. Rarely, patients may exhibit seizures due to low levels of magnesium.

Treatment of mild magnesium deficits that are asymptomatic consists of dietary recommendations. Symptomatic hypomagnesemia warrants replacement. It is important to note that only half of the supplemental intravenous magnesium will remain in the circulation; the remaining half will be excreted in the urine. Replacement of the magnesium will greatly assist in alleviating the symptoms of hypocalcemia and hypokalemia. Ultimately, correction of the underlying cause of electrolyte deficiency is the best objective.

Hypermagnesemia

Increased dietary magnesium intake is virtually unknown to cause hypermagnesemia. Abuse of magnesium-containing laxatives and antacids and excess intravenous magnesium sulfate (such as in the treatment of preeclampsia-eclampsia) can cause magnesium overload. High loads of magnesium are presented to the renal tubules in unbound form and will be excreted provided there is ongoing sodium excretion. Only a set amount of magnesium is reabsorbed; any excess magnesium filtered will be excreted unless the glomerular filtration rate is impaired.

Symptoms and signs of hypermagnesemia are nonspecific: weakness, lethargy, nausea, hyporeflexia. As the level of magnesium rises, the deep tendon reflexes are lost and the patient may exhibit flaccid quadriplegia. Acute, severe hypermagnesemia may also cause respiratory depression, hypotension, bradycardia, and, rarely, complete heart block and cardiac arrest.

Severe, symptomatic hypermagnesemia requires urgent treatment. Calcium is a direct antagonist of magnesium. Intravenous calcium gluconate or calcium chloride will block the effects of magnesium. Once the patient is stabilized, efforts to reduce the level of magnesium are needed. Any excess intake should be discontinued, and magnesium excretion should be maximized. With functional kidneys, furosemide with half-normal saline will increase the urine volume and maintain proper diuresis. In patients with impaired renal function or renal failure, hemodialysis is effective in removing excess magnesium.

BIBLIOGRAPHY

Bennet JC, Plum F (eds): *Cecil Textbook of Medicine,* 20th ed. Philadelphia, Saunders, 1996.

Bongard FS, Sue DY (eds): *Current Critical Care Diagnosis and Treatment.* Norwalk, CT, Appleton-Lange, 1994.

Guyton AC: *Textbook of Medical Physiology,* 6th ed. Philadelphia, Saunders, 1981.

Hafstad L: Evaluation of acid-base disturbances. *Phys Assist.* 16(3):17–45, March 1992.

Isselbacher KJ, Braunwald E, Wilson JD, et al (eds): *Harrison's Principles of Internal Medicine,* 13th ed. New York, McGraw-Hill, 1994.

Kelley WN, DeVita VT Jr, DuPont HL, et al (eds): *Textbook of Internal Medicine,* 2d ed. Philadelphia, Lippincott, 1992.

Kelley WN, Watanabe AM, Yamada T, et al (eds): *Essentials of Internal Medicine.* Philadelphia, Lippincott, 1994.

Marini JJ, Wheeler AP: *Critical Care Medicine—The Essentials.* Baltimore, Williams & Wilkins, 1989.

Marino, PL: *The ICU Book.* Philadelphia, Lea & Febiger, 1991.

Williamson JC: Acid-base disorders: Classification and management strategies. *Am Fam Phys* 52(2):584–590, 1995.

Chapter 4–3
DISORDERS OF FLUID BALANCE
Claire Babcock O'Connell

DISCUSSION

The human body is approximately 60% water, which is able to freely move among body compartments in response to solute concentration. In the average 70-kg man, there is approximately 40 L of water: two-thirds of this water is in the intracellular fluid (ICF) compartment (25 L); one-third is in the extracellular fluid (ECF) compartment (15 L). Within the ECF, two-thirds of the water is interstitial (10 L); one-third is in the plasma (5 L). The average hematocrit is 40 to 45 percent, therefore, leaving about 2.5 L of fluid obtainable by venipuncture—most of which is water.

Daily water intake is about 2500 mL/day, mostly from food and fluid intake. Average daily water loss is about equal (2500 mL/day). Water is lost through skin (500 mL/day), expired air (350 mL/day), urine (1500 mL/day), and feces (150 mL/day). The balance of water intake and loss is maintained within close limits by sensitive thirst mechanisms and kidney regulations. Clinical manifestations occur as a result of problems effecting this balance like inability to swallow, vomiting, diarrhea, excessive urine or perspiration, starvation, and fistulas.

Movement of water among compartments depends on the amount of solute within each compartment. Solute composition includes electrolytes, cells and cellular material, proteins, and organic acids. The ionic state of each compartment is kept in balance by the movement of ions; this requires energy (active transport). Water follows rapidly to balance each compartment following osmotic gradients; no energy is required. The main determinant of ECF volume is sodium concentration. The ICF volume is determined mainly by potassium concentration. Large changes in cell volume can handicap or destroy cells. It is imperative to maintain optimum cell volume; active transport of ions against a concentration gradient and free osmotic movement of water in response to these changes ensures proper cell volume.

In the vascular space, hydrostatic pressure forces water out of the capillaries. The osmotic pressure of plasma proteins and solutes brings water back into the capillaries. Protection of the effective blood volume is key to survival. Disturbances in osmolality cause a response via thirst mechanisms. High osmolality (low water/high solute) increases thirst and stimulates antidiuretic hormone (ADH), which increases tubular water reabsorption; therefore less water is excreted in the urine. Low osmolality (high water/low solute) inhibits thirst and ADH release, resulting in large volumes of dilute urine. Receptors in the kidney and elsewhere also respond to changes in effective blood volume. Low-volume states result in salt retention, thereby retaining water through the renin-angiotensin system. High volume states stimulate release of natriuretic hormones; water is pulled into the urine with the excess sodium through osmosis.

VOLUME EXCESS

Excess fluid volume is essentially excess water. Total body sodium is usually high as well. Volume excess is due to an intake of water and/or salt which exceeds the loss of water and/or salt. Common clinical causes of volume excess include congestive heart failure (CHF), the nephrotic syndrome, hepatic cirrhosis, mineralocorticoid or ADH overproduction, renal insufficiency, and iatrogenic fluid overload. Symptoms of volume excess are dyspnea, orthopnea, paroxysmal nocturnal dyspnea, and rapid weight gain due to edema. Clinical signs reflect the fluid overload in the vascular space and include increased venous pressure, basilar rales, decreased breath sounds, an S_3 heart sound, dependent pitting edema, ascites, anasarca, hepatomegaly, and hepatojugular reflux. The main objective in the treatment of fluid overload states is to treat the underlying cause. Once the cause of the fluid overload is corrected, it is best to monitor the patient and provide supportive measures as needed. The body has tremendous ability to return to hemostatic balance. Fluid and sodium restriction, diuretics, and digitalis are helpful during acute crises as the underlying cause is corrected.

VOLUME DEPLETION

Inadequate volume is a result of inadequate water or salt intake or excessive loss. As depicted in Table 4-3-1, there are three major causes of volume depletion: hormonal deficits, renal deficits, and extrarenal losses. Clinically, symptoms and signs of volume depletion depend on the magnitude, the rate, and the nature of the fluid loss coupled with the responsiveness of the vascular system.

Table 4-3-1. Common Causes of Volume Depletion

Hormonal deficits (loss of ADH or aldosterone)
  Pituitary diabetes insipidus
  Addison's disease
  Interstitial nephritis
  Hyporeninemic hypoaldosteronism
Renal deficits (impaired renal tubular sodium or water conservation)
  Renal tubular nephropathies
    Nephrogenic diabetes insipidus
  Osmotic diuresis
  Diuretic abuse
    Glucose (diabetic ketoacidosis, hyperglycemic hyperosmolar coma, hyperalimentation)
    Urea (burn patients)
    Mannitol, glycerol (iatrogenic)
    Chronic renal failure
Extrarenal losses
  Hemorrhage
  Cutaneous loss
  Gastrointestinal losses
    Fluid loss (vomiting, diarrhea, gastric drainage, GI fistulas)
    Sequestration (peritonitis, ascites)

Water loss is rapidly equilibrated through the ECF and ICF owing to osmosis. Vascular depletion results in circulatory collapse; intracellular loss leads to cellular damage and death, compromising physiologic functions.

It is important to assess the amount of fluid intake in any patient suspected to be volume-depleted. Fluid intake must be assessed in parallel to known fluid losses. On examination, general appearance and mental status are keys to assessing volume status. Vital signs, appearance of skin and mucous membrane, and the ability to cry or sweat are good indicators of the approximate magnitude of loss. A quick patient assessment allows the examiner to decide whether the patient is mildly, moderately, or severely depleted. Table 4-3-2 outlines the general clinical guidelines for the assessment of dehydration.

Tears are lost at approximately 7 percent dehydration. Their presence or absence is the most reliable indicator of fluid status in children. Skin turgor is helpful in assessing children; it is not reliable in adults or the elderly. Pulse, blood pressure, capillary refill, and laboratory measurements are evaluated as a group; none of these measurements should be used alone in assessing fluid status. It is important to examine the complete picture in conjunction with patient history.

Table 4-3-2. General Guidelines of Dehydration Assessment

5% dehydration—mild dehydration
  Mild postural giddiness
  Postural mild tachycardia
  Weakness
  Thirst, +/− dry mucous membranes
  Tears present
10% dehydration—moderate dehydration
  Decreased skin turgor
  Dry mucous membranes
  Tachycardia
  Orthostatic hypotension
  Decreased urine volume
  No tears
15% dehydration—severe dehydration
  Hypotension, shock
  Recumbent tachycardia
  Oliguria, anuria
  Coldness of extremities
  Change in mental status (lethargy, stupor, coma)

Severe volume depletion can result in end organ damage and death. Any comatose patient suspected to be volume-depleted should be challenged with 500 mL of normal saline over 1 to 3 h. This fluid challenge both offers a clue to the underlying diagnosis and helps to maintain effective circulating volume. Mild and moderate volume depletion can be easily remedied. The absolute treatment naturally is treatment of the underlying cause. While definitive diagnosis and treatment protocol is being decided, fluid should be restored to maintain effective circulatory volume and alleviate symptoms. Choice of fluid type, rate of infusion, and route of administration depend on the clinical scenario. Any patient who can be maintained on PO fluids should be. Patients who are more than mildly depleted, are suffering from protracted vomiting or diarrhea, or are candidates for surgical treatment may necessitate intravenous replacement of fluids.

Sodium-free solutions, such as D_5W, are equivalent to solute-free. The fluid will distribute uniformly in all body compartments. One liter of solute-free fluid will result in about 75 to 100 mL of fluid into the intravascular space, a 2 percent increase in intravascular volume.

Sodium-containing solutions preferentially expand the ECF, although much of the water will still flow into the interstitial space and into the ICF. One liter of normal saline will result in about 300 mL of fluid into the intravascular space, a 6 percent increase in intravascular volume.

Colloid-containing solutions (albumin, plasma) preferentially expand the ECF. The oncotic pressure provided by the colloid particles causes an osmotic flow of water from the ICF to the ECF. The large proteins cause a rapid expansion of intravascular volume. However, the solutions have relatively short half-lives and are expensive. They are used primarily in the treatment of burn patients and during acute circulatory collapse with severe fluid depletion.

Blood is the most potent expander of the intravascular space. One liter of packed red blood cells will remain entirely in the vascular space. This will cause an osmotic flow of water into the vessels and a rapid increase in the effective circulatory volume. In acute hemorrhage or severe volume loss with mental status changes, packed cells are administered along with normal saline or a colloid solution to enhance circulatory function.

Amount and rate of fluid replacement is guided by the patient status and weight. Fluid orders must take into account maintenance fluid, any deficit, and any ongoing losses. Maintenance fluid is based entirely on body weight. A simple guide is to provide 100 mL/kg of fluid for the first 10 kg of body weight, 50 mL/kg of fluid for the second 10 kg of body weight, and 20 mL/kg of fluid for every remaining kilogram of body weight. Thus, for the average 70-kg man, 2500 mL/kg of fluid is required per day for maintenance ($10 \times 100 = 1000$; $10 \times 50 = 500$; $50 \times 20 = 1000$; $1000 + 500 + 1000 = 2500$).

Deficits are estimated based on body weight also. If a 70-kg man is assessed clinically as being 5 percent dehydrated, the deficit is estimated to be 3.5 L, or 3500 mL ($70 \times 0.05 = 3.5$). Total fluid requirement for this patient (provided there are no ongoing losses) is 2500 mL + 3500 mL = 6000 mL for the first 24-h followed by maintenance fluid (2500 mL/day) thereafter. Because the patient is dehydrated, fluid replacement is necessary to improve clinical status. Therefore, the objective is to get the fluid in as quickly as possible without overloading the system and risking complications. The general guideline is to infuse one-half of the total fluid needs in one-third of the time. In this case, the orders would be for 3000 mL of fluid in the first 8 h (375 mL/h) followed by 3000 mL of fluid in the following 16 h (188 mL/h). Throughout the replacement time, the patient should be monitored and the fluid rate adjusted according to clinical status. If the patient was admitted without circulatory compromise, indicating the deficit was throughout all body compartments, a dilute

solute-containing solution such half-normal saline would be appropriate. If the patient presented with signs of circulatory compromise, a crystalloid solution such as Ringer's lactate may be the appropriate starting fluid.

BIBLIOGRAPHY

Bennet JC, Plum F (eds): *Cecil Textbook of Medicine,* 20th ed. Philadelphia, Saunders, 1996.

Bongard FS, Sue DY (eds): *Current Critical Care Diagnosis and Treatment.* Norwalk, CT, Appleton-Lange, 1994.

Fauci AS, Braunwald E, Isselbacher KJ, et al (eds): *Harrison's Principles of Internal Medicine,* 14th ed. New York, McGraw-Hill, 1998.

Guyton AC: *Textbook of Medical Physiology,* 6th ed. Philadelphia, Saunders, 1981.

Hafstad L: Evaluation of acid-base disturbances, *Phys Assist* 16(3):17–45, March 1992.

Kelley WN, DeVita VT Jr, DuPont HL, et al (eds): *Textbook of Internal Medicine,* 2d ed. Philadelphia, Lippincott, 1992.

Kelley WN, Watanabe AM, Yamada T, et al (eds): *Essentials of Internal Medicine,* Philadelphia, Lippincott, 1994.

Marini JJ, Wheeler AP: *Critical Care Medicine—The Essentials.* Baltimore, Williams & Wilkins, 1989.

Marino PL: *The ICU Book.* Philadelphia, Lea & Febiger, 1991.

Williamson JC: Acid-base disorders: Classification and management strategies. *Am Fam Phys* 52(2):584–590, 1995.

Chapter 4–4
ANIMAL BITES
Ralph Rice

DISCUSSION

With more than 3 million occurrences every year, animal bites are the cause of 1 percent of emergency room visits.[1] One in every two Americans will be bitten during his or her lifetime by either an animal or another human being.[1,2] The annual health care cost for bite injuries is estimated to be in excess of $30 million.[1] Most animal bites come from dogs and cats. Other animal bites come from snakes, rodents, and other wild and exotic animals. Dog and cat bites are the primary focus of this chapter.

Dog bites account for 80 to 90 percent of all animal bites.[1] Of this, researchers estimate that between 2 and 20 percent will become infected.[1,2] Dog bites occur most frequently in males and in persons between 2 and 19 years of age. The peak incidence of dog bites occurs during the warmer, summer months and between the hours of 4 and 6 P.M.[2,3] The most common site of injury is the hand and upper extremity.[4] However, children are typically bitten on the face. The dog is known by the victim in 70 to 90 percent of reported cases. In the United States, domestic dogs kill 10 to 20 people per year.[5]

With an annual incidence of 400,000 bites per year, cats inflict 5 to 15 percent of all animal bites, the second most common source of bite injury in the United States.[1,2] In contrast to dog bites, cat bites most frequently occur in females. The upper extremity is the site most often bitten. The victim usually knows the cat. The infection rate of cat bites is more than double that of dog bites, with 30 to more than 50 percent becoming infected.

Table 4-4-1. Common Infecting Organisms in Bite Wounds

Streptococcus species
Staphylococcus species
Corynebacterium species
Pasteurella multocida
Bacteroides fragilis
Eikenella corrodens

PATHOGENESIS

In general, animal bites may be classified as contaminated crush injuries or puncture wounds. A dog may generate as much as 450 lb/in^2 of pressure during the bite. As carnivores, their teeth have become adapted to tearing tissue. Their bites may result in devitalization, crushing, tearing, and avulsion of the tissue along with exposure of the victim to the oral flora of the dog.

Because cats' teeth are slender and extremely sharp, inoculation of potential pathogens deep into tissue may occur, along with easy penetration into the bone and joint space. As with any bite, this may result in osteomyelitis, sepsis, septic arthritis, or tenosynovitis.

Cellulitis, lymphangitis, and abscess formation may occur in any animal bite. Possibly the most feared potential consequence of any animal bite is rabies. (See Chap. 9-19, "Rabies.")

A thorough history is vital in assessing a person's risk of infection and in determining optimal wound management. Time of injury is important because treatment delays of more than 12 h increases the risk of infection. The circumstances surrounding the injury (was the attack provoked or unprovoked?), along with the ownership, location, and immunization status of the animal, if known, are important items that should be asked.

MICROBIOLOGY

Reflecting the oral cavity of the mouth, most dog and cat infections are polymicrobial. A mean of 2.8 to 3.6 bacterial species, including one anaerobic species, have been isolated from wound cultures.[1] Although a complete list of organisms recovered from infected dog and cat bites is quite extensive, the most commonly cultured organisms are noted in Table 4-4-1. In infected dog bites, alpha-hemolytic streptococci are the most frequently cultured organisms. In infected cat bites, *Pasteurella multocida* is most commonly isolated.

Pasteurella multocida, along with *Bartonella henselae* and *Capnocytophaga*, deserve special attention. *Pasteurella multocida* is a gram-negative aerobic organism found in the majority of dog and cat mouths. More than 50 percent of cat bites and 30 percent of dog bites that become infected will have *P. multocida* recovered. *Pasteurella* infection causes an intense, rapid inflammatory reaction, normally occurring in less than 24 h, and may be associated with fever and/or a purulent discharge. In addition to osteomyelitis and septic arthritis, peritonitis, meningitis and sepsis have also occurred in *Pasteurella* infections.[5]

Cat-scratch disease (see Chap. 9-5, "Cat-Scratch Disease") is caused by the gram-negative rod *Bartonella henselae* and may be caused by a scratch or bite from either a cat or dog. An erythematous papule forms at the primary site 3 to 10 days after the onset of injury, followed by the development of regional lymph node enlargement and fever. This disease is normally self-limited.

Formally known by the Centers for Disease Control designation DF-2, *Capnocytophaga canimorsus* infection, thought to be rare, is associated with dog bites and has a 28 percent fatality rate.[5] Of those victims who become seriously infected, 80 percent are immunocompromised or asplenic or have alcoholic liver disease. *Capnocytophaga* infection presents with signs of sepsis, characterized by fever, leukocytosis, petechiae, disseminated intravascular coagulation, hypotension, and/or renal failure.

SYMPTOMS AND OBJECTIVE FINDINGS

In most cases, evidence of trauma presents as abrasions, punctures, and/or avulsions. A physical examination should include the description of the injury, including the type (avulsion, puncture, crush), location, and measurement. Diagrams can add clarity to a written description. Exploration of the wound to assess wound depth, to exclude the presence of foreign bodies, and to inspect for damage to underlying structures should be documented. Anesthetizing the area before exploration may be required, but this should be done only after completion of a thorough neurovascular and musculoskeletal examination. If a joint space was penetrated or tendon damage was sustained, limited range of motion and/or decreased motor strength may be noted.

The initial symptoms of infection are inflammation, pain, and swelling in the localized area of the bite. Most infections are associated with a gray, malodorous, serosanguineous discharge along with the cellulitis. Fever may be present in addition to regional lymphadenopathy.

SPECIAL CONSIDERATIONS

Variables that increase the risk of infection are itemized in Table 4-4-2.

LABORATORY TESTS

In general, laboratory tests are unnecessary for most bite injuries. However, if signs or symptoms of infection are present, several tests may be indicated. A complete blood count and sedimentation rate may be useful in suspected cellulitis. A Gram stain, though not useful nor routine in clinically uninfected wounds, may be of value in infected wounds. Whether or not a Gram stain is done, all clinically infected wounds should have aerobic and anaerobic cultures collected. These cultures should be collected from deep in the wound. Due to the slow-growing nature of some pathogens, laboratory personnel should be instructed to hold the cultures for 7 to 10 days. In patients who present with sepsis, liver function and coagulation studies may also be helpful in the management.

RADIOGRAPHIC STUDIES

If there is suspicion of a foreign body, most commonly part of a tooth, a radiograph of the area should be obtained. Some references advocate routine radiographic studies involving "hand bites and any other bites potentially involving deep structures."[6] When a bone or joint space may have been penetrated during the injury, a radiograph will provide a baseline reference for the evaluation of osteomyelitis. When an infection occurs in the proximity of a joint or bone, a radiograph should be obtained. If an infection

Table 4-4-2. Risk Factors for Infection

A bite on the hand or foot
Involvement of bone, joint, or tendon
Prosthetic heart valve
Wound in the proximity of a prosthetic joint
A bite on the face or scalp of an infant
Patient age >50 years
Seeking treatment >12 h after injury
Immunosuppression: immune disorders, asplenism, or corticosteroid use
Underlying medical disorders: diabetes, chronic alcohol abuse, vascular disease, malignancy
Cat bites
Puncture wounds
Severe crush injury and/or edema

is present, the presence of air in the tissue spaces should heighten suspicion for a necrotizing infection.

TREATMENT

The first step in proper treatment is cleaning the wound and the surrounding area. Adding 1% povidone iodine solution to the cleansing solution is acceptable but, because of its tissue toxicity, povidone iodine surgical scrub should be avoided. Wound irrigation with 1 to 2% benzalkonium chloride may have a viricidal activity against rabies.[6] Irrigation of the wound with saline or Ringer's lactate should follow the benzalkonium chloride irrigation or wound cleansing. Wound cleansing using a 18- to 20-gauge angiocatheter and a 35-mL syringe will generate up to 10 lb/in^2 pressure and help remove foreign bodies from the wound. If there is devitalized, crushed tissue present, 1 to 2 mm of debridement of the wound margin should be undertaken. Debridement of puncture wounds, however, is not recommended.

Wound closure remains controversial. In general, all bite wounds without risk factors for infection should be sutured. Because of cosmetic considerations, all facial injuries should be closed by primary intention if less than 12 h old. Wounds that are closed should be loosely approximated to allow for proper drainage to occur. For those injuries not closed by primary intention, delayed primary closure may be considered in the absence of risk factors for infection. The wound(s) should then be loosely bandaged and elevated.

Pharmacologic Treatment

Antibiotics should be used in the treatment of any infected wound and in cases where risk factors for infection are present. Because of the high rates of infection from cat bites, antibiotic prophylaxis is generally recommended. Unless risk factors are present, most dog bites do not require antibiotic prophylaxis. If antibiotics are prescribed, the medication selected should be active against the normal oral flora of the animal, both aerobic and anaerobic, against normal skin flora, and against any possible environmental contaminants.

Because of its broad spectrum of activity, amoxicillin-clavulanate (Augmentin) is an acceptable first choice in the treatment of dog and cat bites.[7] The recommended dose for adults is 500 mg three times per day; in children, 40 mg/kg/day amoxicillin, divided into three equal doses and administered every 8 h. Alternatives include:

- doxycycline   Adults: 100 mg bid
                 Children: >8 years old, 2 to 4 mg/kg/day, divided equally and given every 12 h
- cefuroxime   Adults: 500 mg bid
                 Children: 30 mg/kg/day, divided equally and given bid

Pregnant females and children younger than 8 years old with an allergy to pencillin may require two or more antibiotics to be effective against possible pathogens. This may include a combination of erythromycin and trimethoprim-sulfamethoxazole. In these cases, discussion with the appropriate consultant should help guide proper antibiotic selection.

Prophylactic antibiotics should be given for 3 to 5 days. If cellulitis is noted, antibiotics should be continued for 10 to 14 days. Patients with septic arthritis or osteomyelitis will require intravenous antibiotics and other treatment often longer than 30 days. Hospitalization may be required in these cases.

Analgesics should be considered in the management plan. This is especially important for extensive injuries, injuries to the hands or feet, and injuries to children. Medications may range from over-the-counter anti-inflammatory medications to more potent

Table 4-4-3. Hospitalization Criteria

Complicated wounds
Involvement of bone, joint, or tendon
Severe cellulitis
Rapidly advancing cellulitis
Cellulitis extending beyond one joint
Signs of systemic infection
Failure of outpatient management

agents, such as codeine or oxycodone. The patient profile and extent of the injuries should guide the care giver in this selection.

Tetanus (see Chap. 9-23, "Tetanus"), though rarely acquired from animal bites, has been reported. If no booster injection has been given in the past 5 years, standard of care should include the administration of tetanus toxoid.[8] Those who have never been fully immunized may require tetanus immunoglobulin in addition to the toxoid.

Since the 1940s and 1950s when programs for control of rabies in the United States intensified, the rate of human rabies has been reduced dramatically. From 1994 through May 1996, a total of 11 cases of rabies have been reported to the Centers for Disease Control. Local health departments should be contacted for information regarding rabies. (See Chap. 9-19, "Rabies.")

DISPOSITION

Most animal bite injuries can be treated on an outpatient basis. Clinical follow-up should be done at 24 h after the initial evaluation. In some incidences, additional follow-up at 48 h may be appropriate. An intramuscular or intravenous dose of antibiotic may be instituted in select cases prior to outpatient management. All patients should be educated and advised to seek medical attention on the development of signs and symptoms of infection. Hospitalization should be considered in selected cases, using any of the criteria listed in Table 4-4-3.

PATIENT EDUCATION

Prevention of animal bites is the key to management. Animals should be avoided when they are eating. Strange animals and animals that exhibit erratic behavior should also be avoided. Nursing animals, even if they appear friendly or if they are a pet, should be approached cautiously, if at all. As most bite injuries occur in children, parents should take an active role in educating their children not to tease animals and how to behave properly toward animals. Parents should not leave a child alone with any animal or pet. Simple measures such as these should reduce the incidence of animal bites.

REFERENCES

1. Griego RD, Rosen T, Orengo IF, Wolf JE: Dog, cat and human bites: A review. *J Am Acad Dermatol* 33(6):1019–1029, 1995.
2. Goldstein EJC: Bite wounds and infections. *Clin Infect Dis* 14:633–638, 1992.
3. Doan-Wiggins L: Animal bites and rabies, in *Emergency Medicine. Concepts and Clinical Practice*. Rosen P, Barkin RM, Braen GR, et al (eds). Mosby-Year Book, St. Louis, 1992, pp 864–875.
4. Anderson CR: Animal bites. Guidelines to current management. *Postgrad Med* 92(1):134–147, 1992.
5. Lewis KT, Stiles M: Management of cat and dog bites. *Am Fam Phys* 52(2):479–485, 1995.
6. Hunt RC: Human and animal bites, in *Presenting Signs and Symptoms in the Emergency Department. Evaluation and Treatment*, Hamilton GC (ed). Baltimore, Williams & Wilkins, 1993, pp 186–192.
7. Sanford JP, Gilbert DN, Sande MA: Empirical antimicrobial therapy on clinical grounds, in Sanford JR (ed): *The Sanford Guide to Antimicrobial Therapy*. Dallas, Antimicrobial Therapy, 1995, pp 33–34.

8. Sanford JP, Gilbert DN, Sande MA: Anti-tetanus prophylaxis, wound classification, immunization, in Sanford JR (ed): *The Sanford Guide to Antimicrobial Therapy*. Dallas, Antimicrobial Therapy, 1995, pp 115.

Chapter 4–5
EPIGLOTTITIS: ACUTE SUPRAGLOTTIC LARYNGITIS
Nadine Kroenke

DISCUSSION

Epiglottitis is a true medical emergency. Although relatively rare, failure to accurately and quickly diagnose and intervene can lead to airway obstruction, respiratory arrest, and death.

Anatomically, this infection involves the epiglottis, the supraglottic structures, the lingular tonsillar area, the epiglottic folds, and the false vocal cords.

Until the late 1980s, epiglottitis had been most commonly seen in the pediatric population with a peak incidence in children 2 to 5 years old. Prior to 1990, *Haemophilus influenzae* type b was the most common organism, accounting for almost 80 to 90 percent of cases in both children and adults.

Since the introduction of the Hib-Imune vaccine in 1985, there has been a dramatic decline in the number of cases of epiglottitis. It is now most often seen in children with a median age of seven. Administration of the Hib-Imune vaccine has led to an ever-changing epidemiology with other organisms such as *Streptococcus pneumoniae, Staphylococcus aureus, Candida albicans,* and herpes simplex virus now becoming increasingly documented as the causative agents in adults. *Haemophilus influenzae* now accounts for only 25 percent of all cases.

Classically, epiglottitis is described in children with the acute onset over several hours of sore throat, fever, stridor, and drooling.

Today, epiglottitis is being seen more frequently in adolescents and adults. The course is usually more indolent, progressive over 1 to 2 days. Presentation generally involves a complaint of a sore throat with pain out of proportion to physical findings. Practitioners need to become more suspicious of this disease in the older adult, and in those with less typical symptomatology.

Genetic predisposition leads to prominence in Caucasians and makes it relatively rare in Native American and Inuit populations. There is no agreed seasonal predisposition.

Various pathways are known for the approach and workup with the patient suspected of epiglottitis. The method chosen depends on the clinical stability of the patient and the practitioner's airway expertise. Airway management is key. The diagnosis of epiglottitis remains primarily clinical and does not depend on direct visualization of a "cherry" red epiglottis.

Epiglottitis protocols should be in place to quickly coordinate the appropriate staff to treat the patient. The primary care provider should recognize the disease and transfer the patient appropriately. The emergency physician provides initial care, closely observes the patient's airway, ready to provide an airway if needed while an otolaryngologist and anesthesiologist are notified. A patient with this diagnosis should never be left unobserved without appropriate airway management tools in close proximity.

SIGNS AND SYMPTOMS

Classic presentation of epiglottitis includes the abrupt onset of sore throat, drooling, stridor, anxiety, dysphagia, dysphonia, and high fever. Symptoms develop over several hours and the patient usually appears toxic. Many of the objective findings may be absent in the patients younger than 2 years old.

Adults, because of their larger airways, typically present with complaint of a sore throat, dysphagia, low-grade fever, and pain without significant physical findings.

OBJECTIVE FINDINGS

The textbook appearance of the patient with epiglottitis is an anxious, apprehensive, toxic older child or adult. Most will be febrile with readings approximately 102.2°F (39°C), although up to 25 percent of patients have no documented fever. Respirations are clear and quiet, with little air movement. Absence of spontaneous cough is also important to note.

Tenderness to palpation of the larynx is sometimes found in adults. Adults will have a preference for a sitting position since this is easier on the airway.

The child is typically found in the characteristic "sniffing," or "tripod" position, sitting up with chin forward and neck slightly extended. Children will resist lying prone and should not be laid down. Providers should at all times attempt to reassure and calm the patient. Children should be kept with a parent at all times and should at no time be agitated. Mouth examinations are traditionally avoided in children because of the potential to cause laryngospasm.

Later symptoms are noted by inspiratory stridor, active drooling, or trouble handling secretions by the patient.

DIAGNOSTIC CONSIDERATIONS

The following illnesses should be considered with differential diagnosis:

- Pharyngitis or tonsillitis
- Peritonsillar abscess
- Retropharyngeal abscess
- Croup
- Foreign body obstruction
- Laryngeal tracheitis
- Bronchospasm

SPECAL CONSIDERATION: AIRWAY MANAGEMENT AND INTUBATION

Airway management is the priority whether it be through continuous observation or immediate intervention with intubation. Controversy remains among practitioners regarding the most appropriate management of patients. If a child with symptoms highly suggestive of epiglottitis has a clinically unstable airway, it is necessary to intervene immediately with intubation. If the child has symptoms suggestive of the disease, but has an airway that is patent and well maintained, the child should be transferred, if needed, and closely observed until operating room intervention is performed. Portable radiographs of the lateral neck soft tissues can be obtained, remembering that nothing should be done that would potentially irritate the child.

If airway compromise occurs prior to intervention, bag-mask ventilation will maintain oxygenation. Mask ventilation is easily accomplished in most patients with epiglottitis since airway compromise is usually due to diaphragmatic fatigue and not complete airway obstruction from an enlarged, edematous epiglottis. Generally, unsuccessful mask ventilation means improper head positioning.

The role of intubation in the management of the stable adult is unclear. Successful management is well documented with only observation, antibiotics, and supportive care. The decision to place an airway depends on the need for airway stabilization and availability of personnel skilled in advanced airway management.

While adults can be managed with observation alone, all children with epiglottitis require intubation. The mortality rate is higher in children who are only monitored when compared with the mortality rate in children who are managed with intubation because of respiratory arrest.

LABORATORY TESTS

Laboratory tests should be delayed in children until after airway stabilization. Most practitioners will agree that a complete blood cell count (CBC) with differential and two blood cultures are recommended. A direct culture of the epiglottis may be obtained with intubation, and antigen testing may also be done.

A CBC with differential, will show increased WBC count with many polymorphonuclear leukocytes. Blood cultures will be positive 80 percent of the time in children and about 25 percent of the time in adults.

RADIOLOGIC STUDIES

Radiographs should not delay appropriate airway management or prevent adequate observations of the patient. Portable lateral soft tissue neck radiographs may be obtained in the stable patient. Best results are obtained when the film is taken during inspiration with the neck extended.

When viewing a soft tissue neck film there are four things to consider and examine:

1. The epiglottis
2. The retropharyngeal or prevertebral space
3. The tracheal air column
4. The hypopharynx

In epiglottitis, soft tissue radiographs reveal an enlarged epiglottis and surrounding structures to form the "thumbprint" on the lateral view. In adults, accepted standards that are consistent with epiglottitis are epiglottic width greater than 8 mm, aryepiglottic folds larger than 7 mm, a decrease in the angle of the valleculae, and an increase in the ratio of the hypopharyngeal to tracheal air column (Fig. 4-5-1).

OTHER DIAGNOSTIC CONSIDERATIONS

It is important to look for concurrent infections such as pneumonia, otitis media, and upper respiratory infection (URI). Approximately 25 percent of children will have a secondary infection.

Figure 4-5-1. Lateral soft tissue neck with enlarged epiglottis, "thumbprint" sign, indicative of epiglottitis. *(Photo courtesy Challenger Corporation. Copyright © 1997.)*

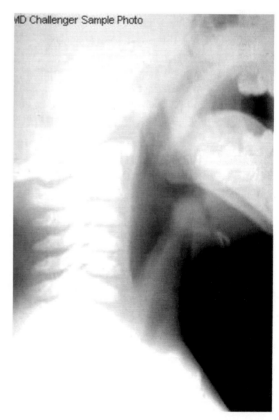

TREATMENT

Supportive Measures

The following should be included in supportive treatment:

- Humidified O_2 administered in accordance with pulse oximetry
- IV hydration

Pharmacological Management

Consideration of *H. influenzae* immunization status is important when planning antibiotic therapy such as the following:

- Cefuroxime (Ceftin) 100 to 150 mg/kg/day divided in three doses
- Chloramphenicol 100 mg/kg/day alternatively to cefuroxime if allergic
- Cefotaxime (Claforan) 50 to 150 mg/kg/day, every 6 to 8 h IV
- Rocephin (ceftriaxone) 50 to 75 mg/kg/day every 12 h IV
- Ampicillin-sulbactam (Unasyn) and trimethoprim-sulfamethoxazole (Bactrim/Septra), also reasonable choices
- In adults, cefazolin (Ancef) 1 g IV, every 6 h often added

IV antibiotics are continued for 48 to 72, followed by a 10-day course of oral medication such as trimethoprim-sulfamethoxazole (Bactrim/Septra) or cefaclor (Ceclor).

Prophylactic antibiotics are recommended in the case of invasive *H. influenzae*. All nonpregnant household contacts over 4 years of age should receive a prophylactic daily dose of rifampin at 20 mg/kg for 4 days.

Racemic epinephrine is not beneficial in reducing stridor. Steroids remain controversial in their role of reducing airway edema and are not recommended.

DISPOSITION

Patients with this diagnosis should be admitted to intensive care for observation, airway management and stabilization, and antibiotic therapy. An ENT and anesthesiologist should be consulted for additional intervention and management. Resolution of symptoms generally takes place over 36 to 48 h.

COMPLICATIONS AND RED FLAGS

Complications involve those that result from airway obstruction secondary to swelling and edema of the epiglottis. If the airway is not managed, there is the potential for respiratory arrest, asphyxia, hypoxic brain damage, and death.

BIBLIOGRAPHY

Barkin R, Rosen P (eds): *Emergency Pediatrics: A Guide to Ambulatory Care.* St Louis, Mosby-Year Book, 1994.

Rothrock S, Perkin R: Stridor: A review, update, and current management recommendations. *Ped Emerg Med Rep* 4:29–40, April 1996.

Ryan M, Hunt M, Snowberger T: A changing pattern of epiglottitis. *Clin Pediatr* 532–535, September 1992.

Saunders, C, Ho M (eds): *Current Emergency Diagnosis and Treatment.* Norwalk, CT, Appleton & Lange, 1992.

Schwartz G, Cayten C, Mangelsen M, Mayer T, Hanke B (eds): *Principles and Practice of Emergency Medicine.* New York, Lea Febiger, 1992.

Tintinalli JE, Ruiz E, Krome RL (eds): *Emergency Medicine: A Comprehensive Study Guide.* New York, McGraw-Hill, 1996.

Wilson JD, Braunwald E, Isselbacher KJ (eds): *Harrison's Principles of Internal Medicine*, 12th ed. New York, McGraw-Hill, 1991.

Chapter 4–6
HEAT STROKE

Jeffrey R. Smith

DISCUSSION

High environmental heat and humidity contribute to a number of heat stress syndromes. It is important to recognize heat injury as a spectrum of disorders ranging from heat cramps to heat stroke, with heat stroke being the most serious and potentially lethal. Heat stroke occurs primarily when the ambient temperature is higher than 95°F for a day or two and the relative humidity is in the range of 50 to 75 percent.[1] High ambient temperature impairs heat loss via radiation, and the high ambient humidity limits heat dissipation by the evaporation of sweat.

The elderly tend to be most susceptible to sudden changes in heat, most likely due to thermoregulatory dysfunction, multiple medications which may inhibit heat control, and socioeconomic factors. The urban poor are particularly susceptible to heat stroke, women are more affected than men, and infants also tend to be at risk. Other factors that may increase the risk of heat stroke include obesity, neurologic and cardiovascular disorders, diuretics, neuroleptic drugs, anticholinergic medications, and alcohol consumption.

A second form of heat stroke is caused by exercising in a hot and humid environment. The primary physiologic mechanism is heat production from exercising skeletal muscle. Affected by environmental factors and dehydration, the potential for heat stroke exists among football players, runners, cyclists, and triathletes. Those athletes who are less fit and/or do not replace fluids during training, races, or games are most likely to succumb to heat stroke. Although dehydration impairs thermoregulatory mechanisms during exercise, the intensity of exercise is a much more accurate predictor of exertional heat stroke.[2] Other factors include exposure to direct sunlight, lack of acclimatization to heat, and inappropriate heavy attire. In the United States, in addition to athletes, exertional heat stroke is seen in industrial workers and military recruits. In Saudi Arabia, both forms of heat stroke are particularly common during the annual pilgrimage to Mecca.[3]

Heat stroke is far from uncommon. Between 1979 and 1991, more than 5200 deaths in the United States were attributed to excess heat exposure.[4,5] In 1980 alone, a severe summer heat wave caused more than 1265 deaths in the United States.[6]

SIGNS AND SYMPTOMS

As with any patient, an accurate and thorough history proves invaluable. In the case of heat stroke, often a source of medical history from someone other than the patient, such as family or friends is more valid. Past medical history, including current medications and doses, is important, as well as possible co-morbid factors. Knowledge of duration and activity during heat exposure is valuable as well.

The major clinical signs and symptoms of both classic heat stroke and exertional heat stroke are similar despite differences in pathophysiology and epidemiology. An abrupt rise in body temperature is universal. In heat stroke, all of the mechanisms for body cooling have failed to the extent that core body temperature above 106°F (40 to 41°C) ensues.[1] Disordered mentation, ranging from lethargy to coma and seizures, soon follows. Irritability, aggressiveness, hysteria, and emotional lability often give way to apathy and a glassy stare. An unsteady gait or inability to ambulate also may occur. Anhidrosis, or failure of perspiration, is commonly seen, although sweating persists in up to 50 percent of exertional heat stroke cases. Pulmonary abnormalities such as pulmonary edema, adult respiratory distress syndrome, and aspiration pneumonia may be seen.

OBJECTIVE FINDINGS

The physical examination is initially focused around the core body temperature and evaluating the cardiovascular and neurologic status of the heat stroke patient. Once a core temperature of above 105°F is determined, attention is given to the patient's cardiovascular status. Nearly all heat stroke victims have sinus tachycardia. Hemodynamic measurements generally reveal hypotension (from a low peripheral vascular resistance and probable low circulating volume) and a high cardiac output. ECG abnormalities include conduction disturbances and ST-segment changes.[7]

Impairment of the patient's neurologic status may range from lethargy to coma, seizures, and nuchal rigidity. It is critical (especially in the elderly patient), to know the baseline mental status of the patient. The important objective finding of pupillary dilation does not always indicate brain death in cases of heat stroke.

Other body systems that give a wealth of information regarding the diagnosis are the hepatic and renal systems; serum glutamic-oxaloacetic transaminase (SGOT) and bilirubin levels are commonly elevated. It is generally considered a poor prognostic sign to have an SGOT level greater than 1000 IU. Coagulation abnormalities are more common in classic nonexertional heat stroke and are clinically evident by the presence of melena, hematuria, purpura, hemoptysis, and even disseminated intravascular coagulation (DIC).

Renal failure is seen in 25 to 30 percent of exertional heat stroke patients but only 5 percent of nonexertional heat stroke patients.[8] Turbid urine, myoglobulinuria, proteinuria, and casts are commonly seen along with oliguria.

DIFFERENTIAL DIAGNOSIS

A meticulous medical history is critically important in developing a complete differential. Since the diagnosis of heat stroke is to a certain extent, a diagnosis of exclusion, ruling out other causes of high temperature and altered mental status is crucial. Encephalitis and meningitis can pass as heat stroke. A lumbar puncture can help differentiate between heat stroke and a CNS infection. If a patient has returned from travel to an area that is endemic for malaria, cerebral falciparum malaria should be considered. A thick and thin blood smear will help in the diagnosis.

Medication-induced heat illness should always be a consideration. Overdoses of such medications as anticholinergics, salicylates, and sympathomimetics like amphetamines and cocaine can all cause hyperpyretic syndromes. Haloperidol therapy is usually the causative agent in neuroleptic malignant syndrome, an uncommon disorder (occurring in fewer than 1 percent of patients receiving neuroleptic therapy) characterized by hyperthermia, severe dyskinesia, diaphoresis, and dyspnea. Phenothiazines, butyrophenones, and thioxanthenes, as well as withdrawal from amantadine, levodopa, and other dopaminergic medications, may also contribute to neuroleptic malignant syndrome.[9] Endocrine disorders like thyroid storm and pheochromocytoma may also present with symptoms that may mimic heat stroke.

LABORATORY TESTS

Laboratory tests used for heat stroke are listed in Table 4-6-1.

TREATMENT

Rapid recognition of heat stroke, followed by aggressive therapy can prevent permanent organ damage and death. Primary therapy

Table 4-6-1. Laboratory Tests for Heat Stroke

Test	Common Findings
CBC	Leukocytosis, hemoconcentration, thrombocytopenia
Electrolytes	Hypokalemia, hypocalcemia hypophosphatemia
Liver panel	Elevated SGOT, hyperbilirubinemia
Renal panel	Elevated BUN and creatinine
Urinalysis	Proteinuria, hematuria, abundant granular casts
Coagulation studies	Prolonged bleeding time, elevated PT/PTT
Arterial blood gases	Respiratory alkalosis followed by a metabolic acidosis
Drug screen	Sympathomimetics, anticholinergics, and salicylates (important for differential)

consists of prompt lowering of the core body temperature. A rectal thermistor probe should be placed for monitoring of core temperature every 5 min. Methods used for lowering the core temperature are varied and somewhat controversial. Immersion in ice water remains the standard approach, although applying ice packs to the body may be just as effective and logistically an advantage. Both techniques produce cutaneous vasoconstriction which potentially could impede the transfer of heat from the skin.

Despite this potential drawback, ice baths remain effective and relatively safe. In a study of 252 marine recruits whose therapy for exertional heat stroke included ice bath immersion, there were no fatalities.[10] Other cooling techniques used include ice water enemas and gastric lavage, and spraying the patient with a cool mist followed by cool air directed over the body from a large fan. Administration of room temperature intravenous fluids should be used as well. The high thermal conductivity of water usually allows reduction of the core temperature to 39°C within a period of 10 to 40 min. At this point cooling measures should be removed to prevent hypothermic overshoot. Use of isopropyl alcohol sponge baths to facilitate cooling, especially in the young patient, should be avoided because of isopropanol poisoning reported in children. Fluid resuscitation is also a crucial element in treating the heat stroke patient. Oral rehydration is preferred, but in cases where that is not possible intravenous fluids with $D_5\frac{1}{2}NS$ at 75 to 100 mL/h is sufficient.

In exertional heat stroke were patients participated in events lasting less than 4 h, the standard fluid replacement is $D_5\frac{1}{2}NS$, and events lasting longer than 4 h, the fluid of choice is D_5NS or lactated Ringer's solution. Administration of mannitol (12.5 g IV initially, followed by 12.5 g/L IV fluid) has been advocated to promote renal blood flow and prevent damage from myoglobinuria; it can also serve to treat cerebral edema. Urinary alkalinization with two ampules (100 meq) $NaHCO_3$ per liter of D_5W, infused at a rate sufficient to maintain output of at least 50 ml per hour, is indicated for myoglobinuria.[8]

In comatose patients, endotracheal intubation for airway protection may be warranted.

Benzodiazepines may be used to control seizures.

As with most medical conditions, prevention is the best treatment. Paying close attention to weather bulletins predicting heat waves, checking on elderly family members and friends regularly, staying cool with fans or air conditioners, maintaining proper hydration, and avoiding strenuous activity in direct heat are recommended.

Acclimatization is an important concept in prevention of exertional heat stroke. Acclimatization is the body's compliance to heat stress over a period of time and involves modification in hormonal, neural, cardiovascular, and pulmonary physiology. Opinions as to optimal amount of time needed for acclimatization varies. Most agree that at least 4 to 7 days with as little as 90 min of exposure to heat each day will allow the body to fully adapt to heat stress. Others claim that full acclimatization does not occur before 2 months of exposure. An informal interview with ultradistance triatheletes arriving in Kona, Hawaii, for a world championship race would probably reveal most athletes arriving for the race 7 to 10 days prior to competition. Appropriate fluid replacement during training and racing and during acclimatization is crucial. The American College of Sports Medicine currently recommends that runners drink 100 to 200 mL after every 2 to 3 km. This is a generality, however. At the extremes, it is interpreted that slow runners drink only 330 mL/h and faster runners should drink up to 2000 mL/h.[11]

DISPOSITION

Even with aggressive therapy, heat stroke has an appreciable mortality rate. However, most patients who do recover have a return to normal thermoregulatory mechanisms and heat tolerance.[12] Despite the dramatic central nervous system manifestation of extreme heat stroke, most patients who survive do not exhibit neurologic impairment.[13]

Patient education of causative factors remains the cornerstone of preventing further episodes of heat stroke.

PEARLS

Beware of athletes on nonsteroidal anti-inflammatory medication. If they exhibit signs and symptoms of heat stroke and yet do not have a core body temperature higher than 105°F, they still may be suffering from heat stroke but cannot register a high core temperature owing to the effects of the NSAID. Treat them as you would any other heat stroke victim, but be judicious in cooling techniques.

REFERENCES

1. American Academy of Orthopaedic Surgeons Editorial Board, Hunter-Griffen LY (chair): *Athletic Training and Sports Medicine,* 2d ed. Rosemont, IL, American Academy of Orthopaedic Surgeons, 1992, p 854.
2. Noakes TD, Myburgh KH, du Plessis J, et al: Metabolic rate, not percent dehydration, predicts rectal temperature in marathon runners. *Med Sci Sports Exerc* 23:443, 1991.
3. al-Harthi SS, Karrar O, al-Mashhadani SA, Saddique AA: Metabolite and hormonal profiles in heat stroke patients at Mecca pilgrimage. *J Intern Med* 228(4):343–346, 1990.
4. Heat-related deaths—United States. *MMWR* 42(28):558–560, 1993.
5. Heat-related deaths—Philadelphia and United States, 1993–1994. *MMWR* 43(25):453–455, 1994.
6. Heatstroke—United States, 1980. *MMWR* 30(23):277–279, 1981.
7. Akhtar MJ, al-Nozha M, al-Harth SS, et al: Electrocardiographic abnormalities in patients with heat stroke. *Chest* 104:1498, 1993.
8. Yarbrough BE: Heat related disorders. *Hosp Med* 27(6):81–91, June 1991.
9. Caroff SN, Mann SC: Neuroleptic syndrome. *Med Clin North Am* 77:185, 1993.
10. Costrini A: Emergency treatment of exertional heatstroke and comparison of whole body cooling techniques. *Med Sci Sports Exerc* 22:15, 1990.
11. Coyle EF, Montain SJ: Benefits of fluid replacement with carbohydrate during exercise. *Med Sci Sports Exerc* 24:325, 1992.
12. Armstrong LE, DeLuca JP, Hubbard RW: Time course of recovery and heat acclimation ability to prior exertional heat stroke patients. *Med Sci Sports Exerc* 22:36, 1990.
13. Sminia P, van der Zee J, Wondergem J et al: Effect of hyperthermia on the central nervous system: A review. *Int J Hyperthermia* 10:1, 1994.

Chapter 4–7
SHOCK
Donald J. Sefcik

DISCUSSION

Shock may be defined as inadequate cellular oxygenation secondary to insufficient tissue perfusion. The result is cellular dysfunction. The manifestations of shock range from subtle, nonspecific symptoms to the classic, clinical presentation of altered mental status, cool extremities, tachycardia, tachypnea, and hypotension.

Although the etiologies of shock are numerous, they may be grouped into four major categories. (See Table 4-7-1.) Inadequate vascular volume, myocardial cellular dysfunction, obstruction of cardiac filling or emptying, and loss of vascular tone may independently or in combination cause the clinical syndrome of shock.

The body employs several compensatory mechanisms (e.g., cardiovascular, respiratory, metabolic) during shock. If they remain unrecognized or suboptimally treated, irreversible cellular injury or death may occur.

PATHOGENESIS

To function normally, tissues require a mechanism to supply necessary nutrients and oxygen. Organ perfusion is determined by two major factors, arterial blood pressure and tissue vascular resistance. If inadequate arterial pressure exists, the driving

Table 4-7-1. Major Categories of the Shock Syndromes

Hypovolemic shock
  Hemorrhage
    Traumatic
    Nontraumatic
      Gastrointestinal hemorrhage
  Nonhemorrhagic
    Volume depletion
      Inadequate intake (e.g., anorexia)
      Excessive losses
        Gastrointestinal (vomiting, diarrhea)
        Urinary (polyuria)
    Extravascular ("third") spacing
      Peritoneal fluid
      Inadequate oncotic pressure
Cardiogenic shock
  Myocardial dysfunction
    Cellular ischemia or infarction
    Dysrhythmias
    Inflammatory disorders (myocarditis)
    Pharmacologic effects (negative inotropic or chronotropic agents)
  Valvular heart defects
    Significant stenotic lesions
    Significant insufficiency
Obstructive noncardiogenic shock
  Pericardial tamponade
  Tension pneumothorax
  Significant pulmonary embolism
  Left ventricular outflow obstruction
Distributive shock
  Septic shock
  Neurogenic shock
  Anaphylactic shock
  Drug-induced shock

Table 4-7-2. Causes of Hypotension

Reduced cardiac output
  Stroke volume
    Preload reduction
      Inadequate intravascular volume
      Inadequate atrial contractile state
    Myocardial cell dysfunction
      Cellular ischemia or infarction
      Dysrhythmias
      Altered heart rate or oxygen demand
      Pharmacologic agents
    Afterload abnormality
      Outflow tract disorder
  Heart rate
    Dysrhythmias
Total peripheral vascular resistance
  Reduction of arterial tone
    Pharmacologic sources (vasodilators)
    Metabolic products
    Exogenous products
      Endotoxins

force behind tissue oxygenation is insufficient. When the vascular resistance is inappropriate (tone is reduced or distribution of blood flow is improper), nutritional and oxygenation demands of tissues are not met. Subsequently, cellular metabolic dysfunction ensues, and the signs and symptoms of the shock syndrome begin.

Arterial blood pressure is the product of the cardiac output (CO) and the total peripheral resistance (TPR). The cardiac output is the product of the stroke volume (SV) and the heart rate (HR). Therefore, the blood pressure is actually determined by three major variables, $BP = SV \times HR \times TPR$. A reduction in any of these variables may diminish systemic blood pressure and produce a relative or absolute state of hypoperfusion. Factors that may exert detrimental effects on systemic arterial pressure are multifactorial and include dysrhythmias, blood loss, myocardial cellular dysfunction, pericardial disorders, and mediators of vascular tone (see Table 4-7-2).

Early stages of shock may be reversible. However, once cellular injury has occurred, the likelihood of irreversible shock increases, and even the most aggressive therapy may not save the patient.

SYMPTOMS

The classic clinical manifestations of shock, hypotension, tachycardia, a weak pulse, cool extremities, tachypnea, an altered mental status (confusion), and a reduced urine output, are well known. The more subtle presentations of shock, however, challenge the diagnostic acumen of even the most experienced clinician.

When presented with an altered mental status, a confusional state, a combative patient, or the comment from a family member that the patient is "just not himself," consideration must be given to a cerebral hypoperfusional state. Complaints of dizziness, especially when assuming an upright position, should be considered a sign of cerebral hypoperfusion and evaluated. Nonspecific complaints of weakness, fatigue, and generalized arthralgias or myalgias might represent a relative hypoperfusional state or metabolic sequelae of inadequate tissue oxygenation.

Shortness of breath at rest, dyspnea on exertion, and palpitations may represent attempts of cardiovascular compensatory efforts. Complaints of reduced urine output or a concentrated-appearing or "strong" odor to the urine may be indications of attempted renal compensation secondary to hypoperfusion.

OBJECTIVE FINDINGS

A common feature in most shock syndromes is hypotension. Sustained systolic blood pressure values lower than 90 mmHg need to undergo diagnostic scrutiny. Keep in mind, however, that although the chronic hypertensive patient may present with what appears to be a normal blood pressure, a relative hypotensive state may, in fact, exist. Recent blood pressure values obtained from prior charts may offer insight.

Tachycardia, especially in a resting state, must be evaluated. This may represent an attempt by the body to compensate for a reduced cardiac output or a reduction of total peripheral resistance. Cool, sometimes cyanotic extremities, are common features of the patient in shock and are manifestations of the body's increasing peripheral resistance through vasoconstriction. Catecholamine release is responsible for both the tachycardia and cool extremities.

Reduced urine output is often noted, a result of nephron hypoperfusion. Renal attempts to elevate perfusion result in fluid reabsorption, which clinically manifests as oliguria. Tachypnea develops in an attempt to increase tissue oxygenation and to compensate for the metabolic acidosis.

DIAGNOSTIC CONSIDERATIONS

Of paramount importance to the appropriate treatment of the patient in shock is discovering the etiology. Initial considerations should be directed toward establishing a general categorical diagnosis. (See Table 4-7-1.)

Hypovolemic causes of shock may be obvious (hemorrhage, trauma, etc.) or less obvious (third spacing of fluids, gastrointestinal losses, or diuresis). Generally, historical information and physical examination (dry membranes, altered skin turgor, reduction of urine output, etc.) will provide diagnostic insight.

Cardiogenic disorders may present more of a challenge. Acute myocardial cellular dysfunction (myocardial ischemia or infarct, valvular alteration, etc.) may be difficult to detect. Cardiac dysrhythmias may be easier to appreciate.

Although obstructive causes of shock may provide clues to their existence, astute diagnostic perception is still required. Pericardial effusions may demonstrate muffled heart tones, jugular venous distention, and hypotension. However, failure to appreciate absent apical breath sounds (often a problem in a setting with significant background noise) may result in a missed diagnosis of tension pneumothorax. The diagnosis of a massive pulmonary embolism is at times elusive, but profound hypoxemia and a widened alveolar-arterial (Aa) gradient provide diagnostic clues.

Distributive forms of shock have many possible causes. After careful evaluation for the other types of shock, the etiologies of this group should be given consideration. The diversity of the causes of distributive shock challenge even the most experienced of clinicians. (See Table 4-7-1.)

LABORATORY TESTING

Critical to the outcome of the patient in shock is hemodynamic monitoring. (See "Treatment," below.) Initial laboratory testing is directed toward those studies that are necessary for early intervention. Studies generally obtained include a complete blood cell count (CBC), serum chemistries (sodium, potassium, calcium, BUN, creatinine, and magnesium), and arterial blood gas (ABG). Additional testing should be directed toward the underlying process. Laboratory selection is guided by history, physical examination, and the patient's response to therapy. Additional tests to consider include cultures (blood, sputum, and urine), toxicology studies, liver enzymes, and cardiac enzymes. Other diagnostic information may be gained by reviewing chest x-rays, ECGs, echocardiograms, CT scans, and nuclear radiologic studies.

Although each of these individual tests may prove useful, the benefit of obtaining serial laboratory studies to optimize patient therapy (assure response to treatment and guide additional therapeutic interventions) cannot be overemphasized.

TREATMENT

As with any medical emergency, basic resuscitative measures are critical in the patient's treatment. Patients need to receive supplemental oxygen, have serial blood pressure measurements obtained, receive intravenous fluids, be placed on cardiac monitors and pulse oximeters, and have a Foley catheter secured. Consideration must be given to an indwelling arterial catheter, both as a monitoring device and as a source for multiple arterial blood specimens, if necessary. A central venous catheter provides important hemodynamic information.

At least two intravenous catheters are placed, preferably large-bore (16 gauge or larger), since rapid fluid administration is a common requirement in the treatment of shock. Normal saline and lactated Ringer's solution are generally the crystalloid fluids of choice. Vasopressors (dopamine or norepinephrine) as well as volume expanders (albumin or dextran) may be required. Pneumatic antishock garments, also known as MAST (military antishock trousers), are useful in selected cases (especially hypovolemia).

Corticosteroids and opioid antagonists (naloxone) have been utilized in some shock situations (to reduce the effects of β-endorphins), but are generally not employed in most cases of shock. As a temporary measure for cardiogenic shock, the intraaortic balloon pump (IABP) is often useful.

COMPLICATIONS AND RED FLAGS

Major complications to anticipate in the course of treatment include the development of adult respiratory distress syndrome (ARDS), DIC, and acute renal failure (ARF).

NOTES AND PEARLS

Be wary of a patient with hypotension and bradycardia. Suspect a primary myocardial disorder or an extracardiac etiology tie (pharmacologic agent) that is inhibiting the normally expected compensatory mechanism to hypotension. Also, be suspicious of the hypotensive patient with warm extremities. This may represent septic shock, also known as warm shock.

PROGNOSIS

If the patient in shock is identified early, the etiology of the problem is determined and aggressive appropriate therapy is instituted, the prognosis is greatly improved. If however, the early symptoms or signs go unnoticed, therapy is not directed at the underlying cause, or therapy is inadequate, the shock syndrome may reach a state of irreversibility and the outcome will be death.

BIBLIOGRAPHY

Ferguson DW: Shock, in *Cecil Textbook of Medicine*, 19th ed. Philadelphia, Saunders, 1992, pp 207–227.

Parrillo JE: Shock, in Fauci AS, Braunwald E, Isselbacher KJ, et al (eds): *Harrison's Principles of Internal Medicine*, 14th ed. New York, McGraw-Hill, 1998, pp 214–222.

Chapter 4–8
POISONING AND OVERDOSE
Karen A. Newell

EPIDEMIOLOGY

It is estimated that more than 4 million cases of poisoning or overdose occur each year in the United States. Most of these occur in children between the ages of 1 and 5 (accidental ingestion). In adolescents and young adults, cases are secondary to drug experimentation and suicide attempts. The majority of the adult cases are intentional, with the remainder from occupational and household accidents.

INITIAL MANAGEMENT

As with any serious emergency, the clinician must address the ABCs of airway, breathing and circulation.

Next, any patient who presents unconscious or with signs of altered mental status should be given 50 mL of 50% dextrose, 0.8 to 1.2 mg of naloxone (1 to 2 mg repeated boluses to a total of 4 mg), and 100 mg of thiamine intravenously. In alcoholic patients, administration of glucose before thiamine can precipitate Wernicke's encephalopathy. Prior to arrival in the emergency department, keeping the patient in the left lateral decubitus position can slow absorption.

HISTORY AND PHYSICAL EXAMINATION

Attention to the identity and amount of the substance, when and why it was taken, association with other substances, and underlying medical conditions can be very helpful; however, this is often unreliable information.

Vital signs Monitor temperature, blood pressure, respiratory pattern and rate, and pulse rate.
General Check for odor on breath.
Skin Assess for needle marks, or "tracks" (linear scarring noted parallel to venous distribution usually located on the forearms), diaphoresis, or color changes.
Pulmonary and cardiovascular systems Auscultate for pulmonary edema or cardiac dysrhythmia.
Abdomen Check for the presence or absence of bowel sounds.
Neurologic signs Give attention to mental status; pupillary size and reaction to light, presence of nystagmus; focal deficits, deep tendon reflexes, and presence or absence of gag reflex.

DIAGNOSTIC STUDIES

These may include the following:

- CBC
- Serum toxicology
- Initial fingerstick glucose
- Electrolytes: blood urea nitrogen (BUN), creatinine, serum glucose, measured osmolality
- Urinalysis and urine toxicology
- ECG
- Chest x-ray

Consideration is also given to arterial blood gases, abdominal x-ray, liver function studies, gastric aspirate or emesis for toxicology.

TREATMENT

Skin Decontamination

Each of the following should be carried out with cutaneous exposure:

- Clothing should be removed and placed in plastic bags.
- Brush off any powder or particulate matter prior to irrigation
- Wash involved skin surfaces thoroughly with mild soap and water
- Protect those in close contact with the patient during the decontamination process with at least gloves, eye protection, and gown.

Gastrointestinal Decontamination

Unless contraindicated, the following three routes are used in GI decontamination: emesis or gastric lavage, treatment with activated charcoal, and use of cathartics.

Emesis

Emesis is still considered useful in many minor cases; however, most authorities realize that seriously poisoned patients require gastric lavage.

Contraindications

Contraindications to using emesis include the following:

- Children younger than 9 months of age
- Patients with lethargy, stupor, coma, or seizures
- Patients who have previously vomited the ingested substance
- Patients without a gag reflex (up to 30 percent of normal people have no gag reflex)
- Patients who have ingested a strong acid or alkali substance
- Patients who have ingested a sharp object
- Patients who have ingested certain hydrocarbons
- Patients who have ingested substances with a rapid onset of toxicity

Dosage

The syrup of ipecac dose is dependent on patient age. The following doses are recommended:

- 10 mL for those between 9 and 11 months of age
- 15 mL for patients between 1 and 10 years old
- 30 mL for patients older than 10 years

Procedure

This procedure should be carried out by using syrup of ipecac only. No other emetic should be used. Remember that *fluid of ipecac* is 14 times stronger than *syrup of ipecac* and can be toxic if not properly used. The procedure includes the following steps:

- Give several glasses of water to the adult after ingesting the syrup of ipecac, less depending on the size and age of the patient.
- Keep the patient supervised and in an upright position.
- The emetic should be effective and induce vomiting within 30 minutes; if not, give a similar second dose; if still no response, then lavage should be considered.

Gastric Lavage

This procedure is indicated for those who have eaten and are unable to protect their airway (altered mental status, seizure activity) or those with a gag reflex who can protect their airway but are unresponsive to syrup of ipecac. The procedure is contraindicated if the patient has a history of ingesting strong acid or alkali.

Procedure

Select the proper size of nasogastric (NG) tube. Use 28 to 40 Fr Ewald orogastric tube (16 to 26 Fr in children), since smaller-bore NG tubes are not effective for lavage.

Confirm tube placement by injecting 60 mL of air while listening over the gastric bubble or aspirate the gastric contents; if unclear, radiologic confirmation is absolutely necessary before lavage.

Typically, these patients are already intubated with either an endotracheal tube or nasotracheal tube. At that point, take the following steps:

- Place the patient in the left lateral decubitus position.
- Withdraw all stomach contents.
- Place 200 to 300 mL of room-temperature tap water (50 to 100 mL in children) into the stomach through the tube.
- Continue to inject and aspirate the fluid until clear; use 2 L in those who are initially clear.
- Send the first 100 mL of aspirate for toxicology.
- Massaging the left upper quadrant can help to dislodge any tablets or large particulate matter during aspiration.

Complications

These include pulmonary aspiration, gastric erosion or perforation, and esophageal tears.

Activated Charcoal

This is the "gold standard" for toxic ingestion. Activated charcoal will bind many toxic substances and is indicated after vomiting or lavage. It is not effective in those who have ingested ethanol, methanol, strong acids or bases, lithium, or cyanide.

Contraindications

In patients that should receive a specific oral antidote, activated charcoal may bind to the antidote and reduce it's effectiveness.

In patients who will require endoscopy (i.e., caustic ingestion), activated charcoal will interfere with the visual inspection.

Procedure

Activated charcoal is diluted in four parts of water or sorbitol and given orally or by lavage. If this is vomited, it should be repeated. It is tasteless, but it is visually unpleasant and gritty.

Select the proper dose: adults or children, 1 g/kg of body weight

May be readministered every 4 to 6 h in those with ingestion of theophylline, phenobarbital, tricyclic antidepressants, phenothiazines, and digitalis to prevent later reabsorption.

Cathartics

The use of cathartics is controversial. Cathartics can be used to expedite elimination of toxic substances through the bowel. Contraindications include the following:

- Infants
- Patients who receive an oral antidote
- Adynamic ileus
- Severe diarrhea
- Intestinal obstruction
- Abdominal trauma
- Recent abdominal surgery
- Sodium sulfate contraindicated in patients with hypertension, severe left ventricular dysfunction or congestive heart failure
- Sodium phosphate (Fleet Phospho-Soda) contraindicated in children and in ethylene glycol ingestion
- Avoidance of magnesium-containing cathartics in patients with renal failure

Cathartic choices and dosages include the following (choose one):

- 30 g magnesium sulfate
- 30 g magnesium citrate (children 4 mg/kg)
- 30 g sodium sulfate
- 100 to 150 mL of a 70% solution of sorbitol
- 15 to 30 mL sodium phosphate, diluted at 1:4 with water

Complications

Avoid oil based-cathartics where there is a risk of pulmonary aspiration. Also, be aware that activated charcoal can bind also to these agents and make them useless.

Enhanced Elimination

Diuresis

Indications

This method may be useful in isoniazid, bromide, or ethanol ingestion.

Contraindications

Patients with hypotension and pulmonary edema should not undergo diuresis.

Dosage

The recommended dose is 20 to 100 g mannitol and intermittent 20 mg furosemide.

Monitor

Electrolytes should be monitored to prevent hyponatremia and hypokalemia.

Alkaline Diuresis

Mechanism

Alkalinization of urine prevents reabsorption by the kidney.

Indications

Diuresis is useful in ingestion of phenobarbital, salicylates, lithium, or isoniazid.

Dosage

Use one or two ampules of IV sodium bicarbonate (slowly), then one or two ampules of sodium bicarbonate in 1 L of 0.25 to 0.45% normal saline constant IV infusion; maintain urine pH at 7.3 to 8.5. Furosemide is also helpful. Keep urine output at 5 to 7 mL/kg/h.

Complications

Complications include metabolic alkalosis, hypernatremia, hyperosmolality, and fluid retention. Make sure to adequately hydrate prior to forcing alkaline diuresis especially in salicylate ingestion.

Acid Diuresis

Mechanism

Acidification of urine prevents reabsorption by kidney.

Indications

Acid diuresis, though controversial, is used in ingestion of amphetamines, phencyclidine, quinidine or quinine, and flufluramine.

Dosage

Use 500 mg to 1 g PO or IV (initially) ascorbic acid repeated every 6 h or ammonium chloride, 4 g every 2 h by nasogastric tube or 1 to 2% solution per normal saline (NS) IV to maintain urine pH between 5.5 and 6.5, or furosemide and 0.45% normal saline IV to keep urine output at 5 to 7 mL/kg/h.

Contraindications

Patients with myoglobinuria (e.g., excessive seizure activity) should not undergo acid diuresis.

Monitoring

Carefully monitor serum electrolytes.

Dialysis

Hemodialysis is the most effective procedure in severe poisonings, especially in nonorganic compounds not well bound by charcoal or peritoneal dialysis.

Indications

Use after ingestion of ethylene glycol, methanol, or paraquat. Dialysis may be considered in severe ingestion of theophylline, lithium, salicylates, phenobarbital, bromide, and ethanol.

Hemoperfusion

Mechanism

The patient's blood is passed through a filter and replaced.

Indication

Use for severe toxicity from substances including barbiturates, glutethimide, methaqualone, ethchlorynol, meprobamate, and chloral hydrate.

Complications

Complications include decreased platelets, plasma calcium, glucose, fibrinogen, or transient leukopenia.

RECOGNITION AND MANAGEMENT OF SPECIFIC DRUGS

This is intended as a review of the more common clinical scenarios encountered and is not complete or exhaustive.

Narcotic Analgesics

These CNS depressants and respiratory depressants are classified as follows:

- *Natural opiates* Opium, morphine, codeine
- *Semisynthetics* Heroin, hydromorphone (Dilaudid), oxymorphone (Numorphan), hydrocodone (Vicodin), oxycodone (Percocet, Percodan, Tylox)
- *Synthetics* Meperidine (Demerol), methadone (Dolophine), butorphanol (Stadol), fentanyl, nalbuphine (Nubain), propoxyphene (Darvon)

Presentation

The patient presents with miotic pupils, bradycardia, decreased respirations, hypotension, hypothermia, decreased gastrointestinal motility, and noncardiac pulmonary edema. Death from respiratory depression may occur.

Treatment

Use naloxone (Narcan) 0.4 to 2.0 mg IV every 5 min to a maximum of 8 to 22 mg (0.03 to 0.1 mg/kg children); consider continuous infusion and/or oxygen.

Heroin Withdrawal

Symptoms occur at about 12 h after the last dose; patients present with restlessness, lacrimation, rhinorrhea, piloerection, diaphoresis, mydriatic pupils, muscle cramps, nausea, vomiting diarrhea, or hyperpyrexia. The condition resolves after 72 to 96 h. Treat with 10 mg PO or IM methadone upon initial symptoms and every 8 to 12 h, taper dose by half every 2 days until resolution.

Barbiturates

These CNS depressants can be long-acting (6 to 12 h), like phenobarbital or barbital; intermediate-acting (3 to 6 h), like amobarbital; short-acting (less than 3 h), like pentobarbital or secobarbital; or ultra-short-acting (20 min), like thiopental.

Presentation

Early there is drowsiness and dysarthria; later there is sedation, hypnosis, or coma. Patients have decreased respiration, hypothermia, decreased gastrointestinal motility, variation in pupillary responses from initially constricted to dilated (often co-ingested with ethanol which potentiates sedation).

Treatment

Use oxygen, gastric lavage up to 8 h after ingestion, activated charcoal, alkaline diuresis, IV fluids, supportive care; consider hemodialysis.

Withdrawal

When seen 2 to 3 days after the last dose, the patient presents with restlessness, agitation, diaphoresis, delirium, auditory hallucinations, tremor, nausea, vomiting hypotension, and seizure (resolves within 3 to 7 days). Treat initially with diazepam then with tapered phenobarbital.

Amphetamines

Presentation

These CNS stimulants may cause agitation, confusion, tremor, diaphoresis, mydriatic pupils, tachypnea, tachycardia, cardiac arrhythmias, nausea, vomiting, hyperpyrexia, seizure, and coma.

Treatment

Use gastric lavage, acid diuresis, and supportive care; benzodiazepine may be helpful.

Marijuana

Route

Marijuana may be smoked or ingested.

Presentation

Marijuana may cause confusion, paranoia, sedation, and ataxia. It may have persisting psychological effects, including depression and apathy.

Cocaine

Route

This CNS stimulant may be taken intranasally, smoked as crack, or taken by IV. Accidental ingestion by body "packers" and "stuffers" may also be seen.

Presentation

The patient presents with agitation, tachycardia, cardiac arrhythmias, hypertension, hyperthermia, seizures, nausea, or vomiting. Death may occur from cardiac ischemia, infarction, and arrest.

Treatment

Give supportive care, benzodiazepine for agitation, and beta blockers for tachyarrhythmias. Consider charcoal.

Hallucinogens (psilocybin/mescaline/STP/LSD)
Route

Hallucinogens like psilocybin, mescaline, STP, and LSD may be sniffed, ingested, or smoked. Onset of action is 20 to 30 min with duration from 1 to 6 h.

Presentation

Acute presentation includes nausea, blurred vision, mydriatic pupils, tachycardia, hyperpyrexia, hyperreflexia, visual distortions, and hallucinations.

Chronic presentation includes flashbacks and intermittent psychosis.

Treatment

Give supportive care and "talk the patient down" with much reassurance; consider benzodiazepine for severe agitation; avoid phenothiazines because they can lessen the seizure threshold; gastrointestinal decontamination procedures are unnecessary; seizures can be treated with diazepam.

PCP

PCP has a 2- to 3-min onset after smoking, with presentation much more violent and bizarre (dissociative); treatment of comatose patients includes gastrointestinal decontamination, charcoal, and acid diuresis.

Benzodiazepines

These include anxiolytics, muscle relaxants, anticonvulsants, and drugs with hypnotic properties. Examples include diazepam (Valium), oxazepam (Serax), chlordiazepoxide (Librium), and lorazepam (Ativan)

Presentation

The patient presents with drowsiness, ataxia, nystagmus, cardiac arrhythmias, and coma; death is possible but uncommon with oral ingestion unless co-ingested with other substances like ethanol.

Treatment

Gastrointestinal decontamination procedures include lavage and charcoal. The antidote is flumazenil, 0.2 mg IV over 30 s; repeat if necessary with 0.3 mg, then increments of 0.5 mg every 60 s to a total dose of 3 mg; it is contraindicated in head injury, in children, and in those who have ingested other substances, since it can precipitate seizure activity.

Withdrawal

Withdrawal is similar to ethanol and barbiturates but less severe.

Ethanol

This sedative-hypnotic can cause the following blood alcohol levels:

- 25 mg/dL blood alcohol from an ounce of whiskey, one glass of wine, or one beer
- 100 mg/dL, which is associated with intoxication in non-chronic user
- More than 400 mg/dL which is associated with lethality, although chronic users can survive with these levels and higher. The level naturally decreases about 20 to 30 mg/dL/h.

Presentation

The patient presents with ataxia, dysarthria, visual impairment, lateral nystagmus, stupor, vomiting, hypotension, seizure, and/or coma.

Treatment

Give oxygen, thiamine, and supportive care. All intoxicated patients must be held in the emergency department until they are not a danger to themselves or others. This may require a physical or chemical restraint.

Withdrawal

Withdrawal can bring on tremor. The patient may have visual or auditory hallucinations. Seizures can occur 12 to 48 h after the last ingestion. Delirium tremens occurs 3 to 4 days after the last alcohol ingestion and is fatal in about 15 percent of cases. Treat with 10 mg diazepam IV followed by 5 mg diazepam every 5 min until sedated. Agitation can be treated with 2 to 5 mg haloperidol IM. Death can occur from respiratory depression.

Methanol

Also known as wood alcohol, methanol is found in paint thinner, antifreeze, and Sterno (fuel for cooking); it is very toxic.

Presentation

Presentation is similar to that with ethanol but with more drowsiness. Toxic metabolites (formaldehyde) can occur from 6 to 36 h after ingestion and can include severe vomiting and upper abdominal pain, diarrhea, headache, dizziness, blurred vision, blindness, and seizures.

Treatment

Use gastric lavage and charcoal administration, bicarbonate IV for acidosis, and continuous IV ethanol (100 to 150 mg/dL) to compete with methanol and decrease amounts of metabolite; consider hemodialysis.

Ethylene Glycol

Colorless, odorless, and having sweet taste, ethylene glycol is used as antifreeze.

Presentation

Between 30 min and 12 h, the patient presents with ataxia, nystagmus, vomiting, hyporeflexia, severe acidosis, seizures, or coma. Between 12 and 14 h, tachypnea, tachycardia, cyanosis, and pulmonary edema appear. From 24 to 72 h flank pain and renal failure secondary to acute tubular necrosis may occur.

Diagnostic Studies

Check for severe acidosis, increased anion gap, hypocalcemia, calcium oxalate crystals in the urine, and hematuria.

Treatment

Treatment is the same as for methanol intoxication; consider calcium gluconate IV for hypocalcemia and seizures.

Isopropyl Alcohol

Rubbing alcohol is used often by alcoholic patients as less expensive and more readily available and produces an intoxicated state more quickly and with less consumption than ethanol.

Presentation

Presentation is similar to that with ethanol toxicity except with increased hemorrhagic gastritis.

Diagnostic Studies

Recommended studies include acetone in urine, elevated anion gap, and elevated osmolar gap.

Treatment

Treatment includes supportive care, gastrointestinal decontamination procedures, and bicarbonate to treat acidosis if noted; hemodialysis should be considered.

Cyanide

Cyanide can be found naturally in apple, apricot, peach, plum, cherry, and almond seeds. It is often used in industry.

Presentation

Giddiness, ataxia, headache, dyspnea, nausea, vomiting, seizures, coma, and death can be signs of ingestion.

Physical Examination

The practitioner may smell bitter almond odor on patient's breath.

Treatment

Initially crush amyl nitrate pearl and have the patient inhale for 15 to 30 s. Once the IV is established, give 10 mg of 3% sodium nitrate IV over 3 to 5 min (0.33 mL/kg in children, maximum of 10 mg) and 50 mL of 25% sodium thiosulfate IV over 10 min (1.65 mL/kg children, maximum of 50 mL). This may be repeated.

Carbon Monoxide

Carbon monoxide is a colorless, odorless gas; 5 percent of automobile exhaust is composed of carbon monoxide; it is also found in furnaces and charcoal fires.

Physical Examination

The practitioner may detect cherry red appearance of skin, mucous membranes, and fingernails since carbon monoxide preferentially binds to hemoglobin molecules limiting oxygen-carrying capacity.

Diagnostic Studies

A rapid initial test detects the presence of carboxyhemoglobin by diluting 1 mL of blood with 10 mL of water and adding 1 mL of 5% sodium hydroxide (color change of straw or pink considered positive, whereas brown is negative).

The blood carboxyhemoglobin level can be assessed definitively. Less than 10 percent of patients is usually asymptomatic, requiring no treatment. Between 10 and 20 percent has mild headache and irritability; treat them with high-flow oxygen (100% nonrebreather mask), which requires medical observation. Between 20 and 40 percent is associated with light-headedness, confusion, dizziness, agitation, nausea, vomiting, and coordination difficulty; these patients require treatment with high-flow oxygen and hospital admission. Between 40 and 60 percent exhibits syncope, dyspnea, lethargy, coma, and respiratory and cardiac arrest; these patients require high-flow oxygen and hospital admission; hyperbaric oxygen may be helpful if available. Cerebral edema may be treated with dexamethasone, 4 to 6 mg IV every 6 h. Transfusion of erythrocytes remains controversial.

Selective Serotonin Reuptake Inhibitors (SSRIs)

Recent development and increase in the utilization of such agents as fluoxetine (Prozac), sertraline (Zoloft), paroxetine (Paxil), and fluvoxamine (Luvox) have contributed to a notable increase in serotonin syndrome usually related to multidrug interactions.

Presentation

Cognitive-behavioral, autonomic nervous system, and neuromuscular changes may occur, including agitation, anxiety, sinus tachycardia, mild hypertension, diaphoresis, diarrhea, and/or muscular rigidity.

Diagnostic Studies

Diagnosis based on clinical suspicion as no definitive confirmatory study.

Treatment

Admission for supportive care. Most symptoms resolve spontaneously within 24 h. Give consideration to benzodiazepines for patient comfort. Cyproheptadine 4 to 8 mg PO may be helpful and may be repeated every 4 to 6 h (maximum of 0.5 mg/kg/d or 32 mg/d).

Tricyclic Antidepressants

Imipramine amitriptyline is a tricyclic antidepressant.

Incidence

Imipramine amitriptyline is dangerous when a patient takes an overdose. The mortality rate is 2 to 5 percent.

Presentation

CNS symptoms include confusion, anxiety, delirium, hallucinations, hyperreflexia, seizures, and coma. Anticholinergic symptoms include mydriatic pupils, hyperpyrexia, skin flushing, blurred vision, tachycardia, dehydration, urinary retention, decreased gastrointestinal motility, and decreased secretions. Cardiac arrhythmia, is characterized by ECG increased intervals, abnormal QRS complexes, bigeminy, fibrillation, and cardiac arrest.

Pearl

"Hot as Hades, blind as a bat, dry as a bone, red as a beet, mad as a hatter" is indicative of anticholinergics.

Diagnostic Studies

The therapeutic dose is 2 to 4 mg/kg; more than 4 mg/kg is considered potentially toxic; more than 10 mg/kg is life-threatening.

Treatment

Aggressive treatment is necessary and includes gastric lavage, charcoal administration, consideration of cathartics, and urinary alkalinization. Physostigmine may be considered (avoid if there are serious conduction delays). The following are contraindicated: quinidine, procainamide, atropine, and digoxin. These may exacerbate abnormal cardiac conduction and may require a central line for careful monitoring.

Lithium

Lithium is a common medication in manic depressive disorders.

Presentation

Mild toxicity is exhibited by sluggishness, drowsiness, tremor, muscle twitching, nausea, vomiting, diarrhea, polydipsia, and polyuria. Serious toxicity is exhibited by muscular rigidity, hyperreflexia, seizures, cardiac arrhythmia, hypotension, renal abnormalities, and coma.

Diagnostic Studies

The practitioner may note hyponatremia and hypokalemia. The ECG may have ST-segment depression and T-wave inversion. There may be a prolonged QT interval if hypokalemic. Obtain serum lithium level where the therapeutic dose is 0.6 to 1.2 meq/L. Mild toxicity is 1.5 to 2.4 meq/L; serious toxicity is 2.5 to 3.5 meq/L; critical toxicity is over 3.5 meq/L.

Treatment

If the patient is hypotensive, give fluids and vasopressors; if the patient is normotensive, give 0.25 to 0.50% normal saline to prevent exacerbation of renal abnormalities and to correct fluids and electrolytes. Consider gastrointestinal lavage if ingestion occurred within 4 h. Charcoal is helpful if there has been co-ingestion of other drugs, since it does not bind lithium. Avoid a magnesium based cathartic since it can exacerbate renal abnormalities. Alkaline diuresis is controversial. Consider hemodialysis in severe cases.

Neuroleptics

Phenothiazines are classified as neuroleptics.

Presentation

Anticholinergic symptoms include muscle rigidity, dystonia, and cardiac abnormalities.

Treatment

Use gastrointestinal decontamination and supportive treatment. Diphenhydramine, 0.5 to 1.0 mg/kg for children (50 mg in adults), or benztropine mesylate, 2 mg IV over 2 min or IM (adults) may help to alleviate extrapyramidal effects.

Acetaminophen

Incidence

Adolescents and young adults may take an intentional overdose. Accidental ingestion is usually found in children, for whom a fatal dose is 7.5 g (23 regular or 15 extra-strength tablets).

Presentation

Within 12 to 24 h, the patient may experience nausea and vomiting, diaphoresis; then may appear to resolve. From 3 to 5 days, there is right upper quadrant pain, anorexia, nausea, coma, and death from hepatic failure.

Diagnostic Studies

Liver function studies and acetaminophen blood level tests are recommended. Obtain acetaminophen blood level at 4 h after ingestion for use with nomograms.

Treatment

Use gastric lavage and charcoal administration if within 2 h of ingestion; use *N*-acetylcysteine (Mucomyst) 140 mg/kg PO, then 70 mg/kg every 4 h for 17 doses, based on the Rumack-Matthews nomogram. For improved taste, give 20% Mucomyst, which has 200 mg/mL of *N*-acetylcysteine diluted 1:3 with fruit juice. If vomited within the hour, repeat dose. This treatment is effective within the first 24 h and best within 8 to 16 h.

Salicylates (Aspirin)

Presentation

CNS stimulation presents as confusion, anxiety, tinnitus, hyperpyrexia, tachypnea, nausea, vomiting dehydration, seizures, and coma.

Diagnostic Studies

Prothrombin time (PT), partial thromboplastin time (PTT), salicylate blood levels 6 h after ingestion and again at 8 to 10 h are recommended. ABGs helpful for acid-base correction.

Treatment

Treatment is based on 6-h salicylate levels, where those with less than 40 mg/dL can be discharged after gastric decontamination, those with 60 to 95 mg/dL admitted for treatment, and those with 110 to 120 mg/dL requiring aggressive treatment. Use gastric decontamination, charcoal administration, cathartics (avoid magnesium-containing cathartics, which increase salicylate absorption), aggressive fluid correction with addition of glucose and potassium, IV bicarbonate for acidosis, oxygen, and alkalinization of urine. Consider hemodialysis. The patient may require a central line for monitoring.

Digitalis (digoxin, digitoxin)

Incidence

Digoxin and digitoxin are common medications used in the treatment of atrial fibrillation and heart failure.

Presentation

The patient may present with mild confusion, anorexia, nausea, vomiting, diarrhea, bradycardia, hypotension, and variable ECG changes.

Treatment

Consider gastrointestinal decontamination; correction of fluid and electrolytes, especially potassium; correction of cardiac arrhythmias. Anti-digoxin Fab fragments are useful in those with severe toxicity.

Theophylline

Incidence

Theophylline is a mild stimulant used in the treatment of asthma.

Presentation

Agitation, tachycardia, cardiac dysrhythmias, and seizures are the most common symptoms.

Treatment

Repeated activated charcoal and dialysis are recommended.

Heavy Metals

Iron

Incidence

Iron is frequently ingested by children because it is readily available.

Presentation

Phase 1 includes vomiting and diarrhea, possible hematemesis (or bloody diarrhea), hypotension, lethargy, seizures, and coma (6 to 24 h after ingestion). Phase 2 includes apparent resolution of initial symptoms; some may skip this stage entirely. Phase 3 includes severe metabolic acidosis and hepatic and renal failure. Phase 4 (weeks later) includes GI obstruction secondary to scarring.

Diagnostic Studies

Draw blood 4 to 6 h after ingestion and test for serum iron and total iron binding capacity (TIBC).

Treatment

Use gastrointestinal decontamination procedures. Charcoal does not bind to iron but is helpful in cases of co-ingestion. Avoid magnesium-based cathartics because they can bind with iron to form gastrointestinal concretions. Consider chelation therapy in severe cases with 25 to 50 mg/kg up to total dose of 1 g deferoxamine IM.

Lead

Lead is ingested inorganically from painted metallic objects or inhaled organically from leaded gasoline.

Presentation

After inorganic ingestion, the patient may have nausea, vomiting, abdominal pain, convulsions, and coma. After organic inhalation, more CNS symptoms appear.

Physical Examination

The practitioner may note lead lines on the gingiva or teeth. Neuropathy may be present.

Diagnostic Studies

Check for anemia and red cell stippling on peripheral smear. Long bone and rib films may demonstrate densities at the ends. Radiopaque material may be seen within the gastrointestinal tract. Obtain blood lead levels and erythrocyte protoporphyrin level.

Treatment

Use gastrointestinal decontamination if there has been recent ingestion or the lead is radiologically evident. Give chelation therapy consisting of dimercaprol, 4 mg/kg IM every 4 h, then calcium disodium edetate (EDTA) begun after the second dimercaprol dose, consisting of 250 mg IV every 6 h. Maintain urine output to prevent renal damage.

Mercury

Route

Mercury used in industry and agriculture can be absorbed cutaneously or by inhalation or ingestion. (Thermometer mercury ingested requires no specific treatment because it is poorly absorbed.)

Presentation

The patient may report a metallic taste. If the mercury was inhaled, symptoms include cough, dyspnea, chest discomfort, weakness, nausea, vomiting, and diarrhea. Ingestion of mercury causes tremor, nausea, vomiting, diarrhea, hematemesis, hematochezia, dehydration, altered mental status, seizure, and renal failure.

Diagnostic Studies

Check blood and urine levels.

Treatment

Use gastrointestinal and skin decontamination procedures and charcoal administration. Avoid cathartics if diarrhea is present. Correct fluids and electrolytes. Perform chelation with dimercaprol (BAL = British Anti-Lewisite), 4 to 5 mg/kg IM every 4 h for 7 to 10 days.

Arsenic

Route

Industrial or agricultural forms of arsenic can be absorbed by inhalation or ingestion.

Presentation

The patient may have garlic-like breath and may complain of metallic taste. Nausea, vomiting, diarrhea, a burning sensation of the oropharynx, cardiac arrhythmias, hypotension, hepatic and renal failure, and coma may occur.

Diagnostic Studies

Test the urinary arsenic level.

Treatment

Use gastrointestinal decontamination and avoid cathartics if there is severe diarrhea. Correct fluid and electrolytes. Perform chelation with dimercaprol, 5 mg/kg IM, then 2.5 mg/kg every 8 h for three doses, then given every 12 to 24 h for 10 days; after 48 h, penicillamine can be given instead at 25 mg/kg PO for 4 to 8 days in those not allergic to penicillin.

Corrosive Household Products

Strong Acids

Strong acid examples include hydrochloric acid, sulfuric acid (battery acid), nitric acid, and hydrofluoric acid.

Skin Contact

When there has been skin contact, which can result in burns, irrigate copiously with water.

Eye Contact

When there has been eye contact, flush copiously with water (pH testing before and after can guide irrigation) and use fluorescein stain for assessment of ocular damage.

Inhalation of Fumes

A patient who has inhaled fumes can present with mild respiratory irritation to complete laryngeal obstruction. Pulmonary edema can be delayed. Give supportive treatment (bronchodilators, oxygen, possibly steroids).

Ingestion

Presentation includes severe pain of oral, pharyngeal, and gastric mucosa, nausea, vomiting, and hematemesis. Avoid neutraliza-

tion with water since this can cause an exothermic reaction. Some authors suggest nasogastric tube placement with aspiration followed by lavage with cold water; others do not wish to risk vomiting during placement of a nasogastric tube, which may expose tissue to further contact with substance.

Strong Alkali

Strong alkali is defined as a substance with a pH greater than 11.5. Included in this category are sodium or potassium hydroxide (detergents, lye, paint removers) and sodium hypochlorite (bleach).

Skin or Eye Contact

If there has been skin or eye contact, irrigate copiously and set up an ophthalmology consultation.

Ingestion

After ingestion of a strong alkali, emesis, lavage, and charcoal are contraindicated; most authors suggest dilution by oral ingestion of milk or water followed by consultation for endoscopy within 12 to 24 h. Chest and abdominal films are needed to assess for perforation.

Hydrocarbons

Petroleum Distillates and Turpentine

Gasoline and kerosene fall into this category.

Ingestion

The patient presents with oral and pharyngeal burning, nausea, vomiting, and diarrhea. Aspiration can produce cough, dyspnea, bronchospasm, and hemoptysis; later, it can cause pulmonary pneumonitis.

Treatment

Intubation is recommended for serious respiratory compromise and terbutaline for bronchospasm. Gastric decontamination is controversial.

Inhalation

The patient presents with euphoria, nausea, vomiting, ataxia, seizures, and coma. The patient may possibly have the odor of the substance involved on breath. Death can result from cardiac arrhythmia or respiratory depression.

Halogenated Hydrocarbons

Carbon tetrachloride and chloroform fall into this category.

Presentation

The patient presents with headache, nausea, vomiting, hepatic and renal dysfunction, and coma.

Treatment

Use gastrointestinal decontamination, oxygen, IV fluids, and vasopressors. Correct electrolytes.

Aromatic Hydrocarbons

Benzene, toluene, and xylene fall into this category.

Acute Toxicity

Acute toxicity is indicated by euphoria, dizziness, weakness, headache, blurred vision, tremor, ataxia, seizures, respiratory depression, and coma.

Chronic Toxicity

Chronic toxicity is indicated by bone marrow depression, leukemia, neoplasm, neuropathy, and renal damage.

Treatment

Treatment is similar to that for halogenated hydrocarbons.

Insecticides

This category includes organophosphates (malathion), carbamates, and organochlorines (DDT and lindane).

Incidence

Eighty percent of all hospitalized cases for pesticide poisoning exposure can have originated through inhalation or absorbed through the skin.

Presentation

Early symptoms include nausea, vomiting, diaphoresis, miotic pupils, blurred vision, abdominal cramping, dyspnea, bradycardia, salivation, lacrimation, urination, and diarrhea. Later the patient may develop mydriatic pupils, restlessness, anxiety, confusion, delirium, headache, ataxia, tremors, muscle fasciculation, weakness, paralysis, seizures, tachycardia, or coma, or even die.

Diagnostic Studies

Test for serum cholinesterase level.

Treatment

Conduct skin, ocular, and gastrointestinal decontamination; give atropine, 2 to 4 mg IV, may repeat every 5 to 10 min depending on severity (0.015 to 0.05 mg/kg children), and pralidoxime (2-PAM), 1 g in 100 mL of normal saline IV given at less than 500 mg/min (children 25 to 30 mg/kg over 15 to 30 min). Dosage can be repeated every 20 min. Treat until symptoms are reversed (may take 12 to 24 h). Avoid atropine toxicity. Do not give morphine, aminophylline, phenothiazines, reserpine, furosemide, or ethacrynic acid to these patients.

Pearl

The mnemonic for cholinergic: salivation, lacrimation, urination, defecation, GI cramping, emesis is SLUDGE.

SUICIDAL ATTEMPTS AND GESTURES

Incidence

Facts about suicide include the following:

Of the general population, 2 percent have seriously considered suicide and 1 percent have attempted it.
Suicide is the ninth leading cause of death in the United States.
Suicide is the second leading cause of death in those younger than age 24.
For every one successful suicide, there are 40 attempts.
Males are two to three times more likely to complete suicide, but women are two to three times more likely to attempt suicide.

Treatment

The practitioner should take every attempt seriously. An attempted suicide necessitates psychiatric evaluation or hospital admission for observation. Remove all potentially lethal items from the patient's vicinity and have the patient supervised at all times. Any patient who wishes to leave the hospital against medical advice must be physically or chemically restrained.

High-Risk Individuals

High-risk individuals fall into the following categories:

- Males (especially those over 45 years of age) often choose a more lethal behavior with less chance of rescue
- Those with a history of previous suicide attempts
- Those with a psychiatric history (10 percent of all schizophrenic patients are eventually successful)
- Excessive alcohol or drug users (alcoholics are at 50 times increased risk; 25 percent of all suicide cases are associated with alcohol)
- Patients with little social support
- Patients having conflict in personal relationships
- Patients experiencing depression or serious medical problems
- Homosexual youths without positive familial or social support
- Patients who are unemployed
- Those of Caucasian and Asian descent

BIBLIOGRAPHY

Jenkins J, Loscalzo J, Braen GR: *Manual of Emergency Medicine,* 1995, pp 435–492, 522, 523.
Rosen P, Barkin R: *Emergency Medicine Concepts in Clinical Practice,* 3d ed. St. Louis, Mosby Year Book, 1992, pp 2470–2689.
Saunders CE, Ho MT: *Current Emergency Diagnosis and Treatment.* 4th ed. Norwalk, CT, Appleton and Lange, 1992, chap 39, pp 730–768, 791–793.
Tintinalli JE, Ruiz E, Krome RL (eds): *Emergency Medicine: A Comprehensive Study Guide,* 4th ed. New York/McGraw-Hill, 1996, pp 735–841, 1337–1340.

Chapter 4–9
HYPOTHERMIA AND OTHER COLD INJURIES
Karen A. Newell

HYPOTHERMIA

DISCUSSION

Hypothermia can be defined as the condition at which human core temperature drops below 35°C, or 95° F. This temperature can be measured through tympanic, esophageal measurements through an endotracheal tube, or through a rectal probe. It is important to recognize that the lowest temperature measured by some standard thermometers is 35°C (95°F), so specialized equipment may be required to accurately measure temperatures and monitor these individuals.

The following list categorizes the severity stages of hypothermia:

- *Mild*   Core temperature above 32°C (89.9°F) but below 35°C (95°F), associated with a 25 percent mortality rate
- *Moderate*   Core temperature between 26 and 32°C (78.8 and 89.6°F), associated with a 50 percent mortality rate
- *Severe*   Core temperature lower than 26°C (78.8°F), associated with a 60 percent mortality rate

Most cases reported in the United States occur in urban areas, especially late summer and early fall nights. Mortality rates can

Table 4-9-1. Susceptible Populations for Hypothermia

Extremes of age (The very young have increased surface area to mass ratio, and the elderly may not sense cold or fail to take necessary adaptive action.)
Individuals with mental or mobility impairment
Intoxicated persons (Ethanol increases heat loss by peripheral vasodilatation and interferes with heat production by inhibiting shivering; barbiturates are sometimes associated.)
Association with certain medications (may interfere with thermoregulation by impairing centrally mediated vasoconstriction); examples: phenothiazines, benzodiazepines, and tricyclic antidepressants
People with endocrine abnormalities (hypoglycemia, hypothyroidism, adrenal insufficiency, hypopituitarism)
Malnourished
People with uremia or sepsis

be greater than 50 percent in those with serious underlying diseases. The susceptible populations are shown in Table 4-9-1. Hypothermia may occur in healthy populations as a result of exposure because of inadequate clothing in an unfavorable environment (e.g., skiers or hikers). These individuals may be inexperienced, exhausted, unprepared, or unknowledgeable with regard to wind chill and their own realistic limitations. Mortality rates in these individuals are significantly less, at about 5 percent. These cases can often be best prevented through education and public awareness including the following recommendations:

1. Encourage recreational activity with a buddy system.
2. Wear layered clothing consisting of natural wool or one of the many newer synthetic products (like Gore-Tex); these materials tend to resist moisture more than down or cotton.
3. Ensure adequate coverage of head, wrists, neck, hands, and feet. (An uncovered head can lose up to 70 to 80 percent of total body heat.)
4. Avoid cold water immersion (increases heat loss by 25 times) and wet clothing (increases heat loss by 5 times).
5. Consider using heat-insulating foils, which may be helpful.

SIGNS AND SYMPTOMS

A person who is found to be *mildly hypothermic* may present with shivering, dysarthria, and ataxia; may exhibit difficulty with judgment; and may appear mildly confused. The shivering mechanism is maximized at 35°C (95°F) and can raise heat production two to five times. It can be effective for several hours until glycogen stores are depleted and fatigue appears. Shivering disappears at temperatures below 32°C (89.6°F).

An individual presenting with *moderate hypothermia* may exhibit progressive mental status deterioration and may appear uncooperative or intoxicated. Many times hypothermia coexists with overdose and intoxication or may mimic other conditions such as cerebrovascular accident. In the elderly it may be confused with septicemia. Other signs may include atrial or ventricular arrhythmias, decreased pulse and respiratory rate, dilated and nonreactive pupils, loss of voluntary motor function, and loss of reflexes. In fact, the knee jerk, if present, may be the last to disappear and the first to reappear during rewarming.

The patient who presents in *severe hypothermia* may exhibit hypotension, ventricular fibrillation, or coma, or even appear deceased. At temperatures below 28°C (82.4°F), ventricular fibrillation occurs. At 19 to 26°C (66.2 to 68°F), the EEG becomes flat line. At 15 to 18°C (59 to 64.4°F), asystole occurs. Because there are reported cases of individuals who were presumed dead who survived, *no one is considered dead until he or she is warm and dead.* Therefore, do not stop resuscitative efforts until the core temperature is greater than 35°C (95°F). Treatment is aimed

at rewarming with attention to identification and treatment of underlying etiology.

Patients may appear cold and pale. They may have stiff to completely rigid or even decomposing extremities. They may appear to be in rigor mortis or opisthotonus (back arched from contraction of major muscle groups). Hands may be fixed in flexion at the interphalangeal joints and wrists with extension at the metacarpophalangeal joints. Mental status varies from mild confusion to coma. Neurologic assessment including the Glasgow coma scale is unpredictable and unreliable for prognosis.

DIAGNOSTIC STUDIES

It is paramount to obtain continuous temperature measurements; most recommend a rectal thermistor probe placed between 5 and 15 cm with care taken not to place it into cold feces. In addition, take careful and frequent vital sign readings (counting pulse for at least 30 to 45 s). Also be aware that the respiratory rate may be asynchronous.

Exercise cervical spine precautions if the history is unknown or if the patient is unconscious until a full cervical spine series can be obtained. Avoid excessive movement of the patient so as to minimize cardiac arrhythmias due to increased cardiac irritability.

Blood work should include initial arterial blood gases (ABG), complete blood cell count (CBC), electrolytes [blood urea nitrogen (BUN), creatinine, glucose, calcium], toxicology screen, liver function studies, and amylase. Also consider obtaining serum cortisol, magnesium, lipase, prothrombin time (PT), partial thromboplastin time (PTT), fibrinogen, thyroid function studies (TFS), cardiac isoenzymes, and blood, urine, and CSF cultures. Realize that the initial unreliability of hematocrit, BUN, and creatinine is secondary to fluid shifts. Also note that most patients will have an elevated glucose (unless the hypothermia is due to hypoglycemia) because there is impairment of insulin secretion, cellular uptake, and effectiveness at low body temperatures. Do not attempt to rapidly correct pH or pCO_2 based on initial blood gases as pO_2 and pCO_2 may be falsely increased and pH may be falsely decreased secondary to the lowered temperature.

Some authors suggest that to correctly reflect true readings, 0.0147 should be added to the measured pH for each degree Celsius below 37°C. However, most current thought supports acid-base treatment without regard for temperature correction.

RADIOLOGIC AND OTHER DIAGNOSTIC STUDIES

Radiologic studies include plain films of the chest and abdomen. Continuous ECG may demonstrate a variety of cardiac arrhythmias including the following:

- Tachycardia.
- Bradycardia, which may be effective in meeting oxygen demands; therefore be cautious since a rapid correction can precipitate ventricular fibrillation and asystole. Atropine is not effective in hypothermic patients. Cardiac pacing is controversial.
- Atrioventricular block.
- Atrial fibrillation, which is common at core temperatures below 32°C (89.6°F) and does not require treatment since it disappears with rewarming.
- Prolonged intervals (may affect all intervals).
- Osborn or J waves, which are sometimes noted at temperatures between 25 and 32°C (77 and 89.6°F). These appear as an extra upward deflection noted at the junction of the QRS and ST segments, especially in leads II and V6. (See Fig. 4-9-1)

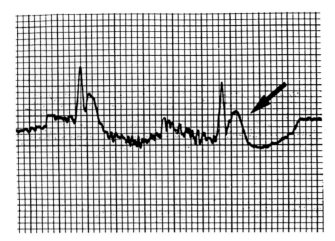

Figure 4-9-1. Rhythm strip from patient with temperature of 25°C (77°F), showing atrial fibrillation with a slow ventricular response, muscle tremor artifact, and Osborn (J) wave (arrow). (*From Tintinalli JE, Ruiz E, Krome RL (eds): Emergency Medicine: A Comprehensive Study Guide, 4th ed. New York, McGraw-Hill, 1996, p. 848. Reprinted with permission from McGraw-Hill, Inc.*)

TREATMENT

Mild Cases

Because these patients are capable of endogenous thermogenesis, passive external rewarming (PER) techniques are employed:

- Remove all clothing, cover the patient with warm blankets to prevent further heat loss, and place in a warm, dry environment.
- Monitor core temperatures carefully; they should rise 0.5 to 2°C/h (0.9 to 3.6°F/h). If core temperatures do not rise, consider giving levothyroxine, 400 to 500 μg IV, and hydrocortisone, 100 mg IV.
- Admission with cardiac observation for at least 24 hours is suggested.

Moderate to Severe Cases

The following treatment is recommended:

- Initially, as with all seriously ill patients, begin with the ABCs: airway, breathing, and circulation.
- Next, as with any unconscious patient, administer thiamine, 100 mg IV, and naloxone hydrochloride (Narcan), 2 mg IV.
- Give 50 to 100 mL of 50% dextrose IV as well if the initial fingerstick glucose is low. The serum glucose level will serve as a guide when results of laboratory work become available.
- An initial fluid challenge of 250 to 500 mL of heated (40 to 42°C or 104 to 107.6°F) normal saline with 5% dextrose may be helpful. This can easily be created with a 1-L bag of fluid placed in the microwave on high power for 2 min. Be sure to shake vigorously to redistribute any "hotspots," and avoid rapid central administration. Fluid warmers are also very helpful.
- The remainder of fluid is given cautiously to avoid fluid overload. Lactated Ringer's solution should be avoided secondary to a potential increased lactate level.
- Central venous pressure or Swan-Ganz monitoring may be necessary.
- An indwelling urinary catheter may also be helpful for fluid monitoring and general assessment of renal function. However,

it is not a reliable indicator of cardiovascular status secondary to "cold diuresis."
- These patients may also require a nasogastric tube secondary to decreased gastric motility.

Although controversy exists, most authorities consider patients with core temperatures below 30°C (86°F) incapable of self-generating heat and requiring some type of active rewarming.

Generally, there are two main types: active external rewarming (AER) and active core rewarming (ACR). AER consists of heated or electric blankets, heated water bottles, and warm water immersion. These methods are applied to the trunk first to prevent extremity vasodilatation and blood pooling which can further exacerbate shock since an already compromised cardiovascular system may not be able to handle the added load of total body rewarming. Similarly, if the entire body is rewarmed simultaneously, shunting cooler blood from the extremities to the trunk, a decrease in core temperature referred to as *afterdrop* can occur. A rapid washout of lactic acid from the periphery can also overload the patient, further complicating acidosis.

ACR may be indicated in those who are hemodynamically unstable and may consist of the following:

- Inhaling heated (43°C or 109.4°F) humidified oxygen by mask or endotracheal tube
- Infused heated (40 to 45°C or 104 to 113°F) crystalloid peritoneal lavage using an isotonic potassium-free dialysate with 1.5% dextrose at a rate of 6 L/h
- Hemodialysis
- GI tract lavage (gastric and colonic)
- Bladder lavage
- Extracorporeal blood rewarming (cardiopulmonary bypass technologies)
- Mediastinal irrigation through chest tubes or open thoracotomy in extreme cases
- Diathermy (Ultrasonic and low-frequency microwave radiation can be employed in those without frostbite, burns, significant edema, metallic implants, or pacemakers.)

Often endotracheal tube placement and ventilatory support may be necessary. However, the patient requires up to 50 percent less than what would normally be suggested. For every 10°C (18°F) decrease in temperature, oxygen consumption decreases two to three times, and similarly for every 8°C (14.4°F), CO_2 production decreases by about half. Attempt to maintain pco_2 at 40 mmHg. Hyperventilation should be avoided to decrease the chance of serious cardiac arrhythmias.

Defibrillation is usually not effective at core temperatures less than 28 to 30°C (82.4 to 86°F). CPR rate is controversial. However, the American Heart Association suggests the same rate as for the normothermic patient. Most believe it should be administered if pulselessness is established, despite the possibility of inducing lethal cardiac arrhythmias in a patient with an undetected yet viable pulse rate.

Most of the cardiac drugs, including lidocaine, may not be effective at lower core temperatures and may even exacerbate cardiac irritability. Therefore, treatment in these situations is aimed at warming the patient first, then treating the specific conditions as they occur. Also be aware that markedly increased doses of medication may be necessary to obtain a response; however, during rewarming the patient may become toxic. Bretylium may be helpful in prevention of ventricular fibrillation.

COMPLICATIONS AND RED FLAGS

Too rapid rewarming can precipitate disseminated intravascular coagulopathy, pulmonary edema, hemolysis, or acute tubular necrosis.

LOCAL COLD INJURIES

DISCUSSION

Local cold injury usually involves the extremities, particularly the hands and feet. At temperatures below 25°C (77°F), tissue metabolism is decreased, producing a cyanotic appearance. At 15°C (59°F), tissue metabolism is markedly decreased and skin may appear pink secondary to dissociation of oxyhemoglobin. It is at and below this temperature that actual tissue damage occurs.

Chilblain, or pernio, results from vasoconstriction which produces dermal edema and mild vasculitis, ultimately resulting in lesions. Anatomic locations commonly include the face and dorsal surface of the hands and feet. It presents more often in women and occurs especially in susceptible individuals (collagen vascular disorders, Raynaud's disease).

SIGNS AND SYMPTOMS

Despite no actual freezing of the tissue, signs and symptoms include erythema, edema, blistering, mild pain, and pruritus. Later, ulcerative lesions may appear and can persist for months. These lesions resolve with warmer weather changes but may recur seasonally.

TREATMENT

Treatment is symptomatic. Some studies suggest nifedipine, 20 mg PO tid, and topical corticosteroids (0.025% fluocinolone cream), or short-course oral corticosteroids (prednisone) may be of benefit. Do not rub or massage the injured tissues and do not apply heat or ice since tissue destruction can be exacerbated. Protect the area from excessive pressure or trauma to prevent further injury (e.g., avoid tight shoewear). Prevention obviously eliminates the need for treatment. Patient education and public awareness may decrease the incidence of this condition.

TRENCH FOOT (IMMERSION FOOT)

DISCUSSION

Trench foot (immersion foot) results from exposure to cold and wet environments. It can occur in 12 to 24 h and is frequently seen in homeless populations. It is important to note that the clinical presentation is not related to outcome. A seemingly minor case may actually be quite severe or vice versa. The initial phase begins with a vasospastic or ischemic period with alternating vasoconstriction and vasodilatation.

SIGNS AND SYMPTOMS

Signs and symptoms include edema, decreased pulse, local pallor, and decreased sensation. The secondary phase begins 12 to 24 h later and consists of a hyperemic or vasodilating phase with bounding pulses which may last between 5 and 10 days.

These patients present with warm or hot, erythematous, edematous, ecchymotic sites, sometimes with blistering and ulceration. They complain of an intense burning or tingling pain. Approximately 2 to 6 weeks later they begin the recovery phase.

TREATMENT

Treatment includes gradual passive rewarming with avoidance of soaking or massage, elevation, avoidance of pressure or further tissue trauma, meticulous local wound care, complete bed rest if a lower extremity is involved, and sometimes hospital admission. Antibiotics are warranted only if infection is present.

COMPLICATIONS

Complication includes hypersensitivity to cold with early cyanosis and permanent injury to vessels and nerves. Other more serious sequelae include lymphangitis, cellulitis, thrombophlebitis, gangrene.

FROSTBITE

DISCUSSION

Frostbite results from excessive cold exposure (−10 to −4°C, or 14 to 24.8°F) with actual freezing of tissues and ischemic necrosis secondary to vasoconstriction. It can be classified into two types:

1. *Superficial* Called first and second degree, reversible injury or frostnip; skin and subcutaneous tissue appears white without blanching (no return of color after mild pressure and no capillary refill) and feels soft and rubbery. Patients report decreased sensation, numbness, paresthesia, and pruritus.
2. *Deep* Called third and fourth degree; this type may involve skin, subcutaneous tissue, muscle, blood vessels, nerves, tendons, and bone. These may appear hard, wooden-like, or edematous. Patients may report mild burning, stinging, numbness, or a feeling of clumsiness of the involved extremity.

Frostbite can be classified into the following grades:

- *First degree* Partial-thickness skin freezing without blistering, erythema, and edema; may peel several days later; hospital admission if extensive; prognosis is excellent.
- *Second degree* Full-thickness skin freezing with blistering (6 to 24 h) and eschar formation (several days); hospital admission; prognosis is good.
- *Third degree* Freezing with skin cell death, hemorrhagic blisters and subcutaneous involvement; hospital admission; prognosis is poor.
- *Fourth degree* Full-thickness freezing including all tissue to bone; little edema; initially mottled, red, or cyanotic; later dry, black, mummified; loss of tissue secondary to necrosis and significant deformity; hospital admission; prognosis is extremely poor.

TREATMENT

Initial treatment of frostnip involves application of constant warmth such as gentle pressure with a warm hand (avoid rubbing) or, in the case of a hand or digit, placed into contralateral axilla. Shoewear should be removed from feet and clean, dry socks or blanket applied. Treatment is aimed at gradual rewarming.

Some authors recommend a rapid rewarming by submersion in a water bath at 40 to 44°C (104 to 108°F) for 15 to 30 min. This can be uncomfortable and require parenteral analgesics secondary to burning pain. Avoid dry heat, such as a stove or open fire, since this is difficult to regulate and burns can develop.

Other contraindications include attempt at rewarming by exercise (e.g., stomping the affected foot on the ground) or by rubbing the body part with snow or immersion in cold water.

To minimize tissue injury, rewarming should be attempted only once; therefore, rewarming should be delayed if possibility of refreezing exists. Minor involvement may require elevation, meticulous local wound care, and tetanus prophylaxis. Clear fluid blisters can be debrided and covered with aloe vera cream placed every 6 h or some suggest silver sulfadiazine cream applied every 12 h. If blisters are left in place, many advise aspiration to minimize contact with fluid containing arachidonic acid cascade and then covering with aloe vera cream. Hemorrhagic blisters should be left in place. Avoid tight or occlusive dressings. Immobilization can be utilized if loose, bulky, dry dressings are carefully applied.

Some authors prescribe whirlpool at 32.2 to 37.8°C (90 to 100°F) twice daily for 30 min.

Antibiotics are usually given only if indicated (penicillin G, 500,000 U IV every 6 h for 2 to 3 days). Ibuprofen, 12 mg/kg/day in divided doses, is helpful even with concurrent narcotic analgesics. The use of low-molecular-weight dextran and anticoagulants have not been consistently documented to be of benefit.

Any serious involvement may require hospital admission and surgical consultation with possibility of amputation. Last, technetium pyrophosphate technicium 99m scanners may be helpful in predicting viability at 5 to 14 days postexposure.

Smoking is a contraindication since it impairs healing.

BIBLIOGRAPHY

American Heart Association: *Advanced Cardiac Life Support.* 1994, pp 10–10 to 10–12.

American Heart Association: *Basic Life Support for Healthcare Providers.* 1994, pp 5–5 to 5–6.

Isselbacher KJ, Braunwald E, Wilson JD, et al (eds): *Harrison's Principles of Internal Medicine,* 13th ed. New York, McGraw-Hill, 1994, pp 2477–2478.

Jenkins JL, Loscalzo J, Braen GR: *Manual of Emergency Medicine,* 3d ed. Boston, Little, Brown, 1995, pp 415–418.

Rosen P, Barkin R: *Emergency Medicine Concepts and Clinical Practice,* 3d ed. St. Louis, Mosby Year Book, 1992, pp 913–937.

Saunders CE, Ho MT: *Current Emergency Diagnosis and Treatment.* 4th ed. Norwalk, CT, Appleton & Lange, 1992, pp 705–709.

Tintinalli JE, Ruiz E, Krome RL (eds): *Emergency Medicine, A Comprehensive Study Guide,* 4th ed. New York, McGraw-Hill 1996, pp 843–850.

Chapter 4–10
ANAPHYLAXIS
Michaela O'Brien-Norton

DISCUSSION

Anaphylaxis is a dramatic, sudden, adverse systemic response to an injected (bee sting), ingested (food, medicine), or inhaled substance in a previously sensitized person. Rarely, it can be from a topical exposure or even exercise. The immune system becomes hypersensitive, releasing chemical mediators, usually IgE, and in anaphylaxis this can cause cardiovascular collapse and respiratory distress. Table 4-10-1 lists some of the many and varied substances that are frequently implicated.

Treatment needs to be rapid and aggressive, initiated by out-of-hospital emergency personnel, if available, and then 24 h observation in hospital to prevent relapse. In severe cases, death can come swiftly from intractable bronchospasm, volume depletion, and/or laryngeal edema, and can be swift.

SIGNS AND SYMPTOMS

Anaphylaxis can be vague initially, with nasal itching, stuffiness, and a lump in the throat. It can rapidly progress to more serious signs and syptoms. See Table 4-10-2.

Table 4-10-1. Common Causes of Anaphylactic Reactions

Drugs
  Penicillin (including penicillin-contaminated milk)
  Cephalosporin (can have cross-reactivity to penicillin because of chemical similarities)
  Aspirin
  Nonsteroidal anti-inflammatory medications
  Sulfa-containing medications
  Vancomycin
  Radiographic contrast dye
  Lidocaine
  Vaccines
  Blood products
Foods
  Milk
  Eggs
  Shellfish: lobster, clams, shrimp, oysters, scallops
  Nuts
  Soybeans, including oleic acid, which is in some metered dose inhalers, and soy lecithin. Soy oil in the United States is highly processed and is not a soy allergen.
  Wheat
  Chocolate
  Citrus: tomatoes, oranges, lemons
  Food additives: monosodium glutamate (MSG), nitrate and nitrite sulfites, tartrazine dyes
  Bee pollen tablets
Environmental Sources
  Hymenoptera venom: honey bee, fire ant, yellow jacket
  Insect parts, especially cockroach
  Molds
  Pollen: trees, grass, plants
  Dander: cat (protein in the saliva)
  Snake venom
Topical Sources
  Spermicidal products
  Latex gloves, condoms, etc.
  Ophthalmic: fluorescein dye

OBJECTIVE FINDINGS

See Table 4-10-3.

DIAGNOSTIC CONSIDERATIONS

Early stages of anaphylaxis could suggest the diseases shown in Table 4-10-4.

SPECIAL CONSIDERATIONS

Be mindful of fluid overload in the elderly and people with renal or cardiovascular disease. Because of vascular permeability, pulmonary edema can develop. Also, a history of heart problems should be elicited before administering epinephrine. However, care cannot be withheld, and the risks versus the benefits need to be assessed.

LABORATORY AND RADIOLOGIC STUDIES

There are no appropriate laboratory and radiologic studies. This is a clinical diagnosis.

TREATMENT

Treatment must be quick and aggressive. A team approach works best. A patent airway is the first priority. Oxygen should be administered via face mask. If the airway is obstructed from bronchospasm, laryngospasm, or edema, then the patient needs endotracheal intubation. At least one, preferably two, intravenous lines should be started, with normal saline or Ringer's lactate, wide open, especially if the patient is hypotensive. Vital

Table 4-10-2. Signs and Symptoms of Anaphylaxis

Respiratory
  Difficulty breathing
  Retrosternal pain
  Cough
Cardiovascular
  Lightheadedness (can be an indicator of vascular collapse)
  Palpitations
  Loss of consciousness
Cutaneous
  Increased warmth of skin
  Oropharyngeal swelling (which can be quite painful)
  Pruritus
Gastrointestinal
  Nausea
  Vomiting
  Diarrhea
  Crampy abdominal pain

Table 4-10-4. Diagnostic Considerations with Anaphylaxis

Respiratory
  Acute asthma
  Pulmonary embolism
  Airway obstruction
Cardiac
  Acute myocardial infarction
  Acute congestive heart failure
  Cardiac dysrhythmias
Cutaneous
  Niacin ingestion
  Hereditary angioedema

signs need to be monitored continuously, and the patient should be on a cardiac monitor. Military or medical antishock trousers can be applied if there is sufficient personnel.

Epinephrine is the drug of choice. The condition of the patient determines the route of administration. If there is no evidence of circulatory collapse, then epinephrine, 0.3 to 0.5 mg of a 1 : 1000 solution, can be given subcutaneously or intramuscularly. (Be sure to draw back on the syringe; inadvertent venous administration can cause severe complications.) This dose can be repeated every 10 to 15 min until the patient improves. If there is no improvement in 30 to 35 min, or if the patient seems to be getting worse, then IV epinephrine is indicated, 0.3 to 0.5 mg of 1 : 10,000 solution. (If not available, dilute 1 mL of 1 : 1000 solution epinephrine with 10 mL of normal saline.) It is important to continually assess patient status. If the patient is hypotensive, then a subcutaneous or IM injection of epinephrine is not going to work.

If the patient is already in shock and has already been intubated, endotracheal administration is possible, with 5 to 10 mL of 1 : 10,000 solution followed by four or five rapid ventilations. Hypotension needs to be closely monitored; expect to administer 2 to 4 L of crystalloid solution. However, pulmonary edema can develop due to vascular permeability, especially in the elderly or in patients with cardiovascular or renal disease. Monitor urine output.

Bronchospasm is treated with inhaled bronchodilators. Aerosolized albuterol, 0.5 mL in 3 mL of saline, should be attached to the oxygen tubing.

Mild hypotension is sometimes assisted with the use of cimetidine (Tagamet), 300 mg IV, or ranitidine (Zantac), 50 mg IV. Theoretically, it is thought to aid in urticaria also, but this is not an approved indication.

Methylprednisolone (50 to 125 mg) administered by IV push helps prevent recurrent symptoms. The body can respond to allergies for up to 72 h, and corticosteroids control this effectively, as well as the administration of an antihistamine, usually diphenhydramine (Benadryl), 50 mg IM.

Supportive measures include hospitalization for 24 h for observation, indicated in moderate to severe reactions. Milder cases that respond quickly in the emergency room can be sent home with corticosteroids, bronchodilators, and antihistamines, after being monitored for up to 8 to 12 h.

PATIENT EDUCATION

Avoid offending substances that cause reactions. The patient will need to carry an emergency epinephrine kit (e.g., EpiPen).

DISPOSITION

Mild cases can be discharged home with an oral prednisone taper, diphenhydramine 25 to 50 mg every 4 to 6 h, rest, and if indicated, especially with first episodes, referral to an allergist for further follow-up and care, including skin testing.

BIBLIOGRAPHY

Austin KF: Diseases of immediate type hypersensitivity, in Fauci AS, Braunwald E, Isselbacher KJ, et al: *Principles and Practice of Internal Medicine*, 14th ed. New York, McGraw-Hill, 1998, pp 1860–1864.
Fontanarosa PB, Blanda M: Management of anaphylaxis. *Phys Assist* 18(8):51–58, 1994.
Salomone JA III: Anaphylaxis and acute allergic reactions, in Tintinalli et al (eds): *Emergency Medicine: A Comprehensive Study Guide*, 4th ed. New York, McGraw-Hill, 1996, pp 209–211.

Table 4-10-3. Objective Findings in Anaphylaxis

General
  Anxiety
  Agitation
Respiratory
  Wheezing
  Tachypnea
  Stridor
  Use of accessory muscles
  Gasping for air
  Cough
Cardiovascular
  Dysrhythmias
  Hypotension
  Tachycardia
Cutaneous
  Generalized erythema
  Edema (orbital, perioral, facial, neck)
  Wheals or flares

Chapter 5–1
DIABETES MELLITUS
Janice Herbert-Carter

DISCUSSION

Diabetes mellitus, often called *sugar diabetes,* is a condition in which the pancreas produces insufficient insulin to meet the body's metabolic needs, leading to hyperglycemia (elevated blood glucose). There may be a total lack of insulin production, decreased insulin production, or even hyperinsulinemia, but in all cases the quantity of insulin is insufficient for effective glucose metabolism. About 5 percent of the U.S. population is affected. The disorder involves a spectrum of abnormalities and encompasses variants that affect primarily children and adolescents (type 1), obese adults (type 2), and pregnant women (gestational). Also included may be "prediabetic," or "latent," states of impaired glucose tolerance in which the person is not overtly ill but laboratory studies indicate abnormal glucose metabolism.

The etiology of primary diabetes is largely unknown, although hypotheses abound. Viruses may be important in type 1. Heredity is clearly involved in type 2, as evidenced by its occurrence in families and high incidence in some ethnic groups. Blacks, Native Americans, and Hispanics are very commonly affected, particularly women.

There are known causes of secondary diabetes. Pancreatic failure with destruction of exocrine and endocrine function as seen in patients with chronic pancreatitis, pancreatectomy, hemochromatosis, and pancreatic cancer is obvious. Other causes include excesses of hormones that oppose the action of insulin, such as Cushing's syndrome (glucocorticoid excess), glucagonoma, pheochromocytoma (catecholamine excess), and acromegaly (growth hormone excess). Drugs such as thiazide diuretics, synthetic glucocorticoids (prednisone), and phenytoin (Dilantin) may induce or unmask diabetes. Obesity is a risk factor in gestational and type 2 diabetes, but the risk factors for type 1 have not been clearly established.

The pathophysiology of type 1 diabetes (approximately 10 to 20 percent of all diabetic patients) is total failure of insulin production. Autoimmune destruction of beta cells in the pancreatic islets of Langerhans occurs. Initially, there may be a symptomatic period caused by failure of insulin production followed by a relatively normal "honeymoon" period. Ultimately, however, all insulin production ceases. In type 2 diabetes (approximately 80 to 90 percent of all diabetics), there is typically inadequate insulin production. However, an obese person may have high circulating levels of insulin that are still inadequate because of insulin resistance. Adipose tissue has fewer insulin receptors than do other tissue types, and this contributes to insulin resistance even in the face of hyperinsulinemia. In gestational diabetes (1 to 2 percent of all pregnancies) the insulin requirement increases, but resistance may also increase, leading to inadequate levels and hyperglycemia.

SIGNS AND SYMPTOMS

Signs and symptoms may be divided into acute presenting findings caused by the hyperglycemia and chronic complications resulting from the systemic effects of the disease. Chronic complications are discussed later in this chapter. Two major acute complications—ketoacidosis and hypoglycemia (insulin shock)—are discussed in Chaps. 5-7 and 5-8, respectively.

Acute signs and symptoms may be the presenting complaints that lead to a diagnosis or may be indications that an established diabetic is out of control. They include thirst (polydipsia), excessive hunger (polyphagia), increased urination (polyuria: large quantities, not simply urinary frequency), blurry vision, fatigue, and weight loss despite increased intake.

DIAGNOSIS

The hallmark of diabetes mellitus is hyperglycemia. For nonpregnant adults, the following criteria are used to establish the diagnosis:

- Random blood glucose >200 with symptoms as above on more than one day or
- Fasting blood glucose ≥126 on more than one day or
- Abnormal glucose tolerance test (GTT) on more than one day

It is important to note that while urine glucose tests may be suggestive, they are never adequate for a diagnosis. Also, GTTs, while diagnostic, are rarely indicated, because most patients are easily diagnosed by one of the first two criteria. The exception is the use of the oral GTT in pregnancy. All pregnant women should have a GTT between the twenty-fourth and twenty-eighth weeks of pregnancy.

The signs and symptoms of diabetes are nonspecific; therefore, taken individually, the differential list would be very long. However, considered together as a symptom complex, the classic signs and symptoms should always prompt a check of the blood glucose. Once the blood glucose is elevated, there is virtually no differential to explore except to determine the cause of the diabetes. This will usually be obvious on the basis of the person's age, weight, and other conditions or medications.

LABORATORY TESTS

Elevated blood glucose is assumed in diabetes. Urine glucose is present when the blood glucose is higher than 175. The kidney normally reabsorbs all filtered glucose, but there is a limit. At about 175, the transport maximum (T_{max}) is reached and any excess glucose is spilled into the urine. Unfortunately, there is no direct relationship between urine glucose levels and blood glucose levels above that point. Therefore, urine levels are not a reliable gauge of treatment efficacy.

Glycosylated hemoglobin (HbA1c) is used to determine long-term glucose control. When blood sugar levels are elevated, hemoglobin irreversibly binds glucose. Thus, the hemoglobin remains glycosylated for the life of the red blood cell (up to 120 days). Patients may have normal glucose levels at the time of their follow-up visits because they have been careful with diet and medications in the hours leading up to phlebotomy but may have been out of control for months at a time. Thus, a random or even fasting blood sugar done during a routine office visit may not accurately reflect their level of control over time. The glycosylated hemoglobin level should not be more than 7 percent.

Other laboratory tests may be abnormal in certain patients (see Chap. 5-7).

RADIOLOGIC STUDIES

No radiological studies are diagnostic or necessary in diabetes. However, some x-rays may give clues to secondary causes. Examples include calcifications in chronic pancreatitis and bony growth in acromegaly. It is unlikely that these studies will be needed for the diagnosis or management of the diabetes itself.

TREATMENT

Diet

There are several basics to remember about the treatment of diabetes. Treatment always involves diet. This may mean weight reduction for a middle-aged obese type 2 diabetic adult, or a high-caloric, low-carbohydrate intake for a thin and growing adolescent. Although referral to a registered dietitian for a specific meal plan and thorough nutritional education is always desirable, it is not always available. The primary care provider must be able to prescribe and explain an appropriate diet for any diabetic patient.

The commonly prescribed diabetic diet provides 55 to 60 percent of calories from carbohydrates (preferably complex carbohydrates, such as starches and fruits), 10 to 20 percent from proteins, and 25 to 30 percent from fats. High fiber is recommended (25 g/1000 kcal) to slow the absorption of sugars. The timing of meals is important. The patient must understand that once an insulin injection is given or an oral agent is taken, he or she must eat. Skipping meals may lead to hypoglycemia, which can be serious (see Chap. 5-8).

Pharmacologic Management

There are two main categories of medications for diabetes mellitus. Insulin is an absolute requirement for type 1 diabetics and is sometimes used for patients with type 2. Oral hypoglycemics (sulfonylureas) are often used for type 2 when diet alone is insufficient but are never used for type 1. Oral agents work by increasing pancreatic insulin secretion. Thus, they are ineffective in a pancreas without islet cells. In addition, sulfonylureas are contraindicated in gestational diabetes, hepatic or renal insufficiency, and patients with an allergy to sulfa drugs. Oral hypoglycemics are *never* appropriate treatment for type 1 diabetics.

Persons who have been taking insulin for years may still be using pork or beef preparations, and "if it ain't broke, don't fix it." There is no reason to change preparations if a person is doing well. However, as a general rule, diabetics starting insulin for the first time should receive one of the human insulin preparations. The use of human insulin affords less risk of allergy, immune-based resistance, and local reactions such as lipoatrophy.

Most commonly used insulin preparations are "regular" (R), which is short-acting, or NPH (N), which is considered intermediate-acting. NPH is mixed with a protein, and the pH is adjusted to provide longer-term coverage. Regular insulin has an onset of action within about 0.5 h when injected subcutaneously, peak action in 2 to 4 h, and a duration of about 6 to 8 h. NPH has its onset in about 2 to 4 h, peaks in 6 to 8 h, and lasts about 18 to 24 h. These numbers are highly variable from individual to individual. A premixed combination containing 70 percent NPH and 30 percent regular is available, but it should be reserved for patients in whom the dose of insulin has been established; it is not appropriate for the initiation of therapy. Most type 1 patients require at least a morning dose and an afternoon dose, commonly totaling 25 to 50 units a day, but this is highly individual. Dosage depends on body size, activity level, and eating habits.

Sulfonylureas may be divided into first- and second-generation agents. First-generation agents include acetohexamide, chlorpropamide (Diabinese), tolazamide, and tolbutamide. The most commonly used is chlorpropamide. The daily dose ranges from 100 to 500 mg given in the morning. It has an extremely long duration of action of 60 h. Adverse effects include an Antabuse-like effect and the syndrome of inappropriate secretion of antidiuretic hormone (SIADH). The long duration of action makes once-daily dosing convenient. When problems occur, such as hypoglycemia in a poorly nourished elderly patient, clearance of the drug is very slow, prolonging the problematic situation.

Second-generation sulfonylureas include glipizide (Glucotrol) and glyburide (DiaBeta, Micronase). These agents are used in doses of 2.5 to 40 mg daily with a duration of action from 12 to 24 h. Their mechanisms of action, contraindications, etc., are similar to those of the first-generation drugs.

The use of sulfonylureas and insulin together in type 2 diabetics when diet and sulfonylureas have failed is controversial. A newer drug that is used when diet and sulfonylureas alone are unsuccessful is acarbose (Precose), an α-glucosidase inhibitor that slows the intestinal absorption of polysaccharides.

The goals of therapy should be a fasting glucose ideally less than 120 but with up to 140 considered acceptable and a postprandial glucose less than 140 but with up to 200 considered acceptable.

Research is ongoing into implanted insulin pumps, which attempt to reproduce the continuous low level of insulin release and its increase in response to blood sugar levels. Research is also progressing on pancreatic tissue transplants.

Exercise

All diabetics need adequate physical exercise, especially obese type 2 diabetic patients. In addition to aiding weight loss, exercise increases insulin secretion and thus is doubly beneficial to these patients. Type 1 diabetics should be encouraged to exercise but must be careful because their insulin supply will be entirely exogenous and must take care not to exercise to the point of hypoglycemia.

Patient Education

Patient and family education is extremely important in diabetes care. Dietary education was discussed above. In addition, for insulin-requiring diabetics, self administration of medication must be taught, along with home monitoring of glucose. Stricter control of blood sugar, which can prevent future complications, depends on frequent measurement of blood sugar levels. Care of the feet and extremities is important. Early recognition of the warning signs of impending hypoglycemia is necessary (see Chap. 5-8).

COMPLICATIONS
Chronic Complications

Diabetes, though considered an endocrine disease, affects every system in the body. It is the number one cause of blindness in the United States, although with proper eye care this often is preventable. It is imperative that every diabetic patient be examined by an ophthalmologist at least yearly. Diabetic retinopathy may take many forms: proliferative disease, microaneurysms, retinal detachment, hemorrhages, infarctions, and exudates. In addition, diabetics have higher rates of cataracts and glaucoma. If the condition is untreated, however, blindness may result from any of these conditions. Blurry vision commonly is due to hyperglycemia, and glasses should not be recommended until glycemic control has been achieved. However, blurry vision may be caused by more serious eye problems and thus should never be taken lightly but always referred to an ophthalmologist.

Diabetes is a major risk factor for atherosclerosis (see Chap. 1-4). This leads to early coronary artery disease as well as peripheral vascular disease (see Chap. 1-9) and cerebrovascular accident (stroke) (see Chap. 1-3). Lipid levels should be checked and managed aggressively in diabetics. Of course, these patients should be advised not to smoke, and hypertension should be managed carefully. The primary care provider should not wait for the appearance of chest pain to screen for atherosclerotic disease. Often diabetics may have silent ischemia, with heart muscle suffering a life-threatening lack of oxygen despite the absence of pain.

Diabetes is a major cause of renal failure (see Chap. 18-1) in the United States. The earliest sign is microalbuminuria too slight to be found by a dipstick check of protein; this will progress to gross proteinuria. Diabetic renal disease can manifest as glomerulosclerosis, with a full nephrotic syndrome; anuric renal failure eventually results. It is therefore very important to treat hypertension and any urinary tract infections aggressively to prevent additional insults to the kidneys. Radiographic contrast agents (CT scan "dye") should be avoided, and if their use is absolutely necessary, the patient must be adequately hydrated. The use of angiotensin-converting enzyme (ACE) inhibitors (captopril, enalapril, lisinopril, etc.) may be beneficial in preventing progression of the microalbuminuria even in the absence of hypertension. Diabetes also may lead to renal tubular acidosis and renal papillary necrosis.

Neuromuscular disorders in diabetics take many forms. Autonomic neuropathy may cause gastroparesis with nausea and vomiting, intestinal motility disorders with diarrhea and/or constipation, vasomotor instability with orthostatic hypotension, bladder dysfunction (urinary retention or incontinence), and impotence. The gastroparesis is of particular concern because it may cause erratic absorption of food, with unpredictable swings in blood glucose levels. Peripheral neuropathy can cause pain and paresthesias or numbness that leads to unnoticed trauma, especially of the feet. The real danger here is that the trauma may lead to infections and ulcerations that fail to heal because of poor vascularization resulting from atherosclerosis and impaired leukocyte function resulting from hyperglycemia. Frequently cultured organisms include *Staphylococcus aureus* and streptococci, but mixed infections including anaerobes and gram-negative bacteria are common. Unfortunately, many diabetics undergo amputations of the lower extremities as a result. Mononeuropathies involve the cranial nerves or larger nerves such as the femoral, sciatic, and peroneal nerves, leading to motor and sensory deficits that manifest as foot drop, wrist drop, or diplopia. Diabetic amyotrophy presents with motor deficits in the absence of sensory problems.

Skin disorders caused by diabetes include necrobiosis lipoidica diabeticorum (waxy scarring of the skin on the anterior lower leg), diabetic dermopathy, skin ulcers, and fungal (*Candida* or *Monilia*) infections. Type 1 diabetes may be associated with vitiligo and acanthosis nigracans.

Acute Complications

Several of the most important acute complications of diabetes mellitus are discussed in Chaps. 5-7 and 5-8.

Diabetics are prone to the same acute infections that affect the general population, but these infections may be more severe as a result of the factors mentioned above. Diabetics are susceptible to several unusual infections as well. Malignant *Pseudomonas* otitis externa may be very serious because it may spread through the mastoid area and infect the sinuses and brain. Rhinocerebral mucormycosis, which is seen in ketoacidotic patients, is a fungal infection that may spread through the nose and sinuses to infect the brain. It begins with a severe headache and nasal discharge but may end in coma and death if untreated. Amphotericin B is the drug of choice, with surgical debridement also being necessary. Other infections seen more frequently in diabetics include emphysematous cholecystitis, necrotizing fasciitis, and chronic osteomyelitis.

PEARLS

An important point to remember in caring for diabetic patients is that controlling the blood sugar is not sufficient. It is easy to chase the numbers and play around with the insulin or sulfonylurea dose, but that alone will not provide adequate care for these patients. Patient and family support and education are crucial. A "normal" blood sugar when the patient is with you for a few minutes a few times a year is no guarantee that there is smooth control the rest of the time. You must be vigilant for complications and not wait for the patient to volunteer symptoms. Preventive care early on can prevent devastating consequences later. Diabetics do not have to go blind, heart attacks are not inevitable, and dialysis is not an assumed fate. A team management approach with frequent appointments; appropriate referrals to nutritionists, podiatrists, and ophthalmologists; and real caring and concern from primary care providers, nurses, social workers, and sometimes psychologists are all important in preventing morbidity and mortality in patients with this chronic disease. This is especially true for type 1 diabetics who face a lifetime of multiple daily injections. This disease may have a major life-style impact in any patient: dietary restrictions, impotence, altered body image after amputation, and embarrassing social situations with unpredictable diarrhea. Always remember that there is far more to diabetes management than glycemic control.

Chapter 5–2
OSTEOPOROSIS
Timothy C. Evans

DISCUSSION

Osteoporosis is a metabolic disease of bone that is characterized by decreased bone mass; that is, both the mineral component and the organic matrix of bone are decreased. This is in contrast to osteomalacia, in which only mineralization is impaired.

Osteoporosis is a major source of morbidity and mortality. Each year in the United States, osteoporosis results in hundreds of thousands of fractures that have enormous personal and financial costs. The risk of death in the elderly from complications suffered after a hip fracture is 12 to 20 percent.

BONE PHYSIOLOGY

Throughout life, bone is formed and resorbed continuously in a finely regulated process known as *remodeling*. The first step in the process is resorption by cells called *osteoclasts,* which form erosion cavities in bone. Next, *osteoblasts* migrate into the erosion cavities and resynthesize the protein matrix of bone. The matrix is composed primarily of collagen with a number of additional minor protein constituents, most notably osteocalcin. Mineralization of the matrix with a salt of calcium and phosphate called hydroxyapatite occurs over the next several weeks.

The processes of bone formation and resorption are coupled so that neither proceeds without the other. During childhood and adolescence, however, formation is faster than resorption, so that bone density increases. During the early adult years, bone density is relatively stable. Peak bone density is reached at about age 30 to 35. Thereafter, resorption is faster than formation so that bone density gradually decreases throughout the rest of life.

Osteoporosis is a clinical disorder in which the bone density falls below a threshold at which susceptibility to fracture increases. An age-related decrease in bone density occurs in all men and women. In women, there is superimposed a period of more rapid loss of bone density for several years around the time of menopause that results from estrogen deficiency. This and the fact that peak bone density is 10 to 15 percent lower in women than in men account for the greater fracture rate from osteoporosis in women.

Although none are completely predictive of symptomatic disease, the factors that have been associated with an increased risk of osteoporosis include female sex, white ancestry, early menopause in women or hypogonadism in men, inactivity, low body weight, low calcium intake during the first three decades of life and again after age 60, smoking, and excessive alcohol intake.

CLASSIFICATION

Primary Osteoporosis

Primary osteoporosis is a condition of reduced bone mass and fractures that occurs in postmenopausal women (postmenopausal osteoporosis) and the elderly of both sexes (senile osteoporosis). Two subcategories have been suggested. Type 1 refers to the loss of trabecular bone that occurs in postmenopausal women and frequently is associated with vertebral compression fractures and fractures of the distal wrist. Type 2 is the age-related loss of cortical and trabecular bone that occurs in both men and women and is associated with hip fractures. Fractures related to type 1 osteoporosis typically begin to occur in women within about 10 years of menopause, while fractures from type 2 begin about 10 years later.

Secondary Osteoporosis

Secondary osteoporosis refers to decreased bone density resulting from other clinical conditions that affect bone remodeling. Glucocorticoid excess causes increased bone resorption and decreased formation. The deleterious effect may result from endogenous Cushing's syndrome or glucocorticoid administration. Thyrotoxicosis, again either endogenous or iatrogenic, causes increased bone resorption. Decreased bone density is a predictable result of long-standing hyperparathyroidism. Certain drugs, such as chronic heparin and anticonvulsants, are associated with osteoporosis. Several malignancies, notably multiple myeloma, may cause diffuse bone density loss.

CLINICAL PRESENTATION

Osteoporosis is asymptomatic, but pain results from its major clinical sequelae, fractures. The fractures most commonly associated with osteoporosis are vertebral compression fractures (primarily of the upper lumbar spine and the middle to lower thoracic spine), Colles' fractures of the distal radius, and fractures of the femoral neck. However, patients with osteoporosis are at increased risk for fractures of all types. Multiple anterior vertebral compression fractures result in the characteristic spine deformity of increased dorsal kyphosis and cervical lordosis known as dowager's hump.

Clinical laboratory tests are typically normal, including calcium, phosphate, and parathyroid hormone. Alkaline phosphatase is usually normal but may be somewhat elevated after a fracture. Abnormalities of blood counts, chemistries, or urine may suggest other underlying disease and should be pursued.

Standard x-rays demonstrate fractures but are insensitive in detecting the loss of bone density (see the material on bone densitometry, below).

DIAGNOSIS

In patients with fractures in a typical setting, osteopenia on x-ray, and no other cause of fracture or loss of bone density, the diagnosis of osteoporosis is likely. Establishing bone density loss, however, requires a bone density measurement.

Several techniques are available for bone densitometry, including single- and dual-photon absorptiometry, quantitative CT scanning, and dual energy x-ray absorptiometry (DEXA). Among these techniques, DEXA is preferred because of its greater precision and lower radiation dose. Bone density determined by DEXA correlates well with the risk of future fracture.

Follow-up and monitoring of osteoporosis are largely clinical, although DEXA performed every 1 to 2 years can show the progression of bone density loss. Several tests are available to measure the rate of bone turnover, including markers of bone resorption such as urinary hydroxyproline and the newer, more specific urinary assays of bone collagen fragments released during resorption. Biochemical serum markers of bone formation include bone-specific alkaline phosphatase and osteocalcin. These indices of bone turnover are being studied for their potential use in identifying patients at risk for osteoporosis and for monitoring treatment, but there has been insufficient validation of their utility to recommend their routine use.

PREVENTION

Bone density decreases continuously after about age 40. Since most bone density, once lost, cannot be regained, prevention of osteoporosis is much more likely to have a satisfactory clinical result than are attempts to treat established osteoporosis. Prevention begins early in life, when adequate calcium in the diet during the first three decades is associated with greater peak bone density and therefore a longer interval of loss later in life before the fracture threshold is reached. This is particularly true for girls, who on average consume significantly less calcium than do boys beginning at puberty. Adequate calcium intake also is particularly important at ages 50 to 60 and should continue thereafter. In general, daily calcium intake for adolescents and adults should be 1200 to 1500 mg.

Regular exercise and avoidance of smoking and excessive alcohol intake also contribute to maximizing peak bone mass and minimizing the rate of loss in later years.

Among the preventive measures for osteoporosis, none is more effective and applicable to the population at greatest risk than the treatment of hypogonadism in either sex, although numerically this applies mostly to women. Estrogen replacement should be offered to all patients with premature menopause to prevent osteoporosis unless there are contraindications. Similarly, estrogen replacement after natural menopause has been well established in preventing rapid bone loss and decreasing the fracture rate. Estrogen is most effective when used at the time of menopause and the following few years of accelerated bone loss. Since bone loss rapidly resumes when estrogens are discontinued, they should be continued in the long term. When estrogen is given to a woman with an intact uterus, a cyclic or continuous progestogen also should be given to prevent endometrial cancer.

TREATMENT

Once a fracture has occurred, osteoporosis can be said to be "established." Several therapies are available for these patients. Intense research efforts are under way to develop this area of pharmacotherapeutics. In all patients, pain control, avoidance of immobility as much as possible, and safety in ambulation (particularly important in the frail elderly) should be attended to.

Drug therapy is directed at decreasing bone resorption and increasing bone formation.

Antiresorptive Agents

Calcium

Dietary calcium supplementation should be provided to ensure 1200 to 1500 mg of elemental calcium intake per day. Several preparations of calcium salts are available. Calcium carbonate is well tolerated and inexpensive.

Vitamin D

The recommended daily allowance of vitamin D of 400 units should be increased to 800 to 1000 units, especially in patients who have limited sun exposure. Calcitriol (active vitamin D, 1,25-dihydroxyvitamin D) also can be used but usually is not necessary and increases the risk of hypercalcemia.

Estrogen

Estrogen slows the rate of bone resorption, slows bone density loss, and prevents fractures. Conjugated equine estrogen at a dose of 0.625 mg per day or its equivalent provides the beneficial effect on bone. Both oral estrogen and transdermal estrogen are effective. When the patient has an intact uterus, a cyclic or continuous progestogen (for example, medroxyprogesterone 2.5 mg per day) also should be given to prevent endometrial cancer.

Calcitonin

Calcitonin inhibits bone resorption by osteoclasts and has an additional beneficial analgesic effect. It appears to be particularly useful in patients with high-turnover osteoporosis: high urinary hydroxyproline and serum osteocalcin. Both salmon calcitonin and human calcitonin are available, and there is less immunologic resistance to the latter. Though effective, calcitonin is expensive and until recently was administered by subcutaneous injection. An intranasal spray is now available.

Bisphosphonates

Bisphosphonates bind to bone mineral and slow osteoclast-mediated resorption. Several agents are now in the latter stages of clinical development for use in osteoporosis. Early studies have shown decreased loss of bone density and fracture rates. Some early analogues may impair bone mineralization, but others appear to have less of this effect. Intense clinical research efforts will further define the place of these agents in the prevention and treatment of osteoporosis.

Bone-Forming Agents

Androgens

Testosterone deficiency in men is a definite cause of osteoporosis and should be treated unless there are contraindications such as prostate cancer. Testosterone treatment increases bone mass, probably by stimulating bone formation. Treatment is with a long-acting testosterone ester (testosterone cypionate or enanthate) 200 mg intramuscularly every 2 weeks. Testosterone also increases bone mass in women, but the virilizing side effects are not acceptable. However, studies are evaluating the potential use in women of testosterone analogues that have less of a virilizing effect while retaining the androgenic effect on bone.

Fluoride

Fluoride has been known for years to increase bone mass. It also has been shown, however, that the increased mass is not associated with decreased fractures and in fact may result in an increased fracture potential, presumably because of an abnormal structure of the bone mineral. Thus, fluoride is not recommended for routine use, but study of its effects continues because it is one of the few agents that increase bone formation.

BIBLIOGRAPHY

Fauci AS, Braunwald E, Isselbacher KJ, et al (eds): *Harrison's Principles of Internal Medicine,* 14th ed. New York, McGraw-Hill, 1998.

Molitch ME, Findling JW, Ladenson PW, et al (eds): *Medical Knowledge Self-Assessment Program in the Subspecialty of Endocrinology and Metabolism.* Philadelphia, American College of Physicians, 1995.

Tierney LM Jr, McPhee SJ, Papadakis MA (eds): *Current Medical Diagnosis and Treatment,* 35th ed. Stamford, CT, Appleton & Lange, 1996.

Chapter 5–3
HYPOTHYROIDISM
Timothy C. Evans

DISCUSSION

Thyroid hormone is required by virtually every cell in the body for normal function. It has effects on multiple metabolic processes, including the production and metabolism of other hormones. Thyroid disease may be manifested by low levels of free thyroid hormone (hypothyroidism), increased free thyroid hormone (hyperthyroidism or thyrotoxicosis), or thyroid gland enlargement (goiter; the enlargement of an isolated portion of thyroid tissue is more commonly referred to as a nodule).

There are two forms of thyroid hormone: thyroxine (T_4) and triiodothyronine (T_3). The active form of the hormone is T_3, which contains three iodines and results from monodeiodination of T_4. The conversion of T_4 to T_3 takes place partly in the thyroid gland but primarily in peripheral tissues such as the liver. The thyroid hormones circulate in the blood bound tightly to serum proteins, particularly thyroid-binding globulin (TBG). Much less than 1 percent of the total thyroid hormone is free and available to interact with target cells. Thus, standard measurements of total T_4 and T_3 give only an incomplete picture of the thyroid state. Additional tests are used to estimate or measure the amount of free hormone.

Thyroid hormone is secreted by the thyroid gland in response to thyroid-stimulating hormone (TSH) from the pituitary. TSH secretion by the pituitary is in turn stimulated by thyrotropin-releasing hormone from the hypothalamus. The secretory activity of both the pituitary and the hypothalamus is controlled by feedback inhibitory effects of free thyroid hormone in the blood such that increased free thyroid hormone results in decreased pituitary secretion of TSH and decreased free thyroid hormone results in increased TSH secretion.

LABORATORY EVALUATION OF THE THYROID

Thyroid Hormone

Both T_4 and T_3 can be measured accurately by radioimmunoassay. It is important to remember, however, that in each case it is the total circulating hormone concentration that is measured, not the free hormone level, which is the physiologically important fraction. Other tests are therefore needed to determine accurately the appropriateness of circulating thyroid hormone levels. The actual free T_4 or free T_3 can be measured, but this is more expensive and not readily available in many clinical laboratories.

T₃ Resin Uptake (T₃ Uptake)

In this test, radioactive T_3 is added to the patient's serum to determine the amount of serum protein binding of thyroid hormone. The result, the T_3RU or T_3U, is multiplied by the total T_4 (or T_3) to derive a calculated free T_4 (or T_3) index (FTI), an estimate of the free thyroid hormone.

Thyroid-Stimulating Hormone

TSH assays have been available for some time, and their sensitivity has increased to the point where so-called third-generation assays can accurately distinguish not only between elevated and normal TSH but also between suppressed and normal TSH levels. Since the hypothalamus and the pituitary, like other tissues, respond to free thyroid hormone, TSH is the single most useful thyroid function test. Sensitive assays of TSH have proved invaluable in assessing free thyroid hormone status.

Antithyroid Antibodies

Autoimmune thyroid disease is common, and it is occasionally useful to measure levels of marker antibodies such as antimicrosomal and antithyroglobulin antibodies. Antibodies directed against the thyroid also can cause thyroid disease, as in the thyroid-stimulating antibody of Graves' disease, which is directed against and activates the TSH receptor, resulting in hyperthyroidism. Measurement of this antibody is occasionally useful in Graves' disease patients when the diagnosis is in doubt and in pregnant women when radioiodine uptake and scan cannot be used to diagnose Graves' disease.

Ultrasound

Ultrasound can be useful to define thyroid size and anatomy, determine if a nodule is solid or cystic, or, occasionally, guide a needle biopsy of a thyroid nodule.

Radioiodine Uptake and Scan

A tracer dose of radioactive iodine will localize in the thyroid gland within hours of administration. The percentage of the administered radioactivity, the radioiodine uptake, that is detected in the thyroid gives an indication of the relative hormone-producing activity of the gland. Scanning the thyroid to determine the pattern of distribution of radioactivity within the thyroid helps determine whether abnormal function is localized or involves the entire gland.

HYPOTHYROIDISM

Causes of Hypothyroidism

Primary

Autoimmune Thyroiditis

Also called Hashimoto's thyroiditis or lymphocytic thyroiditis, autoimmune thyroiditis results from cell-mediated autoimmune damage of the thyroid and is the most common cause of hypothyroidism. Like other thyroid diseases, it is more common in women than in men and may be associated with other autoimmune diseases. The thyroid is typically modestly enlarged and somewhat firm. Antimicrosomal and antithyroglobulin antibodies are elevated.

Postablative Hypothyroidism

Surgical or radioiodine ablation of the thyroid may result in hypothyroidism, depending on the amount of the gland removed or the dose of radioiodine administered.

Subclinical Hypothyroidism

Subclinical hypothyroidism is defined as a normal thyroid hormone level in association with increased TSH. Some but not all cases progress to definite hypothyroidism. The degree of TSH elevation is useful to determine the likelihood of progression and the indication for thyroid hormone replacement therapy. In general, subclinical hypothyroidism with TSH higher than 10 mU/L should be treated.

Drug-Induced Hypothyroidism

A number of drugs can interfere with thyroid hormone synthesis or secretion, including high doses of iodine, the iodine-containing antiarrhythmic agent amiodarone, and lithium.

Transient Hypothyroidism

Hypothyroidism lasting for weeks to months and often preceded by a period of hyperthyroidism occurs commonly during the recovery phase of subacute thyroiditis and after about 5 percent of normal pregnancies.

Iodine Deficiency

Hypothyroidism resulting from deficient dietary iodine content is rare in the United States but occurs in inland isolated parts of the world. The chronic underproduction of thyroid hormone results in long-standing TSH excess and often dramatically enlarged thyroid glands, or endemic goiters.

Secondary

Hypothyroidism secondary to pituitary or hypothalamic dysfunction is unusual. The deficiency in TSH production may be isolated or may be associated with other pituitary hormone deficiencies.

Clinical Presentation

The most severe forms of hypothyroidism are unusual today. Congenital hypothyroidism (cretinism) is associated with severe mental and motor retardation. In adults, myxedema can progress to include respiratory depression and coma.

More commonly, however, hypothyroidism presents insidiously with nonspecific symptoms, such as fatigue and constipation, that may be easily overlooked or ascribed to other causes. Characteristic symptoms and signs of hypothyroidism may be absent or apparent only after careful reexamination of the patient.

The most common symptoms include fatigue, constipation, cold intolerance, mild weight gain, myalgias and arthralgias, dry skin, dry or brittle hair, menorrhagia, and hoarseness. Intellectual vigor decreases. Carpal tunnel syndrome, obstructive sleep apnea, and pericardial effusions are more common in hypothyroidism.

On physical examination the patient may appear lethargic with dry skin, nonlustrous hair, and hoarseness. The face may appear puffy, and the lateral half of the eyebrows thin. Mild diastolic hypertension may be present. A delay in the relaxation phase of the deep tendon reflexes is characteristic. Depending on the etiology, the thyroid itself may be nonpalpable or enlarged.

Laboratory Diagnosis

The diagnosis depends on demonstrating low circulating levels of thyroid hormone. Either free T_4 or total FTI, calculated from T_4 along with a T_3RU, should be measured. TSH should also be measured; except for secondary hypothyroidism, this is the most sensitive test for hypothyroidism. Once primary hypothyroidism is established, only TSH is needed to follow the course of the hypothyroidism and its treatment. Serum T_3 is not helpful in the diagnosis of hypothyroidism.

Other laboratory abnormalities include anemia or increased serum cholesterol, creatine kinase, and prolactin.

Treatment

The treatment of hypothyroidism consists of replacement with thyroid hormone. Since the half-life of T_3 is short, replacement is much easier and safer with T_4, levothyroxine. Administered T_4 is converted naturally in the body to the active form of the hormone, T_3. With few exceptions, therefore, the treatment of hypothyroidism is done with pure synthetic levothyroxine. The average replacement dose for patients with hypothyroidism is 0.1 to 0.125 mg per day given as a single daily dose.

Care should be taken in beginning replacement therapy, especially in frail, elderly patients and those with ischemic heart disease, since thyroid hormone is a cardiac stimulant. In these patients, the starting levothyroxine dose should be 0.0125 to 0.025 mg per day and should be increased slowly over weeks or months.

The replacement dose is monitored by following the TSH level. In this way, the pituitary serves as an internal bioassay for the free thyroid hormone level. After starting or changing the dosage level, a 6-week interval should pass before repeat TSH measurement, since it takes time for pituitary TSH production to reach a new steady state. In general the goal is to normalize but not suppress TSH.

THYROIDITIS

Inflammation of the thyroid occurs in several different settings. All can be associated with hypothyroidism, but none are necessarily associated.

Autoimmune Thyroiditis

As was noted previously, autoimmune thyroiditis, or Hashimoto's thyroiditis, is a result of cell-mediated immune inflammation of the thyroid. Histologic examination of the thyroid shows lymphocytic infiltration. However, the degree of thyroid destruction may not necessarily be sufficient to cause hypothyroidism. If the patient has significant thyroid enlargement or is troubled by the goiter, levothyroxine replacement may be instituted in a euthyroid patient to prevent thyroid growth.

Subacute Thyroiditis

Subacute thyroiditis is a probable viral inflammation of the thyroid associated with fever, myalgias, and a tender enlarged thyroid. The disease is self-limited but may be associated with thyrotoxicosis in the early stages as a result of leakage of stored thyroid hormone from the inflamed gland and a more prolonged hypothyroid phase lasting several months during a later phase of recovery. The symptoms of acute thyroid inflammation usually respond to aspirin or nonsteroidal anti-inflammatory drugs. When it occurs, hypothyroidism should be treated, but since the gland usually reverts to normal function eventually, the replacement levothyroxine should be discontinued and TSH should be rechecked after 6 to 12 months of treatment.

Postpartum Thyroiditis

Thyroid dysfunction occurs after about 5 percent of pregnancies. Most patients with this complication have an underlying autoimmune thyroid disease. It typically presents with an early mild hyperthyroid phase followed by a more prolonged hypothyroid phase. When hypothyroidism occurs, it should be treated with levothyroxine replacement to normalize TSH. In most patients the hypothyroidism resolves after 6 to 12 months, but these patients are at risk for the same sequence after subsequent pregnancies.

BIBLIOGRAPHY

Fauci AS, Braunwald E, Isselbacher KJ, et al (eds): *Harrison's Principles of Internal Medicine,* 14th ed. New York, McGraw-Hill, 1998.

Molitch ME, Findling JW, Ladenson PW, et al (eds): *Medical Knowledge Self-Assessment Program in the Subspecialty of Endocrinology and Metabolism.* Philadelphia, American College of Physicians, 1995.

Tierney LM Jr, McPhee SJ, Papadakis MA (eds): *Current Medical Diagnosis and Treatment,* 35th ed. Stamford, CT, Appleton & Lange, 1996.

Chapter 5–4
HYPERTHYROIDISM
Timothy C. Evans

DISCUSSION

Thyrotoxicosis is the term applied to any condition in which serum levels of the thyroid hormones, thyroxine (T_4) and triiodothyronine (T_3), are excessive. This term often is used interchangeably with *hyperthyroidism,* but strictly speaking, hyperthyroidism applies only to cases in which the excess thyroid hormone comes from the patient's thyroid gland. In almost all forms of thyrotoxicosis, the pituitary secretion of thyroid-stimulating hormone (TSH) is suppressed through feedback inhibition of the pituitary by the increased thyroid hormone levels.

CAUSES OF THYROTOXICOSIS

The causes of thyrotoxicosis can be subdivided in several ways. One useful distinction can be made by considering the intrinsic activity of the thyroid as shown by the radioiodine uptake (RAIU). In this test, a tracer dose of radioactive iodine is administered to the patient and the radioactivity accumulated in the thyroid is counted 2 to 24 h later. A gland that is metabolically active, producing increased amounts of thyroid hormone, has an increased uptake. When the gland is not actively producing excess hormone, the uptake is low. In cases in which RAIU is increased, a next useful step is to scan the thyroid to demonstrate the pattern of distribution of radioactivity within the gland.

High Radioiodine Uptake

In these diseases, the thyroid is overactive, synthesizing and releasing increased amounts of thyroid hormone. The thyroid activity is autonomous of normal control mechanisms or is stimulated by abnormal activators, because pituitary secretion of TSH is appropriately low.

Graves' Disease

By far the most common cause of thyrotoxicosis, Graves' disease is much more common in women than in men. It can be seen at any age but occurs most frequently in the early to midadult years. It is an autoimmune disease and is associated with antimicrosomal and antithyroglobulin antibodies (see Chap. 5-3). It is caused, however, by a unique autoantibody directed against the TSH receptor. When bound to the receptor, this antibody stimulates the thyroid cell just as TSH would when bound to the receptor. The result is diffuse overactivity of the thyroid despite very low levels of TSH. The radioiodine scan shows diffuse increased uptake throughout the gland. There is a familial tendency in Graves' disease, and this disease is associated with an increased incidence of other autoimmune diseases, such as pernicious anemia and myasthenia gravis.

In addition to overactivity of the thyroid gland, Graves' disease is associated with two important clinical manifestations: infiltration of the tissues around the eyes (exophthalmos) and less frequently infiltration of the skin (pretibial myxedema). These manifestations can occur with or without hyperthyroidism and may have a different clinical course than does the thyroid overactivity.

Toxic Multinodular Goiter

Autonomy occasionally develops in long-standing multinodular goiters, with increased thyroid hormone production independent of TSH stimulation. The cause is not understood, but there is no stimulating antibody as in Graves' disease. Toxic multinodular goiter occurs primarily in elderly patients. It is not accompanied by eye or skin infiltrative disease and is not associated with other autoimmune phenomena. The thyrotoxicosis is usually not as severe as in Grave's disease. The radioiodine scan pattern is patchy, with increased uptake throughout the gland.

Autonomous Thyroid Nodule

Also known as a "hot nodule" from its radioiodine scan pattern of a single area of increased uptake surrounded by inactive thyroid tissue, an autonomous thyroid nodule is a variant of toxic multinodular goiter.

Low Radioiodine Uptake

In these cases of thyrotoxicosis, the elevated thyroid hormone levels are not a consequence of increased metabolic synthetic activity of the thyroid. Unlike high-RAIU causes of thyrotoxicosis, these forms of thyrotoxicosis are distinguished by a lack of intrinsic thyroid overactivity, the RAIU is low, and scanning is moot. Since thyroid hormone is increased, however, pituitary TSH secretion is suppressed as it is in high-RAIU thyrotoxicosis.

Thyroiditis

The thyroid contains a large amount of preformed thyroid hormone stored in the colloid space as part of thyroglobulin. In the case of thyroiditis, inflammation in the thyroid gland results in the release of the stored hormone. This occurs most strikingly in the early phase of inflammation of subacute thyroiditis. Mild thyrotoxicosis also occurs occasionally during the course of Hashimoto's thyroiditis, so-called Hashitoxicosis. This occurs commonly after pregnancy and is known as postpartum thyroiditis.

Exogenous Thyroid Hormone

The administration of inappropriately large doses of thyroid hormone also causes low-RAIU thyrotoxicosis. This may result from misunderstanding by the patient, from failure of the prescriber to adjust the thyroid hormone dose on the basis of the TSH, or occasionally from intentional excess dosage by the patient.

Unusual Causes of Thyrotoxicosis

Thyroid tissue contained in ovarian dermoid tumors can function autonomously or in concert with Graves' disease. TSH-secreting pituitary tumors occur rarely and are the only cause of normal or high TSH in association with thyrotoxicosis. High levels of human chorionic gonadotropin (hCG), as seen with trophoblastic tumors or pregnancy, can cause hyperthyroidism, since hCG is similar in structure to TSH. High levels of iodine, as with drugs such as amiodarone and iodine-containing radiographic contrast media, can cause hyperthyroidism or hypothyroidism (see Chap. 5-3).

CLINICAL PRESENTATION

Thyrotoxicosis of any cause may cause nervousness, emotional lability, fatigue, heat intolerance, frequent bowel movements, weight loss despite a good appetite, sweating, menstrual irregularities, proximal muscle weakness, dyspnea, and palpitations. The physical findings include stare and lid lag, fine tremor, warm moist skin, tachycardia or atrial fibrillation, and, when thyrotoxicosis is present chronically, osteoporosis. The thyroid gland may or may not be enlarged, depending on the etiology of the thyrotoxicosis; if it is enlarged, it may be either nodular or diffusely enlarged.

Graves' disease has additional specific physical findings. The thyroid gland in patients with Graves' disease is diffusely enlarged and may be so metabolically active that a bruit is heard on thyroid auscultation. In addition to the stare and lid lag of thyrotoxicosis, Graves' ophthalmopathy occurs in 20 to 40 percent of these patients. This may include chemosis, proptosis, and impaired extraocular muscle movements. When it is severe, exophthalmos can damage vision. Pretibial myxedema occurs in only a small percent of Graves' patients and usually is characterized by raised, thickened lesions on the anterior shins.

Occasionally in the elderly, thyrotoxicosis is asymptomatic, so-called apathetic hyperthyroidism, or presents only with atrial fibrillation.

Thyroid storm is an unusual but life-threatening complication of hyperthyroidism marked by high fever, tachycardia, vomiting, diarrhea, dehydration, and delirium. The mortality rate is high. It can be precipitated by surgery, severe medical illness, or radioiodine treatment.

DIAGNOSIS

A number of tests are available to assess thyroid function and anatomy (see Chap. 5-3). The characteristic laboratory abnormalities include increased T_4 and T_3. Since increased serum protein binding [as commonly seen with estrogen therapy, which increases thyroid-binding globulin (TBG)] results in increased total circulating thyroid hormone but normal free thyroid hormone, it is important to assess the protein binding with a T_3 resin uptake in order to calculate the free thyroid index or to measure free T_4 and T_3 directly. T_3 is a more sensitive indicator of hyperthyroidism than is T_4. Occasionally in mild hyperthyroidism, only T_3 is elevated; this is known as T_3 toxicosis. TSH is decreased in all forms of thyrotoxicosis except the rare circumstance of a pituitary tumor that overproduces TSH.

As was noted above, the RAIU and scan can be helpful in distinguishing between the various causes of thyrotoxicosis.

The level of thyroid-stimulating antibody in Graves' disease can be measured, but this is infrequently necessary or helpful except for diagnostic purposes in cases where Graves' eye or skin disease is present without thyrotoxicosis and in Graves' disease during pregnancy. The thyroid-stimulating antibody does cross the placenta and, when present in a significant amount in maternal blood, is predictive of transient neonatal thyrotoxicosis in the newborn.

TREATMENT

The treatment of thyrotoxicosis is based on RAIU. Diseases characterized by increased RAIU respond to antithyroid drugs and radioiodine ablation. Diseases with low RAIU do not.

Treatment Modalities

Antithyroid Drugs

The thioureas methimazole and propylthiouracil (PTU) inhibit thyroid hormone synthesis by the thyroid gland. Methimazole is more convenient since it can be taken once a day, but PTU inhibits extrathyroidal conversion of T_4 to T_3 and so may be somewhat more effective in patients with marked hyperthyroidism. Each medication has side effects, including rashes and hepatitis. The most dangerous side effect is agranulocytosis, which usually resolves when the drug is discontinued. Patients should be advised to watch for fever, other signs of infection, and oral ulcers. Methimazole has been reported to cause the scalp abnormality aplasia cutis in newborns, and so hyperthyroidism in pregnant women is treated with PTU.

Radioactive Iodine

High-RAIU forms of thyrotoxicosis can be treated with doses of radioiodine sufficient to decrease thyroid activity and eliminate excess thyroid hormone production. It typically takes several months after the dose of radioiodine for the thyroid to slow to a new, lower steady state of activity. During the transition period, antithyroid drugs are continued and the dosage is tapered as the thyroid overactivity resolves. A period of pretreatment with antithyroid drugs is also wise in elderly or medically frail patients and those with very overactive thyroids to deplete the gland of stored thyroid hormone before the radioactive damage is inflicted.

Thyroid Surgery

Surgery for hyperthyroidism is unusual but occasionally is performed for very large thyroid glands or in the second trimester of pregnancy, when Graves' disease cannot be controlled medically. Pretreatment with antithyroid drugs decreases the chance of thyroid storm.

Propranolol

Propranolol is the beta-adrenergic blocking agent of choice to alleviate the symptoms of tachycardia, nervousness, and sweating. Propranolol does not affect the thyroid itself and can be discontinued when the thyroid overactivity is brought under control. It does decrease peripheral conversion of T_4 to T_3, which is beneficial in the early treatment of symptomatic thyrotoxicosis.

High-RAIU Thyrotoxicosis

Graves' disease usually is treated initially with antithyroid drugs and propranolol if necessary. In young patients with small, modestly overactive glands, there is a significant chance of remission if antithyroid drug suppression is continued for a year and then discontinued. The rate of remission may be increased by adding replacement levothyroxine to the methimazole. Most other patients, as well as those in whom remission is not achieved, are treated with radioiodine ablation. After ablation, some patients become hypothyroid and require thyroid hormone replacement. Over the course of the succeeding years additional patients eventually become hypothyroid. Long-term follow-up should monitor for this outcome.

Neither multinodular goiter nor toxic adenoma remits with antithyroid drugs. Therefore, after antithyroid drug pretreatment, definitive treatment with radioiodine ablation usually is carried out.

Low-RAIU Thyrotoxicosis

Adrenergic symptoms of thyrotoxicosis can be relieved with propranolol. The hyperthyroidism of thyroiditis is self-limited and resolves when thyroid inflammation resolves and the store of fcthyroid hormone in the gland is depleted. No other treatment of the hyperthyroidism is necessary or effective.

In patients overtreated with levothyroxine, the daily dose should be decreased. The patient is followed to determine the dose that normalizes the serum TSH.

BIBLIOGRAPHY

Fauci AS, Braunwald E, Isselbacher KJ, et al (eds): *Harrison's Principles of Internal Medicine,* 14th ed. New York, McGraw-Hill, 1998.

Molitch ME, Findling JW, Ladenson PW, et al (eds): *Medical Knowledge Self-Assessment Program in the Subspecialty of Endocrinology and Metabolism.* Philadelphia, American College of Physicians, 1995.

Tierney LM Jr, McPhee SJ, Papadakis MA (eds): *Current Medical Diagnosis and Treatment,* 35th ed. Stamford, CT, Appleton & Lange, 1996.

Chapter 5–5
ADRENAL DISORDERS
Timothy C. Evans

DISCUSSION

The adrenal glands are adjacent to the kidneys and are composed of two distinct types of hormone-secreting tissue: the cortex on the outside and the medulla in the center of each gland. The cortex secretes three classes of steroid hormones: glucocorticoids, mineralocorticoids, and androgens. The medulla secretes catecholamines. Diseases of the adrenal generally are suspected because of clinical evidence of deficiency or an excess of these hormones. On other occasions, adrenal masses are found incidentally on abdominal imaging studies performed for unrelated reasons.

ADRENAL CORTEX

Glucocorticoids

The primary glucocorticoid secreted by the adrenal cortex is cortisol. The stimulus for cortisol secretion is adrenocorticotropic hormone (ACTH) from the anterior pituitary. Cortisol is secreted in a diurnal pattern, with the highest levels on awakening and the lowest at bedtime. Physiologic levels of cortisol have modulatory effects on intermediary metabolism, vascular tone, water balance, and inflammation. Cortisol opposes the action of insulin and is secreted briskly in response to stress, both physiologic and psychological.

Deficiency

Clinical Presentation

Depending on the rate of development, adrenal insufficiency can present as mild chronic fatigue or fulminant cardiovascular collapse. When the deficiency is only partial, the symptoms may be apparent only in times of stress, such as trauma, surgery, and infection. The classic symptoms include weakness and easy fatigability, hypotension with dehydration and postural drop, and gastrointestinal dysfunction with anorexia, nausea and vomiting, diarrhea, abdominal pain, and weight loss. When the insufficiency is primary, ACTH levels are high and are associated with hyperpigmentation.

Laboratory findings may include hyponatremia, hyperkalemia, hypoglycemia, and hypereosinophilia.

Etiology

Adrenal insufficiency may be primary (diseased or absent adrenals) or secondary (insufficient stimulation by ACTH). Primary disease is most commonly an autoimmune phenomenon (Addison's disease), in which case it may be associated with autoimmune disease of the thyroid, gonads, skin (vitiligo), and other tissues. Bilateral adrenal hemorrhage may occur in the setting of anticoagulation or that of critical surgery, trauma, or obstetric illness. Less commonly, disseminated tuberculosis or fungal infections may result in destruction of the adrenal cortices. When the deficiency is primary, mineralocorticoid (see below) as well as glucocorticoid secretion is impaired.

Adrenocortical insufficiency also can be secondary to a lack of ACTH stimulation. By far the most common cause of ACTH deficiency, as well as of adrenal insufficiency overall, is persistent pituitary suppression after the discontinuation of exogenous glucocorticoid administration. It is notable that high-dose glucocorticoid administration for as little as a few weeks can result in prolonged adrenal insufficiency. ACTH deficiency also occurs in the setting of panhypopituitarism, along with deficiencies of other anterior pituitary hormones. In the case of secondary adrenal insufficiency, mineralocorticoid secretion remains relatively normal.

Diagnosis

The diagnosis of glucocorticoid insufficiency is suggested by low morning cortisol levels but is most reliably and reproducibly demonstrated at any time of the day with a cosyntropin stimulation test. In this test, 0.25 mg of cosyntropin is administered intramuscularly or intravenously. The serum cortisol level 30 to 60 min later should be 20 μg/dL or greater. In cases of primary adrenal insufficiency, the ACTH level will be elevated, and in autoimmune disease, antiadrenal antibodies may be elevated.

Treatment

The emergent treatment of patients with cardiovascular collapse from adrenal insufficiency includes immediate intravenous hydrocortisone 100 mg every 6 h, and volume repletion with intravenous saline. Treatment is adjusted over hours and days as the clinical picture evolves.

The long-term management of patients with adrenocortical insufficiency requires physiologic levels of glucocorticoid replacement: 30 mg of hydrocortisone or 7.5 mg of prednisone per day in divided doses with two-thirds in the morning and one-third in the evening. Patients with primary insufficiency also may require mineralocorticoid replacement (see below).

The glucocorticoid dose should be increased temporarily for surgery, trauma, or acute illness, and patients should be educated about the risk of discontinuing treatment.

Excess

Clinical Presentation

Hypercortisolism (Cushing's syndrome) is characterized by central obesity, muscle wasting, thin skin, hypertension, hirsutism, amenorrhea, and osteoporosis. Fatigue and weakness are common, and these patients are subject to infections. Laboratory findings may include hyperglycemia, hypokalemia, and lymphopenia.

Etiology

Hypercortisolism most commonly results from prolonged, high-dose exogenous glucocorticoid administration, such as for asthma or inflammatory rheumatologic disease. Less commonly, an ACTH-producing pituitary tumor (Cushing's disease) results in hypercortisolism and diffuse adrenal hyperplasia. Infrequently, ACTH excess is due to secretion by other tumors, most commonly small cell bronchogenic lung carcinomas. In the remainder, hypercortisolism results from primary hyperfunction of an adrenal tumor, either an adenoma or a carcinoma.

Diagnosis

Iatrogenic glucocorticoid excess is usually apparent from the history. In other patients, the initial diagnosis of hypercortisolism rests on the demonstration of excess, nonsuppressible cortisol production. The best test for this purpose is the 24-h urine free cortisol. More convenient for some patients but less sensitive and specific is the overnight dexamethasone suppression test, in which 1 mg of dexamethasone is taken orally at midnight and a serum cortisol is determined at 8 o'clock the next morning. Normally, the morning cortisol should be suppressed to less than 5 μg/dL. False-positives in these tests occur in patients with exogenous obesity, chronic alcoholism, depression, and acute physiologic or psychological stress.

After hypercortisolism has been established, the evaluation turns to the etiology by establishing patterns of cortisol suppressibility with high-dose dexamethasone and assessment of ACTH secretion. Imaging studies of the pituitary, the adrenals, or, for ectopic ACTH, the chest also may be useful.

Treatment

The guiding principle of exogenous glucocorticoid administration is to use the minimum dose necessary for the shortest time possible. However, when suppressive doses are necessary, it is important that patients be educated about the risks of discontinuing treatment; if treatment is discontinued, the dose should be tapered gradually to allow the return of endogenous adrenal function.

Treatment of the other causes of hypercortisolism primarily consists of surgical removal of the hyperfunctioning pituitary, adrenal, or ectopic tumor. When hypercortisolism cannot be resolved, ketoconazole can be used to inhibit adrenal cortisol production.

Mineralocorticoids

The primary mineralocorticoid secreted by the adrenal cortex is aldosterone. Aldosterone secretion is stimulated by angiotensin II and hyperkalemia. The renin-angiotensin-aldosterone pathway begins with renin secretion by the kidney in response to low perfusion pressure. Renin converts angiotensinogen from the liver into angiotensin I, and this ultimately results in increased levels of angiotensin II from the action of angiotensin-converting enzyme (ACE) on angiotensin I. Aldosterone has its major effect on the renal tubule, where it causes reabsorption of sodium in exchange for potassium and hydrogen ions. In doing so, it helps regulate both volume status and potassium balance.

Deficiency

Clinical Presentation

Hypoaldosteronism is seen most commonly in circumstances of primary adrenocortical insufficiency, in which the clinical presentation is dominated by the signs and symptoms of cortisol deficiency. Hypoaldosteronism itself is the major contributor to hyperkalemia, with resultant neuromuscular and cardiac dysfunction manifested by weakness and ECG abnormalities.

Etiology

Isolated aldosterone deficiency is unusual and occurs most often in the setting of hyporeninism associated with renal insufficiency and diabetes mellitus. More often, hypoaldosteronism is associated with generalized primary adrenocortical insufficiency (see above).

Diagnosis

The specific diagnosis of hypoaldosteronism depends on demonstrating a deficient aldosterone response (with or without a renin response) to sodium restriction and upright posture. In primary hypoaldosteronism, renin is high but aldosterone is low. In secondary hypoaldosteronism, both renin and aldosterone secretion are low.

Treatment

When necessary, mineralocorticoid replacement is accomplished with 0.05 to 0.2 mg oral fludrocortisone daily.

Excess

Clinical Presentation

Hyperaldosteronism can be primary or secondary to excess renin production by one kidney or both kidneys. Primary hyperaldosteronism results in hypertension, weakness, and polyuria. Hyperaldosteronism accounts for about 1 percent of cases of hypertension. In the absence of other abnormalities, these patients do not have edema. Important laboratory abnormalities include hypokalemia and metabolic alkalosis.

A patient with excess renin from renal artery stenosis that causes unilateral renal underperfusion and hypertensive secondary hyperaldosteronism may have a renal artery bruit.

Etiology

In about 70 percent of cases, primary hyperaldosteronism results from a unilateral adrenocortical adenoma (rarely a carcinoma). In most of the remaining cases, the cause is bilateral adrenal hyperplasia. High-renin secondary hyperaldosteronism associated with hypertension results most commonly from renal artery stenosis. Hyperaldosteronism secondary to increased renin secretion also occurs physiologically and without hypertension in circumstances of renal underperfusion, such as hypovolemia and congestive heart failure.

Diagnosis

Hypokalemia in a nonedematous hypertensive patient who is consuming adequate sodium and is not on diuretics is an indication for diagnostic assessment of hyperaldosteronism. The diagnosis rests on demonstrating nonsuppressibility of aldosterone (and renin in the case of renal artery stenosis) in the presence of a high sodium intake. Ideally, drugs that interfere with the renin-angiotensin-aldosterone system should be discontinued before a definitive evaluation is made.

A useful initial screen for primary hyperaldosteronism is an elevated aldosterone/renin ratio. Confirming tests involve the measurement of aldosterone and renin while patients are on a high-salt diet or after the intravenous infusion of normal saline. In primary hyperaldosteronism, aldosterone is high but renin is low. In secondary hyperaldosteronism, both renin and aldosterone are high. Abdominal CT or adrenal vein catheterization studies are used to differentiate adenoma from bilateral hyperplasia in primary hyperaldosteronism.

Treatment

Unilateral adrenalectomy is used to treat an adenoma or carcinoma. In patients with surgical contraindications or bilateral adrenal hyperplasia, medical management of aldosterone-induced hypertension includes spironolactone, calcium channel blockers, and/or ACE inhibitors. Secondary hyperaldosteronism from renal artery stenosis may be treated with angioplasty or revascularization procedures.

Adrenal Androgens

The adrenal androgens are quite weak compared with testosterone and have little physiologic impact in adults. When present in significant excess, however, they can result in abnormalities. The severity and impact of the abnormalities depend on the age of the patient and the degree of androgen excess. In congenital adrenal hyperplasia (CAH), an enzyme in the biosynthetic pathway of cortisol is deficient. In this circumstance, the common precursor accumulates and "spills over" into the adrenal androgen biosynthetic pathway. Adrenal androgens are secreted in excess by some adrenal carcinomas.

Clinical Presentation

In childhood, severe CAH may result in the death of a fetus or infant, sexual ambiguity or a male phenotype in girls, early puberty in boys, accelerated height and bone age, and, depending on the enzyme defect, salt wasting or hypertension. In adult women, a less severe defect of adrenal steroidogenesis can cause hirsutism, oligomenorrhea-amenorrhea, infertility, acne, and temporal balding. In adult women, virilization—clitoromegaly, frontal balding, male-pattern muscularity, and deepening of the voice—suggests adrenal neoplasm.

Etiology

The most common form of CAH results from a deficiency of 21-hydroxylase. Less commonly, 11β-hydroxylase deficiency occurs. In either case, cortisol production is deficient, and the resultant increased pituitary ACTH drives adrenal steroidogenesis, leading to increased androgen secretion. The precursor that accumulates in 11β-hydroxylase deficiency leads to hypertension, while its absence in 21-hydroxylase deficiency leads to salt wasting.

Rarely adrenal androgen excess results from an adrenocortical carcinoma.

Diagnosis

The diagnosis of CAH depends on demonstrating elevation of a precursor to the reaction in the biosynthetic pathway normally catalyzed by the deficient enzymes. The most useful test is serum 17-hydroxyprogesterone. Adrenal androgen excess from hyperplasia, or rarely from carcinoma, is shown by increased levels of dehydroepiandrosterone sulfate (DHEA-S).

Treatment

CAH is treated by replacing the missing adrenal hormone: cortisol. This results in decreased ACTH levels and resolved overactivity of adrenal steroidogenesis. Adrenal carcinoma requires surgery.

ADRENAL MEDULLA

The adrenal medulla secretes catecholamines—epinephrine and norepinephrine—as part of the sympathetic nervous system in response to various stresses. The catecholamines generally result in increased heart rate and force of cardiac contractility, increased glucose production, and central nervous system excitability. The clinical abnormality of the adrenal medulla is pheochromocytoma, a rare tumor that secretes excess amounts of the catecholamines.

Pheochromocytoma

Clinical Presentation

Pheochromocytoma causes less than 1 percent of cases of hypertension. The hypertension may be sustained or paroxysmal. The associated symptoms are variable but classically include paroxysmal headache, palpitations, and diaphoresis in association with acute elevation of blood pressure. There also may be weight loss despite increased appetite and postural hypotension because of volume contraction. Laboratory abnormalities include elevated glucose. Thyroid tests are notably normal.

Etiology

Most pheochromocytomas are solitary benign tumors. About 10 percent are bilateral, 10 percent are extraadrenal, and 10 percent are malignant. In about 5 percent of cases, the pheochromocytoma is part of familial syndromes as an isolated abnormality or as part of the multiple endocrine neoplasia (MEN) syndrome, types 2a and 2b.

Diagnosis

The diagnosis is established by demonstrating increased excretion of the catecholamines or their metabolites—vanillylmandelic acid (VMA) and metanephrines—in 24-h urine collections. Most pheochromocytomas secrete increased catecholamines continuously, but the sensitivity of testing is increased when it is performed during a hypertensive episode. Localization of the tumor usually is possible with CT scanning.

Treatment

The ultimate treatment of pheochromocytoma is surgical removal. However, correct pre- and intraoperative pharmacologic care is critical and is directed specifically toward catecholamine excess. First, α-blockade is established with phenoxybenzamine and volume expansion is carried out over 7 to 14 days. Only after α-blockade is established is β-blockade with propranolol introduced. Isolated β-blockade will result in unopposed α-receptor stimulation and dramatic worsening of hypertension.

ADRENAL INCIDENTALOMA

With the widespread availability and use of CT and MRI scanning, an increasing number of adrenal tumors are being discovered incidentally in patients who are scanned for unrelated reasons. Most of these tumors are nonfunctional, and carcinoma is rare in tumors smaller than 5 cm. The finding of an incidental adrenal tumor should prompt a careful history and physical directed toward findings of adrenal hormone excess and a detailed review of the CT scan, which may suggest the etiology. Laboratory screening for hormone oversecretion may include 24-h urine free cortisol or an overnight 1-mg dexamethasone suppression test, serum potassium, aldosterone/renin ratio, DHEA-S, and urinary VMA/metanephrines/catecholamines. Functional tumors should be treated appropriately. Tumors equal to or larger than 5 cm should be removed. Follow-up CT of smaller nonfunctional tumors should be performed in 6 to 12 months.

BIBLIOGRAPHY

Fauci AS, Braunwald E, Isselbacher KJ, et al (eds): *Harrison's Principles of Internal Medicine,* 14th ed. New York, McGraw-Hill, 1998.

Molitch ME, Findling JW, Ladenson PW, et al (eds): *Medical Knowledge Self-Assessment Program in the Subspecialty of Endocrinology and Metabolism.* Philadelphia, American College of Physicians, 1995.

Tierney LM, Jr McPhee SJ, Papadakis MA (eds): *Current Medical Diagnosis and Treatment,* 35th ed. Stamford, CT, Appleton & Lange, 1996.

Chapter 5–6
ANTERIOR PITUITARY DISORDERS
Timothy C. Evans

DISCUSSION

The pituitary gland is composed of anterior and posterior divisions and is located in the sella turcica, a small bony pocket at the base of the cranial vault. The anterior pituitary consists of several different populations of cells that secrete six different peptide hormones: growth hormone (GH), adrenocorticotropic hormone (ACTH), thyroid-stimulating hormone (TSH), luteinizing hormone (LH), follicle-simulating hormone (FSH), and prolactin. The secretion of these hormones is under the control of the hypothalamus through chemical signals that travel from the hypothalamus to the pituitary via the hypothalamic-pituitary portal circulation. In each case except that of prolactin, the stimulatory signal is a peptide-releasing hormone. Prolactin is unique in that it is under tonic inhibitory control by the hypothalamus. The mediator of this inhibition is dopamine. The posterior pituitary is a direct neuronal extension from the hypothalamus and is discussed in Chap. 5-11.

There are four key anatomic features of the pituitary. The first is its relationship to the hypothalamus, which controls anterior pituitary function through the releasing hormones and dopamine. The second is the location of the pituitary in the sella turcica, which limits the size of the pituitary so that enlargement is generally out of the sella superiorly. The third is the position of the optic chiasm directly above the superior opening into the sella turcica. This means that pituitary enlargement out of the sella results in pressure on or damage to the optic chiasm and characteristic visual field abnormalities. The fourth is the presence of the cavernous sinuses lateral to the sella turcica. Cranial nerves III, IV, and VI pass through the cavernous sinuses, and so lateral extension of a pituitary tumor can result in oculomotor palsies, most frequently of cranial nerve III.

In general, disorders of the pituitary are manifested by the effects of excess secretion of one of the pituitary hormones, a deficiency of one or more pituitary hormones, or pituitary enlargement.

PITUITARY ADENOMAS

Pituitary adenomas are benign pituitary tumors that can be functional or nonfunctional. Functional tumors arise from the cells that secrete pituitary hormones and release excess amounts of the hormone associated with the cells that constitute the tumor. Other tumors are nonfunctional and, like functional tumors, may cause symptoms by compressing the normal pituitary and resulting in decreased secretion of pituitary hormones or through mechanical effects on extrapituitary structures such as the optic chiasm. Small pituitary tumors, less than 1 cm, typically confined to the sella turcica, are termed *microadenomas.* Larger tumors are called *macroadenomas.* When the neurons of the optic chiasm are disrupted, the characteristic visual field defect is bitemporal hemianopia. Other mass effects include headache and cranial nerve III palsy. The most common functional pituitary tumor secretes prolactin. Next in frequency is GH secretion, followed by ACTH secretion. Tumors that secrete excess TSH, LH, or FSH are very unusual.

Prolactin

There are many causes of hyperprolactinemia, including physiologic states such as pregnancy and nursing, many drugs, and diseases such as hypothyroidism and pituitary-hypothalamic lesions or tumors that interfere with the delivery of dopamine from the hypothalamus to the pituitary. Another cause is the most common pituitary tumor: prolactinoma.

Clinical Presentation

Prolactin normally stimulates the production of breast milk after childbirth. Excess prolactin also decreases the pituitary gonadotropins, LH and FSH. Consequently, the symptoms of hyperprolactinemia are those of hypogonadism and infertility. Prolactinomas are more common in women and present with oligo- or amenorrhea and galactorrhea. In men, the symptoms develop gradually and consist of decreased libido and impotence. Because of the menstrual abnormality, prolactinomas tend to be diagnosed in women at an earlier stage than they are in men. In men the tumors are more likely to be macroadenomas.

Diagnosis

Patients with hypogonadism or galactorrhea should have a prolactin measurement. When prolactin is elevated, the various possibilities in the wide differential diagnosis must be considered. The higher the prolactin level, the more likely the diagnosis of prolactinoma. When there is hyperprolactinemia, an MRI should be performed to look for a pituitary tumor.

Treatment

Prolactinoma is the only pituitary tumor for which the treatment is primarily medical. The dopamine agonist bromocriptine effectively inhibits prolactin secretion and results in a decrease in tumor size. The starting dose is 1.25 mg given at bedtime to minimize the side effects of nausea and postural hypotension. Complete inhibition may require 10 to 15 mg per day in two divided doses. Occasionally, large tumors may require surgery.

Growth Hormone

The second most common functional pituitary tumor secretes GH. This hormone has its primary effect on linear bone growth and has a number of metabolic effects, most notably insulin antagonism. The most characteristic consequence of a GH-secreting tumor is excess growth.

Clinical Presentation

In adults GH excess results in acromegaly, and in children it results in gigantism. In addition to the increased rate of bone and soft tissue growth, metabolic abnormalities contribute to the clinical picture. It is more common in males than in females.

Children have increased linear bone growth, and adults show enlargement of the hands, feet, and skull. The hands are broad, and the face is characterized by frontal bossing, coarsening of features, oily skin, and the development of spaces between the teeth. The process is so slow that the changes often are not noticed by the patient and the diagnosis is made only after a long delay. Soft tissue growth results in carpal tunnel syndrome and cardiomegaly with congestive heart failure. Metabolic effects include diabetes mellitus, weight gain, and kidney stones. The tumors have often grown to large size by the time of diagnosis and are associated with headaches and visual field defects.

Diagnosis

The diagnosis is indicated by the physical findings, diabetes mellitus, or glucose intolerance. Comparison with old photographs of the patient can be helpful in showing the change in appearance over time. A useful screening test is the measurement of insulin-like growth factor I (IGF-I, also called somatomedin C), which

is produced by the liver in response to GH stimulation. Unlike GH, it has a long half-life in serum so that levels do not vary from minute to minute.

When IGF-I is elevated, serum GH is measured 60 min after 100 g of oral glucose. Since hyperglycemia has the opposite effect on GH that it has on insulin, the GH level should be suppressed to less than 2 ng/mL. Prolactin, which frequently is cosecreted with GH as well as other pituitary hormones, should be measured, since a large tumor may interfere with the normal secretion of other pituitary hormones. After confirmation of GH excess, an MRI is performed to document the pituitary tumor's anatomy.

Treatment

Treatment of GH-secreting pituitary tumors primarily consists of surgical removal. Since these tumors are often macroadenomas, complete removal is often impossible. Other treatment modalities include high-dose bromocriptine, octreotide (an analogue of somatostatin, a natural hormone that inhibits GH secretion), and radiation therapy.

Adrenocorticotropic Hormone

ACTH is the stimulus for cortisol production by the adrenal cortex. Pituitary tumors that secrete excess ACTH constitute Cushing's disease, a form of Cushing's syndrome. Cushing's disease therefore is characterized by the symptoms of hypercortisolism.

Clinical Presentation

ACTH-producing tumors are typically microadenomas, and so they usually have no local pituitary mass effects. The symptoms are confined to those of hypercortisolism: centripetal obesity, facial plethora, hypertension, thin skin with easy bruising and abdominal striae, osteoporosis, muscle weakness, and glucose intolerance.

Diagnosis

Hypercortisolism is demonstrated by increased 24-h urine free cortisol or nonsuppression of morning serum cortisol in the 1-mg overnight dexamethasone suppression test or after 2 days of low-dose dexamethasone (0.5 mg every 6 h for eight doses). The next step in the identification of the cause of endogenous hypercortsolism is high-dose dexamethasone suppression (2 mg dexamethasone every 6 h for eight doses). Classically, ACTH overproduction by a pituitary tumor is suppressed by high-dose dexamethasone while primary adrenal overproduction and ectopic ACTH-stimulated overproduction are not suppressed.

Since ACTH-producing pituitary tumors are usually small, localization before surgery can be challenging. In addition to MRI, selective catheterization and sampling of ACTH levels in the right and left venous drainage (the petrosal sinuses) of the pituitary gland may help identify the tumor before microsurgery.

HYPOPITUITARISM

Deficient secretion of anterior pituitary hormones can be selective or global: panhypopituitarism. The clinical presentation is determined by the missing hormone or hormones.

Etiology

Isolated Deficiencies

An isolated deficiency of anterior pituitary hormones can be congenital or acquired. An acquired deficiency is more common. The most important acquired pituitary hormone functional deficiency is of ACTH after prolonged glucocorticoid excess, whether from endogenous hypercortisolism or from exogenous glucocorticoid administration. Likewise, TSH levels may remain suppressed for a time after the resolution of hyperthyroidism. Isolated, reversible gonadotropin deficiency and amenorrhea are commonly seen in women who participate in vigorous athletics or suffer from marked weight loss or a serious physical or psychological illness.

Destructive or space-occupying lesions of the pituitary, such as pituitary tumors, may result in a gradual loss of normal pituitary function. The order of loss is typically GH followed by the gonadotropins, TSH, and ACTH.

A congenital isolated deficiency most often involves GH or the gonadotropins. GH deficiency results in decreased growth velocity and delayed bone development. Gonadotropin deficiency results in delayed puberty and infertility.

Panhypopituitarism

Complete loss of pituitary function may be a consequence of pituitary tumors, hypothalamic tumors such as craniopharyngiomas, trauma, pituitary or hypothalamic surgery, vascular insufficiency such as postpartum necrosis or pituitary apoplexy, radiation, and infiltrative or granulomatous lesions such as hemochromatosis and sarcoidosis.

Functional loss may be sudden and catastrophic, as in pituitary apoplexy, or gradual, as with pituitary tumor growth. As was noted above, gradual loss usually occurs in the order GH, LH/FSH, TSH, ACTH.

Diagnosis

The diagnosis may involve various measures to visualize the pituitary, such as MRI, or to document other diseases involving the pituitary, such as hemochromatosis and sarcoidosis. Functional testing of the pituitary, however, is the essence of the diagnosis of hypopituitarism.

Adrenocorticotropic Hormone

A deficiency of ACTH is the most critical life-threatening pituitary deficiency. Testing of chronic deficiency, such as that seen after long-term exogenous glucocorticoid administration, may be carried out by measuring the adrenal cortisol response to stimulation by the synthetic ACTH analogue, cosyntropin (see Chap. 5-5). This test may be normal, however, in the setting of acute pituitary destruction because the adrenal is still capable of producing cortisol when stimulated. Consequently, a test that stimulates the hypothalamic-pituitary axis may occasionally be required, such as the insulin tolerance test, in which 0.05 to 0.1 unit of regular insulin per kilogram of body weight is administered to lower the blood glucose to less than 40 mg/dL. At this level of hypoglycemia, cortisol should be greater than 19 μg/dL. Pituitary production of GH also can be assessed with this test.

Growth Hormone

The adequacy of GH secretion by the pituitary is measured simultaneously with ACTH in the insulin tolerance test described above. At the time of significant hypoglycemia, the serum GH level should be higher than 10 ng/mL. Alternative stimuli for GH secretion include levodopa, arginine, clonidine, and exercise.

Thyroid-Stimulating Hormone

Pituitary TSH production is best tested by measuring serum TSH and free thyroid hormone. Low thyroid hormone with low or inappropriately normal TSH indicates inadequate pituitary TSH secretion. If other pituitary hormones are also deficient, no further thyroid testing is necessary. Before diagnosing isolated TSH deficiency, however, one needs to consider the euthyroid sick syndrome or a deficiency of thyroid-binding globulin.

Gonadotropins

Normal menstruation in women and normal testosterone and spermatogenesis in men rule out gonadotropin deficiency. In patients with amenorrhea, decreased libido, infertility, impotence, or absent or decreasing secondary sexual characteristics, low LH and FSH in the setting of low estrogen or testosterone confirms a gonadotropin deficiency.

Treatment

In most cases, hormone replacement for pituitary hormone deficiency is done with the missing target organ hormone, except for GH and in the case of the gonadotropins when fertility is desired.

Adrenocorticotropic Hormone

Patients require replacement of cortisol but not aldosterone, since the adrenal glands are intact. Glucocorticoid replacement is most often done with 7.5 mg prednisone or 30 mg hydrocortisone per day, with two-thirds given in the morning and one-third given in the afternoon or evening. The dose is temporarily increased during times of stress such as surgery and acute illness. Patients should be carefully educated about the importance of not discontinuing treatment.

Thyroid-Stimulating Hormone

Replacement is done with levothyroxine (0.05 to 0.15 mg per day). Since TSH is absent, clinical signs and the free thyroxine level are used to adjust the dose. It is important to note that thyroid hormone accelerates glucocorticoid metabolism so that treatment with levothyroxine before glucocorticoid replacement can worsen adrenal deficiency and precipitate adrenal crisis. Therefore, glucocorticoid replacement should always precede thyroxine replacement in patients with panhypopituitarism.

Gonadotropins

Estrogen-progesterone replacement in women and testosterone replacement in men relieve symptoms of hypogonadism but do not restore fertility. Ovarian hormone replacement in women can be done with several regimens, such as conjugated estrogens (0.625 mg per day) and medroxyprogesterone (2.5 mg per day). In men, replacement is most often done with testosterone esters given intramuscularly 200 mg every other week. When fertility is desired, ovulation or spermatogenesis stimulation can be attempted with gonadotropin injections over several months.

Growth Hormone

In adults, there is little indication for GH replacement, although research protocols are studying possible benefits on aging and GH has been approved for use in adults with GH deficiency. In children with isolated GH deficiency or panhypopituitarism whose epiphyses have not closed, growth retardation is treated with synthetic GH injections.

BIBLIOGRAPHY

Fauci AS, Braunwald E, Isselbacher KJ, et al (eds): *Harrison's Principles of Internal Medicine,* 14th ed. New York, McGraw-Hill, 1998.

Molitch ME, Findling JW, Ladenson PW, et al (eds): *Medical Knowledge Self-Assessment Program in the Subspecialty of Endocrinology and Metabolism.* Philadelphia, American College of Physicians, 1995.

Tierney LM Jr, McPhee SJ, Papadakis MA (eds): *Current Medical Diagnosis and Treatment,* 35th ed. Stamford, CT, Appleton & Lange, 1996.

Chapter 5–7
DIABETIC KETOACIDOSIS
Janice Herbert-Carter

DISCUSSION

Diabetic ketoacidosis (DKA) is a very serious acute complication of diabetes mellitus, primarily type 1 patients. Nondiabetic causes of ketoacidosis include starvation and alcoholism.

PATHOPHYSIOLOGY

Ketoacids (ketones, or ketone bodies) are formed by the metabolism of fats. The oxidation of fats does not produce carbon dioxide and water, as with carbohydrates. Instead, fats ultimately produce acetic acid, acetoacetic acid, and β-hydroxybutyrate, all of which are ketoacids. Under normal conditions, the body produces few of these, and their excretion is easily handled. In insulin-dependent diabetics, states of insulin deficiency lead to the preferential metabolism of fats because of the inability to utilize glucose. Thus, excessive amounts of ketones are formed. Their accumulation leads to systemic acidemia, ketoaciduria, and electrolyte imbalances. Some of the problems in DKA result from severe hyperglycemia: osmotic diuresis, dehydration, and hyperosmolarity.

The precipitating factors are most commonly infection and/or failure to take insulin. Additionally, trauma, emotional stress, or another serious intercurrent illness may initiate DKA. In older diabetics, myocardial infarction or stroke may precipitate the condition.

SIGNS AND SYMPTOMS

The presentation, especially early, may be nonspecific: abdominal pain, nausea and vomiting, anorexia, malaise, fatigue, thirst, tachycardia, tachypnea, and a fruity odor on the breath. Once the acidosis has progressed, the patient may present obtunded or in coma. In fact, coma may be the initial presentation of an undiagnosed diabetic child.

DIFFERENTIAL DIAGNOSIS

A comatose diabetic should bring to mind three possibilities: DKA, nonketotic hyperosmolar coma (NKHC), and hypoglycemia (insulin shock). Hypoglycemia is discussed in Chap. 5-8. NHKC is more common in type 2 diabetics, and acidosis is not present (unless it is due to another cause, e.g., lactic acidosis in septic shock). Severe hyperglycemia, dehydration, osmotic diuresis, and hyperosmolarity are found. Precipitating factors are similar to those in DKA, as is treatment.

LABORATORY TESTS

Serum ketones are invariably present. Hyperglycemia is also present; it is commonly extreme but sometimes only moderate. Urine ketones may be negative but are present. The common urine tests for ketones check only for acetoacetate, while the predominant one in DKA is β-hydroxybutyrate. Arterial blood gases will demonstrate acidosis (pH <7.4). Usually, there will also be low P_{CO_2} because of tachypnea (a compensatory mechanism caused by the metabolic acidosis). Electrolytes demonstrate an increased anion gap acidosis. Electrolyte abnormalities may be variable because the degree of dehydration and hyperglycemia affects measured values for sodium, potassium, and phosphate. These electrolytes should be monitored, and adjustments should be made as the dehydration and hyperglycemia are corrected.

TREATMENT

The key to therapy for DKA is regular insulin, ideally given by continuous intravenous infusion in an intensive care setting. If this is not available, periodic bolus intravenous injection is acceptable. The absorption of subcutaneous or intramuscular insulin is erratic, and therefore it should not be used. Rehydration is as important as is insulin. Vigorous fluid replacement should be given in a diabetic with normally functioning cardiovascular and renal systems. Fluid replacement must be more carefully attempted in the face of congestive heart failure or renal failure and in any elderly diabetic. Frequent monitoring of acidosis and electrolytes is essential. Insulin therapy should be continued until the acidosis is cleared even if normoglycemia appears first. In such instances, it may be necessary to switch from normal and half-normal saline to dextrose-containing solutions. As acidosis is corrected, potassium and phosphate repletion may be necessary. Bicarbonate therapy is rarely indicated if the pH is >7.1.

PEARLS

Although DKA has a mortality rate of 5 to 15 percent, it can be managed successfully if it is recognized and treated appropriately. The mainstays of treatment are intravenous regular insulin and fluids. These patients benefit from admission to the intensive care unit because frequent monitoring of vital signs, fluid intake and output, electrolytes, and blood gases is important.

Chapter 5–8
INSULIN SHOCK (HYPOGLYCEMIA)
Janice Herbert-Carter

DISCUSSION

Insulin shock is a misnomer because *shock* implies inadequate tissue perfusion. In this case, tissues are perfused but inadequate glucose is delivered. This can occur as a serious acute complication in diabetes mellitus (types 1 and 2). Any cause of an excess of insulin with a deficit of glucose intake may produce hypoglycemia. Thus, injection of too much insulin, ingestion of too much sulfonylurea, excessive exercise, failure of hepatic gluconeogenesis, impaired absorption of food from the intestine, and inadequate food intake may all lead to hypoglycemia.

SIGNS AND SYMPTOMS

A hypoglycemic patient may complain of sweating, palpitations, hunger, tremor, nervousness, and weakness, all of which result from stimulation of the beta-adrenergic system (epinephrine). These signs may be blunted or absent in a patient taking beta blockers such as propanolol (Inderal) for hypertension. Additionally, patients may have light-headedness, diplopia, headache, motor incoordination, confusion, obtundation, seizures, and frank coma resulting from glucose starvation in the central nervous system.

DIFFERENTIAL DIAGNOSIS

The signs and symptoms of hypoglycemia may be nonspecific, but in a known diabetic hypoglycemia must always be suspected.

In general, it does not hurt to err on the side of caution and give a diabetic a dose of glucose that will almost immediately correct the symptomatology if it is due to hypoglycemia. If it is not, little harm has been done. Hypoglycemia in a nondiabetic has varied causes, including insulinoma; hepatic, pituitary, thyroid, renal, or adrenal disease; gastrointestinal surgery; severe malnutrition; drugs and poisons (mushroom poisoning, salicylates, alcohol); sepsis; widespread cancer; and surreptitious insulin use. Surreptitious insulin use is most often seen in health care professionals who have knowledge about and access to drugs and syringes. Nevertheless, hypoglycemia in any nondiabetic is a rare finding.

LABORATORY TESTS

The serum glucose must always be low. How low is controversial. In general, most people have symptoms when serum glucose is less than 50. In known diabetics further laboratory testing is not needed. If surreptitious insulin ingestion is suspected, an insulin level together with a peptide C level (a degradation product produced from the proinsulin molecule) will be useful. In insulinoma, both insulin and peptide C will be high, indicating excess endogenous insulin. When hypoglycemia is due to exogenous insulin, the insulin level will be high but the peptide C level will be low or normal.

TREATMENT

Intravenous glucose (dextrose) is the treatment for hypoglycemia. In early stages, an alert patient may notice tremulousness, hunger, sweating, and palpitations and be able to take oral glucose or simply food. Absorption is not guaranteed, and the onset of action may be delayed. Thus, intravenous glucose is always best when it is available. A comatose patient will awaken quickly if hypoglycemia has not gone on so long that permanent brain damage has occurred. Even with rapid awakening, a hypoglycemic patient must be carefully monitored. One must remember the long half-life of the sulfonylureas. If these agents are the cause of the hypoglycemia, repeat attacks may occur after correction and repeat therapy may be needed.

Chapter 5–9
PAGET'S DISEASE
Timothy C. Evans

ETIOLOGY AND PATHOGENESIS

Paget's disease of bone is a focal bone disease that affects up to 3 percent of individuals over 60 years of age. It is characterized by excess bone lysis followed by replacement initially with vascular fibrous connective tissue and subsequently with bone that has a disorganized structure. Paget's disease resembles a benign bone neoplasm in some respects. Several lines of evidence suggest that Paget's disease may be a consequence of a viral infection.

Paget's disease is initially a localized focal disease and begins with a single site of aggressive bone lysis. After the rapid bone resorption by osteoclasts, fibrous connective tissue is made and bone formation begins, but the osteoblasts are unable to synthesize bone with a normal structure. Instead, the new bone has a disorganized architecture; it is less stable structurally and more liable to fracture.

The process of rapid bone resorption and eventual replacement by abnormal bone may extend from the original focal site, and so the disease may remain localized or extend to involve an entire bone. In some patients, multiple bones may be involved. During the active phase of resorption and bone reformation, pagetic bone is extremely vascular. The rapidity of the process and the microscopic structural abnormality of the new bone result in enlargement or deformity of involved bone.

CLINICAL PRESENTATION

Many patients with Paget's disease are asymptomatic, and the diagnosis is made or indicated by incidental x-ray or laboratory findings. In other patients, however, the symptoms include bone pain or deformity, fractures, deafness, or other neurologic deficits.

Pain is the most prominent symptom. The bones of the pelvis are most commonly involved, followed by the femur, skull, tibia, and spine. Pain may be due to the pagetic process and the development of the abnormal microarchitecture and deformity that result. Pain also may be due to microfractures, especially in weight-bearing bones such as the femur. Gross fractures also occur in pagetic bones and may occur in long bones, vertebrae, or the base of the skull.

Neurologic involvement results from damage to nerves by collapsed or deformed bone. Hearing loss can result from Paget's disease of the bones of the inner ear or from compression of cranial nerve VIII as it passes through the skull. Nerve root or spinal cord compression can result from Paget's disease of the spine.

CLINICAL COMPLICATIONS

In addition to the pain, deformity, fracture, and neurologic consequences of Paget's disease, certain specific complications may arise. When a significant portion of the skeleton is involved, the intense vascularity of pagetic bone during the active phase of resorption and reformation and the vasodilation in surrounding tissues can result in increased cardiac output. In some elderly patients with cardiac compromise, this can result in high-output cardiac failure.

Osteoarthritis commonly develops in joints adjacent to pagetic bones. Arthritis also can develop secondary to abnormal joint stresses caused by deformed or shortened bones.

The hypercalcemia that develops in immobilized patients with Paget's disease can result in kidney stones.

A serious but fortunately uncommon (about 1 percent of patients) complication of Paget's disease is sarcoma of bone. Successful treatment of this malignancy is unusual.

DIAGNOSIS
X-Ray Findings

Radiologic changes in bone are quite specific for Paget's disease. The initial change is the lytic lesion. As bone reformation follows, there is an increased density in the area of new bone. Mixed lesions may show increased thickness, irregular areas of decreased and increased lucency, cortical thickening, and deformity as the bone responds to mechanical stresses during remodeling. Fractures may appear as breaks in long bones or as collapsed bone in vertebrae or at the base of the skull.

The early lytic phase may be difficult to detect radiographically. Bone scans are more sensitive and can be used to locate areas of disease or define the extent of bone involvement.

Bone biopsy is seldom necessary, except in cases where primary or metastatic malignant disease is suspected.

Laboratory Tests

Serum calcium, phosphate, and parathyroid hormone (PTH) are typically normal. However, inactivity or bed rest in a patient with Paget's disease can result in hypercalcemia, sometimes of significant degree. In this circumstance, it is important to eliminate the possibility of primary hyperparathyroidism (by measuring the serum PTH, which would be normal or low in isolated Paget's disease), since coexistent hyperparathyroidism can increase the rate of progression of Paget's disease.

Several markers of the metabolic activity of bone remodeling can be measured. The most commonly measured, and often the initial indication of the presence of Paget's disease, is alkaline phosphatase. Alkaline phosphatase is elevated, often to very high levels, reflecting the activity of osteoblasts synthesizing new bone. A newer serum marker of bone formation is osteocalcin, a minor protein constituent of bone that also is elevated in Paget's disease.

Bone resorption markers, which may also be increased, include urine hydroxyproline and newer, more specific indicators of bone degradation: the terminal fragments of bone collagen excreted in the urine.

The differential diagnosis of Paget's disease includes other lytic or destructive diseases of bone, such as multiple myeloma and primary or metastatic malignancy. Blood and tissue diagnostic tests for these diseases should be carried out when appropriate.

TREATMENT

Treatment is usually instituted for pain, neurologic complications, fractures, hypercalcemia, or high cardiac output. Asymptomatic patients require no treatment, although suggestions have been made that antiresorptives (see below) be used to prevent more severe disease and its complications. Aspirin or nonsteroidal anti-inflammatory drugs may be used for pain in Paget's disease patients.

Appropriate orthotics should be used, and orthopedic measures should be carried out to maintain the functional geometry of bones, especially the weight-bearing bones of the lower extremities. When orthopedic surgery is necessary, it should be preceded by several weeks of antiresorptive therapy to decrease bleeding from pagetic bone and improve the strength of attachment of prosthetic or stabilizing devices. After surgery of any type, patients should be encouraged to ambulate as soon as medically appropriate to minimize the risk of hypercalcemia.

Medical therapy is directed at decreasing bone resorption by osteoclasts. The primary agents for this purpose are the calcitonins and the bisphosphonates. Both salmon calcitonin and human calcitonin are available and are given by subcutaneous injection. Antibody formation and insensitivity to salmon calcitonin develop in about 15 percent of these patients, who then can be treated with human calcitonin. Calcitonin administered by nasal spray is now available, but both the injectable and the nasal calcitonins are expensive.

Like calcitonin, the bisphosphonates decrease osteoclast activity and bone resorption. These new agents also have adverse effects on bone mineralization, but newer agents are being developed that retain potent antiresorptive activity but cause less inhibition of mineralization of new bone. The role of these agents in Paget's disease as well as other metabolic bone diseases is being defined and will continue to evolve as newer analogues are developed and their long-term effects are observed.

When calcitonin and bisphosphonates are unsuccessful, the cytotoxic agent mithramycin can be used. It has serious side effects, however, such as myelosuppression and renal dysfunction, and so it is used only in isolated refractory cases.

BIBLIOGRAPHY

Fauci AS, Braunwald E, Isselbacher KJ, et al (eds): *Harrison's Principles of Internal Medicine,* 14th ed. New York, McGraw-Hill, 1998.
Molitch ME, Findling JW, Ladenson PW, et al (eds): *Medical Knowledge Self-Assessment Program in the Subspecialty of Endocrinology and Metabolism.* Philadelphia, American College of Physicians, 1995.
Tierney LM Jr, McPhee SJ, Papadakis MA (eds): *Current Medical Diagnosis and Treatment,* 35th ed. Stamford, CT, Appleton & Lange, 1996.

Chapter 5–10
PARATHYROID DISORDERS
Timothy C. Evans

DISCUSSION

The four parathyroid glands are behind and partially in the thyroid gland. The function of the parathyroids is regulation of serum calcium through the secretion of parathyroid hormone (PTH). Excessive PTH results in hypercalcemia, and insufficient PTH results in hypocalcemia.

CALCIUM METABOLISM

Calcium is a major body constituent, but only about 1 percent of total calcium circulates in the blood; most is in bone. Calcium in the blood is partly bound to protein, with about 55 percent free as ionized calcium. It is the ionized fraction that is required for proper neuromuscular functioning. Consequently, correct interpretation of serum calcium requires that an adjustment of the normal range of total serum calcium be made on the basis of the serum albumin because of the protein binding of calcium. When the albumin is low, the normal calcium also is low in a ratio of about 0.8 to 1.0 mg/dL calcium for each gram of albumin (less than 4 gm/dL).

The serum calcium level is closely regulated by two hormones—PTH and vitamin D—that act on bone, the kidneys, and the gastrointestinal tract to increase serum calcium. There is no mechanism in humans to lower serum calcium except renal clearance of calcium and the absence of PTH and vitamin D effects.

Parathyroid Hormone

PTH is secreted by the four parathyroid glands in response to hypocalcemia. In turn, PTH raises serum calcium through direct effects on bone and the kidneys and indirect effects on the intestine. PTH stimulates the resorption of bone and decreases the renal clearance of calcium. It also stimulates the renal activation of vitamin D. Each of these mechanisms increases the serum calcium level. When the serum ionized calcium reaches a threshold level, PTH secretion is inhibited.

Vitamin D

The hormone vitamin D is synthesized in the skin and ingested in the diet. With adequate exposure to sunlight, however, vitamin

D is synthesized in adequate amounts and no dietary supplementation is necessary. The critical step in its biosynthesis takes place in the skin under the influence of ultraviolet light. Once it is formed, vitamin D must undergo two hydroxylation steps to become the active agent, 1,25-dihydroxyvitamin D. The first hydroxylation takes place in the liver to form 25-hydroxyvitamin D. The second, rate-limiting hydroxylation to 1,25-dihydroxyvitamin D takes place in the kidney under the influence of PTH. The primary effect of 1,25-dihydroxyvitamin D is increased calcium and phosphate absorption from the intestine.

HYPERCALCEMIA

Hypercalcemia has a wide variety of causes, but 90 percent of cases are caused by primary hyperparathyroidism or malignancy. Other causes include circumstances of high bone turnover such as thyrotoxicosis and immobilization, excess exogenous or endogenous vitamin D, renal disease, and an abnormal upward adjustment of the PTH/calcium set point seen in familial hypocalciuric hypercalcemia (FHH) and lithium therapy.

The PTH in hyperparathyroidism is increased. The PTH in FHH and lithium therapy also may be inappropriately normal or minimally elevated, as is discussed below. All other causes of hypercalcemia are characterized and thus distinguished by appropriately suppressed serum PTH levels. Some malignancies (especially breast cancer) cause hypercalcemia through bony metastasis, others by producing an immunologically distinct protein with PTH-like properties called parathyroid hormone–related protein (PTHrP), and still others by synthesizing vitamin D.

Hypercalcemia of any cause may be associated with symptoms that include anorexia, nausea and vomiting, constipation, weakness, confusion, and polyuria. At higher calcium levels, stupor, coma, and cardiac arrhythmias may occur.

Hyperparathyroidism

Hyperparathyroidism (HPT) is a consequence of excess secretion of PTH. Primary HPT occurs mostly in middle-aged to older adults. It once was thought to be an unusual problem, but an incidence of 0.1 percent has been found in asymptomatic adults since the advent of routine multiphasic serum chemistry analysis. In 80 percent of cases the cause of primary HPT is a single hyperfunctioning benign parathyroid adenoma. In most of the remaining cases all four parathyroid glands are hyperplastic and hyperfunctioning, and in a few patients parathyroid carcinoma is found.

Secondary hyperparathyroidism occurs primarily in the setting of renal disease, in which vitamin D activation is inadequate, leading to decreased intestinal calcium absorption, and in which phosphate retention impairs bone responsiveness to PTH. In this circumstance, the parathyroids respond with excessive PTH secretion in an attempt to normalize serum calcium from the bone reservoir.

Occasionally, primary HPT is familial as an isolated abnormality or as part of the multiple endocrine neoplasia (MEN) syndrome, types 1 and 2a.

Clinical Findings

The clinical presentation of primary hyperparathyroidism is largely dependent on the level of hypercalcemia. Half or more of patients with primary HPT are asymptomatic and are discovered only when hypercalcemia is found on routine blood testing. In other patients the symptoms are due to hypercalcemia, calcium deposition in tissues, and the effects of PTH on bone.

Hypercalcemia has a variety of neuromuscular effects. Anorexia, nausea and vomiting, and constipation are common. Other gastrointestinal effects include an increased incidence of peptic ulcer disease and pancreatitis. Neurologic effects, which may be subtle or profound depending on the calcium level, include fatigue, weakness, confusion, stupor, and coma. Polyuria results from mild renal unresponsiveness to arginine vasopressin. Hypertension is more common in patients with hypercalcemia. Cardiac arrhythmias occur at high calcium levels.

High extracellular calcium can result in the precipitation of calcium salts. This occurs most commonly in the kidney, where about 10 percent of patients with primary HPT present with renal lithiasis. This occurs much less than it did in past years, when hyperparathyroidism went largely undiagnosed until symptoms developed.

Bone pain also occurs in HPT, and in some patients decreased bone density and osteoporosis result from the increased bone turnover. The classic bone disease of HPT, osteitis fibrosa cystica, is now uncommon. This abnormality consists of increased noncalcified space in bones, replacement with fibrous tissue, multiple lytic lesions on x-ray, and subperiosteal resorption seen best in the phalanges of the hands. Bone disease is more pronounced in secondary HPT than in primary HPT.

Diagnosis

The diagnosis of HPT begins with a demonstration of hypercalcemia after correction for serum albumin. When there is doubt about the significance of serum protein-binding effects, ionized calcium can be measured, but this is seldom necessary. The distinction of the cause of the hypercalcemia next depends on the serum PTH level.

The advent of hormone radioimmunoassays has made the differential diagnosis of HPT relatively straightforward. With the exceptions discussed below, only the hypercalcemia of HPT is associated with an increased PTH level, which establishes the diagnosis. In all other cases of hypercalcemia, PTH is appropriately suppressed.

Several assays for PTH are available, but the best is the double antibody immunoradiometric assay (IRMA), which measures the intact PTH molecule. Other assays include the PTH N-terminal and C-terminal assays, which are not as useful. The C-terminal assay in particular is inaccurate in the setting of renal insufficiency, which is a common setting for hypercalcemia.

Clinical evaluation and routine laboratory tests are often sufficient to suggest the correct diagnosis of non-PTH-mediated hypercalcemia, such as malignancy, thyrotoxicosis, or renal disease.

There are two settings in which the cause of hypercalcemia is an abnormal set point of the PTH/calcium threshold. In these patients, the PTH level may not be suppressed in the setting of hypercalcemia and therefore must be distinguished from HPT. These cases are FHH and lithium therapy. In each case, there is an insensitivity of the parathyroid to calcium such that PTH continues to be secreted until the serum calcium level reaches a higher than normal level, at which point PTH secretion is inhibited. The PTH levels are typically normal, which is inappropriate for an increased calcium level, or only slightly increased.

FHH is distinguished from HPT by measuring the urinary excretion of calcium, which is normal to increased in HPT but low in FHH. FHH is a benign condition that does not require treatment and does not respond to parathyroidectomy, and so it is important to exclude it before proceeding to surgery for HPT.

The diagnosis of lithium-induced hypercalcemia is most easily established by demonstrating normalization of laboratory abnormalities when lithium is discontinued.

Treatment

Treatment of significant HPT is surgical. Removal of an adenoma is usually curative. Hyperplasia is treated by removing 3.5 parathyroid glands. Carcinoma is excised with wide margins. Pre- or intraoperative ultrasound can be useful in the localization of a parathyroid adenoma, but other imaging studies are not very helpful in HPT. Though various scanning techniques have been used, none adds much to direct observation carried out by a skilled parathyroid surgeon during neck exploration.

Postoperative hypocalcemia may require large doses of calcium and short-acting vitamin D until the normal function of the remaining parathyroid tissue returns.

Treatment of asymptomatic HPT is more controversial and depends on a number of factors. In general, surgery is recommended for patients less than 50 years old and those with serum calcium more than 1 to 1.5 mg/dL above normal, urinary calcium excretion higher than 400 mg/24 h, renal calcification on x-ray, or bone density more than 2 standard deviations below normal.

Patients who are not operated on should be followed carefully with serum and urinary calcium determinations and periodic radiographic studies.

HYPOCALCEMIA

Like hypercalcemia, hypocalcemia has a wide variety of causes, but it is much less common. Chronic hypocalcemia most often results from hypoparathyroidism, vitamin D insufficiency, or renal disease. Among the many causes of acute or transient hypocalcemia are parathyroidectomy, hypomagnesemia, and pancreatitis.

The symptoms of hypocalcemia include neuromuscular irritability with muscle and abdominal cramps, carpopedal spasm, tingling of the lips and hands, tetany, and convulsions. Chronic hypocalcemia also may be associated with personality changes and cataracts.

The classic physical signs of the neuromuscular irritability of hypocalcemia are Chvostek's sign and Trousseau's sign. Chvostek's sign is a contraction of the facial muscles elicited by tapping the facial nerve at its point of entry into the side of the face. Trousseau's sign is a carpal spasm after the inflation of a blood pressure cuff on the upper arm.

Hypoparathyroidism

Hypoparathyroidism most often follows parathyroid or thyroid surgery. The deficiency may be transient or permanent. There are also several forms of congenital, familial, and autoimmune hypoparathyroidism. Iron can accumulate in and damage the parathyroids in patients with hemochromatosis or iron overload from multiple transfusions.

Serum calcium corrected for albumin is low, and PTH is low. Serum magnesium should be checked, since magnesium is necessary for PTH secretion and hypomagnesemia will result in reversible hypoparathyroidism.

The goal of treatment is to maintain the serum calcium in the low normal range. Transient hypocalcemia may require only brief supplementation with intravenous or oral calcium, vitamin D, and magnesium if they are deficient. Chronic hypoparathyroidism is treated with calcium 1 to 3 g per day and vitamin D. Several forms of vitamin D are available for use, including vitamin D and 1,25-dihydroxyvitamin D. Vitamin D, ergocalciferol, is given in doses of 25,000 to 200,000 units per day. 1,25-dihydroxyvitamin D, calcitriol, is given in doses of 0.25 to 1.0 μg per day. High doses of vitamin D are required because in the absence of PTH, the 1-hydroxylation step in the kidneys is slow. When they are given along with calcium, however, both forms of vitamin D can result in hypercalcemia, and so careful monitoring is required.

BIBLIOGRAPHY

Fauci AS, Braunwald E, Isselbacher KJ, et al (eds): *Harrison's Principles of Internal Medicine,* 14th ed. New York, McGraw-Hill, 1998.
Molitch ME, Findling JW, Ladenson PW, et al (eds): *Medical Knowledge Self-Assessment Program in the Subspecialty of Endocrinology and Metabolism.* Philadelphia, American College of Physicians, 1995.
Tierney LM Jr, McPhee SJ, Papadakis MA (eds): *Current Medical Diagnosis and Treatment,* 35th ed. Stamford, CT, Appleton & Lange, 1996.

Chapter 5–11
POSTERIOR PITUITARY DISORDERS
Timothy C. Evans

DISCUSSION

The posterior pituitary is an extension of neurons from specific areas in the hypothalamus via the pituitary stalk to a position posterior to the anterior pituitary in the sella turcica. The hormones secreted by the posterior pituitary are the peptides arginine vasopressin (AVP) [also known as antidiuretic hormone (ADH)] and oxytocin. AVP acts on the renal tubules, primarily at the collecting duct, to cause water reabsorption that results in urinary concentration. The release of AVP is coordinated with activation of the thirst center in the brain, which causes water-seeking behavior. The stimuli for AVP secretion are hemoconcentration and hypovolemia. Osmoreceptors in the hypothalamus are the primary regulators of AVP secretion. Even a small increase in hemoconcentration will result in increased AVP secretion and strikingly increased urine concentration. Hypotension, which is monitored by stretch receptors in the left atrium, carotids, and aorta, is also a potent stimulus of AVP secretion. A number of drugs can stimulate AVP release, and ethanol has a diuretic effect by inhibiting AVP secretion.

Oxytocin is a similar peptide hormone that has its major effects on the uterus and breast, causing uterine contraction and breast milk ejection, respectively, at the time of parturition.

DIABETES INSIPIDUS

Diabetes insipidus (DI) is an uncommon disease characterized by the inappropriate production of large quantities of dilute urine. It is caused by a deficiency of AVP or renal resistance to AVP. It must be distinguished from other causes of diuresis, such as increased water intake, diuretic use, and osmotic diuresis as in diabetes mellitus.

Clinical Presentation

The hallmark of diabetes insipidus is excess urine volume. In its most severe form, urine output may reach 20 L per day. In an otherwise, healthy, conscious person, the polyuria is accompanied by intense polydipsia. When free access to water is available, there may be no other symptoms. In less severe forms of DI, with only a partial deficiency of posterior pituitary secretion of AVP, the urine output and thirst are less striking.

When water is not available or the patient is unconscious or unaware of thirst (as in the case of destructive lesions of the thirst center), dehydration, hypotension, and vascular collapse can follow rapidly, depending on the degree of AVP abnormality.

When urine loss is unmatched by water intake, the laboratory abnormalities include hypernatremia and hyperosmolality despite a large-volume hypotonic urine.

Etiology

Diabetes insipidus may be due to insufficient secretion of AVP or an inadequate renal response to AVP. Insufficient posterior pituitary AVP secretion—central DI—has several causes. Neoplastic, either benign or malignant, or infiltrative lesions, such as sarcoid granulomas, can result in partial or complete loss of AVP secretion. Pituitary or hypothalamic surgery and head trauma can interfere with AVP synthesis or passage down the pituitary stalk to the posterior pituitary. Idiopathic DI also occurs and can be sporadic or familial. In each of these cases, the abnormality is insufficient secretion of AVP in response to hemoconcentration and hypovolemia.

Inadequate renal sensitivity to AVP is called nephrogenic DI. In this case, AVP is secreted by the posterior pituitary but the urine remains dilute. The causes of nephrogenic DI include intrinsic renal disease, hypokalemia, chronic hypercalcemia, systemic diseases such as sickle cell anemia, and drugs such as lithium and demeclocycline.

Diagnosis

A careful history and physical examination may reveal other causes of polyuria and polydipsia, such as systemic disease, diuretic or other drug use, and excess water intake (oral or intravenous). Serum glucose, potassium, and calcium levels should be checked.

When no other cause is apparent, the essence of DI evaluation is the serum and urine osmolality response to dehydration and AVP administration. Testing should be done under closely monitored conditions. Water intake is withheld, the patient's vital signs are monitored, and serum and urine osmolality are followed frequently. DI is characterized by increasing serum osmolality but persistently low urine osmolality. An injection of AVP (or the synthetic AVP analogue, desmopressin) is then administered. Patients with central DI show an increased urine concentration, while patients with nephrogenic DI have no response. Serum AVP measured before the administration of exogenous AVP is low in central DI patients and elevated in nephrogenic DI patients.

Treatment

Treatment of central or nephrogenic DI secondary to other central nervous system, systemic, or renal disease should include attention to the underlying disease. The water metabolism abnormality of central DI is relatively easily and conveniently treated in most patients with desmopressin given as an intranasal spray 0.05 to 0.1 mL once or twice a day. The less common nephrogenic DI is more difficult to treat and may require thiazide diuretics to decrease the glomerular filtration rate and limit renal water loss.

SYNDROME OF INAPPROPRIATE ANTIDIURETIC HORMONE

The syndrome of inappropriate antidiuretic hormone (SIADH) is characterized by euvolemic hyponatremia. By definition, increased AVP (or ADH) is not inappropriate when it is secreted in circumstances of hypovolemia or hyperosmolality. Thus, SIADH is not present in cases of hypovolemic hyponatremia, such as mineralocorticoid deficiency, or dehydration or diuretic use with free fluid replacement. Similarly, SIADH is not present in conditions of edematous hypervolemic hyponatremia such as congestive heart failure, nephrotic syndrome, and renal disease. AVP secretion rates are also high in hypernatremic dehydration without fluid replacement but again are not inappropriate.

Clinical Presentation

Most often SIADH is discovered by the finding of hyponatremia on electrolyte testing. Since SIADH sometimes is associated with other diseases, the symptoms may be limited to those of the underlying disease. In other cases, the hyponatremia itself, if it is severe enough, may cause symptoms that include lethargy, confusion, stupor, and coma. Neuromuscular excitability, muscle twitches, or even seizures can occur if the serum sodium is very low or if the decrease is rapid. Symptoms are unusual if the serum sodium is higher than 125 meq/L.

Etiology

Since AVP is synthesized in the hypothalamus, the cause of SIADH is often neurologic. In these cases, which include stroke, meningitis, tumors, and trauma, there is presumed to be an abnormality of neural input to the hypothalamus or of the perception of neural input by the hypothalamus that leads to inappropriate AVP release. In other cases, SIADH results from ectopic overproduction of AVP by tumors, primarily small cell lung carcinomas, and is associated with a variety of other pulmonary diseases, such as infections and asthma. Lastly, a wide variety of drugs have been associated with SIADH, including hypoglycemic agents such as chlorpropamide, neuroactive drugs such as amitriptyline and carbamazepine, and antineoplastic drugs, among others.

Diagnosis

The diagnosis is suggested by the finding of hyponatremia. Serum uric acid and blood urea nitrogen are frequently low from increased urinary clearance. The physical examination of volume status is critical in the diagnosis. Dehydration with postural change in pulse and blood pressure and volume overload with edema by definition rule out the diagnosis of SIADH.

Urinary sodium is also helpful in the evaluation of hyponatremia. If the urine sodium is low (less than 20 meq/L) and there is evidence of dehydration, total body sodium is depleted and the treatment consists of normal saline. Dehydration and normal or elevated urine sodium suggest renal disease, diuretic use, or adrenocortical insufficiency. The immediate treatment is normal saline to replete volume. Expanded volume with low urine sodium suggests inadequate renal perfusion such as that which occurs with congestive heart failure, and the correct response is to treat the underlying disease. SIADH is characterized by no edema and elevated urinary sodium resulting from increased renal clearance.

Treatment

Just as DI is treated by administering water, SIADH is treated by water restriction and the provision of adequate sodium in the diet. If there are underlying etiologic features that can be treated, such as CNS or pulmonary disease, they obviously should be addressed. The drugs administered to the patient should be reviewed to see if they may be causative and should be modified if possible. Water restriction results in slow, safe correction of hyponatremia. The patient is typically asymptomatic as long as the serum sodium remains above 125 meq/L.

There are circumstances in which more rapid correction of hyponatremia is indicated, but this treatment entails significant risks to the patient. When the serum sodium has been chronically low, it is often asymptomatic and can be corrected slowly. When the serum sodium is less than 120 meq/L and is associated with symptoms, however, which often occurs when the hyponatremia is very severe or develops rapidly, the correction also should be more rapid. This generally is accomplished by administering hypertonic saline with close monitoring at a rate that leads to a serum sodium increase not exceeding about 0.5 meq/L/h until the serum sodium is above 120 meq/L. More rapid correction can lead to brain swelling and a fatal CNS demyelination syndrome called central pontine myelinolysis.

BIBLIOGRAPHY

Fauci AS, Braunwald E, Isselbacher KJ, et al (eds): *Harrison's Principles of Internal Medicine,* 14th ed. New York, McGraw-Hill, 1998.

Molitch ME, Findling JW, Ladenson PW, et al (eds): *Medical Knowledge Self-Assessment Program in the Subspecialty of Endocrinology and Metabolism.* Philadelphia, American College of Physicians, 1995.

Tierney LM Jr, McPhee SJ, Papadakis MA et al (eds): *Current Medical Diagnosis and Treatment,* 35th ed. Stamford, CT, Appleton & Lange, 1996.

Chapter 5–12
OBESITY

Kimberly Brown Paterson

DISCUSSION

Obesity in America is a multi-million-dollar business. Any amount of time spent examining the popular press or television will reveal dozens of advertisements for weight loss products and programs. There are as many speculations as there are treatments when one ponders the question of what causes obesity and why some individuals are more susceptible to weight problems.

According to a National Institutes of Health (NIH) panel, in the United States 20 to 30 percent of adult men and 30 to 40 percent of adult women are considered obese, with females having a higher risk for obesity. Blacks, especially black women, are more apt to be obese than are whites, and the poor are more often obese than the rich regardless of race.[1]

With these statistics in mind, the question is, What exactly separates ideal body weight from obesity? Ideal body weight can be estimated from a standardized height/weight table or as follows:

- *Women:* 45 kg for first 152 cm of height plus 0.9 kg for each centimeter above 152
- *Men:* 48 kg for first 152 cm plus 1.1 kg for each centimeter above 152

The NIH currently defines obesity as a relative weight over 120 percent, mild obesity as a relative weight of 120 to 140 percent, moderate obesity as a relative weight of 140 to 200 percent, and severe or "morbid" obesity as a relative weight over 200 percent.

However, it is important not only to note weight percentages but also to evaluate weight distribution. Fat distribution patterns are determined by measuring waist and hip circumferences and calculating the waist to hips ratio (WHR).[2]

The android pattern (male pattern or abdominal obesity) has WHR higher than 0.85 for females and 0.95 for males. The gynoid pattern (female pattern or gluteal obesity) has WHR less than 0.85 for females and 0.95 for males. Recent data suggest that excess fat around the waist and flank is a greater health hazard than is fat in the thighs and buttocks. Obese patients with high WHRs have a significantly greater risk of diabetes, stroke, coronary artery disease, and early death than do equally obese patients with lower WHRs (Table 5-12-1).[2]

Table 5-12-1. Weights at Ages 25 to 59 Based on Lowest Mortality

Height in Feet	Height in Inches	Small Frame	Medium Frame	Large Frame
		MEN		
5	2	128–134	131–141	138–150
5	3	130–136	133–143	140–153
5	4	132–138	135–145	142–156
5	5	134–140	137–148	144–160
5	6	136–142	139–151	146–164
5	7	138–145	142–154	159–168
5	8	140–148	145–157	152–172
5	9	142–151	148–160	155–176
5	10	144–154	151–163	158–180
5	11	146–157	154–166	161–184
6	0	149–160	157–170	164–188
6	1	152–164	160–174	168–192
6	2	155–168	164–178	172–197
6	3	158–172	167–182	176–202
6	4	162–176	171–187	181–207
		WOMEN		
4	10	102–111	109–121	118–131
4	11	103–113	111–123	120–134
5	0	104–115	113–126	122–137
5	1	106–118	115–129	125–140
5	2	108–121	118–132	128–143
5	3	111–124	121–135	131–147
5	4	114–127	124–138	134–151
5	5	117–130	127–141	137–155
5	6	120–133	130–144	140–159
5	7	123–136	133–147	143–163
5	8	126–139	136–150	146–167
5	9	129–142	139–153	149–170
5	10	132–145	142–156	152–173
5	11	135–148	145–159	155–176
6	0	138–151	148–162	158–179

Note: Assumes indoor clothing weighing 5 lb for men and 3 lb for women and shoes with 1-in. heels.

SOURCE: Metropolitan Life Insurance Co., New York, NY, 1983.

DIAGNOSIS

Until recently obesity was thought to be related to an excessive intake of calories along with a sedentary life-style. However, strong evidence points toward genetic, medical, and environmental factors as influencing the development of obesity. Specific causes of excessive weight are multifactorial. Rare genetic syndromes have been described, as have more common causes, such as insulinoma, hypothalamic disorders, Cushing's syndrome, and the use of corticosteroid drugs. Idiopathic obesity is generally thought to be due to an imbalance between food intake and energy expenditure (including physical activity and metabolic rate).[3]

The diagnosis of obesity is based largely on the history and complete physical examination. Historic information regarding age at onset is particularly important, as prepuberty and young adulthood appear to be sensitive periods for the development of obesity. Family history, eating and exercise behavior, recent weight changes, occupational history, previous weight loss history, and psychosocial factors also should be addressed. Information related to the use of laxatives, hormones, and nutritional supplements should draw attention.

Physical examination should assess the degree and distribution of body fat, the overall nutritional status, and, as was noted above, possible secondary causes, including hypothalamic disorders and Cushing's syndrome. Hypothyroidism (see Chap. 5-3) can cause obesity secondary to diminished energy needs. Cushing's disease causes obesity involving centripetal fat stores, the face, and cervical or supraclavicular fat deposits. Insulinoma causes obesity from increased energy intake secondary to recurrent hypoglycemia. The Laurence-Moon-Biedl and Prader-Willi syndromes are rare disorders that are thought to be hypothalamic in origin and feature obesity and hypogonadism.

LABORATORY STUDIES

Further study to rule out these possible secondary causes should include serum TSH determination and dexamethasone suppression testing. Laboratory tests of all patients ideally include cardiac risk factors: serum cholesterol, triglycerides, and glucose.[4]

TREATMENTS

Treatment strategies for weight reduction vary widely. The most successful programs include behavior modification, and low-fat, low-calorie eating combined with aerobic exercise. The overall goal must be weight maintenance. Most important, the job of the practitioner is to provide long-term follow-up to prevent further weight gain or regain after weight loss. Recent studies showed that only 20 percent of patients will lose 20 lb and maintain the loss for over 2 years and 5 percent will maintain a 40-lb loss. With this information, it can be a difficult task to develop an appropriate program for weight maintenance. The steps include

1. *Nutritional principles* must apply to obese as well as normal-weight individuals. Low-fat, low-calorie, high-fiber, and complex carbohydrate foods should be the staple of weight loss. Foods that provide large amounts of calories and little nutritional value should be greatly restricted. Special diets that advocate restriction to one or two foods, offer a high protein intake, or limit carbohydrate intake are of little value.
2. *Behavior modification* provides useful techniques. Planning and recording are specific skills that can reveal habits and cues (emotional and situational). They also may provide a source of information that assists the practitioner in problem solving.
3. *Exercise* provides multiple benefits. An aerobic exercise program most importantly can increase daily energy expenditures. It is also helpful in preventing the decrease in basal energy expenditure seen in very low calorie and low-nutrient diets.
4. *Long-term maintenance* should be included. Social support can be drawn from a therapist or from family and peer group involvement to reinforce behavioral change.

Unfortunately for some obese individuals, very low calorie diets may be needed as an aggressive treatment program. These diets (400 to 500 calories per day) are often "liquid" and result in rapid weight loss. Dehydration, hypotension, fatigue, muscle cramps, headaches, and constipation are frequent complaints with these programs. Weight loss of 4 to 5 lb per week is not uncommon; however, very low calorie diets have a high percentage of relapse after discontinuation.

Patients with recent myocardial infarction, a cerebrovascular accident, renal or hepatic disease, cancer, or insulin-dependent diabetes mellitus are not good candidates for these very low calorie diet programs. For all participants, physician monitoring is extremely important.

Medications, both over the counter and prescription, are often the most popular obesity treatments. In the past, various amphetamine-containing medications were commonly prescribed, but they have a high potential for abuse and habituation and have lost favor among practitioners. More recently, the popularity of "phen-fen" (a combination of phendimetrazine and fenfluramine) led to an explosion of medical weight control clinics utilizing those medications as a basis for therapy. The combination

Table 5-12-2. Selected Medications Used in the Management of Obesity

Medications	Dose
Phentermine (Fastin, Ionamin)	30 mg PO every morning
Mazindol (Sanorex)	1 mg up to three times per day with meals
Fenfluramine (Pondimin)	20 mg three times per day up to 120 mg daily*
Phendimetrazine (Prelu-2, Plegine)	105 mg every morning
Phenylpropanolamine (OTC) (Acutrim)	75 mg every morning after breakfast

Contraindications to Some of These Medications Include

Advanced atherosclerosis
Symptomatic cardiovascular disease
Hypertension
Hyperthyroidism
Glaucoma
History of drug abuse
Agitated states
Use of a monoamine oxidase inhibitor[2]

* Removed from the market in 1997.

was removed from the market in late 1997 secondary to claims of heart damage to users. Controversy exists over the efficacy of these products and the specific indications for their use. Some studies show short-term results, but long-term benefit is usually not evident without behavior modification. Common medications and their contraindications are listed in Table 5-12-2.

Surgery is usually considered the last resort. More than 100,000 obese patients have opted for vertical-banded gastroplasty or gastric bypass procedures. Both procedures result in increased weight loss, but surgeons tend to favor the gastric bypass. The perioperative mortality rate generally averages 1 percent but can range from 1 to 4 percent at different centers.

DISPOSITION

The prevention or avoidance of obesity starts with regular exercise and a reasonable diet, especially in children and young adults. Patient education materials along with excellent advice and answers to tough questions can be obtained from[4]

American Dietetic Association
620 N. Michigan Avenue
Chicago, IL 60611

American Heart Association
7320 Greenville Avenue
Dallas, TX 75231

Consumer Nutrition Center
Human Nutrition Information Service
Federal Center Building
Hyattsville, MD 20782

REFERENCES

1. Goodrick GK, Foreyt JP: Why treatments for obesity don't last. *J Am Diet Assoc* 91(10):1243–1247, 1991.
2. Schroeder SA: *Current Medical Diagnosis and Treatment.* Norwalk, CT, Appleton & Lange, 1992, pp 950–959.
3. Fauci AS, Braunwald E, Isselbacher KJ, et al (eds): *Harrison's Principles of Internal Medicine, 14th ed. Companion Handbook.* New York, McGraw-Hill, 1998, pp 227–232.
4. Paterson KB: *Healthweights: A 10-Week Comprehensive Weight Management Program,* 1991, U.S. Copyright TX 489964.

Gastroenterology

Chapter 6-1
ACUTE GASTROENTERITIS
Anne P. Heinly

DISCUSSION

Acute gastroenteritis (AGE) is a common diagnosis that is uncommonly hard to define. Some textbooks do not list it as an entity. Alternative names include viral diarrhea, stomach flu, infectious diarrhea, and rotavirus infection. By consensus, it is a self-limiting viral or bacterial inflammation of the stomach and small intestines producing a characteristic set of symptoms in all human beings at some time in their lives. The colon may be involved with AGE, but diseases involving the colon are usually listed independently as colitis. (See Chap. 6-4, "Colitis.") The vast majority of cases are viral infections (estimated at 40 to 50 percent), and the remainder are probably short-lived, food-borne bacterial infections. Infants and young children have on average two episodes of AGE prior to age 3 and gain immunity to these particular viral pathogens in the process. The vast majority of patients will have a total of two to three episodes of AGE in a lifetime, although environmental factors, like living conditions, widespread food contamination, and travel to developing countries, may increase that dramatically.

PATHOGENESIS

Viral infections of the gastrointestinal tract frequently cause a secretory diarrhea. There is an increase in chloride and water secretion with the inhibition of normal intestinal mucosal sodium and water absorption. The result is copious watery diarrhea without pus or blood. Rotavirus infections are more common in children and can cause an enormous loss of fluids. The Norwalk virus is more prevalent in school-age children and adults. Both viruses and bacteria are found in tainted food or drinking water. They are also spread by the oral-fecal route, which accounts for the majority of community outbreaks. Table 6-1-1 lists the usual causes of acute gastroenteritis. Note the overlap with acute and chronic diarrheal pathogens. (See Chap. 6-7, "Diarrhea.")

SYMPTOMS

The classic symptoms of acute gastroenteritis are the sudden onset of watery diarrhea, one stool about every half hour to hour; nausea and vomiting, every 1 to 2 h; abdominal cramps, malaise (generalized aches and pains), anorexia, fatigue, low-grade fever, dull headache, and chills. Symptoms can appear within 4 h of contamination or as late as 48 h later. The vast majority will start resolving in 6 to 24 h. It is not uncommon to see the patient in the office *after* the worst is over.

The very young, the very old, and the immunosuppressed patient can become quite ill with this usually self-limiting condition. Infants and toddlers can suffer severe dehydration with a history of decreased tears, less urination, poor feeding and/or lethargy, as key points to explore with the parents. The aged may have a change in mental status or become obtunded secondary to dehydration and electrolyte imbalances. In the immunosuppressed (HIV, chemotherapy patients, renal disease) these simple infections can be life-threatening with sepsis and prolongation of symptoms. All these groups deserve special attention and close follow-up.

OBJECTIVE

An ill appearing patient will lie quietly on the examining table, frequently pale and fatigued. Vital signs may reveal a normotensive patient with tachycardia. Orthostatic vital signs may be positive (BP down 10 points, pulse up 20 points) depending on the level of dehydration. Oral mucosa may be dry with slight halitosis. Check the skin and eyes for evidence of dehydration. Abdominal examination usually reveals a nondistended appearance with hyperactive bowel sounds. Palpation may reveal a soft, diffusely tender abdomen without mass effect or rebound tenderness. The area is usually tympanic, and there is no hepatosplenomegaly. Rectal examination is usually negative for findings, including blood.

DIAGNOSTIC CONSIDERATIONS

The danger of an AGE diagnosis is that so many other disease processes can present with similar symptoms. Clues pointing to AGE include the following: severity of symptoms, AGE is usually mild; peak frequency is fall and winter; exposures are usually easily tracked; and the patient should be much improved within 24 to 48 h. On the other hand, AGE symptoms can represent anything from early appendicitis to multiple myeloma (Table 6-1-2). An index of suspicion is required when you are seeing AGE during a community outbreak. A more serious diagnosis may be lurking, and the young, the elderly, and the immunosuppressed may have a more virulent course.

During the last few years, there have been outbreaks of viral gastroenteritis associated with the consumption of raw shellfish—specifically oysters. Besides viral contamination, other pathogens have been *Vibrio* species, *Salmonella*, *Campylobacter*, and hepatitis A.[1]

Also consider a different diagnosis when the patient has had several episodes of AGE in a short period of time. The average adult will have only two or three episodes of AGE in a lifetime because immunity develops to the common viruses and bacteria. If a patient is having frequent episodes, consider chronic infectious disorders, peptic ulcer disease, irritable bowel syndrome, obstruction disorders, Crohn's disease, or ulcerative colitis.

LABORATORY TESTS

Identification of the specific virus causing an episode of AGE is difficult in common practice. There are laboratories that make the diagnosis with immune electron microscopy and enzyme immunoassays. Usually, no laboratory studies are done in the first 24 h of a classic acute gastroenteritis. Stool cultures for bacterial causes can be ordered and are warranted if the patient is very ill, an infant, elderly, or immunosuppressed. Remember, stool cultures can be altered by some usual treatments and by some tests including barium swallow upper gastrointestinal series (UGI), D-xylose absorption tests, and use of antidiarrheal medications. Do cultures first.

Laboratory evaluation should be done if the symptoms have not abated with a clear liquid diet within 24 to 48 h. Laboratory studies should be directed toward the most likely chronic cause of diarrhea, nausea, and vomiting. At the very least that would

Table 6-1-1. Acute Gastroenteritis Pathogens

Rotavirus
Norwalk virus
Astrovirus
Calicivirus
Enteric adenovirus
Parvovirus
Vibrio species
Cryptosporidium
Cyclospora
Staphylococcus
Bacillus cereus
Escherichia coli

include a complete blood cell count (CBC), chemistry studies, urinalysis (UA) and stool for ova and parasite (O & P) analysis, white and red blood cells, and cultures.

RADIOLOGIC (IMAGING) STUDIES

Imaging studies are rarely done for the diagnosis of AGE. A flat and upright plain abdominal radiograph may aid in the differential diagnosis. If symptoms persist, the use of imaging studies increases, depending on what the source is thought to be.

TREATMENT

The patient will expect an antidiarrheal or antiemetic medication. The real objective of treatment is the replacement of fluids and electrolytes, especially in children and the elderly. Any patient unable to tolerate oral fluids requires intravenous fluid replacement. The infant will most likely need hospitalization for rehydration. In children who are able to drink and not severely ill, oral hydration is recommended. The adult may be able to receive 2 L of fluid in an office setting before being sent home under observation. Table 6-1-3 reviews appropriate clear liquid diets and recommended IV replacement fluids. The patient should sip or drink about 8 oz of fluid an hour and can gauge the level of hydration by frequency of urination.

If the patient is using any medication that may add to dehydration (diuretics), consider stopping or decreasing the dose during the acute phase of AGE. Antidiarrheals are not recommended (though commonly given) for the vast majority of patients with AGE. Since AGE is a short self-limiting process and it responds

Table 6-1-2. Differential Diagnosis for AGE

Ulcerative colitis	Diarrhea, blood, pus, LLQ* cramping pain
Crohn's disease	Diarrhea, blood, RLQ* pain
Infectious	Diarrhea, usually lasts longer and/or more severe, associated with blood and pus, leukocytosis
Shigella	
Salmonella	
Campylobacter	
Clostridium difficile	
Hyperthyroidism	Diarrhea, no blood or pus, no abdominal cramping
Irritable bowel syndrome	Diarrhea, usually associated with stress, no systemic symptoms; doesn't wake the patient up
Medication-induced diarrhea	Magnesium antacids, antibiotics, prokinetic agents, laxative abuse
Acute abdomen	
Appendicitis	Diarrhea, nausea, vomiting, fever, abdominal pain; localization of pain, peritoneal irritation; leukocytosis, chemistry changes
Cholecystitis	
Pancreatitis	
Diverticulitis	

* LLQ = left lower quadrant; RLQ = right lower quadrant.

Table 6-1-3. Fluid and Electrolyte Replacement

Oral hydration: water, sodium, potassium, chloride, and citrate
  Gatorade
  Sports drinks
  Pedialyte
  Homemade (can be mixed with Kool-aide or similar mix)
    Half gallon of water, 4–5 teasp sugar, 1 teasp (each) table salt
    and baking soda
Intravenous fluids
  Ringer's lactate with 20–40 meq potassium
    Children: 30 mL/kg in the first hour then
                40 mL/kg in the next 2 h
    Adults: 2 L over first 1-1/2 h and then
              125 mL/h if needed

NOTES

Any food should be avoided until hunger pangs begin, usually 24 h.
Avoid cheese, milk, fried foods, red meats, peanut butter, oils, or
  foods made of these for at least 24 h, preferably 48 h.
Use a progress diet with dry crackers, thin soups, bread, and simple
  fruits.

well to fluid replacement, medications are not essential. The addition of an antidiarrheal may actually prolong the infectious process. Antibiotics are not appropriate and ineffective for a viral illness. Antiemetics are not necessary unless the patient is unable to tolerate sipping fluids.

COMPLICATIONS

By far the most common complication is dehydration. Infants can become severely dehydrated very quickly—within hours of initial symptoms. Signs of dehydration include low urine output, dry mouth and eyelids, orthostatic dizziness, confusion, or change in mentation. In infants look for poor skin turgor and sunken fontanelles as well.

PATIENT EDUCATION

Prevention is first. Educate the patient about good hand washing. The spread of AGE is primarily by oral-fecal route. Patients can diminish the spread of the virus in their home with good, regular hand washing. Convince patients that they don't need antiemetics and antidiarrheals to deal with simple acute gastroenteritis. Proper education on fluid and electrolyte replacement cannot be stressed enough. Additionally, it is cheaper for the patient to use an electrolyte-rich drink for 24 h than to buy two medications. Another important aspect of education is the admonition to return for follow-up if symptoms persist or increase past 24 to 48 h. The expectation is that the nausea, vomiting, and diarrhea should be gone within 24 h. The fatigue, anorexia, and aches and pains should be gone within 48 h. If symptoms persist look for exacerbating sources (like the patient eating a cheeseburger) or at the differential diagnosis.

PEARLS

After upper respiratory infections, acute gastroenteritis may be the next most common diagnosis. The patient is ill but not writhing in pain. The diarrhea and vomiting usually subside within 6 h. Look for the frequency and timing of diarrhea and vomiting—on average, patients report both about every half hour to an hour. Those who have been in the medical office for 1 h and who report their last stool or vomitus was an hour or more earlier are likely well on the way to resolution. Ensure rehydration and electrolyte replacement and encourage the patient to avoid fatty, greasy, milky foods for at least 24 h. Educate rather than medicate.

REFERENCES

1. Multistate outbreak of viral gastroenteritis related to consumption of oysters, 1993, MMWR, *JAMA* 271(3):183, 1994.

BIBLIOGRAPHY

Bad Bug Book. US Food and Drug Administration Center for Food Safety and Applied Nutrition, 1992, Internet: Acute gastroenteritis.
Health Information (Internet): Viral gastroenteritis, June 1996, HTLM-Orbis-AH CN.

Chapter 6–2
ACHALASIA
Anne P. Heinly

DISCUSSION

Achalasia is the most common motor disorder of the esophagus, striking 2 to 3 per 10,000 people in a lifetime. The term *achalasia* literally means "failure to relax." It is actually a twofold process: no peristalsis (or very weak peristalsis) and lack of lower esophageal sphincter (LES) relaxation. This combination leads to the retention of ingested food which then progressively dilates the esophageal body. Although the etiology is still unknown, investigations are pursuing a degenerative lesion within the vagus nerve to explain this lack of neuromuscular response. There is equal distribution between men and women, and it is more commonly seen in older individuals.

PATHOGENESIS

The esophagus is basically a conduit for food intake. The upper esophageal sphincter (UES) is constructed entirely of striated muscle and is an important factor for the motor function of the esophagus. Phase one of the swallowing mechanism begins with the oropharyngeal contraction regulated by an intricate neuromuscular reflex which sends a smooth single peristaltic wave down the entire length of the esophagus. The UES is probably responsible for the sensory input of heartburn and pain arising from a large bolus or tissue irritation. The resting pressure that keeps the UES closed is estimated at 101 mmHg. This is a protective mechanism against regurgitation and can only be overcome by sudden bursts associated with burping or vomiting.

The body of the esophagus begins as striated muscle and converts to smooth muscle at the distal end. Secondary peristalsis is a normal physiologic response to the presence of a bolus. The spreading contraction aids in the continued movement of food to the stomach. The esophagus is lined with squamous epithelium which is easily damaged by pH levels <4. It is the disruption of the squamous epithelium by alcohol, tobacco, chemicals, and the like that predisposes the esophagus to disease.

The final player in achalasia and esophageal disease in general is the lower esophageal sphincter. Its complex neurohormonal muscular activity defines esophageal emptying. If it is too tight, food cannot exit, too loose and gastric juices can reflux. It can malfunction by pure mechanics, such as obstruction, stricture, ulcer, edema, or varices. It can be affected by neuromuscular diseases, infection, medications, tobacco, and alcohol.

Table 6-2-1. Differential Diagnosis for Achalasia

Vigorous achalasia	Simultaneous, high-amplitude contraction in the distal esophagus with increased LES tone. Significant pain and dysphagia, mimics angina.
Diffuse esophageal spasm (DES)	Asynchronous, random contractions. Chest pain, dysphagia exacerbated by hot or cold foods.
Gastric adenocarcinoma	Weight loss, dysphagia, early satiety, pain exacerbated by food, nausea, and vomiting.
Squamous cell carcinoma of the esophagus	Progressive dysphagia, weight loss, lymphadenopathy, cough, hoarseness, GI bleeding.
Chagas' disease	American trypanosomiasis, megaesophagus, often seen in children, cardiomyopathy, periorbital edema, megacolon, myxedema.
Sarcoidosis	Affecting the young, hilar lymphadenopathy (causing achalasia symptoms), pulmonary symptoms with infiltrates, ocular and skin lesions.
Scleroderma	80% will have esophageal symptoms including dysphagia with decreased peristalsis. GERD occurs as well. Diffuse fibrosis and vascular changes to the skin, heart, kidneys, etc.
Myasthenia gravis	A pure motor syndrome, it attacks the UES with subsequent dysphagia and cough. Ocular symptoms and proximal limb weakness are distinguishing.
Angina pectoris	Pressure-like chest pain usually substernal. Not usually associated with dysphagia. Dyspnea and nausea.

SYMPTOMS

Achalasia classically presents as progressive dysphagia with about one-third of patients complaining of chest pain. Patients develop a cough (especially at night) due to regurgitation of material trapped in the esophagus traversing the bronchus. Patients may first present with recurrent pneumonia or frequent upper respiratory infections (URIs). With progression of the disease, patients are not able to vomit or belch without great difficulty because they cannot increase intrathoracic pressures sufficiently to overcome the blockage. Weight loss from malnutrition is common late in the disease (foodstuffs never make it to the stomach). Halitosis and nocturnal regurgitation are common and can be differentiated from gastroesophageal reflux disease (GERD) regurgitation by the lack of oral ulcers. Patient may describe bizarre postures and maneuvers that literally shake the food down.

OBJECTIVE

The physical examination is usually noncontributory. The most likely finding will be evidence of anemia and/or weight loss. Halitosis may be present, and with respiratory complications evidence of pneumonia may be found.

DIAGNOSTIC CONSIDERATIONS

The most common mimickers of achalasia include obstructive diseases. The malignancies and variant achalasia listed in Table 6-2-1 can confuse the picture until definitive biopsies can be done. Some history clues in favor of malignancies include significant weight loss over a short period of time (6 months or less) and chest pain. While achalasia may cause chest pressure or fullness after meals, carcinomas usually have progressive, steady, deep pain.

LABORATORY TESTS

There are no specific laboratory studies that will define achalasia. Standard studies such as complete blood cell count (CBC), chemistries, and *Helicobacter pylori* titers may be helpful in defining anemias and ruling out the differential diagnosis.

RADIOLOGIC (IMAGING) STUDIES

Radiologic studies are the mainstay of diagnosis for achalasia. A simple chest x-ray may reveal a widened mediastinum with air-fluid levels. Barium swallows reveal a distended esophageal body with a beak-like distal LES. The use of amyl nitrite during the barium swallow can help distinguish achalasia from a constricting malignancy—amyl nitrate causes LES relaxation which will not respond in the presence of achalasia. Esophageal manometry can help differentiate the variant types of achalasia. The archetypical finding reveals no primary peristaltic wave and very-low-amplitude secondary waves (bolus type). At the lower esophageal sphincter, resting pressures can be as high as 90 mmHg (normal is 1 to 20 mmHg). The final definitive study is an endoscopic procedure that allows for direct visualization and biopsies. Biopsies may reveal absence of neural plexus in esophageal muscle layers.

TREATMENT

Calcium channel blockers, nitrates of all varieties, hydralazine, and anticholinergics have all been tried to loosen the LES tone. All have been less than successful. Dilatation of the LES can be accomplished with bougienage (for short-term relief) or pneumatic dilators, which can achieve good results for long periods of time. The problem with dilatation is that the more often it is performed the less likely it is to help. The most definitive therapy is an esophagomyotomy, incising the anterior LES extending less than 1 cm into the stomach. The myotomy decreases LES pressure, and with a proper procedure the sphincter competency is preserved, although up to 10 percent of patients may develop reflux esophagitis.

COMPLICATIONS

Weight loss, anemia, and pulmonary complications are common in patients with untreated achalasia. During investigation esophageal rupture can occur. Therapy, however, has its own complications. GERD is the natural consequence of releasing LES tone. The patient may have severe symptoms and require aggressive therapy for control (See Chap. 6-11, "Gastroesophageal Reflux Disease.") The risk of developing esophageal carcinoma from achalasia is unclear. Certainly after myotomy, the risk increases owing to the chronic GERD.

PEARLS

Achalasia and its variants can mimic angina, myocardial infarction, chronic GERD, and other diseases. Esophageal disease warrants careful investigation to rule out malignancies and other systemic diseases. The presentation is quite classic, but it may also present simply as recurrent URI. Medications are limited, leaving dilatation or surgery as the only option for most patients.

BIBLIOGRAPHY

Diamant NE: Physiology of the esophagus, in Sleisenger MH, Fordtran S: *Gastrointestinal Disease*, 5th ed. Philadelphia, Saunders, 1993, pp 319–354.

Chapter 6–3
ANAL FISSURES
Pat C. H. Jan

DISCUSSION

Anal fissures (fissures in ano) are linear tears in the anal mucosa brought on by episodes of diarrhea, constipation, trauma (including anal intercourse), and associated inflammatory bowel disease. Fissures are found in equal numbers in both men and women. They are commonly located in the posterior midline and rarely in the anterior midline.

SIGNS AND SYMPTOMS

Patients will generally present with complaints of severe anal pain with and after bowel movements. They may also relate episodes of bleeding following each bowel movement. The severity of the pain often leads the patient (especially children) to hold back on future bowel movements. This negative reinforcement leads to the vicious cycle of constipation, pain with defecation, and worsening of the preexisting anal fissure.

OBJECTIVE FINDINGS

Typically the diagnosis can be made by history. In cases of severe pain, it may be difficult to examine the anal canal. Gentle exposure by spreading the buttocks along with verbal reassurance to the patient usually allows sufficient exposure of the anal fissure. Anal fissures are generally located in the posterior midline. Pain occurs when the fissure extends beyond the dentate line. The dentate line is the location of the somatic innervation of the anal canal. In chronic fissures, a hypertrophic papilla which is caused by recurrent episodes of infection can be seen. Distal to the hypertrophic papilla, a sentinel pile is found. Sentinel piles are believed to also be a product of infection of the anal canal. The fissure or anal ulcer lies between these two structures and is the first indication of an anal problem. (See Fig. 6-3-1.)

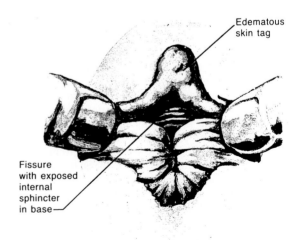

Figure 6-3-1. Anal fissure with hypertrophic papilla and sentinel pile. [*From Schwartz SI, Shires GT, Spencer FC (eds): Principles of Surgery, 6th ed. New York, McGraw-Hill, 1994, p 1226. Used with permission of McGraw-Hill, Inc.*]

Figure 6-3-2. Lateral internal sphincterotomy, open technique. [*From Schwartz SI, Shires GT, Spencer FC (eds): Principles of Surgery, 6th ed. New York, McGraw-Hill, 1994, p 1227. Used with permission of McGraw-Hill, Inc.*]

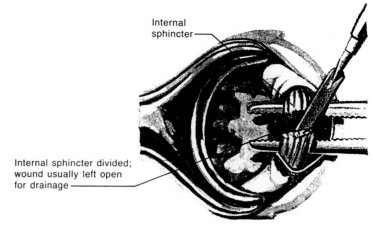

Internal sphincter

Internal sphincter divided; wound usually left open for drainage

DIAGNOSTIC CONSIDERATIONS

Anal fissures from constipation, diarrhea, or trauma need to be differentiated from the following disease processes:

- Carcinoma
- Crohn's disease
- Syphilis, primary state
- AIDS colitis

TREATMENT

Medical Management

Medical management is generally used for acute cases. Treatment consists of dietary fiber and/or the use of stool softeners, topical anal anesthetics, and warm sitz baths for 20 min two or three times daily.

Surgical Management

Surgical treatment is reserved for chronic fissures. The patient is taken into the operating room and placed in the jackknife position. Two surgical procedures are available: lateral internal sphincterotomy and anal advancement flap, with the former being the gold standard. The patient is given intravenous sedation along with local anesthesia of 1% lidocaine with epinephrine; 3 to 6 mL of lidocaine is used. The internal sphincter is identified and divided by any of the following: cautery, scalpel, or scissors. (See Fig. 6-3-2.) The external sphincter and fissure are left alone. If any bleeding is encountered, direct pressure to the wound generally stops the blood flow. The wound is left open and allowed to close by secondary intention. The wound generally heals in about 2 to 4 weeks, and the patient usually does not develop a keyhole deformity if the incision is kept lateral and not in the midline. Bupivacaine hydrochloride (Marcaine) 0.25% with epinephrine, which has a longer duration, can be injected into the wound. The patient will have an easier postoperative recovery. The patient is then instructed on perianal hygiene and dietary modifications to prevent constipation. If the patient is unable to adhere to dietary changes, then Metamucil or other psyllium-based preparation is suggested as an alternative to produce a large, soft, bulky stool. Patients are also instructed to take two or three sitz baths each day to aid in decreasing inflammation and to soothe the wound. Anal advancement flap consists of a rhomboid flap taken at the sentinel pile and placed over the fissure site and sutured in place. The donor site is also sutured closed. Postoperative care instructions consist of good personal hygiene, pain management, stool softener or fiber, and sitz baths.

Supportive Measures

Patients are generally given a prescription for both oral and topical analgesics. Remember, some oral analgesics can cause constipation, so a stool softener or fiber should also be used to prevent constipation. A topical analgesic like dibucaine (Nupercainal) or Hurricane gel can be applied to the wound as needed.

Disposition

Patients are discharged shortly after surgery. They are seen at 1 week, 2 weeks, and 1 month after surgery. Patients are instructed to return earlier if any complications arise.

PATIENT EDUCATION

It is very important for the patient to maintain good perianal hygiene and prevent constipation. Patients are instructed to follow the same postoperative care sheet given to those with hemorrhoidectomies. (See Chap. 6-13, "Hemorrhoids.") If patients do not improve and continue to have pain despite both topical and oral analgesic, they should be reexamined.

COMPLICATIONS

Keyhole deformity and poor wound healing are common complications after a midline sphincterotomy. Lateral internal sphincterotomy is the gold standard for treatment for anal fissures since it does not cause these complications. Anal abscesses may develop and require incision and drainage.

NOTES AND PEARLS

Anal fissures are common among pregnant women and usually respond well to conservative treatment of sitz baths, high-fiber diet, and topical anesthetics. Lateral internal sphincterotomies, if indicated, are delayed until after delivery because of high probability of anal tears during delivery. Anal intercourse should be considered as a possible cause of traumatic or recurrent fissures.

BIBLIOGRAPHY

Mazier WP: Hemorrhoids, fissures, and pruritus ani (Review). *Surg Clin North Am* 74(6):1277–1292, 1994.
Russell TR: Anal fissures, in Way LW (ed): *Current Surgical Diagnosis and Treatment,* 10th ed. Stamford, CT, Appleton & Lange, 1994.
Schwartz SI, Shires GT, Spencer FC (eds): Anal fissures, in *Principles of Surgery,* 6th ed. New York, McGraw-Hill, 1994.

Chapter 6–4
COLITIS

Anne P. Heinly

Colitis

DISCUSSION

Colitis is a term used easily, but it is actually difficult to define. The dictionary says it is "inflammation of the colon," but in general use this could mean anything from acute gastroenteritis to fulminant ulcerative colitis. Most textbooks label an entity *colitis* when there is actual inflammation of the colonic mucosa with structural changes. A brief description of the colon and its anatomy is in order so the clinical practitioner can narrow the differential diagnosis.

The colon (see Fig. 6-4-1) is approximately 1 m in length and frames the intraabdominal contents in an inverted U. Its primary function is the absorption of water and electrolytes, plus it acts as storage area for feces prior to evacuation. Considered to have

five sections, the colon begins in the right lower quadrant with the cecum, which includes the vermiform appendix and the ileocecal valve. The ascending colon is fairly stationary, having a retroperitoneal attachment; it ends at the hepatic flexure. The transverse colon is quite mobile and can be located from xiphoid to pubis, depending on body habitus and position. The descending colon begins at the splenic flexure and blends into redundancy of the sigmoid colon in the left lower quadrant. The descending colon, like the ascending, is relatively stationary in the retroperitoneum. The sigmoid colon with its redundant tissue is actually the most mobile area. The rectum is part of the colon but is often considered separately as is the anal area.

The peristaltic motion of the colon is generated from two sets of muscles, an outer longitudinal set (teniae coli) and the inner circular muscle coat. The teniae coli run (as three bands) the entire length of the colon, cecum to rectum. The teniae coli are just a little shorter than the length of the colon; the ensuing pucker creates the haustra, or outpouchings, that are seen on radiographic examinations of the colon. The presence or absence of the haustra markings can indicate specific disease processes.

Histologically, the colon is fairly simple: there are four basic layers. Disease involvement is often measured by the layer(s) affected. The outermost layer is serosa with attached fatty appen-

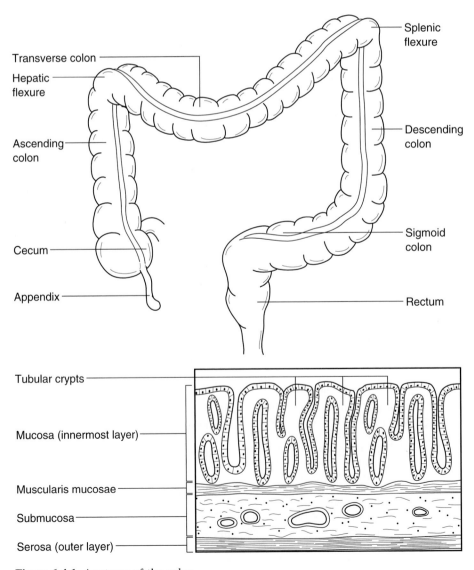

Figure 6-4-1. Anatomy of the colon.

dixes, an extension of peritoneal fat. The muscular coat is composed of a circular layer forming a spiral effect over the entire length of the colon. The submucosa contains many blood and lymph vessels and dense connective tissue. The innermost layer is the mucosa. It has a special layer of smooth muscle cells called the muscularis mucosae between the submucosa and the mucosa. Unlike the small intestine, the absorption surface is flat with numerous straight tubular crypts. The mucosa is lined with a sheet of columnar epithelial cells. Colitis occurs when the mucosa or underlying structures are inflamed or damaged.

SIGNS AND SYMPTOMS

Because of the many types of colitis, it is important for the clinician to perform a thorough history and physical. History questions should include onset, timing, pattern, radiation, and palliative or exacerbating factors of each presenting symptom. Presenting symptoms may include any of the following: nausea, vomiting, diarrhea (its volume and character), melena, hematochezia, hematemesis, pain, cramping, distention, tenesmus, or constipation. A sexual, travel, and dietary history is essential since many causes of colitis are infectious. The review of systems should cover extraintestinal symptoms like joint pain, skin lesions, eye symptoms, and cardiac, pulmonary, hepatic, or renal compromise.

OBJECTIVE FINDINGS

A complete physical examination is a must. Inspect the oral cavity for masses or lesions, the presence or absence of halitosis, or lymph node enlargement. Abdominal examination with digital rectal is done for the evaluation of organ enlargement, mass effect, tenderness, and presence of ascites. Cardiac and pulmonary examination is done for evidence of hypovolemia, cardiomyopathies, or pneumonitis. Skin and musculoskeletal examinations may reveal dehydration, malnutrition, or extraintestinal manifestations of disease. Pelvic examinations in women should be done to rule out a gynecologic etiology for the presenting symptoms.

LABORATORY TESTS

Laboratory evaluation includes three to five separate stool samples for ova and parasite analysis (O &P), culture, and cell counts. Serologic testing should include: complete blood cell count (CBC), liver function studies, basic electrolytes, glucose, hepatitis panel, indirect hemagglutination for amebiasis, and screens for sexually transmitted disease such as Venereal Disease Research Laboratories (VDRL), HIV, RPR, and FTA for syphilis. Antibody titers for cytomegalovirus (CMV), toxoplasma, and herpes simplex virus (HSV) infection may be done. If *Clostridium difficile* is suspected, toxin titers can be done.

RADIOLOGIC (IMAGING) STUDIES

Barium enema may not be indicated in acute situations because of the risk of perforation and should not be done prior to cultures. Sigmoidoscopy and colonoscopy are the definitive tests because they allow visualization of the tissue and access for biopsy and cultures. See Table 6-4-1 for the pathology associated with each type of colitis.

Intestinal Amebiasis

Entameba histolytica is one of the most common forms of amebiasis in the United States. It is also found in the tropics and areas of poor sanitation. Symptoms develop 2 to 6 weeks after the ingestion of the infectious cysts. Acutely the patients will have crampy lower abdominal pain, watery, frequent (10 to 12 stools daily), small-volume stools that contain scant feces, abundant blood, and mucus. Chronic amebiasis leads to significant malaise and weight loss. Sigmoidoscopy reveals mucosal ulceration particularly in the cecal and rectal areas. Fulminant disease can form a large ulcerative granulomatous masses at the flexures and cecum that may be confused for ulcerative colitis. Stool collection for O&P, cultures, and cell identification is generally diagnostic. Endoscopic findings usually reveal friable mucosa with ulcerations. Treatment includes luminal and tissue amebicides. The luminal drugs, iodoquinol, paromomycin and diloxanide furoate, eliminate cysts and trophozoites close to the mucosa. A good tissue amebicide is metronidazole 750 mg tid for 10 days. Several different stools should be checked after therapy to ensure complete eradication.

Infectious Colitis

Clostridium perfringens is a common cause of food poisoning in the United States. Rewarmed food is the usual culprit. Like its bacterial cousins, *C. perfringens* is a spore-forming microbe which can germinate during the reheating process. The type A strains can mature within 8 to 20 h after ingestion. Enterotoxins are produced in the GI tract causing hypersecretions, intestinal epithelium damage, and protein loss into the intestinal lumen. Symptoms include the abrupt onset of watery, profuse diarrhea, and epigastric pain. Fever, nausea, and vomiting are infrequent. Mild infections are self-limiting and need supportive treatment. More persistent or fulminant infections may be treated with penicillin G, 20 million units a day until the infection is cleared.

Infectious causes of colitis include *Shigella, Salmonella, Campylobacter,* and *Yersinia* species. All these are associated with nausea, abdominal cramps, fever, and diarrhea. *Campylobacter* and *Shigella* are associated with bloody diarrhea. *Campylobacter* may produce a liver enlargement. *Shigella, Salmonella,* and *Yersinia* have been associated with Reiter's syndrome, migrating joint pain, and skin symptoms. Diagnosis is confirmed with cultures. Sigmoidoscopy will reveal a red, friable, and ulcerated mucosa. Treatment is supportive with correction of dehydration and electrolyte abnormalities. Of these infectious etiologies for colitis, only *Shigella* requires antibiotic therapy, ampicillin, 500 mg qid, or trimethoprim-sulfamethoxazole bid. The other infections are self-limiting, and in fact, antibiotics given to the patient with *Salmonella* infection tend to lengthen the carrier state of the organism.[1]

Diarrhea is a common first symptom for HIV-positive patients. Immunocompromised patients are more susceptible to unusual infectious colitis including *Candida* spp., *Histoplasma capsulatum*, CMV, HSV, actinomycosis, and tuberculosis. Symptoms may include fever, abdominal pain, weight loss, anorexia, and diarrhea with or without blood. The elderly, the very young, and cancer patients may also be immunocompromised.

Collagenous Colitis

The diagnosis of collagenous colitis can be made only by histology. Often dismissed as irritable bowel syndrome (IBS) it is found in middle-aged (fifth to sixth decade) women who have intermittent diarrhea. The diarrhea is chronic and watery without blood, excessive mucus, or cells. The patient may have evidence of arthritis or connective tissue disorders. Barium enema and endoscope are usually negative. The biopsy, however, reveals a thickened subepithelial layer below the normal-appearing colon mucosa. Linear eosinophilic acellular collagen bands are found.[2] Treatment with oral sulfasalazine, 2 to 3 g daily, yields marked improvement in the majority of patients. NSAIDs should be

Table 6-4-1. Types of Colitis

Types of Colitis	Symptoms	Stool Character	Pathology
Amebiasis	Crampy abdominal pain, rarely perforates	Watery, small volume, streaked with blood or mucus	Mucosal ulcerations, rounded, punched out on x-ray and examination
Clostridium perfringens	Epigastric pain	Watery diarrhea, fecal neutrophils, protein loss	Enterotoxin damages intestinal epithelium
Collagenous	Intermittent abdominal cramping	Chronic, watery, no mucus or blood	Thickened subepithelial layer below colonic mucosa, eosinophilic acellular collagen band
Infectious *Shigella, Salmonella, Campylobacter Yersinia*	Crampy abdominal pain	Profuse, watery with or without blood and mucus, fecal leukocytes	Inflammation without structural changes
Ischemic	Abdominal pain, hypotension	Rectal bleeding	Submucosal hemorrhage and edema
Pseudomembranous *Clostridium difficile*	Fever, abdominal cramps, pain	Profuse, watery with no blood or mucus	Raised plaques 2–5 mm in diameter, interspersed among normal mucosa
Amyloidosis	Diarrhea or constipation	Blood or no blood	Amyloid deposits
Lymphocytic	Vague colicky pain, chronic course	Watery diarrhea, excessive mucus, no blood	Absence of subepithelial thickening. Lamina propria is infiltrated with lymphocytes

avoided because they have been associated with intestinal mucosal inflammation. No evidence of severe progression or increased colon cancer risk has been found.

Ischemic Colitis

Ischemic colitis occurs with the transport of blood away from the intestinal mucosa. This may occur slowly with generalized peripheral vascular disease or acutely with arterial emboli, dissecting aortic aneurysm or abdominal surgeries. Radiation therapy to the abdominal or pelvic regions may also trigger an ischemic reaction. The colon receives the majority of its blood supply from the superior and inferior mesenteric arteries. Compromise of the supply or severe hypotension may lead to ischemia. Transient ischemia involves the mucosa or submucosa. Chronic or prolonged ischemia produces damage to the circular muscle layer. Transmural infarction involves all four layers of the colon and usually leads to perforation, gangrene, or even the death of the patient.

Symptoms include severe lower abdominal pain (abdominal angina) and bloody diarrhea that is quite profuse. The patient will often avoid eating to avoid the pain. When severity increases, vomiting and hypotension are common. Physical examination reveals an acute abdomen with signs of peritonitis. Barium studies have classic "thumbprinting," representing the submucosal hemorrhage and edema.[3] Contrast studies may be hazardous, creating the possibility of perforation. Chronic ischemia may cause stricture formation, ulceration, and granulation tissue. A mesenteric thrombosis is a true life-threatening emergency which needs early lifesaving therapy and surgical consultation.

Pseudomembranous Colitis

Inflammation of the colon associated with the use of antibiotics is the most common cause of pseudomembranous colitis (Table 6-4-2). It has also been seen with mercury poisoning, intestinal ischemia, and bronchopneumonia. Pseudomembranous colitis is characterized by raised plaques of 2 to 5 mm in diameter interspersed among the normal mucosa of the colon.[4] Abscesses appear in one or several adjacent crypts from which exudative

mucus, cellular debris, and leukocytes ooze out into the intestinal lumen. In the case of antibiotic use, *C. difficile* is the pathogen causing the problem. More specifically, *C. difficile* overgrowth results in the release of toxins which in turn cause the symptoms. There are three heat-labile toxins. Toxins A, B, and C cause fluid mobilization. Toxin A causes severe necrosis of the epithelium and bleeding. Toxins A and C cause epithelial cell shedding. The result is a patient with fever, profuse diarrhea, and cramping abdominal pain with a leukocytosis. There is seldom excessive mucus, and there may or may not be bleeding. Physical examination may mimic an acute or surgical abdomen. Plain abdominal radiographs may show irregular mucosal outline with blunting of edematous haustra.

The diagnosis of pseudomembranous colitis is dependent on a history of antibiotic use within the last 4 to 6 weeks. Most colitis will begin 5 to 7 days after antibiotics are begun, but as many as one-third will not develop symptoms until the antibiotic course is completed. Stool cultures for *C. difficile* are not helpful; it is better to confirm by positive *C. difficile* toxin titer. Toxin B may increase 1000-fold and is considered the hallmark of *C. difficile* infections. Contrast studies should be avoided because of perforation risks.

Treatment, of course, includes cessation of the offending antibiotic and providing supportive care. Oral metronidazole or IV vancomycin have been used to combat the *C. difficile*. The fluoroquinalones appear to affective in some patients. Patients show signs of recovery within 24 to 48 h on average. Complications of pseudomembranous colitis include perforation and toxic megacolon, so rapid therapy is recommended. There is no evidence to suggest that the antibiotic that caused the colitis be avoided

Table 6-4-2. Antibiotics Associated with Pseudomembranous Colitis (in order of frequency)

Ampicillin or amoxicillin
Cephalosporins
Clindamycin
Sulfamethoxazole-trimethoprim
Other "cillin" drugs
Rarely seen with tetracycline, sulfonamides

Table 6-4-3. Differential Diagnosis of Colitis

Neoplasm (carcinoma, adenomatous polyps)
Diverticula, diverticulitis
Arteriovenous malformations
Behçet's syndrome
Acute gastroenteritis
Bacillary dysentery: salmonella, *Campylobacter*
Herpes simplex virus
Gonorrhea
Lymphogranuloma venereum (LGV)
Irritable bowel syndrome

in the future. Pseudomembranous colitis can reoccur with any antibiotic use in the future and can be retreated.

PEARLS

With rare exception the many types of colitis have effective treatment options once the type is identified. There is a differential list of processes that might mimic any colitis or contribute to an existing colitis (Table 6-4-3). Ulcerative colitis and Crohn's disease are covered in Chap. 6-15, "Inflammatory Bowel Disease."

REFERENCES

1. Schmitt S, Wexner S: Bacterial, fungal, parasitic, and viral colitis. *Surg Clin North Am* 73(5):1055–1062, 1993.
2. Brady S, McKee D: Collagenous colitis: A cause of chronic diarrhea. *Am Fam Physician* 48(6):1081–1083, 1993.
3. Bower T: Ischemic colitis. *Surg Clin North Am* 73(5):1037–1051, 1993.
4. Turkiewicz D: Colo-rectal diseases—Pseudomembranous colitis. Department of Surgery, Mather Hospital, February 1996, Internet: http://qmec.herston.uq.oz.au

Chapter 6–5
COLORECTAL POLYPS
Marquitha S. Mayfield

DISCUSSION

Polyps are soft tissue mucosal lesions that protrude into the lumen of the intestines. They result from excessive proliferation of normal mucosal cells (hyperplastic changes) or neoplastic changes of glandular epithelial cells (adenomatous growths). Polyps can occur anywhere in the intestinal tract. Most occur in the colon and rectum, with 70 to 80 percent of polyps located in the rectosigmoid colon. Polyps may be sessile (broad-based growths), or pedunculated (attached to a stalk), singular or multiple, and vary in size from smaller than 0.5 cm in diameter to larger than 4 cm in diameter. The average polyp is equivalent to 1 cm in diameter. Most polyps are benign; however, some are considered to be premalignant. There is a strong association between adenomatous polyps and the subsequent development of adenocarcinoma of the colon. Dietary factors such as high fat, low fiber, and low calcium may promote malignant transformation. Genetic factors also play a role in the development of colorectal polyps.

The incidence of polyps increases with age. By age 40 years, 20 percent of the adult population will have developed some form of polypoid lesions. Adult males are at greater risk than females (2 : 1 ratio). There are two primary pathologic groups of polyps:

1. *Nonneoplastic polyps* Hyperplastic, hamartomas, and inflammatory (pseudopolyps) and juvenile polyps. These benign lesions have no potential for malignant transformation. Hyperplastic polyps are the most common benign tumors. More than 80 percent are located in the rectosigmoid colon, and they are usually <4 mm in diameter. Hamartomas are developmental malformations resulting in tumors from the overgrowth of normal tissue. Cells do not reproduce once they reach maturity; therefore the growths are self-limiting and benign. Pseudopolyps are commonly associated with inflammatory changes seen with ulcerative colitis and Crohn's disease. Juvenile polyps are benign colonic growths detected primarily in children and young adults. These polyps are often large, vascular, and attached to long stalks and may bleed or prolapse rectally.

2. *Neoplastic polyps* Primary adenomatous polyps, which have significant potential for malignant transformation to adenocarcinoma of the colon. Dysplastic changes are slow to develop in adenomatous polyps, and it may take 5 to 10 years for malignant changes to occur. Approximately 25 percent of polyps are found to be adenomatous on histologic report. The prevalence of adenomatous polyps increases with age with a peak incidence after age 50. Adenomatous polyps may be classified as tubular, tubovillous, or villous adenomas. Malignant potential correlates with the size of the polyp, degree of dysplastic changes, and villous features. Villous adenomas have the greatest potential for malignant transformation (>50 percent), and tubular adenomas, the least potential (20 percent). Tubovillous lesions have a risk for malignant transformation between 20 and 50 percent. Lesions larger than 1 cm in diameter have a 10 percent risk of harboring malignant cells, whereas polyps >2 cm have a 46 percent risk. Sessile adenomas are more likely to harbor malignant changes than pedunculated adenomas. Approximately half the patients with adenomatous polyps have more than one lesion.

SIGNS AND SYMPTOMS

Most patients with colorectal polyps are asymptomatic, with lesions detected on routine endoscopy. Symptoms, when they do occur, consist primarily of intermittent rectal bleeding from ulcerated large polyps. Physical examination findings are uncommon. Digital rectal examination might reveal a palpable rectal mass with large rectal polyps. Gross rectal bleeding may be present. Usually only a positive test for occult bleeding is noted.

DIFFERENTIAL DIAGNOSIS

The differential diagnosis for rectal bleeding includes the following:

- Hemorrhoids
- Upper GI bleeding
- Angiodysplasia
- Diverticular disease
- Infectious diarrhea
- Colorectal cancer
- Ischemic colitis
- Inflammatory bowel disease

SPECIAL CONSIDERATIONS

Familial polyposis is an autosomal-dominant inheritable disorder in which hundreds to thousands of adenomatous polyps form throughout the colon. Lesions often appear during childhood and have a high rate of malignant transformation by age 50.

A colectomy is often performed prophylactically. Peutz-Jeghers syndrome is another inherited disorder in which hamartomatous polyps predominate. Lesions are distributed throughout the GI tract, mostly in the small intestine. Although hamartomas are usually benign, patients with Peutz-Jeghers are prone to develop other forms of GI cancer (e.g., gastric, pancreatic, or duodenal malignancies).

Patients with a family history for either of these disorders require enhanced surveillance for early detection of malignant transformation and management of polypoid growths.

LABORATORY AND RADIOLOGIC TESTS

Stool for occult blood is a common screening test used for colorectal cancer. However, it is less sensitive and specific for detecting polyps. Sigmoidoscopy is a better screening test because most colorectal polyps are accessible by the flexible sigmoidoscope. Double-contrast barium enema is also useful and can detect up to 90 percent of polyps >1 cm. On radiograph, polyps appear as rounded filling defects with sharply defined margins. Colonoscopy is the most reliable method for diagnosing polyps detecting up to 98 percent of polyps. The entire colon can be visualized and polyps can be removed for histologic evaluation at the same time.

TREATMENT

The mainstay of treatment for colorectal polyps is endoscopic removal. Routine removal of adenomatous polyps significantly reduces the incidence of subsequent development of colorectal cancer. If possible, all colonic polyps should be excised and sent for tissue pathology. A polypectomy using electrocautery techniques can be safely completed through the colonoscope for many sessile and pedunculated lesions. Lesions larger than 3 cm in diameter may require surgical resection. Patients with adenomatous polyps should undergo a repeat colonoscopy within 3 years to detect and remove any additional lesions or residual tissue.

Patients with a family history for inheritable polyposis syndromes may require regular screening sigmoidoscopy beginning at an early age (10 to 20 years).

SUPPORTIVE MEASURES

Adopting a diet that is low in saturated fat (<30 percent of total calories), high in fiber (at least three servings daily of fruit and vegetables), as well as limited in the amount of red meat (fewer than three servings per week) and alcohol (fewer than two drinks daily) consumed, may reduce the risk for dysplastic changes of the colorectal mucosa.

PATIENT EDUCATION

The risk for colonic cancer should be explained to all patients with adenomatous polyps. These patients should be encouraged to return for routine follow-up colonoscopy. Instructions on instituting a low-fat, high-fiber diet should also be given.

DISPOSITION

Patients with polyps detected on barium enema or sigmoidoscopy should be referred to a gastroenterologist for diagnostic and therapeutic colonoscopy. Recommendations for repeat "surveillance" colonoscopy vary and are based on pathologic type of the removed polyp and individual risk for cancer. Generally, benign hyperplastic polyps do not require additional follow-up. Patients with adenomatous polyps should have repeat colonoscopy in 3 years. Patients with large polyps, polyps with very dysplastic features, or a strong family history of colon cancer should have repeat colonoscopy sooner.

COMPLICATIONS AND RED FLAGS

Large polyps may precipitate intussusception or cause bowel obstruction. Additionally, polyps may ulcerate and bleed. The major complication, however, is the development of invasive adenocarcinoma of the colon.

OTHER NOTES AND PEARLS

Epidemiologic data from recent studies suggest that the use of NSAIDS (e.g., aspirin and Sulindac) on a daily basis may significantly reduce the incidence of adenomatous polyps and the associated risk for dysplastic changes in some patients.

BIBLIOGRAPHY

Alberts DS, Hixson L, Ahnen D, et al: Do NSAIDS exert their colon cancer chemoprevention activities through the inhibition of mucosal prostaglandin synthetase? *J Cellular Biochem* (Suppl) 22:18–23, 1995.

Barker LR, Burton JH, Zieve PD (eds): *Principles of Ambulatory Medicine,* 4th ed. Baltimore, Williams & Wilkins, 1995, pp 472–475.

Ceabert JG: Colorectal cancer: Reducing mortality through early detection and treatment. *Physician Assist* 17(1):25–42, 1993.

Goroll AH, May LA, Mulley AG Jr (eds): *Primary Care Medicine: Office Evaluation & Management of the Adult Patient,* 3d ed. Philadelphia, Lippincott, 1995, pp 353, 441–442.

Greenberger NJ: How best to screen for colorectal cancer. *Clin Focus Supple Contemp Nurse Practit* 25–31, Summer 1995.

Martinez ME, McPherson RS: Aspirin and other nonsteroidal anti-inflammatory drugs and risk of colorectal adenomatous polyps among endoscoped individuals. *Cancer Epidemiol Biomarkers Prev* 4(7):703–707, 1995.

Neugut AI, Horvath K, Whelan RL, et al: The effect of calcium and vitamin supplements on the incidence and recurrence of colorectal adenomatous polyps. *Cancer* 78(4):723–728, 1996.

Tierney L, McPhee SJ, Papadakis MA: *Current Medical Diagnosis and Treatment.* Stamford, CT: Appleton & Lange, 1996, pp 567–569.

Chapter 6–6
CONSTIPATION
Anne P. Heinly

DISCUSSION

For many people it is a constitutional right to have at least one bowel movement a day. Failing that, these same people will complain of constipation and self-medicate with a laxative. Constipation is a pervasive symptom affecting women more than men and the majority of people at least once in a lifetime. As a symptom, constipation may herald a disease process but is not a disease in and of itself. The presence of constipation is highly subjective: a patient may be anxious if the daily routine of three stools a day drops to one; others may go several days with no stool evacuation without concern. Constipation is a problem at the extremes of life, affecting infants and toddlers and the elderly most adversely.

PATHOGENESIS

The elimination of stool from the intestinal tract should occur on average three to five times a week and is dependent on multiple

Table 6-6-1. Causes of Constipation

General
 Diet: high fat, low fiber, minimal fruits and vegetables
 Poor bowel habits: ignoring the urge, avoidance of public toilets, avoidance of pain
 Poor exercise habits: sedentary lifestyle, prolonged bed rest
 Travel: change in schedule or diet, absence of good drinking water
Metabolic
 Hypercalcemia: malignancy, thryotoxicosis, sarcoidosis, theophylline toxicity
 Hypokalemia: chronic laxative abuse, diuretic therapy, metabolic alkalosis
 Hyponatremia: vomiting, burns, diuretic therapy, cirrhosis, congestive heart failure
 Diabetes: polyuria, thirst, weight loss, ketoacidosis
 Dehydration: excessive heat, lack of thirst mechanism, illness, fever, vomiting
Mechanical
 Redundant, copious bowel
 Pregnancy
 Scarring from radiation therapy
 Surgical adhesions or anastomosis
 Extrinsic or intrinsic tumors or other masses
Neuromuscular
 Hirschsprung's disease: congenital aganglionic bowel
 Spinal cord injury
 Paraplegia
 Cerebral vascular accidents
 Muscular dystrophy
 Dementia, e.g., Alzheimer's disease
 Parkinsonism
 Depression
Medications
 Smooth-muscle relaxants: dicyclomine hydrochloride (Bentyl), verapamil, belladonna
 Antiparkinsonism medications: carbidopa-levodopa (Sinemet), bromocriptine mesylata (Parlodel), amantadine hydrochloride (Symmetrel), levodopa
 Antidepressants: tricyclics, chlorpromazine, benzodiazepines
 Calcium- and aluminum-based antacids
 Diuretics: hydrochloratriazide (HCTZ), furosemide (Lasix), bumetanide (Bumex), spironolactone (Aldactone)
 Iron supplements
 Tranquilizers: chlorpromazine (Thorazine), fluphenazine hydrochloride (Prolixin), haloperidol (Haldol), lithium, trifluoperazine hydrochloride (Stelazine)
 Narcotics and sedatives: morphine, meperidine hydrochloride (Demerol), codeine, chloral hydrate (Noctec), hydroxyzine (Vistaril), zolpidem tartrate (Ambien)

elements. The first factor is mobility; slow transit allows the stool to become compact, making it difficult to move. Chronic constipation is usually secondary to slow transit time and redundant colon. Water intake and absorption is another key mechanism. Water and electrolytes are normally reabsorbed from waste products, but if a person has inadequate fluid intake, hard stools develop since the body is conserving fluids. Water also acts as a lubricant. Dietary intake of fiber allows for frequent bulky stools. The average American stool is small and weighs 75 to 150 g, which can be exhausting to move. Fiber adds bulk, increasing the weight (200 to 500 g) and size of the stool. Other elements that slow stool evacuation include prolonged bed rest, lack of exercise, and medication use (Table 6-6-1). Constipation in the elderly is probably multifactorial—a combination of aging changes, poor diet, lack of exercise, and medication effects.

SYMPTOMS

Variable is the key word. Constipation is defined by the patient's perception of what is normal with regard to frequency, consis-

tency (harder than normal), and size. Cramping abdominal pain that comes in wavelike spasms can be described as mild to severe. The pain may be localized or generalized. It is not unusual to have flank pain or pain in the lateral upper quadrants as the stool turns the corner of the hepatic or splenic flexure. With an impaction, patients may have tenesmus, with watery diarrhea escaping around the stool (encopresis). With rare exceptions, the patient does not have systemic symptoms. In addition, there is no weight loss or bleeding. This helps differentiate constipation from an acute abdominal event like appendicitis.

OBJECTIVE

A good history and physical examination may be sufficient to make the diagnosis. Generally, the patient presents with intermittent pain and normal vital signs. Abdominal examination may reveal a rounded mass effect in the flanks, which follows the tract of the colon. Rectal examination is necessary. There may be an impaction. (See Chap. 6-9, "Fecal Impaction.") An empty vault does not exclude constipation since stool may be filling the entire colon but not have reached the rectal vault. Generally, there is no rebound tenderness or other peritoneal signs.

DIAGNOSTIC CONSIDERATIONS

Risk factors for constipation should be explored: injury, illness, dehydration, sedentary lifestyle, multiple medications. (See Table 6-6-2 for differential diagnosis.) In infants, congenital Hirschsprung's disease (small rectal vault, aganglionic colon) presents with constipation, abdominal distention, and vomiting. Toddlers can get into a constipation cycle, delaying defecation because it hurts, and then have exceptional difficulty with evacuation, which leads to further avoidance.

The elderly can present with a change in mentation and anorexia. Because of normal physiologic aging changes and/or concomitant illness, the older patient may experience transient blood supply loss to the heart and brain while straining to evacuate stool. Some elderly can strain so long that rectal prolapse and severe hemorrhoids develop. Urinary retention and fever may complicate the picture in an elderly person.

LABORATORY TESTS

Laboratory testing is only necessary when other disorders are being considered. If tests are ordered, include: complete blood cell count (CBC) (anemias), electrolytes (hypokalemia, hypercalcemia), thyroid function studies (hypothyroidism), and glucose (diabetes). If the constipation is functional or due to dehydration, poor diet, or lack of exercise, the laboratory results are usually within normal limits.

RADIOLOGIC (IMAGING) STUDIES

Plain films of the abdomen are useful in acute constipation. They may reveal gaseous distention of the colon with fecal material throughout the colon. The diagnosis of chronic constipation may be made if eight or more radiopaque markers are found on plain films 3 days after ingestion of 20 markers.

Table 6-6-2. Differential Diagnosis for Constipation

Irritable bowel syndrome
Hirschsprung's syndrome
Small bowel obstruction
Colon carcinoma
Colonic polyposis
Rectal disease: ulcerative colitis, fistulas
Foreign body obstruction
Acute abdomen: appendicitis, diverticulitis

Table 6-6-3. Medical Therapy for Constipation

Agent	Mechanism of Action	Common Name	Dose
Increased dietary fiber	Natural bulk agents	Fresh fruits, whole grains, vegetables	10–35 g daily
Bulking agents	Adds bulk to stool, but increased water intake essential		
Psyllium		Metamucil	1 tbs 1-3 × daily with lots of water
Methylcellulose		Citrucel	
Calcium polycarbophil		FiberCon	
Osmotic agents	Draws water into the colonic lumen, inducing peristaltic movement	No special trade names	15 g in water
Magnesium sulfate			15–30 mL daily
Milk of magnesia			240 mL on ice
Magnesium citrate			4–8 g in water
Sodium phosphate			15–30 mL daily
Lactulose		Chronulac	
Stimulants	Increases intestinal peristalsis by direct action on the colon		325–650 mg q HS
Cascara sagrada			12–24 mg q HS
Calcium salts			
Senna		Senokot	2 tablets q HS
Castor oil			15–60 mL q HS
Bisacodyl		Dulcolax	10–15 mg q HS
Lubricants	Coats the intestinal walls and the stool and aides in mobility		
Mineral oil			5–30 mL at bedtime
Fecal softeners	Promotes water retention thereby softening stool (Not a laxative)	Colace, Surfak	
Docusate sodium			50–240 mg with water
Docusate calcium			240 mg daily
Docusate potassium			100–300 mg daily

A barium enema remains the study of choice in the evaluation of constipation, since it can confirm obstructive lesions, redundant colon, megacolon, congenital aberrations, and other problems. Endoscopy is performed to rule out organic lesions, especially in the older patient where colon cancer may present with constipation. A full colonoscopy may be beneficial.

TREATMENT

Pharmacologic Management

Medications are separated into classes based on their action in the colon (Table 6-6-3). Almost all these medications are available over the counter in some form, so it is critical to find out what the patient has been using for self-medication prior to recommending a new regimen.

Supportive Measures

These include regular exercise, increased fluid intake (preferably water), and the intake of at least 5 to 15 g dietary fiber daily. Fiber is essential for increasing the bulk of the stool (making it easier to move). Fruits like dates and prunes, raw or steamed vegetables, and whole grains are considered natural bulking agents. A consultation with a nutritionist is needed in chronic constipation to establish total fiber intake and recommend ways to increase fiber up to between 30 and 35 g/day. Additional measures include a comfortable and private place for defecation. Children and the elderly are not always afforded the privacy they feel is necessary for comfortable evacuation. Steps should be taken to prevent constipation if the patient is placed on a medication regimen that is likely to cause constipation (narcotics, verapamil).

COMPLICATIONS

Ordinarily, constipation does not produce serious complications. Constipation may be a symptom of a serious problem; therefore new onset constipation should be evaluated completely. The most common complication of constipation is hemorrhoids. (See Chap. 6-13, "Hemorrhoids.") Hard stools and extended periods of time on the toilet lead to venous pooling. Hemorrhoids may bleed and/or cause pain. Painful fissures and cracks (see Chap. 6-3, "Anal Fissures") can develop and rectal prolapse can occur especially in the elderly. Excessive straining can create poor blood flow to the heart and brain due to the prolonged increase in abdominal pressure and may exacerbate cardiac and cerebral vascular disease.

Chronic constipation can lead to laxative abuse. The more often an osmotic or irritant cathartic is used, the more "lazy" the colon will become. Eventually, the intestines become insensitive and fail to work on their own; the result is megacolon with loss of haustration and peristalsis.

PATIENT EDUCATION

Judging from pervasive laxative advertisements, constipation is a common problem. Young and old need to be educated on what "normal" bowel habits are and how to avoid constipation. A diet high in fiber and low in fat with adequate fluid intake is the first, best step. Regular exercise, regular times, and a comfortable location for evacuation will help the patient avoid constipation and laxative abuse.

PEARLS

A good history is essential when dealing with constipation. Care should be taken to establish the patient's "normal" bowel habits prior to their perception of the constipation. Investigate the activities of daily living to evaluate mobility, exercise, usual diet, and medication use (over the counter and prescription). Encourage the natural fix for constipation—exercise, fiber, water—before recommending a laxative or similar intervention. Encourage all patients to respond to the natural urge to defecate as soon as possible; delaying evacuation can exacerbate the situation.

BIBLIOGRAPHY

Yasko J: *Constipation—Guidelines for Cancer Care: Symptom Management.* Reston, VA, Reston Publishing, 1983. Updated for Internet 1995: "Etiology of Constipation."

Chapter 6–7
DIARRHEA
Anne P. Heinly

DISCUSSION

Diarrhea is one of the most common human symptoms. Caused by a myriad of diseases or medications, it spares no one in any country. The widely held definition of diarrhea is an increase of daily stool weight by more than 250 g with a change in usual bowel habits. Most patients complain of diarrhea when their stool becomes softer, watery, and/or more frequent. Although most sources of diarrhea are acute and self-limiting, there are other etiologies that can be chronic and potentially life-threatening. A logical and knowledgeable approach is required to discern the differences.

PATHOGENESIS

The gastrointestinal tract functions on fluid, on average a total of 9 L of fluids per day pass through the system, mouth to anus (Table 6-7-1). The GI tract churns ingested food with hydrochloric acid, and the subsequent chyme moves through the pyloric sphincter into the small intestine, where absorption of nutrients, electrolytes, and water take place. The small intestines have an absorption surface equivalent to the size of an outdoor tennis court. Disease can render it ineffective, reducing the surface activity to the size of a ping-pong table.

The small intestine has a dynamic flux of absorption and secretions. Approximately 20 ft long, the small intestine includes the C loop of the duodenum, the jejunum, and the ileum. The mucosal layer contain millions of villi whose fingerlike projections gives the small intestine its incredible absorptive surface. The microvillous membrane absorbs disaccharides, peptides, and amino acids, and is responsible for the co-transport of sodium and D-glucose. Diarrhea is an interruption of this absorption-secretion cycle in the small intestine and the colon.

Most of the fluid (H_2O) is reabsorbed in the distal ileum and the large intestine, with an average final stool weight of 100 to 150 g containing 60 to 65 percent water. Diarrhea occurs when the water weight increases due to either decreased absorption or increased fluid secretions. Table 6-7-2 defines the five different mechanisms of diarrhea and their common etiology. Not all causes of diarrhea fit neatly with a mechanism but may be a combination of factors.

SYMPTOMS

The approach to evaluating a patient with diarrhea should include a good history. First, elicit a description of the onset, duration, timing between stools, color, consistency, and quantity of stool. The presence of blood, mucus, or floating stools are valuable clues to etiology.

- Large, watery, soupy, or greasy stools with cramping and periumbilical pain suggest small bowel.

Table 6-7-1. Daily Fluid Input to GI System

Oral intake	2000 mL
Salivary secretions	1500 mL
Gastric juices	2000 mL
Pancreatic juices	2500 mL
Biliary secretions	500 mL
Small intestinal secretions	1000 mL

- Frequent, small quantities of mushy brown stool with mucus or blood, tenesmus, and achy pain suggest left colon.
- Blood suggests inflammatory, vascular, infectious, or neoplastic etiologies.

The next set of questions should be a good diet history. Does the diarrhea occur before, during, or after meals or at night? Define exposures to others with similar symptoms, travel, camping, and HIV risk factors. Third, explore medication use (Table 6-7-3), especially antibiotic use in the last 2 weeks (see "Pseudomembranous Colitis," Chap. 6-4, "Colitis"). Laxative abuse may cause diarrhea or constipation with a watery diarrhea flowing around an impaction (see Chap. 6-6, "Constipation," and Chap. 6-9, "Fecal Impaction").

OBJECTIVE

Because diarrhea can have so many causes, a complete physical examination may be necessary. Every examination should begin with a complete set of orthostatic vital signs and skin inspection for hydration: dry lips, dry eyes, dry oral mucosa, or skin tenting. Severe dehydration may present with a mental status change: disorientation or altered consciousness. Fever is common with infectious etiologies. The abdominal examination usually reveals mild distention; hyperactive bowel sounds, especially with infectious etiology; and diffuse, poorly localized tenderness. There is usually no mass effect except with Crohn's (right lower quadrant) and diverticulitis (left lower quadrant). Peritoneal signs suggest perforation or toxic megacolon. A digital rectal examination should be done noting fecal impaction, pain, bleeding, fissures, or fistula. An occult blood card (Hemoccult) should be used; the presence or absence of blood helps with the differential diagnosis. Extragastrointestinal symptoms may shed light on the diagnosis as well (Table 6-7-4).

DIAGNOSTIC CONSIDERATIONS

Complications from diarrhea have two basic mechanisms. The first is water and electrolyte losses and their consequences: dehydration, vascular collapse, and potentially death (i.e., epidemic cholera). The second is malabsorption, which can lead to anemias and weight loss.

Acute Diarrhea

Acute diarrhea is generally secondary to an infectious origin or dietary imprudence. Common viral etiologies are due to the rotavirus and Norwalk virus. Bacterial causes are listed in Table 6-7-5. Parasitic causes include *Giardia lamblia, Cryptosporidium, Cyclospora,* and *Entamoeba histolytica.* The signs and symptoms include loose, watery stools, fever, headache, malaise, anorexia, vomiting, myalgia, and abdominal discomfort. The majority of these sources of diarrhea are short-lived, about 24 to 48 h, and require only supportive home care.

Chronic Diarrhea

Chronic diarrhea is defined as a diarrhea that lasts longer than 2 to 3 weeks or appeared as acute, ebbed, and reoccurred within 2 weeks. Persistent diarrhea requires thorough scrutiny. If the diarrhea contains fat (steatorrhea), malabsorption syndromes should be investigated (Chap. 6-18). Chronic diarrhea with blood indicates the need to evaluate for inflammatory bowel disease (Chap. 6-15) or colon cancer (Chap. 13-5). Watery diarrhea without blood is more likely due to a systemic disease like hyperthyroidism, diabetes, or pheochromocytoma. Recent antibiotic use may give clues leading to the diagnosis of pseudomembranous colitis (Chap. 6-4). Complications of any cause for chronic diarrhea include electrolyte and fluid imbalances and malnutrition.

Table 6-7-2. Types of Diarrhea

OSMOTIC

Excess water soluble molecules in bowel lumen causes water influx into the lumen; watery diarrhea is the consequence. Responds to a clear liquid diet.

  Carbohydrate overload
  Magnesium products
    Antacids
    Food supplements
  Lactose deficiency (milk intolerance)
  Sorbitol use
    Sugar-free products
    Diet sodas

SECRETORY

An increase in chloride and water secretion with inhibition of normal active sodium and H$_2$O absorption, copious watery diarrhea without pus or blood ensues. May or may not respond to fasting or clear liquid diet.

  Enterotoxins
    Vibrio cholerae
    Enterotoxigenic *Escherichia coli*
    Aeromonas species
  Hormonal secretagogues
    Cholecystokinin
    Substance P
    Insulin
    Glucagon
  Gastric hypersecretions
    Peptic ulcer disease
    Zollinger-Ellison syndrome
    Carcinoid syndrome
  Laxatives
    Bisacodyl
    Docusate sodium
    Senna
    Cascara
    Phenolphthalein
  Bile salts malabsorption
    Ileum resection
    Primary biliary disease
  Fatty acid malabsorption
    Celiac sprue
    Bacterial overgrowth

EXUDATIVE

Exudation of protein, mucus, and blood from sites of active inflammation of the bowel wall into the intestinal lumen. There is an abnormal mucosal permeability of the intestinal mucosa.

  Idiopathic
    Crohn's disease
    Ulcerative colitis
    Collagen colitis
    Whipple's disease
  Infectious
    Shigella
    Salmonella
    Campylobacter
  Ischemic
    Mesenteric angina or infarction
  Radiation enteritis: (a form of ischemic diarrhea from local radiation therapy
    Abscess formation from any source)

Fast transit causes reduced contact; slow transit may cause diarrhea from bacterial overgrowth.

  Reduced contact with fast transit
    Hyperthyroidism
    Postgastrectomy patients or short bowel syndrome
    Carcinoid syndrome
    Pheochromocytoma
    Irritable bowel syndrome
    Postcholecystectomy

ABNORMAL INTESTINAL MOTILITY

DECREASED MOTILITY WITH SLOW TRANSIT AND BACTERIAL OVERGROWTH

  Diabetes (especially insulin-dependent diabetes mellitus)
  Hypothyroidism
  Addison's disease
  Scleroderma
  Amyloidosis
  Postgastrectomy (blind loop syndrome and afferent loop syndrome)

Traveler's Diarrhea

Traveler's diarrhea affects approximately 10 million travelers a year. The vast majority complain of three or four unformed stools daily with classic acute diarrhea symptoms. Anywhere from 50 to 80 percent of cases are caused by dietary ingestion of diarrhea-producing bacterias (see Table 6-7-5). The mechanism of traveler's diarrhea is usually secretory and caused by enterotoxins. *Escherichia coli* and *Salmonella* are relatively common with travelers in Asia, Africa, and Latin America. Travelers to Russia or campers in the United States may encounter *G. lamblia*. Traveler's diarrhea is a major nuisance on a trip but is rarely life-threatening.

HIV and Diarrhea

Diarrhea may be the presenting symptom of an active HIV infection. The organisms that cause diarrhea in the immunocompromised patient are commonly the opportunistic type (Table 6-7-6). Because of the patient's diminished immune status, symptoms may be more severe and recurrent. Bacteremia and sepsis are often seen, and antibiotic therapy is almost always required.

LABORATORY TESTS

Acute diarrhea without blood may not require any laboratory tests. If the acute diarrhea is causing severe symptoms (e.g., dehydration) or is bloody, it is evaluated as a chronic diarrhea. Begin with a complete blood count, electrolyte panel including

Table 6-7-3. Medications and Diarrhea

There is hardly a medication that does not have diarrhea listed as possible side effect. These are the most common in no particular order:
  Magnesium antacids
  Sulfa drugs
  Antibiotics: Augmentin, Erythromycin
  Antineoplastic: Nolvadex, Adriamycin, Efudex
  Prokinetic agents: Reglan, Propulsid
  Sorbitol: sweetener in many diet foods
  Theophylline products

Table 6-7-4. Extragastrointestinal Symptoms Associated with Diarrhea

Polyarthritis	Ulcerative colitis, Crohn's disease, Reiter's syndrome, Whipple's disease, AIDS, sarcoidosis
Fever	Amebiasis, lymphoma, tuberculosis, inflammatory bowel disease, carcinoid syndromes
Bruising, purpura	Celiac sprue, tropical sprue, acetaminophen overdose
Conjunctivitis or episcleritis	Crohn's disease, ulcerative colitis, thyroid disease, Reiter's syndrome
Erythema nodosum	Sarcoidosis, acute or chronic pancreatitis, ulcerative colitis, Crohn's disease, radiation therapy, *Campylobacter*, *Salmonella*, *Shigella*

Table 6-7-5. Bacterial and Viral Source of Diarrhea

Type/Cause	Characteristics	Remarks
ACUTE DIARRHEA		
Norwalk virus, enterovirus	Watery diarrhea, usually no fever	Supportive hydration, lasts 24–48 h.
Vibrio cholerae	Watery diarrhea, usually no fever	Fluid replacement; tetracycline may shorten course.
Bacillus cereus	Starts with vomiting, then watery diarrhea, rarely fever	Supportive hydration; usually lasts only 24–48 h.
Clostridium perfringens	Profuse, watery diarrhea	Supportive hydration; lasts 24–48 h.
Clostridium difficile	Crampy abdominal pain followed by bloody diarrhea	Cultures not helpful; toxins levels elevated; treat with oral metronidazole (Flagyl) or vancomycin and fluid replacement.
Salmonella spp.	Diarrhea, but usually not profuse, vomiting, low-grade fever	No antibiotics (prolongs carrier stage) unless sepsis is present; fluid replacement.
Shigella spp.	Diarrhea with blood and protein, cramps, fever	Severe cases can be treated with sulfa drugs; mild cases are self-limiting; replace fluids.
CHRONIC DIARRHEA		
Campylobacter jejuni	Fever, diarrhea, blood, and proteins	Intermittent diarrhea over weeks; treat with erythromycin.
Giardia lamblia	Relapsing watery diarrhea, flatulence, bloating, and nausea	Can last for months; treat with metronidazole.
Entamoeba histolytica	Intermittent bloody diarrhea, abdominal pain, weight loss, flatulence	Can be asymptomatic to fulminant; intraluminal, treat with iodoquinol; systemic, treat with metronidazole.
Cyclospora	Relapsing, watery diarrhea, weight loss, anorexia	Self-limiting in most patients; life-threatening in AIDS patients.

blood urea nitrogen (BUN) and creatinine, sedimentation rate, and total protein evaluation. Culture the stool and check for cells, ova, and parasites. *Escherichia coli* 0157:H7 should be specifically sought, because it is implicated in hemolytic uremic syndrome (HUS), which can be life-threatening. *Clostridium difficile* is difficult to culture, so the toxin levels can be evaluated instead (Chap. 6-4, "Colitis").

When looking for the cause of chronic diarrhea, the blood count may indicate malabsorption of folate, niacin, or iron. Liver function studies and thyroid studies may be helpful. Hypersecretion states can be associated with elevated gastrin levels. A Sudan black B fat stain can assess malabsorption syndromes (Chap. 6-18). Check two or three different stools for culture, ova, and parasites, since the organisms or their by-products may not be present in every stool. Be sure to obtain all cultures prior to antibiotic use or barium studies, since both may change the results.

RADIOLOGIC (IMAGING) STUDIES

Plain abdominal films rarely reveal a definitive cause for diarrhea. The one exception is the presence of epigastric calcifications secondary to chronic pancreatitis. Barium studies may reveal the results of exudative diarrhea, neoplasm, diverticulitis, inflammatory bowel disease (IBD), or the spastic colon of irritable bowel syndrome (IBS).

The best study is sigmoidoscopy. This allows direct visualiza-

tion, cultures, and biopsies. Sigmoidoscopy should be done *prior* to barium studies and without the usual hyperosmotic preparation to avoid disturbing the bowel architecture. If no diagnosis is forthcoming, a colonoscope is recommended with multiple biopsies to evaluate the patient for IBD, amebiasis, or amyloidosis. Finally, a CT scan or MRI may be helpful in defining occult carcinomas, pancreatic pseudocysts, or similar problems.

TREATMENT

The patient comes to a provider because of annoying symptoms, and diarrhea tops the list with most people. Try to treat the underlying source of the diarrhea rather than just the symptom. Since dehydration is a common side effect of diarrhea, rehydration is a fundamental part of treatment. Oral hydration solutions include glucose solution with a combination of essential salts: sodium, potassium, chloride, and citrate. Many of the sports drinks, like Pedialyte, are excellent choices in the first 24 h. A homemade rehydration solution can be made with 1/2 gallon of water, 4 to 5 teasp of sugar, and 1 teasp each of table salt and baking soda. Osmotically induced diarrhea and some secretory diarrhea will diminish or cease completely within 24 h of clear liquids only.

Antidiarrheals like loperamide (Imodium), 4 mg initial dose, followed by 2 mg every 4 to 6 h, should be used with care. Loperamide slows the transit time of the intestine and inhibits some intestinal secretions. It does not increase water absorption or change electrolyte balances. Loperamide should not be used in exudative causes of diarrhea like ulcerative colitis, pseudomembranous colitis, or acute dysentery, because the gut slows down too much and the disease process may be exacerbated.

Diphenoxylate hydrochloride (Lomotil) is very effective in slowing intestinal motility, allowing for increased contact of contents with the mucosal surface. This in turn may increase fluid reabsorption. Like loperamide, diphenoxylate should be used with care and never in a patient with fever, bloody diarrhea, or the potential of enterotoxin-producing organisms.

Kaolin and pectin are absorbents and gels used in over-the-counter antidiarrheal medications (Kaopectate). For acute cases, these have not been proved to decrease diarrhea and are not recommended for the treatment of diarrhea of any source.

Table 6-7-6. HIV and Diarrhea

Protozoans
Cryptosporidium
Cyclospora
Entamoeba histolytica
Giardia lamblia
Isospora belli
Microsporida
Strongyloides stercoralis
Viruses
Cytomegalovirus
Epstein-Barr
Herpes simplex

The use of antidiarrheals is not recommended in children under 2 years or the elderly because of potential side effects. Treatment of the underlying cause remains the best choice with adequate fluid and electrolyte replacement regardless of age.

COMPLICATIONS

Acute diarrhea is associated with dehydration with patient complaints of headache, body aches, and anorexia. Electrolyte imbalances may occur with fulminant diarrhea and demand immediate attention to avoid mental status changes or cardiac events. Chronic diarrhea may result in malabsorption of nutrients and vitamins leading to anemias, muscle atrophy, bone loss, failure to thrive, and other symptoms.

PATIENT EDUCATION

Traveler's diarrhea is preventable if proper care is taken. Travelers should avoid tap water when drinking, brushing teeth, using ice cubes, or rinsing drinkware, fruits, and vegetables. Tell patients to drink only bottled water or carbonated drinks from containers that are factory sealed. They should avoid fresh fruits and vegetables unless they peel this food themselves. Foods that have been rewarmed, street food, rare meat, raw seafood, doubtfully boiled foods, or food that appears undercooked should not be eaten.

Prophylaxis with antibiotics may be recommended for trips shorter than 2 weeks in certain populations: the elderly, patients with concomitant GI disease, diabetes, renal disease, cancer, or immunosuppression. Currently, trimethoprim-sulfamethoxazole (Bactrim DS) once daily is the recommended prophylaxis. The fluoroquinolones (Cipro, Noroxin) may be used as an alternative.

PEARLS

The most common cause of diarrhea, virus, and bacteria, are easily treated with fluids, bed rest, and time. Encourage the patient to rest and sip fluids all day, avoid milk products and greasy foods for at least 48 h, and follow a clear liquid diet for at least 24 h. Do not overprescribe antidiarrheals; they are not innocuous and can be abused. This author never gives a patient more than six tablets for control of acute diarrhea. This prevents overuse, and if the diarrhea persists, it forces them to seek follow-up care and further workup. Remember, diarrhea is a symptom, not a disease. Look for the underlying cause and treat it appropriately.

BIBLIOGRAPHY

Almroth S, Latham MC: Rational home management of diarrhea. *Lancet* 345:709–711, 1995.

Talal A, Murray J: Acute and chronic diarrhea. *Postgrad Med* 96(3):30–35, 1994.

Chapter 6–8
DIVERTICULAR DISEASE
Anne P. Heinly

DISCUSSION

Diverticular disease appears to be an unwanted by-product of industrialization, specifically, the milling of whole grains into processed breads and cereals. Virtually, unheard of prior to 1900, diverticular disease may be found in up to half the population in the United States by the age of 70 to 80 years. The development of diverticulosis is unusual before age 40, but the risk increases approximately 5 to 10 percent per decade of life. Of those patients with diverticulosis, perhaps one-fifth will develop diverticulitis, with equal distribution between men and women. Diverticular disease has two components: *diverticulosis,* the presence of diverticula—usually asymptomatic, and *diverticulitis,* inflammation of diverticula—usually symptomatic.

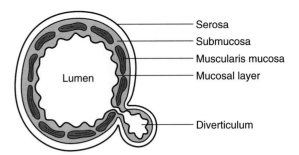

Figure 6-8-1. Diverticular disease.

PATHOGENESIS

Diverticula can occur anywhere along the gastrointestinal tract. However, by convention, the term, when used independently, refers to colonic diverticula. The colon has four layers, the serosa (the outer layer), the muscular layer, the submucosa, and the mucosa (the innermost layer). Diverticulum (singular) and diverticula (plural) are actually pseudodiverticula or herniations of the two inner layers through a defect in muscular band enveloped by the encircling serosa (Fig. 6-8-1). The mechanism of formation appears to be a function of ambient intraluminal pressure in the colon. Because of the low-fiber diet of Americans and other westernized countries, the circular muscles of the colon must contract more forcefully to expel smaller and harder stool products. This leads to an increased intraluminal pressure in segments of the colon, especially the descending and sigmoid colon. Over time, the strength of the colonic connective tissue appears to weaken, and defects in the muscular layer allow for the herniation.

SYMPTOMS

Diverticulosis

More than 80 percent of patients with diverticulosis have no symptoms. Diagnosis is made incidentally during other examinations. Those with symptoms may have left lower quadrant (LLQ) crampy abdominal pain, often described as "gripping"—a short, sharp pain followed by 1 to 2 h of dull, achy pain. This is most likely caused by increased intraluminal pressure during colonic peristalsis. With diverticulosis there is no inflammation, so fever, chills, nausea, and peritoneal signs are absent.

The second symptom in patients without inflammation is painless rectal bleeding, which can be quite extensive. The source is usually a single colonic diverticulum in the ascending colon that has enlarged sufficiently to erode or tear the vast arterial supply in the right lower quadrant (RLQ). The blood may be bright red or maroon (seldom black) and may stop spontaneously or continue intermittently for days. Once a bleed has occurred, there is a 50 percent chance of recurrent bleeds.[1]

Diverticulitis

Diverticulitis is the inflammation of the diverticula. Patients will present with acute abdominal pain, generally persistent and localized to the LLQ. Anorexia, fever, chills, nausea, and vomiting may accompany the pain. A change in bowel habits is common and ranges from sudden onset of constipation to profuse diarrhea. With severe inflammation (multiple microperforations) or frank colonic perforations, peritoneal signs will be present.

OBJECTIVE

With diverticulosis, the patient may have a mass effect in the LLQ. This is most likely in the sigmoid colon, which presents as a firm and tender mass. There may be abdominal distention and increased tympany. Diverticulosis seldom presents with peritoneal signs, fever, or vital sign changes.

Diverticulitis, on the other hand, presents as an acute abdomen with quiet or sluggish bowel sounds, distention, rebound tenderness, fever, and vital sign alterations. Peritoneal irritation is often present with positive psoas, obturator, or heel-tap sign. A tender, firm mass effect is common in the LLQ and can be confirmed with pelvic and/or rectal examination. In the elderly, signs may be blunted owing to decreased immune response.

DIAGNOSTIC CONSIDERATIONS

A differential diagnosis for symptomatic diverticulosis would include constipation, lactose intolerance, or irritable bowel syndrome. Painless bleeding may be secondary to a variety of sources, but it is important to rule out colonic carcinoma, Crohn's disease, or ulcerative colitis, especially in the elderly.

Diverticulitis may mimic any other acute abdomen: appendicitis, colitis, acute gastroenteritis, ulcerative colitis, Crohn's disease, and gynecologic or urologic complaints. The most consistent distinguishing factor is the presence of the a mass effect in the LLQ in the majority of diverticulitis episodes.

LABORATORY TESTS

Laboratory findings for diverticulosis are usually normal. Diverticulitis commonly reveals an elevated white blood cell count with a left shift [prevalence of polymorphonuclear neutrophil leukocytes (PMN)]. Sedimentation rate is elevated, and serum amylase may also climb. In the elderly, the immune response is often blunted, so laboratory signs of inflammation may be less dramatic. A urinalysis may reveal hematuria and/or leukocytosis if there has been compromise of the ureters or bladder.

RADIOLOGIC (IMAGING) STUDIES

During acute episodes of diverticulitis, a plain abdominal film may reveal colonic ileus or air-fluid levels of a perforation. The best examination to define diverticulosis is a barium enema. Diverticula on a barium enema may appear as solitary lesions or in clumps of pedunculated mushroom-like appendages. A barium enema can also demonstrate paracolic abscesses, leaking sacs, fistulas, and strictures caused by the diverticula. The debate still continues on the value of a barium enema during acute diverticulitis. The degree of inflammation may distort the findings, and there is risk of perforating a swollen diverticulum or contaminating the peritoneum with contrast medium if a perforation exists.

Computer tomography has been successfully used to diagnosis acute diverticulitis. The benefit is that it is noninvasive and can detect subtle differences in the colonic walls, fistulas, paracolic abscess, and perforations. Ultrasound and MRI may also be used to define the presence of diverticula. Sigmoidoscopy is not recommended during acute episodes and is limited in its ability to diagnosis diverticulum. Endoscopy is valuable to rule out the

Table 6-8-1. Antibiotics for Diverticulitis

Oral
  Metronidazole (Flagyl), 500 mg every 8 h, with amoxicillin, 500 mg every 8 h
  Ciprofloxacin (Cipro) 500 mg bid
  Norfloxacin (Noroxin) 400 mg bid
Intravenous
  Amikacin (Amikin), 15 mg/kg/day divided dose every 8 h, with metronidazole (Flagyl), 500 mg every 8 h
  Gentamicin (Garamycin), 1 mg/kg every 8 h, with clindamycin, 1.5–2.5 mg/kg/day in divided doses every 8 h
  Cefoxitin, 1–2 g every 12 h

differential diagnosis of cancer, ulcerative colitis, Crohn's disease, or similar illness. Arteriograms can locate the bleeding source from an asymptomatic diverticulum.

TREATMENT

Conservative treatment for diverticulosis is aimed at decreasing intraluminal pressure. The best therapy for this is a high-fiber diet consisting of whole grains, legumes, fruits, and vegetables. The older recommendation of avoiding foods with small seeds and popcorn has not been shown to affect the disease process. Mild analgesics (acetaminophen) and anticholinergics (Bentyl, 10 mg every 6 h) can relieve symptoms of cramping.

Diverticulitis, if mild, can be treated as diverticulosis with the addition of antibiotics (Table 6-8-1). Additionally, the initial diet should be a clear liquid diet to allow for gut rest. After acute symptoms subside, the diet can progress slowly to a high-fiber diet. Many patients can be cared for as outpatients, and elective colon resection is done only for recurrent attacks, fistula formation, or obstruction.

More severely ill patients will require hospitalization and intravenous antibiotics (Table 6-8-1). Surgery is done only for frank perforation, obstruction, or paracolonic abscesses that do not improve with 3 to 7 days of hospital therapy. The optimal situation is to have decreased inflammation prior to surgery to decrease blood loss and surgical risks. There are two approaches: laparotomy with colectomy and resection (when possible) and the newer percutaneous abscess drainage under CT visualization. Obviously, the abscess drainage presents less risk to an acutely ill patient and allows for a delay in the colectomy in 6 to 8 weeks. Delay in colectomy is expedient because it permits immediate resection (anastomosis) at the time of surgery versus the placement of a colostomy during emergency surgery for perforations. In the elderly, the prospect of one surgery versus two (repair of the colostomy) and the attendant anesthesia risk is an important consideration.

COMPLICATIONS

Diverticular abscess, perforation, fistulas, scarring, obstruction, and bleeding are all complications of diverticular disease. Death occurs rarely but is associated with the infirm elderly and immunocompromised patients. Emergency surgery complications occur in about 10 percent of patients ranging from cardiac events and pulmonary embolisms to sepsis.

PEARLS

A diet high in fiber is probably one of the best things to recommend for patients. Diverticular disease is a direct result of low fiber in the diet. Colon cancer has been related to low fiber, and constipation is a chronic problem for many Americans. Encourage patients to add 15 to 20 g of fiber daily to their diet, and diverticular disease may not be the only ailment they avoid.

REFERENCES

1. Sleisenger MH, Fordtran JS: *Gastrointestinal Disease*, 5th ed. Philadelphia, Saunders, 1993, vol 2, p 1353.

BIBLIOGRAPHY

Elfrink R, Miedema B: Colonic diverticula. *Postgrad Med* 92(6):97–105, 1992.

Table 6-9-1. Medications That Cause Constipation and Often Contribute to Impaction

Opiate analgesics (codeine)
Tricyclic antidepressants (amitriptyline)
Phenothiazines
Antihypertensives (alpha- and beta-adrenergic blockers, Ca channel blockers)
Diuretics (furosemide, thiazides)
Antacids (aluminum containing)
Sucralfate
Iron

Chapter 6–9
FECAL IMPACTION
Freddi Segal-Gidan

DISCUSSION

Fecal (stool) impaction is a common and often overlooked disorder, particularly among the elderly and immobilized. It has a variable presentation and many potential complications. It is generally thought to be the end result of unrecognized and untreated constipation. (See Chap. 6-6, "Constipation.") Masses of hard feces accumulate in the rectum, which distends to accommodate the enlarging mass that may back up into the sigmoid colon. It can cause discomfort, pain, delirium, and rarely, in extreme cases, bowel perforation.

Fecal impaction primarily involves the rectum and colon. Changes in the absorption of salt and water from the colon lead to a hardening of the stool. Slowing of peristaltic activity causes packing of fecal matter. The rectum is distendible and able to accommodate an enlarging fecal mass, but the anal canal has limited distensibility and therefore the feces becomes too large to pass.

In hospitalized and immobilized individuals the common presentation is as diarrhea or urinary incontinence. The hard stool of a fecal impaction acts as an irritant against the rectum or colon wall. This then causes production of mucus and fluid, which leaks around the mass and causes small amounts of diarrhea, often associated with fecal incontinence. Irritation by the fecal mass can also lead to bleeding.

SYMPTOMS

Impaction usually presents as a subtle and nonspecific finding. Typical symptoms include abdominal pain, anorexia, nausea, and vomiting. It may be associated with complaints of constipation, diarrhea, and incontinence, either urinary or fecal. Often it is the underlying problem in an elderly person who presents with diarrhea or new-onset urinary incontinence, particularly when accompanied by fecal incontinence. Acute confusion (delirium), especially in an elderly or debilitated individual, may also be due to fecal impaction. Elevated temperature, dysrhythmias, and tachycardia due to impaired motility of the diaphragm from fecal impaction have also been reported.

Whenever the frequency of bowel movements is less than one every other day, a diagnosis of fecal impaction should be considered. There may be a history of no bowel movement for several days or up to a week or more. History of a prior impaction is also a useful clue.

Medications that delay gastric motility are often a contributing factor (Table 6-9-1). Depression and psychosis can themselves be associated with constipation. Ironically, the agents that treat these conditions may worsen the problem and produce impaction as a result of their anticholinergic properties. Fecal impaction occurs at high incidence in association with neurologic conditions that are complicated by immobility such as stroke, Parkinson's disease, multiple sclerosis (MS), and amyotrophic lateral sclerosis (ALS). Rectal impaction is frequently associated with lumbosacral spinal cord injuries, whereas cervical and thoracic spinal cord injuries tend to cause proximal impactions.

OBJECTIVE FINDINGS

A digital rectal examination is essential to assess for impaction of the distal bowel. The lack of stool in the rectal ampule or only loose, watery fecal material may be a tip-off to the presence of impaction higher up. Sphincter tone is usually present. The abdominal examination is often completely normal. There may be decreased or few bowel sounds throughout the abdomen or there may be increased sounds over one region. Fullness may be palpable if a large amount of stool causes distention, especially in thinner individuals. Abdominal mass may be palpated and can be misinterpreted for a tumor or abdominal aorta aneurysm. Urinary retention may be evident, especially when there is urinary incontinence (usually overflow type).

DIAGNOSTIC CONSIDERATIONS

Fecal impaction should be considered to be the underlying cause or a contributing factor in an older adult with diarrhea, urinary incontinence, fecal incontinence, constipation, and any patient presenting with delirium. Patients with chronic renal failure are predisposed to impaction when there is a disturbance of fluid volume and electrolyte imbalance.

SPECIAL CONSIDERATIONS

The geriatric population is particularly prone to develop fecal impaction as a result of a combination of aging changes in the bowel, low dietary fiber, limited fluid intake, and decreased mobility. Hospitalized and immobilized elderly individuals are especially at risk. Patients with a long history of laxative use (dependency) are also at higher risk for both constipation and fecal impaction.

LABORATORY TESTS

Leukocytosis on a complete blood cell count (CBC) may indicate associated sepsis, usually urinary in origin. Electrolyte abnormalities, particularly hyponatremia and hypokalemia, may also be associated with impaction and/or underlying dehydration. Stool samples should be assessed for occult blood, which may reflect mucosal irritation of an impaction or be a sign of an underlying colon tumor.

RADIOLOGIC STUDIES

A flat-plate x-ray of the abdomen (KUB) is useful for documentation of the presence of an impaction, particularly when high in the sigmoid colon. The abdominal x-ray may demonstrate colonic dilatation and unusual air-fluid level in the small bowel due to masses of stool or obstruction.

TREATMENT

Disimpaction is essential. This should be initiated manually by rectal examination and stimulation to break up the impaction, followed by an enema (oil retention or Fleet saline). Further manual disimpaction may be necessary. Gentle, progressive dilatation first with one, then two fingers and a scissoring action is used to fragment the impaction and aid its expulsion. Lidocaine jelly for local anesthesia and lubrication may be used. Transvaginal pressure with the other hand in women may also be helpful. Do not use irritant laxatives as they may irritate the rectal mucosa and cause bleeding. Attempts to remove an impaction from above by catharsis are useless, may worsen the pain, or may contribute to complications.

Normal bowel function should then be restored to prevent reimpaction. An essential component of this is review of the patient's daily food and fluid intake. A diet high in fiber, preferably obtained from fruits, vegetables, and whole grain cereals and with adequate liquids (2 L/day at minimum) is ideal. Dietary fiber can be supplied by Miller's bran added to foods or the use of bulk-producing products (e.g., Metamucil). Stool softeners and lubricants may be required daily in the individual with chronic constipation, but contain risk. If there is no stool for 2 days, a glycerine suppository should be administered. If this fails to produce any stool, a saline enema on the third day may be required.

COMPLICATIONS AND RED FLAGS

Fecal incontinence is the most common complication of impaction. Seepage of mucus and stool may lead to decubitus ulceration around the anus. Urinary tract infections may also be caused by fecal contamination from incontinence associated with an impaction. Ulcerations with occult bleeding may occur from the pressure and ischemic necrosis on the colon wall caused by the fecal mass. Perforation is rare and has a high mortality rate. In the spinal cord–injured, autonomic dysreflexia, a potentially life-threatening condition, may be provoked by fecal impaction. Fecalomas may be caused by tumors as well as mimic them.

PEARLS

In the elderly, immobilized, and institutionalized always keep a high suspicion for underlying fecal impaction. Impaction high in the colon is often associated with an underlying adenocarcinoma.

BIBLIOGRAPHY

Read NW, Celik AF, Katsinelos P: Constipation and incontinence in the elderly. *J Clin Gastroenterol* 20(1):61–70, 1995.
Wrenn K: Fecal impaction. *New Engl J Med* 321(10):658–662, 1989.

Chapter 6–10
GALLBLADDER DISEASE
Anne P. Heinly

ANATOMY

The gallbladder is a small pear-shaped organ tucked beneath the liver in the right upper quadrant, protected by the anterior rib cage. Its primary function is the storage and subsequent release of bile. Holding approximately 40 mL of bile, the gallbladder releases bile in response to meals, especially fatty meals. The bile is released through the cystic duct into the common bile duct, traveling to the sphincter of Oddi and into the duodenum, aiding in the digestion of fats. (See Fig. 6-10-1.) Bile is a conglomeration of bile salts (acids), phospholipids, unconjugated bilirubin, and cholesterol held in suspension. Bile acids are detergents which, above a critical concentration, form aggregates called *micelles*. These micelles are essential for normal intestinal absorption of dietary fats.

Cholelithiasis
DISCUSSION

Between 10 and 20 percent of the general population develops gallstones. Women are twice as likely to develop stones; the acronym "4Fs = female, fat, forty, and fertile" is most likely secondary to the estrogen factor. The likelihood of stone development increases with age. Stones are rare in the Far East and Africa but common in Native Americans and in women in Chile and Sweden. Although four-fifths remain asymptomatic, found only when abdominal studies are done for other reasons, a small percentage (1 to 4 percent) of patients per year will develop symptoms if stones are present.

PATHOGENESIS

Choleliths, or gallstones, are formed when the concentrations of bile salts and cholesterol change. Eighty percent of all gallstones are cholesterol stones, formed when there is a relative increase in cholesterol biosynthesis and a decrease in bile acid synthesis.[1] A bile acid concentration greater than half keeps cholesterol in solution. Supersaturation of bile with cholesterol, gallbladder hypomotility, and crystal nucleation all promote stone formation. Table 6-10-1 reviews risk factors for the formation of cholesterol stones.

Black pigment stones are more common in patients with cirrhosis or chronic hemolytic conditions like hereditary spherocytosis and sickle cell disease, commonly found in the pediatric population. The stones are made up of polymers of bilirubin. Brown pigmented stones are composed of calcium salts of bilirubin and may be associated with infection. *A special note concerning ceftriaxone (Rocephin):* this drug can cause ceftriaxone-calcium sludge and may present as cholelithiasis. The condition appears to be transient and reversible with the discontinuation of the medication.

SIGNS AND SYMPTOMS

Typical signs and symptoms include biliary colic, which is described as a steady, severe pain that takes several hours to resolve. (Colic is a misnomer because it implies an intermittent process; biliary pain is generally steady.) Pain is frequently located in the right upper quadrant (RUQ) and/or epigastrium and it may

Table 6-10-1. Risk Factors for Cholesterol Stones

Risk Factors	Mechanism
Estrogens (childbearing age, OC, HRT)	Reduces synthesis of bile acid, increased cholesterol
Obesity	Increased hepatic secretion of cholesterol
Very-low-calorie diet	Changes in biliary lipid profile and gallbladder hypomotility
Decreased high-density lipoprotein	HDLs break up cholesterol
Ileal disease (Crohn's)	Decreased bile acid retrieval
Clofibrate (Atromid S) therapy	Increased hepatic secretion of cholesterol
Hypertriglyceridemia	Change in lipid concentrations
Increasing age	Increased hepatic secretion and decreased bile acids
Non-insulin-dependent diabetes mellitus	Mechanism not well understood

NOTE: OC = oral contraceptives; HRT = hormone replacement therapy; HDL = high-density lipoprotein.

radiate to the right shoulder, right scapula, or back. Anorexia and nausea with or without vomiting is common. Attacks are often precipitated by a fatty meal but not always. Bile excretion follows a diurnal pattern, peaking at midnight, so the patient may awaken with pain. Symptoms often attributed to the presence of gallstones, including belching, bloating, chronic pain and fatty food intolerance, are not necessarily exclusive to cholelithiasis.

OBJECTIVE

Right upper quadrant and/or epigastric tenderness without rebound may be noted. The gallbladder may be palpable. Murphy's

Table 6-10-2. Complications of Cholelithiasis

Cystic duct obstruction
Acute cholecystitis
Cholangitis (sepsis)
Perforation and peritonitis
Fistulization to other abdominal structures
Provoked acute pancreatitis

sign is when there is an inspiratory arrest with deep palpation under the midpoint of the right costal margin. Vital signs may show tachycardia with no fever. Jaundice is rarely seen. Complications of cholelithiasis (Table 6-10-2) reveal more physical findings and should be considered with any examination.

DIAGNOSTIC CONSIDERATIONS

It is good to remember that the differential diagnosis can work in reverse. Gallstones may present atypically and manifest as a lactose intolerance or gastroesophageal reflux disease. Conversely, the presence of stones may be blamed for symptoms that are actually associated with a totally different disease process. See Table 6-10-3 for the differential diagnosis.

A special note about gallbladder cancer: the vast majority of patients with gallbladder cancer have choleliths. The choleliths are often solitary and large (3 cm), though no concrete connection has been made between the presence of stones and the development of cancer. It is worth an index of suspicion when evaluating a patient with symptoms. Native Americans are at high risk of gallbladder cancer, and with cholelithiasis that risk increases. Large stones or a calcified gallbladder wall (porcelain gallbladder) should ring alarm bells for continued evaluation and treatment.

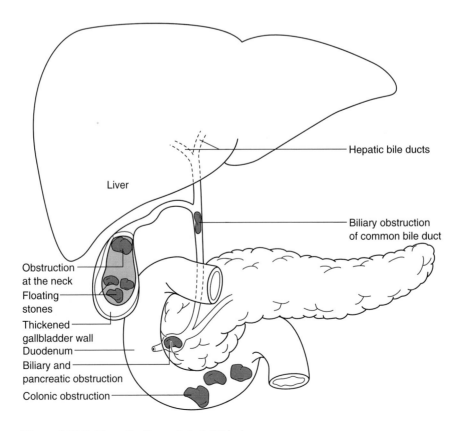

Figure 6-10-1. Complications of cholelithiasis.

Table 6-10-3. Differential Diagnosis of Cholelithiasis*

Disease	Helpful Lab Differential
Pancreatitis	Amylase five times normal, ↑ lipase
Acalculous cholecystitis	Leukocytosis, mild LF abnormalities
Hepatitis (any type)	Elevation of liver enzymes
Peptic ulcer disease	CBC may reveal anemia, ± LFS changes
Colon disease	CBC may reveal anemia, ± LFS changes
Gastroesophageal reflux disease	CBC may reveal anemia, ± LFS changes
Lactose intolerance	No lab changes
Drug-induced cholestasis	Liver function changes, mild to severe
Calcium channel blockers	
Oral hypoglycemics	
Antibiotics	
Tricyclic antidepressants	
Anticonvulsants	
Tranquilizers	

* Limited list, represents the most common differentials.

NOTE: LF = liver function; CBC = complete blood cell count; LFS = liver function studies.

LABORATORY TESTS

Laboratory studies do not diagnose the presence of choleliths but may help differentiate their potential complications. Liver function tests may show an increase in conjugated bilirubin and increased alkaline phosphatase out of proportion with the mild elevation seen with the other liver enzymes. A serum amylase may be elevated with a common bile duct obstruction causing an acute pancreatitis. Complete blood cell count (CBC) may reveal a leukocytosis consistent with inflammation or infection.

RADIOLOGIC (IMAGING) STUDIES

Some choleliths may be radiopaque and easily seen on plain abdominal films. The oral cholecystogram (OCG) has been around for years and has a predictive rate of 90 to 95 percent. However, an OCG may not visualize small stones, takes longer to perform (not good in emergent care), and is contraindicated in pregnancy and iodinate contrast allergies. The study of choice today is the ultrasound.

The gallbladder ultrasound can be done rapidly, accurately identifies stones (even a small one) with a predictive rate of >95 percent, and can give a real-time assessment of gallbladder volume and contractility. Additionally, other abdominal structures are easily visualized and ruled out as a source of pathology. The ultrasound may not be diagnostic in the setting of obesity, ascites, excessive bowel gas, or recent barium studies.

Technetium iminodiacetic acid 99m (IDA) cholescintigraphy (HIDA, DIDA scans) has a predictive value in excess of 95 percent and is especially helpful in revealing a nonfunctional gallbladder with or without stones. This examination is generally done when gallbladder ultrasound has failed to reveal stones but symptoms of gallbladder disease persist. It is not used as the initial diagnostic tool.

TREATMENT

Management of asymptomatic stones is still controversial but it is generally accepted for the following conditions: nonfunctioning gallbladder, calcified gallbladder wall, history of pancreatitis or diagnosis of non-insulin-dependent diabetes mellitus (NIDDM). Studies do not support the presumption that all choleliths require treatment.

There are three treatment choices for symptomatic cholelithiasis: dissolution therapy, laparoscopic cholecystectomy, and open cholecystectomy. Dissolution therapy is a noninvasive medication option indicated in approximately one-third of symptomatic patients. Criteria[2] for use are listed in Table 6-10-4. Ursodiol (ursodeoxycholic acid) increases the bile acid concentration and over 6 months to 2 years can dissolve stones up to 15 mm in size. Complete dissolution occurs in less than half of patients with free-floating stones. The primary side effect of the medication is a transient diarrhea. Unfortunately, the reoccurrence of stones is likely, and patients may have complications due to cystic duct obstruction and inflammation. Smaller stones are still stones and can cause trouble.

Methyl-*tert*-butyl ether (MTBE) has been used for direct-contact solvent of choleliths. Again, only one-third of symptomatic patients are candidates for this type of dissolution. The agent is instilled into the gallbladder through a percutaneous catheter placed through the liver using endoscopic retrograde cholangiopancreatography (ERCP). Dissolution can occur within 24 h. Cholesterol stones are the only ones affected by this solvent, and reoccurrence of stones is common. Currently, this procedure is available only at large medical teaching facilities.

Laparoscopic cholecystectomy is a new procedure. It was first performed in 1988, and it has now become commonplace. The most dramatic results of the laparoscopic cholecystectomy are the reduction of hospital days, decreased postoperative pain, and a quick return to routine for the patients. Patients who should not be considered for laparoscopic surgery include those with widespread peritonitis, severe pancreatitis, septic shock from cholangitis, end-stage liver disease, and gallbladder cancer and those in the third trimester of pregnancy.[3]

Open cholecystectomy remains a safe and effective therapy for symptomatic cholelithiasis. Unlike the dissolution therapy, cholecystectomy considerably decreases the reoccurrence of stones and gallbladder cancer. Additionally, the open approach facilitates bile duct exploration for choledocholithiasis (bile duct stones) which are a potential complication in up to one-fourth of patients. Severe complications of open cholecystectomy are rare, but the cost in hospital days, pain, and time off from work have made this procedure second choice to the laparoscopic approach.

Gallstone lithotripsy is being investigated. In countries using this method of extracorporeal shock wave lithotripsy, the stone clearance is as high as 95 percent. Solitary stones up to 20 mm in diameter have been shattered. Complications include transient liver enzyme elevations, pancreatitis, and hematuria. As with dissolution therapy, reoccurrence is a problem. Currently, the U.S. Food and Drug Administration (FDA) has not approved gallbladder lithotripsy in the United States.

Several recommendations may help diminish the occurrence of gallstones. Slow weight loss versus drastic weight loss diets may help. Studies found that women who lost 10 kg in a 2-year period had a higher incidence of cholelithiasis then those who lost 4 to 9 kg.[4] A vegetarian diet decreases the incidence rate and can be recommended for prevention of other disease processes as well. Avoidance of medications that are known to precipitate gallstones is a reasonable idea where possible.

Table 6-10-4. Ursodiol (Actigall) Criteria

Functional gallbladder
Stones are less than 15 mm in diameter
Stones are shown to float
Patient is poor candidate for surgery or refuses surgery

SPECIAL CONSIDERATIONS

Three special groups deserve mention when discussing cholelithiasis. The first is North American Indians, who are at high risk for the development of stones and subsequent complications. Although the pneumonic, "fat, forty, female, and fertile" is generally true, North American Indians sometimes develop stones in the first and second decade. Additionally, normal-weight women may form gallstones. The rationale for this has been linked to slow intestinal transit time; constipation seems to change the composition of the bile.

The second group is made up of children who are incidentally diagnosed with choleliths (often associated with hemolytic anemia, cystic fibrosis, and sickle cell disease). These children should be considered for prophylactic cholecystectomy because they will almost always develop symptoms. The geriatric population is the third group frequently plagued with cholelithiasis. Unfortunately, the normal aging process dulls signs and symptoms owing to a decrease in immune responses. The geriatric patient with a gangrenous or ruptured gallbladder secondary to stones may not run fever or reveal a significant leukocytosis. A good history, good physical, and healthy suspicion are required to pick up the source of an acute abdominal event in the elderly.

PEARLS

The majority of people with cholelithiasis will never have symptoms, but those who do will have pain and nausea. Since pain and nausea are common to many other gastrointestinal disease processes, evaluation for stones or the acalculous nonfunctioning gallbladder is worth the time and effort. Potential complications, especially in the elderly, can be debilitating and life-threatening.

Cholecystitis

DISCUSSION

Cholecystitis is inflammation of the gallbladder. Affecting more than 15 million people a year, the vast majority are associated with the presence of choleliths (gallstones). Initially, there may be obstruction to the neck of the gallbladder or the cystic duct by stones. (See Fig. 6-10-1.) This leads to distention and inflammation. The inflamed gallbladder wall is then colonized by opportunistic bowel flora and infection ensues. The pathogens most often found include *Escherichia coli*, *Klebsiella* species, group D *Streptococcus*, *Staphylococcus* species, and *Clostridium* species.[5] Factors that may predict a serious course include the presence of diabetes, stones more than 2 cm in diameter, a nonpacifying gallbladder, or a calcified gallbladder.

About 10 percent of cholecystitis is caused by an acalculous gallbladder. The incidence is rising, especially in the elderly. Failure to diagnose and treat it early can result in gangrene and perforation of the gallbladder. Reported death rates range for 6 to 67 percent, compared with 3 percent for ordinary acute cholecystitis.[6] One possible etiology is decreased blood flow through the cystic artery secondary to CHF, arteriosclerosis, diabetes, lymphadenopathy, shock, or metastasis. See Table 6-10-5 for the setting of acute gallbladder inflammation complicating severe underlying illnesses.

SIGNS AND SYMPTOMS

The trio of RUQ pain, fever, and leukocytosis is extremely suggestive of acute cholecystitis. The pain is steady and unremitting, increasing in intensity over 24 h in the RUQ and/or epigastrium. Radiation of pain may be to the right scapula, back, or shoulder. Nausea with vomiting is frequently seen, and the patient may present with evidence of dehydration. A low-grade fever

Table 6-10-5. Etiology of Acalculous Cholecystitis

Decreased gallbladder function ($\downarrow$ motility)
Starvation (very-low-calorie diets)
Major trauma
Severe burns
Nonbiliary surgery
Prolonged labor
Total parental nutrition
Anesthesia induction
Narcotic use
Unusual bacteria
Leptospira
Vibrio cholerae
Salmonella
Parasites: *Isospora billi* found in some AIDS patients
Immunosuppressed patients
Severe atherosclerotic heart disease (AHD) and peripheral vascular disease

($<103°F$) is common. Mild jaundice is present in some patients. The presenting symptoms are the same with calculous and acalculous nonfunctioning gallbladder disease.

OBJECTIVE

Physical examination may show an acutely ill patient, often preferring the fetal position with fever, mild tachycardia, and shallow respirations. Abdominal examination reveals mild distention, hypoactive bowel sounds, and RUQ tenderness with guarding. Rebound tenderness may occur if there is peritoneal irritation. Murphy's sign is often positive (inspiratory arrest with steady compression of the right costal margin in the midclavicular line). Jaundice and evidence of dehydration may be evident.

DIAGNOSTIC CONSIDERATIONS

The elderly often present differently. As many as half do not have a fever, and one-third may have a nontender abdomen. The differential diagnosis can include every "-itis" possible in the abdomen and many pulmonary or cardiac diagnoses as well. Table 6-10-6 reviews the most common differentials.

LABORATORY TESTS

Laboratory studies should include a complete blood count, which will frequently reveal a leukocytosis (10,000 to 15,000) with a left shift. Serum bilirubin may be mildly elevated as will the alkaline phosphatase.

RADIOLOGIC (IMAGING) STUDIES

The gallbladder ultrasound is the diagnostic choice because it is rapid, easily accessed at the bedside, and noninvasive. Although the following findings are not exclusive to acute cholecystitis, they do help in the diagnosis:

- Gallbladder wall thickening (greater than 4 mm)
- Distention of the gallbladder

Table 6-10-6. Differential Diagnosis for Cholecystitis*

Perforated peptic ulcer
Retrocecal appendicitis
Right lower lobe pneumonia
Myocardial infarction
Pancreatitis
Hepatitis

* Partial list—most commonly seen.

Table 6-10-7. Postcholecystectomy Complications

Early
    Atelectasis or other pulmonary events
    Subphrenic abscess formation
    Biliary enteric fistula
    Bile leak
    Hemorrhage
    Mechanical obstruction by retained calculi
Late
    Biliary strictures
    Retained biliary calculi
    Cystic stump syndrome
    Stenosis of the sphincter of Oddi
    Bile-salt–induced diarrhea or gastritis

- Dependent echogenic bile sludge or stones
- A sonographic Murphy's sign (focal tenderness directly over the visualized gallbladder)

There are several ultrasound findings that are consistent with an acalculous cholecystitis with gangrene:

- There is no sonographic Murphy's sign (nerve fibers have been destroyed).
- The inner layer sloughs in the presence of necrosis and may reveal thick mucus within the lumen.
- A frayed or irregular gallbladder wall indicates hemorrhage and microabscesses.

Radionuclide scans (HIDA, DIDA) can diagnose acute cholecystitis or a nonfunctioning gallbladder when bilirubin levels or acute disease precludes the usefulness of other examinations.

COMPLICATIONS

Emphysematous Cholecystitis

This is an acute cholecystitis with ischemia and infection by gas-producing organisms like *Clostridium welchii* and *Clostridium perfringens*. It is common in elderly men and patients with diabetes. Plain films will reveal gas within the gallbladder lumen and dissection with the gallbladder wall forming a gaseous ring. Mortality rate is high, and surgical intervention is essential.

Chronic Cholecystitis

Cholelithiasis is almost always responsible for chronic cholecystitis. Repeated bouts of subacute cholecystitis lead to a chronic colonization of bacteria in the gallbladder. Surgery is the preferred treatment with intraoperative and postoperative antibiotic therapy.

Acute cholecystitis left untreated can lead to gallbladder rupture and gangrene, hepatitis, and pancreatitis. Prompt treatment of this acute abdomen is essential to avoid life-threatening sequelae. Table 6-10-7 reviews complications associated with postcholecystectomy patients.

TREATMENT

Pharmacologic Management

Antibiotic therapy is aimed at gram-negative organisms. One of the commonly used combination antibiotics is ampicillin sodium–sulbactam sodium (Unasyn), 1.5 g every 6 h by IV piggyback. Single-therapy choices include ampicillin, 500 mg qid; cefoperazone (Cefobid), 2 to 4 g/day in divided doses; or amikacin sulfate, 15 mg/kg/day in divided doses.

Surgical Management

Surgical management is a cholecystectomy within a few days of the first attack. Early surgery in those without anesthesia risk has limited complications and precludes additional attacks if surgery is delayed for several months. One-fourth of patients who decline surgery will have another significant attack. Seriously ill patients with concomitant disease who have not responded to antibiotics may not be eligible for cholecystectomy. The alternative therapy, done under local anesthesia, is the ultrasound-guided percutaneous puncture of the gallbladder.

Laparoscopic cholecystectomy is revolutionizing therapy for cholecystitis. An appropriate patient is prepped for surgery. A single trocar needle is inserted through the umbilicus, and the abdomen is distended with CO_2. Once the structures are visualized and judged approachable, two other small incisions are made to essentially triangulate on the gallbladder. With three laparoscopic or trocar devices, the gallbladder is teased away from the liver and the cystic duct cut and clamped simultaneously. The entire procedure can take as little as 20 min compared with an average of 1 1/2 h for the standard open cholecystectomy. Only a small number of laparoscopic surgeries are converted to open cholecystectomy intraoperatively.

The recovery expectations are excellent. Some centers are doing the laparoscopic procedure as a day surgery versus open cholecystectomy hospital stays of 2 to 5 days. The patient is often back to work (without limitations) in 1 week compared to 4 to 6 weeks. The most common complaint of patients is a feeling of pressure in the abdomen and chest secondary to the CO_2.

Supportive Management

Supportive management of acute cholecystitis begins with bed rest and GI tract rest. The patient should be kept NPO (nothing by mouth) or if necessary (to ensure gastric decompression) use a nasal gastric tube. IV therapy for replacement of fluids and electrolytes should be maintained and adjusted to the patient's needs. Caution is required because the elderly can develop CHF and pulmonary edema with fluid overload. Pain relief should not include morphine, which may cause spasm at the sphincter of Oddi. Ketorolac (Toradol), 60 mg IM every 8 h, is good alternative to narcotic use. Improvement is generally seen within 24 h, at which time surgical intervention is considered.

PEARLS

Cholecystitis is the most common complication of cholelithiasis and presents with classic symptoms of RUQ pain, fever, and leukocytosis. The pattern of pain is the practitioner's best clue to the source of this acute abdomen: constant, unremitting, and progressive pain in the RUQ. Colonic pain tends to be colicky and pancreatic in the left upper quadrant (LUQ). Additionally, history helps with the common presentation of symptoms in females who are fertile, older than 40 years, and obese. Remember the special circumstances of the North American Indian, children, and the elderly, where a healthy index of suspicion is required to make the diagnosis.

REFERENCES

1. Johnston D, Kaplan M: Pathogenesis and treatment of gallstones. *New Engl J Med* 348(6):412–418, 1993.
2. Shaw M: Current management of symptomatic gallstones. *Postgrad Med* 93(1):183–187, 1993.
3. NIH releases consensus statement on gallstones, bile duct stones and laparoscopic cholecystectomy. *Am Fam Physician* 46(5):1571–1574, 1992.
4. Everhart J: Contributions of obesity and weight loss to gallstone disease. *Ann Intern Med* 119(10):1029–1034, 1993.
5. Greenberger NJ, Isselbacher KJ: Diseases of the gallbladder and bile

ducts, in Fauci AS, Braunwald E, Isselbacher KJ (eds): *Harrison's Principles of Internal Medicine,* 14th ed. New York, McGraw-Hill, 1998, chap 302.

6. Chung, SC: Acute acalculous cholecystitis. *Postgrad Med* 98(3):199–204, 1995.

Chapter 6–11
GASTROESOPHAGEAL REFLUX DISEASE

Anne P. Heinly

DISCUSSION

Commercial programming on television gives a hint about the prevalence of gastroesophageal reflux disease (GERD). It is estimated to occur monthly in at least one-third of the adult population with equal distribution between men and women. A low estimate of 10 percent of the population has GERD symptoms once a week. Unlike acute illness, gastroesophageal reflux disease tends to be chronic and reoccurring, with many patients reporting 10 or more years of intermittent symptoms. It is by far the most common esophageal disease process, known to the public as heartburn, indigestion, or dyspepsia. It is often self-treated with over-the-counter medications for years prior to patients' bringing complaints to their health care provider.

PATHOGENESIS

Lined by stratified squamous epithelium, the esophagus acts as a conduit for food transport. The outer longitudinal layer of muscle is primarily striated, skeletal muscle, and the inner circular layer is smooth muscle, especially over the distal half of the esophagus. Food is transferred from the mouth to the stomach in three phases: swallowing, esophageal peristalsis, and passage through the lower esophageal sphincter (LES). The main culprit in gastroesophageal reflux disease seems to be the lack of LES tone.

The lower esophageal sphincter is a physiologic phenomenon functioning at the distal esophagus. The LES relaxes to a pressure of zero in response to swallowing a bolus of food with a combination of muscular attributes and active neural tone regulated by a complex interaction of neural and hormonal factors. Lower esophageal sphincter pressure is easily changed by many different mechanisms, as listed in Table 6-11-1.

Gastroesophageal reflux disease is secondary to a low or absent resting LES pressure, allowing gastric contents to contaminate the esophageal mucosa. The other part of the equation is the gastric contents; the longer hydrochloric acid, bile salts, and pepsin contact the esophageal mucosa, the greater the chance of injury. Injury to the basal cell layer of the esophagus requires pH level < 4. The body's natural protective mechanism is to replace the injured areas with tissue better suited to low pH levels. Persistent irritation can lead to change of the squamous cell structure to a metaplastic columnar epithelium, a condition called Barrett's esophagitis. Table 6-11-2 reviews the protective mechanisms for the esophagus against the elements that cause GERD.

Table 6-11-1. Lower Esophageal Sphincter Tone

LES Pressure Increased by = Tighter Tone	LES Pressure Decreased by = Looser Tone
Hormones: Tighter tone occurs during gastric churning, preventing reflux.	Hormones: Loosen tone in response to pyloric antrum chemoactive agents; allow the pyloric sphincter to relax and food to pass to the duodenum; lower LES pressure.
Gastrin	Secretin
Substance P	Cholecystokinin
Pancreatic polypeptides	Glucagon
Prostaglandin $F_{2\alpha}$	Progesterone
	Birth control pills
	Hormone replacement therapy
	Adenosine
Foods	Foods
High-protein foods	Fats
	Chocolates
	Alcohol
	Peppermint
	Coffee (caffeine)
Medications and miscellaneous	Medication and miscellaneous
Antacids	Beta adrenergics (Alupent, Proventil)
Metoclopramide (Reglan)	Alpha adrenergics (Minipress, Hytrin)
Cisapride (Propulsid)	Theophyllines
Histamine	Anticholinergic agents
Raised intraabdominal pressure	Antihistamines
	Antidepressants
	Antipsychotics
	Calcium channel blocking agents
	Diazepams and barbiturates
	Dopamine and nitrates
	Meperidine (Demerol), morphine
	Smoking
	Obesity and pregnancy (prolonged increased abdominal pressure

SYMPTOMS

The severity of symptoms does not necessarily translate into level of tissue injury. The most classic symptom of GERD is heartburn, which is translated variously as burning substernal pain, sternal pressure, uncomfortable chest, or crushing chest pain. The pain may radiate to the neck, back, or left shoulder. Thus it often confuses a cardiac workup. The pain is ordinarily worse with bending over or lying down, especially after a meal. The pain is improved with antacids, sitting up, or standing. The pain is seldom described in the epigastric area.

Associated symptoms include increased belching and regurgitation, which leave a bitter (gastric contents) or salty taste (water brash) in the mouth. Symptoms consistent with complications from GERD include progressive dysphagia (strictures, tumors); chronic cough or recurrent pneumonia (aspiration); exacerbation of asthma (GERD is found in up to 70 percent of asthma patients); and hoarseness and mouth and gingival ulcers (possibly due to acidic reflux, especially with nighttime regurgitation). In infants, symptoms include failure to thrive, recurrent upper respiratory infections, and frequent regurgitation. Another unusual indication of possible GERD in children is Sandifer's syndrome, which is intermittent torticollis or peculiar posturing.

"Red flag" symptoms should prompt rapid evaluation of the patient's disease process. When a patient has red flag symptoms, clinical treatment without investigation is not appropriate. Evaluate GERD as soon as possible with any of the following symp-

Table 6-11-2. Esophageal Protection and Injury Mechanisms

Protection Mechanisms	Injury Mechanisms

Antireflux barrier: The lower esophageal sphincter, closes with gastric churning and in response to other stimulants. Average resting pressure 20 mmHg.	Weak or incompetent LES: Loss of resting tone, pressures as low as 0–10 mmHg.
	    Transient LES relaxation secondary to foods, medications, or hormones
	    Disruption of the anatomy—hiatal hernia
	    Loss of neural/hormonal tone—etiology unknown

Luminal clearance: Primary and secondary peristaltic waves sweep down the entire esophagus, emptying out the LES each time, leaving limited acidic residue.	Poor luminal clearance: Esophagus unable to clear properly.
	    Mechanical: Strictures, tumors, diverticuli, hiatal hernia, volume of food, poor gastric emptying
	    Tertiary peristalsis: Ineffective, random peristalsis of the esophagus
	    Neuromuscular disorders: Chagas disease, myasthenia gravis, etc.

Saliva: Salivary bicarbonate neutralizes acid pH. It takes 7–10 mL of saliva to neutralize 1 mL of 0.1 N HCl.*	Gastric refluxant: HCl, pepsin, bile acids, and trypsin cause mucosal injury or facilitate susceptibility to injury.

Epithelial resistance: Mucous layer, unstirred water layer (just adjacent to cell surface with pH 5), and bicarbonate protect the immediate surface.
Tyrosine kinase, an epidermal growth factor, promotes buffering and swift cell replication and replacement.
	Tobacco use:
	    Decreased mucosal blood flow
	    Decreases LES tone
	    Depresses gastric mucosal prostaglandin synthesis
	    Interferes with the action of H_2 blockers

Rich blood supply and tissue acid-base status allow for waste removal and intact cell-mediated healing factors.	
LES/stomach anatomy: The acute angle at which the esophagus enters the stomach creates a type of flap valve	Gastric volume: The fuller the GI tract is, the more likely the acute angle of the LES and stomach will be lost, increasing reflux.
Gastric emptying time: Along with appropriate esophageal clearance, keeps food on its way.	Increased volume from large meals, especially if patient lays down after meal. Pyloric obstruction (ulcers, strictures). Obesity, pregnancy, and ascites increase intraabdominal pressure.

* Kahrilas P, Hogan P: Physiology of the Esophagus, in Sleisenger MH, Fordtran JS: *Gastrointestinal Disease,* 5th ed. Philadelphia, Saunders, 1993, p 384.

toms: progressive dysphagia, recurrent pneumonia, persistent cough, failure to thrive (in children), or evidence of bleeding.

OBJECTIVE

Physical examination is often disappointing. A thorough examination of the mouth, pharynx, lungs, heart, and abdomen is indicated, in addition to a rectal examination. Occasionally, gingival erosion or oral mucosal ulcers are seen. Halitosis may be present. Skin changes such as thickening, Raynaud's phenomenon, sclero-

dactyly, and telangiectasia may suggest scleroderma, which is commonly associated with esophageal diseases.

Infants and children should be examined for evidence of growth retardation or failure to thrive. Measure height, weight, and head circumference on each visit to track any trends. Stools in both adults and children should be checked for occult blood.

DIAGNOSTIC CONSIDERATIONS

The differential diagnosis includes the skin and all the systems in the chest: respiratory, cardiac, musculoskeletal, gastrointestinal, and neurologic (Table 6-11-3). Of primary concern is the similarity of cardiac pain with esophageal pain. Angina pectoris and myocardial infarction can mimic GERD and vice versa. In emergent situations, cardiac sources must be ruled out first. Few people die of acute GERD, but they do of acute myocardial infarction (MI).

LABORATORY TESTS

No routine laboratory testing defines GERD since it is a structural problem, not a systemic one. Routine laboratory tests, ECG, and chest x-ray may be done to help rule out the differential diagnosis.

The most definitive test is esophageal pH monitoring. A probe is placed near the LES area and pH is monitored over a 24-h period. A low esophageal pH is conclusive for GERD. Unfortunately, pH monitoring is not available to all providers and is expensive. The Berstein test can be done readily in most areas. It is the infusion of a measured amount of hydrochloric acid into the esophagus. It is considered positive if there is reproduction of patient symptoms. Esophageal manometry will show decreased LES pressure. Esophagogastroduodenoscopy (EGD) is a useful procedure for direct visualization of lesions, evaluation of strictures and masses, and retrieval of tissue for biopsies.

RADIOLOGIC (IMAGING) STUDIES

The imaging modality of choice for any esophageal disease is a barium swallow. The barium swallow can highlight mucosal injury, ulcerations, strictures, or hiatal hernias. The barium swallow can help define a relaxed LES or tertiary peristalsis, which may

Table 6-11-3. Differential Diagnosis of GERD

Achalasia	LES tone too tight, full chest, weight loss, unable to vomit
Defuse esophageal spasm	Strong, random peristalsis: severe stabbing substernal pain, short lived, exacerbated by hot or cold foods
Infectious esophagitis	Severe, persistent odynophagia, drooling
Chemical ingestion	Severe dysphagia, odynophagia, bleeding
Cardiac pain—MI, angina	Substernal chest pain with radiation to arm or neck, associated with exertion, dyspnea, diaphoresis
Costochondritis	Substernal-sternal chest pain, worse with deep respiration and movement
Pneumonia, pleurisy	Chest pain, generally no radiation pattern, worse with respiration, cough, fever
Biliary tract disease	Epigastric to right upper quadrant pain, radiating to chest, colicky in nature, associated with fat intake
Peptic ulcer disease	Epigastric pain with radiation to chest and back, associated with food intake, stress induced
Postherpetic syndrome	Dermatome involvement, persistent pain over area, no relation to food intake

Table 6-11-4. General Measures for Control of GERD

Things to Do	Things to Avoid
Small or reasonably sized, well-chewed meals	Lying down within 3 h of a meal Smoking
High-protein diet, low fat	Fatty foods, chocolate, acidic foods
Elevate the head of the bed 3–6 in.	Alcohol, coffee, and peppermints
	Obesity and lack of exercise
Weight control and regular exercise	Medications that cause loss of LES tone

contribute to GERD. A radionuclide scintigraphy uses ^{99m}Tc-sulfur to help indicate esophageal reflux and measure gastric emptying time. Both tests are noninvasive and are readily available to most patients.

TREATMENT

Because many patients treat themselves without a definitive diagnosis, a clinician can make a presumed diagnosis of GERD by history and treat empirically. The mainstay of therapy is the elimination of precipitating factors. This is best done by good patient education on lifestyle changes (Table 6-11-4). If lifestyle changes are not enough, medications can be used to decrease acidity, decrease refluxant contact, or tighten LES tone.

Antacids are by far the most common over-the-counter medications used. They neutralize the gastric acid and promote healing, but only with frequent dosing. Magnesium-based antacids are the most potent, but 2 Tbs five times a day tend to cause diarrhea. Aluminum antacids work well but produce constipation and bind tetracyclines and other medication. Calcium types do neutralize acid but can induce rebound HCl secretions, creating a vicious cycle. The best antacid is a combination magnesium-aluminum product to get maximum antacid effect with minimal side effects. Many patients like liquid antacids because they relieve symptoms quickly.

Histamine is a potent stimulant of gastric acid. H_2 receptor antagonists (Zantac, Axid, Tagamet, Pepcid) are designed to decrease the acidity of the gastric refluxant by blocking production at the parietal cell. The intermittent use of over-the-counter H_2 blockers will diminish symptoms in patients who commit dietary indiscretions like eating a huge and/or a fatty meal or lying down after eating. However, for persistent symptoms, the OTC strength is not sufficient for healing erosive esophagitis.

For more severe GERD, high-dose H_2 blockers or a proton pump inhibitor is recommended (Table 6-11-5). Omeprazole (Prilosec) inhibits the proton pump within the parietal cell and can create achlorhydria with long-term use. It is an effective therapy for healing esophagitis with the convenience of a single daily dose. Omeprazole can also be used for maintenance therapy to prevent reoccurrence of the GERD symptoms and its sequelae. Yearly follow-up is required when a patient is using omeprazole because persistent achlorhydria can cause pernicious anemia (intrinsic factor, vitamin B_{12} absorption is dependent on parietal cell activity) and may predispose to gastric carcinoma.

Table 6-11-5. Medication Regimens for GERD

Mylanta or Maalox, 2 Tbs 4–5 times a day	Ranitidine (Zantac), 150 mg bid or tid
Zantac 75 (OTC), 75 mg bid	Cimetidine (Tagamet), 300 mg qid
Tagamet HB (OTC), 150–200 mg qid	Famotidine (Pepcid), 20 mg qd
	Nizatidine (Axid), 150–300 mg qd
Pepcid AC (OTC), 5 mg bid	Omeprazole (Prilosec), 20 mg qd, add if needed
Axid AR (OTC), 75 mg qd	Cisapride (Propulsid), 10 mg tid
	Metoclopramide (Reglan), 10 mg qid

Other therapeutic alternatives are the prokinetic agents Reglan and Propulsid. Both tighten LES tone (decreasing reflux contact) and promote rapid gastric emptying. The addition of either to a regimen of H_2 blockers can be helpful in resistant cases of GERD.

Finally, when all preventive and medication regimens are exhausted, surgery may be done to correct the anatomic defect. If Barrett's esophagitis or carcinoma is present, a partial removal of the esophagus may be accomplished. Surgery is the last resort because sequelae include esophageal clearance problems with regurgitation, weight loss, dumping syndrome, anemia, and other conditions.

COMPLICATIONS

Since most people have episodes of GERD at some time in their life, it is important to recognize severe symptoms and complications. Being a mechanical problem, GERD will be recurrent, so complications can occur at any time and may be exacerbated with age or concomitant disease. The most common complication of GERD is esophagitis with subsequent stricture formation (scarring), which decreases lumen clearance. Perforation, ulceration, hemorrhage, aspiration pneumonia, and obstruction are all possible results of severe GERD.

The most ominous complication of persistent GERD is Barrett's esophagitis. The squamous cell structure changes to a metaplastic columnar epithelium, which is considered a premalignant state (adenocarcinoma). The intestinal metaplasia progresses slowly up the esophageal mucosa and is associated with ulcerations, bleeding, and stricture formation. An EGD is required for definitive diagnosis of Barrett's esophagitis, and follow-up includes yearly EGDs for life.

PATIENT EDUCATION

Table 6-11-4 includes all the preventative measures that can be taken to avoid or treat GERD. Patient education should be directed to these measures. Medications are short-term fixes for the most part and carry their own risk factors with continued use. The commercial media seem to give people permission to eat anything they want, in any quantity, because they can take a pill to solve subsequent problems. Better to teach the patient good eating habits and avoid medication use completely.

PEARLS

Gastroesophageal reflux disease is a common problem and for the most part easily resolved with good habits. The trick is to have an index of suspicion for increasing severity. Unfortunately, severe disease may exhibit limited symptoms, and mild disease may bother a patient tremendously. Any increase or change in symptoms justifies investigation. A patient who seeks medical help has probably tried all the OTC medications, so evaluation is warranted. In an elderly patient with no previous history of GERD or ulcer disease, evaluation should be done for carcinoma. A common disorder should not lull a good diagnostician into a false sense of security.

BIBLIOGRAPHY

Martin JC: Primary Health Care for People with GERD, Judy C, July, 1995 (Internet). GERD_Pri.Care@utmgopher.utmem.edu.
"Therapeutic Management of GERD," Annual Meeting of the ASCP, 1995 (Internet). Medical Association communication.

Chapter 6–12
GASTROINTESTINAL BLEEDING
Anne P. Heinly

DESCRIPTION

Between 1 and 2 percent of Americans will be hospitalized for bleeding in the next year, the vast majority from gastrointestinal sources. Blood loss can occur in eight different ways; five are common to the GI system. Bloody vomitus is called *hematemesis*; it may be bright red or have the "coffee-ground" appearance of older, accumulated blood. *Melena* is the presence of 50 to 100 mL of blood in stool causing black, tarry, and foul smelling stools. *Hematochezia* denotes rapid bleeding, usually from the lower GI tract with the presence of bright red or maroon blood from the rectum or mixed with stool. *Occult* bleeding can occur anywhere, but in the GI tract it can be identified with a chemical reagent like Hemocult cards. Finally, there is *presumption of bleeding* because of physical findings but no overt or occult bleeding can be identified. This can happen with hemorrhagic pancreatitis.

PATHOGENESIS

The gastrointestinal tract from the mouth to the anus can bleed anywhere, anytime. The challenge is to try to define the location, severity, and cause of bleeding. Traditionally, upper GI bleeding comes from any location above the ligament of Treitz, and lower GI bleeding originates below the ligament of Treitz (Fig. 6-12-1). The gastrointestinal tract has a complex blood supply with a lot of redundancy to ensure proper digestion and absorption of food. At any given time, up to 25 percent of the blood supply may be involved in digestion. When bleeding occurs due to injury or disease, it can be rapid and devastating (chemical ingestion or Boerhaave's syndrome) or it can slowly ooze from a carcinoma or ulceration.

SYMPTOMS

A good history is essential. If bleeding is obvious, questions should include history of NSAID use; previous history of bleeding; illnesses that may predispose the patient to bleeding like cirrhosis, vitamin deficiency, and malabsorption syndromes; use of medication that might effect coagulation, like warfarin (Coumadin) or long-term omeprazole use; recent surgeries or instrumentation; use of alcohol or tobacco products; presence of pain or indigestion prior to bleeding; sexual orientation (HIV syndromes); and family history of bleeding dyscrasias.

Most people can handle a 10 percent volume loss without symptoms. With overt blood loss, the patient may present with sudden fatigue, heart palpitations, increased respiratory rate, dizziness, diaphoresis, nausea, thirst, and/or agitation. As blood volume is lost, the body tries to compensate with an increased pulse in an effort to maintain blood pressure to supply vital organs with needed oxygen and nutrients. In slow, occult blood loss, the patient will probably come to a routine appointment with a history of progressive fatigue, increasing thirst, persistent nausea, inability to maintain usual physical activities without shortness of breath, or palpitations. In children, a failure to thrive may occur. The elderly patient may present with a change in mentation, constipation and/or diarrhea, or loss of appetite.

OBJECTIVE

Quantifying blood loss is quite difficult. Where and what is the source? Is it actively bleeding? If so, how fast? Is there more than one bleeding source or a chronic blood loss overlaying an acute bleed? Even today, orthostatic vital signs are still used to judge the effect of blood loss and estimate cardiac reserve. Orthostatic vital signs include blood pressure and pulse determinations from a supine to sitting to standing position over a period of 3 to 6 min. Orthostatic vital signs are considered positive when there is a 20-point rise in the pulse rate and a drop in blood pressure of 10 to 15 mmHg from one position to the other. Patients with severe blood loss will appear pale or gray, be diaphoretic, and exhibit hypotension, tachycardia, tachypnea, and progressive loss of sensorium.

The obvious bleeding source should not be ignored, but the provider should also do a thorough inspection for other sources or disease processes that may complicate therapy. A complete physical should be done looking for signs of dehydration (dry mucous membranes), evidence of underlying cirrhosis (jaundice, hepatomegaly), skin lesions (Kaposi's sarcoma), and vascular anomalies (deep vein thrombosis, spider angiomas). Abdominal tenderness with and without peritoneal signs may indicate ulcer disease or rupture of a diverticulum. Back pain and tenderness may be secondary to an abdominal aneurysm. Rectal examinations are mandatory with investigation of GI bleeding to evaluate for blood, hemorrhoids, and polyps.

DIAGNOSTIC CONSIDERATIONS

Upper GI bleeding is usually manifested in two ways. Esophageal and stomach lesions usually cause hematemesis because the blood is an irritant and because of changes in gastric volume. The blood can be bright red, or if it has been accumulating, it may have a dark coffee ground appearance. Bleeding from ulcer disease, hiatal hernias, or esophageal varices does not necessarily cause hematemesis but may cause melena instead. The blood darkens and mixes with the stool on its 8- to 14-h transit through the small intestines and colon. It is possible to have hematochezia from the upper GI tract, but it is usually associated with massive blood loss (Table 6-12-1).

Lower gastrointestinal bleeding can present as melena (slow bleed and transit) common to carcinomas, polyps, or diverticuli irritation. Inflammatory bowel disease and ischemic bowel disease may cause hematochezia with frank, bright red blood through the rectum. Some researchers attribute maroon-colored stools to lower GI bleeding, estimating the bleeding location to be in the ascending colon because the darker color denotes some transit time but not an extended period in the colon. Occult bleeding can occur from any location, and massive bleeding may produce melena, hematochezia, and hematemesis all at the same time (Table 6-12-2).

LABORATORY TESTS

Blood loss is reflected in hematocrit. With chronic, slow GI bleeding from an ulcer or similar problem, iron stores are depleted over time and the hematocrit decreases. A complete blood cell count (CBC) will reveal a microcytic, hypochromic anemia. If the anemia is macrocytic, it is most likely secondary to a vitamin deficiency. Rapid blood loss may not register accurately for the first 12 to 72 h because the plasma volume has to return to normal before the hematocrit is valid. Better to follow orthostatic vital signs, cardiac monitoring, and clinical picture initially.

The remainder of the laboratory tests are designed to evaluate the organs affected by blood loss. Chemistries should be done to check renal status (uremia can cause GI blood loss) and electrolyte balance. An elevated blood urea nitrogen (BUN) with a normal creatinine indicates blood in the GI tract (BUN is a byproduct of hemolysis). Liver enzymes should be done because cirrhosis, portal hypertension, and hypoproteinemia may all be implicated in GI bleeding. Coagulation studies are a must. The

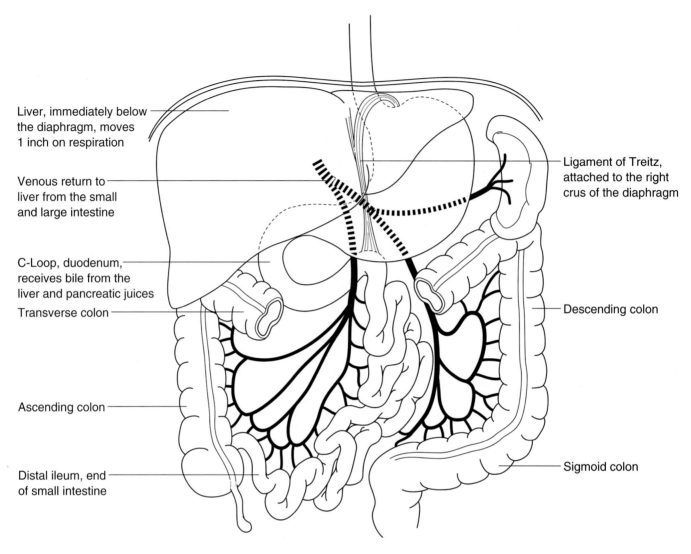

Liver, immediately below the diaphragm, moves 1 inch on respiration

Venous return to liver from the small and large intestine

C-Loop, duodenum, receives bile from the liver and pancreatic juices

Transverse colon

Ascending colon

Distal ileum, end of small intestine

Ligament of Treitz, attached to the right crus of the diaphragm

Descending colon

Sigmoid colon

Figure 6-12-1. GI anatomy in relation to GI Bleeding.

Table 6-12-1. Sources of Upper GI Bleeding

Disease	Symptoms	Treatment of Bleed
Peptic ulcer disease		
Gastritis or ulcer	Epigastric pain, worse with empty stomach, usually	Endoscopic hemostasis most successful with le-
Duodenitis or ulcer	progressive. The occasional patient can have a si-	sion 1-2 cm. Surgical removal is considered for
Zollinger-Ellison	lent ulcer with bleeding as the first clue.	severe or numerous bleeding sites.
Esophageal disease		
Esophagitis (GERD)	GERD presents with substernal pyrosis, increased	Varices may be treated with balloon tampon-
Hiatal hernia	burping, cough, hoarseness. Varices and Mallory-	ade, but reoccurrence is high. More common:
Varices	Weiss tears common to alcohol abuse, liver cir-	variceal sclerotherapy done weekly until vari-
Mallory-Weiss tears	rhosis—presents with pain and hematemesis.	ces are obliterated. Endoscopic ligation is un-
Boerhaave's syndrome	Boerhaave's is sudden massive bleeding with	der investigation as a valid alternative.
	poor prognosis.	
Carcinomas		
Esophageal	Depending on location: progressive dysphagia,	Surgical resection is the optimal (and hopefully
Gastric	early satiety, weight loss, cough, epigastric pain.	curative) care. Palliative therapy may include
Duodenal	Duodenal may present with jaundice and gallblad-	endoscopic hemostasis.
	der symptoms. Bleeding is usually occult.	
Overdoses		
Warfarin	Widespread bruising, hematuria, hematochezia, he-	Empty the stomach by lavage after protecting
Heparin	moptysis and even joint bleeding. PTT increased	the airway. Activated charcoal is recom-
Acetaminophen	within 12–24 h. Acetaminophen presents with	mended. Vitamin K, 5–10 mg subcutaneously
Rodent killers	fine petechiae.	with a unit of fresh frozen plasma for warfarin.
		Watch for relapse.

Table 6-12-2. Sources for the Lower GI Bleeding

Disease	Symptoms	Treatment

Anal disease
  Hemorrhoids
  Anal fissures
  IBD fistulas
  Anal carcinoma
	Hemorrhoids are by far the most common. The blood is seen on the stool versus mixed with the stool; usually intermittent. Bleeding often painless.	Sitz baths and high-fiber diet with stool softeners for hemorrhoids and fissures with topical treatments. Surgery only if recurrent. IBD fistulas and carcinoma are surgical referrals.

Carcinoma
  Small intestinal CA
  Colonic CA
	Especially in the elderly, a change in bowel habits, weight loss, and occult bleeding may indicate cancer.	Resection of the lesion with lymph biopsy and evaluation for metastasis.

Inflammatory
  Crohn's disease
  Ulcerative colitis
  Infectious colitis
	Symptoms are disease-specific, but bleeding is usually obvious with lots of diarrhea. Especially ulcerative colitis and infectious colitis can bleed briskly.	Treatment of all these begin with medical therapy; surgery is used as a last resort in most cases.

Vascular anomalies
  Bowel ischemia
  Aortoenteric fistula
  Hereditary
    telangiectasia
  Colonic varices
	Bowel ischemia may be due to obstruction, carcinoma, infection. Bleeding is usually brisk with extreme pain. Other anomalies may be seen on endoscope.	Bowel resection is done for ischemia and fistula bleeding. Sclerotherapy or coagulation by endoscope may contain varices and anomalies.

Diverticuli
  Diverticulitis
 	
  Solitary ascending
    diverticulum
	May present with LLQ pain, fever, chills, peritoneal signs, and bleeding.
	May present as abundant, sudden, painless bleeding (hematochezia with bright red or maroon stools).
		Depending on severity and response to medical therapy, colon resection may be done.

NOTE: IBD = inflammatory bowel disease; CA = cancer; LLQ = left lower quadrant.

bleeding time and prothrombin time with a platelet count can help judge the severity of blood loss or the likelihood of more bleeding. A partial thromboplastin time (PTT) double normal has a poor prognosis. If circumstances warrant it, look for a drug overdose, especially acetaminophen, warfarin, or heparin, as possible etiologies.

RADIOLOGIC (IMAGING) STUDIES

The decision to be made is: What is the presumed severity of GI bleeding? If bleeding is occult, in a young person with limited symptoms, then a barium study is acceptable. Depending on the presumed location of the bleeding, a barium swallow for esophageal lesions, upper gastrointestinal (UGI) series for stomach and duodenal etiologies, small bowel follow-through for midgut lesions, or barium enema for colonic lesions can be recommended.

With massive bleeding, slower bleeding causing significant symptoms, or bleeding in the very young or elderly, the recommended study is endoscopy. The advantages of an esophagogastroduodenoscopy (EGD) with upper GI bleeding or a colonoscopy, sigmoidoscopy, or anoscopy with lower GI bleeding have increased over the years with better tools and better trained practitioners.

The well-trained endoscopist can usually locate the bleeding source and in most cases administer therapeutic modalities. Therapies available with the endoscope are quite impressive. They include monopolar electrocoagulation, essentially cauterizing the lesion, but it does produce a fair amount of tissue damage. Laser therapy, when available, is the more precise choice for endoscopic hemostasis. Sclerosing therapy uses epinephrine, absolute ethanol, or polidocanol to control bleeding. Epinephrine produces less tissue damage while causing localized vasoconstriction.

The other option for evaluation of a GI bleed is arteriography. Arteriography is probably still superior to endoscopy when there is massive bleeding because even skilled surgeons cannot see through blood. The arteriogram can localize the bleeding if the blood loss is more than 0.5 mL/min and can often determine the cause—a diverticulum and angiodysplasia. Arteriograms are also better when looking for a vascular lesion or anomaly.

Finally, more providers are turning to nuclear scans to localize bleeding. Technetium 99m scintigraphy has a reasonably good record of finding slow bleeding that arteriograms do not pick up. The drawback to nuclear scans, however, is that they are good only for active bleeding sources; they will miss intermittent bleeding and are not sufficiently site-specific.

TREATMENT

The first step is to stabilize the patient. Nasogastric tube placements, arteriogram, and even endoscopy all have to wait for a hemodynamically stable patient. For the orthostatic or shocky patient, two large-bore intravenous lines should be started with rapid fluid resuscitation with either Ringer's solution or normal saline. Replace fluids to compensate for fluids lost. Monitor the patient's cardiovascular status and urine output.

The next step is blood product replacement. Blood transports oxygen better than intravenous fluid. Blood products should be used to replenish the supply for patients who are down to one-fourth of their normal reserve or for patients with evidence of poor tissue perfusion (angina, cyanosis, renal failure, loss of consciousness). Packed red blood cells (PRBC) should be used if improving systemic oxygen delivery is the goal. Fresh frozen plasma or platelets are used to replenish clotting factors or in the presence of severe thrombocytopenia. The rule of thumb is one unit of platelets to every five units of packed RBCs. While evaluating a patient for transfusion, consider whether the bleeding has stopped. Is it likely to reoccur? Are there other disease processes that may complicate fluid or blood resuscitation (CHF, polycythemia)? After the patient's plasma volume is replaced, it will take 12 to 72 h for stabilization. Hematocrit may fluctuate as the volume load settles down. Hematocrit taken right after transfusions may underestimate actual RBCs present.

Once fluid and blood replacements are underway, the patient should be evaluated often for vital signs, mentation changes, blood transfusion reactions, urine output, and regular ECG. The use of nasogastric tubes (NGT) in upper GI bleeding is falling out of use. An NGT may be helpful in washing the upper gastrointestinal areas prior to endoscopy, but cold or warm water lavage has not been proved to curtail bleeding.

COMPLICATIONS

Slow or occult bleeding can lead to anemia and fatigue, which may mask or exacerbate other disease processes. Depending on the etiology, the bleeding may be a signal of a more serious problem like carcinoma. Massive bleeding can cause organ failure due to poor perfusion, which may not be reversible with the resuscitation effort. The ultimate complication is death, which occurs in approximately 14 to 20 percent of those hospitalized with bleeding.

PATIENT EDUCATION

The best way to avoid GI bleeding is to prevent the disease processes that predispose a patient to bleeding. A healthy diet, regular exercise, limited alcohol and NSAID use, and abstention from tobacco go a long way in limiting the possibility of GI bleeding.

PEARLS

Bleeding can occur at any location in the gastrointestinal tract. If the nasogastric lavage is negative for blood, it does not preclude upper GI bleeding. A negative Hemocult card does not exclude GI bleeding. Sometimes it may seem easier not to notice low hematocrit on the routine laboratory test, but an investigation may save a life. Be alert for GI bleeders, especially in the elderly. If they progress to massive bleeding, their chances of recovery are quite bleak.

BIBLIOGRAPHY

Books

Isselbacher KJ, Braunwald E, Wilson JD, et al: Gastrointestinal bleeding, in *Harrison's Principles of Internal Medicine,* 13th ed. New York, McGraw-Hill, 1994, pp 223–226.
Sleisenger MH, Fordtran JS: Gastrointestinal bleeding, in *Gastrointestinal Diseases,* 5th ed. Philadelphia, Saunders, 1993, pp 162–169.

Internet Selections

"GI Bleeding," indy.radiology.uiowa.edu/Pr...lectricGiNucs/Text/GIBleeding.html. National Institutes of Health Consensus Development Conference Statement, 1980, updated 1996.
"Endoscopy in Upper GI Bleeding," isis.nlm.nih.gov/nih/cdc/www/26txt.html.

Chapter 6–13
HEMORRHOIDS
Pat C.H. Jan

DISCUSSION

Hemorrhoids, a common anal disease, affects individuals as early as in their mid-twenties to as late as in their sixties and seventies. Men and women are equally affected. The leading predisposing factor in the formation of both internal and external hemorrhoids is constipation. In addition, many women relate a worsening of existing hemorrhoids after childbirth.

Table 6-13-1. Classification of Internal Hemorrhoids

Degree	Physical Findings
First degree	Bleeding
Second degree	Prolapse and spontaneously reducible
Third degree	Prolapse and requires digital manipulation
Fourth degree	Prolapse and unable to reduce

PATHOGENESIS

Hemorrhoids are commonly located in the right anterolateral, right posterolateral, and left lateral positions in the anal canal. The anal canal normally has hemorrhoidal tissues, or cushions, that aid in anal continence. Intraluminal pressure caused by straining or pushing from hard stools causes the hemorrhoidal plexus to become engorged and form internal and external hemorrhoids.

SIGNS AND SYMPTOMS

Internal hemorrhoids cause bleeding and prolapse without pain. They can be classified into four types. (See Table 6-13-1.) External hemorrhoids, on the other hand, thrombose and cause pain. They are located below the dentate (pectinate) line. The dentate line has somatic innervation. Thus, structures like external hemorrhoids located below this line also have sensory innervation.

OBJECTIVE FINDINGS

Thrombosed external hemorrhoids are tender, hard, and bluish structures located at the anal verge. In acute thrombosed external hemorrhoid, gentle spreading pressure by the examiner to the buttocks allows enough exposure of the anal verge. Internal hemorrhoids are located above the dentate line in the anal canal. They have a strawberry appearance and can prolapse outside the anal canal. Occasionally, a patient presents with a complex hemorrhoid with both an external and internal component. Internal hemorrhoids can easily be seen by the insertion of an anoscope which has been lubricated with petroleum jelly.

DIAGNOSTIC CONSIDERATIONS

When a patient presents with a complaint of rectal bleeding and anal examination does not reveal hemorrhoids, the following should be considered in the differential diagnosis:

- Carcinoma
- Diverticulitis
- Trauma
- Inflammatory bowel disease
- Colon polyps
- Portal hypertension from liver disease

TREATMENT
Medical Management

First- and second-degree internal hemorrhoids respond well to conservative treatment of a high-fiber diet or stool softener and decreased time in the bathroom. If patients do not follow the hemorrhoid care protocol, then the hemorrhoids may need to be ablated by rubber band ligation or by Endo-Lase. Endo-Lase or heat cautery and rubber band ligation can be performed in the office. (See Fig. 6-13-1.) The tip of the Endo-Lase is applied to the base of the hemorrhoid. Care must be taken to avoid the dentate line to prevent pain to the patient. Several treatments may be required in some patients. Rubber band ligation is used for second- and sometimes third-degree hemorrhoids. (See Fig. 6-13-2.) The patient is placed in the right lateral decubitus position

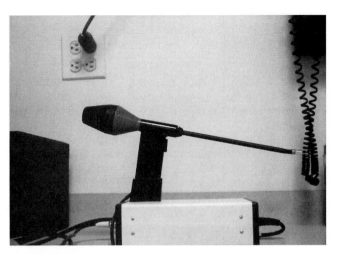

Figure 6-13-1. Endo-Lase instrument used for first- and second-degree hemorrhoids.

Table 6-13-2. Hemorrhoid Care Protocol

Keep stool soft
  Eat 3 or more servings of fruits and vegetables each day.
  Drink at least 6 to 8 glasses fluid per day.
  If feeling constipated, take milk of magnesia (15–30 mL twice daily).
  If difficult to eat enough fruits and vegetables, try to take psyllium hydrophilic mucilloid (Metamucil), 1–2 tsp every day.
Limit time on toilet
  Do no spend reading time on toilet.
  Go to the toilet when definitely ready; do not sit on toilet and wait for bowel movement.
  If bowel movement is not coming, do not sit on toilet and strain. Get up and come back later.
Keep anal area clean
  Wash anal area with hand, not wash cloth, gently after each bowel movement (soap and water).
  Sitz bath, 2–3 times daily for 20 min.
  If tissue comes out around the anus, use a product like Preparation H or Anusol to help push the tissue back into the anal canal with a finger.

with legs flexed and the head of the bed bent as in Trendelenburg's position. An anoscope is inserted, and the hemorrhoid is identified. The hemorrhoid is then grasped up and outward as the rubber band ligature is pushed toward the base of the hemorrhoid. The hemorrhoid will atrophy and fall off in about 5 to 7 days. Patients should not feel any pain as long as the rubber band is well above the dentate line. If symptoms continue, then excisional hemorrhoidectomy is the next alternative.

Surgical Management

Third- and fourth-degree hemorrhoids require excision. Patients are brought into the operating suite and placed in the jackknife position. The patient is placed under either intravenous sedation with local anesthesia or epidural or general anesthesia. If the patient is placed under intravenous sedation, lidocaine 1% with epinephrine is injected into the base of the hemorrhoids. An elliptical incision is made by either a scalpel or cautery. Care is taken to remove the hemorrhoid from the internal sphincter. The sphincter must be identified and preserved. A single surgical gut (chromic) suture is used to approximate the edges. The remaining incision is left open and allowed to heal by secondary intention. The wound is infiltrated with bupivacaine (Marcaine) 0.25% with epinephrine, and dibucaine ointment is applied into the anal canal.

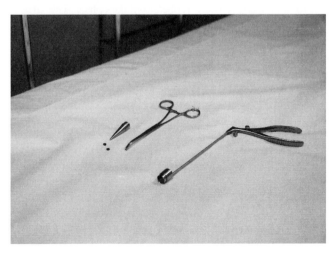

Figure 6-13-2. Rubber band ligature used for second- and third-degree hemorrhoids.

Uncomplicated external thrombosed hemorrhoids can be removed in the office. They are anesthetized with lidocaine 1% with epinephrine. An incision is made with a scalpel, and a hemostat is used to remove all the thrombus which is purplish. A single inverted suture using either chromic or Vicryl is used to approximate the edges while allowing the remaining incision to heal by secondary intention. Oral analgesics are used for pain management. Patients are given the hemorrhoid care protocol. (See Table 6-13-2.)

PATIENT EDUCATION

Patients are instructed to increase their dietary intake of both fruits and vegetables. If they are unable to make these dietary modifications, then stool softeners and fiber are added into the diet. Patients are reminded not to strain or push during bowel movements and not to spend prolonged time in the bathroom. After each bowel movement, patients should wash the anal area with soap and water. If any tissue prolapses, it should be gently pushed back into the anal canal with the aid of a lubricant like Anusol or Preparation H. Warm sitz baths are suitable for all postoperative hemorrhoidectomy patients.

DISPOSITION

Patients are seen 1 week after medical or surgical procedure. If satisfactory healing has occurred, then patients are seen on an as-needed basis. In case of poor wound healing or prolonged pain, patients are seen weekly until postoperative symptoms have subsided.

COMPLICATIONS AND RED FLAGS

Common postoperative complications of Endo-Lase, rubber band ligation, and excisional hemorrhoidectomy are urinary retention, bleeding, infection, anal stenosis, and incontinence. Bleeding can be controlled with adequate coagulation and pressure dressing. Infections are prevented with a single-dose second-generation cephalosporin, which is given preoperatively. Anal stenosis can be avoided if complex hemorrhoids are removed in stages instead of attempting to remove them all at once.

Postoperative edema and excessive excision of the anal derm can lead to stricture. Incontinence is avoided by careful separation of the hemorrhoid off the internal sphincter muscle and limiting the intravenous solution given during the procedure to 400 mL or less.

NOTES AND PEARLS

Since constipation is common among pregnant women, preventive care as well as conservative therapies should be utilized. As mentioned earlier, high-fiber diet or stool softeners, topical analgesics and sitz baths should be the recommended therapy until after childbirth. If at that time, the hemorrhoids are still painful or bleeding, then surgical management would be the next step.

Patients who are immune-compromised should definitely receive conservative treatment because performing surgical procedures on this group of patients may lead to sepsis.

BIBLIOGRAPHY

Mazier WP: Hemorrhoids, fissures, and pruritus ani (Review). *Surg Clin North Am* 74(6):1277–1292, 1994.
Russell TR: Hemorrhoids, in Way LW (ed): *Current Surgical Diagnosis and Treatment,* 10th ed. Stamford, CT, Appleton & Lange, 1994.
Schwartz, SI, Shires GT, Spencer FC (eds): Hemorrhoids, in *Principles of Surgery,* 6th ed. New York, McGraw-Hill, 1994.

Chapter 6–14
HEPATITIS
JoAnn Deasy

DISCUSSION

Hepatitis is an inflammatory and necrotic disease of liver cells. The hepatitis viruses, which are specific for the liver, can cause acute hepatitis and sometimes chronic hepatitis. Five hepatitis viruses are generally recognized (hepatitis A, B, C, D, and E). Molecular technology is uncovering further hepatotropic viruses. Hepatitis G, GB-A, GB-B, and GB-C have been characterized as bloodborne viruses. Chronic hepatitis is defined as elevated liver enzymes for longer than 6 months. Hepatitis B, C, D, and probably G, GB-A, and GB-B viruses can cause chronic disease. (See Table 6-14-1.)

SYMPTOMS: ACUTE VIRAL HEPATITIS

The clinical course of acute viral hepatitis is variable. It may be asymptomatic, symptomatic but anicteric, or symptomatic and icteric. Rarely, it is very severe and can cause a prolonged illness with a high mortality rate or fulminant hepatitis that progresses to death in a few days or weeks. The onset of symptoms may be gradual or sudden. Early symptoms are usually nonspecific and include anorexia, nausea, vomiting, abdominal discomfort, fatigue, headache, and low-grade fever. The clinician may not be overly suspicious of hepatitis when the patient presents with these symptoms, until it is realized that the liver enzymes are elevated. Patients who present with right upper quadrant (RUQ) abdominal pain and jaundice are easier to diagnose. Some patients also have skin rashes, myalgias, arthralgias, diarrhea, and/ or itching.

OBJECTIVE FINDINGS

Physical findings may include skin and scleral icterus and mild hepatomegaly with tenderness to percussion and palpation. In a small number of patients, the spleen is palpable. Some patients may have acute arthritis with local pain, redness, and swelling. Joint symptoms and signs are usually associated with hepatitis B and hepatitis E viruses. Dark urine and light stools are also signs of acute viral hepatitis. Clinical signs and symptoms cannot be used to determine the specific virus responsible for hepatitis. Identification of the etiologic virus depends on serologic testing.

LABORATORY FINDINGS

Liver enzymes, specifically alanine aminotransferase (ALT) and aspartate aminotransferase (AST), are released into the blood by damaged liver cells. During acute viral hepatitis, these enzymes may rise to 10 to 20 times their normal values. ALT will usually be elevated out of proportion to AST. However, the levels of these enzymes do not correlate with the functional capacity of the liver. The prothrombin time and serum albumin level are used as indicators of hepatic function. Every patient with acute hepatitis needs a prothrombin time done on a same-day basis. Prolongation of the prothrombin time is an ominous sign. Both the conjugated and unconjugated bilirubin may become elevated, resulting in jaundice.

HEPATITIS A

Hepatitis A virus (HAV) is an RNA virus that is transmitted via the fecal-oral route or through contaminated shellfish. The virus is resistant to gastric acid and travels from the gastrointestinal tract to hepatocytes, where replication takes place. The virus is shed in bile and excreted in the stool. Large amounts of HAV accumulate in the stool before symptoms occur, resulting in the

Table 6-14-1. The Five Generally Recognized Hepatides

	Hepatitis A	Hepatitis B	Hepatitis C	Hepatitis D	Hepatitis E
Transmission	Fecal-oral, shellfish	Percutaneous venereal perinatal	Percutaneous venereal	Percutaneous	Fecal-oral
Incubation, days	20–40	60–110	40–60	?	40
Diagnosis	IgM anti-HAV	Acute = HBsAg and HBcAb-IgM; Chronic = HBsAg for >6 months	Anti-HCV appears in 5–30 weeks	Anti-HDV	Neg. serologies for all hepatitis viruses
Course	Acute disease only	Acute and chronic	Acute and chronic	Acute and chronic	Acute disease only
Vaccine	Yes	Yes	No	No	No
Prevention after exposure	Immune globulin	HBIG + vaccine	Uncertain	Unknown	Uncertain

spread of the disease unknowingly. In a significant number of persons, HAV infection never becomes clinically apparent. Older adults tend to have worse symptoms than young adults and children. Diagnosis is made by detection of serum IgM anti-HAV, which is present at the onset of symptoms in most patients. IgG anti-HAV reaches a high titer during convalescence and persists indefinitely, conferring immunity. Most cases of hepatitis A resolve over several weeks. In some persons, malaise persists for many months. There is a less than 1 percent incidence of fulminant hepatitis and death from HAV. There is no progression to chronic hepatitis.

Strategies for prevention of hepatitis A include handwashing and not eating raw shellfish. HAV is likely to spread when there is close and prolonged contact with infected individuals. Those at risk include household contacts and individuals in settings such as day-care centers. Persons who have been exposed to HAV in these settings should be given passive immunoprophylaxis with immune globulin as soon as possible after exposure.

An inactivated hepatitis A vaccine became available in 1995. The vaccine is indicated for persons over age 2 years who are traveling to areas endemic for HAV. The vaccine confers protection 4 weeks after the initial dose; therefore, persons traveling sooner than 4 weeks should receive a simultaneous injection of immune globulin. Other than travelers, the vaccine is indicated for homosexual men, users of injectable drugs, persons who have chronic liver disease and persons at occupational risk, such as day-care and food service workers. Two injections of hepatitis A vaccine are required; one at time zero and a booster 6 to 12 months after the first.

HEPATITIS E

Hepatitis E is similar to hepatitis A. It is transmitted fecal-orally and has been associated with contaminated food and water. It produces only acute disease, and the clinical course is usually mild and self-limiting. However, in pregnant women hepatitis E causes a high rate (20 percent) of fulminant disease with a high risk of disease. Hepatitis E is rare in the United States, but is endemic in Southeast Asia, and there have been reported outbreaks in Mexico. The clinician should suspect hepatitis E in a patient with signs and symptoms of hepatitis who has traveled to an endemic area and who has negative serologies for hepatitis A, B, and C. There is no commercially available test for hepatitis E at this time; a serologic test is available from the Centers for Disease Control.

HEPATITIS B

Hepatitis B virus (HBV) is a DNA virus that causes both acute and chronic disease. The virus is spread by direct contact with infected blood or body fluids. It is transmitted mainly by sexual contact, both heterosexual and homosexual, and by the sharing of needles among intravenous drug users. It is also transmitted to babies at birth by infected mothers. In a substantial number of persons, no risk factor is identified; 90 to 95 percent of adults infected with HBV recover completely. The other 5 to 10 percent become asymptomatic carriers or develop chronic hepatitis B. Persons with chronic hepatitis B may go on to develop cirrhosis and are at increased risk for developing hepatocellular carcinoma (HCC). The younger a person is when infected with HBV, the greater likelihood of becoming chronically infected. Fifteen to twenty percent of infected children develop chronic hepatitis B, and more than 90 percent of infected neonates develop chronic infection. The infection becomes chronic if the virus is not eliminated during acute disease by the immune system and continues to replicate. The damage done to the liver in HBV infection is thought to be due to the immunologic response of the host rather than to the cytopathic effect of the virus. Some symptoms, such as rash and arthritis, are more common in hepatitis B than other types of hepatitis and are thought to be due to the deposition of immune complexes.

The diagnosis of acute hepatitis B can be made with two serologic tests: hepatitis B surface antigen (HBsAg) and IgM hepatitis B core antibody (HBcAb-IgM). If both are positive, the patient has acute hepatitis B. HBsAg is the predominant viral envelope protein. The test for this antigen is the first serologic marker to become positive, appearing as early as 2 to 12 weeks after exposure and preceding symptoms. HBsAg concentration reaches a peak during acute disease and then usually becomes negative in 3 to 6 months. The persistence of HBsAg beyond 6 months indicates chronic infection. HBcAb-IgM also becomes negative and is replaced by the total hepatitis B core antibody (HBcAb). There is no available test for HBcAb-IgG. A positive HBcAb with a negative IgM fraction indicates prior infection. Antibody against HBsAb appears approximately 6 months after the initial infection. The loss of HBsAg and the presence of HBsAb indicate immunity. HBsAb also appears and may persist after hepatitis B vaccination.

Hepatitis B e antigen is another viral antigen. It is released during active viral replication and is associated with infectivity. In acute disease it appears at approximately the same time as HBsAg and then declines shortly before HBsAg. Persons with chronic hepatitis B should be tested for HBeAg. Hepatitis B DNA (HBV-DNA) is another test of viral replication. It is very sensitive, but also expensive. "Healthy carriers" of HBV are positive for HBsAg for longer than 6 months, but have undetectable levels of HBeAg. The rate of viral replication in these persons is very low, and therefore their infectivity is probably low. These individuals usually show no or minimal evidence of liver damage. Patients who are positive for HBsAg and HBeAg have active viral replication and probably high infectivity. Hepatic injury is more likely to occur in these individuals; liver enzymes may or may not be elevated.

To summarize the serologic diagnosis, the presence of HBsAg and HBcAb-IgM indicates acute hepatitis B. HBeAg is also positive in acute hepatitis B. The loss of HBsAg (and HBeAg) and the development of HBsAb indicates immunity. Chronic hepatitis B (or carrier state) is diagnosed when the HBsAg is positive for longer than 6 months. The presence of HBeAg (or HBV-DNA) indicates ongoing viral replication.

Recombinant vaccines against HBV are available and safe and have been incorporated into the childhood immunization schedule. Adolescents should be vaccinated, as well as other persons at risk. This includes those who are sexually active with multiple partners, abusers of injectable drugs, and healthcare workers. All pregnant women should be screened for HBsAg to identify neonates at risk for perinatal infection.

HEPATITIS D (DELTA HEPATITIS)

Hepatitis D virus (HDV) is a defective RNA virus that causes hepatitis only in persons who are already infected with hepatitis B virus. The delta virus is dependent on the continuing presence of hepatitis B surface antigen to replicate. If an individual becomes coinfected with the hepatitis B and hepatitis D virus at the same time, the risk of fulminant hepatitis is high. Patients with stable chronic hepatitis B who become infected with HDV usually exhibit an exacerbation of their condition with rapid deterioration of liver function. HDV is diagnosed by the serologic test for hepatitis delta antibody. A positive result in a person with HBsAg indicates infection with the delta hepatitis virus. HDV is endemic in Mediterranean countries, in the Middle East and parts of South America. In nonendemic countries it should be suspected in persons from high-risk groups, such as intravenous drug users and recipients of multiple blood products.

HEPATITIS C

Hepatitis C virus (HCV) has emerged as the major cause of non-A, non-B hepatitis. HCV is a RNA virus that causes both acute and chronic disease. There are at least six HCV genotypes. Although the exact mechanism is not understood, HCV produces disease by cytopathic effects. Until 1986, blood transfusion was responsible for most cases of hepatitis C. In the 1990s, injectable drug use is the predominant risk factor. Although spread of HCV is primarily via the parental route, sexual, familial, and maternal transmission may rarely occur. As with hepatitis B virus, a significant number of patients with HCV have no identifiable risk factor. The clinical course of acute hepatitis C is generally milder than hepatitis A or hepatitis B. A large percentage of cases are asymptomatic.

The association between HCV, chronic hepatitis, and hepatocellular cancer (HCC) is well established. It is estimated that approximately 70 percent of persons with hepatitis C infection will go on to develop chronic hepatitis. Patients with chronic hepatitis C are at increased risk for cirrhosis and HCC. During the time from infection with HCV to the development of cirrhosis, the patient may be asymptomatic.

HCV infection is diagnosed by ordering the hepatitis C antibody test by the second-generation enzyme-linked immunoabsorbent assay (ELISA-2). The time from infection to seroconversion is approximately 6 weeks (range 5 to 30 weeks). Patients with a risk factor for HCV infection and persons with abnormal liver enzymes should be tested for the antibody. The hepatitis C antibody test is associated with false positives in persons with autoimmune disease or any disease that might increase gamma globulins. If a false-positive result is suspected, a confirmatory test for the hepatitis C antibody by the recombinant immunoblot assay second generation (RIBA-2) method should be done. Serum levels of HCV RNA can be measured by polymerase chain reaction (PCR) or branched-chain DNA assays.

TREATMENT OF ACUTE VIRAL HEPATITIS AND PATIENT EDUCATION

There is no specific treatment for acute viral hepatitis. Recommended supportive measures include adequate hydration and reduced physical activity. Absolute bed rest is not necessary. A low-fat and high-carbohydrate diet may cause less nausea. Hygiene and stool precautions should be emphasized for hepatitis A and E, and blood and body fluid precautions for hepatitis B, C, D, and G. Hepatotoxins, including alcohol and drugs, should be avoided.

INDICATIONS FOR HOSPITALIZATION

Patients with severe nausea and vomiting require hospitalization because of the risk of dehydration and hypoglycemia. Patients with a prolonged prothrombin time or other signs of deteriorating hepatic function should be hospitalized.

TREATMENT OF CHRONIC VIRAL HEPATITIS

Hepatitis B, C, and D can cause chronic disease. The natural history of infection with hepatitis B and C is variable, but both viruses can cause serious liver disease, cirrhosis, and hepatocellular carcinoma. Chronic hepatitis should be considered in patients with elevated liver enzyme levels persisting for greater than 6 months. Interferon alfa-2b is approved for treatment of chronic hepatitis B and C. Generally, therapy is indicated when chronic infection is present with viral replication occurring and there are histologic changes on liver biopsy. Treatment is limited by the side effects of interferon. For chronic hepatitis B, there is a 50 to 60 percent cure rate, with cure being defined as no evidence of virus 1 year after stopping treatment. For hepatitis C, the

Table 6-14-2. Differential Diagnosis

Acute Hepatitis	Chronic Hepatitis
Viral hepatitis	Viral hepatitis
Toxic, drug-induced, alcoholic	Drug-induced and alcoholic
Bacterial hepatitis	Wilson's disease
Biliary obstruction	Hemochromatosis
	Autoimmune hepatitis
	Primary biliary cirrhosis
	Primary sclerosing cholangitis

record is not as good. Less than 50 percent improve, and only 20 percent are cured. The dosing and frequency of interferon for hepatitis C are still being investigated. Patients with chronic hepatitis B or C and replicating virus should be referred to a hepatologist or gastroenterologist for consideration of interferon therapy.

DIFFERENTIAL DIAGNOSIS

The differential diagnosis of acute hepatitis includes viral hepatitis, toxic hepatitis (including drug and alcoholic hepatitis), bacterial hepatitis, and biliary obstruction. (See Table 6-14-2.) Viruses, other than the hepatotropic viruses, that cause hepatitis include Epstein-Barr virus (infectious mononucleosis), cytomegalovirus, herpes simplex, and less commonly varicella, rubella, mumps, and yellow fever. All medications, prescription and nonprescription, should be considered potential hepatotoxins. An ALT greater than 5000 suggests a toxic hepatitis, such as that caused by acetaminophen or other medications. Alcoholic hepatitis is suggested by an AST higher than the ALT (ALT is usually < 500). Bacteria, such as *Salmonella, Campylobacter,* and *Listeria,* can cause hepatitis and should be considered when the patient has acute hepatitis and a fever higher than 101°F. A bilirubin of 10 or higher suggests biliary obstruction as the cause of the hepatitis. The differential diagnosis for chronic hepatitis includes viral hepatitis, drug-induced hepatitis, alcoholic hepatitis, Wilson's disease, hemochromatosis, autoimmune hepatitis, primary biliary cirrhosis, and primary sclerosing cholangitis.

BIBLIOGRAPHY

Bowden DS, Moaven LD, Locarnini SA: New hepatitis viruses: Are there enough letters in the alphabet? *Med J Aust* 164(2):87–89, 1996.

Franklin D, Becherer PR, Bacon BR: Hepatitis C virus: What recent studies can tell us. *Postgrad Med* 95(6):121–130, 1994.

Mandell GL, Douglas RG, Bennett JE: *Principles and Practices of Infectious Diseases.* New York, Churchill Livingstone, 1995.

Chapter 6–15
INFLAMMATORY BOWEL DISEASE
Anne P. Heinly

DISCUSSION

When Inflammatory bowel disease (IBD) is discussed, it is inclusive of two similar but essentially different disease processes: ulcerative colitis and Crohn's disease. Both cause chronic in-

Table 6-15-1. Comparison of Ulcerative Colitis and Crohn's Disease

Ulcerative Colitis	Crohn's Disease
Symptoms	Symptoms
Acute onset	Insidious onset
LLQ pain	Fatigue
Bloody diarrhea	Weight loss
Fever	Anorexia
Fatigue	RLQ pain
Weight loss	Diarrhea with or without
Anorexia	blood
Rectal tenesmus	Crampy relieved with defe-
	cation
Objective	Objective
Tachycardia	Thin, undernourished
Volume depletion	RLQ tenderness, mass effect
Pale, anemia	Perianal fissures
Fever	Fistula and abscess formations
Abdominal tenderness, perito-	Pale, anemia
neal signs	
Heme positive	
Systemic manifestations	Systemic manifestations
Inflammatory arthritis	Inflammatory arthritis
Ankylosing spondylitis	Osteoarthritis
Sacroiliitis	Ankylosing spondylitis
Digital clubbing	Sacroiliitis
Episcleritis	Digital clubbing
Pyoderma gangrenosum	Episcleritis
(common)	Erythema nodosum
Erythema nodosum (less	(common)
common)	Pyoderma gangrenosum (less
Aphthous ulcers	common)
Cirrhosis (common)	Aphthous ulcers (common)
Pericholangitis (common)	Cirrhosis
Renal stones	Pericholangitis
Growth retardation	Renal stones (common)
	Gallstones (common)
	Growth retardation

flammation or ulceration of the intestinal tract. Both are chronic debilitating diseases with systemic manifestations that may have long periods of remission. Both are of unknown etiology. One of the major distinguishing factors between the two diseases is the underlying tissue pathology; ulcerative colitis affects the mucosa and submucosa of the colon, whereas Crohn's disease affects all four layers of the colon and/or small intestine. (See Table 6-15-1.)

PATHOGENESIS

Maintaining a stable environment in the intestinal tract is dependent on several factors: the presence of friendly bacteria, dietary intake, inflammatory triggers, and the host's immune defenses. Inflammatory bowel disease disrupts this process in an idiopathic manner. There are theories on the cause, but it essentially remains unknown.

Genetics seem to play a role in both branches of IBD. There is a consistent presence of human leukocyte antigen HLA-B27 in patients with IBD. Ulcerative colitis is associated with HLA-DR2 and Crohn's is associated with HLA-A2. Both are associated with autoimmune disease, autoantibodies, immunoglobulin, and complement deposition. Possible etiologies range from a viral or bacterial trigger of the immune system to abnormal mucosal immunoreactivity, but nothing has been proved. The end-point is the activation of the inflammatory cells of the gastrointestinal tract whose products cause varying degrees of tissue damage.

Ulcerative Colitis

DISCUSSION

An estimated 250,000 Americans have ulcerative colitis (UC); it is more common than Crohn's disease. A disease of the young, it is seen from ages 10 to 40 with equal prevalence for men and women. Genetic predisposition may increase likelihood of developing UC up to 10 times normal. There is a concordance rate for UC in identical twins of 6.3 percent.[1] Ulcerative colitis is more common in the Jewish populations and in industrialized countries than in other populations.

PATHOGENESIS

Ulcerative colitis causes the inner lining of the large intestine to die and slough off. Only the mucosal and submucosal layer of the colon are affected, and only rarely will the ileum (distal small intestine) be involved. The inflammation predictably will start in the rectum and sigmoid area, which manifests uninterrupted mucosal friability with a propensity to bleed and ulcerate. Ulcerations seldom cause fissures or fistulae. Over time the chronic mucosal dysplasia deteriorates to adenocarcinoma in many patients.

SYMPTOMS

Typical symptoms include abdominal pain, usually in the left lower quadrant, but it may be generalized, bloody and/or mucus-containing diarrhea, fever, fatigue, weight loss, and anorexia. Approximately one-fourth of patients have tenesmus and rectal bleeding. Ulcerative colitis is generally an acute process and can become fulminant over a 24- to 48-h period. These patients are often quite ill. A small percentage (<10 percent) of patients develop pancolitis with involvement of the entire colon. Of all the possible systemic manifestations, some sort of arthritis is most likely. Twenty percent will have either a migratory, inflammatory, or peripheral arthritis with a predilection to the hips, ankles, wrists, and elbows.[2] See Table 6-15-1 for systemic manifestations of UC.

OBJECTIVE

A patient with UC appears quite ill. Patients may be pale, tachycardic, and hypotensive owing to volume depletion and blood loss. Fever is frequently elevated (>103°F), and there may be increased skin turgor. Abdominal examination reveals distention, slow to absent bowel sounds, firm abdomen (not rigid unless perforation occurs), tender to light and deep palpation in the left lower quadrant (LLQ) with or without rebound, depending on the level of peritoneal irritation. Rectal examination may reveal exaggerated tenderness and a positive heme check. A complete physical should be done to evaluate for other systemic manifestations.

DIAGNOSTIC CONSIDERATIONS

The list of differential diagnosis in UC is listed in Table 6-15-2. When sorting out the possibilities it is helpful to remember, pain, bleeding, and age range. These help the provider differentiate quickly. Infectious diseases should always be ruled out initially and reconsidered in a patient with known UC. The colon is a warm, dark moist place, and bacteria love to take advantage; an exacerbation of UC may have a bacterial trigger.

LABORATORY TESTS

The standard tests for the evaluation of an acute abdomen should be done initially: complete blood cell count (CBC), a chemistry panel for electrolytes, urinalysis, amylase, and plain abdominal films. Stool for ova and parasite analysis (O & P), fecal leukocytes, and cultures are a must to rule out infectious colitis (Chap. 6-4, "Colitis"). The CBC may reveal a mixed anemia from blood loss and iron deficiency. Liver function studies may be abnormal, and there may be hypoalbuminemia from protein leakage from the ulcerative mucosa. Additional tests may include a sedimentation rate, antinuclear antibodies (ANA), and C-reactive protein.

RADIOLOGIC (IMAGING) STUDIES

A barium enema will reveal the extent and severity of the UC. The classic finding of UC on a barium study is loss of haustral markings, giving a "cobblestone" appearance which represents ragged mucosal ulcerations and narrowing of the intestinal lumen. During the acute fulminant phase, the barium enema should be done with great care because the colon is quite friable and perforations are a distinct possibility.

The preferred definitive study is an endoscopic examination with biopsies. Direct visualization during a sigmoidoscopy or colonoscopy will reveal an irregular mucosal surface with a granular appearance and shallow ulcerations.

TREATMENT

Pharmacologic Management

Pharmacologic management is directed at the control of symptoms, since there is no definitive cure for ulcerative colitis. Sulfasalazine has been the mainstay of therapy for years. Split by colonic bacterial activity, the effects appear to be topical versus systemic. The active ingredient is mesalamine, with sulfapyridine as the transport mechanism. The probable mechanism of action is an increase in colonic oxidation of glucose.

The pH-dependent 5-amino salicylic acids (5-ASA) are the newer oral formulations, which deliver mesalamine directly to the colonic tissue. Their advantage is the delivery system and the absence of sulfapyridine, which can cause hypersensitivity and decreased sperm counts in men. Another option is the microsphere formulations, which slowly release medication beginning in the duodenum and extending to the colon. Rectal 5-ASA

preparations have been very successful in the control of UC. Rectal instillation leads to high concentrations in the descending colon (up to the splenic flexure). Efficacy is essentially the same. Side-effect profile and cost determines which medication a patient will tolerate (Table 6-15-3). Sulfasalazine is used for control of mild to moderate disease, but avoided in acute and severe ulcerative colitis since it might cause exacerbation of symptoms.

First-line therapy for fulminant UC is adrenal steroids. Absorption factors include the level of inflammation, total dosing, and efficiency of delivery. The greater the inflammation, the more steroidal absorption. Steroidal systemic side effects will thus depend on the level of colonic uptake. The most common dosing is oral prednisone, 45 to 60 mg/day. Intravenous prednisolone, 40 to 60 mg/day, is used if there is a problem with absorption. Improvement is seen in 7 to 10 days, and steroids can be tapered slowly over 4 to 16 weeks.

Cyclosporine inhibits immune response, which is regulated by T lymphocytes, and is used for refractory UC (nonresponsive to steroids). The vast majority of refractory cases will respond to IV therapy of 4 mg/kg/day. Cessation or slowing of rectal bleeding is usually the first clinical sign of improvement.

Additional therapy includes IV fluids and electrolyte replacement. It may be prudent in the acute situation to type and crossmatch blood products. Total parenteral nutrition (TPN) is a time-honored treatment for fulminant UC since it gives complete bowel rest. Patients are kept nothing by mouth (NPO) until improvement is seen, then progress to low-roughage meals and elemental diet drinks like Vivonex, Tolerex, and Vital. Patients who do not respond to any of the above are surgical candidates for partial or complete colectomy.

Surgical Management

Approximately one quarter of patients with UC will require a colectomy at some point in their disease. Surgery is performed for the complications of UC: persistent bleeding, perforations, cancer risks, toxic megacolon, and debilitating illness. Three basic surgeries may be done:

- *Proctocolectomy* Removal of colon and rectum with ileostomy.
- *Proctocolectomy with continent ileostomy* A pouch is formed with the ileum inside the abdominal wall. The patient inserts a tube through a small opening in the flank for evacuation of stool.
- *Ileoanal anastomosis* Called a "pull-through" operation, the ileum is pulled down and secured to the anus for close to normal evacuation of stool. Unfortunately rectal tone is lost and the patient will most likely have dumping syndrome.

COMPLICATIONS AND RED FLAGS

As many as one-third of ulcerative colitis patients will develop colon cancer. Cancer surveillance is recommended with any exacerbation of the UC and 10 years after diagnosis with or without remission. Colonoscopy with biopsies is recommended once a year to every 2 years. Some gastroenterologists advocate total colectomy as a prophylactic measure against cancer risks. It is best to educate the patient as to risk of cancer and the side effects of a total colectomy.

Crohn's Disease

DISCUSSION

Seen in all countries of the world, Crohn's can present at any age. Like UC it has a peak between ages 10 and 40 but has another peak in the elderly, ages 60 to 80. The idiopathic inflammatory process that can effect any GI mucosa (mouth to anus)

Table 6-15-2. Differential Diagnosis of Inflammatory Bowel Disease

Disease	Common Symptoms
Intestinal tuberculosis	Fever, anorexia, nausea, constipation, RLQ pain
Tropical sprue	Profuse, frothy diarrhea, anemia, paresthesias, muscle cramps
Amebic colitis	Crampy abdominal pain, watery diarrhea, malaise, weight loss
Infectious colitis *Campylobacter, Shigella, Salmonella, Yersinia*	Bloody diarrhea, generalized abdominal pain, fever, chills
Ischemic colitis	Severe abdominal pain, profuse bloody diarrhea, vomiting, hypotension
Diverticulitis	Elderly, LLQ pain, mass effect, constipation
Whipple's disease	Middle-aged men, steatorrhea, abdominal pain, lymphadenopathy, polyarthritis, GI bleeding
Acute abdomen	Abdominal pain, peritoneal symptoms, fever, tachycardia
Irritable bowel syndrome	Abdominal pain, constipation or diarrhea, ↑ mucus, anxiety component
Colon carcinoma	Altered bowel habits, bloody stools, anemia, sudden weight loss
Pseudomembranous colitis	Profuse watery diarrhea (rarely bloody), tenesmus, antibiotic-related

Table 6-15-3. Medical Management of Inflammatory Bowel Disease

Medication	Dose	Side Effects	Drug Interactions
Sulfasalazine (for control of mild disease)	4–6 g daily in divided doses	Nausea or vomiting, anorexia, headache, dyspepsia, megaloblastic anemia, male infertility	Inhibits folic acid ↓ Digoxin ↓ Antibiotic metabolism
pH-dependent 5-ASA analogues (Asacol, Claversal)	1.5 to 3 g daily in divided doses	Infrequent headache, nausea, indigestion	No known drug interactions
5-ASA microsphere (Pentasa)	Up to 4 grains/day in divided doses	Avoid in the presence of renal or hepatic failure; diarrhea, headache, nausea	No known drug interactions
Bond 5-ASA (Dipentum)	1.0 g/day in divided doses	Infrequent diarrhea, nausea, abdominal pain	Increased PTT with warfarin
Corticosteroids	Severe disease: hydrocortisone, 300–400 mg/day, or prednisolone, 60–80 mg/day, or methylprednisolone, 60–80 mg/day, or ACTH, 120 U/day	Peptic ulcer disease, hypertension, psychiatric disturbances, facial mooning, acne, ecchymosis, cataracts, osteopenia, growth retardation (limited list)	
Cyclosporine (ulcerative colitis)	4 mg/kg/day continuous infusion	Renal damage, hypertension, hyperkalemia, hepatotoxicity	Extensive drug interactions with any drug associated with hepatic P450 system
Metronidazole (Flagyl) (Crohn's)	750–2000 mg/day in divided doses	Glossitis, headache, ataxia, vertigo, paraesthesias, neutropenia	Alcohol agonist: increase warfarin action; cimetidine lowers clearance; decrease dilantin clearance

has had different names over the years: skip colitis, regional colitis, granulomatous colitis, and transmural colitis.

PATHOGENESIS

Crohn's disease effects all four layers of the intestinal mucosa (transmural) with ulcerations and distinct noncaseating granulomas filling the crypts. Once the process is ingrained, the bowel wall thickens and becomes inflexible and stenotic. Because the disease is transmural, fistulas and perirectal fissures are common. These can invade other intraabdominal structures like the bladder and ureters. Unlike UC, Crohn's is characterized by "skip" lesions; there may be a lesion in the ascending colon and another in the jejunum. Approximately one-third of patients will have small bowel or colon lesions exclusively, but as many as half will have lesions in both areas. The vast majority will develop ileal disease at some point, affecting the reabsorption of bile salts.

SYMPTOMS

An insidious onset is characteristic with vague complaints of fatigue, malaise, weight loss, and low-grade fever. Pain in the right lower quadrant (RLQ) with diarrhea is the most common presentation. The abdominal pain is described as crampy in nature and generally relieved by defecation. The majority of patients will have watery diarrhea. Mild cases may present with occult bleeding while more severe cases may have gross GI bleeding. This wide spectrum of disease activity can result in a diagnostic delay. Steatorrhea is possible with small bowel involvement. Perianal disease is prevalent with perianal fistulas, fissures, and abscesses. (Systemic symptoms are listed in Table 6-15-1). It is important to note that Crohn's patients are much more likely to develop gallstones and oxalate kidney stones. Chronic Crohn's disease may present with obstructive symptoms, including nausea and vomiting.

OBJECTIVE

The general appearance of a patient with Crohn's disease is that of a thin and undernourished individual with a low-grade fever. Aphthous ulcerations may be seen in the mouth. A tender mass in the RLQ is common and may be confused with acute appendicitis. A careful rectal examination may reveal perianal scarring, skin tags, fissures, or abscesses. Systemic signs may include erythema nodosum, nail clubbing, and joint inflammation.

DIAGNOSTIC CONSIDERATIONS

The differential diagnosis is essentially the same as that for ulcerative colitis (Table 6-15-2). The elderly are often misdiagnosed with diverticulosis or ischemic bowel disease.

LABORATORY TESTS

A complete blood count usually reveals a mixed anemia (iron deficient, B_{12} deficient), and increased WBC count. An elevated sedimentation rate is common. Chemistries may reveal low albumin, calcium, and sodium. Alkaline phosphatase and gamma globulins usually increase. C-reactive proteins are most closely related to clinical disease activity and are good markers to judge the recovery process.

RADIOLOGIC (IMAGING STUDIES)

Barium studies are essential in the evaluation of Crohn's disease. Since the lesions can be anywhere, a complete examination includes a barium swallow, upper gastrointestinal (UGI) series with small bowel follow-through, and barium enema. Obviously, these should be done in sequence, with the barium enema being the preferred first examination. Radiographic features may include rectal sparing, long longitudinal ulcerations, and mucosal edema appearing as blunting, flattening, thickening, or straightening of the normal bowel patterns. Fibrotic stenosis will cause distortion of landmarks and may appear pipe-like. Fistulization, perforations, and abscess formation may also be seen.

Endoscopy is used as a compliment to the barium studies, allowing for biopsies of the strictures, masses, or filling defects. Computed tomography (CT) can demonstrate the transmural thickening and track the fistula formation to the skin, bladder, and retroperitoneum.

Table 6-15-4. Parenteral Nutrition*

Total Parenteral Nutrition (TPN)†	Ingredients‡
Proteins (amino acids 4.25%)	42.5–50 g
Dextrose (25–50%)	250 (25%) or 125 g (50%)
Calcium	4–5 meq
Magnesium	5–8 meq
Potassium	20–50 meq
Sodium	20–50 meq
Acetate	30–75 meq
Chloride	20–55 meq
Phosphorus	10–20 mM
Multivitamins with biotin, B_{12}, and folic acid	10–15 mL
Heparin: helps prevent venous thrombosis	1000 U

* Daily laboratory tests include full electrolyte set, glucose, CO_2, BUN, weight, and fluid input and output.
† Give through a central line to those who need total bowel rest.
‡ These are recommended starting ranges. They must be adjusted for patient needs by a multidisciplinary team.

TREATMENT

Pharmacologic Management

Medical treatment of Crohn's is similar to that for ulcerative colitis with a few differences. Sulfasalazine and its analogues have been quite helpful for the control of inflammation in the colon, but their efficacy in the small bowel is debated. Corticosteroids have been highly successful in treating Crohn's disease at a dose of 0.25 to 0.75 mg/kg/day. Oral budesonide, 9 mg daily, can induce remission in patients with ileal disease. Cyclosporine does not improve symptoms or reduce requirements for other forms of therapy. Another anti-inflammatory that has enjoyed some success is methotrexate, 12.5 to 15 mg daily. Unfortunately, long-term use may predispose the patient to hepatic fibrosis, pneumonitis, and pulmonary fibrosis.

Metronidazole (Flagyl), 750 to 2000 mg/day, has been shown to be at least as effective as sulfasalazines. This reduces or eliminates the need for corticosteroids. Unfortunately, the side-effect profile is not good over the long term, with paresthesias being quite common. Relapse frequency is increased with metronidazole versus sulfasalazine.

Supportive therapy includes good nutrition (high-protein diet) with the addition of fat-soluble vitamins and B_{12}. Severe cases of Crohn's will require total parenteral nutrition (TPN) (Table 6-15-4). Abdominal cramping can be treated with antispasmodics like dicyclomine (Bentyl) or Donnatal. Diarrhea may be controlled with Imodium, 2 to 4 mg every 6 h or Lomotil, one or two tablets every 6 h. It is important to rule out ulcerative colitis and bacterial colitis prior to the use of either antispasmodics or antidiarrheals, since both can exacerbate these conditions. Bile acid binding resins (Questran or something similar) may be helpful with absorption problems and steatorrhea. Conservative local treatment of perianal disease is recommended, since surgical revisions can lead to worsening fistulas and abscesses.

Surgical Treatment

Surgery is reserved for perforations, abscess drainage, obstructions, intractable disease, and some fistulas. Some fistulas are "innocent," causing no major symptoms or complications. More nuisance fistulas (perianal) are treated with good skin care and topical and/or oral antibiotics. Unfortunately, recurrence of the disease is high after partial intestinal removals, and some patients return to the surgical service on a recurrent basis.

COMPLICATIONS AND RED FLAGS
Cancer Risk

Crohn's is recognized for increasing a patient's chances of developing colon cancer fivefold. There may also be an increased risk of small bowel carcinomas. Cancer surveillance should begin about 15 years after the initial diagnosis of Crohn's with routine colonoscopy with biopsies every 1 to 2 years. A sudden change in a patient's usual bowel pattern should prompt an early evaluation. Since colon cancer and Crohn's are both possible in the elderly, it is important not to delay investigation of new symptoms.

Other Inflammatory Bowel Disease Complications

Ulcerative colitis and Crohn's disease predispose the patient to electrolyte imbalances and dehydration, especially in hot weather. Hypoalbuminemia may cause varying levels of fluid retention. Weight loss is common to both processes, as is persistent anorexia. One-forth of children may experience growth retardation. (See Table 6-15-5.)

SUPPORTIVE MEASURES AND PATIENT EDUCATION

Both ulcerative colitis and Crohn's are chronic, often debilitating disease processes that strike patients in the prime of their lives. The diseases are bad enough in and of themselves, but the therapies used can cause at least as much if not more debilitation. Patients with ileostomies must deal with the mechanical needs of emptying an ostomy bag daily, dumping syndrome with malabsorption and dehydration, and psychosexual difficulties to name a few. Crohn's patients with persistent diarrhea and perianal disease can develop embarrassing rectal incontinence. Rectal or vaginal fistulas can affect sexual activities and complicate birthing in women. Children may suffer growth retardation and vitamin deficiency syndromes. These problems plus the ever-present risk of colon cancer make IBD a difficult disease to live with.

Providers must form a trusting relationship with these patients, so they feel free to call when symptoms or concerns overwhelm them. Like the proverbial "headache" patient, chronic disease can test the patience of all concerned. Each new symptom should be approached with the same fervor exhibited when investigating an unknown process. Having IBD does not preclude having a viral acute gastroenteritis (AGE) or appendicitis.

It is essential that patients understand the disease process and the expectations of the course, progress, chance of remission, and overall prognosis. Good nutrition is key; both UC and Crohn's patients struggle with iron deficiency and low protein, whereas Crohn's patients contend with B_{12} deficiencies. Diet should be high-protein, low-fat (especially after colectomy), and low-residue (avoid raw foods). Ensure that a dietitian follows the patient and tailors a meal plan conducive to individual tastes.

Patients may suffer anxiety and/or depressive episodes due to loss of self-image, loss of job, and marriage difficulties. Psychological needs should be met with appropriate consultation and referral to support groups and professionals.

Table 6-15-5. Complications of Inflammatory Bowel Disease

Colon cancer: ulcerative colitis > Crohn's
Toxic megacolon: ulcerative colitis > Crohn's
Hemorrhage: ulcerative colitis > Crohn's
Perforation: Crohn's > ulcerative colitis
Fistulas and fissures: Crohn's > ulcerative colitis
Growth retardation: Crohn's > ulcerative colitis
Malabsorption syndromes: Crohn's > ulcerative colitis

PEARLS

Diagnosis of IBD is usually not made in the first visit. As with any disease process, the patient should always be instructed to return for care if diarrhea persists more than 24 to 48 h. Past medical history is particularly important in IBD, because the systemic symptoms of IBD may present well ahead of the gastrointestinal symptoms. Take care in the elderly to keep IBD in the differential, since its treatment is radically different from that for diverticulitis or ischemic bowel disease. The vast majority of these patients are initially cared for by the internal medicine department, but their follow-up care is often monitored by primary care providers. Keep that index of suspicion high with changes in disease pattern and remember to do cancer surveillance.

REFERENCE

1. Hasting, Glen, Weber, Richard: Inflammatory bowel disease: Part I. Clinical features and diagnosis. *Am Fam Phys* 47(3):598–606, 1993.

BIBLIOGRAPHY

Lightiger S, Present D, Kornbluth A, et al: Cyclosporine in severe ulcerative colitis. *New Engl J Med* 330:1840–1845, 1994.
Medical Science Bulletin (Internet): Ulcerative Colitis. National Institute of Diabetes and Digestive and Kidney Diseases, NIH publication no 95-1597, April 1992.
Rectal approach to treatment of distal ulcerative colitis. *Lancet* 346:520–521, 1995.
Rodgers A, Coelho-Borges S: Medical therapy in Crohn's disease. *Postgrad Med* 92(8):169–183, 1992.

Chapter 6–16
INTESTINAL OBSTRUCTION
Anne P. Heinly

DESCRIPTION

Intestinal obstruction is simply something either inside or outside the intestinal tract stopping or blocking the progress of food or waste. Obstruction is a common phenomenon and accounts for about 20 percent of the emergency surgeries performed each year. *Mechanical obstruction* is something physically in the way or something pressing on the intestine blocking the path. *Nonmechanical obstruction* (also known as pseudoobstruction) occurs when intestinal peristalsis stops and nothing moves forward or backward. Young people are more likely to have mechanical obstruction in the form of an incarcerated hernia and intussusception (bowel telescoping on itself). The elderly are more likely to have obstruction from carcinomas, volvulus, and diverticulosis. Men and women have an equal chance of having an obstruction, and there is no age group safe from the possibility of obstruction.

PATHOGENESIS

Traditionally, intestinal obstruction refers to a partial or complete blockage of the small or large intestine. Esophageal and gastric obstructions are different entities. As seen in Chap. 6-18, "Malabsorption," the small intestine is in charge of digesting and absorbing nutrition, and the colon is responsible for continued water

and electrolyte retrieval. When obstruction slows or stops this process, harmful things start to happen. The small intestine, the most common location for obstruction, receives or produces up to 4000 mL of fluid a day. An obstruction allows all that fluid to accumulate, the subsequent pooling causes intestinal wall edema, and vasodilatation ensues causing even more fluid to pour in. The result is liters of slush backing up with little or no absorption until vomiting is the only path out. Fluid deficits are amassed from intestinal secretions, vomiting, and poor oral intake, and soon there is a dehydrated, hypotensive, ill patient presenting to the emergency department.

Obstruction over time can cause bowel necrosis, which adds the possibility of bleeding, sepsis, electrolyte imbalances, and surgical consequences. Bowel necrosis is more likely to occur when there is a "closed loop" obstruction, or more simply an obstruction that blocks two or more points. A volvulus (twisted intestine) is an example, resembling a sausage twisted into a loop, with the stool going nowhere. The result is increasing fluid, increasing pressure, bacterial endotoxins at work, and ultimately bowel wall injury and necrosis.

SYMPTOMS

Small bowel obstruction or proximal obstructions usually present with abdominal pain. The pain usually waxes and wanes as the intestinal peristalsis tries to clear the obstruction. The higher the obstruction, the faster vomiting occurs, often with bile and partially digested food products. The vomitus is usually copious, and it has a foul (fecal) smell due to bacterial overgrowth. The lower the obstruction is in the tract, the more likely abdominal distention may be a presenting symptom (trapped gas and fluids).

A colonic obstruction more commonly presents with distention, borborygmi, and pain. The pain has a tendency to be a dull, steady pain versus the cramping pain in higher obstructions. It takes longer to get to a vomiting stage because the fluid backup has farther to go and the small intestine can stand a fair amount of distention. When the patient does vomit, it is feculent. Patients often complain of constipation or may have "obstipation," which is the passage of stool below the obstruction or watery diarrhea that is able to sneak through. In the elderly, the only symptoms may be distention and constipation because of changes in immune and neurologic status.

OBJECTIVE

Physical findings fluctuate with location and duration of the obstruction. An early obstruction or partial obstruction reveals less distention and more bowel sounds like rushes and gurgles as the bowel tries to clear the obstruction. As the obstruction persists, the abdominal distention can be impressive. The protuberant abdomen can make the patient look 10 months pregnant. Strangulation, peritonitis secondary to necrosis, sepsis, or complete obstruction can present with absent or very slow bowel sounds and increasing tympany.

The pseudoobstruction patient is less likely to have distention but will have absent bowel sounds due to the lack of peristalsis (adynamic or paralytic ileus). All patients may have evidence of dehydration: poor turgor, dry oral and eye mucosa, orthostatic vital signs, and/or poor urinary output. A rectal examination is necessary; it may reveal impacted stool, mass, fistula, or blood. Bleeding is not unusual with diverticulitis, carcinoma, ischemia, or intussusception.

DIAGNOSTIC CONSIDERATIONS

Table 6-16-1 reviews the possible causes of obstructions. By far the most common cause is the presence of abdominal adhesions especially with the small intestine. Colonic obstructions are more

Table 6-16-1. Cause of Obstruction

INTRALUMINAL MECHANICAL OBSTRUCTION	
Tumors: carcinoma, lymphoma Crohn's disease Diverticulosis, diverticulitis Foreign body: sexual or deviant behavior Gallstones Parasites, worms Intussusception	These occur within the lumen of the intestine, physically blocking the progress of food. In the case of intussusception, the intestine telescopes in on itself, creating an intrinsic blockage.

EXTRALUMINAL MECHANICAL OBSTRUCTION	
Volvulus Hernias: inguinal, umbilical, ventral Pregnancy Uterine, ovarian enlargement Adhesions: postsurgical, endometriosis, Pseudocysts, abscesses Abdominal aneurysm	Extraluminal obstruction occurs from outside the intestinal lumen. A hernia or volvulus is an extrinsic process caused by the bowel twisting on itself or getting caught in a tight spot. Any enlarged or shifted abdominal structure can compress the bowel, squeezing it closed.

ILEUS OR PSEUDOOBSTRUCTION	
Peritoneal insult: trauma, abdominal and nonabdominal surgery, burns, stress Peritonitis: appendicitis, cholecystitis, diverticulitis, ruptured viscous, etc. Electrolyte imbalance, especially potassium, sodium, or magnesium disturbances Ischemia: blood loss from any source, abdominal angina, MI, CVA Renal failure, uremia, liver failure, CHF Renal stones, fractures Infection: sepsis, cellulitis, pneumonia, pancreatitis, ulcerative colitis, glomerulonephritis Medications: narotics, anesthetics, etc.	The intestines are sensative to multiple stimuli with activity or inactivity triggered by nerves, hormones, or mechanical distention. Ileus occurs because of an insult to the system as a whole, usually effecting the sympathetic nervous system, and the intestinal tract literally stops. Depending on the severity of the stress or insult and the subsequent treatment, the ileus can last only a few hours or for several days.

CHRONIC PSEUDOOBSTRUCTION	
Scleroderma Dermatomyositis Amyloidosis Muscular dystrophy Myxedema Diabetes mellitus Parkinson's disease	A chronic problem with slow intestinal transit or propulsion, these patients are prone to develop megacolon. The mechanism seems to be a loss of smooth-muscle control, connective-tissue loss and/or neurologic disconnect. The result is relative immobility with chronic constipation, bloating, anorexia, and cramping.

NOTE: MI = myocardial infarction; CVA = cardiovascular accident; CHF = congestive heart failure.

likely due to carcinoma or diverticuli. Constipation (Chap. 6-6) is sometimes referred to as the most common type of obstruction. Certainly it is common, but it is generally a temporary condition that seldom causes distention or vomiting.

LABORATORY TESTS

Volume depletion and electrolyte derangement are the most common findings on laboratory evaluation. The complete blood cell count (CBC) may show a high hematocrit owing to volume loss and a mild elevation in white blood cells. The leukocytosis may be more dramatic if necrosis, peritonitis, or sepsis is present. Amylase may be elevated, but like the sedimentation rate, it is nonspecific for the etiology of the obstruction. Urinalysis usually demonstrates the patient's poor fluid status with a high specific gravity. Chemistries may show a metabolic acidosis with a rising blood urea nitrogen (BUN) and creatinine. Severity is dependent on the duration of the obstruction, age of the patient, and concomitant disease processes.

RADIOLOGIC (IMAGING) STUDIES

The plain abdominal film, supine and upright, is usually enough to make the diagnosis of obstruction. Table 6-16-2 reviews possible findings. If the plain films are not sufficient for diagnosis, a barium study is recommended. Barium versus a water-soluble contrast is preferred because it does not add to the osmotic fluid confiscation that the obstruction is already causing. The study generally defines the location of the obstruction and often its probable cause. In the case of intussusception or colonic volvulus, the heavy barium may actually help resolve the obstruction.

TREATMENT

Despite the large number of obstruction patients who end up in surgery, the first step is medical management. Correction of electrolyte imbalances and fluid replacement is essential. Stabilizing the cardiac and renal status of the patient is required prior to any operative therapy. Up to 80 percent of patients with proximal small intestinal obstructions will resolve with early decompression with a nasogastric tube and strict oral fluid restriction (at least for a while). With the postoperative paralytic ileus, nasogastric tube (NGT) decompression and fluid restriction may be required for weeks or even months. In these cases total parenteral nutrition has to be implemented as well. NGT decompression is recommended for all types of obstruction because it puts the intestines at rest and removes secretions.

Table 6-16-2. Radiologic Findings in Obstruction

Supine and Upright Abdominal Films
 Multiple air-fluid levels—small bowel obstruction
 Dilated bowel loops, folded over on themselves—small bowel obstruction
 Bird's beak appearance, classic for a volvulus
 A loop of bowel displacing normal appearing colonic gas—closed loop obstruction
 Blurred haustral markings with large loops (may indicate edema and ischemic injury)
 Evidence of gallstones, pancreatic calcifications, renal stones, or aortic aneurysm

For about 50 percent of obstruction patients, surgery is the solution. The goal of surgery is to relieve the obstruction with as little disruption of the abdominal contents as possible. Since adhesions frequently cause obstruction, it is important to minimize trauma to the peritoneal tissue during surgery. The second goal is to limit the bowel resection and achieve a clean anastomosis. Laparoscopic abdominal surgery is making new inroads to reaching both goals.

The key to therapy for an obstruction is knowing when to wait and when to operate. Medical therapy may relieve an obstruction for a time, but recurrence is common. A trial of medical therapy may put the bowel at risk for strangulation, necrosis, and bleeding. Since there is an increased risk of complications, including death with delayed surgery, the decision and timing of surgery can be critical. Serial radiographs, laboratory studies, and physical examinations should be carefully followed to catch subtle progression of the obstruction.

COMPLICATIONS

Prior to the relief of an obstruction, the complications include volume loss (decreasing cardiac and renal reserves); electrolyte imbalances that can cause acidosis and cardiac arrhythmias; perforation of the bowel at a weak spot (diverticulosis or ulcer), causing a peritonitis, bleeding, shock, or sepsis; and bowel necrosis.

Postsurgical patients are susceptible to wound infection, especially with perforations or in cases of bowel necrosis. In the elderly, the risks are higher because of decreased organ reserve (they cannot take the hypotension and insult as well) and concomitant diseases. Small intestinal obstructions are less likely to end in death, but as many as 20 percent of colon obstructions result in death, despite aggressive therapy and early surgery.

PATIENT EDUCATION

Prevention of obstruction is difficult. Adhesions may form even without a history of previous abdominal surgery. Intrinsic problems like hernias, volvulus, and intussusception are not avoidable. Pancreatic pseudocyst and carcinomas may be preventable with alcohol restriction and a low-fat diet. Postsurgical education should include the likelihood of another obstruction in the future.

PEARLS

An obstruction is a sign of an underlying problem. Stabilize the patient with fluids, decompression, and bowel rest. Look for the underlying cause; an adynamic ileus can be caused by pneumonia or even otitis media in children. Watch for progression of the obstruction, and do not delay surgery if there is risk of strangulation or necrosis.

BIBLIOGRAPHY

Sleisenger MH, Fordtran JS: Intestinal obstruction, in *Gastrointestinal Disease,* 5th ed. 1993. pp 989–993.
Winslow B, Westfall J, Nicholas R, et al: Intussusception. *Am Fam Phys* 54:213–217, 1996.

Chapter 6–17
IRRITABLE BOWEL SYNDROME
Anne P. Heinly

DISCUSSION

A common diagnosis, prevalent among young women, irritable bowel syndrome (IBS) continues to defy definition. A syndrome and not a disease, IBS is a collection of typical symptoms generally associated with aberrant colonic motility. Table 6-17-1 lists the alternative names given to IBS over the years. Although the set of symptoms varies from race to race, there appears to be no specific ethnic predilection for irritable bowel syndrome. Making a diagnosis of exclusion, the clinician must first rule out physiologic disease. The reason IBS is not classified as a disease is that its etiology has long eluded researchers. There is no evidence of anatomic or physiologic components to explain the set of symptoms.

PATHOGENESIS

The primary function of the colon is threefold. First, it moves waste products out of the system through slow peristaltic movements which for most patients are imperceptible. The second is the retrieval of essential electrolytes like potassium, sodium, calcium, and magnesium. The third is the reabsorption of water. As the fecal material is propelled through the gastrointestinal tract, it is condensed, molded, dehydrated, and evacuated by the colon.

The motility of the colon is a mixture of muscle action, hormonal triggers, and nervous system control. Stimulation of the colon may occur with distention, stress, dietary intake, chemical factors, and/or medications. Patients with IBS appear to have a heightened sensitivity to colonic motion and perceive it as crampy abdominal pain. For years, IBS research looked for a motility anomaly to explain the set of symptoms. To date, none has been found. New research is examining "visceral hyperalgesia" (increased sensitivity to pain in an organ). The peripheral nervous system of the gut is composed of multiple nerve terminals. Blocking three (in particular, mu, delta, and kappa) may diminish the neuronal excitability of the colon. Although this information

Table 6-17-1. Alternative Names for Irritable Bowel Syndrome

Spastic colon
Spastic colitis
Psychogenic colitis
Irritable colon
Nervous stomach
Mucous colitis
Functional bowel disease

Table 6-17-2. Differential Diagnosis for Irritable Bowel Syndrome

Amebic colitis	Crampy abdominal pain, profuse watery diarrhea, malaise, and weight loss
Infectious colitis	Bloody diarrhea, generalized abdominal pain, fever and chills, positive laboratory studies
Inflammatory bowel disease (Crohn's and ulcerative colitis)	RLQ or LLQ pain (seldom both), fever, weight loss, diarrhea (with or without blood); peritoneal signs, perianal fissures, biopsy changes
Ischemic colitis	Severe abdominal pain, profuse bloody diarrhea, vomiting and hypotension
Whipple's disease	Middle-aged men, steatorrhea, abdominal pain, polyarthritis and GI bleeding
Acute abdomen Appendicitis Cholecystectomy Diverticulitis Ruptured viscous, etc.	Acute onset, not chronic, steady abdominal pain, fever, tachycardia, peritoneal symptoms, positive laboratory studies
Colon carcinoma	Altered bowel habits, bloody stools, anemia, sudden weight loss; positive endoscopic findings
Lactose intolerance	Abdominal cramping, bloating, and diarrhea 20 to 30 min after a milk or cheese meal; increased flatulence, lasts 4 to 6 h; no fever, no systemic symptoms

may help with therapeutic modalities, it really has not accounted for the symptom cycle that IBS patients suffer.

SYMPTOMS

Usually a chronic and recurrent problem, the three most common symptoms of IBS are crampy abdominal pain, associated with gas and bloating, and loose, frequent stools. The pain is usually described as intermittent, mild to moderate, and localized in the lower abdominal quadrants. It is often short-lived (30 min to 1 h) and normally relieved with defecation. Patients complain of bloating and increased flatulence. Three to four stools will occur in a short period of time (2 to 6 h). They are semiformed, brown, and usually nonodorous. Some patients describe stools with mucus. This should not be confused with steatorrhea, which floats and is yellow to gray.

Patients may have the "diarrhea" cycle with alternating constipation. This is manifest by 1 to 2 days of loose stools followed by 5 to 10 days of constipation. Still others have the diarrhea episodes with persistent sensation of incomplete evacuation. These patients seldom have systemic manifestations such as dehydration, fever, chills, night sweats, nocturnal awakening, or weight loss. Stools are without blood or bacterial overgrowth.

OBJECTIVE

One of the frustrations of this diagnosis is that the physical examination is normal. If the patient is seen during a painful episode, there may be some evidence of abdominal bloating and diffuse, nonspecific abdominal tenderness. The physical should be thorough with at least a full cardiac, pulmonary, and abdominal examination and a rectal examination.

DIAGNOSTIC CONSIDERATIONS

The differential diagnosis for IBS is enormous. Table 6-17-2 addresses the most likely probabilities. It is vital to rule out anatomic

and physiologic disease because of the severe consequences associated with some diagnoses. Although it is tempting at times to make a clinical diagnosis based on history and physical alone, it is inappropriate with IBS. A complete workup is required for the diagnosis of irritable bowel syndrome to avoid missing a potentially life-threatening disease.

LABORATORY TESTS

No laboratory test will define IBS. Laboratory studies are directed toward the differential diagnosis. Standard tests should be done, but additional tests may be necessary to exclude disease. Stool for ova and parasite (O & P) analysis, cell counts, and cultures are the first steps. Complete blood cell count (CBC), sedimentation rates, antinuclear antibodies (ANA), and chemistries are all helpful in finding physiologic disease.

RADIOLOGIC (IMAGING) STUDIES

Radiology studies usually include a full gastrointestinal workup including an upper gastrointestinal (UGI) series, small bowel follow-through, and barium enema. The barium studies may reveal an increase in spasticity. Patients should also have (at the very least) a flexible sigmoidoscopy examination to rule out the differential diagnosis. A full colonoscopy may be necessary before a final diagnosis of IBS is made.

TREATMENT

Stress Reduction

Many medical providers can relate to IBS symptoms, remembering a critical test or the moments before an important speech. The colon is responsive to stress. The process is incompletely understood but may be related to cranial nerve X (vagus stimulation). Anxiety increases blood pressure, pulse, and other functions; the flight-or-fight adrenal surge seems to trigger colonic motility. Given that, IBS patients may benefit from stress reduction. First, map the patient's stress pattern and its relationship to IBS symptoms. If significant correlation exists coping mechanisms may be helpful. Be careful not to make this a "psychiatric" diagnosis, since it will not benefit the patient and there is truly more to IBS than mind control. Biofeedback, exercise, adequate sleep, and stress reduction classes are all recommended if there is an anxiety component.

Diet

Diet is by far the mainstay of therapy. The cephalic-gastrointestinal connection has been well established. The mere thought or smell of food can trigger GI secretions and motility. An IBS patient needs to first keep a food diary to establish which foods trigger or exacerbate their symptoms. Fats, milk, and size of the meal are often culprits in an IBS episode and may define its length and severity.

Although it is difficult to make generalized dietary recommendations owing to individual needs, there are two basic goals. The first goal is to regulate (normalize) bowel habits. Regular fiber intake can help achieve this. Increased fiber in the diet will help reabsorb water in the diarrhea-prone patient and add softening bulk to those prone to constipation. The fiber also keeps the colon slightly distended, which decreases the severity of any spasms that might occur.

Patients can add fiber to their diet with whole grain breads and cereal, legumes, fresh or dried fruits, and vegetables. Whether adding fiber naturally or with over-the-counter bulking agents like Metamucil, it is important to go slowly. Inform the patient that the initial use of these may actually cause more symptoms

Table 6-17-3. Medications for Irritable Bowel Syndrome

Bulking agents		
Metamucil	Begin with 1 tbsp/day	Requires regular use,
Citrucel	and increase up to 3	and increased water
FiberCon	tbsp until regular bowel	intake; may cause
	habit is established.	increased gas and
		cramping initially.
Antispasmodic		
Bentyl	10–20 mg every 6 h as	May cause mild
	needed for cramping;	sedation.
	may diminish diarrhea	
	as well.	
Anticholinergic, anxiolytic		
Librax	One or two tablets at	
Donnatal	meals and bedtime;	
	slows the gut and dimin-	
	ishes diarrhea.	
Lactose intolerance		
Lactase supplements	One to two tablets 20–30	Increase gas produc-
	min prior to milk in-	tion and flatulence.
	gestion	

for 1 to 2 weeks because gas production will increase. A slow start and small portions will minimize this problem.

The second goal is small regular meals, avoiding fatty over-loads. Large meals (especially fatty ones) can cause cramping and diarrhea due to an osmotic overload. A high-carbohydrate, low-fat diet is suggested with pastas, rice, grainy breads, vegetables, and fruits. Both dietary suggestions come with the recommendation of adequate water intake and regular exercise to promote good bowel habits.

Pharmacologic Management

OTC and prescription medications should be used for acute symptom control or as a therapy of last resort (Table 6-17-3). The medications are usually aimed at decreasing abdominal cramps versus slowing the diarrhea. It is imperative to remember that these medications may decrease symptoms, but do not impact the disease process. Use them judiciously. Better to use lifestyle changes like diet, exercise, and stress relief than to become dependent on medications and risk their side effects.

COMPLICATIONS

Although IBS plagues millions of people a year with an annoying set of symptoms, it has no known major complications. It is not related to inflammatory bowel disease (Chap. 6-15) or any other type of colitis (Chap. 6-4). Research has not shown any increase in cancer risk due to the diagnosis of IBS.

PEARLS

Patient education is key with irritable bowel syndrome. Tell patients what they don't have and reassure them that IBS has no known permanent sequelae. Diet and stress are major components in the vast majority of cases and should be addressed at length with patients. Medications can help but should *not* be relied on for long-term control of symptoms.

It is dangerous, once a diagnosis of IBS is made, to blame all subsequent GI complaints on IBS. The patient should always be reevaluated. Irritable bowel syndrome is a problem of young women. The very young, elderly, and men are not likely to have IBS, so it is important to look for a differential diagnosis. The young woman who has a change in the usual symptoms deserves

another look. Providers should not miss disease because they get too comfortable with an ill-defined problem such as irritable bowel syndrome.

BIBLIOGRAPHY

Dapoigny M, Fraitag B, Abitbol J-L, et al: "Kapping" visceral pain in patients with IBS: Does it work? *Gastroenterology* 3(2):531–533 (1996).

Medical Science Bulletin (Internet): "Irritable Bowel Syndrome." National Institute of Diabetes and Digestive and Kidney Disorders, NIH No. 95-693, October 1992.

Chapter 6–18
MALABSORPTION
Anne P. Heinly

DESCRIPTION

Malabsorption refers to the body's inability to digest or absorb necessary nutrients from its daily food intake. There are numerous disorders that can cause a malabsorption syndrome (Table 6-18-1). Malabsorption, to the point of weight loss or vitamin deficiency, is usually associated with chronic, long-standing problems. Its prevalence and severity is dependent on cause. It is best to approach it with a clear understanding of the mechanisms of digestion and nutrient absorption of the GI tract.

PATHOGENESIS

The small intestine, located loosely in the middle of the abdominal cavity, is about 15 ft long, but it has an absorption surface about the size of a basketball court. The duodenum receives digestive enzymes from the pancreas and gallbladder (bile), which continues the breakdown of fats, proteins, and carbohydrates that begins in the stomach. Bile salts produced by the liver are essential for the digestion and absorption of fats. Great detergents, bile salts wash the ingested fats and allow the formation of micelles. The micelles then enter the mucosal layer, and the fatty acids and monoglycerides are absorbed by diffusion. The proximal small intestine is responsible for most fat digestion and absorption. The distal ileum is responsible for the re-uptake of bile salts, which are returned to the liver in enteral feedback loop.

The pancreatic enzymes help break down carbohydrates and proteins. Protein polypeptides are disassembled by pancreatic trypsin and chymotrypsin into amino acids that are easily absorbed by the proximal and middle jejunum. Amylase breaks down the starches and maltose, sucrose, fructose, and lactose. Glucose is readily absorbed by the microvilli of the small intestine, but the other disaccharides have to be split enzymatically prior to absorption.

The small intestine is also responsible for the absorption of iron, calcium, vitamins A, D, E, and K (Table 6-18-2), and water. The distal bowel (ileum) absorbs vitamin B_{12} and bile salts. The ability of the small intestine to absorb nutrients is critical to good health. After the absorption process, the final step is into the portal or lymphatic circulation. The portal circulation carries the absorption products to the liver, where protein production, detoxification, and storage take place.

Table 6-18-1. Causes of Malabsorption

Disease	Mechanism of Malabsorption	Symptoms	Tests	Treatment
Pancreatic insufficiency Chronic pancreatitis Cystic fibrosis Pancreatic cancer Ductal stricture Zollinger-Ellison	Loss or destruction of enzyme activity affecting protein and carbohydrate digestion. With ductal strictures the enzymes may be produced but cannot be delivered.	Watery diarrhea; may have concomitant IDDM	Low serum albumin; glucose changes	Treat underlying problem. Replace enzymes: 8000 U lipase, 30,000 U protease, 30,000 U amylase before meals and at bedtime.
Bile salt insufficiency Liver disease Gallbladder disease Bacterial overgrowth Intestinal obstruction Zollinger-Ellison Crohn's disease with illeum involvement Ileal resection Intestinal vascular disease Intestinal bypass	Absence of or decreased bile acids limit fat digestion and absorption. In the case of vascular disease or postsurgical cases, there is limited contact with available bile salts. Loss of fats and B_{12} ensues in all cases.	Steatorrhea, weight loss, anemia, glossitis, neurological deficits	Low-serum B_{12}, macrocytic anemia, positive fecal fat	Cholestyramine can bind colonic bile salts, decreasing diarrhea, not loss of fats. There are no functional bile acid replacements that help with fat digest. Diet of medium-chain triglycerides recommended.

Mucosal defects
Amyloidosis
Radiation enteritis
Celiac sprue
Collagenous sprue
Tropical sprue
Lymphoma
Scleroderma
Crohn's disease
Infectious disease
  Whipple's disease
  Samonella
  Tuberculosis
  CMV
  HIV-induced
	After digestion, mucosal changes limit the absorption of carbohydrate products. The monosaccharides and disaccharides cannot cross the brush border. Severe mucosal disease will affect absorption of all products: fat, proteins, vitamins, carbohydrates, and minerals.	Gaseous distention, borborygmi, and osmotic diarrhea are the result. Steatorrhea dependent on degree of disease.	Mixed anemia acid stools with or without fat; vitamin deficiencies	Correction of underlying disease: e.g., gluten-free diet for celiac sprue; antibiotic therapy for Whipple's disease and tropical sprue.

Protein-losing enteropathies Intestinal lymphangiectasis Mechanical blockage of lymphs by extralymph masses Lymphomas	Obstruction of the lymphatics prevents the absorption of the chylomicron and lipoproteins required for production of protein complexes.	Edema, ascites, anasarca, steatorrhea, abdominal pain, and fever	Hypoproteinemia, serum albumin decreased	Treat underlying disease.

NOTE: IDDM =insulin-dependent diabetes mellitus; CMV = cytomegalovirus.

SYMPTOMS

Despite its variety of etiologies, malabsorption almost always present with one common characteristic: frequent, large, loose, foul-smelling stool. With rare exception fat metabolism is upset, causing elevation of fecal fat. Additionally, many patients complain of crampy abdominal pain (bloating), and with time, all have weight loss from the loss of calories. Vitamin and mineral deficiencies may be exhibited by bone pain, tetany, and weakness (calcium); night blindness and peripheral neuropathies with vitamin A; and purpura and poor clotting with vitamin K.

OBJECTIVE

Physical examination almost always reveals evidence of weight loss and muscle wasting from poor nutrition. Pallor and bruising may be present owing to anemias. Skin dryness, coloration, or texture changes may give clues to specific etiologies like Crohn's disease, Whipple's disease, or scleroderma. Patients with protein-losing enteropathy may have edema and in the worst cases ascites or anasarca. A complete and thorough physical examination is required to help define the cause of malabsorption.

DIAGNOSTIC CONSIDERATIONS

Simple acute gastroenteritis or diarrhea from any source can cause a mild steatorrhea. The difference between an acute diarrhea state and malabsorption syndrome is time. Most malabsorption etiologies are chronic illnesses that predispose the patient to weight loss and multiple systemic complications. Pancreatic insufficiency can present with watery diarrhea and excessive flatulence just like irritable bowel syndrome (Chap. 6-17), but the difference is a persistent intolerance to carbohydrate or lactose meals and weight loss encountered with malabsorption. Chronic diarrhea (a type of malabsorption) may be confused with other malabsorption syndromes. Investigate for infectious origins, especially in patients at risk for immune deficiencies.

LABORATORY TESTS

Of all the areas of the gastrointestinal system, the small intestines is perhaps the hardest to access. The definition of malabsorption is dependent on laboratory testing. First, the basic laboratory tests should be done to evaluate anemia and vitamin deficiencies: complete blood cell count (CBC), iron studies, vitamin B_{12} level, folate level, calcium level, alkaline phosphatase levels, and protein electrophoresis.

Fecal fat measurement is an unpleasant but necessary mainstay of diagnosis. The average person will eliminate 6 g of fat in stools over a 24-h period. The test is conducted by 72 h of stool collection (the unpleasant part) while the patient maintains a high fat diet (100 g daily); a measurement of more than 15 g of fat in 24 h is considered significant steatorrhea.

Another method is to measure carbohydrate absorption with a D-xylose test. The patient ingests 25 g of D-xylose and then has blood xylose levels checked 2 h after ingestion. If a blood level of 30 mg/dL or more is found, there is normal carbohydrate absorption by the proximal small bowel. If the blood level is low, the urine concentration is examined in 5 h; 4 g or less in the urine indicates mucosal malabsorption.

The Schilling test is used to evaluate B_{12} deficiency. It has two parts. First the patient ingests a measured dose of radioactive B_{12} and receives an injection of nonlabeled B_{12}. If urinary secretion of the radioactive B_{12} is less than 8 percent of the measured dose, then B_{12} malabsorption is confirmed. The next step is to administer intrinsic factor. If the malabsorption rectifies itself, then the small bowel is not the problem but an intrinsic factor deficiency exists. The Schilling test is especially helpful with diagnosis of Crohn's disease (Chap. 6-15) but may be positive because of bacterial overgrowth and renal failure.

These are the standard first tests when malabsorption is suspected. Borderline tests or tenacious symptoms may warrant further analysis which may include small intestinal mucosal biopsy (Crohn's disease, celiac sprue, Whipple's disease); culturing intestinal aspirate to rule out bacterial overgrowth; and any number of breath tests. Breath tests for glycocholic acid, D-xylose, and glucose hydrogen depend on the metabolic leftovers of absorption-liberating CO_2. The expired breath is examined for radiolabeled CO_2 for each specific test. These may be helpful, but their reliability is limited.

IMAGING STUDIES

Imaging studies are of limited value. Small bowel barium studies may reveal jejunal dilatation, fold thickening, or segmentation with malabsorption. Sprues will typically cause dilatation. Small intestine imaging may reveal jejunal polyps or intestinal pseudo-obstruction due to sclerosis. Imaging for probable causes may be beneficial, for example, CT scan for pancreatic pseudocysts, abscesses, or carcinoma may define the malabsorption etiology.

Pancreatic Exocrine Insufficiency

Pancreatic exocrine insufficiency is usually concurrent with a diagnosis of chronic pancreatitis or recurrent episodes of acute pancreatitis. The most common etiology is alcohol abuse, but it can occur secondary to trauma, viral infections, and pancreatic carcinoma. With the absence of pancreatic enzymes, digestion and absorption of fats, proteins, and carbohydrates are severely limited. Weight loss, watery diarrhea, and abdominal pain are presenting symptoms. X-ray evaluation may reveal pancreatic calcification in the epigastrium.

Treatment includes trying to reduce chronic pancreatitis symptoms. Stop all alcohol ingestion, and prescribe pain control, which may require narcotics. Replacement of pancreatic enzymes is

Table 6-18-2. Vitamin and Mineral Deficiency

Vitamin or Mineral	Symptoms	Tests	Treatment
Vitamin B_{12}	Megaloblastic anemia, weakness, fatigue, glossitis, stomatitis, paresthesias	Decrease serum B_{12} with macrocytic anemia	B_{12} injection 1000 μ monthly
Vitamin B_1 (thiamin)	Anorexia, muscle cramps, paresthesias, loss of reflexes	Decreased serum thiamin	Thiamin injection 100 mg/day for 1 week, then oral dose of 5 mg/day
Vitamin B_6 (pyridoxine)	Aphthous ulcers, anemia, glossitis, weakness, neuropathy, and seizures	Decreased pyridoxal phosphate levels	Vitamin B_6, 10–20 mg/day
Folic acid	Aphthous ulcers, anemia, glossitis, stomatitis	Normal serum B_{12} with reduced folate level in RBC, megaloblastic anemia	Folic acid, 1 mg/day
Vitamin A	Night blindness, xerosis, poor wound healing, corneal abrasion, blindness	Serum levels below 30 mg/dL	Vitamin A, 30,000 IU for a week
Vitamin D	Rickets osteomalacia, osteoporosis, muscle weakness	Decreased serum calcium and phosphate and vitamin D	Vitamin D, 10 mg/day
Vitamin E	Areflexia, disturbances of gait, decreased proprioception and vibrating sensation	Decreased vitamin E (less than 0.5 mg/dL) in relation to lipid profile	Vitamin E, 100 IU/day
Vitamin K	Bruising, bleeding	Prothrombin time prolonged	A single dose of subcutaneous vitamin K, 15 mg
Calcium	Rickets, osteomalacia, osteoporosis, paresthesias, tetany	Low serum calcium and phosphorus	1200 mg calcium daily
Magnesium	Paresthesia, tetany, weakness, cramps	Low serum magnesium	400 mg magnesium daily
Zinc	Dermatitis, poor wound healing, poor taste	Low serum zinc	15 mg zinc daily

essential, though normalization is not achievable. Commercial products like Viokase and Cotazym S contain enough lipase, protease, and amylase to enhance protein and carbohydrate absorption and alleviate at least some of the steatorrhea. Dosing is generally two or three tablets before each meal and at bedtime.

Bile Acid Insufficiency

Bile acid insufficiency can occur secondary to liver disease, gallbladder disease, faulty ductal delivery, intestinal obstruction, bacterial overgrowth or disorder of the terminal ileum that interferes with reabsorption. The result in all cases is malabsorption of fat with significant steatorrhea (20 g in 24 h). Protein and carbohydrate absorption usually are maintained. Watery diarrhea because of colonic irritation from bile salts is common.

Treatment is directed to the cause. In the case of bacterial overgrowth, a course of tetracycline or similar broad-spectrum antibiotic for 10 to 14 days may do the trick. In the presence of ileum disease (Crohn's), monthly B_{12} injection and cholestyramine, 2 g bid is recommended. The cholestyramine helps bind the bile salts, decreasing the diarrhea but not the fat loss.

Celiac Sprue

Celiac sprue is a disease of the small bowel mucosa and effects the absorption of fat, protein, carbohydrates, iron, fat-soluble vitamins, and water. The peak incidence is in the first year of life and again in the sixties. It is seen in women more often than men. In infants and children the malabsorption can cause failure to thrive, weight loss, infantilism, dwarfism, tetany, mouth ulcers, and angular stomatitis. In adults there is vertigo, weakness, fatigue, large appetite with weight loss, explosive flatulence, and diarrhea.

The cause of celiac sprue is still not clearly understood, but the gliadin fraction of gluten seems to be the problem. The treatment is the elimination of all gluten from the diet. A gluten-free diet includes the removal of all wheat, rye, barley, and oat products. Patients may require calcium and vitamin D supplements. As they reach their teen years, children may be able to resume a regular diet, but they should be counseled on the possible recurrence of symptoms in later life.

Tropical Sprue

Despite the lack of a specific pathogen, tropical sprue appears to be an infection of the small intestinal mucosa. Endemic to most of Asia and some Caribbean islands and parts of South America, epidemics of sprue can last 2 to 10 years. Symptoms may emerge years after leaving a tropical area. The chief symptom is explosive watery diarrhea followed by pale, frothy, foul-smelling greasy stools. Severe malnutrition and water loss cause electrolyte imbalances. Weakness, anemia, paresthesias, glossitis, stomatitis, dry rough skin, flatulence, muscle cramps, night blindness, purpura, and severe weight loss may be seen.

Since megaloblastic anemia is common, vitamin B_{12} 1000 μg IM is given daily for a week and then monthly for 6 months. Folic acid, 5 mg a day, and tetracycline dosing of 250 mg qid for 1 to 2 months is recommended. Tetracycline dosing may need to be extended for 6 months at half-strength (250 mg bid).

Whipple's Disease

Whipple's disease is a rare disorder found in middle-aged men presumably secondary to an infection of *Tropheryma whippleii.* The onset is insidious, and it can be fatal if not found and treated. Patients have diarrhea with mild steatorrhea, gastrointestinal bleeding, fever, lymphadenopathy, polyarthritis, edema, and anemia. With progression of the disease, peripheral and finally central neuropathies become evident.

Treatment is with penicillin G, 600,000 U IM bid for 10 days, or penicillin VK, 250 mg qid for 4 months. About 50 percent of patients may relapse. In relapsing cases, the current recommendation is trimethoprim-sulfamethoxazole for 6 to 12 months. Supplements of B_{12}, folate, iron, and calcium are also recommended for correction of vitamin deficiencies.

COMPLICATIONS

Certainly the most common complications with any of the malabsorption syndromes is weight loss, electrolyte imbalances, vitamin deficiencies, and dehydration. Without correction the patient, especially young children and the elderly, can suffer permanent damage to vital organs and even death. Celiac sprue left untreated leads to marked neurologic deficits which may not be reversible.

PATIENT EDUCATION

Depending on the cause of the malabsorption syndrome, patient education is tailored to the needs of the patient. In the case of bile acid insufficiency or pancreatic exocrine insufficiency, dietary changes are recommended. Generally, a high-protein, low fat diet is advocated to decrease steatorrhea and diarrhea. A medium-chain triglyceride diet (high in coconut oil) is easier to digest and may help patients tolerate fat intake. Mineral and vitamin supplementation is recommended, including vitamin D (necessary for calcium processing) and magnesium.

PEARLS

Malabsorption may be caused by a variety of diseases affecting the intricate balance of the small intestine. Pancreatic enzymes, bile salts, and intact mucosal surfaces are required to keep the delicate balance. Identification of these diseases is important to help avoid weight loss, chronic fatigue, anemia, and systemic manifestations. Virtually all malabsorption syndromes can lead to neurologic deficits and organ failure. It is imperative that a clinician define the cause of recurrent or chronic diarrhea and attempt to ameliorate the symptoms if not the disease.

BIBLIOGRAPHY

Sleisenger MH, Fordtran JS: *Gastrointestinal Disease,* 5th ed., Philadelphia, Saunders, 1993, pp 1009–1023, Maldigestion and malabsorption; pp 1078–1092, Celiac sprue; pp 1097–1103, Tropical sprue; pp 1118–1125, Whipple's disease.

Chapter 6–19
NAUSEA AND VOMITING
Anne P. Heinly

DISCUSSION

Nausea and vomiting are often associated, yet a patient can be nauseated without vomiting and vomit without first being nauseated. Common to a myriad of diverse conditions, nausea and vomiting are symptoms known to every man, woman, and child at some point in life. Nausea and vomiting can be the early signals of significant disease processes and should be investigated. Nausea is a sensation, described variously as queasy, uneasy, churning, gnawing, agitated, or nervous stomach or abdomen. Nausea may be "anticipatory," caused by an odor, sight, or sound that the patient associates with a bad experience (e.g., chemotherapy). Nausea and vomiting may have mechanical, chemical, or hormonal triggers. There are few diseases or medications that do not have some level of nausea or vomiting associated with them.

PATHOGENESIS

Nausea and vomiting are probably part of the basic regulatory mechanisms of the body, as natural as a pulse or respiration. The presumed location of the nausea chemoreceptor trigger zone (CTZ) is near the fourth brain ventricle and the vomiting center is on the dorsum of the medulla oblongata. The CTZ seems to be most responsible for the nausea sensation, which is mediated by the vagus nerve (cranial nerve X) and sympathetic pathways. The vagus enervates multiple areas including the baroreceptors of the heart, aortic arch, and carotid sinuses; the pharynx; the esophagus; and the GI tract to the splenic flexure. The extent of vagus involvement explains why nausea is a symptom in so many processes.

Another association appears to involve vasopressin, a hormone released by the posterior pituitary which is most sensitive to changes in osmotic pressure (those baroreceptors mentioned above). Research has shown a marked increase in vasopressin during even brief episodes of nausea. Thus a disease process that interrupts blood pressure (e.g., infections, medications, motion, etc.) can trigger nausea.

Nausea is the sensing side of the equation and vomiting is the action side. Vomiting is a complex patterned response involving the skeletal muscles and visceral organs of the chest and abdomen. As nausea progresses, at a point of no return, the pyloric sphincter loses tone, allowing for bile reflux into the churning stomach. The early retching causes lower esophageal sphincter tone loss, and finally there is a forceful sustained contraction of the diaphragm and abdominal muscles. The force ejects duodenal, gastric, and esophageal contents through the esophagus and out the mouth.

SYMPTOMS: AN APPROACH TO NAUSEA

Given the mechanism of nausea and vomiting and the association with many disease processes, it is important to treat the cause. A thorough history can be quite helpful, especially eliciting timing and character. If the symptoms have been over hours or days consider the following:

- Infectious processes like acute gastroenteritis (AGE), appendicitis, cholecystitis, otitis media, cellulitis, streptococcal pharyngitis
- Ingestion of toxins, poisons, or nausea-inducing medications (Table 6-19-1)
- Pregnancy
- Chronic diseases like peptic ulcer disease (PUD), myocardial infarction (MI), angina, Crohn's disease

If the nausea has been present a week to months consider partial obstructions, carcinoma, brain tumors, visual or auditory sources, motility disorders, or psychogenic causes (anorexia nervosa).

Timing may give vital clues to etiology. It is actually unusual to vomit during or immediately after a meal. Psychiatric disorders and esophageal disease are possible culprits. Esophageal diseases like Zenker's diverticulum, cancer, and strictures are characterized by regurgitating undigested food usually without nausea.

Vomiting one or more hours after a meal is associated with infections (any source), gastric outlet obstruction (especially in

Table 6-19-1. Medications and Nausea (Representative List)

Dopamine agonists	
Dopamine (Levodopa)	Dopamine receptors seem to induce nausea, used for hypotension.
Bromocriptine (Parlodel)	Dopamine receptor used in parkinsonism, acromegaly.
Narcotics	
Morphine	Reduces gastric motility; used for severe pain control; nausea usually subsides with regular use.
Codeine	Reduces gastric motility; nausea worse with increasing doses in most patients.
Antibiotics	
Erythromycin	Most likely due to gastric irritation; nausea worse with increasing doses; commonly used antibiotic.
Augmentin	Clavulanic acid is probably the culprit; Nausea and diarrhea are common.
Chemotherapy	
Cisplatin	Most chemotherapy induces some level of nausea probably from a variety of sources: neurologic toxicity, renal toxicity, and gastric retention. Used in the treatment of hormonal tumors; considered the worst for causing nausea.
Dacarbazine	Used for the treatment of metastatic melanoma and Hodgkin's disease.
Mithracin	Potent antineoplastic used in treatment of testicular cancers.
Procarbazine	Used as part of a regimen of vincristine, prednisone, and mustard for treatment of Hodgkin's disease.
5-Fluorouracil	Used widely for treatment of colon, rectal, breast, gastric, and pancreatic carcinomas.
Methotrexate	An antimetabolite used in the treatment of adult rheumatoid arthritis, severe psoriasis, breast cancer, acute lymphocytic leukemia, osteosarcoma, and small cell carcinomas.

infants), and decreased gastric motility (illness, chemotherapy). Morning vomiting is most associated with pregnancy but occurs with alcohol toxicity, uremia, peptic ulcer disease, and intracranial tumors.

The character of vomit may be telling as well. Old food suggests gastric retention (gastric outlet obstruction, PUD). The presence of bile implies duodenal reflux from cholecystitis, PUD, liver disease, or pancreatitis. Blood may be present as a result of vomiting (Mallory-Weiss tears) or may be the cause of nausea and vomiting (gastric ulcers, PUD, and carcinomas). Fetid breath and emesis may indicate bacterial overgrowth, obstruction, bowel ischemia, or necrosis.

OBJECTIVE

The physical examination should focus on the possible cause of nausea or vomiting. Orthostatic vital signs should be accomplished. Dehydration can cause nausea but seldom vomiting. Infectious disease from any source commonly causes nausea and vomiting. Look for the bottom line with a thorough physical examination, including a rectal or pelvic/prostate examination when indicated.

DIAGNOSTIC CONSIDERATIONS

Table 6-19-2 reviews the differential diagnosis for nausea and vomiting. The commonality of the symptoms defies true classification, and there may be more than one source of the problem. Nausea is often seen with malignancy and may be exacerbated by chemotherapy. Morphine is used for pain control but is well known for its ability to cause nausea. All possible factors should be explored and treated when possible.

LABORATORY TESTS

Laboratory assessment is aimed at the presumed cause of the nausea and vomiting and the potential complications. At the very least an electrolyte survey should be obtained to find evidence of dehydration or electrolyte aberrations.

RADIOLOGIC (IMAGING) STUDIES

Imaging studies, like the laboratory studies, are focused on the presumed cause of the nausea and vomiting. It is not wrong to do plain abdominal films to ascertain colonic ileus, free air, renal and gallbladder calculi, or obstructions.

TREATMENT

Key to the treatment of nausea and vomiting is determining the source. There are several medications (Table 6-19-3) helpful in controlling symptoms, but they should not be used in place of definitive treatment of the underlying cause of nausea.

COMPLICATIONS

The complications of vomiting can be serious. By far the most common is water and electrolyte loss. Sodium, potassium, hydrogen, and chloride are lost readily, creating a metabolic alkalosis. If diarrhea is present, fluid losses can be impressive and deadly, especially in the elderly and infants. Fluid and electrolyte replacement is essential.

Table 6-19-2. Causes of Nausea and Vomiting

Infectious origins	
Abdominal	Appendicitis, cholecystitis, ruptured viscous, glomerulonephritis, colitis, diverticulitis, pancreatitis, AGE
Systemic	Especially in infants and children or elderly Otitis media pneumonia, sinusitis, cellulitis, herpes zoster, PID, prostatitis, epididymitis, meningitis
Hormone-induced	Pregnancy, menses, hypo- or hyperthyroidism, uremia, diabetic ketoacidosis, renal failure, Addison's disease, hypoglycemia
Gastrointestinal sources	Dystonia due to obstruction, ulcers, strictures, hiatal hernia, volvulus, malignancy, hepatitis, cirrhosis, postsurgical syndromes (afferent loop, dumping), gastric retention, decreased gastric motility from medications
Vascular sources	Acute MI, congestive heart failure, abdominal vascular disease (abdominal angina), headaches, hypotension
Esophageal sources	Zenker's diverticulum, malignancy, GERD, achalasia, strictures, ulcer, candidiasis, CMV
Ear to eye to brain	Meniere's disease, otitis media, labyrinthitis, motion sickness, intracranial pressure from tumors, aneurysms, hydrocephalus, or encephalitis.
Medications	See Table 6-19-1

NOTE: AGE = acute gastroenteritis; PID = pelvic inflammatory disease; MI = myocardial infarction; GERD = gastrointestinal reflux disease; CMV = cytomegalovirus.

Table 6-19-3. Treatment of Nausea and Vomiting

Drug	Use	Side effects
Antihistamines Meclizine (Antivert) Hydroxyzine (Vistaril)	Helpful for motion sickness, mild AGE or similar, postoperative nausea. Hydroxyzine good when there is a psychological component to nausea.	Sedation, additive effects with other CNS depressives, rare extrapyramidal symptoms
Phenothiazines Prochlorperazine (Compazine) Thiethylperazine (Torecan) Chlorpromazine (Thorazine) Promethazine (Phenergan)	Control of severe nausea, postoperative nausea, used commonly after radiation and chemotherapy.	Sedation, interaction with other CNS depressives, extrapyramidal symptoms, blood dyscrasias
Selective 5-HT$_3$ receptor antagonist Ondansetron (Zofran)	Control of severe nausea from chemotherapy and prevention of postoperative nausea.	Headache, dizziness, musculoskeletal aches
Butyrophenones Droperidol (Inapsine) Haloperidol (Haldol)	Inapsine is used for pre- and postoperative nausea. Haldol is used for nausea associated with anxiety states.	Tardive dyskinesia, neuroleptic malignant syndrome, hypotension
Prokinetics Metoclopramide (Reglan) Cisapride (Propulsid)	Increases lower esophageal sphincter tone and promotes gastric emptying. Used widely for many types of nausea.	Extrapyramidal symptoms (Reglan); Arrhythmias (Propulsid)
Benzquinamide (Emete-Con)	Used in patients who do not tolerate the phenothiazines for postsurgical nausea or chemotherapy.	Low side-effect profile; drowsiness most common
Treat underlying cause Dehydration Tube decompression for obstruction (NGT or rectal tube) Adrenal crisis— hydrocortisone Drug-induced: reduce or stop drug	Oral or IV fluid replacement with electrolytes.	

NOTE: AGE = acute gastroenteritis; NGT = nasogastric tube.

PEARLS

Pay close attention to the timing of the nausea and vomiting. AGE nausea and vomiting occurs every 1 to 2 h on average but usually subsides within 6 to 8 h and requires fluid replacement only. Do not medicate unless necessary. On the other hand if it is known that an essential medication like chemotherapy or morphine will be used, premedicate with an antiemetic to avoid undue hardship on the patient. Remember to treat the underlying condition.

BIBLIOGRAPHY

"Nausea and Vomiting," Health Information (Internet). HTLM< 1996, Orbis-AHCN.

"Nausea and Vomiting," National Cancer Institute, No. 208-04466 (Internet). University of Bonn Medical Center, June 1996.

Chapter 6–20
PANCREATIC DISEASE
Anne P. Heinly

ANATOMY

Not many providers have concluded a visit with, "Oh, it's just your pancreas," because the pancreas is a rather unassuming but vital gastrointestinal organ. Considered a retroperitoneal organ, the pancreas is about 6 in. long and resembles a long, thin chunk of Roquefort cheese. This friable organ is tucked in snugly under the body of the stomach and sits in the curve of the C loop of the duodenum. (See Fig. 6-20-1.) There is a central duct which connects with the bile duct at the ampulla of Vater, entering the C loop of the duodenum where it dumps its products. Unlike the liver and the spleen, the pancreas does not have an adhesive capsule. The absence of a capsule allows cysts or tumors to grow with relative impunity, at least until they encroach on other abdominal structures.

The importance of the pancreas to normal body function is reflected in its huge blood supply: branches of the celiac, superior mesenteric, gastroduodenal, and splenic arteries all supply the pancreas. The venous drainage is straight to the portal system as part of the continuous feedback loop between the stomach, liver, and intestines. As with most of the gastrointestinal tract, the vagus nerve (cranial nerve X) innervates the pancreas.

PHYSIOLOGY

The pancreas has one basic function, the excretion of hormones or enzymes which deal with the digestion and absorption of nutrients from daily food intake. The primary endocrine function is located within the islets of Langerhans, which secrete insulin, glucagon, pancreatic polypeptides, and somatostatin, which are essential for glucose utilization. (See Chap. 5-1.)

The exocrine side of the pancreas is made up of billions of acinar cells which can bud from tiny ductules, which eventually become larger ducts and join to a central duct. The secretory ducts of the acinar cells contain the centroacinar cells. Between the acinar and centroacinar cells the pancreas secretes between 2 and 3 L of digestive enzymes a day. Table 6-20-1 reviews the different enzymes and their functions in regard to digestion and absorption. Because the cells that produce the enzymes also form the transportation system (most other ducts, like the bile duct, only transport), disease arises when infection, cancer, or medication triggers stimulate the autodigestion of the tissues themselves.

The enzyme secretions are dependent on complex feedback loops involving the stomach, liver, and small intestines. Between meals there is relative pancreatic rest with minimal enzyme secretions that provide for basic cleanup duties. The meal phase is the connection between the brain thinking about food, the nose smelling the food, and the mouth chewing and tasting the food. This "cephalic" phase prepares the bicarbonate brew to be dumped into the duodenum to alkalinize the chyme. The digestion and absorption of food stuffs is best done at a pH of 7 to 8.[1] The mediators appear to be cholecystokinin (CCK) and enkephalins in the stomach and liver.

The intestinal phase begins as the chyme is passed into the duodenum. Secretin secretion apparently turns off the gastrin in the stomach and turns on the pancreatic secretions. The amount of secretions is dependent on the fat content of the chyme. The higher the chyme fat content, the more pancreatic and bile secretions occur. Again, CCK seems to play a major role in this neural and hormonal balancing act. The CCK is then regulated by the very enzyme it has released, trypsin. Intraluminal trypsin turns the CCK production down or off as needed. So the interaction of secretin, volume, fat, bicarbonate secretions, and finally trypsin operate in an intricate pattern to achieve proper digestion and absorption. Disruption of this balance results in malabsorption at the very least and destruction of the pancreas at worst.

LABORATORY TESTS

The serum amylase test is the most frequently performed test. Care must be taken when interpreting an amylase alone. Amylase is not unique to the pancreas; it is found in the mouth, liver, kidneys, and small intestine and may be produced by a variety of carcinomas. Given that, a serum amylase level over 300 U is highly indicative of pancreatic disease. To further localize the pancreas, P isoamylase (specific to the pancreas) remains elevated longer, whereas the total amylase is likely to drop rapidly (within 2 to 5 days). Lipase, has been increasingly relied on for a clear indication of acute pancreatic disease. Lipase levels rise slowly but are maintained on average 7 to 14 days. Conditions that can confuse elevated lipase findings are renal failure, bowel obstruction, bowel necrosis, or perforated ulcer disease.

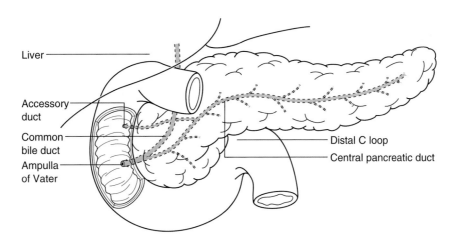

Figure 6-20-1. Pancreatic anatomy.

Table 6-20-1. Pancreatic Enzymes

Amylase	Saliva contains amylase, which starts the digestion of starch and glycogen, and the pancreatic amylase continues the job. The small intestinal brush border enzymes convert the final product to glucose.
Trypsinogen, proteolytic	Attacks the peptide bonds of protein molecules in the duodenum resulting in free amino acids, which are then absorbed by the brush border of the jejunum.
Chymotrypsinogen, proteolytic	Works with trypsinogen to break catalyzed protein bonds.
Proelastase, proteolytic	Cleave specific protein bonds to liberate amino acids.
Procarboxypeptidase A, proteolytic	Continues the protein breakdown at the end of the protein chains resulting in free amino acids.
Procarboxypeptidase B, proteolytic	Continues the protein bond breakdown.
Lipase, lipolytic	Breaks down the triglyceride molecule into 2 fatty acids and a monoglyceride. The presence of bile acids and colipase are essential to the process.
Prophospholipase A_2, lipolytic	Breaks down the fatty acids, leading to the formation of free fatty acids, which are absorbed to the portal circulation
Carboxylesterase lipase, lipolytic	This enzyme can do a little of everything, cleaving cholesterol ester, lipid-soluble vitamins, triglycerides, monoglycerides, and diglycerides. Bile is required for smooth function.
Deoxyribonuclease	Two isozymes which are specific to protein DNA.
Ribonuclease	Up to 5 isozymes which are specific to protein RNA.
Procolipase	The mediator between lipase and bile acids to aid in triglyceride breakdown.
Trypsin inhibitor	A group of 56 amino acids that essentially neutralize trypsin. A protective mechanism from autodigestion

Testing exocrine pancreatic function is usually done to determine the consequence of disease or injury. Persistent nonfunctioning may result in a malabsorption syndrome hypertriglyceridemia, vitamin B_{12} loss, hypercalcemia, ascites, or other condition. (See Chap. 6-18, "Malabsorption.") Direct stimulation of the pancreas is the gold standard to determine function. It analyzes the duodenal contents before and after a challenge of secretin and cholecystokinin. This should cause enzyme production; absence of production indicates widespread, chronic pancreatic disease. See Table 6-20-2 for laboratory findings.

Additional tests include complete blood cell count (CBC) with possibilities of megaloblastic anemia, chronic blood loss anemia, and/or a leukocytosis. Liver function studies and chemistries may reveal a hyperglycemia, hypoproteinemia, hypertriglyceridemia, hypocalcemia, increased blood urea nitrogen (BUN), and creatinine. Blood gases may show hypoxia.

RADIOLOGIC (IMAGING) STUDIES

Plain abdominal films are valuable about half of the time. They may reveal the "sentinel loop," which is a localized ileus involving the jejunum, or a "colon cutoff sign," which is distension of the transverse colon.[2] In chronic pancreatitis, especially with exocrine insufficiency, the plain film may reveal epigastric calcifications.

Quick, easy, and useful diagnostic information can be gained by using ultrasound. It can delineate edema, pseudocysts, masses, and calcifications. Acute pancreatitis usually presents with enlargement and blunting of the shape owing to edema. Cancer distorts the architecture, and a pseudocyst (common to acute or chronic pancreatitis) is a rounded mass with fluid levels. Ultrasound has drawbacks in that the ileus (bowel gas) can obscure findings, as can obesity, pregnancy, or recent barium studies.

Computerized tomograms (CT scan) are helpful in the diagnosis of pancreatic disease. Tumors and pseudocyst show up with contorted structures with or without fluid levels. The endoscopic retrograde cholangiopancreatography (ERCP) utilizes the cannulization of the pancreatic duct. This provides definitive information on stenosis, abscesses, tumor size, location, and biopsy potentials.

Acute Pancreatitis
DISCUSSION

Pancreatitis is an inflammatory disease that is probably grossly underdiagnosed. In the past, especially in the United States, most pancreatitis was thought to be due to alcohol abuse. New studies are finding that infections and drugs induce pancreatitis much more commonly than previously realized. See Table 6-20-3 for the causes of acute pancreatitis. About 1 percent of both men and women have at least one episode of acute pancreatitis.

Table 6-20-2. Laboratory Findings in Pancreatic Disease

Findings	Acute Pancreatitis	Chronic Pancreatitis	Pancreatic Cancer
Amylase	>300; elevated 2–12 h after onset; diminishes over 3–5 days	May be normal or only mildly elevated	Rarely elevated
Lipase	>300; elevated 24–72 h after onset; diminishes slowly	May be normal or only mildly elevated	May be normal to mildy elevated
AST	Up to 15 times normal	Mildly elevated	Mildly elevated
ALT	Usually only minimally effected	Usually only minimally effected	Progressive elevation with hepatic metastasis
Bilirubin	Mild elevation	Mild to moderate elevation due to liver congestion	Progressive elevation
Leukocytosis	15,000–20,000 in most cases; may be lower in the elderly	May be normal	Normal
Hyperglycemia	Less insulin production; usually mild	Glucose intolerance or diabetes may occur	Possible occurrence of glucose intolerance or diabetes
Hypocalcemia	Mild; mechanism unknown	Mild to moderate; changes in the parathyroid secretions	
Alkaline phosphatase	Normal	Mildly elevated	>5 times normal in many cases, but still not specific

NOTE: AST = aspartate aminotransferase; ALT = alanine aminotransferase.

Table 6-20-3. Possible Triggers for Acute Pancreatitis

Gallstones	Bile stasis, bile is essential for lipid breakdown.
Alcohol abuse	Mechanism poorly understood, but there is high correlation to disease.

Medications
  Sulfonamides
  Estrogens
  NSAIDs
  ACE inhibitors
	Most are dose-related, with mild to severe pancreatitis possible. Certainly rare, the mechanism seems to be an interruption of fat digestion and degeneration of liver function as well.

Trauma-surgery	Loss of architecture is secondary to trauma or change in blood supply.
Hyperlipidemias	The breakdown of large amounts of triglycerides seems to cause a cytotoxic level of free fatty acids.
Pregnancy	Most often associated with concomitant gallstones.
Obstruction of the ampulla of Vater	Ductal tumor, choledocholithiasis, Crohn's disease, peptic ulcer disease block secretions.

NOTE: ACE = angiotensin converting enzyme.

PATHOGENESIS

Though still the subject of intense study, the prevailing theory is that the condition of "autodigestion" causes pancreatitis. Trypsin appears to be stimulated inside the pancreas, allowing the other proteolytic enzymes (chymotrypsin, elastase, carboxypeptidase, and phospholipase) to be activated as well. Since these enzymes are designed to break down cell walls, the enzymatic actions literally "eat the hand that feeds them." The result is edema (inflammatory reaction), vascular injury (hemorrhage), and finally tissue loss and necrosis. Additionally, systemic reactions of bradykinin and histamines cause vasodilation not only in the pancreas but in pulmonary tissue, which accounts for the pulmonary edema seen in fulminant acute pancreatitis.

SYMPTOMS

As with all disease, there are classic signs (Virchow's triad); with acute pancreatitis they are midepigastric to left upper quadrant (LUQ) pain, severe nausea and vomiting, and progressive severity. The pain is described as constant, deep, boring pain often with radiation to the back. Patients may avoid laying supine to avoid increased pain. Fever, fatigue, and dizziness may also be noted by patients. The not-so-classic symptoms occur in the elderly. In the elderly the pain may be muted or absent, and there is less nausea and vomiting. This is presumably due to the poor immune response of the aging patient. In the elderly, the presenting symptoms may be a change of mentation, shock, or coma.

OBJECTIVE

The physical examination often finds the patient sitting on the table with knees pulled to the chest, rocking. One of the differentiating signs of severe pancreatitis is that the onset is sudden, so the abdomen is slightly distended and exquisitely tender without peritoneal signs initially, and the stomach is soft and painful. With increasing severity, dehydration and hypotension are evident. With hemorrhagic pancreatitis, a bruising or ecchymosis may develop on the flanks (Turner's sign) or periumbilically (Cullen's sign). A quiet abdomen is indicative of an ileus caused by the inflammation. Pulmonary signs may include pneumonitis (crackles), pleural effusion (rhonchi), or frank respiratory distress.

DIAGNOSTIC CONSIDERATIONS

Any source of an acute abdomen is suspect: appendicitis, cholecystitis, perforated ulcer, perforated diverticulitis, severe acute

gastroenteritis (AGE), or hepatitis. Another consideration of great importance is an abdominal aortic aneurysm (AAA), which can present with exactly the same symptoms with the addition of a pulsating, expanding mass on examination. Bowel and duct obstruction can also masquerade as acute pancreatitis.

TREATMENT

Monitoring is very important. Progression or abatement of disease should be followed by serial vital signs (dehydration) and frequent blood gases or pulse oxygenation measurements (pulmonary complications). Serial chemistries and possibly ECGs should be monitored for electrolyte changes like hypocalcemia, hypokalemia, hyperglycemia, and renal functions. With severe pancreatitis, coagulation profiles should be done because disseminated intravascular coagulation (DIC) is a possibility.

To date there is no definitive treatment for acute pancreatitis. Steroids, H₂ blockers, anticholinergics, glucagon, and antibiotics have been found to be of little or no use in shortening the course of the disease. *Fluid and electrolyte replacement is essential.* Total parenteral nutrition may be an option if the episode lasts more than 5 days and should be accomplished with a multidisciplinary team. (See Chap. 6-15, "Inflammatory Bowel Disease," Table 6-15-4.) In the past a nasogastric tube (NGT) has been placed to obtain full intestinal rest. If nausea and vomiting are controllable, it is not absolutely necessary, but the patient should be kept strictly NPO.

Pain control is the second part of supportive therapy. Traditionally meperidine (Demerol) has been used, but ketorolac (Toradol) is a great alternative to avoid narcotic loads and side effects. Morphine is generally avoided because it may cause ductal spasm.

Antibiotics may be used if an infectious origin is identified, but the vast majority of acute pancreatitis cases are purely inflammatory; therefore there is no rationale for the indiscriminate use of antibiotics. Finally, while supporting the patient look for a treatable etiology like alcohol abuse, gallstones, choledocholithiasis, or Crohn's disease.

Surgical excision of the pancreas is technically challenging and questionably useful. The drainage of large pseudocysts, persistent pain, hematoma, and abscesses are about the only reasons most surgeons attempt the process. Postoperative complications are common, and the mortality rate is high.

COMPLICATIONS

Acute pancreatitis is not a benign process; it kills people. Complications include cardiovascular collapse from hypovolemia or hy-

Table 6-20-4. Ranson-Imrie Criteria

Upon admission	48 h after Admission	Number Criteria
Age over 55 years	Hematocrit drops 10%	0–2 items, 1% mortality rate
White blood count of 16,000	BUN rises >5 mg/dL with adequate hydration	3–4 items, 16% mortality rate
Serum glucose >200 mg/dL	Arterial PO₂ <60 mmHg	5–6 items, 40% mortality rate
Serum LDH >350 IU/L	Serum calcium <8 mg/dL	7–8 items, 100% mortality rate
Serum AST >250 IU/L	Fluid sequestration >4–5 L Serum albumin <3.2 g/dL	

SOURCE: Modified from Isselbacher KJ, Braunwald E, Wilson JD, et al: *Harrison's Principles of Internal Medicine,* 13th ed. New York, McGraw-Hill, 1994, p 1522.
NOTE: LDH = Lactate dehydrogenase; AST = aspartate aminotransferase; BUN = blood urea nitrogen.

poproteinemia and even sudden death. Pulmonary complications are usually evident on examination: pleural effusions, pneumonitis, atelectasis, and in severe disease, adult respiratory distress syndrome. The electrolyte imbalances can cause oliguria and azotemia with progressive renal failure. The pancreatic debris can embolize to the renal artery, brain, or heart. Finally, damage to the pancreas itself can cause diabetes, exocrine insufficiency (with malabsorption), pancreatic pseudocysts, or chronic pancreatitis. Used for years, the Ranson-lmre criteria for prognosis are quite useful (Table 6-20-4).

PATIENT EDUCATION

Since alcohol abuse is still the number one trigger for acute pancreatitis, it is a good idea to recommend limited alcohol use to all patients. Other than that, there is really no preventive education available for patients. After acute pancreatitis, the patient should be instructed to avoid all alcohol use. Diet should be tailored to the residual function of the pancreas. Fortunately, a patient can lose up to 90 percent function before nutrition is severely affected. Most patients do well on a low-fat diet (usually less than 40 g/day) with moderate amounts of carbohydrates and proteins. The diet may need to address diabetic needs as well. Reoccurrence is common, and severity is generally progressive.

PEARLS

Acute pancreatitis is a wait-and-watch process. It is important to be clinically alert to progression of the disease. Pseudocyst can enlarge, hemorrhage can progress, and bacterial infection can ensue. Monitor and support the patient. The average hospital stay for most patients is 7 days, so be patient and vigilant.

Chronic Pancreatitis

DISCUSSION

About 10 percent of patients with acute pancreatitis will progress to the chronic phase. It is not clear whether the patient has a series of acute episodes that progressively destroys tissue or there is a continuous loss of tissue without significant inflammation. The end result is the same: the incremental loss of pancreatic architecture leads to exocrine insufficiency and diabetes.

SYMPTOMS

Chronic pancreatitis can present as acute but most commonly does not. It often presents with insidious deep pain, steatorrhea (reflecting malabsorption) and insulin-dependent diabetes mellitus. Weight loss owing to malabsorption and jaundice owing to hepatic complications may be evident. Pulmonary symptoms may or may not be present.

OBJECTIVE

Physical examination may reveal a thinning patient with mild jaundice. Mild epigastric or even diffuse abdominal tenderness without distention is the most common finding. Vitamin deficiency anemia is rarely found.

DIAGNOSTIC CONSIDERATIONS

Diagnostic considerations are the same as for acute pancreatitis.

TREATMENT

Pain and malabsorption are the focus. Pain can be diminished by strict restriction of alcohol products and in some cases a low-fat diet. Some patients may require narcotics for pain control,

which can lead to addiction. Adequate enzyme replacement may diminish the pain syndrome. When all medical therapies are not sufficient to control pain, surgery is considered. But as a surgeon once said, "The pancreas is a skunk you don't want to poke." Surgery is the last resort.

Most chronic pancreatitis patients need enzyme replacement for exocrine dysfunction. Viokase, Cotazym-S or a similar substance can be used to try to address the malabsorption. Unfortunately, it is difficult to deliver the active enzyme intact to the duodenum at the perfect time. Therefore, the dosing is large and frequent (Table 6-20-5).

COMPLICATIONS

The long-term life expectancy of the chronic pancreatitis patient is limited; if alcohol is continued, death is likely in 5 to 15 years after diagnosis. As pancreatic dysfunction progresses, the manifestations and complications of malabsorption become more apparent with weight loss and vitamin deficiencies.

PATIENT EDUCATION

Same as "Acute Pancreatitis."

PEARLS

Chronic pancreatitis is also a watching and waiting game. Monitor the nutritional status of the patient. A chemistry profile should be examined for changes in glucose, calcium, magnesium, potassium, and proteins. Adjust diet and supplements to meet the needs of each patient. Involve a multidisciplinary team to ensure maximum results for the patient. Given proper care and alcohol abstinence, these patients can live a long life.

Pancreatic Cancer

DISCUSSION

About 0.001 percent of the U.S. population is diagnosed with pancreatic cancer each year. Only 2 percent of those patients are likely to survive more than 5 years. Pancreatic cancer is called "the silent cancer" because it is seldom found early. Recognized as the fifth most common cancer killer in the United States, black men seem to have the highest risk, but men in general have pancreatic cancer with a 2 : 1 ratio over women.[1] The aged are the most likely to develop cancer, but pancreatic cancer may occur at any age (See Chap. 13-8.)

PATHOGENESIS

Adenocarcinoma of the pancreas has no proven etiologies. There appears to be an increased risk with tobacco smoking and/or heavy beer consumption, but no specific triggers have been identified. Gallbladder disease and acute or chronic pancreatitis does not appear to predispose to pancreatic cancer. The vast majority of cancers arise from the exocrine tissue (ductal system), and symptoms are dictated by the location of the tumor. Periampullary lesions encroach into the common bile duct, duodenum, and liver. The tumors arising in the body or tail of the pancreas are usually found later because encroachment causes less trouble initially. The absence of an adhesive capsule allows the tumors to enlarge unchecked with minimal symptoms. The rich lymphatics and blood supply of the region disseminate the cancer before a patient is aware of the tumor.

SYMPTOMS

A slow and insidious presentation is the usual for pancreatic cancer. Weight loss is common and a dull aching pain may be

Table 6-20-5. Treatment of Pancreatic Enzyme Deficiency

Preparation	Lipase	Trypsin	Proteolytic Activity	Amylase	Dose
Cotazym	8000 U	0	30,000	30,000 U	1–3 tablets prior to each meal or snack
Arco-Lase	25 mg	38 mg	6 g	30 mg	1 tablet with or immediately after meals
Donnazyme	1000 U	0	12,500 U	12,500 U	2 tablets with meals and snacks
Kutrase or Ku-zyme	1200 U	0	6 mg	30 mg	1–2 tablets with meals and snacks
Viokase	8000 U	0	30,000 U	30,000 U	1–2 tablets with meals and snacks or every 2 h after pancreatectomy

noted in the epigastrium or left upper quadrant. The patient may believe it is a muscle pull. With tumors in the body or tail, the nerves of the retroperitoneal areas are invaded and the pain may become much more severe. Patients may complain of a vague nausea and persistent anorexia. With tumors near the ampulla of Vater, painless jaundice may be the presenting symptom with pruritus, nausea, and perhaps vomiting. Though rare in an adult patient, the development of insulin-dependent diabetes mellitus may signal early pancreatic cancer.

OBJECTIVE

The physical examination is usually negative initially. With metastasis of the carcinoma, weight loss with muscle wasting is evident. Jaundice and hepatomegaly are common findings. Evidence of malnutrition may be present: pale (anemia); nail bed changes (vitamin deficiency); and fractures (metastasis and calcium changes).

DIAGNOSTIC CONSIDERATIONS

Pancreatic cancer can masquerade as almost any abdominal complaint. In fact, valuable time is often lost looking for gallstones, ulcers, or malabsorption syndromes in these patients. Still worse, most patients may have gallbladder disease or peptic ulcer disease concomitantly, and the clinician may stop investigations with the presumed diagnosis. The most significant clue is weight loss and malnutrition. Malnutrition syndromes are almost always accompanied by diarrhea with steatorrhea. Significant weight loss is cancer until proved otherwise. Gallbladder, Crohn's, and similar diseases do not usually involve major weight loss.

LABORATORY

The most important test to be done is a biopsy. A tissue biopsy can be obtained by endoscopic retrograde cholangiopancreatography (ERCP) or by exploratory surgery. The importance comes from the possibilities of nonmalignant ductal tumors and chronic pancreatitis. Both can present as hard masses in the pancreatic area with similar symptoms. Obviously, the treatment and prognosis are quite different.

TREATMENT

Treatment is unfortunately limited to palliative care in the vast majority of patients. Surgery (Whipple's procedure) is an option for only about 10 percent of patients, and the life expectancy beyond 5 years is very poor.[2] Treatment is aimed at quality of life—for the approximately 5 months the majority of patients have left, the provider should make every effort to keep the patient comfortable, awake, and functional. As with all terminal diagnoses, the inclusion of a hospice team can be a great help to patient and family.

Chemotherapy with 5-fluorouracil (5-FU) and radiation therapy can shrink the tumor size and provide symptomatic relief of ductal obstruction and jaundice. Morphine or its adjuncts should be titrated to maximum pain relief with minimal sedation effects. The morphine should not be limited for fear of respiratory compromise or addiction. Neither occur in the vast majority of patients. Patient will need nutritional support and nausea and constipation control as well.

PATIENT EDUCATION

It is important to be honest. Pancreatic cancer (with rare exception) is a grave, terminal diagnosis. The patient and family should be educated on expectations and what can be done to make the patient comfortable. One item of specific concern to most families is the ability of the patient to eat. Pancreatic cancer causes profound anorexia. Additionally, as the carcinoma progresses the ability of the body to process and absorb nutrition slows and eventually stops. Families must be educated about the process so they will not become petulant with a sick family member for not eating.

PEARLS

Diagnosis of pancreatic cancer is very difficult. It is an index of suspicion that leads to early diagnosis. Once diagnosed, be cognizant of the needs of the patient and family. Support and manage symptoms to provide the best quality of life for the patient.

REFERENCES

1. Sleisenger MH, Fordtran JS: *Gastrointestinal Disease.* Philadelphia, Saunders, 1993, vol 2, pp 1585, 1682.
2. Isselbacher KJ, Braunwald E, Wilson JD, et al: *Harrison's Principles of Internal Medicine,* 13th ed. New York, McGraw-Hill, 1994, pp 1519, 1533.

BIBLIOGRAPHY

"Pancreatic Cancer." (Internet). National Cancer Institutes Cancer Information Service, 208/00046. www.graylab.ac.uk/cancernet/20046.htm 4

Chapter 6–21
PEPTIC ULCER DISEASE
Anne P. Heinly

DESCRIPTION

Peptic ulcer disease (PUD) encompasses diagnoses of gastritis, duodenitis, and gastric and duodenal ulcers. Zollinger-Ellison (ZE) syndrome is included under the PUD umbrella, although its etiology is quite different from that of the average PUD. It is estimated that 2 of 10 adults have peptic ulcer disease at some point in their life. PUD is rare before age 6 and becomes apparent in many people in their twenties. In some countries the estimate is near 100 percent in the elderly. Men are more likely to have episodes of PUD, but it is by no means a sex-specific problem. A previously recurrent disease that was poorly understood, PUD may be well on its way out the door as a chronic illness. The reason is the discovery of *Helicobacter pylori* and its impact on the gastric and duodenal areas of the GI tract.

PATHOGENESIS

Gastric physiology has everything to do with peptic ulcer disease. The stomach has several jobs: mixing and churning foods into a chyme; secretion of pepsinogen, which becomes pepsin and initiates protein digestion; secretion of HCl and an intrinsic factor, essential for B_{12} absorption; and secretion of gastrin, which helps regulate stomach, hepatic, and pancreatic enzymes and lowers pyloric, Oddi, and ileocecal sphincter pressures.

The parietal cells of the stomach secrete up to 2 quarts of hydrochloric acid a day. The physiologic triggers are a complex set of chemical, neural, and hormonal factors that participate in feedback loops to turn acid production on and off. The hormone gastrin stimulates the HCl production triggered by thoughts of food, smells, ingestion of food, ingestion of calcium, alcohol use, and medications.

The stomach's defense against the excess HCl and the corrosive effect of even normal levels of acid is impressive. A pH level below 1.5 turns the HCl production off. Feedback from secretin, cholecystokinin, or glucagon can shut HCl production down. The mucous-producing cells protect the gastric mucosa and prevent back-diffusion of the HCl. Bicarbonate ions in the "unstirred" water layer, a gel-like line separating parietal cells and mucous cells, provides an alkaline environment perfect for healing. Prostaglandin, which is abundant throughout the gastrium, protects the cells and promotes good blood flow that engenders rapid healing when needed.

Given all this physiology, providers used to look for exogenous stimulation to upset the natural balance of the gastric environment (Table 6-21-1). Although all these are players, *H. pylori* seems to be a key factor for recurrent ulcer disease (in the absence of NSAIDs use or ZE). *Helicobacter pylori* is an S-shaped bacterium which finds a home between the cells under the stable layer of mucus in the antrum of the stomach. It is currently estimated that this bacterium is responsible for up to 90 percent of all PUD and is found worldwide. How people are infected with *H. pylori* is still debated, but it is thought to be waterborne. To date, reinfection is rare, so treatment of *H. pylori* is considered curative in the vast majority of patients. *Helicobacter pylori* is thought to cause gastritis or ulcers by producing an urease that causes deterioration of the protective barriers of the mucous layer. Since many people are infected with *H. pylori* and do not have PUD, more research is required to get the complete picture on this organism.

SYMPTOMS

The classic symptom of PUD is a deep, gnawing, or burning epigastric pain 1 to 3 h after meals (empty stomach) with nocturnal awakenings. Typically this pain is relieved by food intake and antacids. Some patients may not complain of pain, but a careful diet history may reveal that they nibble to the point that their stomach is never empty, providing a buffer to excess acid. The pain may radiate to the back, "straight through me" or may be

Table 6-21-1. Causes of Peptic Ulcer Disease

Triggers for PUD	Mechanism
Helicobacter pylori	Bacterium hidden in the gastric mucosal layer; urease secretion causes chronic inflammation and ulcerations.
Medication	
Alcohol	Damages the mucous lining and interferes with healing mechanisms.
Aspirin or NSAIDs	Antiprostaglandins; damage to mucous lining and disruption of blood supply occurs.
Tolazoline	Stimulates gastric secretion and stress ulcers in children treated for pulmonary hypertension.
Corticosteroids	The mechanism is poorly understood; probably a feedback interruption.
Tobacco	Decreases pancreatic bicarbonate secretion (feedback loop) and mucosal blood flow hampering healing. Inhibits the actions of H_2 blockers.
Stress ulcers	
Burns (Curling's ulcer)	Stress ulcers can occur within hours to days of severe trauma or burns and are most likely due to an ischemic phenomenon. As blood is shunted to damaged area or lost, gastric protection mechanisms are retarded and feedback loops are interrupted. Prophylactic therapy should be undertaken to avoid complications.
Intracranial trauma	
Shock	
Hypoglycemia	
Dehydration	
Renal failure	
Vasculitis	
Disease	
Cystic fibrosis	Any disease process that changes the feedback mechanism of acid secretion, blood supply, or mucous layer integrity could cause PUD.
Gastrinoma (ZE)	
Type 1 MENS	
COPD	
Cirrhosis	
Polycythemia	

NOTE: MENS = multiple endocrine neoplasia syndrome; COPD = chronic obstructive pulmonary disease.

simply described as an "acid stomach." Many patients have already self-treated with over-the-counter antacids and H_2 blockers, so symptoms may be dulled.

Nausea with or without vomiting is also a common symptom, especially with severe pain. If occult bleeding is occurring with "itis" or ulceration, the patient may present with or without pain in an orthostatic state. Patients complain of dizziness, thirst, syncope and/or melenic stools. It takes 50 mL of blood to make a melenic stool, so several stools usually represent a hemoglobin drop of 2 to 4 points.

The symptoms may wax and wane, with several pain episodes over a short period of time followed by long periods of remission. Patients with PUD often have concomitant histories consistent with gastroesophageal reflux disease (GERD, Chap. 6-11) as well. Symptoms of concern, especially in the young or the elderly, include weight loss, anorexia, early satiety, nausea, and vomiting or regurgitation. These symptoms suggest an obstruction due to stricture formation, gastric outlet syndrome, or carcinoma and merit immediate workup.

OBJECTIVE

The physical examination may reveal point tenderness in the epigastric to right upper quadrant (RUQ) area in adults. With children the pain may present periumbilically or be poorly localized. If the patient has eaten recently, this may be muted. There is no guarding, peritoneal signs, ascites, or percussion changes unless a perforation has occurred. If bleeding has occurred, the patient may have positive orthostatic signs, evidence of dehydration, or in the worse case, stupor or loss of consciousness. The elderly can present without pain with a change in sensorium or frank shock. A rectal examination with an occult blood examination should be done. Absence of blood in the stool does not preclude PUD or bleeding.

DIAGNOSTIC CONSIDERATIONS

Table 6-21-2 reviews the differential diagnosis for PUD. Zollinger-Ellison syndrome is caused by a hypersecretion state in the presence of gastrinomas with a marked increase in severity and recurrence of symptoms. In children ulcers may present as chronic abdominal pain or gastric outlet syndrome. With outlet syndrome a gastric succession splash may be found. Congenital pyloric stenosis is generally identified in early infancy as a mass in the RUQ and should not be confused with PUD. Whereas nearly 70 percent of older Americans are likely to have *H. pylori* present, the most common etiology of ulcers is the use of nonsteroidal anti-inflammatory medications because of their antiprostaglandin effects. In the elderly, as with so many diseases, the symptoms may be muted or absent due to aging changes. Orthostatic changes from blood loss may be the first signal of trouble.

LABORATORY TESTS

There are those who still propound the use of imaging studies first in the diagnosis of PUD. But, with time, the hunt for *H. pylori* will probably become the most valuable method. There are three ways to potentially identify *H. pylori* in the laboratory. The *H. pylori* serum titer searches for immunoglobulin G antibodies to its antigen and is considered a fairly sensitive test. The second is the breath test for urease response using C-labeled urea. The sensitivity of the breath test is still under debate, but with time this may become a mainstay. The final laboratory test involves *H. pylori* cultures obtained during endoscopic evaluation. One would think a culture would be the gold standard, but

H. pylori is a finicky organism and is not easily cultured. As the cost and convenience of the serum and breath tests decrease, they will probably become the first diagnostic tool.

Additionally, a complete blood count and chemistries should be run to rule out PUD-induced anemia and other differential diagnoses. Hemocult cards should be done on three separate occasions to rule out occult bleeding. Since duodenitis or an ulcer may bleed intermittently, stools may not be consistently positive. A negative guaiac does not preclude PUD. When ZE is suspected because of severity or reoccurrence, a serum gastrin level (usually over 500 pg/mL) and secretin stimulation test can be done.

RADIOLOGIC (IMAGING) STUDIES

Certainly a mainstay for years, the upper gastrointestinal (UGI) series with small bowel follow-through can be used to diagnose PUD. The barium study can potentially identify ulcer craters, webs, hiatal hernia, strictures, incompetent sphincters, masses, and contour changes. The distinction between duodenitis or gastritis and ulcer craters is harder to see because GI contour is not as drastically affected. This probably accounts for the almost one-third of false-negatives reported with UGIs in the presence of classic symptoms. On the flip side, those who appear to have an identifiable lesion on UGI often have negative endoscopic results because of the mobile and foldable nature of the intestinal tissue itself.

The most definitive diagnosis for PUD and ZE is the endoscopic evaluation. Despite being an invasive test, it does allow direct visualization of all the tissue, permits biopsies and cultures, and provides therapeutic opportunities in the case of bleeding. In the presence of severe symptoms that are marginally responsive to medications, endoscopic evaluation may be considered a first-line diagnostic procedure, especially if ZE or cancer is suspected.

TREATMENT

As with all diseases, treatment is tailored to etiology. For a stressed-out smoker, lifestyle changes may be all that is required. If *H. pylori* is the culprit, a strict medication regimen should do the trick. If the PUD is NSAID-induced, medications are used to heal and prevent future ulcers. Table 6-21-3 reviews treatment plans in detail. Keep in mind that it may be necessary to address more than one etiology in most patients.

COMPLICATIONS

By far the most common complication of PUD is bleeding. Up to one-fourth of PUD patients have occult blood loss, and about 10 percent have frank bleeding episodes. This can be life-threatening in the very young and the old because of dehydration and organ perfusion problems. Perforation occurs in about 5 percent of patients and presents as a typical acute abdomen with peritoneal signs. Remember, in the elderly, the only "typical" sign may be change in sensorium—keep that index of suspicion. Duodenal scarring and gastric outlet syndrome may occur, especially with the diagnosis of ZE, which is seen in men more than women. Finally, chronic gastric irritation can lead to atrophic changes of the gastrum, predisposing the patient to gastric carcinoma. Research is slowly making the link between chronic *H. pylori* infections and gastric cancer, especially in Asia where gastric carcinomas are quite common. Gastric lymphoma may also be a result of chronic *H. pylori* infection; thus the lesson learned is eradicate *H. pylori* when possible.

PEARLS

Like GERD, peptic ulcer disease is (1) common and (2) self-treated with over-the-counter medications. Inadequate dosing for

Table 6-21-2. Differential Diagnosis of PUD

Gastric carcinoma	Weight loss, early satiety, persistance of pain despite food or medication, anemia.
Pancreatitis	Usually associated with alcohol, severe epigastric to LUQ pain, radiating to or from the back, fever, chills, elevated amylase and lipase.
Gallbladder disease	Episodic, colicky pain in the RUQ to epigastrium with radiation to the right shoulder, worse with fatty meals, not relieved with antacids.
Abdominal angina (mesenteric insufficiency)	Severe, debilitating epigastric or umbilical pain 5–15 minutes after meals. Patient will starve rather suffer the pain. Weight loss, bleeding are common; seen in the elderly.
Acute gastroenteritis	Sudden onset of nausea, vomiting, often associated with diarrhea, fever, chills, and aches; short-lived, not recurrent.
Corrosive ingestion (accidental in children or suicidal)	Ingestion of strong alkali or acids, sudden onset, burns to lips, mouth, pharynx; epigastric pain with vomiting and hematemesis.
Liver disease	Constant deep RUQ and right chest pain, jaundice, ascites; may have evidence of right heart failure.

NOTE: LUQ = left upper quadrant; RUQ = right upper quadrant.

Table 6-21-3. Treatment Regimens for PUD

Regimen	Dose	Side Effects
Lifestyle changes		
Stop tobacco use	These are outstanding recommendations for any patient.	None known.
Stop alcohol use		
Low-fat diet		
Avoid stress		
Avoid offending medications		
Helicobacter therapy	Taken concurrently (approximately 90% cure rate)	
Bismuth compound	2 tablets qid for 14 days	Allergies, drug resistance, diarrhea, pseudomembranous colitis, noncompliance.
Metronidazole (Flagyl)	250 mg tid for 14 days	
Tetracycline or amoxicillin	500 mg tid for 14 days	
H$_2$ blocker or omeprazole may be used for control of symptoms		
or		
Omeprazole	Taken concurrently (approximately 80% cure rate)	As above.
Clarithromycin	20 mg bid for 14 days	
	500 mg tid for 14 days	
Relief therapy	To heal an ulcer	Side effects
Antacids (representative)		
Mylanta	2 tbsp qid for 6 weeks	Diarrhea and/or constipation, noncompliance.
Maalox	2 tbsp qid for 6 weeks	
Riopan	2 tbsp qid for 6 weeks	
Avoid calcium products, owing to rebound hyper-acidity		
H$_2$ blockers		Cimetidine has the most warnings with drug interactions. It may also cause disorientation in the elderly.
Ranitidine (Zantac)	150 mg bid for 12 weeks	
Cimetidine (Tagamet)	200 mg qid for 12 weeks	
Famotidine (Pepcid)	20 mg bid for 8 weeks	
Nizatidine (Axid)	150 mg bid for 12 weeks	
Cytoprotective		
Sucralfate (Carafate)	1 g 30 min before meals and at bedtime	Won't work in the presence of concomitant H$_2$ blockers; it needs an acid environment to work; constipation.
Misoprostol (Cytotec) (not a first-line medication)	100 μg qid with food to start, may increase to 200 μg as tolerated.	Diarrhea, dehydration, use with care in the elderly.
Proton pump inhibitor		
Omeprazole (Prilosec)	20 mg qd for 4–8 weeks	Prolong elimination of phenytoin, warfarin and diazepam. Suppression of B$_{12}$ mechanism; megaloblastic anemia with long-term use.

healing purposes and the likelihood of muted symptoms leading to a chronic problem that goes undetected for years is a concern. The provider's job is to educate patients about ulcer disease and specifically about *H. pylori.* With full treatment many patients will never spend money on antacids again, and the serious consequences of under-treated disease are eradicated. Lifestyle changes remain important, so help patients stop smoking, encourage proper diet and exercise, and avoid ulcer-inducing medications when possible.

BIBLIOGRAPHY

Textbooks

Fauci AS, Braunwald E, Isselbacher KJ, et al: Peptic ulcer and gastritis, in *Harrison's Principles of Internal Medicine,* 14th ed. New York, McGraw-Hill, 1998, pp 1596–1616.
Sleisenger MH, Fordtran JS: Gastric, duodenal, and stress ulcer, in *Gastrointestinal Disease,* 5th ed. Philadelphia, Saunders, 1993, pp 580–652.
Young, Renee L: *Peptic Ulcer Disease: What's New.* Lecture handout, UNMC, Omaha, NE, 1996.

Internet Selections

Dyspepsia/peptic ulcer disease, in "Family Practice Handbook," 1996. chap 4, indy.radiology.uiowa.edu.
Focus on peptic ulcer disease, in "Medical Sciences Bulletin," 1996. pharminfo.com/pubs/msb/peptic.html.
Helicobacter pylori in peptic ulcer disease, "National Institutes of Health Consensus Development Conference Statement," 1994. text.nlm.nih.gov/nih/cdc/www/94txt.html.
Peptic ulcer disease, in "PEDBASE," 1996. icondata.com/health/pedbase/files/pepticul.html.

Chapter 6–22
PILONIDAL DISEASE
Pat C. H. Jan

DISCUSSION

Pilonidal disease is caused by epithelial tissues trapped in the natal cleft. It was once thought to have congenital origin but is currently regarded as an acquired lesion. Young adults have the highest incidence of occurrence, with prevalence in males over females and a peak age of 30 years. Patients with a tendency toward hirsutism are predisposed to pilonidal cysts.

PATHOGENESIS

Pilonidal cysts and abscesses are caused by infections of the hair follicles in the natal cleft. The hair which normally grows at a 90° angle comes out at 100°. The epidermis forms a tunnel-like structure about the hair follicle. There is an increased chance of cyst formation and infection with elongated tunnels. In addition, midline follicles become obstructed by keratin or hair, which leads to a foreign-body reaction. The patient subsequently develops an abscess which can spontaneously drain in the acute case with no further recurrence. Recurrence, however, is extremely common if the hair acting as a foreign body is not removed.

SIGNS AND SYMPTOMS

Patients generally present with pain in the affected areas in acute cases. In chronic states, patients may complain of drainage from the gluteal area. In cases of pilonidal abscess, patients may relate a history of chronic "boils." As mentioned above, the abscess may spontaneously drain.

OBJECTIVE FINDINGS

Physical examination may reveal multiple midline sinus at the natal cleft with tufts of hair from each sinus. If an abscess is present, the area is generally indurated with mild to severe erythema in the surrounding subcutaneous tissue. There is tenderness to palpation. (See Fig. 6-22-1.)

DIAGNOSTIC CONSIDERATIONS

Identifying pilonidal disease is straightforward and can be determined by history and physical examination alone. Gluteal abscess of other origin can easily be ruled out by identification of a pilonidal sinus and tufts of hair. Other diseases which may appear similar to pilonidal disease are hidradenitis suppurativa, infection of the sweat glands; perianal abscess located close to the anus, which should be differentiated from pilonidal abscess; and furuncle, which is an infection of a single hair follicle leading to a pustule and simply requires drainage and antibiotics.

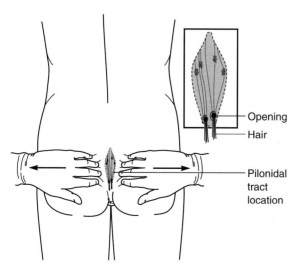

Figure 6-22-1. Pilonidal sinus tract.

TREATMENT

Medical Management

The most current management of noninfected pilonidal disease is focused on good personal hygiene with weekly shaving of all hairs in the sinus. It is believed that by removing the hairs in the sinus tracts, a foreign body reaction is prevented. In acute pilonidal abscess, incision and drainage are the current mainstays of treatment. Once the infection has subsided, the patient may undergo elective excision of the pilonidal sinus for a more definitive treatment.

Surgical Management

To prevent an acute pilonidal abscess from becoming a chronic infection, excision of the offending sinus needs to be performed. Two treatment options are available. This first technique consists of excision and primary closure of the sinus tract. This is performed under general anesthesia, and the patient is given a broad-spectrum antibiotic. The sinus tract is excised down to the fascia layer. Another technique is to marsupialize the wound. Marsupialization requires excision of the offending tissues down to the epithelized tract of the lowest hair follicle. Skin edges on either side are then sutured to the epithelized tract instead of the fascia. The open area is then cleaned daily. Another technique seldom used today but worth mentioning is healing by secondary intention. The patient requires frequent dressing changes and close monitoring for any signs of potential infection. Good personal hygiene is the key.

PATIENT EDUCATION

Recurrence is common and can be minimized by remembering a few principles. First, personal hygiene and shaving of all hairs in the gluteal folds helps to decrease the foreign-body reaction caused by the hairs. Second, good postoperative care by keeping the wound clean and dry helps to facilitate wound healing. Last, prevention of constipation decreases straining and decreases pressure to the surgical wound.

DISPOSITION

Postoperative care is extremely important, and patients should be seen weekly until the wound is completely healed. There is always a possibility of poor wound healing and occurrence of drainage, with local infection leading to more sinus tracts. Therefore any drainage or signs of infection (i.e., swelling, erythema, or increased pain) should be reported. Care should be taken to avoid chronic wetness by the overuse of topical ointments.

COMPLICATIONS AND RED FLAGS

The most common complication of pilonidal disease is the development of an abscess with further damage of the surrounding tissue secondary to inflammation. As mentioned, early recognition leads to early treatment with minimal postoperative care and recurrence.

NOTES AND PEARLS

There is no current universal treatment protocol for pilonidal disease. Recommendations are aimed at good personal hygiene and weekly shaving of hairs in the sinus tract. Marsupialization has the advantage of a rapid postoperative recovery. After multiple recurrences, frustration leads to wide excisions with closure by secondary intention. The drawback is constant monitoring of wound for drainage and infection.

BIBLIOGRAPHY

Armstrong JH: Pilonidal sinus disease: The conservative approach. *Arch Surg* 129:914–918, 1994.
Jones DJ: Pilonidal sinus. *Brit Med J* 305:410–412, 1992.
Surreal JA: Pilonidal disease. *Surg Clin North Am* 74(6):1309–1315, 1994.

Chapter 6–23
PROCTITIS

Marquitha S. Mayfield

Table 6-23-1. Differential Diagnoses of Proctitis

Infectious etiology
Sexually transmitted disease
Gonorrhea
Herpes simplex
Chlamydia
Syphilis
Condyloma acuminata
Other
Shigellosis
Campylobacter
Amebiasis
Noninfectious etiology
Inflammatory bowel disease
Ulcerative colitis
Crohn's disease
Other
Trauma
Radiation therapy
Chemical irritants
Ischemic bowel

DISCUSSION

Proctitis is a nonspecific term used to describe a variety of inflammatory diseases involving the rectal portion of the colon. Most of these diseases have an infectious etiology. Other causes include trauma, radiation therapy of the pelvis, and irritative rectal medications. Ulcerative colitis can also present with strictly rectal involvement as an inflammatory proctitis in some patients. About 90 percent of these cases never advance beyond the rectum. There is a high incidence of proctitis associated with sexually transmitted disease (STD), particularly in adult, homosexual males with multiple sexual partners.

Proctitis may manifest as an acute or chronic inflammatory process and affects 10 to 30 per 100,000 patients in the United States. Adult males are more commonly affected than females.

SYMPTOMS

Symptoms vary depending on the etiology and may range from none to severe anorectal pain, bleeding, tenesmus, and/or mucopurulent anal discharge. Some common symptoms associated with specific disorders include:

* *Gonococcal and Chlamydia proctitis* Mucopurulent rectal discharge associated with anal discomfort.
* *Syphilitic proctitis* Mucopurulent discharge initially, tenesmus and transient nontender perianal ulcer(s).
* *Herpes simplex proctitis* Severe rectal pain, tenesmus associated with constipation, and draining rectal ulcers. Additionally, if the sacral nerve roots are involved, paresthesias of the buttocks and lower extremity bladder dysfunction, and impotence may also occur.
* *Amebiasis, Campylobacter, or Shigellosis proctitis* Diarrhea is the hallmark symptom. Fever, rectal bleeding, and abdominal pain may also occur.
* *Inflammatory proctitis* Bloody diarrhea, tenesmus, and rectal pain occur. Patients with Crohn's disease or ulcerative colitis may also present with fever, malaise, abdominal pain, arthralgias, skin rash, and/or weight loss.
* *Radiation proctitis* Rectal pain, tenesmus, diarrhea, and rectal bleeding or discharge are present.

OBJECTIVE FINDINGS

Physical examination findings also vary according to etiology, stage of disease, and severity of inflammatory response. Unless the anus is involved, few physical examination findings may be noted. Nevertheless, anal skin should be examined for ulcerations, erythema, and other inflammatory changes, nodules, vesic-

ular lesions, condyloma, fissures, fistulas, patches of psoriasis with secondary IBD, hemorrhoids, and/or discharge. A digital rectal examination may elicit tenderness and/or palpable nodules. Stool should be checked for occult blood loss. Classic findings for specific disorders include the following:

* *Herpes proctitis* Perianal vesicular lesions that later ulcerate and become secondarily infected.
* *Inflammatory bowel disease (Crohn's disease) and radiation therapy* Perianal, fistulous tracts, perirectal abscesses. Anal skin tags noted on examination have a strong association with Crohn's disease.
* *Gonorrhea and Chlamydia* Mucopurulent anal discharge.
* *Syphilis* Mucopurulent anal discharge, nontender, indurated ulcers (chancres).
* *Amebiasis, Campylobacter, or Shigellosis proctitis* Possible fever, abdominal tenderness or distension, positive occult blood in stools.

DIFFERENTIAL DIAGNOSIS

Because many cases of proctitis are caused by STD, a detailed sexual history should be obtained to help establish a working differential diagnosis. Most cases of proctitis caused by STD are seen in patients engaging in receptive anal intercourse. Also common in this group is an allergic proctitis caused by chemical irritants in enemas or anal lubricants. Additionally, trauma from rectal intercourse can result in anorectal tears and fissures which can become secondarily infected. The differential diagnosis for the etiology of proctitis is included in Table 6-23-1. The most common pathogens isolated by laboratory studies are *Neisseria gonorrhea*, *Chlamydia* species, and herpes simplex virus.

SPECIAL CONSIDERATIONS

Proctitis in pediatrics is rare. When it does occur, the disease can have a fulminant course with extension to the sigmoid and more proximal areas of the colon. Consider sexual abuse in any child with STD-related proctitis. Geriatric patients with severe proctitis should be evaluated for ischemic bowel.

LABORATORY AND RADIOLOGIC TESTS

Anoscopy in the office is an effective screening tool. The provider can visualize the anorectal vault for signs of inflammation and obtain specimens of any discharge. Sigmoidoscopy is indicated in any patient with rectal bleeding, fistula, fissures, or diarrhea.

The rectal mucosa in proctitis appears friable and inflamed, and ulcers may be noted. The architecture of the rectal crypts may also be disrupted. In 15 percent of cases, inflammatory changes may extend beyond the rectal vault to involve the sigmoid colon and/or anus.

Additional laboratory studies help determine the etiology of proctitis and include viral cultures of vesicular lesions to detect herpes simplex, biopsy of anorectal nodules or ulcers to rule out occult malignancy, and tissue histology to confirm the presence of ulcerative colitis or Crohn's disease. Rectal Gram stains for gonorrhea have low yield. Cultures of the anus are preferred and should be taken from the rectal wall to diagnose *Chlamydia.* Also obtain stool cultures for shigellosis and *Campylobacter,* and serologic studies for syphilis and amebiasis.

TREATMENT

Medication

Inflammatory or Radiation Proctitis

Topical steroids (retention enemas or foam) are the treatment of choice for proctitis caused by inflammatory bowel disease or radiation therapy. One applicator full, taken rectally, of Cortifoam (at bedtime or bid) or ProctoFoam (tid or qid) is prescribed for 2 to 3 weeks. A course of oral steroids (prednisone or SoluMedrol Dose Pak) may be used when the proctitis is unresponsive to the above agents. An infectious cause, however, must be ruled out before initiating any steroid therapy. 5-ASA (Rowasa) is an alternative to steroid use and may be given orally [in varying doses depending on agent used: mesalanine (Asacol), olsalazine sodium (Dipentum), or mesalanine (Pentasa)] or in suppository form (1 rectally bid, retained for 1 to 3 h). Treatment is continued for 3 to 6 weeks.

Chlamydia Proctitis

Use doxycycline, 100 mg bid, or tetracycline, 500 mg tid, both given orally for 14 days.

Gonorrhea Proctitis

Use a single dose of ceftriaxone, 250 mg IM (preferred). Alternative drugs given in single dose include spectinomycin, 2 g IM, or ciprofloxacin, 500 mg PO. A 7-day course of doxycycline, 100 mg PO bid, follows. Rectal gonorrhea is difficult to treat, and up to 35 percent of cases may be resistant.

Herpes Proctitis

Use acyclovir (Zovirax), 200 to 400 mg PO five times per day, or valacyclovir (Valtrex), 500 mg PO bid. Both are given for 7 to 10 days.

Amebiasis

Use iodoquinol (Yodoxin), 650 mg PO tid for 21 days for noninvasive intestinal infections. Use metronidazole (Flagyl), 750 mg PO tid for 5 to 10 days, followed by iodoquinol (21-day course) for cases of severe invasive proctocolitis.

Shigellosis/*Campylobacter*

Give ciprofloxacin, 500 mg PO bid for 5 to 7 days.

Supportive Measures

Patients with anal involvement may benefit from hot sitz baths 3 to 4 times a day. Topical anesthetics may help with acute anorectal pain.

PATIENT EDUCATION

Provide instruction on safe sex for STD and HIV prevention. Anal intercourse should be avoided during active treatment.

DISPOSITION

Patients should be reevaluated in 2 to 4 week intervals until completely healed as documented by follow-up sigmoidoscopy.

COMPLICATIONS AND RED FLAGS

Rectal abscess, anorectal fistulas, chronic ulcerative colitis, perforation of bowel wall, and treatment failure are the most common complications seen. Suspect these disorders in patients with severe rectal pain, tenesmus, or fever.

BIBLIOGRAPHY

Barker LR, Burton JH, Zieve PD (eds): *Principles of Ambulatory Medicine,* 4th ed. Baltimore, Williams & Wilkins, 1995, pp 1359–1361.

Bassford T: Treatment of common anorectal disorders. *Am Fam Phys* 45(4):1787–1794, 1992.

Goroll AH, May LA, Mulley AG Jr (eds): *Primary Care Medicine: Office Evaluation and Management of the Adult Patient,* 3d ed. Philadelphia, Lippincott, 1995, pp 372–423.

Griffith W, Dambro MR: *5 Minute Clinical Consult.* Philadelphia, Lea & Febiger, 1996, pp 848–850.

Jayanthi V, Chuah SY, Probert CS, et al: Proctitis and proctosigmoiditis—A need to identify the extent of disease in epidemiological surveys. *Digestion* 54(1):61–64, 1993.

Tierney L, McPhee SJ, Papadakis MA: *Current Medical Diagnosis and Treatment.* Stamford, CT, Appleton & Lange, 1996, pp 422–424.

Chapter 6–24
ABDOMINAL HERNIAS
Karen A. Newell

DISCUSSION

Hernia can be defined as the defect through which an organ or part of an organ protrudes from its cavity. Abdominal hernias are the second most common cause of bowel obstruction, trailing postoperative adhesions. This chapter covers primarily those defects located in the abdomen that protrude externally.

Incidence

The incidence of hernia is as follows:

- 75 percent groin (direct, indirect, femoral)
- 10 percent incisional and ventral
- 3 percent umbilical

Predisposing Factors

Owing to increased intraabdominal pressure and/or decreased muscle strength, a variety of medical problems can cause a hernia:

- Chronic obstructive pulmonary disease (COPD)
- Obesity
- Pregnancy

- Benign prostatic hypertrophy (BPH) secondary to chronic urination strain
- Straining during defecation
- Excessive lifting and exercise
- Trauma to transversalis fascia (e.g., from weightlifting)
- Smoking
- Systemic illness
- Ascites
- Aging (related to decreased muscle tone)
- Heredity (connective tissue strength associated with direct inguinal hernia)

TYPES OF HERNIAS

Hernias may be congenital or acquired and are divided into the following types:

- *Reducible hernia* Contents return to the abdomen spontaneously with supination or with light manual pressure by the patient or examiner.
- *Incarcerated or irreducible hernia* Contents are "stuck"; they do not return to the abdomen. If acute, it may be accompanied by crampy abdominal pain and severe localized tenderness, nausea, vomiting (can be feculent), constipation or other change in bowel habits, fever. There is an impending surgical emergency, if the jejunum is involved. This type exhibits more acute symptoms than ileum or large bowel.
- *Strangulated hernia* The caught tissue has its blood supply compromised; ischemia and necrosis ensue, bringing about a surgical emergency.
- *Sliding hernia* Part of the hernia sac is a portion of an organ (e.g., sigmoid colon or cecum).
- *Interparietal hernia* This lies between abdominal wall layers.
- *Inguinal hernia* This is the most common site of all hernias, can be direct or indirect, and occurs in males nine times more often than in females; 5 percent of all males will have an inguinal hernia at some point in their life.
- *Direct inguinal hernia* Typically affecting males over 40 years of age, this type is rare in females. The defect is through the floor of the inguinal canal (Hesselbach's triangle) where the lateral border is the inferior epigastric artery, the inferior border is the inguinal ligament, and the medial border is the lateral edge of the rectus abdominis. These tend not to strangulate as they present as a wide defect visibly noted as a bulge at the external inguinal ring. Usually they are easily reduced, rarely migrate into the scrotum; recurrence after surgical correction is variable, up to about 30 percent.
- *Indirect inguinal hernia* Most common of the inguinal hernias, these have a tendency to strangulate secondary to narrow defect. Seen often in the first year of life, they are again common between 10 and 30 years of age. Both males and females can be affected, with males affected four times more often than females, often occur bilaterally. There is a defect in the internal inguinal ring as it is the weakest site of the abdominal wall secondary to the descent of the gonads during embryonic development. The abdominal contents follow a patent processus vaginalis through the spermatic cord (hernia sac lies anteromedial to cord structures) into the scrotum. Therefore, all these are considered congenital: 80 percent of newborns have a patent processus vaginalis; 40 to 50 percent of 1-year-olds have a patent processus vaginalis; 20 to 25 percent of adults have a patent processus vaginalis.

The processus vaginalis usually closes by 2 to 3 months after birth. Actual herniation occurs in 60 percent of premature male infants and 1 to 4 percent of young children, with 45 percent of these occurring during first year of life. Sixty percent occur on the right since the right gonad is last to migrate and close, 25 percent left, and 15 percent bilateral. In children, 10 percent of those that herniate become incarcerated, and 30 percent of these go on to strangulate. In girls, the hernia sac can include the ovary, fallopian tube, and/or uterus. Recurrence rate after surgery varies realistically between 5 and 10 percent.

The differential diagnosis of a *strangulated inguinal hernia* includes the following:

1. Testicular torsion of an undescended testicle (absence of a testicle in the scrotum; may have vomiting but not feculent material).
2. Inflamed inguinal lymphadenopathy usually associated with erythema, edema of the skin and soft tissue, fever; absence of vomiting and abdominal pain. Usually presents with associated genitourinary infection.
3. Thrombosis of the spermatic cord usually presents with marked localized testicular swelling.

Pantaloon Hernia

Combined direct and indirect inguinal hernias are called pantaloon hernias.

Femoral Hernia

These account for 2 percent of groin hernias in men and one-third of groin hernias in women. Therefore, most are found in females (thought to be associated with a wider pelvis and pregnancy). Right side hernias are more common than the left, may be asymptomatic until incarceration or strangulation, and are located below the inguinal ligament in the femoral triangle (inguinal ligament superiorly), sartorius muscle (laterally), and adductor longus muscle (medially). The highest risk of incarceration or strangulation is secondary to a narrow defect in the transversalis fascia that is usually irreducible. Postsurgical recurrence is about 5 to 10 percent.

The differential diagnosis of a *femoral hernia* includes the following:

1. Inflamed inguinal lymphadenopathy (absence of vomiting or abdominal pain, more local skin and soft tissue edema, and erythema)
2. Thrombosis of a saphenous vein branch (absence of vomiting and abdominal pain; may palpate a thrill when the patient coughs)

Ventral Hernia

Incisional, umbilical, and epigastric hernias are all considered ventral hernias, which are identified by protrusion through the abdominal wall, usually in the midline through the linea alba. These are common after repeated pregnancies or multiple abdominal surgeries that weaken the abdominal musculature; therefore, prevention can be obtained with careful closure of the anterior rectus sheath, since this is the strength of the closure. Usually the small bowel is involved. Patients with incarceration present with abdominal pain, vomiting, constipation, and localized tenderness.

Incisional Hernia

These hernias are marked by protrusion through a previous incision site by a defect in the fascial closure, a result of 10 percent of all abdominal surgeries. They are associated with poor surgical technique, increased age, infection, serious systemic illnesses, obesity, smokers or those with COPD who cough frequently, and surgical drain tracts. Postsurgical recurrence rates vary depending on the incision size: small 2 to 5 percent, medium 5 to 15 percent, and large 25 percent. Recurrence can be up to 50 percent in some cases.

Umbilical Hernia

In umbilical hernias, the abdominal contents protrude through the umbilicus. The GI tract developmentally begins outside of the abdomen and enters the abdomen at 10 weeks in utero through the umbilicus. This remnant passage is usually partially closed at birth but may not be completely sealed until age 4 (higher incidence seen in those of African descent). This usually closes spontaneously if smaller than 1.5 cm. Surgery is indicated in those with greater than a 2-cm defect or if not completely closed by age 3 to 4 years old to prevent incarceration in adulthood. Adult females are more often affected than males. These hernias are associated with marked obesity; therefore, they are often hidden in abdominal fat. Usually the large bowel or omentum is involved, so symptoms are less acute. If the hernia is incarcerated, the patient may present with abdominal pain, vomiting, and localized tenderness with possible palpable swelling.

Epigastric Hernia

Epigastric hernias affect 3 to 5 percent of the population and men more than women. Common ages are 20 to 50; 20 percent are multiple; 80 percent occur on the midline, located above umbilicus through the linea alba. They are often found on routine examination. Most are painless but can present with mild tenderness to deep, burning pain, which can radiate to the back; other symptoms may include bloating, nausea or vomiting. These hernias are exacerbated by large meals and palliated with supination. With an increased incidence of incarceration and strangulation, the postsurgical recurrence rate is 10 to 20 percent.

Parastomal Hernia

Parastomal hernias are those that develop at a stomal site.

Richter's Hernia

This is an incarcerated antimesenteric portion of bowel (the side opposite that which is attached to the mesentery); therefore, bowel lumen may remain unaffected and subacute symptoms may occur until perforation and peritonitis develop.

Spigelian Hernia

This is a rare protrusion through the point of intersection of the linea semilunaris and the semicircularis. It is usually not visible externally, because it is hidden in the abdominal fatty layer.

Perineal Hernia

This is a rare protrusion through the pelvic floor, usually secondary to previous surgical procedure, such as a prostatectomy.

Lumbar or Dorsal Hernia

This is a protrusion through the lateral abdominal wall at either the inferior lumbar triangle (Petit's: anterior border = external oblique, inferior = iliac crest, and posterior = latissimus dorsi muscle) or superior triangle (Grynfeltt's). Patients describe a "lump" in the flank and a dull, heavy sensation. Incarceration is found in 10 percent, and the postsurgical recurrence rate is low.

Obturator Hernia

This rare internal hernia follows the obturator vessels and nerve. It is seen in cachectic elderly females who complain of inner thigh pain with radiation to the knee as the obturator nerve is compressed. Crampy abdominal pain with vomiting may accompany the presenting complaint. Rectal examination may reveal a tender, palpable mass in the obturator canal. The mortality rate ranges from 13 to 40 percent in those that present acutely.

Sciatic Hernia

The rarest of all the abdominal hernias, this is an internal hernia which protrudes through the greater sciatic foramen.

Littre's Hernia

This hernia contains a Meckel's diverticulum. It is associated with inguinal region 50 percent, femoral region 20 percent, umbilical region 20 percent, and other regions 10 percent. It is seen more often in males and on the right side.

Diaphragm Hernia

This is an internal protrusion through the diaphragm.

Traumatic Hernia

This type of hernia is secondary to direct blunt abdominal trauma.

SIGNS AND SYMPTOMS

Many patients have no symptoms and learn they have a groin hernia only through a routine sports or preemployment physical. Some may experience gradual onset of discomfort, reported as a dull ache with radiation into the scrotum. If swelling is present, it is typically maximized at the end of the day and disappears with supination. Occasionally a patient will report acute onset of swelling and discomfort after a particularly strenuous straining or lifting episode. In infants who have acutely incarcerated hernias, presentation may consist only of irritability.

PHYSICAL EXAMINATION

A symmetric, circular bulge located just superior to the pubic tubercle can often be seen on inspection in the patient who presents with a direct hernia. This can be visually exacerbated by coughing or Valsalva maneuver. Patients with a large indirect hernia may present with scrotal enlargement. Otherwise there may not be any visible findings.

The best examination maneuver for detecting an inguinal hernia consists of placing the gloved index finger of the examiner into the external inguinal ring of the patient during standing. Start low by imaginating loose scrotal skin (in the case of the male), aiming superior, then lateral toward the patient's anterior superior iliac spine (ASIS). Once the examiner's digit is in position, the patient can turn his or her head and cough or perform the Valsalva maneuver. This increase in intraabdominal pressure may force abdominal contents into the inguinal canal secondary to abdominal wall weakness and may allow palpation by the examiner's finger. This is performed bilaterally. When the right index finger is placed in the patient's right inguinal canal and directed at the ASIS, touching of abdominal contents to the fingertip may indicate an indirect inguinal hernia and touching the side of the digit suggests a direct hernia. This is not a completely reliable finding, since it may be very difficult to distinguish between the two, but it may be useful in some cases. The same situation is reversed, using the examiner's left index finger aimed toward the patient's left ASIS within the left inguinal canal. The patient then can be examined in the supine position to determine reducibility. In the patient who is suspected of having a hernia that is incarcerated or strangulated, auscultation of the scrotum can yield bowel sounds if detected early. Later, bowel sounds may cease on further ischemia and necrosis.

Attempting to get fingers above a scrotal mass can help to differentiate between a hernia (cannot get above) and a hydrocele (which typically can get above). Transillumination of the mass can also help to distinguish between hydrocele that typically transilluminates and hernia that does not. Hydroceles are usually described as nontender.

DIAGNOSTIC STUDIES

Vitals signs may demonstrate elevated temperature and slight tachycardia in those who are strangulated. Use complete blood cell count (CBC) for evidence of leukocytosis and left shift in those suspected of strangulation. Electrolytes may be abnormal if strangulation is secondary to dehydration and toxicity. Flat and upright plain films of the chest and abdomen help assess for bowel obstruction and/or perforation. Ultrasound may be helpful in differentiating scrotal masses. Urinalysis may be helpful in differentiating genitourinary involvement. CT is sometimes helpful in difficult cases (internal pelvic and spigelian hernias). Herniography (which consists of intraperitoneal injection of contrast material, then a plain film obtained while the patient performs the Valsalva maneuver) may also be used.

TREATMENT

Some patients benefit from the use of a daytime truss and avoidance of heavy straining or lifting; however, this is temporizing in most and actually contraindicated in those with femoral hernia. Surgical repair (herniorrhaphy or hernioplasty) to reduce the sac and close the defect is the only method of treatment and should be done to prevent possibility of incarceration or strangulation. This can usually be accomplished electively with local anesthesia and same day surgery. Most can return to a sedentary job within several days or 3 to 6 weeks for a heavy manual worker. Surgical consideration should be given based on health, activity level, and life-style of the patient. Surgical benefits should outweigh the risks. In acute cases, gentle attempts at manual reduction of the incarceration using the Trendelenburg position can be implemented. However, surgical consultation should be instituted quickly. The patient should be given IV fluids and kept NPO; a nasogastric tube should be placed. Many types of surgical repair are utilized. It is important to be familiar with some of the more common types.

- *Bassini repair* Most widely used method (originally described in 1887); sew conjoined tendon (internal oblique aponeurosis and transversus abdominis aponeurosis, transversalis fascia) to the inguinal ligament also called Poupart's ligament.
- *Halstead repair* Sew external oblique fascia beneath the spermatic cord; of historical significance only.
- *Lotheissen-McVay repair/Cooper's ligament repair* This useful indirect hernia repair always requires a relaxing incision in the rectus sheath to relieve tension. It is also effective for femoral hernia repair.
- *Shouldice repair* The technique of running suture closure of transversalis fascia; the strength in the groin is the transversalis fascia, also known as the shelving margin or iliopubic tract.
- *Lichtenstein repair* A polypropylene mesh (Marlex) or other synthetic patch is used to repair the transversalis fascial effect.
- *Mercy repair* Tighten the internal ring.
- *Laparoscopic repair* This newer closed technique involves stapling and mesh; the long-term results are unknown.

HERNIORRHAPHY AND HERNIOPLASTY COMPLICATIONS

Complications include hemorrhage and severed vas deferens. There can be resection or entrapment of the ilioinguinal nerve: altering skin sensation of upper thigh, root of the penis and scrotum (in males), mons pubis and labia majora (in females), or entrapment of the genitofemoral nerve disrupting skin sensation of the groin and upper thigh. Other possibilities are testicular

swelling if closure of ring is too tight, recurrence, infection, and failure in diabetic patients secondary to decreased healing and in obese patients secondary to weight. Ischemic orchitis, testicular atrophy, bladder injury, and bowel injury can also occur.

BIBLIOGRAPHY

Bates B: *A Guide to Physical Examination and History Taking.* Philadelphia, Lippincott, 1995, chap 12, pp 361–375.

Jenkins J, Loscalzo J, Braen GR: *Manual of Emergency Medicine.* Boston, Little, Brown, 1995, chap 24, pp 197, 218, 265–267.

Schwartz SI, Shires GT, Spencer FC (eds): *Principles of Surgery,* 6th ed. New York, McGraw-Hill, 1994.

Silen W: *Cope's Early Diagnosis of the Acute Abdomen.* New York, Oxford University Press, 1996, pp 198–205.

Tintinalli J, Ruiz E, Krome R (eds): *Emergency Medicine: A Comprehensive Study Guide.* New York, McGraw-Hill, 1996, chap 80, pp 466–468.

Way L (ed): *Current Surgical Diagnosis and Treatment.* Norwalk, CT, Appleton & Lange, 1994, chap 33, pp 712–724.

Zollinger RM Jr, Zollinger RM (eds): *Atlas of Surgical Operations.* New York, McGraw-Hill, 1993, pp 424–447.

Chapter 6–25
ABDOMINAL PAIN
Pat C. H. Jan

DISCUSSION

Abdominal pain is the most common complaint at the emergency room and outpatient clinic. It is important to identify those disease processes involving abdominal pain which require immediate surgical intervention and those which require a complete medical workup.

Common surgical emergencies include small and large bowel obstruction, appendicitis, mesenteric ischemia, cholecystitis, perforated duodenal ulcer, incarcerated inguinal hernia, and ectopic pregnancy.

It is very important to obtain a complete history on each patient. Be sure to ask for the following information: onset (early morning, afternoon, dinner, bedtime), duration (minutes, hours, days), radiation (from left upper quadrant to the shoulder, right lower quadrant to lower extremities), aggravating factors (does food or movement make the pain worse), relieving factors (what makes the pain less or what alleviates the pain), quality (sharp, dull, burning, gnawing), and location of pain.

SIGNS AND SYMPTOMS
Left Upper Quadrant Pain

Pain in this area can be from a myocardial infarction, duodenal ulcer, splenic injury, or gastroenteritis. The pain can present as sharp, burning, or gnawing. Kehr's sign may be present with splenic injury. It is referred pain to the left shoulder from the splenic area. (See Chap. 6-21, "Peptic Ulcer Disease," and Chap. 6-1, "Acute Gastroenteritis.")

Left Lower Quadrant Pain

Diverticulitis, inflammatory bowel disease, pelvic inflammatory disease, and rupture of ovarian cyst are common causes of abdominal pain in this area. A careful history of bowel habits, sexually transmitted diseases, and menstruation should be obtained. (See Chap. 6-8, "Diverticular Disease"; Chap. 6-15, "Inflammatory Bowel Disease"; Chap. 12-8, "Pelvic Inflammatory Disease"; and Chap. 12-9, "Polycystic Ovarian Syndrome.")

Right Upper Quadrant Pain

Palpation of the right upper quadrant for Murphy's sign indicates cholecystitis. (See Chap. 6-10, "Gallbladder Disease.") Pneumonia and pulmonary embolism can cause pain at the costal vertebral angle and should be differentiated from abdominal causes. (See Chap. 17-7, "Pneumonia.")

Right Lower Quadrant Pain

Pain may be diffuse, as in early appendicitis, or crampy and nonradiating, as in ectopic pregnancy. Colon obstruction secondary to colon cancer and ureterolithiasis are common causes of pain in this area. (See Chap. 6-26, "Appendicitis.")

OBJECTIVE FINDINGS

Inspection

Begin by lying the patient flat with arms placed at the side. Put the bed in the supine position and look at the abdomen for distention. If there is dropoff at the costal margins, then the abdomen is not distended. Look to see what area of the abdomen is distended. Right upper quadrant distention can be gastric outlet obstruction in a patient with a gastrostomy tube. Left upper quadrant distention can be caused by hepatomegaly. Abdominal distention with bowel sounds may be due to a fecal impaction from prolonged narcotic or laxative abuse leading to constipation. Abdominal distention without bowel sounds is ileus. Bowel obstruction and perforation are common causes.

Auscultation

Hypoactivity to absence of bowel sounds can be heard with ileus. Hyperactive bowel sounds are generally heard in gastroenteritis. High pitch with crescendo-decrescendo is common with bowel obstruction.

Percussion

Percuss over each quadrant for tympany and dullness. Patients with liver disease may have a distended abdomen filled with ascites. Perform the fluid wave and shifting dullness to determine if the patient has ascites.

Palpation

Always start from an area of nontenderness to the area of pain. Palpate lightly and then deeply to locate the source of the abdominal pain. Locate the abdominal aorta and determine approximate size, since it can be a source of abdominal pain. Some special maneuvers can be used to help with the diagnosis of abdominal pain. Cutaneous hypersensitivity is caused by pain from gentle squeezing of the skin in the abdominal area between the thumb and index finger. Deep palpation of one quadrant with peritoneal irritation to the opposite quadrant is a positive Rovsing's sign. Psoas sign is elicited by resistance with extension of the right

thigh. It is used as a diagnostic aid in appendicitis. The obturator sign causes pain with flexion and extension of the flexed right thigh. Murphy's sign is tenderness with palpation of the gallbladder with inspiration. A rectal examination should be performed as well.

DIAGNOSTIC CONSIDERATIONS

Common causes of abdominal pain are listed in Table 6-25-1.

Cholecystitis

This presents as right upper quadrant pain, worse after a fatty meal. Pain is worse with obstruction of the common bile duct by a gallstone. Common risk factors are female, fat, forty, and fertile. Ultrasound is the gold standard. (See Chap. 6-10, "Gallbladder Disease.")

Mesenteric (Intestinal) Ischemia

Findings are out of proportion to physical examination with mesenteric ischemia. Utilize angiography to aid in the diagnosis.

Diverticulitis

Diverticulitis presents as left lower quadrant pain. Patients have mild leukocytosis, fever, and chills with perforation. Plain films may illustrate multiple diverticula in the left colon. (See Chap. 6-8, "Diverticular Disease.")

Pancreatitis

Epigastric pain with radiation to the back is the typical presentation of pancreatitis. Patients are often found in the fetal position. The abdomen may be distended and tender to palpation. Cullen's sign (periumbilical ecchymosis) or Grey Turner's sign (flank ecchymosis) are late findings. Since a history of alcohol abuse is a common cause of pancreatitis, the patient should be placed on delirium tremens (DT) prophylaxis. (See Chap. 6-20, "Pancreatic Disease.")

Duodenal Ulcers

Epigastric pains that are relieved with food denote duodenal ulcers. Perforations are seen on plain abdominal films as free air under the diaphragm. Endoscopic biopsy may reveal *Helicobacter pylori* as the cause of the ulcers. (See Chap. 6-21, "Peptic Ulcer Disease.")

Other diseases to keep in mind are ectopic pregnancy, bowel obstruction, endometriosis, inflammatory bowel disease, and biliary disease. (See Fig. 6-25-1.)

LABORATORY STUDIES

Complete Blood Cell Count

Decreased as well as elevated WBC indicates an inflammatory process. This is seen in abdominal abscess formation, perforated viscus, carcinoma, and gynecologic infections. Occasionally, a patient will present with an elevated WBC with no significant findings other than recent surgery or resolution of a recent infection. This is termed a leukemoid reaction. A follow-up WBC will be within the reference range. Steroids can also cause a falsely elevated WBC. If a differential is included in the CBC, left shift caused by increased polymorphonuclear leukocytes and increase bands indicate acute bacterial infection. Elevations in lympho-

Table 6-25-1. Common Causes of Abdominal Pain

Disease	Signs and Symptoms	Physical Findings	X-ray and Lab Tests	Treatment	Etiology
Duodenal ulcers	Epigastric pain; relieved with food; burning sensation	Epigastric tenderness	EGD; (+) CLO; *H. pylori*	BMT (peptobismol 525 mg tid, flagyl 250 mg tid, amoxicillin 500 mg bid, or tetracycline 500 mg qid) × 14 d or clarithromycin 500 mg tid + omeprazole 40 mg qd × 14 d, then omeprazole 20 mg qd × 14 d	*H. pylori*
Pancreatitis	Initially midepigastric pain; radiating pain to back; nausea and vomiting	Epigastric tenderness; may have abdominal distention; in fetal position; Cullen sign; Grey Turner's sign	Chem profile (watch glucose, calcium, magnesium); amylase (*p*-isoenzyme); lipase	NPO (allow for pancreas to rest); NG tube (for abdomen distention and nausea, vomiting); pain control (demerol or morphine); Delirium Tremens (IV w/MVI 10 mL, thiamine 100 mg)	Alcohol; gallstone; drugs
Acute cholecystitis	RUQ pain; nausea, vomiting; fever, chills; pain worse after fatty meal	(+) Murphy sign; RUQ tenderness	Ultrasound; HIDA scan; plain abdominal x-ray; chemistry profile (watch for increased alkaline phosphatase in obstruction)	Laparotomy; laparoscopic cholecystectomy	Gallstone obstruction; bile stasis (TPN, drugs—rocephin, dehydration)
Small bowel obstruction	Nausea, vomiting; crampy abdomen pain	Abdomen distention; crescendo-decrescendo bowel sound; absent bs; abdomen scar;	4 views of abdomen (look for air-fluid levels, dilated loops of bowel)	NG tube; pain control; laparotomy	Previous surgery (adhesions); inflamatory bowel disease (strictures); hernia
Large bowel obstruction	Nausea, vomiting; obstipation; abdomen pain	Abdomen distention; high pitched bowel sound with rushes	Plain abdominal x-ray (look for dilated loops of bowel); barium enema (stricture)	Laparotomy	Carcinoma; volvulus; diverticular disease
Appendicitis	Periumbilical pain; localized RLQ pain; anorexia; fever/chill	Rebound tenderness; Rosving's sign; psoas sign; obturator sign; heel sign	Plain abdominal x-ray (psoas shadow); barium enema (nonvisualization of appendix); CBC (increased WBC)	Laparotomy; Laparoscopic appendectomy	Lymphoid tissue; fecal/fecalith; tumor (carcinoid)
Mesenteric ischemia	Acute abdominal pain; melena	Abdomen distention; shock; minimal PE findings	WBC > 15,000; elevated amylase; elevated CPK; elevated inorganic phosphate; mahogany color peritoneal fluid; ^{133}Xe scan (retained xenon in ischemic bowel); ^{111}In scan (infarcted bowel); angiogram	Surgery; heparin administration	Mitral stenosis; connective tissue disease; drugs; trauma
Diverticulitis	LLQ pain; fever, chill; bleeding; crampy abdominal pain	LLQ tenderness; abdomen distention; LLQ mass	Plain film abdominal (mass, obstruction); CT scan (abscess, fistula); barium enema (abscess, stricture, diverticular sac)	Medical treatment; (NG tube, IV fluids, pain control, broad-spectrum antibiotic); surgical treatment: primary resection with or without anastomosis	Low dietary fiber; weakness in colon wall
Ectopic pregnancy	Amenorrhea; pelvic pain; sudden nonradiating back pain	Enlarge uterus; Adnexal mass; Cervical tenderness; Abdominal peritoneal signs	Quantitative beta HCG (look for doubling q 48 h); serum progesterone (<30 nm/L); pelvic sonogram (empty gestational sac)	Medical treatment: methotrexate; surgical treatment: salpingectomy, laparoscopic salpingectomy	Pelvic inflammatory disease; IUD use; previous induced abortions
Abdominal aortic aneurysm	Vague abdomen pain	Palpation of abdomen mass	Ultrasound (measure size of aorta); plain film abdominal (calcification); CT scan (size of aorta)	Laparotomy (replace segment of aneurysm wall with graft)	Atherosclerosis

NOTE: EGD = esophagogastroduodenoscopy; CLO = campylobacter-like organism test; BMT = Pepto Bismol + metronidazole + tetracycline; MVI = multivitamin; bs = bowel sound; HIDA = 99mTc iminodiacetic acid scan; TPN = total pareneteral nutrition; PE = physical exam; CPK = creatine phosphokinase; HCG = human chorionic gonadotrophin; IUD = intrauterine contraceptive device.

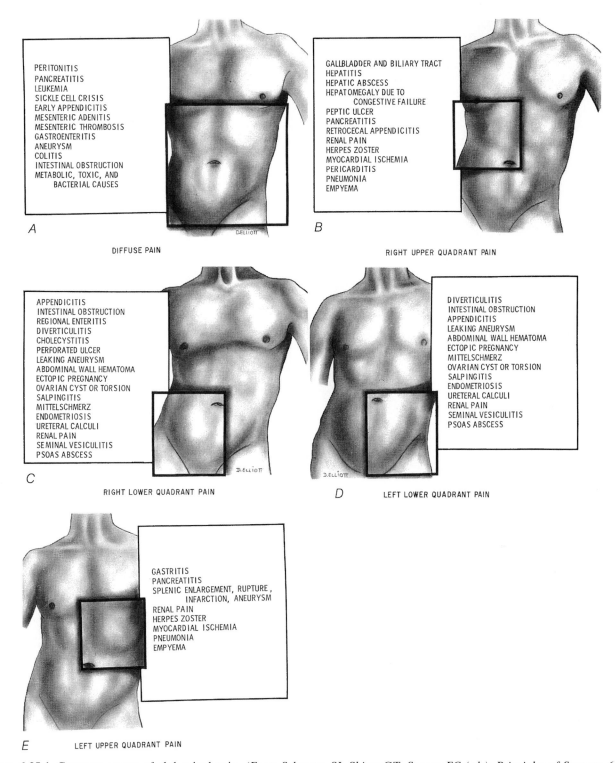

A

PERITONITIS
PANCREATITIS
LEUKEMIA
SICKLE CELL CRISIS
EARLY APPENDICITIS
MESENTERIC ADENITIS
MESENTERIC THROMBOSIS
GASTROENTERITIS
ANEURYSM
COLITIS
INTESTINAL OBSTRUCTION
METABOLIC, TOXIC, AND
    BACTERIAL CAUSES

DIFFUSE PAIN

B

GALLBLADDER AND BILIARY TRACT
HEPATITIS
HEPATIC ABSCESS
HEPATOMEGALY DUE TO
    CONGESTIVE FAILURE
PEPTIC ULCER
PANCREATITIS
RETROCECAL APPENDICITIS
RENAL PAIN
HERPES ZOSTER
MYOCARDIAL ISCHEMIA
PERICARDITIS
PNEUMONIA
EMPYEMA

RIGHT UPPER QUADRANT PAIN

C

APPENDICITIS
INTESTINAL OBSTRUCTION
REGIONAL ENTERITIS
DIVERTICULITIS
CHOLECYSTITIS
PERFORATED ULCER
LEAKING ANEURYSM
ABDOMINAL WALL HEMATOMA
ECTOPIC PREGNANCY
OVARIAN CYST OR TORSION
SALPINGITIS
MITTELSCHMERZ
ENDOMETRIOSIS
URETERAL CALCULI
RENAL PAIN
SEMINAL VESICULITIS
PSOAS ABSCESS

RIGHT LOWER QUADRANT PAIN

D

DIVERTICULITIS
INTESTINAL OBSTRUCTION
APPENDICITIS
LEAKING ANEURYSM
ABDOMINAL WALL HEMATOMA
ECTOPIC PREGNANCY
MITTELSCHMERZ
OVARIAN CYST OR TORSION
SALPINGITIS
ENDOMETRIOSIS
URETERAL CALCULI
RENAL PAIN
SEMINAL VESICULITIS
PSOAS ABSCESS

LEFT LOWER QUADRANT PAIN

E

GASTRITIS
PANCREATITIS
SPLENIC ENLARGEMENT, RUPTURE,
    INFARCTION, ANEURYSM
RENAL PAIN
HERPES ZOSTER
MYOCARDIAL ISCHEMIA
PNEUMONIA
EMPYEMA

LEFT UPPER QUADRANT PAIN

Figure 6-25-1. Common causes of abdominal pain. *(From Schwartz SI, Shires GT, Spence FC (eds): Principles of Surgery, 6th ed, New York, McGraw-Hill, 1994, p 1018. Used with permission of McGraw-Hill, Inc.)*

cytes can indicate viral infection. Eosinophils can be elevated in a number of disease processes such as neoplasm, Addison's disease, allergic reaction, collagen vascular disease, and parasitic infections.

Urinalysis

This may be useful in demonstrating an urinary tract infection in a female patient presenting with low abdominal pain.

Prothrombin Time and Partial Thromboplastin Time

An elevated PT and PTT will signify worsening liver function. Remember all coagulation factors are made by the liver except for factor VIII.

Chemistry Profile

Electrolyte abnormalities can be related to small bowel obstruction or gastroenteritis secondary to a bacterial infection. Hyper-

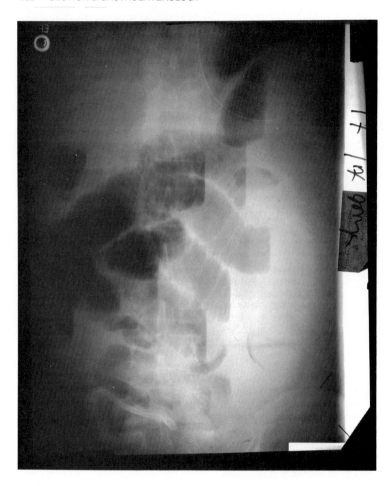

Figure 6-25-2. Air-fluid levels in left lateral position as seen in small bowel obstruction.

glycemia may be related to a patient presenting with alcoholic pancreatitis. Elevations in liver function profile may represent disease processes in the liver or indicate a mesenteric infarction. High levels of alkaline phosphatase are seen in common bile duct obstructions and bone diseases. Amylase and lipase are high in acute pancreatitis. Total bilirubin elevation is associated with liver disease. Creatine phosphokinase (CPK) isoenzymes will help to differentiate between cardiac, skeletal muscle, and liver pathology.

RADIOLOGIC STUDIES

Plain Abdominal Films

These are used to identify perforated viscus by looking for free air under the diaphragm. Small bowel obstruction can be confirmed with visualization of air-fluid levels and distended loops of small bowel. (See Figs. 6-25-2 and 6-25-3.) Radiopaque gallstones can be seen in the upper right quadrant of the abdominal film. Loss of psoas shadow can indicate appendicitis.

Ultrasonography

Ultrasonography is the gold standard test for gallstones. It is very useful in pelvic pain to identify fibroids, ovarian cysts, empty gestational sacs in ectopic pregnancy, and aortic aneurysms.

CT Scan

A CT scan is very useful in identification of abscess formations, diverticular disease, pancreatic cancer, liver cancer, gallstones, and perforated viscus.

Barium and Gastrografin Studies

These studies are useful in locating diverticular disease, fistula formations from inflammatory bowel disease, appendicitis with nonfilling appendix, stenosis, or edema at surgical anastomosis sites.

HIDA Scan

Technetium 99 is injected into the patient. Acute cholecystitis is confirmed when the gallbladder is not visualized.

Angiography

Use an angiogram to demonstrate arterial bleeding, infarction, and stenosis.

NOTES AND PEARLS

Patients with short bowel syndrome secondary to bowel resection from inflammatory bowel disease, may present to the emergency room with the complaint of abdominal pain and vomiting. Plain abdominal x-ray films reveal distended loops of small bowel which are seen in small bowel obstruction. The patient is taken into the operating room, and the abdomen is benign. It is common for the small bowel to become distended in this group of patients because the intestine is adapting. Patients with a history of narcotic abuse may present with a distended abdomen and constipation. Rectal examination usually reveals fecal impaction, or they may have a "lazy bowel" from laxative abuse.

BIBLIOGRAPHY

Nyhus LM: *Abdominal Pain: A Guide to Rapid Diagnosis.* Stamford, CT, Appleton & Lange, 1994.

Figure 6-25-3. Distended loops of bowel.

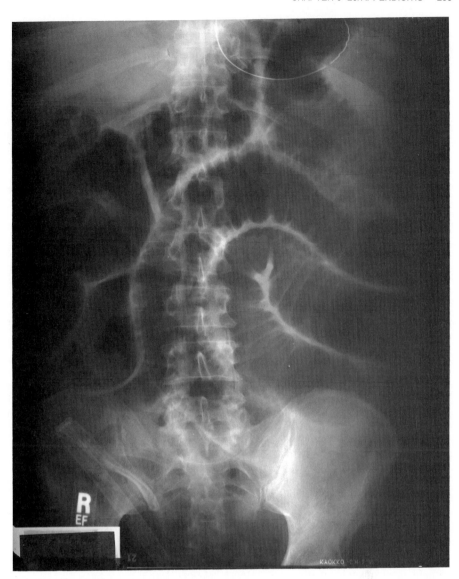

Schwartz SI, Shires GT, Spencer FC (eds): *Principles of Surgery,* 6th ed. New York, McGraw-Hill, 1994.
Seller R: *Differential Diagnosis of Common Complaints.* Philadelphia, Saunders, 1996.

Chapter 6–26
APPENDICITIS

Pat C. H. Jan

DISCUSSION

Acute appendicitis continues to remain a common cause of abdominal pain, often requiring surgical management. Appendicitis occurs equally in males and females until puberty. After puberty, the occurrence rate is greater in males by a ratio of 2 : 1. Overall the incidence of appendicitis has decreased since the 1940s. Some say the decline is attributed to such things as better nutrition and better diagnostic abilities of the clinician.

PATHOGENESIS

Appendicitis is caused by obstruction of the appendiceal lumen. Lymphoid follicle tissue generally appears in the appendix 2 weeks after birth. Hyperplasia of this tissue can be a result of GI infection from bacterial or viral organisms. These follicles can then obstruct the lumen of the appendix. Fecal stasis and fecalith formation are caused by entrapment of small amounts of vegetable fiber in the appendiceal lumen which stimulate mucous secretion. The mucus surrounds the fiber causing the irritation of the walls of the appendix, which stimulates further mucous secretion, and the appendix becomes obstructed. Foreign bodies and strictures of tumors of the appendix account for a small percentage of appendicitis cases. The common tumor type is carcinoid.

SIGNS AND SYMPTOMS

Patients with acute appendicitis present with abdominal pain as their initial complaint. The abdominal pain starts out as a generalized abdominal discomfort or periumbilical pain which is poorly localized. Patients may complain of crampy abdominal pain or gastroenteritis. As the disease progresses, the pain may shift from the periumbilical area to the right lower quadrant.

Prior to the onset of abdominal pain, the patient may relate a history of decreased appetite or anorexia and general malaise for a few days. Therefore, patients with good appetites are less likely to have appendicitis. Patients may complain of nausea and vomiting as the lumen of the appendix becomes obstructed and distended. An elevated white count of greater than 12,000 and low-grade temperature may or may not be present. Patients may also present with pain to the lower back or flank, and suprapubic pain. Lower back or flank pain may indicate a retrocecal appendix. A pelvic appendix may present as suprapubic pain.

OBJECTIVE FINDINGS

Typically patients are found in bed with guarding of the right lower quadrant. They may even have the right leg flexed to prevent irritation and pain. If patients are seen walking about or sitting comfortably in bed, appendicitis is probably unlikely. The first step is to observe the abdomen for distention. This is best accomplished with the bed placed in the supine position and the patient lying flat with hands at the side. The abdomen is inspected for a dropoff at the costal margins. If the dropoff is seen, the patient is not distended. The costal margin dropoff can also be readily seen in obese patients as well. Auscultation for hypoactive, normoactive, and hyperactive bowel sounds is the next step. Hypoactive to absent bowel sounds can be heard with ileus secondary to inflammation of the appendix. Acute appendicitis may present with normoactive bowel sounds. Meanwhile, hyperactive bowel sounds are generally more common in intestinal obstruction and gastroenteritis.

When performing percussion for tympany or dullness, it is important to start from an area of nontenderness and slowly work toward the place of tenderness. The same principle goes for palpation. If, during palpation, abdominal rigidity is encountered, perforation should be suspected. Additional maneuvers, sometimes called special tests, can be utilized in the diagnosis of appendicitis. Cutaneous hypersensitivity is pain caused by gentle squeezing of the skin in the abdominal area between the thumb and index finger. McBurney's point is located approximately one-third the distance between the anterior superior iliac spine and the umbilicus. This is the point of maximum tenderness. Patients have a positive rebound when they complain of pain after a sudden release from a deep palpation at McBurney's point. Rovsing's sign consists of deep palpation of the left lower quadrant of the abdomen to elicit peritoneal irritation in the right lower quadrant. Sometimes, the appendix when inflamed will cause irritation of the psoas muscle. The psoas sign is elicited by resistance with extension of the right thigh. The obturator sign consists of flexion and extension of the flexed right thigh. If positive, consider the pelvis as the location of the appendix. In the heel drop test, the patient or child is asked to stand up on the toes and drop down on the heels. This will cause peritoneal irritation. A modified heel drop can be done with the patient in the supine position. In this case, the examiner hits the bottom of the heel and transmits a vibration to the right lower quadrant. A more reliable test is performed by asking the patient to cough. Coughing can cause peritoneal irritation in an inflamed appendix. The patient indicates the right lower quadrant as the source of pain and discomfort. Lastly, a rectal examination should be performed for tenderness from a suprapubic appendix.

DIAGNOSTIC CONSIDERATIONS

Pain in the right lower quadrant has a myriad of potential etiologies, including but not limited to appendicitis. The following common diseases should be considered in the differential diagnoses.

Enteritis

Patients present with diffuse crampy abdominal pain and episodes of diarrhea. If patients have consumed any food toxins, they may present with fever, chills, and dehydration secondary to diarrhea. (See Chap. 6-1, "Acute Gastroenteritis.")

Pelvic Inflammatory Disease

The patient may relate a worsening of abdominal pain after menstruation. Usually both salpinxes are inflamed, and the patients may present with fever, chills, nausea, and vomiting. Physical examination generally demonstrates cervical motion tenderness, and a vaginal discharge may be noted. Sexual history should be ascertained. (See Chap. 12-8, "Pelvic Inflammatory Disease.")

Ectopic Pregnancy

Heterosexually involved women of childbearing age, especially those with a past history of pelvic inflammatory disease (PID), may have an ectopic pregnancy. Even in cases where sexual activity is denied (e.g., adolescent females), a pregnancy test should be performed or a pelvic ultrasound ordered. (See Chap. 12-6, "Ectopic Pregnancy.")

Ovarian Cyst

Patients may complain of lower quadrant pain at the start of each month's menstrual cycle. Physical examination can reveal adnexal tenderness. A pelvic sonogram can be used to confirm the diagnosis. (See Chap. 12-9, "Polycystic Ovarian Syndrome.")

Mesenteric Adenitis

Patients may present with a history of a recent bout of infection causing enlargement of regional lymph nodes. Patients have diffuse abdominal pain.

Diverticulitis

Although diverticula are more common in the left colon, inflamed right colon diverticula can be difficult to distinguish from appendicitis. Questions should be directed at bowel habits, signs of diarrhea, and blood in the stool. (See Chap. 6-8, "Diverticular Disease.")

Acute Cholecystitis

Acute cholecystitis usually presents with right upper quadrant pain. Pain may be worse after a fatty meal. Signs and symptoms also include fever and chills. Palpation will reveal right upper quadrant tenderness. Ultrasound is the gold standard confirmatory test. (See Chap. 6-10, "Gallbladder Disease.")

Ureteral Stones

Sharp, stabbing pains to the right quadrant and back, and hematuria are common signs and symptoms of ureteral stones. Intravenous pyelography usually demonstrates kidney stones. (See Chap. 18-5, "Renal Lithiasis and Pyelonephritis.")

Other diseases to keep in mind are perforated ulcers, inflammatory bowel disease, and aortic aneurysm.

SPECIAL CONSIDERATIONS

Appendicitis in Children

It is often difficult to get accurate histories from children regarding onset of abdominal pain and radiation of pain to the right lower quadrant. Parents may unknowingly delay treatment of what they presume is gastroenteritis. Physical examination and special tests may be limited secondary to fear of the clinician. Children usually present with episodes of diarrhea, fever, chills, and dehydration.

Appendicitis in the Elderly or Mentally Challenged

This is another population of individuals where accurate histories may be limited secondary to poor attention to detail and difficulty with memory retention. These patients often present initially with adverse behavioral changes that may be misinterpreted. Unfortunately, diagnostic laboratory findings may be normal or borderline abnormal. Physical examination findings may be unremarkable. Therefore, it is no surprise that many elderly or mentally challenged patients have perforated appendix when taken into the operating room.

Appendicitis and Pregnancy

Appendicitis is common during the first trimester of pregnancy. Signs and symptoms associated with appendicitis are very similar to those of a normal pregnancy. Physical examination findings may not be helpful because the appendix may shift location during pregnancy. Quite often, there is a delay in surgery because of the concern of inducing premature labor.

LABORATORY TESTS

There may be a mild to moderate elevation of the WBC in the range of 10,000 to 17,000. A mild left shift is also common. A urinalysis may be useful in ruling out a bladder infection. Occasionally, if an inflamed appendix rests on the ureter, white cells may be seen in the urine.

RADIOLOGIC STUDIES

Plain Abdominal Films

Abdominal x-rays may demonstrate distended loops of bowel localized around the site of inflammation, loss of the psoas shadow, or gas in the appendix.

Barium Enema Study

If the appendix is completely filled with the barium, then appendicitis is unlikely. On the other hand, nonfilling of the appendix can suggest appendicitis. (See Figs. 6-26-1 and 6-26-2.)

Figure 6-26-1. Filling of the appendix on barium enema study.

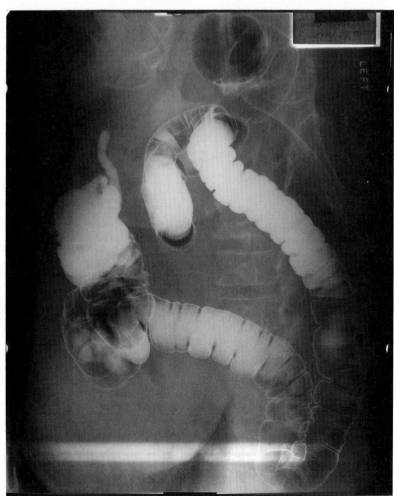

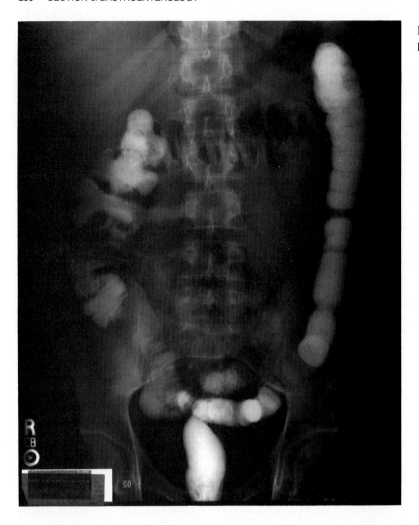

Figure 6-26-2. Nonfilling of the appendix on barium enema study.

Ultrasonography

Ultrasonography may demonstrate an inflamed appendix or rule out a pelvic disease.

CT Scan

A CT scan can be useful in finding appendiceal abscess.

TREATMENT

Laparotomy

An incision is made over McBurney's point in classic appendicitis. If there is doubt, a midline incision is used, so that other procedures are feasible if needed. (See Fig. 6-26-3.) In case of perforation, the subcutaneous layer is left open and allowed to close by secondary intention to minimize infection.

Laproscopic Appendectomy

This procedure can be used when there is doubt from objective and subjective findings. It can also be used to rule out gynecologic pathology. Four ports are inserted into the abdomen, and the appendix artery is divided. The appendix is separated from the cecum and removed from one of the ports. If there is perforation or pus, a Jackson-Pratt drain should be placed.

DISPOSITION

Patients are initially followed 1 week after discharge from the hospital and in uncomplicated appendectomy, they can be reeval-

uated in 2 to 3 weeks. In case of perforation or abscess formation, weekly visits are recommended until the abdominal wound is completely healed. Patients are then reevaluated in 3 weeks.

COMPLICATIONS AND RED FLAGS

Perforation

Postoperative monitoring for shock and sepsis is required in case of perforation. Patients should be placed on broad-spectrum antibiotics like clindamycin, plus an aminoglycoside or a second-generation cephalosporin (Mefoxin) or an aminopenicillin (Unasyn) or antipseudomonal penicillin (Timentin) for an additional 5 to 7 days. The subcutaneous layer should be left open to close by secondary intention, and a drain should be left behind.

Appendiceal Abscess

There is some controversy regarding treatment. Some advocate percutaneous radiologic guided drainage with a scheduled appendectomy at a later date, whereas others recommend immediate appendectomy with evacuation of the abscess. Patients are also placed on broad-spectrum antibiotics for 5 to 7 days postoperatively.

Fecal Fistula

Fistula may occasionally occur secondary to loosening of surgical ties, and generally these spontaneously close.

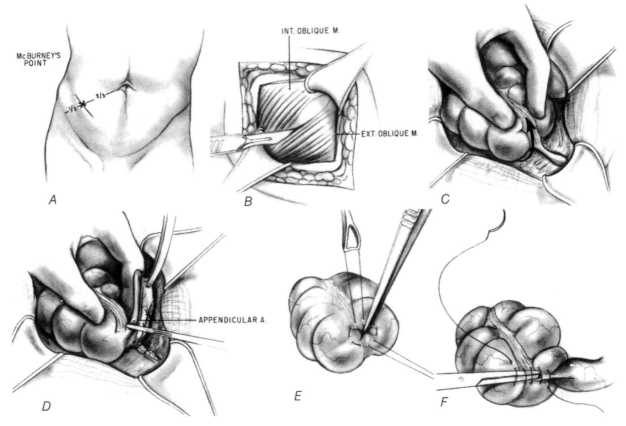

Figure 6-26-3. Appendectomy by laparotomy. (*From Schwartz SI, Shires GT, Spencer FC (eds): Principles of Surgery, 6th ed. New York, McGraw-Hill, 1994, p 1315. Used with permission of McGraw-Hill, Inc.*)

Intestinal Obstruction

This occurs secondary to ileus. A nasogastric tube should be inserted to prevent vomiting and aspiration until normal bowel movements have returned.

PEARLS

The diagnosis of appendicitis is more often a clinical decision. Quite often, the physical examination and laboratory and radio-logic studies are inconclusive. Sometimes the clinician has to make the determination of appendicitis by history alone.

BIBLIOGRAPHY

Schwartz SI, Shires GT, Spencer FC (eds): Appendicitis, in *Principles of Surgery,* 6th ed. New York, McGraw-Hill, 1994.

Vitello JM: Appendicitis, in Nyhus LM (ed): *Abdominal Pain: A Guide to Rapid Diagnosis.* Stamford, CT, Appleton & Lange, 1995.

Way LW (ed): Appendicitis, in *Current Surgical Diagnosis and Treatment,* 10th ed. Stamford, CT, Appleton & Lange, 1994.

Chapter 7–1
CYSTIC FIBROSIS (MUCOVISCIDOSIS)
William A. Mosier

DISCUSSION

Cystic fibrosis (CF) is the most common debilitating autosomal recessive disease that presents in persons of white European ancestry. It has been estimated that 30,000 Americans are afflicted by this lethal condition. It occurs in over 1 in every 2500 live births. An estimated 4 percent of the white population (about 9 million Americans) are carriers of the defective gene. Approximately 1200 new cases of CF are diagnosed annually in the United States. CF usually manifests within the first year of life. The respiratory tract is the organ system that generally determines the prognosis and survival of a CF patient. However, 90 percent of patients with CF also have pancreatic insufficiency and require pancreatic enzyme supplements. Most patients with CF have severe difficulty breathing and maintaining a clear airway. In fact, respiratory tract involvement is responsible for over 90 percent of the morbidity rate of CF. The median survival of patients with CF is only 30 years.

PATHOGENESIS

CF is a genetic-based protein defect. The disease consists of a defect in the protein product of the CF gene called the cystic fibrosis transmembrane conductance regulator (CFTR). The CF gene is a relatively large gene on chromosome 7 that encodes a protein containing 1480 amino acids. The CF gene has 27 subregions (exons) that code for the processed messenger ribonucleic acid (mRNA), which in turn is translated into the protein CFTR. The basic biochemical defect in CF is an abnormality of chloride ion (Cl^-) transport across airway epithelial cells. It has been hypothesized that there is an impaired ability of airway cells to secrete Cl^- through CFTR. CFTR serves as a Cl^- channel in response to cyclic $3',5'$-adenosine monophosphate (cAMP)–mediated secretagogues. An enhanced rate of sodium ion (Na^+) absorption also occurs as a result of increased amiloride-sensitive Na^+ conductance on the luminal membrane and increased Na^+, K^+-ATPase sites on the basolateral membrane. The result is a water imbalance caused by this decreased Cl^- permeability and excessive Na^+ reabsorption. The resulting electrolyte and transport abnormality leads to abnormal airway secretions, impaired mucociliary clearance, and persistent airway infections (predominantly bacterial). Human alveolar macrophage (AM)–derived cytokines are the key to the pathogenesis.

MICROBIOLOGY

The persistent infections that occur with CF cause neutrophils to migrate to the sites of infection. Neutrophils release large amounts of the viscous polyanion deoxyribonucleic acid (DNA) and actin during their routine disintegration. The lysosomal protein elastase also is released at this time. The DNA is present in CF sputum at a concentration of approximately 1 to 15 mg/mL. The DNA, actin, and elastase debris then mix with already present airway secretions. The secretions are retained because of apparently impaired mucociliary clearance in patients with CF. The secretions display increased viscosity and elasticity and decreased pourability. These properties tend to hinder the upward flow of respiratory tract secretions and inhibit the patient's ability to expectorate sputum. Thus, these secretions are associated with airway obstruction, shortness of breath, and exacerbation of infections. This process also causes an increase in the inflammatory response, which leads to a vicious cycle of further accumulation of leukocyte-derived debris mixing with airway secretions, resulting in more airway obstruction. The retention of these secretions in the airways predisposes CF patients to persistent *Staphylococcus aureus*, *Pseudomonas aeruginosa*, and *Haemophilus influenzae* infections. Once *P. aeruginosa* becomes established in the lungs of a patient with CF, it is extremely difficult to eradicate. Progressive lung destruction can then result in bronchiectasis, respiratory failure, and eventually premature death. The fungal pathogens found in CF are *Candida* and *Aspergillus* spp. Other gram-negative pathogens are occasionally isolated from CF cultures, including *Escherichia coli*, other *Pseudomonas* spp., and *Klebsiella*, *Proteus*, *Enterobacter*, and *Citrobacter* spp. Rarely, *Burkholderia cepacia* may appear. In addition to bacteria, some viruses have been responsible for respiratory tract infections in CF patients, most notably respiratory syncytial virus (RSV) and influenza A virus.

SYMPTOMS

The most common symptoms are chronic cough with sputum production and dyspnea. Symptoms observable in infants include foul-smelling fatty stools, severe constipation in a newborn, weight loss, wheezing, and a salty taste on a baby's skin. The salty taste is due to the blockage of chloride channels, which causes the abnormal sodium balance, resulting in a discharge of excess sodium excreted through the pores. Flatulence also may be a prominent symptom. The typical patient with CF will have 9 days of hospitalization annually related to CF complications from exacerbation of respiratory tract infections.

OBJECTIVE FINDINGS

CF can have varying clinical manifestations. The initial findings in 10 percent of newborns with CF are intestinal obstruction and meconium ileus. The mortality rate among these infants is between 20 and 60 percent. The meconium from babies with CF is high in albumin and lactase and is extremely viscous. The first signs are usually a persistent cough and wheezing with a rapid respiratory rate. Gagging, vomiting, and difficulty sleeping as well as recurring respiratory infections are suggestive of CF. Failure to gain weight and passing large, frequent bowel movements in association with an excessive appetite are also characteristic features in early childhood (Table 7-1-1).

DIAGNOSTIC CONSIDERATIONS

Although most cases of CF are diagnosed in childhood, 20 percent of CF patients are not diagnosed until after age 15. Therefore, any young adult who presents with interstitial infiltrates plus chronic sinopulmonary infections with a mucoid variant of *P. aeruginosa*, bronchiectasis, symptoms of asthma, unexplained gastrointestinal complaints, or a family history of similar complaints should receive a sweat chloride test. Rare alternative

Table 7-1-1. Clinical Manifestations of Cystic Fibrosis

Respiratory tract complications
  Viscous secretions causing small duct obstruction
  Bronchitis
  Sinusitis
  Atelectasis
  Emphysema
  Bronchopneumonia
  Bronchiectasis
  Lung abscesses
  Aspergillosis
  Nasal polyposis
  Hemoptysis
  Pneumothorax
  Pulmonary hypertension
  Cor pulmonale
  Respiratory failure
Pancreatic complications
  Steatorrhea
  Deficiencies of vitamins A, D, E, and K
  Diabetes mellitus
  Pancreatic calcifications
  Nutritional and growth failure
Intestinal complications
  Delayed meconium passage at birth
  Peritonitis
  Meconium ileus
  Volvulus
  Ileal atresia
  Rectal prolapse
  Intussusception
  Fecal impaction
  Pneumatosis intestinalis
Hepatobiliary complications
  Mucus hypersecretion
  Cholelithiasis
  Loss of bile salts
  Bile plugging of ductules
  Portal hypertension
  Esophageal varices
  Hypersplenism
  Atrophic gallbladder
  Cirrhosis
Skeletal complications
  Demineralization
  Hypertrophic osteoarthropathy
  Bone retardation
Reproductive system
  Males: sterility and absence of vas deferens, epididymis, and seminal
  vesicles
  Females: decreased fertility, increased viscosity of vaginal secretions
Miscellaneous complications
  Salt depletion
  Heat stroke
  Salivary gland hypertrophy
  Retinal hemorrhage
  Apocrine gland hypertrophy

diagnoses that may be confused with CF on chest radiography include eosinophilic granuloma and lymphangiomyomatosis.

SPECIAL CONSIDERATIONS

Malabsorption leading to malnutrition is a complication of considerable importance in CF. Because of mucus plugs in the pancreas that block pancreatic enzymes from passing into the small intestine, undigested food passes out of the body in the stool. To control this problem, digestive enzymes must be taken daily as supplements.

LABORATORY TESTS

To confirm the diagnosis of CF, a sweat test with pilocarpine iontophoresis is performed. Sweat chloride concentrations exceeding 60 meq/L are found in 98 percent of patients with CF. A level of 60 meq/L confirms the diagnosis in patients under age 20 years. A value of 80 meq/L is required for the diagnosis in persons age 20 years or older. Gene testing can be used to clarify the diagnosis in equivocal cases or when it is not possible to obtain an adequate sweat collection.

RADIOLOGIC STUDIES

A chest x-ray containing diffusely increased markings with cystic spaces, upper lobe predominance, and hyperinflation is highly characteristic of CF.

OTHER DIAGNOSTICS

Imaging procedures, including magnetic resonance imaging (MRI), CT, and ultrasonography, are useful for identifying pancreatic abnormalities in CF patients. They also can be useful in identifying liver complications.

TREATMENT

The standard of care for CF includes chest physical therapy (CPT), a procedure in which the patient's chest is pounded on to mechanically dislodge lung secretions); enzyme therapy; and antibiotic therapy (Table 7-1-2).

Medications

Current treatment includes the utilization of medications to hydrolyze extracellular DNA to improve the clearance of airway secretions. Deoxyribonuclease I (DNase) is a natural occurring enzyme produced by the pancreas and salivary glands that is responsible for this function. Recombinant human DNase I (rhDNase) has been cloned from human pancreatic complementary DNA (cDNA) to be used as a treatment to alter sputum viscoelasticity and improve the clearance of secretions. This medication is referred to commercially as dornase alfa (Pulmozyme). This drug improves forced expiratory volume in 1 second (FEV_1) and helps decrease dyspnea. Its use has also been shown to reduce cough, congestion, and the frequency of respiratory infections. It is available in single-use ampules administered by nebulizer. A typical starting dose is 2.5 mg a day. Possible side effects related to aerosol use include chest pain, dyspepsia, facial edema, laryngitis, pharyngitis, rash, conjunctivitis, and hoarseness. However, these adverse effects are uncommon, mild, and self-limiting.

    Another important mainstay of treatment is replacement therapy with pancreatic enzyme preparations, preferably in the form of enteric-coated microspheres. The enzymes are taken with meals and snacks. The enzymes provide only partial relief from maldigestion and diarrhea. Doses vary with the age and weight of the patient, the severity of the deficiency, and the contents of any given meal. High doses of the enzymes are associated with an increased risk of uricosuria.

Table 7-1-2. The Goals of CF Treatment

Improve lung function
Reduce respiratory symptoms
Delay bronchiectasis
Reduce frequency of exacerbations of respiratory tract infections
Reduce use of parenteral antibiotics
Optimize patient's sense of well-being
Minimize number of lost school and/or work days caused by CF-
  related illness

Chronic endobronchial infection with *P. aeruginosa* is a major cause of morbidity rate and mortality rate in CF patients. Therefore, antibiotic therapy is aimed at controlling its progression. Because *P. aeruginosa* is rarely eradicated once it is established, the chronic production of immune mediators tends to result in a slow progression of the lung disease. For this reason, the efficacy of current antibiotics is limited. Multidrug-resistant *P. aeruginosa* is a consequence of frequent and prolonged antibiotic therapy. Slowing the emergence of resistance by pairing antibiotics from different classes has been tried with some success. Oral ciprofloxacin plus aerosolized colistin may reduce chronic infection. However, this has not been confirmed in controlled trials. Short-term, high-dose aerosol administration of tobramycin in patients with clinically stable CF has proved to be an efficacious and safe treatment for endobronchial infection with *P. aeruginosa*. Additional drug therapy includes bronchodilators and anti-inflammatory agents such as inhaled corticosteroids, ibuprofen, and antipseudomonal intravenous immunoglobulin (IVIG).

SUPPORTIVE MEASURES

Airway clearance techniques (ACTs), also referred to as CPT, are the primary nonpharmacologic therapies for clearing airway secretions and improving pulmonary function in patients with CF. Although anti-inflammatory agents may aid in reducing inflammation, the physical removal of purulent secretions appears to be more effective in slowing the progression of CF airway disease. Therefore, ACTs are essential for the preservation of pulmonary function in CF patients. However, because traditional CPT can be uncomfortable, alternative ACTs are available, including the following:

1. High-frequency chest percussors, such as inflatable vests, that deliver compression pulses to the chest
2. Oral oscillators
3. Masks used to deliver a back pressure to the lungs during expiration

These therapies can combine controlled breathing, autogenic drainage, and a positive expiratory pressure to facilitate airway clearance. Physical exercise is also a valuable adjunct to ACTs in prolonging pulmonary function and improving the patient's quality of life.

Nutritional support and diet therapy are of vital importance in the overall treatment program for CF patients. Because of the malabsorption, the diet should include sufficient calories and protein to provide for normal growth. This usually includes a higher than normal total fat intake to increase the caloric density of the diet. Taking multivitamin and mineral supplements in megadoses, especially the lipid-soluble vitamins such as vitamin E, is usually necessary. Salt supplements during periods of thermal stress or increased sweating are also advised. Great attention must be paid to emotional support issues. CF care centers are available in many communities to implement the specialized care required.

PATIENT EDUCATION

Families should be encouraged to seek a CF support group. These support groups can provide valuable self-help information for both parents and victims of CF. The Cystic Fibrosis Foundation at HTTP:/WWW.CFF.ORG/NEWINDEX.HTM has a wealth of materials for families facing this debilitating disease. If there is a family history of CF, couples should be referred for genetic counseling before attempting a pregnancy. Accurate prenatal diagnosis and carrier detection have been available since 1985. Gene testing can be performed to determine the relationship between genotype and phenotype. Because most patients with CF have digestive problems, nutrition support services also must be provided.

DISPOSITION

Diffuse bronchiectasis leading to pulmonary hypertension and its complications are the typical terminal events. The only curative therapy currently available for end-stage bronchiectasis resulting from CF is lung transplantation.

COMPLICATIONS AND RED FLAGS

Two important complications of lower respiratory tract involvement in patients with CF that must be watched for are hemoptysis and pneumothorax. Although antibiotic therapy often is able to eradicate *S. aureus*, *H. influenzae*, and other bacteria from the respiratory tract, it seldom is able to permanently clear *P. aeruginosa* from the endobronchial space. Because of this resistance, a pulmonary consultation is strongly advised at the first sign of pneumonia.

OTHER NOTES OR PEARLS

In the future, the possibility of recombinant CFTR replacement therapy and recombinant CF gene therapy may allow correction of the basic disease mechanism. Testing is being done using the potassium-sparing diuretic amiloride to block the uptake of sodium ions in airway epithelia. This may suppress the inflammatory milieu in the distal airways of CF patients through its action on AM-derived cytokines, reducing the subsequent injury caused during the release of neutrophil-derived products. Studies are also under way using uridine triphosphate (UTP) to induce chloride ion efflux via aerosolized nucleotides. The current strategy in gene therapy for CF is to use recombinant adenoviruses, adeno-associated virus, and liposomes as gene delivery methods. The plasma protein gelsolin, which severs actin filaments, is also being explored as a mucolytic agent. Anti-inflammatory therapy research is under way to study the role of pentoxifylline and antiproteases in the treatment of CF. Investigators also are studying the feasibility of an antipseudomonal vaccine.

BIBLIOGRAPHY

Collins FS: Cystic fibrosis: Molecular biology and therapeutic implications. *Science* 256:774–779, 1992.

Davis PB: Cystic fibrosis: New perceptions, new strategies. *Hosp Pract* 27:79–118, 1992.

Dodge JA, Brock DJH, Widdicombe JH (eds): *Cystic Fibrosis: Current Topics*. New York, Wiley, 1993.

Eigen H, Rosenstein BJ, FitzSimmons S, et al: A multi-center study of alternate-day prednisone therapy in patients with cystic fibrosis. *J. Pediatr* 126:515–523, 1995.

FitzSimmons SC: The changing epidemiology of cystic fibrosis. *J Pediatr* 122:1–9, 1993.

Fuchs HJ, Borowitz DS, Christiansen DH, et al: Effect of aerosolized recombinant human DNase on exacerbations of respiratory symptoms and on pulmonary function in patients with cystic fibrosis. *New Engl J Med* 931:687–642, 1994.

Hodson ME: Aerosolized dornase alfa (rhDNase) for therapy of cystic fibrosis. *Am J Respir Crit Care Med* 151:S70–S74, 1995.

Knowies MR, Olivier K, Noone P, Boucher RC: Pharmacologic modulation of salt and water in the airway epithelium in cystic fibrosis. *Am J Respir Crit Care Med* 151:S65–S69, 1995.

Koch C, Hoiby N: Pathogenesis of cystic fibrosis. *Lancet* 341:1065–1069, 1993.

Schuster A, Fahy JV, Ueki I, Nadel JA: Cystic fibrosis sputum induces a secretory response from airway gland serous cells that can be prevented by neutrophil protease inhibitors. *Eur Respir J* 8:10–14, 1995.

Warner JO: Immunology of cystic fibrosis. *Br Med Bull* 48:893–911, 1992.

SECTION 8
Hematology

Chapter 8–1
IRON-DEFICIENCY ANEMIA
JoAnn Deasy

DISCUSSION

Iron-deficiency anemia (IDA) occurs when the body's iron supply is inadequate to meet the iron requirement of the red blood cells (RBCs) and body tissues. RBCs are responsible for oxygen transport and can be thought of as containers for hemoglobin. The hemoglobin molecule in the RBC releases oxygen to body tissues. The nutritional factors necessary for the RBC to go through proliferation and maturation in the bone marrow are iron, folic acid, and vitamin B_{12}. Iron and protoporphyrin form the heme portion of the hemoglobin molecule. Globin is the protein portion of the hemoglobin molecule.

The most immature RBC in the bone marrow is the pronormoblast. It divides and matures through various stages, forming the nucleated red blood cell (NRBC) in the bone marrow. The nucleus of this cell disintegrates, forming the immature RBC called the reticulocyte. Some reticulocytes are released into the bloodstream where after 1 or 2 days they mature into red blood cells. The reticulocyte count is an indicator of RBC productivity. The RBC has a life span of approximately 120 days; "old" red blood cells are removed by the spleen.

A state of negative iron balance can first be detected by a low ferritin level that falls as iron stores are depleted. As long as some iron stores remain, other laboratory parameters remain in the normal range, including serum iron level and transferrin (total iron-binding capacity). At this point, the hemoglobin level is normal and there is no change in the red cell morphology. When all the iron stores are completely exhausted, the serum iron becomes decreased, the total iron-binding capacity rises, and the percent saturation falls. This state, when anemia has not yet developed, can be labeled iron-deficient erythropoiesis. The poor iron supply has an impact on the developing RBC, and finally iron-deficiency anemia develops.

Anemia is clinically defined as a reduction in hemoglobin or hematocrit concentration. Although normal values may vary with different laboratories, anemia is usually present when the hemoglobin is less than 14 g/dL in adult males, less than 12 g/dL in menstruating females, and less than 11 g/dL in pregnant women. In IDA, in addition to a lowered hemoglobin, the red blood cells become progressively microcytic and hypochromic. Microcytosis is defined as a mean corpuscular volume (MCV) of less than 80 femtoliters. Iron deficiency anemia is the most common cause of microcytic anemia.

PATHOGENESIS

The causes of IDA include blood loss, inadequate dietary intake, and inadequate absorption of iron. In adults, chronic blood loss is the most common cause. This most often occurs from gastrointestinal bleeding or from menstrual loss. A diet deficient in iron is the most common cause in children. In infancy, a diet consisting predominantly of cow's milk may lead to IDA. After age 4 to 6 months, growth requirements are so great that without iron supplementation iron deficiency is common. Later in childhood, as the caloric intake increases, the diet usually supplies an adequate amount of iron.

SYMPTOMS

The symptoms of IDA, and anemias in general, depend on the severity of the anemia, the abruptness of onset, age, and the ability of the body to compensate. Until the hemoglobin falls below 10 (hematocrit less than 30 percent) the patient usually does not experience any symptoms. With a hemoglobin below 10 g/dL, the symptoms of IDA are nonspecific and common to anemia in general. These include fatigue and dyspnea on exertion, faintness, vertigo, palpitations, and a headache with exertion. In obtaining the patient's history, a detailed review of systems (ROS) is essential. The possibility of blood loss may be detected by a careful review of the gastrointestinal system and the menstrual and pregnancy history in females. In the ROS, information regarding frequent blood donations, recurring epistaxis and toxic exposure should also be ascertained. The patient's nutritional habits, including alcohol intake, merit special attention. Patients with severe IDA may crave ice, or less frequently have a sore mouth.

OBJECTIVE FINDINGS

Pallor is an indicator of anemia because mucous membranes and skin color reflect hemoglobin levels. In severe anemias, there is an increase in cardiac output, resulting in a rapid pulse and systolic murmur. With iron loss, there is epithelial cell shedding. Epithelial atrophy results in signs that are specific to IDA: atrophic glossitis, cheilitis, and koilonychia with spooning.

A complete physical examination is necessary. Special attention should be paid to skin color and the color of the mucous membranes. Examinations of the conjunctiva, nailbeds, and palmar creases of the hand are usually best for detecting pallor. In severe IDA, the cardiac examination may reveal a forceful apical pulse, hyperactive heart sounds, and a systolic murmur. The abdominal examination and rectal examination with a test of occult blood in the feces are important, as is the pelvic examination in the female.

DIFFERENTIAL DIAGNOSES

When microcytic anemia is present, the differential diagnosis includes iron deficiency anemia, thalassemia trait, anemia of chronic disease, sideroblastic anemia, lead poisoning, and copper deficiency. (See Table 8-1-1.)

DIAGNOSTIC STUDIES

A laboratory diagnosis is necessary to validate the diagnosis of iron-deficient anemia. The most important tests are the complete

Table 8-1-1. Differential Diagnosis of Microcytic Anemias

Anemia	MCV	RBC count	RDW	Serum Fe	TIBC
IDA	Low	Low	High	Low	High or normal
Thalassemia	Low	Normal or high	Normal	High or normal	Normal
Chronic disease	Normal or low	Normal		Low	Low
Sideroblastic	Normal or low			Normal or high	Normal

NOTE: IDA = iron-deficiency anemia; MCV = mean corpuscular volume; RBC = red blood cell; RDW = red cell distribution width; TIBC = total iron-binding capacity.

blood cell count (CBC) using an automated counter, the red cell morphology, and the evaluation of the iron supply by measuring the serum iron, the total iron-binding capacity (TIBC), and the serum ferritin. The CBC and red cell morphology yield a considerable amount of information. If anemia is present based on the hemoglobin, the RBC indices should first be examined. If microcytosis is present (MCV < 80), IDA is a definite consideration. The mean corpuscular hemoglobin (MCH) usually moves in the same direction as the MCV. Pay attention to the red cell distribution width (RDW). The RDW is a parameter that expresses the degree of variation in cell size (anisocytosis). IDA results in small red blood cells whose size is highly variable, and therefore the RDW is elevated. The RDW discriminates IDA from thalassemia. With thalassemia, the red cells are uniformly small and the RDW is normal. The tests needed to evaluate the iron status are serum iron, TIBC, and ferritin. As explained in the physiology section, the serum ferritin, which measures iron stores, is the first measure to fall. This is followed by a decrease in the serum iron and an elevation of the TIBC. The measurement of serum iron reflects iron bound to serum proteins. Most iron is bound to transferrin. Normally transferrin is about one-third saturated. Serum total iron binding capacity is an approximate estimate of serum transferrin. Bone marrow aspiration is not usually necessary to make the diagnosis of IDA, but if done, the bone marrow would reflect diminished iron stores.

Once the diagnosis of IDA is established, a search for the underlying cause must be undertaken. The history may indicate which further tests need to be done. In the iron-deficient male and postmenopausal female, there is a strong possibility of occult bleeding from the gastrointestinal tract, and therefore endoscopic and possibly radiographic investigations of the GI tract should be done.

TREATMENT
Oral Route

This is the preferred treatment. Administer a ferrous iron salt (ferrous gluconate, sulfate, or fumarate, or ferrous sulfate syrup) and calculate the dosage according to the amount of elemental iron in the salt. For adults, administer 200 mg of elemental iron daily in three divided doses; for children, give 6 mg/kg of elemental iron daily in three divided doses. The maximum dose for children ages 1 to 5 years is 45 mg/day and for ages 6 to 12 years is 120 mg/day. Most iron tablets contain 60 to 70 mg of elemental iron, so that three tablets a day provide adequate iron therapy for an adult. Absorption is improved by giving between meals.

The most common side effect of iron therapy is gastrointestinal (GI) intolerance, particularly heartburn, nausea, and gastric discomfort. If GI intolerance occurs, lower the dose of iron. Iron therapy should be continued until anemia is corrected and then for an additional 6 months to replenish iron stores. During therapy, stools are black.

Parenteral Iron

In situations where oral iron is ineffective because of malabsorption, parental iron can be administered in the form of iron dextran, which can be given by intramuscular or intravenous routes. IV is the preferred route. Dosage (in mL) is based on the observed hemoglobin, desired hemoglobin level, and patient's lean body weight. A dosage chart comes with most product inserts. Anaphylaxis and other hypersensitivity reactions have been reported, and therefore parental iron should be used only when effective oral therapy is clearly impossible. As with oral iron, gastrointestinal side effects are not uncommon.

Transfusion

Indications for transfusion require individual evaluation of the patient. Generally, persons with a hemoglobin less than 6 g/dL require a blood transfusion. Patients with heart disease may require a transfusion at a higher hemoglobin measurement.

PATIENT EDUCATION

Instruct the patient on iron-rich foods. The patient should be informed as to the possible causes of the IDA. If the patient is experiencing symptoms, such as fatigue or depression, the clinician should tell the patient to what extent the anemia accounts for the symptoms. In the person without heart disease, it is unlikely that these symptoms can be attributed to anemia unless the hemoglobin is below 10.

DISPOSITION

Unless bleeding is acute, appropriate follow-up is to see the patient in 3 weeks to check on compliance and side effects from the iron therapy, and to do a reticulocyte count and CBC. An increased reticulocyte count indicates a response to treatment. At 3 weeks, a 2-g increase in hemoglobin is an adequate response. Failure to respond may indicate continued bleeding, malabsorption of iron, noncompliance, or incorrect diagnosis. The CBC must be monitored at frequent intervals until the anemia is corrected, and then at increasingly longer intervals.

PROGNOSIS

Iron-deficiency anemia due to dietary factors has an excellent prognosis. When the cause of IDA is bleeding, the prognosis depends on the ability to correct the underlying cause responsible for the bleeding.

BIBLIOGRAPHY

Deasy JA: Clinical interface: Three anemic patients. *Physician Assist* 15(6):58–62, 1991.

Hillman RS, Finch CA: *Red Cell Manual*, 5th ed. Philadelphia, Davis, 1985.

Leiner S, Mays M: Diagnosing microcytic anemia in adults. *Physician Assis* 20(3):24–26, 32–38, 56, 1996.

Ravel R: *Clinical Laboratory Medicine*, 6th ed. St Louis, Mosby, 1995.

Chapter 8–2
LEUKEMIA
Diane S. Wrigley

DISCUSSION

Discussion of leukemia can be lengthy, confusing, and highly complex. For purposes of this book and the relevance to the practicing physician assistant in clinical medicine, the information is concise and as practical as possible. Leukemia occurs as an acute or chronic disease. Leukemia is classified by type of blast or blood cell progenitors, and according to the course as follows:

- Acute lymphoblastic leukemia (ALL)
- Acute nonlymphoblastic leukemia (ANLL)
- Chronic myelocytic leukemia (CML)
- Chronic lymphocytic leukemia (CLL)

The yearly incidence is 13.2 in 100,000 in males and 7.7 in 100,000 in females. Seventy percent of leukemias occur in adults, mostly CLL and ANLL, 30 percent in children, mostly ALL. Leukemia is the 20th most common cause of cancer deaths. The type of leukemia defines the treatment and the prognosis.

With the current cure rate, especially good for childhood ALL, estimates predict that by the year 2010, 1 in 1000 young adults, between 15 and 45 years of age will be a childhood ALL survivor.

PATHOPHYSIOLOGY

Malignant clonal expansion of the hematopoetic stem cells leads to an accumulation of abnormal immature blood cell progenitors, or blasts, in the bone marrow and in other tissues. This process leads to marrow failure. It can be aggressive and rapidly fatal if not treated. The normal differentiation of stem cell maturity is interrupted, and immature cells occur. Systems affected are the heme, lymphatic, and immune systems. Genetics are unknown, but some forms appear to be familial. Precise cause is unknown.

SIGNS AND SYMPTOMS

Many of leukemia's signs and symptoms are nonspecific, relating to marrow failure or infiltration. There may be fever, bleeding as evidenced by petechiae, easy bruising, oozing, bone pain, pallor, fatigue, lymphadenopathy, hepatosplenomegaly, gingival swelling, or anemia with neutropenia and/or thrombocytopenia.

DIAGNOSTIC CONSIDERATIONS

Considerations here are very broad. All forms of bone marrow failure or invasion must be considered. Often a viral-induced cytopenia with lymphadenopathy and organomegaly can mimic a leukemia. Immune and drug-induced cytopenias must also be considered. A large number of patients may have low or normal white blood cell (WBC) counts, so a thorough examination of the peripheral blood for abnormal cells such as circulating blasts should be done. A careful history should document the onset of symptoms, date of the last normal blood count, family history, and exposure to chemicals or radiation. Ask whether the patient has had transfusions or a history of disseminated intravascular coagulation (DIC). Assess renal, cardiac, and hepatic function in preparation for possible chemotherapy.

RISK FACTORS

Genetic and chromosomal abnormalities, trisomy 21, and translocations are risk factors for leukemia. Other factors include radiation exposure; immunodeficiency states; chemical and drug exposure, such as nitrogen mustard and benzene; preleukemia; and cigarette smoking.

LABORATORY

A complete blood cell count (CBC) with differential should be done. Look for a reticulocyte count < 0.5, an elevated sedimentation rate, elevated lactate dehydrogenase (LDH) or uric acid chemistries, and low immunoglobulins (IgG). The coagulation profile may be abnormal or prolonged. *Caution*: Corticosteroid use may alter laboratory results.

DIAGNOSTIC PROCEDURES

In bone marrow studies, aspirates are stained for cell morphology, which is important for correctly identifying the type of leukemia, since this will have a direct bearing on treatment and prognosis. Biopsy of the marrow then provides information on cellularity, architecture, and megakaryocytic series. A marrow cell suspension is used for cytochemistries, such as Sudan black, confirming positive myeloblasts. The suspension can also be used for immunophenotyping to differentiate monoclonal versus polyclonal, B lymphocytes or T lymphocytes, early or late. Chromosome studies show the ploidy or presence of a translocation (Philadelphia chromosome), which is of prognostic value.

TREATMENT

Consult with a chemotherapist, and use inpatient care for acute leukemia treatment. The overall focus is recognizing and treating signs of infection, bleeding, CNS involvement, or tissue invasion. Respiratory difficulties, change in vision, and abdominal pain are examples of the latter. Chemotherapy is used to induce a marrow aplasia; if and when successful, hematopoiesis from the surviving stem cells lead to repopulation. This stage is called remission, not to be confused with cure or eradication. Advances in supportive care, indwelling central venous catheters, broad-spectrum antibiotics, antifungals, and blood product support improvements have decreased treatment-related deaths.

PATIENT EDUCATION

Patients need an adequately balanced diet and close follow-up on weight checks. There is a need for psychological support for children with leukemia and for their families. The emotional reaction of children is age-dependent, but a team approach with providers, nurses, social workers, and psychologists should help with the emotional as well as economic impact on the families.

Platelets and packed red blood cells (RBCs) for transfusion may be given. Isolation may be necessary. Watch for DIC.

Surgical measures include allogenic bone marrow transplants.

NOTES AND PEARLS

The overall prognosis for childhood leukemias continues to improve with 70 percent of patients achieving long-term disease-free survival. The following factors have prognostic significance:

- The higher the WBC at diagnosis, the poorer the prognosis.
- 2- to 10-year-olds fare best, adolescents less well, and infants under 1 year have only a 25 to 30 percent survival rate.
- Presence of CNS disease at diagnosis increases subsequent relapse.

BIBLIOGRAPHY

Hoffman R, Benz EJ, Shattil SJ, et al: *Hematology Principles and Practice.* New York, Churchill Livingstone, 1991, chap 58.

Rakel R (ed): *Conn's Current Therapy.* Philadelphia, Saunders, 1995, pp 390–412.

Schrier S, McArthur J: *Hematology.* Seattle, University of Washington School of Medicine, Education Program of the American Society of Hematology, 1993, pp 38–44.

Williams WJ, Beutler E, Erslev AJ, Lichtman MA: *Hematology,* 4th ed. New York, McGraw-Hill, 1990, chap 25.

Wood ME, Bunn PA Jr: *Hematology/Oncology Secrets.* Philadelphia, Hanley & Belfus; St. Louis, Mosby, 1994, chap 27.

Chapter 8–3
SICKLE CELL ANEMIA
Diane S. Wrigley

DISCUSSION

Sickle cell anemia is a chronic hemoglobinopathy transmitted genetically through an autosomal recessive gene, mostly found in persons of African-American descent. The result is a moderately severe chronic hemolytic anemia.

The homozygous form has a variant of sickle hemoglobin (Hb S). The heterozygous state carries one gene for the normal hemoglobin state (Hb A) and one for Hb S, thereby connoting a carrier state or exhibiting what is known as *sickle cell trait*. Between 8 and 10 percent of African Americans carry the trait. About 1 in 500 have the full disease, known as *sickle cell disease*. There is a 1 in 164 chance that two carriers will mate, and the chance of their offspring having the disease is 1 in 4. The illness affects all ages, males and females equally. It is also referred to as Hg S disease or S/S disease.

PATHOPHYSIOLOGY

There is a direct correlation between the concentration of Hb S and the susceptibility of sickling. Carriers, who have 50 percent Hb S, are symptom-free. The fact that infants carry a high concentration of hemoglobin F in the early months often hides the effect of the S hemoglobin. A high index of suspicion should exist when dactylitis appears in the 6- to 12-month age group, often a sign of sickle cell.

Red blood cells, which are normally biconcave or Frisbee-shaped, take on a sickle shape when deoxygenated. This may occur through oxygen tension less than 66 mmHg under such circumstances as high altitude, anesthesia, or scuba diving. A drop in temperature with subsequent vasoconstriction may affect the cells. An acidotic state with increase of hydrogen ions produces a right shift in the oxygen dissociation curve. Conversely, alkalosis helps retard sickling. Sickle-shaped cells are inflexible; hence, the rigidity causes increased blood viscosity, stasis, and mechanical obstruction of small arterioles, leading to distal ischemia. They are also more fragile, rendering them likely to hemolyze. The vasoocclusive crisis, or painful crisis, results in pain secondary to occlusion and tissue hypoxia and even necrosis. Progressive organ failure and acute tissue damage can be the result. Crisis may occur as frequently as once a day to less than once a year.

There appears to be an advantage in malarial endemic countries where infection is diminished due to the sickling effect of the cell. Evidence of cerebral malaria and death is low.

SIGNS AND SYMPTOMS

Sickle cell anemia is often asymptomatic in early months of life. The patient may present with pallor; symmetric, painful swelling of hands and feet, known as hand-foot syndrome; painful crises in bones, joints, abdomen, and back; and scleral icterus. There is increased susceptibility to infections, such as pneumococcal sepsis and *Salmonella* osteomyelitis. There may also be delayed physical or sexual maturation. Many multisystem complications may appear in later childhood and adolescence.

OBJECTIVE FINDINGS

Findings may include delayed puberty, but growth late into adolescence; dactylitis in about 50 percent of children on the dorsum of hands and feet; and bone manifestations mimicking osteomyelitis or arthritis. There can be other findings, like pulmonary emboli, jaundice, hepatomegaly, priapism with serious complications, tachycardia during crisis, retinal vessel obstruction, and cerebrovascular accidents.

LABORATORY FINDINGS

Hemoglobin is between 5 and 11 g/dL. The patient is normochromic and normocytic. There are elevated reticulocytes and a detectable presence of Hb S.

DIAGNOSTIC CONSIDERATIONS

Consider other hemoglobinopathies such as sickle cell hemoglobin C disease (Hb SC) disease, or sickle cell–β-thalassemia. The sickle cell anemia term is used for the homozygous state of the sickle cell gene. In a painful crisis, consider other etiologies, such as infections.

LABORATORY STUDIES

In hemoglobin electrophoresis, Hb S predominates and no Hb A is present. The sickle cell trait has both Hb S and Hb A. Screening can be done by Sickledex test or a sodium metabisulfite reduction test. Hemoglobin is about 8 g/dL, and there are normal indices, but mean corpuscular volume > 75. Look for reticulocytes to 10 to 20 percent; leukocytosis with normal bands; thrombocytosis; peripheral smear, a few sickled RBCs, nucleated RBCs, and polychromasia; elevated bilirubin; low erythrocyte sedimentation rate; elevated lactate dehydrogenase; and absent haptoglobin.

RADIOLOGIC STUDIES

Use a bone scan to rule out osteomyelitis and CT and MRI scans to rule out cerebrovascular accident.

NOTES AND PEARLS

Infections and other anemias may alter laboratory results.

TREATMENT

Treat infections and fevers with antibiotics. Minimize factors that enhance sickling. Use hydration for painful crises—twice the normal dose of maintenance fluids. Use transfusion with aplastic crisis, and hospitalize for most crises and complications. Assess the patient's growth and development and give regular immunizations, including Pneumovax.

With advancing molecular techniques in the '90s, multiple trials of hydroxyurea, given 10 to 30 mg/kg/day to patients with severe clinical cases of sickle cell, have been performed. The mechanism is unknown, but the drug does increase Hb F levels from three to five times. A concentration of 20% Hb F results in greatly reduced clinical symptoms. Long-term effects are unknown, and concerns about giving it to growing children remain. New Hb F stimulating agents such as butyrates are being studied. There is a prospect of using chemotherapeutic regimens to obtain Hb F levels with minimal toxic side effects.

HLA compatible donors as transplants have eradicated sickle cell in 80 percent of severely affected patients.

PATIENT EDUCATION

Tell patients they need bed rest during a crisis and a well-balanced diet with a folic acid supplement. Stress the importance of good hydration, and teach early recognition of possible complications. Genetic counseling may be valuable.

BIBLIOGRAPHY

Hoffman R, Benz EJ, Shattil SJ, et al: *Hematology Principles and Practice.* New York, Churchill Livingstone, 1991, chap 60.

Lusher JM, Sarnaik S: Hematology. *JAMA* 275(23):1815–1816, 1996.

Williams WJ, Beutler E, Erslev AJ, Lichtman MA: *Hematology,* 4th ed. New York, McGraw-Hill, 1990, chap 60.

Wood ME, Bunn PA Jr: *Hematology/Oncology Secrets.* Philadelphia, Hanley & Belfus; St Louis, Mosby, 1994, pp 46–48.

Chapter 8–4
APLASTIC ANEMIA
Diane S. Wrigley

DISCUSSION

In aplastic anemia the loss of the hemopoietic cells in the bone marrow fails to produce adequate numbers of peripheral blood elements. Aplastic anemia may also be referred to as pancytopenia. It can be acquired or genetic. The marrow becomes hypocellular, and hemopoietic cells may occupy as many as 25 percent of the marrow or as little as 0 to 5 percent. The injury to the marrow can be initiated by toxic, radiation, or immunologic etiologies to the erythroid elements. A single blood cell line may be involved at the beginning, followed by a full line of erythroid elements. Although the acquired form can be seen at all ages, it is usually a disease of the young, with the median age being 25 years. The genetic or constitutional form is limited to children and young adults.

PATHOPHYSIOLOGY

Bone marrow failure results from damage to the hemopoietic stem cells. This can occur because of damage to the DNA from exposure to radiation, chemicals such as benzene, or drugs such as chloramphenicol and cytotoxic drugs used in chemotherapy. Viruses have been known to be cytotoxic to stem precursors; 50 to 75 percent of cases of stem cell damage are idiopathic.

Radiation damage is dependent on the amount of energy absorbed and the radiosensitivity of the tissue. To put this in terms of visualization, doses of radiation are measured in sievert (Sv). At 0 to 1.0 Sv there are few if any symptoms. At 100 Sv there is 100 percent mortality rate. Cosmic rays give 0.001 Sv compared with a radioactive isotope such as a thyroid scan, which gives 0.001 Sv.

In this industrialized society potentially toxic compounds are limitless: insecticides, fertilizers, food additives, and benzene radicals for both household and commercial uses. All hydrocarbons are suspected in the etiology of aplastic anemia, as are insecticides such as pentachlorophenol, lindane, and DDT.

Introduced over 40 years ago, chloramphenicol has an inherent risk of 1 in 20,000 to 30,000 of causing aplastic anemia, but that still is 10 to 20 times the idiopathic risk. The anemia is reversible when the drug is withdrawn. Specifically, the chloramphenicol affects the maturation and proliferation of the marrow precursor cells, then irreversibly damages the genetic structure of the stem cells. Stem cells produced without the influence of the drug return to normal. Other drugs implicated are the nitrobenzene compounds. As many as 75 drugs have been implicated, but the hydantons, pyrazoles, sulfonamides, and gold have an unusual affinity for this relationship. No specific genetic pattern is detected in acquired aplastic anemia. However, there may be a genetic defect in the ability to handle drug elimination or detoxification, leaving stem cells vulnerable.

Infections, such as hepatitis viruses commonly cause up to 5 percent of marrow failures, while Epstein-Barr virus, rubella, and parvovirus have also been implicated. Paroxysmal nocturnal hemoglobinuria has been associated with pancytopenia.

Immunologic changes, such as graft-versus-host disease, or other states of immune status change, such as pregnancy, can cause damage to these stem precursors. Presence of antibodies to stem cells is a phenomenon in the immunologic or autoimmune etiology. Suppression of normal stem cell function can also be caused by the action of abnormal stem cells.

Another form of aplastic anemia is inherited; called Fanconi syndrome or constitutional anemia, it was first described in 1927. There is an autosomal recessive gene in constitutional Fanconi syndrome.

A considerable loss can take place in the marrow before peripheral blood is affected. Pure red cell aplasia is a related syndrome caused by selective failure of the erythroid elements, leaving leukocyte and platelet counts unaffected.

SYMPTOMS

Patients look and feel well. The onset is usually insidious. Symptoms caused by anemia, infections exacerbated by neutropenia, and cutaneous bleeding associated with thrombocytopenia are frequently treated symptomatically until purpura, with its more serious connotations, forces a more complete hematologic evaluation. The less severe form of aplastic anemia is striking in that the symptoms are restricted to the hematologic system. Prognosis is dependent on the degree of anemia. When neutrophil counts are <500/mm^3, platelets < 20,000, and reticulocyte count < 1 percent, it is considered severe. In acquired aplastic anemia, bleeding is an early symptom of a severe level, as are fatigue, weakness, shortness of breath (SOB), pounding sensation in ears, pallor, and weight loss.

OBJECTIVE FINDINGS

Physical examination may be very unremarkable. Ecchymoses, petechiae, melena, occult stool blood, retinal flame hemorrhage, systolic ejection murmur, menorrhagia, and purpura may all be present. In short, many of the objective findings have to do with hypovolemia and hypoxia from lack of circulating cells. In constitutional anemia, short stature, microcephaly, and renal anomalies prevail.

DIAGNOSTIC CONSIDERATIONS

Beware of other causes of pancytopenia. Lack of peripheral elements can be due to destruction after the marrow has produced them. A bone marrow biopsy will rule this out. A mean corpuscular volume (MCV) of greater than 100, indicating a possible megaloblastic anemia from deficiencies that are easily reversible, is a good clue to normal marrow elements. Splenomegaly and lymphadenopathy are conspicuously absent in true aplastic anemia. Other myelodysplastic disorders may be mistaken for aplastic anemia.

SPECIAL CONSIDERATIONS

Persons with early very severe aplastic anemia that is not treated may have a median survival of only 3 to 6 months. Patient history taking should include careful attention to exposure to drugs and conditions in the workplace and home.

LABORATORY

Do a complete blood cell count (CBC) with evidence of pancytopenia, specifically anemia, leukopenia, neutropenia, and thrombocytopenia, but normochromic RBCs. Check for increased bleeding time, decreased reticulocyte count, normal total iron-binding capacity (TIBC), high MCV (>104), and hematuria. Erythropoietin levels increase up to 500 to 1000 times normal values. Check liver function tests (for hepatitis). Check for increased fetal hemoglobin (Fanconi syndrome). Other diagnostic tests include a bone marrow biopsy. Check for increased iron stores, decreased cellularity (<10 percent), and decreased megakaryocytes, myelocytes, and erythroid precursors.

RADIOLOGIC STUDIES

X-ray radius and thumbs; do a renal ultrasound if constitutional anemia is suspected.

TREATMENT

Admit the patient to a facility with experienced practitioners. Consider a bone marrow transplant. Eighty percent are done in those <20 years of age, with severe anemia and a human leukocyte antigen (HLA) compatible donor. If the patient has been transfused, then the risk of graft-versus-host reaction increases. For patients older than 40 years, give antithymocyte globulin therapy (AGT) at 40 mg/kg/day for 4 days. Use cyclosporine at 12 mg/kg/day for adults and 15 mg for children. Consider androgen therapy. Signs of infection are treated aggressively with parental or broad-spectrum antibiotics. Treatment is empiric. Do not wait

for cultures. Ensure scrupulous hand washing. Do platelet transfusions with leukocytes removed for platelet counts of <10,000 because of risk of intracranial bleed. Suppress menstruation in females. Avoid aspirin and nonsteroidal anti-inflammatory drugs. Transfuse with RBCs to get the Hb at 7.0 g or better at 2 U every 2 weeks. If transfusions are to be chronic, then an iron chelation, deferoxamine, by the 50th unit may be necessary to avoid a secondary hemochromatosis or iron overload.

SUPPORTIVE MEASURES

Give oxygen therapy to help with SOB and lack of hemoglobin transport of O_2. Isolation precautions may be indicated. Encourage a nutritious diet and good oral hygiene.

PATIENT EDUCATION

Avoid likely causative agents, and prepare for a search of unrelated donor transplants if other therapies fail.

BIBLIOGRAPHY

Griffith CJ: Evaluation and management of anemia. *Adv PA* 4(5):33–38, May 1996.

Hoffman R, Benz EJ, Shattil SJ, et al: *Hematology Principles and Practice.* New York, Churchill Livingstone, 1991, chap 18.

Williams WJ, Beutler E, Erslev AJ, Lichtman MA: *Hematology*, 4th ed. New York, McGraw-Hill, 1990, chap 18.

Wood ME, Bunn PA Jr: *Hematology/Oncology Secrets*. Philadelphia, Hanley & Belfus; St Louis, Mosby, 1994, pp 43–46.

Chapter 8–5
HEMOCHROMATOSIS
Diane S. Wrigley

DISCUSSION

Hemochromatosis, or iron overload disease, is caused by increased iron absorption from the gut. The nature of this defect is unknown. Since the body cannot excrete iron, the excess is stored in organs such as liver, pancreas, and heart. The condition is genetic, with the homozygote occurring as frequently as 1 in 200 to 1 in 600 persons, with an incidence of clinical disease of 8 to 13 percent of the homozygous population. Normally two-thirds of the total body iron is found in red blood cells, making up about 2 g of iron. The remaining one-third is found in storage iron that is in the form of iron storage protein, ferritin. The term *hemochromatosis* is used for the state of iron overload with resultant tissue damage.

The heterozygote state occurs in approximately 1 in 10 people, making it the most abnormal gene in the U.S. population. The clinical disease is often detected between ages 40 and 60, with the incidence of males to females being 8 : 1. The biggest risk of untreated hemochromatosis is formation of hepatomas. Once established, the treatment of the disease does not affect the clinical outcome of the malignancy. The goal of treatment is early identification and treatment, thereby reducing morbidity and mortality rates.

PATHOPHYSIOLOGY

Iron that is in the reticuloendothelial cells is harmless, but if iron is stored in parenchymal cells, it is a noxious agent. Consequences of untreated iron overloading are increased skin pigmentation and hepatomegaly with increased risk of hepatoma. Iron metabolism appears normal in this disease, but there is a higher level of circulating iron. Iron usually is stored as ferritin, but in this case can be stored as hemosiderin. Ferritin levels may be as high as 700 and into the thousands. Twenty grams of excess iron is necessary to cause clinical disease.

The signs and symptoms of hemochromatosis are much the same as diabetes, arthritis, impotence, and congestive heart failure (CHF). The disease is probably underdiagnosed because the incidence of these diseases is so common.

RISK FACTORS

Loss of blood delays onset of symptoms, so menstruating and pregnant women exhibit lag in time of presentation. Intake of iron in supplement form with not only the iron but also vitamin C enhances iron absorption. Increased alcohol consumption enhances iron absorption.

SIGNS AND SYMPTOMS

Look for weakness; abdominal pain; arthralgia, particularly in large joints and metacarpal phlangeal joint (MCP); loss of libido or sexual potency; amenorrhea; increased skin pigmentation; hepatomegaly; and diabetes mellitus symptoms.

OBJECTIVE FINDINGS

Hepatomegaly, splenomegaly, jaundice, hepatic tenderness, and increased skin pigmentation can be appreciated on physical examination. Testicular atrophy and gynecomastia, found in alcoholism are also often present. A good physical examination with positive confirmation of appropriate laboratory tests exclusively looking for hemochromatosis will result in a proper diagnosis.

DIFFERENTIAL DIAGNOSIS

The differential diagnosis includes repeated transfusions, hereditary anemias with ineffective erythropoiesis, alcoholic cirrhosis, and excessive iron ingestion (rare).

LABORATORY TESTS

Ferritin >300 μg/L for men and >120 for women is diagnostic. If the saturation is >62 percent, then the homozygous state can be predicted with 92 percent accuracy. Once it is suspected, the firm diagnosis can be made by liver biopsy, staining specifically for iron and identifying excess iron deposition in hepatocytes. Quantitative iron on the hepatic tissue as well as evidence of cirrhosis can also be checked. Also look for urinary iron; decreased follicle-stimulating hormone (FSH), luteinizing hormone (LH), testosterone, albumin as indications of hemochromatosis; oral glucose tolerance test to rule out hyperglycemia; and increased serum glutamic-oxaloacetic transaminase (SGOT).

DIAGNOSTICS

Use an echocardiogram to rule out cardiomyopathy. Consider a liver biopsy for iron particles when there is evidence of cirrhosis.

TREATMENT

The best treatment is phlebotomy. One unit of blood contains 250 mg of iron. At least 80 phlebotomies will be necessary to normalize total body iron. Once patients have achieved normal iron levels, then only two to four phlebotomies a year will be required for maintenance. Patients with induced (not hereditary) hemochromatosis associated with transfusion therapy should receive treatment with an iron chelating agent. An iron-free diet is not necessary.

Patients with mild clinical disease have a normal life span. Patients with diabetes mellitis (DM), cardiac damage, or hepatic cirrhosis have decreased survival rates. Phlebotomy at that stage does not decrease the risk of developing a hepatoma.

NOTES AND PEARLS

Hepatic computer tomography and MRI and magnetic susceptibility measurements (MSM) are in the future.

PATIENT EDUCATION

Teach patients to avoid alcohol and iron-fortified foods. Restrict vitamin C to small doses between meals. Tea chelates iron, so the patient may drink tea with meals. Once a firm diagnosis of hemochromatosis is made, immediate family members should also be screened for the disease. The best treatment is early intervention. Patients may enjoy full activity unless there is evidence of significant heart disease.

BIBLIOGRAPHY

Williams WJ, Beutler E, Erslev AJ, Lichtman MA: Disorders of iron metabolism, in *Hematology,* 4th ed. New York, McGraw-Hill, 1990, pp 752–758.
Wood ME, Bunn PA Jr: *Hematology/Oncology Secrets.* Philadelphia, Hanley & Belfus; St Louis Mosby, 1994, chap 15.

Chapter 8–6
HEMOLYTIC ANEMIA
Diane S. Wrigley

DISCUSSION

Hemolytic anemia can be acquired or inherited. In this disease red blood cell destruction occurs prematurely as a result of immunologic, physical, or chemical injury. The mechanism of the destruction is the binding of autoantibodies and/or complement to the red cells. Physical injury may result from cardiac pathology, narrowed heart valves, pathologic shunts, valve prosthesis, and increased tissue temperatures. Chemical causes include exposures to arsenic or copper or inappropriate water exposure. A drop in Hb of >1 g/week should be suspicious for excessive blood loss or hemolysis. The congenital form involves intrinsic defects of the RBC membrane. The clinical manifestations of the acquired versus the inherited forms are the same. The hereditary anemia is a common autosomal dominant disease of varying severity.

PATHOGENESIS

Three components of the red blood cell that are involved in hemolytic anemia are the membrane, the Hb, and the intracellular erythrocyte enzymes that provide adenosine triphosphate (ATP) energy and reducing equivalents. Patients who once had a normal hematocrit and normal reticulocyte can be diagnosed as having the acquired form as opposed to inherited. The mechanism of hemolysis or rupture of the normal RBCs is the same as in persons with intrinsic red cell defects. The integrity of the RBC can be overcome when exposed to sufficiently severe stress. In hereditary spherocytosis (HS), the RBC intrinsic defect plus the intact spleen selection in retaining the abnormal cells contribute to the pathophysiology. In accelerated HS, RBC destruction is a multistep process resulting from dysfunction of the skeletal proteins of the membrane.

RISK FACTORS

Acquired hemolytic anemia is idiopathic in 50 percent of cases. Risk factors include warm and cold antibodies, neoplasias (leukemias, myelomas, lymphomas, thymomas), collagen vascular disease, viral infections, and drugs such as methyldopa, quinidine, penicillin, sulfasalazine, phenazopyridine hydrochloride, and sulfonamides. Additionally, insect venoms, excessive water inhalation in drownings, excessive distilled water in the circulation such as in dialysis or surgical procedures and increased heat >47°C (extensive burns) may cause hemolysis.

OBJECTIVE FINDINGS

Vital sign findings include increased pulse and change in blood pressure with postural changes. These occur with marked blood loss. There is pallor of skin and/or palpebral conjunctival pallor in dark-skinned patients. Splenomegaly and lymphadenopathy are also found.

LABORATORY

Spherocytes, schistocytes, and helmet cells are found in the peripheral smear in the complete blood cell count (CBC). There is elevation of the mean corpuscular hemoglobin concentration (MCHC) indices and elevated reticulocyte count. Do an indirect hyperbilirubinemia test and a CBC, noting RBC indices values and laboratory comments on cells. Also do an osmotic fragility test, which tests the integrity of the RBC membrane. Cells that are susceptible to easy damage will hemolyze at hypertonic saline concentrations. A Coombs' test is positive direct in 90 percent of autoimmune hemolytic anemia patients since it measures immunoproteins; the indirect Coombs' measures antibodies that are formed with the glucose-6-phosphate dehydrogenase (G6PD), deficiency. This is an enzyme abnormality resulting in the RBC's inability to defend itself against oxidative assaults. The oxidants damage vital cell constituents. Patients lacking the enzyme exhibit signs of hemolysis if exposed to oxidant drugs such as the nitrofurantoin or even ingest fava beans. Looking at the laboratory's comments and finding "Heinz" bodies should raise the suspicion of G6PD insufficiency. The gene for the G6PD deficiency is on the X chromosome. Look for suspicious drug levels of antimalarials, sulfonamides, nitrofurantoins, chloramphenicol, aspirin, and ascorbic acid, which all may be measured if suspected in a case of hemolytic anemia. Other tests include indirect bilirubin, haptoglobin, IgG and IgM antibodies, and lactate dehydrogenase (LDH).

SYMPTOMS

Symptoms of hemolytic anemia include weakness, fatigue, dyspnea on exertion, dizziness, palpitations, malaise, pallor, splenomegaly and hepatomegaly, anemia, hemoglobinemia, and jaundice.

SUPPORTIVE MEASURES

Ensure rest until the patient is asymptotic; no special diet or restrictions are required. Check family history for any hemolytic anemias.

TREATMENT

Give 1 to 1.5 mg/kg/day of prednisone for rapid hemolysis or IV cortisone at 400 to 800 mg/day. Consider a splenectomy. Give large amounts of IV gamma globulin 0.5 to 1.0 g/kg infused for 5 days. Prescribe daily chlorambucil, 2 to 4 mg orally to decrease the rate of cold agglutinin. Remove offending causes.

PATIENT EDUCATION

Make patient aware of potentiating factors, if identified, and talk about avoidance in the future. A screening is recommended for the congenital form if one relative is identified.

BIBLIOGRAPHY

Griffith CJ: Evaluation and management of anemia. *Adv PA* 4(5):33–38, May 1996.

Hoffman R, Benz EJ Jr, Shattil SJ, et al: *Hematology Principles and Practice.* New York, Churchill Livingstone, 1991, chap 37.

Williams WJ, Beutler E, Erslev AJ, Lichtman MA: *Hematology,* 4th ed. New York, McGraw-Hill, 1990, chaps 55, 65, 66.

Chapter 8–7
HENOCH-SCHÖNLEIN PURPURA
JoAnn Deasy

DISCUSSION

Henoch-Schönlein purpura (HSP) is a vasculitis that is more common in childhood, but may affect adults. Vasculitis is an inflammatory and often destructive process affecting the arteries and veins. The median age of onset of HSP is 6 years, and males are affected twice as often as females.[1] The cause of this condition is unknown. An association has been shown with a preceding exposure to an infectious disease agent (particularly viruses causing upper respiratory infections) and drugs.

HSP is considered an IgA-mediated vasculitis of small vessels. The most commonly involved organs are the skin, joints, gastrointestinal tract, and kidneys. It has been postulated that there is a trapping of immune complexes in the vessel wall and activation of complement which results in the production of complement breakdown products that are chemoattractants to polymorphonuclear leukocytes (PMNs). These PMNs accumulate at the site of inflammation and release various enzymes and free radicals, resulting in damage to the vessel wall.[2] Histologically, granulocytes are seen in the walls or perivascular cuff of arterioles or venules.

SIGNS AND SYMPTOMS

The most characteristic manifestation of HSP is the typical rash, which occurs primarily over the buttocks and lower extremities, but may involve the entire body. The skin lesions may consist of urticarial wheals, erythematous macules and papules, petechiae, and palpable purpura. New lesions may continue to occur in crops. Arthritis of the large joints and acute abdominal pain may occur. When arthritis occurs before the rash of HSP, diagnosis can be difficult. The knee and ankle joints are most commonly involved, and the arthralgias may be migratory. When abdominal pain is present, it is usually diffuse and may be severe, presenting as an acute abdomen. The pain is often described as crampy and is thought to be due to hemorrhage and the accumulation of fluid primarily in the small intestine. Other gastrointestinal symptoms include bloody or nonbloody diarrhea, nausea, and vomiting. If there is renal involvement, hematuria may be present but usually is a later symptom occurring during the second or third week of the illness.

OBJECTIVE FINDINGS

Petechiae and purpura involve blood that is extravascular, and therefore the color does not blanch with pressure. If swelling of the joints is present, the swelling is often periarticular and not a true joint effusion. The findings on abdominal examination may be inconsistent with the severity of the abdominal pain. The tenderness to palpation is often diffuse, and signs of peritoneal irritation are usually absent. However, intussusception may occur as a complication with associated abdominal distension, and a tubular mass may be palpable.

COMPLICATIONS

Glomerulonephritis and nephrotic syndromes may occur. It is thought that the glomerulonephritis is due to deposition of immune complexes in the glomeruli. Approximately 20 percent of children have renal involvement during the acute attack.[2] Only a small number go on to have persistent renal disease. Death from renal failure has occurred. Intussusception of the small bowel, testicular torsion, and involvement of the central nervous system are other possible complications.

DIAGNOSTIC CONSIDERATIONS

Conditions which may present similarly to HSP include systemic lupus erythematosus, thrombocytopenia purpura, the rash of meningococcemia, subacute bacterial endocarditis, rickettsial diseases, and Walderstom's hyperglobulinemic purpura.

LABORATORY TESTS

A platelet count, platelet function tests, and a bleeding time are ordered. Results should be normal. Urinalysis may show hematuria and proteinuria. Stool occult blood may be positive. IgA may be elevated.

RADIOGRAPHIC STUDIES

If intussusception is suspected, ultrasonography or barium enema should be ordered to confirm this complication.

TREATMENT

There is no specific treatment for HSP. In severe cases, a short course of corticosteroids may provide relief of symptoms but does not alter the course of the disease.

PROGNOSIS AND DISPOSITION

The disease is usually self-limited, and the prognosis for complete recovery is excellent. Attacks may recur in some patients for months to a year after the initial onset. In patients with renal involvement, hematuria and proteinuria may persist and regular periodic follow-up is essential.

REFERENCES

1. Schaller JG, Szer IS: Systemic lupus erythematosus, dermatomyositis, scleroderma, and vasculitis in childhood, in Delley WN, Harris ED Jr, Ruddy S, et al (eds): *Textbook of Rheumatology*, 3d ed. Philadelphia, Saunders, 1989, pp 1340–1341.

2. Athreya BH: Vasculitis in children. *Pediatr Clin North Am* 42(5):1239–1261, 1995.

BIBLIOGRAPHY

Patrignelli R, Sheikh S, Shaw-Stiffel TA: Henoch-Schönlein purpura. *Postgrad Med* 97(5):123–134, 1995.

Chapter 8–8
PERNICIOUS ANEMIA
Diane S. Wrigley

DISCUSSION

Pernicious anemia (PA) is a disease of unknown origin in which the basic defect, atrophy of the gastric mucosa (parietal cell), eventually leads to the lack of intrinsic factor (IF) and hydrochloric acid (HCl) secretion. PA is categorized under the megaloblastic macrocytic anemias: mean corpuscular volume (MCV) > 95 percent in the RBC indices. The incidence of PA is about 25 cases per 100,000 per year. Average age of onset is 60. The predisposition to developing PA may have a genetic basis, but precise information is lacking. There is a positive family history in up to 30 percent of patients with clinical PA.

PATHOPHYSIOLOGY

Since vitamin B_{12} can be absorbed only by binding to IF, the end result is B_{12} deficiency. These macrocytic anemias account for about one-third of the anemias because ability to incorporate B_{12} into new RBC synthesis, impairing DNA synthesis, results in a dissociation between the maturation of the nucleus and cytoplasm in developing cells. An RBC with an immature nucleus has open chromatin and is enlarged or megaloblastic.

There is a significant association of PA with other autoimmune diseases such as Graves', Hashimoto's, hypoparathyroidism, vitiligo, and adult-onset hypogammaglobulinemia.

PA may affect up to 10 percent of the population older than 70 years. Achlorhydria and partial, subtotal gastrectomies are contributing factors in the elderly, in addition to the loss of pepsin. Total gastrectomy leads to removal of IF producing cells. Ninety percent of patients with PA have anti-IF-antibodies in either the serum or gastric juice. Although a genetic predisposition is shown, the full expression of pathology, which appears to be autoimmune, may be modified by acquired environmental influences.

RISK FACTORS

Alcoholism with or without liver disease can cause B_{12} deficiency. Drugs such as ascorbic acid, colchicine, cholestyramine, neomycin, cimetidine, and oral contraceptives have been implicated. Folate deficiency and lack of dietary B_{12} ingestion, as well as strict vegetarianism, with no dairy products and bacterial overgrowth syndromes in the gut competing for vitamin B_{12}, all play a role in macrocytic, megaloblastic anemias.

LABORATORY

Look for complete blood cell count (CBC) > 95 MCV, decreased reticulocytes, low hemoglobin and hematocrit, and hypersegmented polymorphonuclear sites. Check vitamin B_{12} and folate levels. Do a Schilling test. Radioactive B_{12} is given orally. The amount excreted in the urine is measured. Patients lacking IF do not absorb B_{12}; therefore, they do not excrete it. Serum methylmalonic acid is increased in >95 percent of B_{12}-deficient patients. Values may be as high as 2,000,000; normal is between 70 and 270. B_{12} is essential in mammals as a cofactor in two enzymes. Reduced activity of these critical enzymes leads to an increase in methylmalonic acid.

SYMPTOMS

Symptoms of severe anemia include weight loss, GI symptoms like bloating and diarrhea, infertility, orthostatic hypotension, loss of proprioception, ataxia, memory loss, abnormal smell or taste, and listlessness or hallucinations.

OBJECTIVE FINDINGS

Objective findings include glossitis, stomatitis, premature gray hair, and neurologic symptoms from pareathesias and dysesthesias of extremities (particularly lower extremities) and depression to frank psychosis.

TREATMENT

Give IM or subcutaneous vitamin B_{12} once per week for 8 weeks, then one time per month for the rest of the patient's life. Use oral treatment with B_{12} at a dose of 10 μg/day for strict vegetarians.

PATIENT EDUCATION

Response to therapy is the ultimate determination of existence of deficiency, regardless of the etiology. Screen of symptomatic family members. Get the general family history.

BIBLIOGRAPHY

Griffith CJ: Evaluation and management of anemia. *Adv PA* 4(5):33–38, May 1996.
Wood ME, Bunn PA Jr: *Hematology/Oncology Secrets.* Philadelphia, Hanley & Belfus; St Louis Mosby, 1994, pp 34–39.

Chapter 8–9
POLYCYTHEMIA VERA
Diane S. Wrigley

DISCUSSION

Polycythemia vera is one of a group of myeloproliferative disorders with resultant excessive erythroid, myeloid, and megakaryocytic elements in the bone marrow. It is considered a clonal disorder, which means there is an unregulated growth of a malignant cell. Patients with polycythemia have increased numbers of CFU-GEMM (colony-forming units—granulocytes, erythroids, macrophages, megakaryocytes). These units have demonstrated unregulated proliferation in culture in the absence of erythropoietin. The prevalence in the population is 0.5 per 100,000, males slightly outnumber females, and the predominant age is middle to late years, the mean being 60 years of age. Untreated patients have a median survival rate of about 18 months from diagnosis. Treated patients may live 10 to 15 years.

Individuals with relative or spurious polycythemia have normal red blood cell mass and conditions that reduce the plasma volume, causing hemoconcentration. Real polycythemia or polycythemia vera has an elevated RBC mass (>36 mL/kg for males or >32 mL/kg for females). Generally the hematocrit is >60 percent without any evidence of dehydration.

PATHOPHYSIOLOGY

The increased blood volume leads to generalized vascular expansion and venous engorgement. The increased blood viscosity is reflected in the characteristic ruddy cyanosis of the skin and mucous membranes. These factors are magnified by the significant decrease in cerebral blood flow that goes with an elevation of the hematocrit and contributes to the symptoms of headaches, tinnitus, and an often described feeling of fullness or light-headedness in the head and neck. The consequence is an increase in thrombotic complications, particularly in the cerebrovascular circulation. Epistaxis and upper GI hemorrhage also may occur. The resultant hypervolemia may result in decreased cardiac output, ultimately impairing tissue oxygenation.

The proliferative phase, which is the initial phase, has ineffective hematopoiesis. The bone marrow biopsy may reveal a trilinear hyperplasia; that is, hemoglobin, platelet, and white blood cell production are increased. The peripheral smear may also mirror this. Vascular congestion, splenomegaly, bleeding, and thrombosis are seen in this stage.

The spent phase is seen after about 10 years in a small percentage of patients (5 to 15 percent). Now extensive bone marrow fibrosis and ineffective hematopoiesis are evident. Anemia is due to splenic sequestration, iron deficiency, and excessive bleeding due to platelet dysfunction. Between 20 and 50 percent of cases at this stage transform into acute leukemia, carrying a poor survival prognosis of 70 percent mortality within 3 years.

DIAGNOSTIC CONSIDERATIONS

Consider secondary polycythemias. Affected individuals have evidence of tissue hypoxia or erythropoietin-secreting tumors. High erythropoietin levels will be detected. This increased level may be appropriate in chronic obstructive pulmonary disease (COPD), sleep apnea, and cardiovascular shunts. Renal disease such as hydronephrosis, cysts, and renal transplants can also account for this level.

LABORATORY

Do a complete blood cell count (CBC), looking for increased RBC mass, WBCs > 12,000. Check for iron-deficiency anemia (check total iron-binding capacity (TIBC) and percent iron saturation), leukocytosis, elevated leukocyte alkaline phosphatase (LAP) score, increased vitamin B_{12}, increased uric acid and lactate dehydrogenase (LDH), increased platelet >500,000, and a normal erythropoietin level.

OBJECTIVE FINDINGS

In the early stages there are no objective findings. Then headaches, tinnitus, vertigo, blurred vision, and epistaxis may appear. There is plethora of hands, face, and feet. There may be arterial and venoocclusive events, sweating, weight loss, splenomegaly or hepatomegaly, bone tenderness and pain, gout, pruritus, and ruddy cyanosis of complexion. There may be evidence of peripheral vascular disease. However, signs of infection are *not* present.

Table 8-10-1. Select Gene Combinations in α-Thalassemia

Hemoglobin Genes*	Diagnosis	Implications
$\alpha\alpha/\alpha\alpha + \beta/\beta$	Normal adult hemoglobin	None
$-\alpha/\alpha\alpha + \beta/\beta$	α-Thalassemia silent carrier	None
$-\alpha/-\alpha + \beta/\beta$	α-Thalassemia trait	Moderate microcytic anemia, more common in African Americans
$--/\alpha\alpha + \beta/\beta$	α-Thalassemia minor	Moderate microcytic anemia, more common in Asians
$--/-\alpha + \beta/\beta$	Hemoglobin H disease	Moderate to severe anemia
$--/-- + \beta/\beta$	α-Thalassemia major (Bart's disease)	Hydrops fetalis, stillbirth, high-risk pregnancy

* Minus sign indicates missing gene.

TREATMENT

Use phlebotomy to reduce hemoglobin to <14 g for males and <12 g for females. Cytoreductive drugs such as hydroxyurea or interferon can be used adjunctively with phlebotomy. ^{32}P and chlorambucil have been effective in the past, but the high incidence of leukemia developing precludes usage except as a last resort.

NOTES AND PEARLS

When a patient shows increased hemoglobin levels, always search for a secondary and reversible causes. Consider high altitude, excessive smoking, medications (particularly anabolic steroids and corticosteroids), burns, and stress such as the elusive pheochromocytoma. An iron deficiency may mask an increased RBC volume as may a folate or B_{12} deficiency. RBC volumes in the obese are imprecise. The hypoxic smoker may have polycythemia as well—look for elevated WBC or an elevated platelet count. Splenectomy during the proliferative phase of polycythemia vera carries a high thrombolytic risk from the release of a large volume of pooled platelets.

BIBLIOGRAPHY

Dale DC, Federman DD: *Sci Amer Med* 5:1–10, 1997.
Williams WJ, Beutler E, Erslev AJ, Lichtman MA: *Hematology,* 4th ed. New York, McGraw-Hill, 1990, chap 21.
Wood ME, Bunn PA Jr: *Hematology/Oncology Secrets*. Philadelphia, Hanley & Belfus; St Louis Mosby, 1994, pp 50–56.

Chapter 8–10
THALASSEMIA
JoAnn Deasy

DISCUSSION

Thalassemias are common hereditary hemoglobinopathies. Patients are classified as having *thalassemia trait (minor)*, *thalassemia intermedia*, or *thalassemia major*, depending on the severity of their anemia. Thalassemia trait is underdiagnosed and frequently misdiagnosed as iron-deficiency anemia. An alert practitioner who recognizes the potential for prevention of congenital disease and who watches for microcytosis on electronic blood counts, can identify persons with thalassemia trait. Working toward the prevention of homozygous thalassemia, an invariable fatal condition, can be accomplished through the detection and education of heterozygous carriers.

The thalassemias constitute a group of congenital disorders in which there is defective production of the globulin chains, alpha or beta. α-Thalassemia is due to gene deletion. (See Table 8-10-1.) Normal individuals inherit two alpha-chain genes from each parent. Deletion of one of the four genes results in a silent carrier state with no hematologic abnormalities. Persons with deletion of two alpha-chain genes have α-thalassemia trait (also referred to as α-thalassemia minor), causing microcytosis with or without anemia. Deletion of three genes causes a compensated hemolytic, microcytic anemia, called hemoglobin H disease. Deletion of all four genes (Bart's disease) is incompatible with fetal survival as a result of hydrops fetalis. The diagnosis of homozygous disease is also important because of associated serious obstetric complications to the mother. α-Thalassemia syndromes primarily affect persons from Southeast Asia and China and African Americans.

The β-thalassemias are usually caused by mutations rather than deletions. Individuals inherit only one beta chain from each parent. Therefore β-thalassemias are either heterozygous, homozygous, or compound heterozygous, such as, sickle β-thalassemia. The heterozygous state, β-thalassemia trait (β-thalassemia minor), results in a hematologic picture similar to α-thalassemia trait. The homozygous state, β-thalassemia major, produces a severe, life-threatening anemia sometimes called Cooley's anemia. β-Thalassemia affects persons of Mediterranean origin, African Americans, Chinese, and other Asians. Thalassemia intermedia patients may have a combined α- and β-thalassemia defect, or a milder form of homozygous beta thalassemia, or beta thalassemia with high production levels of hemoglobin F.

SYMPTOMS

Thalassemia trait (minor) is generally asymptomatic, since the degree of anemia is usually mild. Most often thalassemia trait is diagnosed in asymptomatic persons who undergo an evaluation for microcytosis detected on a routine electronic blood count. In differentiating thalassemia trait from iron-deficiency anemia (IDA), the medical history should include questions regarding diet and the possibility of blood loss. Inquiry as to the duration of the anemia and previous hemoglobin determinations should be made, as well as to racial origin and the presence of anemia in other family members. Persons with thalassemia intermedia and β-thalassemia major have symptoms referable to their anemia; fatigue, dyspnea on exertion, faintness, and palpitations. The presentation of a patient with hemoglobin H disease is clinically that of an α-thalassemia intermedia.

OBJECTIVE FINDINGS

There are no characteristic physical findings associated with α- or β-thalassemia trait. Hemoglobin H disease can vary in its severity. Physical examination of some patients with hemoglobin H disease may reveal pallor and splenomegaly. α-Thalassemia major results in stillbirth. Children affected with β-thalassemia major (Cooley's anemia) develop a severe anemia during the first year of life with numerous subsequent clinical abnormalities. On physical examination, jaundice and hepatosplenomegaly are usually present. There may be sexual and growth retardation and skeletal abnormalities. The findings in thalassemia intermedia vary with the severity of the anemia; hepatosplenomegaly may be present. Transfusion therapy leads to cardiomyopathy and

Table 8-10-2. Types of Hemoglobin

Adult Hb—Hg A	$\alpha_2\beta_2$	>95% of the adult Hb	
Fetal Hb—Hb F	$\alpha_2\gamma_2$	70% of the Hb at birth	
		<1% of adult Hb	
Hb A$_2$	$\alpha_2\delta_2$	<3% of adult Hb	

other dysfunctions. Death from cardiac failure generally occurs between ages 20 and 30.

DIFFERENTIAL DIAGNOSIS

The α- and β-thalassemia trait must be differentiated from other causes of microcytosis and is frequently confused with IDA. (See Table 8-10-1.)

LABORATORY DIAGNOSIS

In persons with uncomplicated α- and β-thalassemia trait, the microcytosis is striking [mean corpuscular volume (MCV) is 60 to 75] and more prominent than the anemia. This is because the red blood cell (RBC) count is relatively high, resulting in only a slight decrease in the hemoglobin level, or even a normal hemoglobin. This is in contrast to patients with IDA, in whom the anemia is usually more prominent with a lesser degree of microcytosis and with lower RBC counts. The red cell distribution width (RDW) that is generated by an electronic blood count tends to be normal in thalassemia trait because of the uniform microcytosis. IDA produces more anisocytosis (degree of variation in cell size), and thus the RDW tends to be elevated. The peripheral blood smear will reveal microcytic cells with possible hypochromasia and target cells. In β-thalassemia trait, basophilic stippling may be present.

β-Thalassemia trait can be diagnosed by ordering hemoglobin electrophoresis, which will demonstrate an increase in Hb A$_2$ (normal = <3.5 percent). If IDA and β-thalassemia trait coexist, the Hb A$_2$ will not be elevated. Once the IDA is successfully treated, the elevated Hb A$_2$ will be exposed. β-Thalassemia major (Cooley's anemia) is suggested by a severe anemia that becomes evident at 2 to 3 months of age with hypochromic RBCs, target cells, many nucleated RBCs, and a high-risk ethnic origin. Diagnosis is made by demonstrating elevation of Hb F on hemoglobin electrophoresis. In addition, an alkali denaturation test can be done. Hb F is more resistant to denaturation than is Hb A. (See Table 8-10-2.)

Currently, there is no easy laboratory test to diagnose α-thalassemia trait. It is usually a diagnosis of exclusion. However, the cord blood of a baby with thalassemia trait or hemoglobin H disease will show the presence of Bart's hemoglobin by electrophoresis in approximate proportion to the severity of the anemia. By the age of 4 to 6 months Bart's hemoglobin generally disappears. After that age, globulin chain synthesis studies or the DNA probe technique can be used, but these are available only in research laboratories.

TREATMENT

Usually, no treatment is indicated for thalassemia trait. Chronic transfusions are the mainstay of treatment for β-thalassemia major (Cooley's anemia). Iron chelation therapy is used to prevent iron overload. Some individuals with thalassemia intermedia also require transfusion.

PATIENT EDUCATION

Once individuals are diagnosed with thalassemia minor, they should be informed so that they are not unnecessarily treated with iron in the future. Patient education should include partner screening and preconception counseling.

BIBLIOGRAPHY

Deasy JA: Clinical interface: Three anemic patients. *Physician Assist* 15(6):58–62, 1991.

Hillman RS, Finch CA: *Red Cell Manual*, 5th ed. Philadelphia, Davis, 1985.

Lops VR, Hunter LP, Dixon LR: Anemia in pregnancy. *Am Fam Physician* 51(5):1189–1197, 1995.

Ravel R: *Clinical Laboratory Medicine*, 6th ed. St Louis, Mosby, 1995.

Chapter 8–11
THROMBOCYTOPENIA
Diane S. Wrigley

DISCUSSION

Thrombocytopenia is a decrease in the number of platelets to <100,000/mL due to platelet destruction, decreased production, sequestration of platelets in the spleen, or a combination of any of the three.

PATHOPHYSIOLOGY

The clinical presentation varies depending on the presence or absence of pancytopenia and the etiology. The hallmark is petechiae, which reflect bleeding at the level of the capillary venule. Usually petechiae develop over the lower extremities, because of elevated hydrostatic pressure and constrictive clothing, and in the oral mucosa, because of the masseter's force on the surface while chewing. Decreased platelets may be due to decreased numbers of megakaryoblasts and replacement of the bone marrow by abnormal tissue. Abnormal maturation of megakaryocytes may also contribute. Deficiency of vitamin B$_{12}$ or folate can result in thrombocytopenia due to ineffective thrombopoiesis or hematopoietic dysplastic syndromes. Increased destruction of platelets can be secondary to immune disorders such as idiopathic thrombocytopenic purpura (ITP) or systemic lupus erythematosis (SLE); chronic lymphocytic leukemia; infectious diseases such as mononucleosis, cytomegalovirus (CMV), or AIDS; and drugs such as heparin, sulfa, quinidine, acetaminophen, and gold salts. Nonimmune disorders of destruction include disseminated intravascular coagulation (DIC), sepsis, malaria, paroxysmal nocturnal hemoglobinuria (PNH), acute renal transplant rejection, and congenital cyanotic heart disease. Disorders of distribution may occur because of hypersplenism and increased sequestration of platelets.

SYMPTOMS

Patients feel well, but may have menorrhagia, easy bruising, petechial rash, excessive bleeding with cuts or dental work, purpura, or splenomegaly.

OBJECTIVE FINDINGS

There are skin and oral mucosal changes. A complete blood cell count (CBC) peripheral smear establishes presence of decreased platelets as well as abnormal morphology.

DIAGNOSTIC CONSIDERATIONS

It is necessary to look for the cause.

LABORATORY

Recommended tests include CBC and reticulocytes, vitamin B_{12} and folate levels, a direct Coombs' test, and a coagulation panel including bleeding time. Prothrombin time (PT) and partial thromboplastin time (PTT) are normal.

RADIOLOGIC STUDIES

Use a CT of the head to rule out intracranial bleeding.

OTHER DIAGNOSTICS

Do a bone marrow biopsy if hypoplastic marrow is suspected. A normal marrow with only decreased numbers of megakaryocytes suggests drug ingestion rather than a neoplastic process. A platelet associated antibody (PA-IgG) test may be useful.

TREATMENT

Remove the offending agent. Replace vitamin B_{12} and folate if indicated. Consider doing a platelet transfusion: 1 U = 10,000 platelets that will circulate approximately 24 h. Give prednisone, 20 to 30 mg/day, to maintain vascular integrity. Supportive measures include outpatient management, unless actively bleeding. Recommend minimal activity to prevent bruising. Tell the patient to avoid contact or collision sports and avoid aspirin and other platelet-inhibiting drugs.

BIBLIOGRAPHY

Hoffman R, Benz E, Shattil S, et al: *Hematology Principles and Practice.* New York, Churchill Livingstone, 1991, chaps 15, 123, 125.

Wood ME, Bunn PA Jr: *Hematology/Oncology Secrets.* Philadelphia, Hanley & Belfus; St Louis, Mosby, 1994, pp 64–67.

Chapter 9–1
HIV/AIDS

Claire Babcock O'Connell

DISCUSSION

In the early 1980s, the first clusters of opportunistic infections and neoplasms in gay men were reported to the Centers for Disease Control and Prevention (CDC). This often fatal syndrome of immune breakdown was designated gay-related immune disease (GRID) and prompted a strong public outcry and fear (the "gay plague"). In the ensuing years, the number of persons with this acquired immune deficiency state grew exponentially, affecting people from all walks of life around the world. In 1984, after massive epidemiologic analysis and biologic research, the etiology of AIDS (acquired immunodeficiency syndrome) was isolated, and the agent was later named the *human immunodeficiency virus* (HIV).

Today an estimated 15 million people worldwide are believed to have been infected with HIV, two-thirds of whom have met the criteria for the diagnosis of AIDS; over half these patients have died. Spread of the virus continues in all segments of society despite ongoing public education. Much has been learned about the biology and clinical spectrum of HIV disease. Treatment options have undergone a substantial evolution; reactive treatment against opportunistic infections and neoplasia is being replaced by proactive treatment against the virus. The most recent advances in the treatment of HIV involving triple therapy with nucleoside analogues and protease inhibitors have provided the first glimpse of a possible cure or at least chronic control of disease progression. However, despite preliminary work on treatment and vaccines, education and public health efforts aimed at controlling the spread of the virus remain the only effective method of halting the epidemic.

BIOLOGY OF HIV

HIV is a single-stranded RNA virus in the retrovirus family. It is an icosahedral that has a significant ability to mutate. The biology of HIV has been studied extensively; the development of new drugs and vaccines is a direct result of increased understanding of the virus. The virus attaches to the host cell, predominantly the CD4+ (T-helper) lymphocytes, fuses with the host cell membrane, and enters the cell. The virion contains reverse transcriptase, which is required to produce DNA from RNA, and the DNA then gets integrated into the host nucleus, seizing control of the cell and dictating replication and integration of virus. The infected host cell can no longer function. Loss of functioning T-helper cells, to which HIV has the greatest affinity, as well as loss of monocytes, macrophages, Langerhans cells, and other members of the human immune system, leads to the profound deficiency state that is characteristic of AIDS.

TRANSMISSION

HIV does not survive well outside cells. It quickly dies when exposed to air, heat, or a variety of chemicals. Transmission occurs through body fluids: parenteral exposure to blood or blood products (including exchange through contaminated intravenous drug paraphernalia), exchange of sexual fluids through sexual contact, and vertical transmission between an infected mother and her child perinatally or through breast milk. There has been no documented transmission of HIV through casual contact, tears, saliva, respiratory droplets, or insects. Public health and preventive efforts have highlighted these facts of transmission in an attempt to allay public fear and stem the growth of the epidemic. Barrier methods are effective against sexual transmission. All blood and blood products have been screened for the virus since 1985. Occupational risk among health care workers is minimized through the practice of universal precautions. Infected pregnant women receive antiviral treatment to reduce the incidence of vertical transmission.

SYMPTOMS

HIV disease should be viewed as a continuum of initial exposure, asymptomatic infection, symptomatic disease, and end-stage AIDS. Progression along the continuum cannot be predicted; the rate of decline varies significantly. Each patient must be evaluated as an individual, and, together with the health care team, decisions for assessment and treatment can be made throughout the course of the disease.

The Acute HIV Syndrome

More than half the individuals who contract HIV experience an acute syndrome 3 to 6 weeks after the primary infection. However, many individuals do not recall symptoms, or the symptoms are thought to result from other infections or bodily stress. The typical scenario is a constellation of flulike symptoms similar to mononucleosis, including fever, pharyngitis, arthralgias and myalgias, headache, lethargy, and anorexia. These patients also may have lymphadenopathy and nausea, vomiting, and diarrhea. The flulike syndrome is associated with the initial dramatic rise in the viral count. Less often, patients may experience signs of meningitis, encephalopathy, peripheral neuropathy, or dermatologic conditions.

Unless a clinician maintains a suspicion for HIV infection, the syndrome may be misdiagnosed and the infection may go undetected. Clinicians should be alert for the acute HIV syndrome in any patient presenting with fever and mononucleosis-like symptoms, especially if the patient is sexually active or is known to inject drugs. The syndrome persists up to 2 to 3 weeks and gradually wanes. The decline in symptomatology accompanies the immune response. In most patients, the immune system begins to produce antibodies to different sections of the virus. The level of immunity is inversely proportional to the level of virus.

Clinical Latency

After the acute HIV infection, the virus is sequestered in lymph tissue and the body mounts a response. Viral load declines, antibodies to the virus appear, and molecular changes in the immune system are detectable. Clinically, there is a variable period of freedom from symptoms. This period may last many years (median, 10 years). There are several documented cases of symptom-free periods continuing after two decades of infection. However, there is no true latent period. It is now known that even in the face of normal immune function and low levels of virus detectable in the blood, the virus continues to multiply. The level of activity and the speed of decline in the immune system vary among individuals, ranging from a few weeks to decades, but occur in all untreated infected patients. Antiretroviral therapy is aimed at halting this progression. A cure is still not available.

Symptomatic Disease

The onset of clinical symptoms may begin any time after the initial infection with HIV. The median length of time between infection and clinical disease is 10 years. The CDC has compiled a list of clinical diseases or states that qualify a patient for a diagnosis of AIDS (Table 9-1-1). This list has been reevaluated and expanded in response to increased epidemiologic and biologic information throughout the history of the HIV epidemic. A diagnosis of AIDS (symptomatic HIV disease) is important for surveillance and gives the patient access to treatment and government-funded community and psychosocial resources.

The most frequent manifestation of HIV disease after the acute syndrome is a generalized lymphadenopathy without another cause. The nodes are multiple, found in more than two locations, larger than 1 cm, smooth, mobile, and persistent. They are caused by a follicular hyperplasia in response to the virus. Biopsy is not indicated unless another separate or confounding pathology is suspected. In general, the lymphadenopathy occurs early in the course of HIV disease, although it may occur after symptoms of neoplasia or opportunistic infection. Reduction in nodal size or quantity late in HIV disease may be a poor prognostic sign that indicates further loss of immune capacity and function.

As the decline in immune function progresses, the clinical manifestations become more apparent and frequent. When the CD4+ count falls below 500, patients begin to exhibit clinical signs of oral thrush, herpes simplex or zoster, and oral hairy leukoplakia and declining numbers of platelets, leukocytes, and erythrocytes. Patients may have weight loss, unexplained fevers, dementia, and diarrhea. Below a count of 200, opportunistic infections and neoplasia are very likely to occur. In general, the more common manifestations of advanced HIV disease can be predicted from the CD4+ count (Figs. 9-1-1 and 9-1-2), although exceptions in either direction are possible. Patients can be diagnosed with a disease or condition with higher than predicted CD4+ counts, and some patients with very low CD4+ counts do not show any clinical disease.

HIV disease encompasses myriad clinical presentations. The clinical syndromes may be due to HIV itself, opportunistic infection, neoplasia, psychosis, or depression (Table 9-1-2).

HIV may manifest clinically in any body system or systems. The presentation is widespread and varied. Table 9-1-3 provides a list of conditions grouped by system that are typically encountered in patients with HIV disease.

PATIENT HISTORY

The medical history is an important tool in the initial evaluation of suspected HIV infection and for the monitoring of known HIV-positive individuals. Careful attention to behavioral factors is paramount. A complete sexual history should be obtained in all patient encounters, with special emphasis on behaviors known to be of high, intermediate, and low risk (Table 9-1-4).

The sexual history must be completed free of judgments and assumptions. A prior history of sexually transmitted diseases, hepatitis B, sexual trauma, or prostitution should alert the practitioner to HIV risk. The use of alcohol and recreational drugs also must be assessed; the common correlation with the use of mind-altering substances and unsafe sex is well documented.

Table 9-1-1. Centers for Disease Control and Prevention Surveillance Case Definition for AIDS, 1993

A. Indicator diseases diagnosed definitively in the absence of other causes of immunodeficiency and without laboratory evidence of HIV infection
   1. Candidiasis of the esophagus, trachea, bronchi, or lungs
   2. Cryptococcosis, extrapulmonary
   3. Cryptosporidiosis with diarrhea persisting >1 month
   4. Cytomegalovirus disease of any organ excluding liver, spleen, and lymph nodes in a patient >1 month of age
   5. Herpes simplex virus infection causing a mucocutaneous ulcer persisting >1 month or bronchitis, pneumonia, or esophagitis in a patient >1 month of age
   6. Kaposi's sarcoma in a patient <60 years of age
   7. Lymphoma of the brain (primary) in a patient <60 years of age
   8. Lymphoid interstitial pneumonia and/or pulmonary lymphoid hyperplasia in a child <13 years of age
   9. *Mycobacterium avium* complex of *Mycobacterium kansasii* disease (disseminated)
   10. *Pneumocystis carinii* pneumonia
   11. Toxoplasmosis of the brain in a patient >1 month of age
B. Indicator diseases diagnosed definitively regardless of the presence of other causes of immunodeficiency and in the presence of laboratory evidence of HIV infection
   1. Any disease listed in section A
   2. Bacterial infections (multiple or recurrent) in children <13 years of age caused by *Haemophilus, Streptococcus,* or other pyogenic bacteria
   3. Coccidioidomycosis, disseminated
   4. HIV encephalopathy
   5. Histoplasmosis, disseminated
   6. Isosporiasis with diarrhea persisting >1 month
   7. Kaposi's sarcoma at any age
   8. Non-Hodgkin's lymphoma of B-cell or unknown phenotype having the histologic type of small noncleaved lymphoma or immunoblastic sarcoma
   9. Any mycobacterial disease, disseminated, excluding *Mycobacterium tuberculosis*
   10. *M. tuberculosis,* extrapulmonary
   11. *Salmonella* (nontyphoid) septicemia, recurrent
   12. HIV wasting syndrome
C. Indicator diseases diagnosed presumptively in the presence of laboratory evidence of HIV infection
   1. Candidiasis of the esophagus
   2. Cytomegalovirus retinitis with loss of vision
   3. Kaposi's sarcoma
   4. Lymphoid interstitial pneumonia and/or pulmonary lymphoid hyperplasia in a child <13 years of age
   5. Mycobacterial disease, disseminated
   6. *P. carinii* pneumonia
   7. Toxoplasmosis of the brain in a patient >1 month of age
D. Indicator diseases diagnosed definitively in the absence of other causes of immunodeficiency and in the presence of negative results for HIV infection
   1. *P. carinii* pneumonia
   2. Other indicator diseases listed in section A and CD4+ T-lymphocyte count <400/μL
E. The 1993 expanded definition includes
   1. All HIV-infected persons who have <200 CD4+ T-lymphocyte counts per microliter or a CD4+ T-lymphocyte percentage of total lymphocytes <14
   2. Pulmonary tuberculosis
   3. Recurrent pneumonia
   4. Invasive cervical cancer

Sharing needles and trading sex for drugs are strong indicators of risk. A patient who is HIV-positive must continue to be counseled regarding behaviors that carry a risk of transmission of HIV to others and contact with potentially fatal pathogens in the face of the patient's compromised immune system function.

Figure 9-1-1. Major opportunistic infections in advanced HIV infection.

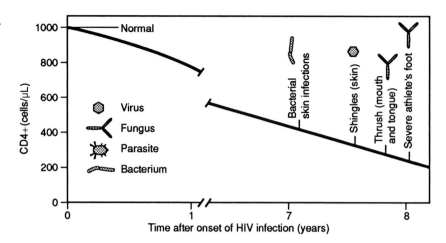

Portions of the review of systems in each patient encounter also warrant special emphasis. Constitutional symptoms such as fever, fatigue, and weight loss can be caused by HIV or by infection. Skin changes, respiratory complaints, gastrointestinal or genitourinary symptoms, and changes in mental status also may herald disease progression.

OBJECTIVE FINDINGS

A thorough physical examination is warranted in all patients; specific areas are of particular importance in assessing HIV disease. The respiratory examination and the examination of the skin may uncover the first signs of HIV disease; *Pneumocystis carinii* pneumonia and Kaposi's sarcoma remain the most common initial case-finding conditions in HIV disease. The skin examination also may reveal signs of herpes infection, molluscum contagiosum, syphilis, or staphylococcal infection.

Examination of the oral mucosa may reveal signs of candidiasis, herpes, oral hairy leukoplakia, and Kaposi's sarcoma. Patients with oral candidiasis and dysphagia are presumed to have esophageal candidiasis and do not need to be endoscoped before the initiation of treatment. Lymphadenopathy should be recorded in terms of size, number, location, and tenderness; correlation to HIV disease and/or an opportunistic infection is necessary. Biopsy should be reserved for cases in which the nodes are associated with fever or weight loss to assess for lymphoma or mycobacteria.

The genital examination may reveal the lesions or ulcers of sexually transmitted diseases. Pap smears should be performed every 3 months in HIV-positive women to detect cervical dysplasia. The rectum and anus may exhibit signs of sexually transmitted diseases or cancer.

A complete neurologic examination should be performed on all new HIV-positive patients and any patients who present with changing symptoms. Changes in mental status may be subtle; caregivers or companions may provide insight into changes in personality or behavior. Motor and sensory examinations and assessment of reflexes will aid in the analysis of neurologic diseases or possible drug side effects such as peripheral neuropathy.

LABORATORY TESTS

HIV Testing

The standard test for HIV infection is an enzyme-linked immunosorbent assay (ELISA) for antibodies to the HIV virus. The "HIV test" has been available since March 1985. It has high sensitivity and is relatively inexpensive. False-positive ELISA tests may occur in patients with systemic lupus erythematosus or pregnancy and in conditions that produce rheumatoid factor or

Figure 9-1-2. Major opportunistic infections in advanced HIV infection *(continued)*.

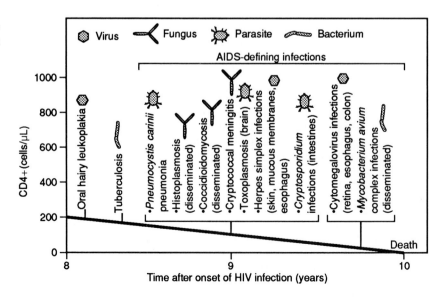

Table 9-1-2. Grouping of Common HIV Clinical Conditions by General Etiology

    I. HIV proper
        AIDS dementia
        Aseptic meningitis
        Sensory neuropathy
        AIDS enteropathy
        Renal failure/AIDS nephropathy
   II. Opportunistic infections
        A. Bacterial
            Mycobacterium
            Streptococcus
            Haemophilus
            Staphylococcus
            Pseudomonas
            Neisseria
            Shigella
            Salmonella
            Campylobacter
        B. Fungal
            Cryptococcus
            Cryptosporidium
            Coccidioides
            Histoplasma
            Aspergillus
            Microsporidium
            Candida
            Isospora
            Toxoplasma
        C. Viral
            Herpes simplex
            Herpes zoster
            Epstein-Barr
            Cytomegalovirus
        D. Protozoan
            Toxoplasma
            Pneumocystis
  III. Neoplasia
        Kaposi's sarcoma
        Non-Hodgkin's lymphoma
        Hodgkin's lymphoma
        Cervical cancer
        Anal cancer
   IV. Psychosis and depression

Table 9-1-3. Manifestations of HIV Disease by System

Pulmonary
    Pneumocystis carinii pneumonia
    Bacterial pneumonia
    Tuberculosis and other mycobacterial diseases
    Lymphoid interstitial pneumonia
    Disseminated histoplasmosis
    Disseminated coccidioidomycosis
    Aspergillosis
    Cytomegalovirus
    Kaposi's sarcoma
    Lymphoma
Gastrointestinal
    Candidiasis ("thrush")
    Esophagitis
    Acute and chronic diarrhea
        Cryptosporidium
        Microsporidiosis
        Mycobacterium
        Cytomegalovirus
        Isosporosis
        Other bacterial (shigella, shigellosis, campylobacter infection)
    AIDS enteropathy
    Wasting syndrome
    Lymphoma
Ophthalmologic
    Retinal disease (cotton-wool spots)
    Cytomegalovirus retinitis
    Toxoplasmosis chorioretinitis
    Necrosis (herpes simplex, varicella)
    Optic neuropathy
Hematology/oncology
    Cytopenia
    Thrombocytopenia
    Anemia
    Neutropenia
    Hematopoietic suppression
    Kaposi's sarcoma
    Non-Hodgkin's lymphoma
    Hodgkin's lymphoma
    Cervical cancer
    Anal cancer
Neurologic
    Toxoplasmosis
    Cryptococcal meningitis
    Progressive multifocal leukoencephalopathy
    Cytomegalovirus meningitis
    Syphilis
    Lymphoma
    AIDS dementia
    Aseptic meningitis
    Sensory neuropathy
Renal
    Fluid and electrolyte imbalances
    Acid-base disorders
    Renal failure
    HIV nephropathy
Cardiac
    Ventricular dysfunction
    Myocarditis
    Pericarditis
    Endocarditis
    Arrhythmias
Endocrine
    Adrenal dysfunction
    Hypogonadism
    Hypothyroidism
Rheumatology
    Arthralgia
    Myopathy
    Reiter's syndrome
    Sjögren's syndrome
    Arthropathy
    Vasculitis

cryoglobulins. False-negative ELISA tests occur in the early "window" period after infection (up to 12 months; average period, 3 months) and also in the later stages of symptomatic AIDS. The most common cause of false-positives and false-negatives is laboratory error. Any positive ELISA test is repeated; if it is again positive, a confirmatory Western blot (immunoblot) test is performed. If the Western blot is also positive, the patient is diagnosed as HIV-positive. If either of the ELISA tests is positive and the Western blot is negative or if the ELISA is negative but a strong suspicion is held, the patient is retested in 3 months. Meanwhile, all patients should be counseled regarding risk factors and educated to reduce any possible impending risk of transmission to the patient and the patient's contacts. A patient with a negative ELISA or Western blot may indeed be positive for the virus but not yet mounting an immune response.

Laboratory tests are available for detecting various parts of the virus, such as the p24 antigen and the β_2-microglobulin; other tests measure antibodies to other parts of the virus but generally are confined to the research arena. Recent scientific advances show the potential for some of these testing methods to become part of the standard diagnostic protocol. Direct culture of the virus is a very slow process that is performed exclusively in research trials. Several virus particles are undergoing testing in the hope of developing a vaccine; to date no preventive or therapeutic vaccine is available.

Table 9-1-4. Sexual Practices and Risk for HIV/AIDS

Safe
  Massage
  Hugging
  Stroking
  Mutual masturbation (no skin cuts or breakage)
  Self-masturbation
  Dry kissing
  Monogamous relationship between two uninfected partners
  Abstention
Possibly safe
  French (wet) kissing
  Anal intercourse using a latex condom
  Vaginal intercourse using a latex condom
  Urine contact (not with mouth, rectum, or any broken or cut skin)
Possibly unsafe
  Cunnilingus
  Fellatio
  Fellatio without ejaculation
  Sharing of sexual devices
Unsafe
  Receptive anal intercourse without a condom
  Vaginal intercourse without a condom
  Anilingus
  Unprotected anal penetration with the hand
  Anal douching with oral sex
  Multiple sex partners

SOURCE: From Cohen.

Routine Laboratory Analysis

When a patient is known to be HIV-positive, several laboratory tests should be performed on a scheduled basis. Baseline counts of leukocytes, erythrocytes, and platelets are important for prognosis, disease state, and detection of changes resulting from drug therapy. Anemia is very common in HIV disease patients, as is neutropenia, especially if a patient is receiving antiretroviral therapy. Clinicians should monitor cell counts and initiate therapy as is appropriate. Renal function and liver enzymes also should be recorded before the initiation of any therapy, and as monitoring tools, serum glucose, protein, and albumin are important in assessing overall health and nutritional status. Changes in liver enzymes may indicate hepatitis or drug toxicity.

Serologic tests for syphilis are recommended; positive screening results should be followed with specific treponemal testing and appropriate antisyphilis therapy. Patients with latent syphilis should have the CSF examined for organisms in light of the high risk of neurologic involvement with syphilis in HIV-positive patients. Skin testing for tuberculosis is mandatory in all HIV-positive patients. Any reaction >5 mm in a patient who is HIV-positive should be treated with a minimum of 1 year of isoniazid. In geographic areas with a high prevalence of multidrug-resistant tuberculosis, treatment should be adjusted accordingly.

The CD4+ Count

HIV has a particular affinity for CD4+ cells. The virus can attach to the surface of these cells like Velcro, enter a cell, and begin the cycle of viral replication and dysfunction and the death of immune cells. A normal CD4+ count is above 500; most people have above 1000/μL. The CD4+ count has become the most widely used method to track HIV disease progression. As the disease progresses, the number of CD4+ cells declines, indicating continuing destruction of the immune system. Parameters of CD4+ counts have been established for use in diagnosing HIV disease and in predicting the risk of acquiring an opportunistic infection and therefore assisting in the decision for prophylaxis. A CD4+ count below 200/μL meets the CDC criteria for AIDS

regardless of symptom status. It is also the level at which prophylaxis against the most common opportunistic infections (*P. carinii* pneumonia and toxoplasmosis) and treatment with retrovirals [azidothymidine (AZT)] has generally been recommended, although these recommendations have been controversial and are undergoing renewed analysis in light of the introduction of newer anti-HIV medications.

Viral Load

The most recent advance in HIV laboratory testing is direct viral load measurements. These tests encompass polymerase chain reactions (PCRs) to detect viral RNA by augmenting viral replication in the lab and a branched DNA (bDNA) test that detects viral RNA via a light-producing reaction in the lab. Viral load may offer an excellent marker of disease progression. Studies have shown an inverse relationship between viral load and CD4+ count and therefore the probability of clinical symptoms. As the CD4+ count is a marker of change in the immune system and its ability to function, viral load is a marker of viral progression. Together, the tests may prove to be powerful indicators of disease status with or without clinical symptoms. However, it is also widely believed that only about 2 percent of the virus circulates in the blood at any time. Therefore, a very low or even negative viral load test does not guarantee a virus-free state even in a patient with a high CD4+ count.

TREATMENT

The goals of treatment in HIV disease are multiple. First and foremost is to identify patients infected with HIV and ensure their access to medical treatment and monitoring. Once HIV is identified, a variety of services are needed to manage the complex medical and psychosocial needs of HIV-positive patients. Medical management starts with a full history and physical examination to assess the patient and the status of the HIV infection as well as any preexisting non-HIV-related diseases or conditions. Control of HIV replication and enhancement of immune function are a constant struggle; the development of new drugs is aimed at solving this conflict. The ultimate goal is to have zero HIV units and a fully functional immune system. This goal has not been met, but research is ongoing.

Throughout the course of HIV disease, the prevention, diagnosis, and management of opportunistic infections and malignancies are key to patient survival. Death more commonly is due to overwhelming infection or malignancy than to HIV itself. As patients progress through the stages of HIV disease and end-stage AIDS, simple needs such as housing, transportation, nutritional supplements, emotional counseling, bereavement counseling, legal services, and financial assistance for medical costs and living expenses become important. Health care practitioners must work with other service providers to provide effective and efficient care.

There are four broad areas of treatment: conventional care (prophylaxis and treatment of opportunistic infections, prevention of HIV transmission, antiretroviral and protease inhibitors), preventive care and wellness (nutrition, exercise, stress reduction, and elimination of smoking, alcohol excess, and drug abuse), psychological counseling (suicide prevention, management of anxiety and depression, grief and loss counseling), and nontraditional approaches (hypnosis, biofeedback, physical manipulation, unorthodox therapies). This chapter emphasizes conventional care.

Several drugs have been approved for use against HIV. The first drugs developed were reverse transcriptase inhibitors that act by blocking the ability of the virus to transcribe viral RNA into host DNA. The latest drugs are the protease inhibitors, which act by blocking the protease enzyme that is active further in the cycle of HIV replication. The new viral copies that are manufactured in the host cell are thus rendered unable to infect new host cells.

Reverse Transcriptase Inhibitors (Nucleoside Analogues)

AZT (Retrovir, Zidovudine, ZDV)

AZT was the first anti-HIV drug approved. It is often recommended to begin therapy with AZT when the CD4+ count drops below 500/μL, presumably before irreversible damage has occurred in the immune system, but many clinicians believe that the earlier any therapy is started, the better the outcome will be. Other practitioners reserve treatment until symptoms appear or the CD4+ count drops below 200/μL. Monotherapy with AZT has been replaced with combination therapy, which has proved to be much more effective and to delay the emergence of resistance. The success of the most recent clinical trials combining AZT with another reverse transcriptase inhibitor and/or protease inhibitor has caused combination therapy to become the norm in HIV treatment.

AZT has been shown to delay the decline in CD4+ cells, reduce viral load (previously assessed via the p24 antigen test but now measurable through newer PCR methods), decrease opportunistic infections, prevent or reduce HIV-associated dementia, and significantly alter the risk of vertical transmission. The usual dose is 200 mg orally tid; the minimum effective dose is 300 mg/d. Side effects include nausea, headache, and fatigue; these symptoms usually abate after the first few weeks of therapy. Myelosuppression is a serious side effect. The complete blood count (CBC) should be monitored every 3 months. Some patients can survive with seriously low blood cell counts; others may benefit from the addition of granulocyte-stimulating factor (G-CSF) or erythropoietin.

ddI (Videx, Didanosine)

Another nucleoside analogue, ddI, also inhibits reverse transcriptase. It is indicated in patients with advanced infection, prolonged therapy with AZT, or intolerance to or progression of disease in the presence of AZT. It has been used as monotherapy as well as in combination with AZT. This drug also delays the decline in the CD4+ count, reduces the viral burden, and reduces the rate of disease progression. The usual dose is 200 mg orally bid. This drug must be taken on an empty stomach, and the taste is not well tolerated. Side effects include pancreatitis and peripheral neuropathy as well as nausea and fatigue. Some clinicians monitor amylase levels every 1 or 2 months. Vitamin B complex therapy may help manage the peripheral neuropathy.

ddC (HIVID, Zalcitabine)

ddC was first introduced as monotherapy for patients who could no longer tolerate AZT or had developed resistance to AZT. These patients had advanced disease (CD4+ below 300/μL). ddC reduces the rate of CD4+ decline and reduces the viral burden. The usual dose is 750 μg tid. About 20 percent of patients on ddC suffer from peripheral neuropathy; pancreatitis has also been problematic.

d4T (Zerit, Stavudine)

d4T was developed for use as another alternative in patients with advanced disease who could not tolerate AZT or were progressing despite AZT. The usual dose is 40 mg orally bid, and the most common side effect is peripheral neuropathy.

3TC (Lamivudine)

3TC was the fifth reverse transcriptase inhibitor developed. It is most efficacious when used with AZT to reduce the viral load and slow the decline in the CD4+ count. The usual dose is 150 to 300 mg orally bid. Side effects are minimal.

Protease Inhibitors

Invirase (Saquinavir)

Invirase was the first protease inhibitor approved for anti-HIV therapy. It is a complex synthetic peptide that is very expensive. It has poor oral bioavailability and high first-pass metabolism, making it the least potent of the protease inhibitors. Invirase has been shown to be effective when used in combination with at least two other antiretrovial medications. It is fairly safe and well tolerated. Diarrhea and abdominal pain are the most common side effects; patients also may exhibit elevated liver enzymes. Invirase may limit the effects of rifampin and may cause arrhythmias in patients taking terfenadine (Seldane), astemizole (Hismanal), or cisapride (Propulsid) because of interaction within the cytochrome P450 pathway. Invirase is available in 200-mg tablets; three tablets every 8 h with a fatty meal is the recommended dose. Resistance develops quickly, especially when Invirase is used along. Cross-resistance to other protease inhibitors also develops very rapidly after the induction of resistance to Invirase. A newer formulation of Invirase with higher bioavailability may improve the clinical value; until such time, Invirase is not recommended unless a patient has exhausted all other protease inhibitors.

Ritonavir (Norvir)

Ritonavir is a potent protease inhibitor that has been shown to be effective against HIV. Patients have exhibited a substantial reduction in viral load; in some cases the viral load has dropped below detection. Ritonavir also has caused increases in CD4+ cells and CD8+ cells. Patients receiving Ritonavir have demonstrated significant drops in short-term mortality and progression to advanced disease, especially when it is used in combination therapy. Gastrointestinal side effects are common, including moderate to severe nausea, vomiting and diarrhea, anorexia, taste disturbance, and circumoral paresthesia. An improved gel cap formulation of the drug, as well as the practice of dose escalation, has helped reduce the side effects. Interactions with terfenadine, alprazolan (Xanax), meperidine (Demerol), cisapride (Propulsid), and many other drugs occur through the shared cytochrome P450 metabolic pathways; this is a serious consideration in patients with advanced disease who may be taking many different drugs. Ritonavir is available in 100-mg tablets; six tablets every 12 h is recommended.

Indinavir (Crixivan)

Indinavir has shown the most profound and durable impact on viral load in clinical trials. It also has resulted in significant increases in CD4+ counts. Early trials showed a sustainable reduction of viral load in some patients, although many patients on monotherapy or lower doses reverted back to increasing viral loads after 6 months of therapy. Resistance is also more likely to develop with less than optimal dosing. There is a low rate of gastrointestinal side effects, including abdominal pain, nausea, and reflux; indinavir may exacerbate preexisting elevation of liver enzymes. The drug produces a sludgelike effect, causing kidney stones in about 5 percent of patients; aggressive hydration is important. Indinavir should be kept away from moisture and should not be taken with a full meal, although it may be taken with a smaller low-fat, low-protein meal. It is available in 400-mg tablets; two tablets every 8 h is recommended.

Nelfinavir (Viracept)

Nelfinavir is the newest protease inhibitor. It is the first protease inhibitor that has a pediatric formulation and the first to be tested in pregnant women. It has good bioavailability (80 percent) and is well tolerated. There may be some loose stools, but they are easily treated with over-the-counter measures. It may limit the effects of rifampin and rifabutin and also interacts with many drugs through the cytochrome P450 pathway (terfenadine, astemizole, cisapride, etc.). It is available in 750-mg doses and is taken three times per day with or without meals.

Combination Therapy

The most promising result of the recent advances in HIV medical treatment has been the introduction of combination therapy. The most potent increases in CD4+ counts and the longest-lasting reduction in viral load have been achieved through three-drug regimens that include AZT, a second reverse transcriptase inhibitor, and a protease inhibitor. Not everyone has responded to the newer therapy. For some patients, the newer regimens have not provided any further benefit compared with previous attempts at treatment. However, there have been reports after three-drug regimens of reductions of viral load to below detectable levels along with substantial increases in CD4+ counts. For the first time, AIDS advocates have begun to speak of a "cure"; however, this may be premature, as the final verdict will not be available for some time. There are many questions still to be answered: Are the newly produced CD4+ cells truly functional? Will they continue to be produced after discontinuation of the drugs? Can we develop a method to detect virus in tissue or a fluid other than serum? How long should the drugs be maintained after a viral load drops below the level of detection? What are the chances of recurrence once the drugs are discontinued? What is the risk of further transmission at this level? Are there long-term risks inherent in the drugs themselves? How can these expensive drugs regimens be made available to every patient?

The remarkable ability of the HIV virus to mutate should encourage practitioners to adhere to strict guidelines in treating infected patients. Similar to the management of tuberculosis, optimal dosing of each drug and acute awareness of impending resistance are warranted to provide the best chances of prolonging survival and to avoid the development of virus resistance and cross-resistance between drugs. Noncompliance with recommended dosing regimens, subtherapeutic levels, interactions with other drugs, and the use of monotherapy, intermittent therapy, and sequential therapy all may contribute to the development of resistance. The fear of an emerging multidrug-resistant HIV is very real. It is imperative that practitioners involved in the care of HIV-positive patients remain attuned to current and evolving knowledge and recommendations regarding treatment with anti-HIV drugs. Patient education is also a crucial element; open communication regarding the need for compliance, the risks of drug-drug interactions, the progression of disease and resistance, and the need for thorough follow-up on all recommendations is paramount to maximizing the benefits of treatment.

SUPPORTIVE MEASURES

HIV-infected individuals have shown great support for and claim benefit from nontraditional medical approaches to disease.

Proper nutrition and nutritional supplements, exercise, stress management, and avoidance of unhealthy habits such as smoking and drug abuse certainly have a beneficial effect on any disease state. A strong investment in nutritional awareness has been evident in HIV disease; research has shown that proactive nutritional management can prevent or slow the HIV wasting syndrome and reduce the chances of gastrointestinal manifestations of the disease. Optimum healthy living has proved to increase the efficiency of the immune system and thus slow the progression of HIV disease.

HIV advocates have also been in the forefront of other nontraditional or complementary therapies. Hypnosis, biofeedback, acupuncture, imagery, and physical manipulation are just a few of the practices that have been widely used through the years by the general public and have received attention and increased acceptance as a result. Further research is needed before recommendations for alternative or complementary therapies can be made.

WOMEN AND HIV/AIDS

In the United States, women constitute one of the fastest growing segments of the HIV population; HIV is the third leading cause of death in women age 25 to 44 years. Heterosexual transmission and injection of drugs account for the vast majority of HIV-infected women. The manifestations of HIV disease in women include all the opportunistic infections and neoplasms seen in men, with the addition of vaginal infections, pelvic inflammatory disease (PID), and cervical dysplasia and cancer. Many of the infections are more aggressive and less responsive to treatment in women, including syphilis, herpes, human papillomavirus, and tuberculosis. In general, infection in women is not detected as early in the course of the disease and treatment is not sought as aggressively as it is in men. Increased public awareness and patient education are needed.

HIV disease in pregnancy is a major concern. The virus can be transmitted in utero, during delivery, and through breast milk. There is no way to predict the chances of vertical transmission in any individual pregnancy. The results of clinical trials have shown a significant reduction (from 30 to 13 percent) in the risk of transmission to the fetus with the use of AZT prenatally, at delivery, and in the neonate. Research is ongoing on the role of protease inhibitors in pregnancy and the long-term effects of treatment on the infant and the mother. Studies have shown that routine cesarean section does not reduce the risk of infection; however, the use of artificial rupture of membranes, fetal electrodes, and episiotomies may increase the risk. Practitioners need to be aware of the risks of infection and the benefits of treatment. They should counsel all pregnant patients that they be tested for HIV and should never withhold treatment for HIV or its manifestations because of pregnancy.

PEDIATRIC AND ADOLESCENT HIV

Children are at risk of HIV through perinatal transmission from an infected mother, sexual abuse, contaminated drug-injection equipment, and the reception of infected blood or blood products. Since the introduction of blood testing in the United States in 1985, the risk from infected blood and blood products has been extremely low. The majority of cases result from perinatal transmission and can be detected at birth. The expansion of the use of antiretroviral therapy during pregnancy and the neonatal period should result in a reduction in pediatric cases. However, at this time not all pregnant women and neonates are monitored for HIV infection.

Infants born to infected mothers will be positive for HIV antibodies; continued positivity or positive viral antigen testing confirms infection in a baby. Failure to thrive, continued or recurrent bacterial infections, chronic diarrhea, development delay, persistent thrush, diffuse lung disease, lymphadenopathy, and hepatosplenomegaly constitute the usual manifestations of HIV disease in infants and children.

Lymphoid interstitial pneumonia is the most common AIDS-defining illness in children. It presents with nonproductive cough, wheezing, and respiratory distress. The presumptive diagnosis is common, and there is no specific treatment; symptomatic treatment includes oxygen, bronchodilators, and steroids. Pediatric dosing with antiretroviral medication is recommended.

OCCUPATIONAL EXPOSURE IN HEALTH CARE WORKERS

Health care providers are at risk of contamination from blood-borne pathogens such as hepatitis and HIV. HIV is far less likely to be transmitted from such contaminations than is hepatitis, but HIV produces greater fear and anxiety. HIV carries a greater degree of social discrimination and ostracism and a far more likely death sentence. The fear of contracting HIV through needle stick injuries, open skin exposure, and splash accidents prompted the development of universal precautions that were formalized by the CDC in the 1980s and have been updated and maintained since. They are now known as standard precautions, and the main objective is to view each patient encounter as a potential source of contamination and use the same commonsense precautions in every situation. The precautions include wearing gloves and protective equipment whenever exposure to bodily fluids is likely, never recapping needles, and using the proper tools to clean up spills and dispose of waste. All health care practitioners should be fully cognizant of and adamantly adhere to all Standard Precautions.

The risk of transmission of the virus from patient to practitioner when the source patient is known to be HIV-positive is less than 0.3 percent after a percutaneous exposure (needle stick injury) and even lower after mucous membrane or skin exposure. If contamination with bodily fluids does occur, regardless of the status of the source, the first step is to copiously wash the involved area. Hands and other skin surfaces should be washed with soap and water, letting the injury bleed; mucous membranes should be irrigated with water. All such accidents must be reported to the institutions at which they occurred, and proper counseling and follow-up must be initiated. Baseline HIV testing of the health care worker and the source patient should be performed after consent is obtained. Testing should be repeated 6 weeks, 12 weeks, and 6 months after the incident.

Prophylaxis against HIV after occupational exposure has undergone several changes since the advent of AZT and the development of additional anti-HIV drugs. The current recommendations offer guidance according to the status of the source and the nature of the injury. In all such occupational accidents, the risk of disease must be balanced against the risk and benefits of treatment. For percutaneous injuries, prophylaxis is encouraged for any deep intramuscular puncture and is recommended for superficial injuries and accidental skin prick with a used bloody sharp object if the source has end-stage AIDS. Health care workers who sustain superficial percutaneous injuries associated with an asymptomatic patient can be offered prophylaxis, but it is not recommended or encouraged.

Mucous membrane exposure occurs with accidents such as a splash to the eyes or mouth with bodily fluids or tissue. Prophylaxis is encouraged if the source has end-stage AIDS and the exposure is large and prolonged and is recommended if the contact is either large or prolonged regardless of the source's status.

Prophylaxis can be offered in the case of small and brief contact if the recipient strongly desires it.

Surface cutaneous exposures involve the presence of body fluids on skin that is abraded or chronically chapped or that contains a moderate to severe dermatitis without the protection of gloves. Prophylaxis is recommended if the exposure is large and/or prolonged and may be offered in small and brief contact if the exposure occurs on skin that is nonintact.

Current prophylaxis regimens advise the use of combination drug therapies. AZT should be included in all regimens at the recommended dose of 200 mg orally tid. The addition of another reverse transcriptase inhibitor as well as a protease inhibitor completes the regimen. Four weeks of the full triple regimen is the minimum recommended therapy for serious injuries. One such regimen in use in the major teaching hospitals in New York City is AZT (Retrovir) 200 mg orally tid, 3TC (Lamivudine) 150 mg orally bid, and indinavir (Crixivan) 800 mg orally tid or saquinavir (Invirase) 600 mg orally tid; all three drugs are continued for 4 weeks and should be prescribed in conjunction with ongoing counseling. HIV testing is done at baseline, 6 weeks (2 weeks after completion of the drug therapy), 12 weeks, and 6 months. The cost of this therapy is quite high: over $700 for the full recommended doses.

BIBLIOGRAPHY

AMA Physician Guidelines No. 511: HIV blood test counseling. American Medical Association, Division of Health Science, Atlantic Information Services, January 1993.

Bartlett JG: *Pocket Book of Infectious Disease Therapy.* Baltimore, Williams & Wilkins, 1995.

Bennet JC, Plum F, eds: *Cecil Textbook of Medicine,* 20th ed. Philadelphia, Saunders, 1996.

Carmichael CG, Carmichael JK, Fischl MA: *HIV/AIDS Primary Care Handbook.* Norwalk, CT, Appleton & Lange, 1995.

Cohen PT: Safe sex, safer sex and prevention of HIV infection, in Cohen PT, Sande MA, Volberding PA (eds): *The AIDS Knowledge Base.* Waltham, MA, Medical Publishing Group, 1990.

Delaney M: Protease inhibitors: Choices and analysis. *Project Inform Perspect,* May 3, 1996, pp 1–5.

Diaz E (moderator): Primary care physician's role in treating patients with early HIV infection: A round table discussion. *Prim Care Cancer,* July 1990, pp 11–23.

Isselbacher KJ, Braunwald E, Wilson JD, et al (eds): *Harrison's Principles of Internal Medicine.* New York, McGraw-Hill, 1994.

Lewis JE: History of the acquired immunodeficiency syndrome (AIDS) epidemic, in Hopp JW, Rogers EA (eds): *AIDS and the Allied Health Professions.* Philadelphia, Davis, 1989.

Managing early HIV infection: A quick reference guide for clinicians. *AIDS Patient Care,* June 1990, pp 144–163.

Mascolini M: Can new HIV assays put more science and less art in antiviral prescribing? *J Phys Assoc AIDS Care,* August 1994, pp 8–15.

Mayer-Quezada D: Guidelines for occupational exposure. Lecture, New Jersey Academy of Medicine, Mount Laurel, NJ, December 5, 1997.

Miles SA: Diagnosis and staging of HIV infection. *Ann Fam Pract* 38(4):248–256, 1988.

Muma RD, Lyons BA, Borucki MJ, Pollard RB: *HIV Manual for Health Care Professionals.* Norwalk, CT: Appleton & Lange, 1994.

1993 Revised Classification System for HIV Infection and Expanded Surveillance Case Definition for AIDS among Adolescents and Adults. *MMWR,* Centers for Disease Control and Prevention, Atlanta, GA, December 12, 1992.

Shacker T, Collier A, Hughes J, et al: Clinical and epidemiologic features of primary HIV infection. *Ann Intern Med* 125(4):257–264, 1996.

Weiss W: Current guidelines in the diagnosis and treatment of HIV disease; lecture. Piscataway, NJ, December 9, 1996.

Wright M: Guide to the management of opportunistic infections. *Project Inform,* November 14, 1995.

Chapter 9–2
KAPOSI'S SARCOMA
Claire Babcock O'Connell

DISCUSSION

Until the advent of HIV disease, Kaposi's sarcoma (KS) was a malignancy of Mediterranean and Jewish elderly men, residents of certain endemic areas of central Africa, and persons undergoing immunosuppressive therapy after a transplant. Since the emergence of HIV disease, KS has become the most frequently encountered neoplasm in infected patients. KS is 20,000 times more common in HIV-positive persons than in the general population of the United States. In the early 1980s, KS was reported in 40 percent of patients diagnosed as HIV-positive. The frequency has declined in recent years; KS is now seen in 15 percent of HIV-positive persons. It is much more common in homosexual and bisexual males, supporting the theory that an infectious agent or cofactor is responsible for KS. The exact cause of KS remains unknown.

Histopathologically, KS demonstrates a mixture of different cell types. The lesions predominantly consist of endothelial cells and spindle cells that are enveloped in erythrocytes, altered lymphocytes, and macrophages. The cell of origin is not known, but it is most likely of mesenchymal origin.

SYMPTOMS

KS most commonly affects the skin and mucous membranes, although other systems, such as the lungs and gastrointestinal (GI) tract, also may be affected. The lesions usually first appear as small violaceous macules that are not painful or pruritic. The lesions commonly have a surrounding ring of erythema. As the disease progresses, the lesions may enlarge, and become nodular and/or confluent. Large plaquelike areas may develop, particularly on the lower legs. The rate of growth and the pattern of progression are highly variable.

It is not unusual to find lymphatic involvement in KS presenting as tender lymphadenopathy or painful lymphedema. Pulmonary disease results in respiratory distress and pulmonary effusion and is commonly mistaken for *Pneumocystis carinii* pneumonia (PCP). KS of the oral cavity is most commonly asymptomatic and must be specifically searched for in any HIV-positive patient. Oral lesions may become painful and interfere with eating. Other lesions along the gastrointestinal tract may cause malabsorption, bleeding, and diarrhea. KS lesions are found in the large intestine at autopsy in over 40 percent of patients with known cutaneous lesions.

OBJECTIVE FINDINGS

KS most commonly appears as nonblanching cutaneous lesions that are red to purple and painless. They are cosmetically worrisome but do not cause major morbidity. Nodular lesions often are brown. Suspicion of visceral involvement necessitates biopsy for confirmation.

DIAGNOSTIC STUDIES

The diagnosis of KS is based on physical findings and patient risk: HIV-infected or otherwise immunocompromised. Punch biopsy findings show a typical mixed pattern. Cutaneous lesions are readily identified, and the diagnosis is not difficult. Bacillary angiomatosis is caused by the microbe *Rochalimaea* and may present with similar lesions; the diagnosis is achieved by Warthin-

Table 9-2-1. National Institute of Allergy and Infectious Diseases AIDS Clinical Trials Group TIS System for Kaposi's Sarcoma

Parameter	Good risk (stage 0): all of the following	Poor risk (stage 1): any of the following
Tumor (T)	Confined to skin and/or lymph nodes and/or minimal oral disease	Tumor-associated edema or ulceration Extensive oral lesions Gastrointestinal lesions Nonnodal visceral lesions
Immune system (I)	CD4+ T-cell count ≥200 cells/μL	CD4+ T-cell count <200 cells/μL
Systemic illness (S)	No B symptoms* Karnofsky performance status >70 No history of opportunistic infection, neurologic disease, lymphoma, or thrush	B symptoms* Karnofsky performance status <70 History of opportunistic infection, neurologic disease, lymphoma, or thrush

* B symptoms include unexplained fever, night sweats, >10% involuntary weight loss, and diarrhea persisting more than 2 weeks.

Starry staining of the biopsy, and treatment consists of antibiotics. Oral KS lesions must be differentiated from lymphoma.

Pulmonary disease and KS generally necessitate bronchoscopy for an adequate diagnosis. Often bronchoscopy is ordered in search of PCP, and KS is found. Respiratory distress and pulmonary effusions carry a wide differential; the diagnosis is assisted by patient history and the index of suspicion and confirmed by bronchoscopic evidence of submucosal lesions with characteristic biopsy results. Symptoms of GI involvement also present a diagnostic difficulty; KS is usually first suspected after other, more common causes of the symptoms (bacterial, parasitic, wasting syndrome) are ruled out; confirmation is achieved through endoscopy and biopsy.

LABORATORY TESTS

No laboratory tests are necessary.

RADIOLOGIC STUDIES

Chest x-rays in patients with pulmonary KS show thickened bronchial walls and nodularity. Lesions are commonly found centrally and at major bifurcations. Kerley B lines, pleural effusions, and hilar or mediastinal adenopathy also are seen. Bronchoscopy reveals typical flat red to purple lesions that may appear similar to hemorrhagic lesions produced by bronchoscopic trauma. Intestinal endoscopy reveals typical raised red nodules in KS of the GI tract.

OTHER DIAGNOSTICS

The National Institute of Allergy and Infectious Diseases AIDS Clinical Trials Group has developed a TIS staging system for Kaposi's sarcoma (Table 9-2-1). The system is based on *t*umor (location and extent), *i*mmune system (CD4+ T-cell count), and *s*ystemic illness. The classification divides patients into two broad categories and is used to predict the prognosis.

TREATMENT

Small, nonpainful lesions that do not involve lymphatics or other organ systems can be simply observed. Excision is possible for small lesions that are cosmetically bothersome. Local radiation, intralesional chemotherapy (vinblastine), and local cryotherapy have been successful, but recurrence is typical. In patients with disseminated disease or extensive cutaneous advancement, systemic combination chemotherapy provides a 50 percent response rate within the first few weeks. However, the treatment must be continued chronically, as the lesions will recur when the chemotherapy is stopped. It is wise to consult an expert before initiating chemotherapy. Severe pulmonary KS also may respond to radiation therapy.

Patient Education

Although KS commonly occurs on sun-exposed areas, there is no evidence that avoidance of sun exposure helps prevent KS. Patients should be made aware of the myriad patterns of development and prognosis. Involvement of the viscera does not imply a poor response to therapy.

COMPLICATIONS

Extensive organ involvement, although rare, can be life-threatening. Extensive pulmonary involvement may be clinically silent for a prolonged period and may occur without cutaneous involvement. Respiratory distress and parenchymal or pleural involvement may cause severe respiratory compromise. Lymphatic involvement may cause severe lymph blockage and the threat of vascular compromise of the extremities or groin.

BIBLIOGRAPHY

Bennet JC, Plum F (eds): *Cecil Textbook of Medicine,* 20th ed. Philadelphia, Saunders, 1996.

Isselbacher KJ, Braunwald E, Wilson JD, et al, (eds): *Harrison's Principles of Internal Medicine,* 13th ed. New York, McGraw-Hill, 1994.

Muma RD, Lyons BA, Borucki MJ, Pollard RB: *HIV Manual for Health Care Professionals.* Norwalk, CT, Appleton & Lange, 1994.

Chapter 9–3
LYME DISEASE
Anne P. Heinly

DISCUSSION

Borrelia burgdorferi is the spirochete that is known to cause Lyme disease. Named for the town of Old Lyme, Connecticut, the disease has been around since the turn of the century but was not identified as a single infectious disease process until 1975. Well known in the northeastern, midwestern, and Pacific coast areas of the United States, Lyme disease may infect up to 10,000 patients a year. People become a vector for ticks carrying *B. burgdorferi* when hiking through wooded or grassy areas populated by deer. Ticks emerge when the weather warms up, and so infections are most common from May through September, when temperatures are above 2°C (35°F).

PATHOGENESIS

Spirochetes are slender, undulating motile bacteria that form spirals or helixes about 15 μm long. There are three recognized pathologic spirochete classes: *Borrelia* (Lyme disease), *Treponema* (syphilis), and *Leptospira* (leptospirosis). *Borrelia burgdorferi* gains entry to the skin through the bite of an infected deer tick (east and midwest) or a western black-legged tick (Pacific coast). The ixodid tick is very small and populates the growing herds of deer that are spreading throughout the United States. Because the tick lives up to 2 years, there are three distinct growth phases that require a blood meal (biting humans and deer). First, the larvae hatch in the spring and feed on ground hosts (rodents, including mice and rats), and birds that may also act as reservoirs. A year later the young ticks (the size of a typed period) feed on rodents, and finally in the fall they attach to a deer, where they may grow to an impressive 5 mm in size.[1] The small size is important in that most patients never see the tick; the larger pet tick is accused unjustly. *Borrelia burgdorferi* can be transmitted during any blood meal. The spirochete then slowly replicates in the skin and eventually spreads via the lymphatics or bloodstream to other organs. Infection is improbable if the tick is removed within 24 to 36 h of attachment. Lyme disease cannot be transmitted from human to human.

Pregnant women who contract Lyme disease do not appear to have adverse fetal outcomes.

SYMPTOMS

Lyme disease is a continuum. By far the most common initial symptom (stage 1) involves the skin rash (>50 percent[2]) erythema migrans (EM). The rash typically appears 10 to 14 days after a bite. The lesion initially appears as a red macule that expands into a red, raised plaquelike round (annular) lesion with central clearing. EM migrates relatively quickly and has no scaling. The rash may appear vesicular or even ulcerative. The final lesion (at 2 to 4 weeks) may be up to 40 cm in size.

Systemic symptoms appear early but may be diagnosed as a viral illness with fever, headache, myalgias, malaise, and vague joint pain. Up to 80 percent of patients with multiple EM lesions have systemic manifestations early.[1]

Stages 2 and 3 can be somewhat blurred. It is accepted that stage 2 symptoms generally occur weeks to months after stage 1, usually involving the skin, CNS, and joints. Stage 3 is the chronic state of untreated Lyme disease, succeeding stage 2 after months or even years. The disseminated phase of the infection tends to be exhibited in three areas.

The joint pain is common (>80 percent[2]) and migratory and almost always includes some neck or back pain. The later stages of the disease involve more arthralgias. There seems to be a predilection for the knees, the temporomandibular joint (TMJ), and large joints. Swelling without heat or erythema is common and usually is not associated with eye symptoms. Polyarticular involvement is seldom seen. In the chronic stage, patients may complain of recurrent bursitis, synovitis, and tendinitis.

With progression of the disease, neurologic symptoms (>15 percent[2]) become evident. Patients may present with meningeal symptoms, facial nerve palsies, peripheral neuropathies, and even radiculopathy. In stage 2, patients may present with classic viral meningitis symptoms, including headaches, stiff neck, and mild photophobia.

Cranial neuropathies are quite prevalent, usually presenting in stage 2. Any patient presenting with a facial palsy (Bell's palsy) should be investigated for Lyme disease. The palsies usually subside in 6 to 8 months. Peripheral neuropathies are manifested by intermittent paresthesias and weakness that may be confused with diseases such as Guillain-Barré. Fortunately, it is rare for a patient to progress to encephalomyelitis (stage 3) or spastic parapareses. Encephalopathy may cause persistent memory loss, dementia, headache, and difficulty with concentration. Some patients suffer chronic fatigue, confusion, depression, mood changes, and sleep changes.

Other symptoms may include cardiac arrhythmias (<5 percent[2]), most frequently heart blocks. The most common heart

Table 9-3-1. Differential Diagnosis for Lyme Disease

Disease	Characteristics
Rocky Mountain spotted fever	*Rickettsia rickettsii,* transmitted by ticks. Sudden onset of fever, headache, and chills for 2–3 weeks. Red rash seen on palms, soles, ankles, and wrists, progressing to a red maculopapular rash on the trunk, buttocks, and axilla. Cough and CNS symptoms occur
Relapsing fever	A *Borrelia* spirochete infection from a louse or tick. Louse-borne is endemic to Africa, China, and Peru; tick-borne is seen worldwide. Characterized by relapsing fever and neurologic symptoms, including deafness, unilateral blindness, and neuropathies
Typhus fever	*Rickettsia typhi,* transmitted by fleas. It causes shaking chills, headache, and fever. Rash begins in the axilla and becomes a dull macular rash involving the entire body eventually. Cough and rales are common. Neurologic effects may include dementia and coma
Juvenile rheumatoid arthritis	Insidious onset of arthralgia (polyarticular), fever, fatigue, myalgia with a fine rash. Sedimentation rate elevated with positive RF in some patients. ANA may be elevated as well
Systemic lupus erythematosus	Insidious onset of myalgia, fever, arthritis symptoms, eye pain and vision changes, and weight loss. Rash is usually erythema nodosum over the legs plus a "butterfly" macular rash over the cheeks and nose. Positive ANA and elevated sedimentation rate
Scleroderma	Insidious onset of joint stiffness, arthralgia, myalgia, and skin changes, including swelling, dryness, and cracking. Dyspnea, weakness, weight loss, and proximal muscle weakness all possible. Increased sedimentation rate and ANA
Tinea corporis	Scaling plaque with well-demarcated annular red rings. Maximum size for most lesions is 5 cm with no central clearing and mild itching. No systemic symptoms
Erythema multiforme	A self-limiting skin sensitivity characterized by sudden onset of rash on palms, soles, and all extensor surfaces. Oral mucosa vesicles and ulcers are common. The lesions may have central clearing and a burning sensation
Encephalitis, viral	Sudden onset of malaise, fever, and neck pain followed by meningeal irritation with stiffness and headache. Myalgias and arthritis symptoms may increase with fever. No rash generally
Meningitis, bacterial	Fever, headache, and neck pain and stiffness, usually after an upper respiratory infection. Rigor, seizures, dementia, loss of concentration, weakness, and photophobia common. A maculopapular rash initially, then petechial with mild pruritus

block is a simple first-degree block. Complete heart block can occur on occasion but rarely remains past 1 to 2 weeks. Third-stage disease rarely includes chronic cardiomyopathy and pericardial effusions. Patients also may present with tachycardia, bradycardia, myocarditis, and pericarditis.

OBJECTIVE FINDINGS

The rash of Lyme disease is the first clue. The erythema usually is red but may be a mottled blue-red with central clearing without scaling. The rash progresses rapidly over days, ranging in size from 20 to 40 cm around. As the lesions become larger, the central clearing may be bright red, ulcerative, or papular (resembling a burn). The rash is typically nontender. A single large lesion is common to the trunk. When there are multiple lesions, EM may be confusd with erythema multiform. A distinguishing feature is that EM typically spares the palms, soles, and mucous membranes. Systemic manifestation may include a low-grade fever, diaphoresis, and mild dehydration.

DIAGNOSTIC CONSIDERATIONS

The differential diagnosis for Lyme disease includes several dermatologic, rheumatologic, and neurologic processes, depending on when the patient is seen (Table 9-3-1). If the rash is not present on examination, the diagnosis can be hard to establish and a thorough evaluation is essential to rule out major cardiac, neurologic, and arthritic conditions. If a tick-borne disease is considered, one must be sure to rule out Rocky Mountain spotted fever and relapsing fever, as the treatment is quite different. A vital clue is the presence of arthritic symptoms with a normal rheumatoid factor (RF) or antinuclear antibodies (ANA) and the lack of associated symptoms as seen in Reiter's syndrome.

LABORATORY TESTS

Laboratory testing is the mainstay for confirming the diagnosis. A standardized flagellin–enzyme-linked immunosorbent assay (ELISA) serologic test is used in edemic areas. Timing is everything, as testing a day after a presumed bite will yield nothing. The optimal testing time is between 3 and 6 weeks after the

bite, when circulating IgM levels are at their peak.[3] An antibody response may take up to 8 weeks to be measurable. False-positives may occur because other *Borrelia* spp. may contaminate the serologic antigens or react to other spirochetal diseases (e.g., syphilis). If the ELISA is borderline, a Western blot can help detect antibody bands and decrease the number of false-negative and false-positive reports. Because of the imperfections in serologic testing, the final diagnosis is as dependent on the history and clinical presentation as it is on the laboratory findings.

Cultures of the EM skin lesions can yield *B. burgdorferi* but take several days to weeks to incubate. Research continues on ways to isolate the spirochete. Culturing of CSF, blood, and synovial fluid has been disappointing as a method of diagnosis. Complete blood count (CBC), RF, ANA, and other laboratory parameters are usually normal or negative in Lyme disease patients.

RADIOLOGIC (IMAGING) STUDIES

Imaging studies are not generally helpful in diagnosing Lyme disease but may be useful in ruling out various arthritides. In the chronic phase, some joint erosion may be noted, but it is not consistent with the usually joint stiffness and elevated RF or ANA common with rheumatoid arthritis.

TREATMENT

Lyme disease can be treated at any phase after discovery, with a variable cure rate. Certainly if the history and clinical findings are supported by positive serology, therapy should be started immediately. If the diagnosis is unconfirmed but highly suspected by history and examination, therapy also should be started. Table 9-3-2 reviews the current therapeutic options. Supportive measures should be tailored to the stage of the disease, the age of the patient, and concomitant diseases. Joint pain may be treated with anti-inflammatories and joint rest. A pacemaker may be necessary for temporary relief of heart blocks. Persistent neuralgias may require antidepressant serotonin reuptake inhibitors therapy.

Table 9-3-2. Treatment of Lyme Disease

Symptom	Medication	Timing and Considerations
Erythema migrans (EM)	Doxycycline 100 mg bid or amoxicillin 500 mg tid or cefuroxime 500 mg bid or clarithromycin 500 mg bid Azithromycin 500 mg day 1, then 250 mg × 4 days	Give for 2–3 weeks with the exception of azithromycin; use amoxicillin in children and pregnant or lactating women
Facial palsies CNS disease Cardiac disease Arthritis	Doxycycline 100 mg bid or amoxicillin 500 mg tid or ceftriaxone 2 g/d IV or cefotaxime 2 g/d IV or penicillin G 20–24 million units IV daily	Early symptoms can be treated for 2–3 weeks. Late or severe symptoms should be treated for 3–4 weeks and may require IV therapy

SOURCE: Modified from Sanford J, Gilbert D, Moellering R, et al: *The Ranford Guide to Antimicrobial Therapy.* Vienna, VA: Antimicrobial Therapy, Inc., 1997.

COMPLICATIONS

As many as 50 percent of patients with untreated Lyme disease may develop recurrent synovitis and migratory arthritis symptoms. The infection may be a trigger for fibromyalgia and/or chronic fatigue syndrome. Peripheral neuropathies and parasthesias are also common complications. Encephalopathies may include memory loss, dementia, poor concentration, and stroke-like symptoms. Some patients treated late in the course of the disease (>60 months) may have permanent damage to the CNS, heart, or joints.

Patient Education

The best treatment is prevention. The recommendations for endemic areas include wearing long sleeves and long pants tucked into the socks. Light-colored clothing is a must, as black ticks then show up better and are more easily removed. A repellent may be helpful (DEET) but should be used with care in children and the elderly. One should never use repellent near the eyes and should try to avoid thick brush and high grasses, as the ticks do not jump well. After finishing a hike or work, it is necessary to inspect the body for ticks. Removal is accomplished with a tweezer and a gentle but firm tug. One should try not to crush the tick because the body fluids may contaminate the bite area. One must wash the area well, save the tick for inspection, and watch for the development of the rash and/or flulike symptoms.

In endemic areas, it may be wise to clear the property of ticks, especially for farmers and hunters. Several over-the-counter insecticides are available to treat soil and lawns. All these products should be used with care and according to the manufacturer's instructions. Another measure may include special baits for the field mice and rodents that act as vectors for the ticks. The rodents carry the insecticides into their burrows and kill existing ticks.

PEARLS

On any given day in the spring or summer in an endemic area, parents worry about tick bites. Remember, ticks usually wander over the body for a few hours to find a cozy spot to feed at, and so inspection and brushing off the skin and clothing are the key to prevention. Additionally, the tick needs to be attached for 24 to 36 h before transmission of *B. burgdorferi* occurs. Prophylaxis for even confirmed bites is generally avoided and has not proved to be effective. Watch for the rash. If you have the rash, systemic symptoms, and the tick, treat it. With today's rapid transit, anyone

can present with Lyme disease. If the rash has receded before you see a patient, a high index of suspicion is required to order the serology.

REFERENCES

1. Lyme Disease: Clinical Update for Physicians. American Lyme Disease Foundation, with the CDC of the U.S. Public Health Service, fall 1993.
2. Infectious disease: VII. Leptospirosis. *Scientific American,* 1996, pp 7–15.
3. Steere AC: Lyme borreliosis, in Fauci AS, Braunwald E, Isselbacher KJ, et al (eds): *Harrison's Principles of Internal Medicine,* 14th ed. New York, McGraw-Hill, 1998, pp 1042–1044.

INTERNET RESOURCES

Consensus Conference on Lyme Disease. *Can Med Assoc J* 144:1627–1632, 1991.
Lyme disease. American College of Rheumatology. Internet article, 1996.
Lyme disease, tertiary. Internet article supplied by Applied Medical Informatic, 1996.

Chapter 9–4
ASCARIASIS
JoAnn Deasy

DISCUSSION

Ascariasis, or roundworm infection, is the most common helminthic infection worldwide. In the United States, approximately 4 million people are infected with *Ascaris lumbricoides,* mostly in the southeast. *Ascaris* eggs reach the soil in feces and in 2 to 3 weeks develop into embryos that are infectious. The eggs can persist for years in the soil. Transmission is usually from hand to mouth. In dry, windy climates, the eggs may become airborne and then be inhaled and swallowed.

The larval worms hatch in the small intestine and migrate through the gut wall into the bloodstream. They are carried through the liver to the alveoli of the lungs. In the course of this migration, the larvae increase in size. By the time they reach the pulmonary capillaries, they are too large to pass through to the left side of the heart. Since their route is blocked, they rupture through the alveolar spaces and are coughed up and swallowed. When they return to the upper intestine, they complete their maturation and mate. The adult worms are white or reddish-yellow and are 15 to 35 cm in length, a little longer than a pencil. Each female produces a daily output of approximately 200,000 ova.

SYMPTOMS

The symptoms are dependent on the intensity of infection and the organ involved. If the worm load is small, infections may be completely asymptomatic. In the lungs, the worms may cause a pneumonitis known as Löffler's pneumonia. Transient symptoms of fever, cough, substernal burning, wheezing, and shortness of breath are associated with the pneumonia. The presence of adult worms in the intestines may cause vague abdominal discomfort or nausea. Heavier worm loads may result in abdominal pain and malabsorption. Occasionally, a mass of worms may develop and cause intestinal obstruction or an adult worm may migrate to the appendix, bile duct, or pancreatic duct, causing inflammation and obstruction of that organ.

OBJECTIVE FINDINGS

In a patient with pulmonary involvement, wheezes and rales may be heard on auscultation of the lungs. Oxygen desaturation may occur. Occasionally the collection of worms in the intestine may be large enough to be palpated on abdominal examination. In an asymptomatic individual, the only indication of infection may occur when the adult worms are vomited up or passed in the stool.

DIAGNOSTIC CONSIDERATIONS

During the pulmonary stage, ascariasis must be differentiated from asthma and pneumonia caused by bacteria or a virus. The gastrointestinal symptoms must be differentiated from other parasitic infections and other causes of intestinal obstruction.

LABORATORY AND RADIOLOGIC TESTING

To make the diagnosis, a stool examination for ova and parasites should be ordered. Characteristic eggs are seen in the feces. The peripheral blood may exhibit eosinophilia. The pulmonary phase of ascariasis is diagnosed by the finding of larvae and eosinophils in the sputum. Perihilar infiltrates may be seen on chest x-ray.

TREATMENT

The treatment of choice is mebendazole (Vermox) 100 mg twice daily for 3 days. Pyrantel (1 mg/kg, maximum dose 1 g) may be prescribed for pregnant patients. Drug treatment may fail to kill the larvae, and so a follow-up examination of the stool for ova and parasites should be done 2 months after treatment. Ultimately, eradication requires adequate sanitation facilities.

BIBLIOGRAPHY

Juckett G: Common intestinal helminths. *Am Fam Phys* 52(7):2039–2048, 1995.
Mandell GL, Douglas RG, Bennett JE: *Principles and Practice of Infectious Diseases,* 4th ed. New York, Churchill Livingstone, 1995.
Sherris JC (ed): *Medical Microbiology.* New York, Elsevier, 1990, pp 734–736.

Chapter 9–5
CAT-SCRATCH DISEASE
Katherine Adamson

DESCRIPTION

Anyone who sees children in his or her daily practice will see cat-scratch disease. Cat-scratch disease (CSD) can best be described as a generally benign and self-limiting type of lymphadenitis. CSD is most often encountered in the pediatric population, with an estimated 22,000 cases occurring annually in the United States.[1]

PATHOGENESIS

As one might infer from its name, CSD is transmitted by contact with cats that have picked up the offending organism from the soil. Typically, an immature animal is infected with the causative agent, a small, pleomorphic gram-negative bacillus known as *Bartonella henselae.* The cat remains asymptomatic as it carries the organism in its mouth and paws. CSD is most often transmitted by a scratch or bite, though a lick or even contact with infected secretions has been known to inoculate the disease. Within a few days of contact with an infected cat, the affected individual presents with a small papule that rapidly becomes a vesicle and just as rapidly (2 to 3 days) resolves, leaving a macule that may persist for weeks. This prodromal skin lesion appears at the site of inoculation, whether it is a bite, a scratch, or mucous membrane contact with previously broken skin. Days to weeks may go by before the characteristic sign of lymphadenopathy appears.

MICROBIOLOGY

The causative organism of CSD, *B. henselae,* has been isolated from the lymph nodes of affected patients. This organism, formerly known as *Rochalimaea* and briefly called *Alfipia felis,* has been associated with bacillary angiomatosis in immunocompromised individuals.[2] An immunocompetent patient generally presents with a limited, occasionally regional lymphadenopathy with no pathologically distinct diagnostic changes. If the lymph tissue is excised in an effort to rule out a more serious etiology, the pathologist will report changes "consistent with" CSD. Grossly, granulomatous changes occur in the affected lymph tissue, which then may go on to suppurate.

SYMPTOMS

Typically, a patient with CSD presents to the clinic 2 weeks or so after inoculation. The symptom that prompts parents to bring their children for medical care is invariably a tender enlarged lymph node. The associated symptoms are not unlike those of many infectious disorders: malaise, low-grade fever [39°C (102°F)], appetite disturbances, and vague generalized aches and pains. Rarely, conjunctival inoculation may lead to an oculoglandular syndrome known as Parinaud's syndrome, which is striking in appearance but actually carries a very good prognosis.

OBJECTIVE FINDINGS

The lymphadenopathy of CSD is found proximal to the site of inoculation. Typically one or two nodes are involved, with disseminated disease reported in patients with an immune deficiency. Since the site of inoculation is most often an upper extremity, the location of the adenopathy probably will be epitrochlear, axillary, or cervical. A small minority of these nodes progress to suppuration, with the vast majority slowly regressing over several weeks. Parinaud's oculoglandular syndrome is notable for preauricular adenopathy, conjunctival granuloma formation, and surprisingly minimal local discomfort and purulent discharge.

DIAGNOSTIC CONSIDERATIONS

Of paramount importance in the diagnosis of CSD is a history of exposure to a cat in the setting of limited lymphadenopathy. Careful questioning will elicit a history of contact with a cat in the vast majority of cases. The clinician should inquire carefully for the presence of the premonitory papule, which may have been forgotten or overlooked. At the same time, the clinician must be aware that this papule is seen in only about one-half of cases of CSD. Other, more devastating etiologies of lymphadenopathy must be included in the differential. It is this need to rule out malignancy of the lymph node that often leads a clinician

Table 9-5-1. Common Causes of Lymphadenopathy

Infectious
  Viral
    Cytomegalovirus
    Ebstein-Barr virus
    Herpes family (varicella, zoster, simplex)
    Human immunodeficiency virus
    Mycobacteria
    Rubella
  Bacterial
    Streptococci
    Staphylococci
    Chlamydia (lymphogranuloma venereum, trachoma)
    Spirochetes (syphilis, leptospirosis)
    Mycobacteria
  Fungal
    Coccidioidomycosis
    Histoplasmosis
  Malignancy
    Lymphomas (Hodgkin's and non-Hodgkin's)
    Leukemias
    Metastatic carcinomas (breast, lung, gastrointestinal tract, head, and neck)
  Hypersensitivity reactions
    Drug reactions (phenytoin)
    Foreign body
    Vasculitis (systemic lupus erythematosus, rheumatoid arthritis)
  Endocrinopathy
    Hyperthyroidism
  Other
    Sarcoid

to search for a definitive diagnosis. Table 9-5-1 includes a partial list of the more common diagnoses that must be included in the differential.

SPECIAL CONSIDERATIONS

The key to preventing CSD lies in limiting opportunities for infected cats to transmit the infection. Parents and children should be warned to avoid stray and unknown animals. Family pets, particularly kittens, should be kept indoors and handled carefully. If a break in the skin occurs, immediate cleansing and wound care will minimize disease transmission. One must also remember that other organisms are transmitted by a cat bite or scratch, particularly *Pasturella multocida,* which presents very differently with a rapidly developing cellulitis.

LABORATORY TESTS

Standard laboratory investigations are not helpful. One can expect to find a mildly elevated white blood cell count, though this is too nonspecific to be of assistance.

RADIOLOGIC STUDIES

Radiographic investigations generally are reserved for investigating other etiologies of lymphadenopathy. For instance, this includes a chest CT in the workup of lymphoma or a mammogram if axillary adenopathy may be due to breast carcinoma.

OTHER DIAGNOSTICS

A skin test for CSD exists, but there is controversy about its safety. The antigen used in the skin test is derived from human lymph node aspirate. This has given rise to concerns about viral contaminates that may be present in the antigen.[3] A reasonably reliable diagnosis can be made on the basis of the time-honored methods of a suggestive history and physical findings. The clinical situation of the patient will dictate the clinician's comfort level in choosing between watchful waiting and a more invasive approach (node biopsy).

TREATMENT

Medications

Antibiotic therapy is rarely indicated in the treatment of CSD. A variety of antibiotics, including trimethoprim-sulfamethoxazole, rifampin, amoxicillin, and tetracycline, have shown in vitro effectiveness against *B. henselae,* but no clear benefit has been demonstrated from using these antibiotics in clinical treatment.[1] Most authors recommend treating only the rare patient who is severely ill. A commonly suggested regimen for an unusually ill patient is combination therapy with a third-generation cephalosporin and an aminoglycoside.

Supportive Measures

Treatment with analgesics is often helpful in controlling the associated symptoms. In addition, the patient should be advised to rest and avoid any activity that may traumatize the involved lymph tissues. In the rare instance when affected nodes painfully suppurate, it can be comforting to aspirate the involved nodes using sterile technique and a large bore (16-gauge) needle.

Patient Education

Once the diagnosis has been confirmed, it is important to review the pathogenesis and prognosis with the patient. The patient needs to know that some degree of malaise and activity limitation probably will occur over the recovery period of weeks to a few months.

Disposition

It is vital that all instances of lymphadenopathy be followed at regular intervals until complete resolution has occurred. Early in the course of CSD, this may mean weekly or even biweekly visits to the office. Once the patient is obviously recovering, it is reasonable to follow the affected nodes every few weeks until they are no longer enlarged.

COMPLICATIONS AND RED FLAGS

In a patient with an intact immune system, complications are fortunately rare. It is possible to see involvement of the central nervous system (encephalitis), liver, spleen, lung, bone, and skin.[2]

NOTES AND PEARLS

It is of the utmost importance that affected lymph nodes be followed sequentially until resolution has occurred. The difficulty of obtaining an accurate node measurement can be minimized through the use of commonly available ECG calipers, measuring the node in both the horizontal and the vertical planes.[4]

In the not too distant future a serologic test utilizing indirect fluorescent antibody technology will be widely available and may limit the need for invasive lymph node excisions to obtain a definitive diagnosis of CSD.

REFERENCES

1. Encephalitis associated with cat scratch disease—Broward and Palm Beach counties, Florida. *MMWR* 43:909, 915–916, 1994.
2. Adal KA, Cockerell CJ, Petri WA: Cat scratch disease, bacillary angiomatosis, and other infections due to Rochalimaea. *New Engl J Med* 330:1509–1513, 1994.

3. Breeling JL, Weinstein L: Cat-scratch disease, in Isselbacher KJ, Braunwald E, Wilson JD, et al (eds): *Harrison's Principles of Internal Medicine,* 13th ed. New York, McGraw-Hill, 1994, p 570.
4. Carithers HA: Cat-scratch disease, in Dershewitz RA (ed): *Ambulatory Pediatric Care,* 2d ed. Philadelphia, Lippincott, 1993, pp 758–761.

Table 9-6-1. Differential Diagnosis of Cervicitis/Urethritis

Chlamydia trachomatis
Neisseria gonorrhoeae
Trichomonas vaginalis
Ureaplasma urealyticum
Bacterial vaginosis
Candidiasis
Herpes simplex virus
Allergic urethritis/cervicitis (latex)

Chapter 9–6
CHLAMYDIA
Meredith Hansen

DISCUSSION

The etiologic agent of chlamydia is *Chlamydia trachomatis,* an obligate intracellular parasite that is currently the most common bacterial sexually transmitted disease in the United States. *Chlamydia trachomatis* is responsible for more than 4.6 million infections annually in the United States; 20 to 40 percent of sexually active American women show serologic evidence of exposure. Reported prevalence rates range from 4 to 9 percent in primary care settings to as high as 30 percent in sexually transmitted disease (STD) clinics.

Risk factors that have been shown to increase the incidence of infection include multiple sexual partners, a new sexual partner (within the last 2 months), age below 25 years, being unmarried, inconsistent use of barrier contraceptives, poverty, and being African-American. The incubation period is 7 to 21 days after exposure.

SIGNS AND SYMPTOMS AND OBJECTIVE FINDINGS

Uncomplicated infections

Studies show that up to 80% of infected women display no apparent signs or symptoms. In symptomatic women, a mucopurulent discharge and a friable cervix are the most common clinical findings. Dysuria and urinary frequency occur in women with chlamydial urethritis.

Asymptomatic infection is also common in men (studies show up to 25 percent). The most common infection sites in men are the urethra and the rectum. Urethritis presenting with a clear or mucopurulent urethral discharge is the most common clinical finding in symptomatic men.

Complicated infections

In women, a chlamydial infection may migrate into the upper genitourinary (GU) tract and present as a bartholinitis, an infection of Bartholin's ducts; salpingitis; or perihepatitis (infection of the hepatic capsule), also known as the Fitz-Hugh–Curtis syndrome. This syndrome should be suspected in any sexually active woman who presents with right upper quadrant abdominal pain, fever, nausea, and vomiting. A concurrent salpingitis is generally present. Asymptomatic or symptomatic chlamydial infections may persist for months, during which time sexual transmission and complications may occur. Other complications that occur in women include chronic pelvic pain, infertility, and ectopic pregnancy.

Complications in men include the following:

1. Epididymitis presenting as unilateral scrotal pain, swelling, tenderness, fever, and associated urethritis
2. Proctitis
3. Prostatitis
4. Reiter's syndrome

Chlamydia rarely produces systemic infections.

DIAGNOSTIC CONSIDERATIONS

A variety of genital pathogens, many of which are sexually transmitted, may cause urethritis or cervicitis (Table 9-6-1).

SPECIAL CONSIDERATIONS
Management of Sexual Partners

The sexual partners of infected patients must be evaluated and treated. A patient should be instructed to refrain from intercourse until the patient and his or her partners are cured.

HIV Infection

Treatment of chlamydia infections in HIV-infected patients is identical to the treatment regimens listed below.

Pregnancy

The prevalence of *C. trachomatis* infection exceeds 5 percent among pregnant women. There are specific treatment regimens for pregnant patients (see "Treatment," below).

Chlamydial Infections in Infants

Each year more than 155,000 infants are delivered to mothers infected with chlamydia. Infants exposed to *C. trachomatis* during passage through an infected birth canal may have conjunctivitis (ophthalmia neonatorum) and/or pneumonia. Chlamydia is the most common cause of infectious conjunctivitis in infants up to 30 days of age. Chlamydia also may produce a subacute pneumonia in infants, commonly presenting up to 90 days of age.

Diagnostic Testing

Serologic testing is not useful in the diagnosis. A laboratory diagnosis of chlamydia relies on culture and nonculture diagnostic testing. Many cases are treated empirically.

Cell culture is reliable but expensive. Nonculture tests are DNA probing of samples and enzyme-linked immunoassay (EIA) (Chlamydiazyme). A number of rapid tests are now available, taking about 10 to 30 min to yield results. The advantages of office testing include ease of processing, rapid results, and more cost-effectiveness. The main disadvantage of these tests is lower specificity.

TREATMENT

Pharmacologic Management

The recommended regimens are as follows:

Doxycycline 100 mg orally two times a day for 7 days
Azithromycin 1 g orally in a single dose

Alternative regimens include the following:

Ofloxacin 300 mg orally two times a day for 7 days
Erythromycin base 500 mg orally four times a day for 7 days
Erythromycin ethylsuccinate 800 mg orally four times a day for 7 days
Sulfisoxazole 500 mg orally four times a day for 10 days (least effective)

The recommended regimen for pregnant women is erythromycin base 500 mg orally four times a day for 7 days. Alternative regimens for pregnant women include

Erythromycin base 250 mg orally four times a day for 14 days
Erythromycin ethylsuccinate 800 mg four times a day for 7 days
Erythromycin ethylsuccinate 400 mg four times a day for 14 days
Amoxicillin 500 mg orally three times a day for 7 to 10 days

The recommended regimen for infants with ophthalmia neonatorum or pneumonia caused by chlamydia is erythromycin 50 mg/kg/d orally in divided doses for 10 to 14 days.

PATIENT EDUCATION

Patients must be advised to abstain from sexual activity until they and their partners are cured. Concurrent treatment of partners is essential, even if they are asymptomatic. All sexual partners within the last 60 days should be treated. A history of an STD places a patient at risk for subsequent STDs. When used consistently, condoms are effective in preventing STDs. Patient education in the proper use of condoms should occur during every patient visit for STDs.

DISPOSITION

A follow-up test to cure is not mandatory since treatment failures (if medication is taken properly) are uncommon. Retesting should be performed if symptoms persist or reinfection is questionable. Owing to higher treatment failure rates with sulfisoxazole and erythromycin, test to cures should be considered. Nonculture follow-up testing at less than 3 weeks after the completion of therapy may be a false-positive because of the excretion of dead organisms.

COMPLICATIONS AND RED FLAGS

Many, but not all, states trace and notify the sexual partners of patients with a chlamydial infection. Physician assistants should be knowledgeable about reporting procedures for communicable diseases in their states.

Routine screening for asymptomatic infection in women during the annual pelvic examination is recommended, particularly in high-risk patients. Physician assistants should be aware of clinical findings that are suggestive of asymptomatic infection (friable cervix, mucopurulent discharge). Routine screening of asymptomatic infection in men is not recommended at this time.

BIBLIOGRAPHY

Centers for Disease Control and Prevention: 1993 sexually transmitted diseases treatment guidelines. *MMWR* 42:3–7, 47–56, 1993.
Majeroni BA: Chlamydial cervicitis: Complications and new treatment options. *Am Fam Phys* 49:1825–1828, 1994.
Preventive Services Task Force: *Guide to Clinical Preventive Services,* 2d ed. Alexandria, VA, International Medical Publishing, 1996.
Tierney L, McPhee SJ, Papadakis MA: *Current Medical Diagnosis and Treatment,* 34th ed. Stamford, CT, Appleton & Lange, 1995, pp 1194–1195.

Chapter 9–7
COCCIDIOIDOMYCOSIS
Diane S. Wrigley

DISCUSSION

Coccidioidomycosis is a pulmonary fungal infection that is endemic in the southwestern United States. The common names are "cocci" or "valley fever." Found only in the western hemisphere and in specific areas of Argentina and Central America, cocci is largely seen in the San Joaquin Valley of California and in southern Arizona. It is the oldest of the major pathologic mycoses. The first case was described in 1892 in an Argentine soldier. A major dust storm in California in 1977 resulted in large amounts of spores being transported to northern and coastal areas several hundred miles away. In 1978, the incidence of cocci had a fourfold increase in the state and a 20-fold increase in the San Joaquin Valley.

PATHOGENESIS

Cocci or valley fever is caused by the fungus *Coccidioides immitis*, which is a normal inhabitant of the sandy and saline soil of the lower Sonoran Desert life zone. Infection occurs when liberated spores are inhaled from disturbed soil through digging, building construction, dust storms, spelunking, archaeological digging, and rodent burrowing. It cannot be transmitted from person to person. After exposure to the spores, with or without symptoms, the body develops immunity. Although the lung is the primary site of infection as spores are inhaled, cocci can become progressive and spread hematogenously to involve extrapulmonary sites such as bone, skin, and CNS. This process is referred to as *dissemination*. It can affect people of all ages without regard to sex, but the very young, the very old, and the pregnant have the worst clinical outcomes. The incidence in the United States is 100,000 cases a year, with 0.5 percent of cases being extrapulmonary (Table 9-7-1).

Table 9-7-1. Risk Factors for Increased Morbidity of Coccidioidomycosis

Age group: very young and very old
Race: Filipino, black, Native American, Hispanic, Oriental, White, in order of most to least susceptible
Negative skin test
Serum complement fixation >1:64
Pregnancy: second half and postpartum
Immunosuppression: HIV, diabetes mellitus, chemotherapy, malignancies

SIGNS AND SYMPTOMS

About 65 percent of these infections are asymptomatic, with no complications. Evidence of exposure to *C. immitis* infection is detected by means of a positive skin test. The cocci spherule antigen is applied in exactly the same manner as a purified protein derivative (PPD) skin test. The results show whether a patient has been exposed to cocci much as a tuberculin skin test shows exposure to mycobacterium. Many symptomatic patients pass the illness off as the "flu" or an uncomplicated upper respiratory infection (URI) (Table 9-7-2).

The other 35 percent of infections present as a primary pneumonia, often with pleuritic chest pain. Eventually 95 percent of all cases progress to full resolution without complications. The other 5 percent advance to pulmonary complications such as acute respiratory disease (ARD), a pulmonary nodule or cavity, empyema, and progressive pulmonary involvement with skin lesions, abscesses, arthritis, osteomyelitis, and meningitis. The most common skin manifestations are erythema nodosum and erythema multiforme. The arthritis is experienced mostly in the knees and ankles and is symmetric. It is a result of immune complexes, not dissemination.

OBJECTIVE FINDINGS

Ear, nose, and throat (ENT) examination may reveal minimal to marked congestion with otherwise normal findings. The lungs are clear to auscultation and normal to percussion in asymptomatic or moderately symptomatic individuals. Rales may be heard in those who present with pneumonia. An inspection of the skin that reveals evidence of erythema nodosum or erythema multiforme should increase suspicion of cocci. Any rash that does not fit a particular pattern in a symptomatic patient should raise the consideration of cocci. Cocci is known as a great "imitator," just as syphilitic rashes are. If a skin test has been administered, any evidence of induration or erythema after 48 h constitutes a "positive." Chest x-rays may range from normal to showing infiltrates that abut fissures and exhibit hilar adenopathy. Paratracheal and superior mediastinal infiltrates or mediastinal widening may signal dissemination.

DIAGNOSTIC CONSIDERATIONS

Cocci is not easily distinguished from other respiratory tract illnesses. The index of suspicion for cocci should increase with the chance of exposure to endemic regions, an erythrocyte sedimentation rate (ESR) >28, signs of erythema nodosum, an absolute lymphocyte count <1.6, and pediatric and adolescent patients with complaints of chest pain.

LABORATORY TESTS

In the complete blood count (CBC), the white blood cell count (WBC) is usually below 10,000 in 27 percent of cases of eosinophilia. The ESR is elevated above 28. In sputum cultures, *C. immitis* will grow as thin strands of cotton on blood agar plates.

Antibodies titers or complement fixation titers

Tube precipitin antibodies (TPs) yield IgM or early signs of infection within the first 30 days after exposure to the spores. This is not a prognostic test, but it is useful as a screen for the presence or absence of possible disease. The complement-fixing antigen or IgG is proportional to the disease. These are quantitative antibodies determined by serial dilutions. The titers are reported as <1:2, 1:2, 1:4, 1:8, 1:16, 1:64, 1:132, and 1:264. Titers >1:16 suggest extrapulmonary infections, and titers that increase by more than twofold over 2 to 3 weeks increase the suspicion of dissemination. Titers should be followed until the level is <1:2.

Table 9-7-2. Symptoms of Coccidioidomycosis

Symptom	Prevalence, %
Fatigue	77
Fever	46
Cough	64
Headache	22
Arthralgia	22
Chest pain	53
Dyspnea	17
Rash	23

Often the symptoms disappear as the antibody level drops. Biopsies of lung and skin may have cocci spherules present. A lumbar puncture may show persistent headache, changes in mental status, or neurologic symptoms.

TREATMENT

Most cases resolve without therapy. One must remember that 65 percent of these cases are asymptomatic. Rest and time are the recommended treatment for those who are symptomatic but are not at risk for extrapulmonary disease or dissemination. There is no evidence that treatment can shorten the course of illness or prevent more serious problems.

Immunodeficient patients and those who exhibit signs of extrapulmonary disease or are at risk of dissemination on the basis of x-ray, risk factor, or rising titers may be treated with

- Fluconazole (Diflucan) 400 mg/d
- Itraconazole (Sporanox) 400 mg/d
- Ketoconazole (Nizoral) 400 to 800 mg/d
- Amphotericin B (dose of cumulative therapy to maximum of 1.0 g intrathecally until improved, followed by ketoconazole at 800 mg/d)

SUPPORTIVE MEASURES

Patients who develop bronchospasm may be treated with β_2-agonists delivered orally or by medidose inhalers and inhaled corticosteroids. Caution must be exercised in using systemic corticosteroids. Malaise and arthralgias may be treated with nonsteroidal anti-inflammatory drugs (NSAIDs) unless specific contraindications exist.

PATIENT EDUCATION

Patients must limit physically exhausting activities. For the most part, the body's own defense system is the best treatment. One should remove physical education from the school curriculum for students and heavy labor from the work of adults, encouraging bed rest as much as possible until the patient is asymptomatic and/or titers are <1:2. The patient must know the importance of following up on laboratory work for serial titers every 2 to 3 weeks.

Once a person is infected, lifelong immunity should persist. There is no need to repeat skin testing once a positive has been determined.

NOTES AND PEARLS

Medical and indirect costs for the most benign cases are $300 to $5000 per patient. The most severe cases cost $30,000 to $300,000, with physician office visits accounting for 18 percent, lost wages for 12 percent, drugs for 6 percent, and hospitalization for 63 percent of the bill. Kern County in southern California in 1991–1994, a period of an epidemic with the specific etiologies unknown, had 8434 cases of cocci at a cost of $66.6 million. The annual cost to the county is $4.8 million.

Currently a vaccine is being worked on in Kern County. The hope is to eliminate the personal and financial burden of the disease. Expectations are that the vaccine will be developed over the next 7 years at a cost of $6 million.

BIBLIOGRAPHY

A Vaccine for Valley Fever. Bakersfield, CA, Rotary America's Valley Fever Research Foundation, 1996.
Clin Infect Dis 16:349–356, 1993.
West J Med, Conferences and Reviews, John Galgiani, MD. Tucson, AZ, pp 153–171, August 1993.

Chapter 9–8
CRYPTOCOCCOSIS
Claire Babcock O'Connell

DISCUSSION

Cryptococcus neoformans is a common yeastlike fungus that is found in the soil. The fungus becomes aerosolized and is inhaled by humans. It does not cause disease unless the host is immunocompromised. There is no evidence that cryptococcus is transmitted from human to human or from animal to human. In HIV-positive patients, cryptococcus is the leading cause of fungal meningitis, with an incidence of 6 to 12 percent. Cryptococcal meningitis is often an indolent process, causing symptoms for a period of weeks or months before being diagnosed. However, it is not uncommon to have a fulminant course of the disease that rapidly leads to death. Cryptococcus generally presents in patients with a CD4+ T-cell count below $100/\mu L$.

SIGNS AND SYMPTOMS

The majority of HIV-positive patients with cryptococcal infection present with subacute meningoencephalitis. The symptoms are often subtle and nonspecific. All these patients have fever. Approximately 40 percent have nausea and vomiting. One-quarter complain of changes in mental status (depression, dementia, delirium), headache, and meningeal signs. Seizures and focal neurologic signs occur but are less common. A few patients with central nervous system (CNS) infection with cryptococcus develop cryptococcomas that show multiple ring-enhancing lesions on MRI.

Cryptococcal pulmonary disease occurs in about 40 percent of HIV-positive patients with cryptococcal infection; over 90 percent of these patients have concurrent infection of the CNS. Fever, cough, and dyspnea with a focal or diffuse interstitial infiltrate aid in the diagnosis of cryptococcal pneumonia.

About half the HIV-positive patients with cryptococcal infection experience fungemia and complain of fatigue and malaise. Also, about 4 to 8 percent may present with fungemia as the only manifestation of cryptococcal infection. Other, less common manifestations of cryptococcal infection are seen more commonly in the disseminated fulminant infection and may include skin lesions, lymph node involvement, oral ulcers, gastroenteritis, hepatitis, splenic dysfunction, arthritis, and prostatitis.

OBJECTIVE FINDINGS

Altered mental status is the most useful physical finding. The Folstein Mini-Mental Status Exam can be used as a screening examination to detect subtle changes in mental status. Subtle changes in personality may be revealed during attentive interviewing. Photophobia and neck stiffness are rare.

DIFFERENTIAL DIAGNOSIS

The manifestations of cryptococcal infection are often subtle and nonspecific. A high index of suspicion and early examination of the cerebraospinal fluid (CSF) are necessary to avoid missing the diagnosis. Other diseases in the differential diagnosis include AIDS dementia complex, toxoplasmosis, progressive multifocal leukoencephalopathy, cytomegalovirus, tuberculosis, syphilis, and lymphoma.

LABORATORY AND RADIOLOGIC STUDIES

A presumptive diagnosis of cryptococcal meningitis is made by identifying the fungus on India ink staining of the CSF. The diagnosis is further justified if cryptococcal antigen is measured in the CSF or blood. A definitive diagnosis is confirmed by culturing the fungus from the CSF, blood, bone marrow, sputum, or tissue specimen. Any positive culture, regardless of site, is considered significant and should prompt treatment against cryptococcus.

In almost all cases of cryptococcal meningitis, CSF antigen testing is positive. In almost all cases of non-HIV cryptococcal meningitis and in the majority of cases of HIV-positive cryptococcal meningitis, the CSF also shows an increased white blood cell count (WBC), elevated protein, and a low glucose concentration. In about 20 percent of HIV-positive cases, the antigen is positive but all other CSF findings are normal.

The radiologic findings in cryptococcal meningitis are usually normal. Nonspecific changes, such as cortical atrophy, ventricular enlargement, and enhancement of the meninges, may be seen on CT. Mass lesions that may be ring-enhancing on MRI (cryptococcomas) must be differentiated from toxoplasmosis. Pulmonary cryptococcal infection appears as a focal or diffuse interstitial infiltrate but also may cause a lobar or cavitary lesion with pleural effusion and possible hilar or mediastinal adenopathy. Some (up to 40 percent) of these patients present with pulmonary cryptococcal disease without meningitis.

TREATMENT
Medication

Amphotericin B given intravenously at a dose of 0.5 to 0.8 mg/kg/d until the patient shows clinical improvement is the first line of therapy against cryptococcal meningitis. Treatment should be initiated in any patient suspected of having cryptococcal meningitis and continued for a minimum of 2 weeks. After the patient shows clinical improvement, amphotericin is continued at a lower dose of 0.3 mg/kg/d for an additional 4 weeks. Many clinicians add flucytosine (5-FC, Ancobon) at a dose of 100 to 150 mg/kg/d and lower the dose of amphotericin B to 0.3 mg/kg/d given orally until clinical improvement occurs.

An alternative therapy is fluconazole (Diflucan) 400 mg a day given orally. Fluconazole is not as effective as amphotericin B with or without flucytosine but is better handled by patients and may be chosen as the initial therapy in patients with milder disease.

Because of the high recurrence rate (approximately 40 to 60 percent in successfully treated patients), chronic therapy is recommended in any patient with a history of cryptococcal infection. Fluconazole is the drug of choice for suppression therapy. Itraconazole 200 mg per day given orally may be an alternative in patients who are unable to tolerate fluconazole, but its penetration into CSF is not as effective as that of fluconazole. Prophylaxis against cryptococcal infection with fluconazole is recommended for HIV-positive patients with CD4+ T-cell counts below $200/\mu L$. Prophylaxis with fluconazole is also effective against candida.

Amphotericin B is fraught with side effects. Patients complain of headache, fever, chills, nausea, vomiting, hypotension, malaise, muscle and joint pain, and anorexia. It also can cause renal damage. Flucytosine can be very toxic to the bone marrow, causing anemia and neutropenia; approximately one-half of patients who are started on flucytosine must discontinue the drug because of its toxic effects on bone marrow. Peak serum levels of flucytosine should not rise above 100 $\mu g/mL$. Fluconazole generally is better tolerated but may cause gastrointestinal upset, including nausea and vomiting, elevated liver enzymes, and a rash.

Patient Education

Patients and their caretakers should be alert to any changes in mental status or personality. Any subtle changes or reports of headache should prompt a consultation with a health care provider in regard to the possibility of cryptococcal meningitis.

Disposition

All patients with CD4+ T-cell counts below $200/\mu L$ should be monitored for cryptococcal infection. Most clinicians advocate prophylaxis at this level; some clinicians postpone prophylaxis until the CD4+ T-cell count drops below $100/\mu L$. Once infection is suspected, treatment is initiated and must be continued indefinitely because of the high recurrence rate. Patients must be monitored for the toxic effects of treatment. Regardless of treatment, about one-quarter of patients ill with cryptococcus will die.

COMPLICATIONS AND RED FLAGS

Patients who do not demonstrate a successful response to therapy may develop cryptococcomas, which are mass lesions within the brain parenchyma and/or spinal cord. In these patients, CSF antigen testing and fungal cultures may be negative; biopsy confirmation is needed. Other possible complications of cryptococcus include hydrocephalus, encephalitis, brainstem vasculitis, and optic nerve involvement.

OTHER NOTES AND PEARLS

Further research is being done to develop alternative medications with fewer side effects and toxicities. Oral medications, including newer azoles (itraconazole, etc.), are under investigation.

BIBLIOGRAPHY

Bennet JC, Plum F (eds): *Cecil Textbook of Medicine,* 20th ed. Philadelphia, Saunders, 1996.

Dobkin JF: Opportunistic infections and AIDS. *Infect Med* 12(Suppl A):58–70, 1995.

Fauci AS, Braunwald E, Isselbacher KJ, et al (eds): *Harrison's Principles of Internal Medicine,* 14th ed. New York, McGraw-Hill, 1998.

Gallant JE, Moore RD, Chaisson RE: Prophylaxis for opportunistic infections in patients with HIV infection. *Ann Intern Med* 120:932–944, 1994.

Lane CH (moderator): Recent advances in the management of AIDS-related opportunistic infections. *Ann Intern Med* 120(11):945–954, 1994.

Chapter 9–9
CYTOMEGALOVIRUS INFECTION
Claire Babcock O'Connell

DISCUSSION

Cytomegalovirus (CMV) is a double-stranded DNA virus in the herpes family. Infection results in a characteristic enlargement of cells and large intranuclear inclusions with clear halos referred to as "owl's eyes." CMV is found worldwide; it can be detected in urine, feces, saliva, milk, semen, and sexual fluids. It is transmitted through prolonged intimate or close contact.

Initial contact with the virus causes a mononucleosis-like illness with atypical lymphocytes and T-cell proliferation. Newly infected neonates display an often fatal disseminated cytomegalic inclusion disease. Most infected individuals recover and continue to harbor the virus in multiple tissue sites as a latent infection. Immune compromise, most commonly HIV disease, results in a reactivation of the infection, leading to pneumonia, gastrointestinal disease, sight-threatening retinitis, or disseminated illness.

Evidence of infection is apparent in over 90 percent of HIV-positive patients, and clinical disease is apparent in over 40 percent. CMV disease becomes a statistically higher risk in patients with advanced HIV disease when CD4+ T-cell counts drop below $100/\mu L$. It is rarely the presenting or AIDS-defining infection in HIV-positive patients. CMV also may act as a cofactor that furthers the immune system compromise in addition to the impact of HIV.

SIGNS AND SYMPTOMS

CMV causes many symptoms; colitis, esophagitis, pneumonia, and retinitis are the most common manifestations in HIV-positive patients. Retinitis is the most devastating presentation and the most common cause of blindness in patients with HIV disease. CMV retinitis usually appears with a CD4+ T-cell count of $40/\mu L$. Patients present with painless visual loss, blurriness, and visual field defects ("floaters"). One eye usually is affected first, but most cases progress to bilateral infection. Without treatment, the disease can cause complete retinal detachment and permanent blindness.

Gastrointestinal (GI) infection with CMV can present anywhere along the GI tract. Difficult and painful swallowing accompanied by substernal chest pain is typical of CMV esophagitis. The most common manifestation of CMV in the GI tract is colitis, which presents with diarrhea (with or without blood in the stools), crampy abdominal pain, and weight loss. CMV colitis may follow an indolent, prolonged course or, less commonly, a fulminant, abrupt course, resulting in perforation and bacteremia.

CMV is commonly isolated from the lungs of HIV-positive patients but is rarely thought to be the primary agent of lung disease. Although rare, CMV pneumonia presents with dyspnea and dry cough. The diagnosis is made if inclusion bodies are found, the virus is cultured from tissue, and no other etiology for the pneumonia can be discovered.

CMV also can cause other, less common manifestations, including carditis, pancreatitis, thyroiditis, pyelonephritis, hepatitis, biliary disease, and CNS involvement.

OBJECTIVE FINDINGS

A definitive diagnosis of CMV disease is confirmed by a demonstration of CMV inclusion bodies, which can be found in virtually all tissues that may be infected. Viral cultures also can verify the presence of CMV but are not particularly sensitive. Most patients with a CD4+ count below $100/\mu l$ shed CMV, but it may not necessarily be the cause of a patient's symptoms.

Funduscopic changes in retinitis characteristically consist of white to yellow cheesy retinal exudates with or without hemorrhage. Lesions are commonly found on or near vessels. Involvement of the macula quickly leads to visual loss. Examination of the retina shows inclusion bodies and full-thickness necrosis. All patients with CD4+ counts below 100 should be examined and followed by an experienced ophthalmologist.

Endoscopy reveals characteristic multiple shallow ulcers along the mucosa. In the large intestines, it is common to see edema and erythema with erosions and hemorrhage. Biopsy specimens will reveal the inclusion bodies and may confirm the presence of the virus. Stool cultures are not sensitive; barium enemas are usually normal. Chest x-rays in patients with CMV pneumonia are not well defined; a diffuse interstitial pattern is more common but is not easily distinguished from other causes of interstitial lung disease.

DIAGNOSTIC CONSIDERATIONS

CMV retinitis must be differentiated from cotton-wool spots, retinal hemorrhages, choroidal granulomas, retinal necrosis syndromes, and retinitis caused by toxoplasmosis or syphilis. The physical appearance should be confirmed by an expert.

Esophagitis and colitis caused by CMV can be confused with many other causes of GI inflammation, including candida, other viruses, bacteria, inflammatory bowel diseases, chronic illness, and reaction to medications. Endoscopy findings and inclusion bodies in biopsy specimens are needed to establish diagnostic certainty. CMV pneumonia is diagnosed only after other causes of the respiratory symptoms are ruled out [*Pneumocystis carinii* pneumonia (PCP), other pathogens, and injury from drugs or radiation].

LABORATORY TESTS

Viral cultures are not highly correlated with patient symptomatology. The demonstration of CMV inclusion bodies (owl's eyes) is the key to the diagnosis. Patients with CMV disease will have other laboratory findings, including low CD4+ counts, leukopenia, thrombocytopenia, and abnormal liver enzymes, but these findings could be due to the CMV or other pathologies associated with the immunocompromised state.

OTHER DIAGNOSTICS

Early retinal involvement in susceptible patients can be detected through the use of an Amsler grid. The patient is instructed to stare at the central dot in the middle of a blocked grid. If any part of the grid appears distorted or disappears, the patient is instructed to call his or her health care practitioner.

TREATMENT

Pharmacologic Management

Ganciclovir and foscarnet are the two drugs used in the treatment of CMV. Ganciclovir (dihydroxypropoxymethyl guanine, DHPG) was the first U.S. Food and Drug Administration (FDA)-approved drug for CMV retinitis and colitis. The dose is 5 mg/kg intravenously bid for 14 to 21 days. The drug is static to the virus and halts progression of the disease in 90 percent of patients. The virus is not eradicated, and thus treatment cannot be stopped. Oral ganciclovir (Cytovene) has proved to be as effective as intravenous ganciclovir for the prophylaxis and prevention of recurrence after the disease has been stabilized. The dose is 1000 mg orally tid.

Foscarnet offers equivalent efficacy against CMV and is useful against ganciclovir-resistant strains. It is given in doses of 60 mg/kg intravenously tid for 14 to 21 days. Foscarnet therapy also must be continued chronically in a dose of 120 mg/kg/d intravenously. Clinical trials have indicated that foscarnet therapy may improve survival through its action against HIV and may be the drug of first choice for CMV retinitis in patients with good renal function.

Both drugs have potentially severe side effects. Ganciclovir is toxic to bone marrow, especially when given with zidovudine (AZT), and often is given with granulocyte colony stimulating factor or granulocyte-macrophage colony stimulating factor to offset leukopenia. Ganciclovir also has caused nausea and vomiting, renal toxicity, and rash. Foscarnet can be very toxic to the kidneys; adequate hydration is very important to minimize toxicity. Foscarnet also can cause rash, fevers, and abnormal electrolytes, including calcium, phosphorus, magnesium, and potassium; it also can induce seizures. Hypocalcemia is very likely to occur with foscarnet in the presence of intravenous pentamidine.

Patient Education

Patients are the most important players in the monitoring of sight. They can be instructed in the use of the Amsler grid and should be strongly counseled to report to their health care providers if they suspect any change in vision.

Disposition

Close monitoring of blood chemistries and hematologic function is warranted during treatment. CD4+ levels that start to drop to 100 or less should alert a practitioner to begin prophylaxis against CMV.

NOTES AND PEARLS

The recent introduction of intraocular implants of ganciclovir in a sustained-release form has offered promising results. The FDA has approved the marketing of Vitrasert, manufactured by Chiron Vision and Roche Laboratories. The FDA also has recommended the approval of Vistide (cidofovir) for CMV. Cidofovir has a longer duration of action and can be given once every 2 weeks after induction. Rapidly progressing disease or resistant strains of CMV may be treated with combinations of foscarnet and ganciclovir.

BIBLIOGRAPHY

Bennet JC, Plum F (eds): *Cecil Textbook of Medicine,* 20th ed. Philadelphia, Saunders 1996.
Dobkin JF: Opportunistic infections and AIDS. *Infect Med* 12(Suppl A):58–70, 1995.
Fauci AS, Braunwald E, Isselbacher KJ, et al (eds): *Harrison's Principles of Internal Medicine,* 14th ed. New York, McGraw-Hill, 1998.
Lane HC (moderator): Recent advances in the management of AIDS-related opportunistic infections. *Ann Intern Med* 120:945–955, 1994.
Muma RD, Lyons BA, Borucki MJ, Pollard RB: *HIV Manual for Health Care Professionals.* Norwalk, CT, Appleton & Lange, 1994.
Sharp V, Ferri RS: AIDS update. *Clin Rev* 6(5):115–119, 1996.

Chapter 9–10
DIPHTHERIA
Richard Dehn

DISCUSSION

Diptheria is a localized acute infectious disease of the upper respiratory tract mucous membranes or skin caused by the toxin-producing organism *Corynebacterium diphtheriae.* Typically, the primary site of infection is the mucosa of the throat, larynx, or nose; however, in developed countries, cutaneous presentations have become more common. The infection typically is local, and the site of infection is characterized by the formation of a fibrinous pseudomembrane. Serious consequences can result from the pseudomembrane, which can contribute to airway obstruction, and from the production of exotoxin, which can cause myocarditis, neuropathy, and renal failure.

In the 1920s it was discovered that treating diphtheria exotoxin with formaldehyde converts it to a nontoxic substance called diphtheria toxoid and that the vaccination of individuals with diphtheria toxoid results in the production of an antibody known as antitoxin. The antitoxin can neutralize the diphtheria exotoxin but cannot prevent *C. diphtheriae* infection or the carrier state. Immunized individuals tend to have a lower susceptibility to infection by *C. diphtheriae* and, if infected, have a less severe illness.

Before the development of the diphtheria toxoid vaccine in the 1920s, diphtheria was common. In 1921 more than 206,000 cases were reported in the United States, compared with only 22 cases reported from 1980 to 1987. This decrease in incidence in immunized populations has been accompanied by a shift in the age of infected individuals from children to adults. In unvaccinated populations diphtheria is primarily a disease of children. Mortality rates of 30 to 50 percent have been reported in patients with untreated disease. Treatment with antitoxin can reduce the mortality rate to 5 to 10 percent.

PATHOGENESIS

Diphtheria is caused by the organism *C. diphtheriae,* a gram-positive slender rod that lacks spores or a capsule. The organism has clubbed ends and has a tendency to branch, producing a cuneiform appearance. In the 1920s *C. diphtheriae* was classified into the three subtypes—*gravis, intermedius,* and *mitis*—according to the severity of the disease thought at that time to be caused by each subtype. It is now recognized that the severity of clinical diphtheria is dependent on the quantity of exotoxin produced, and all three subtypes of *C. diphtheriae* are capable of producing exotoxin. The organism's ability to produce exotoxin is conferred by a lysogenic bacteriophage that transmits the gene for toxin production. Infection of a nontoxic strain occurs after the introduction of the bacteriophage, converting the organism to a toxin-producing strain. The toxin produced is a cytotoxic protein that interferes with cell protein synthesis.

C. diphtheriae usually is transmitted to the host by intimate contact with an infected patient or carrier. The infection source is often discharges from the nose, throat, eye, or skin lesions of an infected person. Humans are the major reservoir for *C. diphtheriae.* The organism can survive for long periods outside a host and has been known to be transmitted through contaminated food routes. The incubation period is typically 2 to 3 days but can be up to 1 week. Most commonly the organism colonizes the tonsil or nasopharynx; however, other sites can include the larynx and the skin. The infection tends to remain local; however, toxo-genic strains produce exotoxin, which kills adjacent host cells. The destruction of a layer of epithelium and the resulting exudate coagulate to form a pseudomembrane containing bacteria, fibrin, leukocytes, and necrotic epithelial cells; the pseudomembrane at first appears yellowish white but turns gray after about 5 days. The exotoxin is absorbed locally and carried by the blood systemically and can damage cells in distant organ systems. The most common sites of damage are the nervous system and the myocardium, although occasionally the kidneys are affected.

As the disease progresses locally, pharyngeal and laryngeal edema as well as obstruction from the pseudomembrane can contribute to airway compromise. A sudden detachment of the membrane can result in complete airway obstruction. If exotoxin diffuses into the neck tissue, a severe edema known as "bull neck" can result that carries a grave prognosis. If the membrane extends into the bronchi, a virtual cast will result, which is almost always fatal. Nasal diphtheria is usually the mildest upper respiratory form of the disease and usually does not produce toxicity. Cutaneous diphtheria generally is not known to be toxin-producing and rarely exhibits a pseudomembrane.

The exotoxin is capable of damaging the heart, nervous system, and kidneys. Clinical myocarditis develops in about 10 percent of patients with diphtheria, usually within the first week of the illness. Involvement of the nervous system occurs in 5 to 10 percent of patients with diphtheria. The symptoms vary from an isolated nerve palsy to a Guillain-Barré-appearing syndrome. Nervous system involvement can occur in the first week of the illness but more commonly presents between the second and sixth weeks. Patients who survive diphtheria involving the nervous system do not have residual damage after recovery. A rare but fatal complication of diphtheria is renal failure, which is caused by a toxic nephropathy.

An infection with diphtheria will not necessarily stimulate a patient's natural immunity.

SIGNS AND SYMPTOMS

An infection with *C. diphtheriae* can range from an asymptomatic carrier state, to a single localized lesion without systemic symptoms, to rapidly progressive fatal systemic disease. The severity of the symptoms is a function of the quantity of exotoxin produced, the site and extent of the primary infection, the patient's age, and any preexisting disease. *C. diphtheriae* infections of the anterior nasal area, middle ear, and skin rarely produce exotoxins; consequently, these patients usually have no symptoms other than purulent drainage from the involved site. Infections from these sites can become chronic, and the discharge can transmit the organism to others.

Infection of the respiratory tract is usually exotoxin-producing, with the exception of the anterior nasal area. The most common site is tonsillopharyngeal, followed by laryngeal and tracheobronchial. The onset of symptoms is typically insidious, progressing so rapidly that patients seek care within a few days after the start of symptoms. The initial symptom is often a sore throat in adults and nausea and vomiting in children. Half these patients have a moderate fever, and 25 percent have cough, hoarseness, and dysphagia. Other symptoms include chills and rhinorrhea. While patients without toxicity may have only localized symptoms, patients with severe toxicity may be listless and pale and have a tachycardia that can quickly progress to vascular collapse. Diphtheria should be suspected in a patient presenting with tachycardia and a low-grade fever.

The affected local respiratory mucosa initially appears erythematous; this is quickly followed by the appearance of a yellowish white or gray exudate. These lesions often grow and coalesce within the next 24 h to form a pseudomembrane that progressively thickens, adheres more tightly to the mucosa, and turns a darker gray color. Attempts to dislodge the membrane will cause bleeding. Extensive pseudomembrane formation usually is associated with more severe toxicity.

A particularly malignant form of pharyngeal diphtheria called "bull neck" presents with a rapid onset of extensive pseudomembrane formation, massive edema of the neck, cervical lymphadenopathy, foul-smelling breath, and thick speech. Extension of the pseudomembrane to the larynx or beyond can produce airway obstruction with stridor and cyanosis.

As many as half of at least moderately toxic patients exhibit myocarditis from the direct effect of toxin on myocardial cells. The effect of toxin on neural tissue occurs in 10 to 20 percent of patients and usually presents as a progressive palsy.

Skin lesions rarely produce exotoxin and are most commonly found on the extremities. These infections are usually secondary to a preexisting wound, and the lesions have a "punched-out" well-demarcated ulcerative character with necrotic sloughing of membrane.

DIFFERENTIAL DIAGNOSIS

Diphtheria pseudomembrane should be differentiated from other pharyngeal exudates, such as those caused by beta-hemolytic streptococcal infection, infectious mononucleosis, viral infections, and fungal infections. Diphtheria should be considered early on in patients with sore throat, low-grade fever, tachycardia, and edema, since prompt antitoxin treatment will reduce the toxic complications. Suspicion of infection with *C. diphtheriae* justifies the initiation of treatment before the results of cultures are available.

LABORATORY TESTS

Because of the importance of early treatment, therapy often is begun before the diagnosis can be confirmed. The diagnosis of diphtheria is made by culture, and the organisms are evaluated for exotoxin production. The preferred culture medium is Löffler's medium or tellurite agar, and the laboratory should be informed that diphtheria is suspected. A presumptive diagnosis can be supported by staining exudate with methylene blue, and the presence of deeply staining metachromatic granules is strongly suggestive of infection with *C. diphtheriae*. Beta-hemolytic streptococci are present in 20 to 30 percent of diphtheria infections.

TREATMENT

Hospitalization is advised for symptomatic patients, and those with an infection of the respiratory system should be placed in strict isolation until two cultures from the nose and throat are negative for *C. diphtheriae*. Respiratory, neurologic, cardiac, and renal complications should be monitored carefully. It is important that antitoxin be given as soon as possible to neutralize the toxin that is not yet bound to cells. Antitoxin usually is given as soon as the clinical diagnosis of diphtheria is seriously entertained instead of waiting for the results of cultures.

Since diphtheria antitoxin is derived from horse serum, the patient must be tested for sensitivity before administration. This can be done with a 1:10 antitoxin dilution to the conjunctiva or a 1:100 dilution intradermally. Antitoxin is administered intravenously, with the dose determined by the characteristics of the infection. Suggested dosages are 20,000 to 40,000 U for pharyngeal or laryngeal disease that has lasted 48 h, 40,000 to 60,000 U for nasopharyngeal lesions, and 80,000 to 100,000 U for extensive disease lasting more than 3 days or bull-neck characteristics. Although antitoxin has no proven value in cutaneous diphtheria, some consultants advise using 20,000 to 40,000 U, since a few cases of toxin-producing cutaneous strains have been reported. Individuals sensitive to antitoxin need to undergo a desensitization procedure before antitoxin administration.

Antimicrobials are required to eradicate the organism and stop further toxin production but should not substitute for antitoxin therapy. Erythromycin 40 to 50 mg/kg/d for 14 days is the drug of choice, and eradication of the organism should be documented after treatment by two negative cultures. Asymptomatic carriers also should receive antibiotics, eradication of the infection should be documented. A single intramuscular injection of benzathine penicillin, 600,000 U for those less than 30 kg and 1,200,000 U for those over 30 kg, is an acceptable alternative therapy.

Diphtheria toxoid vaccination will stimulate the host to produce antitoxin for at least 10 years. Most diphtheria cases occur in unvaccinated or inadequately vaccinated individuals. Unvaccinated survivors of diphtheria should begin and complete the immunization series after recovery. Inadequately vaccinated survivors should complete the vaccination regimen. Unvaccinated carriers should begin or complete the immunization series immediately.

Close contacts of a suspected patient or carrier should be cultured, should receive antimicrobial therapy, and should receive a diphtheria toxoid booster if the last vaccination occurred over 5 years earlier. Those with incomplete immunization should immediately resume and complete their immunizations. The administration of antitoxin to unvaccinated close contacts is not recommended.

Vaccination of the population is the key to preventing diphtheria. Children should be vaccinated at 2, 4, and 6 months with a combined diphtheria, tetanus, and pertussis (DTP) vaccine and again at 18 months and 4 to 6 years of age with a DTP or a DTaP vaccine. The first three doses should be at least 4 weeks apart, and the fourth dose should follow the third by at least 6 months. A fifth dose is necessary at school entry if the fourth dose was given before age 4. Children under 7 years of age who did not receive any vaccination in the first year of life should have two vaccinations at least 4 weeks apart and a third vaccination at least 6 months after the second and a fourth before school entry unless the third dose was given after age 4. Those receiving the vaccination series after age 6 should get a Td, which has a smaller quantity of diphtheria antitoxin. The first two doses should be administered at least 4 weeks apart, and a third dose should be administered at least 6 months after the second. Booster vaccinations of Td should be administered every 10 years. DTP, DT, and Td vaccinations can be given concurrently with other vaccinations.

Inadequately immunized teenagers and adults are thought to constitute a large pool of individuals susceptible to diphtheria infection. Practitioners should identify all inadequately protected individuals in the population and immunize them.

BIBLIOGRAPHY

Berkow R (ed): *Merck Manual of Diagnosis and Therapy*, 16th ed. Rahway, NJ, Merck Sharp & Dohme, 1992.

Chambers HF: Diphtheria, in Tierney LM Jr, McPhee SJ, Papadakis MA (eds): *Current Medical Diagnosis and Treatment*, 35th rev. Norwalk, CT, Appleton & Lange, 1996.

Committee on Infectious Diseases, Peter G (ed): *1994 Red Book*. American Academy of Pediatrics, Elk Grove Village, IL, 1994.

Cunningham GF, MacDonald PC, Gant NR, et al (eds): *William's Obstetrics*, 19th ed. Norwalk, CT, Appleton & Lange, 1993.

Hewlett EL: *Cecil Textbook of Medicine*, 19th ed. Philadelphia, Saunders, 1992.

Holmes RK: Diphtheria, Other Coryebacterial Infections, and Anthrax, in Fauci AS, Braunwald E, Isselbacher KJ, et al (eds): *Harrison's Principles of Internal Medicine*, 14th ed. New York, McGraw-Hill, 1998, pp 892–899.

Ogle JW: *Current Pediatric Diagnosis and Treatment*, in Hay WW Jr, Groothuis JR, Hayward AR, et al (eds): 12th ed. Norwalk, CT, Appleton & Lange, 1995.

Overturf GD: *Conn's Current Therapy, 1995*, in Rachel RE (ed): Philadelphia, Saunders, 1995.
Ryan JL, Grossman M: *Basic and Clinical Immunology*, in Stites DP, Terr AI, Parslow TP (eds): 8th ed. Norwalk, CT, Appleton & Lange, 1994.

Chapter 9–11
ENTEROBIASIS (PINWORMS)
JoAnn Deasy

DISCUSSION

Pinworms (*Enterobius vermicularis*) are the most common helminthic infection seen by clinicians in the United States. They are intestinal nematodes whose life cycle is confined to humans. The eggs of *E. vermicularis* hatch in the small intestine, where the larvae differentiate into adults and then migrate to the colon. The adult worms are small (about 1 cm in length), whitish in color, and threadlike in appearance. In the colon, mating occurs, and then at night the female worms migrate from the anus to deposit thousands of fertilized eggs on the perianal skin that then may be transferred to clothes, bedding, and the air. Within 6 h the eggs develop into infectious larvae.

Reinfection can occur when the larvae return to the colon or eggs can be carried to the mouth on the fingers after anal scratching. Microscopic eggs that have contaminated bedding and other surfaces in the home promote the spread of infection to entire families.

SYMPTOMS

The most common presenting symptoms of pinworms are perianal and perineal pruritus and restless sleep caused by the itching. Many infections with *E. vermicularis* are asymptomatic.

OBJECTIVE FINDINGS

The physical examination may be entirely normal, or evidence of scratching with excoriations may be present. Examination of the anus very late at night or early in the morning with a light source may reveal the presence of the glistening adult worms. A heavy infestation with *E. vermicularis* may cause vulvovaginitis.

DIAGNOSTIC CONSIDERATIONS

The differential diagnosis includes dermatologic problems that may present with localized pruritus.

SPECIAL CONSIDERATIONS

The prevalence of pinworm infections is greatest in children under 12 years of age. Spread in institutionalized settings may be quite rapid.

LABORATORY TESTS

The diagnosis is made by recovering the eggs of *E. vermicularis* from perianal skin by using the "Scotch tape" technique and then examining the specimen microscopically. To recover the eggs, a tongue blade covered with a segment of clear cellulose tape is placed sticky side down on the unwashed perianal skin

in the morning. The specimen is transferred to a glass slide and then examined microscopically for the colorless eggs, which are flattened on one side. The collection of several specimens on separate mornings increases the detection rate. These eggs are not found in stools, but occasionally the adult worm can be found in feces.

TREATMENT

Pinworm infection is treated with mebendazole (Vermox) in a single oral dose of 100 mg. A second dose 10 days later often is recommended to ensure effectiveness. Reinfection is very common. The entire family should be treated to ensure eradication.

PATIENT EDUCATION

Clothing and bedding should be washed in hot water. Personal cleanliness is a useful, general principle, but there is no good means of preventing pinworm infection.

BIBLIOGRAPHY
Juckett G: Common intestinal helminths. *Am Fam Phys* 52(7):2039–2048, 1995.
Mandell GL, Douglas RG, Bennett JE (eds): *Principles and Practice of Infectious Diseases*, 4th ed. New York, Churchill Livingstone, 1995.

Chapter 9–12
GIARDIASIS
JoAnn Deasy

DISCUSSION

Giardia lamblia is the most clinically significant protozoal pathogen in the United States. *Giardia* possesses both a trophozoite form and a cyst form. The mature cysts are the infective form of the parasite and generally are transmitted fecally-orally or through the ingestion of contaminated food or water. Sexual transmission, usually homosexual, has been reported. In the duodenum of a new host, the cyst divides into trophozoites. The trophozoites flourish in the duodenum and jejunum, absorbing nutrients from the intestinal tract. Disease manifestations appear to be related to intestinal malabsorption, particularly of fat and carbohydrates. The trophozoites may be carried by the fecal stream to the large intestine, where some trophozoites encyst. The infective cysts are passed in feces and can survive in cold water for more than 2 months; they are resistant to the concentration of chlorine generally used in municipal water systems.

SYMPTOMS

Infection with *Giardia* may result in asymptomatic passage of cysts, an acute case of often self-limited diarrhea, or a chronic syndrome of diarrhea, malabsorption, and weight loss. The presence of symptoms and their severity most likely are related to the number of cysts and the strain of *Giardia* ingested and the individual's immune response to the parasite. The incubation period from the ingestion of the cysts to the development of symptoms is 1 to 2 weeks.

Acute giardiasis is characterized by diarrhea, foul-smelling stools, abdominal cramps or pain, bloating, and flatulence. The patient may experience fatigue, nausea, and anorexia. Acute symptoms generally resolve within several weeks. Patients who go on to have chronic symptoms often experience a more profound fatigue, and have upper abdominal pain and flatulence. Diarrhea is usually present but may be interrupted by periods of constipation or normal bowel movements. Malabsorption and weight loss may develop.

OBJECTIVE FINDINGS

The physical examination may be entirely unremarkable, or mild epigastric tenderness may be present.

DIAGNOSTIC CONSIDERATIONS

Giardiasis may be confused with diarrhea caused by other parasites or with diarrhea caused by viral or bacterial gastroenteritis. Other diseases that should be considered in the differential diagnosis include irritable bowel syndrome, malabsorption syndromes, peptic ulcer disease, lactase deficiency, inflammatory bowel disease, and cholecystitis.

SPECIAL CONSIDERATIONS

All ages and economic groups may become infected with *G. lamblia,* but there is a higher incidence in young children and young adults. Giardiasis is common among non-toilet-trained young children who attend day-care centers, and person-to-person transmission to their families may occur. The ingestion of fecally contaminated water accounts for many cases of traveler's diarrhea. Waterborne outbreaks of giardiasis have been reported in the United States. The sources have included untreated stream water, sewage-contaminated municipal water supplies, and chlorinated but inadequately filtered water. It is thought that wild mammals, particularly beavers, have been the reservoir hosts of *Giardia* in some of these outbreaks. Persons with IgA deficiency are more likely to develop symptomatic giardiasis.

LABORATORY TESTS

The diagnosis of giardiasis should be considered in patients who present with prolonged diarrhea, abdominal crampy pain, or malabsorption. Recent travel to an endemic area or the presence of children in the home who attend day-care centers should raise the index of suspicion. The diagnosis is confirmed by ordering a stool examination for ova and parasites and finding the cyst in semisolid or formed stool specimens or the trophozoite in liquid stool. In acutely symptomatic patients, the parasite usually can be demonstrated by examining one to three stool specimens. In chronic cases, passage of the parasite is often intermittent, making confirmation more difficult. Duodenoscopy with biopsy and duodenal fluid sampling for *Giardia* trophozoites are reserved for diagnostically difficult cases. Detection of anti-*Giardia* IgM is compatible with the diagnosis of acute infection. Testing for fecal *Giardia* antigen by enzyme-linked immunosorbent assay (ELISA) has been shown to be sensitive and specific.

TREATMENT

Giardiasis may be treated with metronidazole (Flagyl) 250 mg three times a day for 5 days (pediatric dose, 15 mg/kg/d in three doses). Metronidazole may cause nausea, vomiting, and a metallic taste in the mouth. It also is known to cause a disulfiram-like (Antabuse) reaction with alcohol. As an alternative, furazolidone (Furoxone) 100 mg four times a day for 7 to 10 days for adults or 6 mg/kg/d in four doses for children may be prescribed. Furazolidone comes in a suspension form and therefore is especially useful for treating children under age 5 years. Paromomycin is less effective but may be used during pregnancy in a very symptomatic woman. Although treatment of asymptomatic persons is not clinically required, it should be considered to prevent person-to-person transmission of *Giardia*.

PATIENT EDUCATION

The prevention of giardiasis includes attention to good personal hygiene, particularly hand washing, especially in day-care settings. Hikers and travelers should use caution when drinking local water. Adequate disinfection of water can be accomplished by using portable purification systems, available from outdoor supply stores, that filter out *Giardia*.

DISPOSITION

Once a diagnosis of giardiasis is made, consideration should be given to testing other household members. Patients should be reevaluated if their symptoms persist.

BIBLIOGRAPHY

Juckett G: Intestinal protozoa. *Am Fam Phys* 53(8):2507–2516, 1996.
Mandell GL, Douglas RG, Bennett JE (eds): *Principles and Practice of Infectious Diseases,* 4th ed. New York, Churchill Livingstone, 1995.
Sherris JC (ed): *Medical Microbiology.* New York, Elsevier, 1990, pp 734–736.

Chapter 9–13
GONORRHEA
Meredith Hansen

DISCUSSION

Etiology

The etiologic agent of gonorrhea is *Neisseria gonorrhoeae,* a gram-negative diplococcus. It is found intra- and extracellularly.

Epidemiology

Gonorrhea is considered the most prevalent sexually transmitted disease (STD) in the United States. It has been estimated that gonorrhea infects more than 2.5 million people annually. Although gonorrhea is reportable in all states, it has been estimated that only 20 to 30 percent of cases are reported. The risk factors for the development of gonorrhea are multiple sexual partners, young age, early onset of sexual activity, lack of barrier contraceptive use, and a history of a previous STD. The average incubation period of gonorrhea is 2 to 5 days.

Multidrug resistance is common with gonococcal infections. Penicillinase-producing *N. gonorrhoeae* (PPNG) has been detected in the United States since 1976. PPNG is currently implicated in 5 to 20 percent of all gonococcal infections in the United

States. Tetracycline- and spectinomycin-resistant gonococcal infections have been documented since the mid-1980s.

SIGNS AND SYMPTOMS AND OBJECTIVE FINDINGS

The clinical syndrome of gonorrhea is broad, ranging from patients who are asymptomatic or superficially symptomatic to patients who have complicated infections at multiple sites or disseminated disease.

Uncomplicated infections remain localized to the site of inoculation. Gonorrhea rarely causes disabling symptoms or sequelae. Eighty to 90 percent of treated cases in the industrial world are uncomplicated.

Uncomplicated Infection in Men

Acute urethritis is the most common clinical manifestation of gonorrhea in men. The incubation period ranges from 1 to 14 days, with 2 to 5 days being the average. Symptoms include dysuria, urethral discharge, and meatal erythema. The discharge may be scanty and mucoid or mucopurulent, becoming frankly purulent and profuse within 24 h. Anorectal symptoms include proctalgia, anal pruritus, purulent discharge, and tenesmus. Gonococcal pharyngitis commonly is asymptomatic but may present with a sore throat and an acute tonsillopharyngitis. Pharyngeal infections carry an increased risk of dissemination. Studies have demonstrated that 3 to 7 percent of men with gonorrhea are asymptomatic.

Complicated Infection in Men

Gonorrhea in men may ascend from the lower genital area to an upper tract site, presenting as an acute epididymitis, an acute or chronic prostatitis, an inguinal lymphadenitis, or urethral stricture formation.

Uncomplicated Infection in Women

Cervicitis is the most common clinical manifestation in women. The incubation period averages 2 to 10 days. Common symptoms include vaginal discharge, dysuria, dyspareunia, dysmenorrhea, and irregular menstrual bleeding. The physical examination may be normal or may show an abnormal cervix with purulent or mucopurulent discharge, erythema, and friability. A high prevalence of coexisting infections has been demonstrated. Female anorectal and pharyngeal clinical manifestations are identical to the male presentations. Studies have demonstrated that 10 to 20 percent of women with gonorrhea are asymptomatic.

Complicated Infection in Women

Gonococcal infection in women migrates from the lower genital area and ascends to the fallopian tubes in approximately 15 percent of infections. This spread may result in endometritis or salpingitis. Chronic salpingitis may lead to scarring in the fallopian tubes, resulting in sterility. Gonorrhea may migrate into the abdomen and create a perihepatitis that also is called the Fitz-Hugh–Curtis syndrome. The symptoms of Fitz-Hugh–Curtis syndrome are right upper quadrant abdominal pain, fever, and nausea. A concurrent salpingitis is common with Fitz-Hugh–Curtis syndrome.

Skene's and Bartholin's glands are commonly infected, resulting in abscess formation. A unilateral Bartholin's abscess is strongly suggestive of gonorrhea. In pregnancy, spontaneous abortion and premature membrane rupture may occur.

Table 9-13-1. Differential Diagnosis of Cervicitis/Urethritis

Neisseria gonorrhoeae
Chlamydia trachomatis
Ureaplasma urealyticum
Candidiasis
Bacterial vaginosis
Trichomonas vaginalis
Herpes simplex
Allergic urethritis/cervicitis (latex)

Disseminated Disease

Disseminated gonococcal infections result from a gonococcal bacteremia, resulting in a triad. All three presentations of the triad rarely occur together:

1. Skin lesions: papular, pustular, or necrotic
2. Asymmetric arthralgias or septic arthritis
3. Tenosynovitis

Two-thirds of disseminated disease occurs in women. The symptoms of disseminated infection tend to appear immediately after a menstrual cycle. This is thought to occur secondarily from sloughing of the endometrium, exposing blood vessels to the infectious agent. Strains of *N. gonorrhoeae* that cause disseminated disease tend to produce limited genitourinary symptoms.

Disseminated gonococcal infections are uncommonly complicated by hepatitis, endocarditis, or meningitis.

DIAGNOSTIC CONSIDERATIONS

A variety of genital pathogens, most of which are sexually transmitted, may cause urethritis or cervicitis. A differential listing is provided in Table 9-13-1.

SPECIAL CONSIDERATIONS
Management of Sexual Partners

The sexual partners of infected patients must be evaluated and treated. Patients should refrain from intercourse until they and all their partners are cured.

HIV Infection

Treatment of gonorrhea in HIV-infected patients is identical to the treatment regimens listed below.

Pregnancy

The treatment regimens used in pregnancy are listed below. Pregnant women should not be treated with quinolones or tetracyclines.

Gonococcal Infections in Infants

During delivery, the conjunctiva, pharynx, or rectum of the newborn may be infected. Infants at high risk for gonococcal ophthalmia are those whose mothers did not receive prenatal care or have a history of STDs or drug use. Prophylaxis for the prevention of gonococcal ophthalmia is the standard of care in U.S. hospitals. Topical therapy alone is inadequate if the infant has a documented gonococcal infection. Treatment for gonococcal infections in infants should consist of ceftriaxone 25 to 50 mg/kg intravenously or intramuscularly in a single dose.

LABORATORY TESTING

Isolation of *N. gonorrhoeae* is the diagnostic standard. Gram's stain of exudate (men) represents a presumptive diagnosis when gram-negative diplococci are identified within polymorphonuclear cells. Culture using Thayer-Martin medium is indicated when Gram staining is negative or equivocal. *N. gonorrhoeae* is a fastidious organism that dies quickly. Cultures should be plated immediately and incubated as soon as possible. The existence of coinfection with other STDs is common. All patients should be tested for chlamydia and syphilis. Patients also should be counseled about HIV testing.

TREATMENT

Pharmacologic Management

The recommended regimen is ceftriaxone 125 mg intramuscularly in a single dose. Alternative regimens include cefixime 400 mg orally in a single dose, ofloxacin 400 mg orally in a single dose, spectinomycin 2 g given intramuscularly in a single dose, and ciprofloxacin 500 mg orally in a single dose.

Since coinfection with chlamydia is common, these regimens should be followed by a 7-day course of doxycycline or erythromycin. A single 1-g dose of azithromycin is also effective.

The recommended regimen in pregnant women is ceftriaxone 125 mg given intramuscularly in a single dose. This regimen should be followed with a 7-day course of erythromycin.

The recommended regimen for disseminated infection consists of ceftriaxone 1 g intramuscularly or intravenously daily* or ceftizoxime 1 g intravenously every 8 h.†

Patient Education

Patients must be advised to abstain from sexual activity until they and their partners are cured. Concurrent treatment of all partners is essential even if they are asymptomatic. All sexual partners within the last 30 days should be tested and treated.

A history of an STD places a patient at risk for subsequent STDs. When used consistently, condoms are effective in preventing STDs. Patient education in the proper use of condoms should occur during every patient visit for STDs.

DISPOSITION

A follow-up test to cure is not mandatory, since treatment failures are uncommon. Retesting, including drug sensitivity, should be performed if symptoms persist; reinfection is questionable.

COMPLICATIONS AND RED FLAGS

Gonorrhea is a reportable communicable disease in all states. Physician assistants should be knowledgeable about the reporting procedures in their states.

Routine screening for asymptomatic infection in women during the annual pelvic examination is recommended, particularly for high-risk patients. Physician assistants should be aware of clinical findings that are suggestive of asymptomatic infection (friable cervix, mucopurulent discharge, and chronic pelvic pain). Routine screening for asymptomatic infection in men is not recommended at this time.

BIBLIOGRAPHY

Centers for Disease Control and Prevention: 1993 sexually transmitted diseases treatment guidelines. *MMWR* 42(No. RR-14):3–7, 40–45, 1993.

Fauci AS, Braunwald E, Isselbacher KJ, et al (eds): *Harrison's Principles of Internal Medicine,* 14th ed. New York, McGraw-Hill, 1998, pp 915–922.

Preventive Services Task Force: *Guide to Clinical Preventive Services,* 2d ed. Alexandria, VA, International Medical Publishing, 1996.

Tierney L, McPhee SJ, Papadakis MA (eds): *Current Medical Diagnosis and Treatment,* 36th ed. Norwalk, CT, Appleton & Lange, 1997, pp 1214–1216.

Chapter 9–14
GRANULOMA INGUINALE
Meredith Hansen

DISCUSSION

Granuloma inguinale (GI) is also called donovanosis and is associated with the presence of an intracellular organism known as a Donovan body.

Etiology

The etiologic agent of GI is *Calymmatobacterium granulomatis,* a gram-negative rod.

Epidemiology

GI is uncommon in developed countries. The greatest incidence of GI occurs in tropical and subtropical areas, where endemic clusters are found. The reported incidence is 10:1 male:female. Demonstrated HIV coinfection has been found in Africa. The incubation period is broad, falling between 8 and 90 days.

SIGNS AND SYMPTOMS AND OBJECTIVE FINDINGS

The most common initial presentation is a painless granulomatous ulcer at the inoculation site. The lesion may become quite disfiguring as the ulcer enlarges. Enlargement of the lesion or lesions occurs by autoinoculation or continuous spread. Regional lymphadenopathy is uncommon unless there is a secondary bacterial infection.

Dissemination with bony, splenic, or hepatic involvement has been reported. Perianal GI may mimic the condylomata lata of secondary syphilis. Complications of GI include urethral, vaginal, or anal stenosis and lymphatic obstruction that produces a genital edema. A causal relationship involving the development of genital carcinomas secondary to GI has not been proved.

---

* This regimen should be given until 24 to 48 h after the resolution of symptoms; then cefixime should be given at 400 mg daily to complete a 7- to 10-day course.

† This regimen should be followed with a 7-day course of erythromycin or doxycycline or a single 1-g dose of azithromycin.

DIAGNOSTIC CONSIDERATIONS

A variety of genital pathogens, most of which are sexually transmitted, cause genital ulcer disease. A differential listing is provided in Table 9-14-1.

SPECIAL CONSIDERATIONS

Management of Sexual Partners

The sexual partners of infected patients must be evaluated and treated. Patients must be told to refrain from intercourse until they are cured. Studies document increased coinfection with HIV and syphilis. Patients must be counseled about HIV testing and tested for syphilis.

HIV Infection

Current studies do not recommend a different treatment regimen for GI when the patient has HIV infection.

LABORATORY TESTING

Serologic testing is not useful in diagnosing GI but is essential in ruling out syphilis and HIV. The most successful method used to identify the Donovan bodies in GI patients is a punch biopsy of the granulation tissue from the border of the lesion or lesions. With the use of Wright-Giemsa staining techniques, the Donovan bodies can be seen within the cytoplasm of large mononuclear cells.

TREATMENT

Pharmacologic Management

Four commonly used antibiotics are effective in the management of GI. However, because of the uncommon nature of GI in the United States, clinical efficacy trials have not been performed.

The recommended regimen is tetracycline 500 mg orally four times per day, doxycycline 100 mg orally twice per day, erythromycin 500 mg orally four times per day, or trimethoprim (160 mg)-sulfamethoxazole (800 mg) orally twice per day.

Regardless of the antibiotic used, the regimen must be continued until the lesions resolve.

Patient Education

A history of sexually transmitted disease (STD) places a patient at risk for subsequent STDs. Patients should be advised of their increased risk status and counseled on methods to reduce the risk of subsequent STDs. When used consistently, condoms are effective in preventing STDs. Patient education in the proper use of condoms should occur during every patient visit for an STD. Patients need to be advised about sexual abstinence while undergoing treatment for GI.

Table 9-14-1. Differential Diagnosis of Genital Ulcers

Treponema pallidum
Herpes simplex
Leishmaniasis
Haemophilus ducreyi
Granuloma inguinale

DISPOSITION

A follow-up test to cure is not necessary in GI. Patients who are unresponsive to antibiotic therapy should be reassessed on their diagnosis.

COMPLICATIONS AND RED FLAGS

Because of the uncommon nature of GI in the United States, few states include it in their reportable disease lists. GI should be reported to the appropriate health authorities.

BIBLIOGRAPHY

Centers for Disease Control and Prevention: 1993 sexually transmitted diseases treatment guidelines. *MMWR* 42(No. RR-14):4–7, 19–21, 1993.

Goens JL, Schwartz R, DeWolf K: Mucocutaneous manifestations of chancroid, lymphogranuloma venereum and granuloma inguinale. *Am Fam Phys* 49(2):415–425, 1994.

Hoffman I, Schmitz J: Genital ulcer disease. *Postgrad Med* 98(3):67–80, 1995.

Preventive Services Task Force: *Guide to Preventive Clinical Services,* 2d ed. Alexandria, VA, International Medical Publishing, 1996.

Tierney L, McPhee SJ, Papadakis MA (eds): *Current Medical Diagnosis and Treatment,* 36th ed. Norwalk, CT, Appleton & Lange, 1997, p 1168.

Chapter 9–15
INFLUENZA
JoAnn Deasy

DISCUSSION

Influenza is a common respiratory pathogen of humans caused by RNA viruses of the Orthomyxoviridae family. There are three antigenically different groups of influenza viruses, designated as A, B, and C. Influenza A and influenza B are clinically indistinguishable, while influenza C causes a milder illness. Influenza is spread by respiratory droplets. The incubation period is 1 to 3 days.

Outbreaks of influenza occur virtually every winter but vary considerably in extent and severity. The major determinants for morbidity and mortality are the virulence of the circulating strain of virus and the preexisting immunity in the population in which the infection occurs. In the United States, 10,000 to 20,000 people die annually from influenza-related illness in nonpandemic years. Influenza virus causes large economic losses from disruption of the workforce and high health care costs.

SYMPTOMS AND SIGNS

Influenza is characterized by an abrupt onset of fever [38–41°C (101 to 106°F)]; myalgias, especially of the back and thighs; headache; and a nonproductive cough. Coryza and a sore throat are also usually present. Influenza can cause severe malaise lasting several days. Physical examination may reveal no signs or minimal signs such as mild pharyngeal injection.

DIFFERENTIAL DIAGNOSIS

In absence of a community outbreak, influenza can be difficult to diagnose. The differential diagnosis includes other febrile illnesses and other viral respiratory infections.

COMPLICATIONS AND SPECIAL CONSIDERATIONS

Influenza causes damage to the respiratory epithelium that predisposes an individual to a secondary bacterial infection. The most common complications of influenza are acute sinusitis, otitis media, bronchitis, and bacterial pneumonia. Secondary pneumonia most often is caused by *Streptococcus pneumoniae. Haemophilus influenzae* and *Staphylococcus aureus* also may cause pneumonia. Staphylococcal pneumonia is less common but is the most serious form. A primary pneumonia caused by the influenza virus itself occurs but is rare.

Reye's syndrome can be a hepatic and central nervous system (CNS) complication of influenza and other viral infections. It occurs almost exclusively in children. Because of the association between Reye's syndrome and aspirin, the administration of aspirin should be avoided. Myocarditis and pericarditis are other rare complications of influenza. In addition to the complications of individual organ systems listed above, elderly and chronically ill persons may experience multisystem deterioration. Persons at high risk for the complications of influenza include those over age 65 and persons with chronic cardiopulmonary or metabolic diseases.

DIAGNOSTICS

A clinical diagnosis of influenza can be made with a high degree of certainty if typical "influenza-like illness" is encountered in the middle of a documented outbreak. The white blood cell (WBC) count may show leukopenia or may be normal. Proteinuria may be present. A chest x-ray will be normal in a patient with uncomplicated pneumonia. A specific laboratory diagnosis is established by isolating the virus in cell culture from oropharynx or respiratory secretions. A serologic diagnosis can be made retrospectively by comparing antibody titers in acute and convalescent serums obtained 10 to 14 days apart.

TREATMENT

The treatment of uncomplicated influenza is largely symptomatic and includes antipyretics-analgesics. Aspirin should be avoided because of the risk of Reye's syndrome. Patients should be advised to rest and maintain hydration during acute illness.

Amantadine can be used for the treatment of influenza A but is not effective against influenza B. The administration of amantadine within 48 h of the onset of illness has been shown to reduce the signs and symptoms of influenza by 50 percent. The usual dose is 200 mg/d in two divided doses for adults. Because the drug is excreted largely by the kidneys, the dose should be reduced in patients with decreased renal function as well as in the elderly (over age 65), for whom the usual dose is 100 mg/d. Amantadine is associated with mild CNS side effects, including jitteriness, anxiety, insomnia, and difficulty concentrating. An increased incidence of seizures has been reported in persons with a history of seizure disorder taking amantadine.

The antiviral rimantadine (200 mg/d in two divided doses) also may be used and is associated with fewer side effects. Rimantadine is preferred in patients with renal failure. It has not been approved for the treatment of influenza in children.

Table 9-15-1. High-Risk Groups in Which Yearly Influenza Vaccine Is Recommended

Persons 65 years of age or older
Residents of nursing homes and other chronic care facilities that house persons of any age with chronic medical conditions
Adults and children with chronic disorders of the pulmonary or cardiovascular system, including children with asthma
Adults and children who have required regular medical follow-up or hospitalization during the preceding year because of chronic metabolic diseases (including diabetes mellitus), renal dysfunction, hemoglobinopathies, or immunosuppression (including immunosuppression caused by medications)

SOURCE: Centers for Disease Control and Prevention: Prevention and control of influenza: Recommendations of the Advisory Committee on Immunization Practices. *MMWR* 45(RR-5):1–24, 1996.

Antibacterial antibiotics should be prescribed only when bacterial complications occur. The persistence of fever beyond 4 days, leukocytosis, or a cough that becomes productive should precipitate a workup to verify or rule out a secondary bacterial infection.

PREVENTION

Prevention may be accomplished by immunoprophylaxis with inactivated (killed-virus) vaccine or chemoprophylaxis with amantadine or rimantadine. Vaccination of persons at high risk each year is the most effective measure for reducing the impact of influenza. Each year's vaccine contains three virus strains (usually two type A and one type B). The vaccine's antigenic formulation changes yearly and is based on the prevalent strains of the preceding year. Influenza vaccine is recommended for any person 6 months of age or older who is at increased risk for influenza-related complications (Table 9-15-1), health care workers and others in close contact with people at high risk for influenza, and individuals who wish to reduce their chances of becoming infected with influenza. Vaccination provides partial immunity (efficacy depends on age, immunocompetence, and how well the vaccine matches circulating influenza strains) for a few months to 1 year. It takes up to 2 weeks for the development of antibodies. Influenza vaccine should be administered in October or November each year. Immunosuppressed individuals may have a decreased antibody response to influenza vaccine but should still be immunized. Two doses 1 month apart may be necessary to achieve a satisfactory antibody response in previously unvaccinated children less than 9 years old.

Influenza vaccine is contraindicated in persons who are known to have anaphylactic hypersensitivity to eggs or other components of the vaccine. Since influenza vaccine contains only noninfectious viruses, it cannot cause influenza. The most common side effect of vaccination is soreness at the vaccination site. Myalgias and fever occur rarely.

For persons in high-risk groups for whom the influenza vaccine is contraindicated, chemoprophylaxis with amantadine or rimantadine may be indicated throughout the influenza season. The dose is the same as that used for treatment.

PROGNOSIS

The duration of uncomplicated influenza is 1 to 7 days, and the prognosis is excellent. The mortality rate is highest in debilitated persons. In influenza epidemic years in the United States, more than 90 percent of the deaths attributed to pneumonia and influenza have occurred among persons over 65 years of age.

BIBLIOGRAPHY

Centers for Disease Control and Prevention: Prevention and control of influenza: Recommendations of the Advisory Committee on Immunization Practices. *MMWR* 45(RR-5):1–24, 1996.

Mandell GL, Douglas RG, Bennett JE: *Principles and Practice of Infectious Diseases,* 4th ed. New York, Churchill Livingston, 1995.

Small PA Jr: Influenza: Pathogenesis and host defense. *Hosp Pract,* 25(11):51–54, 1990.

Chapter 9–16
MEASLES/RUBEOLA
Richard Dehn

DISCUSSION

Measles, also known as rubeola and the seven-day measles, is a highly contagious viral illness that is characterized by a prodromal phase consisting of high fevers, cough, malaise, coryza, anorexia, and conjunctivitis. The prodromal phase begins 7 to 14 days after exposure, and 2 to 4 days later Koplik's spots appear on the buccal and labial mucosa. A day or two after the appearance of Koplik's spots, the characteristic rash begins, first around the ears and then spreading downward to the trunk and extremities. It begins as irregular macules that rapidly progress to maculopapular lesions. By the time the rash reaches the extremities (usually about 2 days), the earliest lesions have begun to fade to a brownish color, which eventually desquamates.

Before the routine vaccination of American children beginning in 1963, virtually everyone acquired measles, usually before age 10, and this conferred a lifelong immunity. In the prevaccination era, measles epidemics 3 to 4 months long occurred every 2 to 5 years. The justification for vaccination of the nonimmune population is based on the morbidity and mortality rates of the complications that occasionally result from a measles infection.

Vaccine products currently in use produce immunity in about 95 percent of the population immunized. After the introduction of widespread immunization in 1963, the annual number of reported cases in the United States decreased from about 500,000 before 1963 to 1497 in 1983. More recently the annual number of measles cases in the United States has increased to more than 27,000, resulting in more than 60 deaths in 1990. The increase in cases has been attributed to populations of nonimmunized preschool children, the immigration of nonimmunized individuals to the United States, and a population of nonimmune but previously vaccinated individuals. The recent rise in measles cases has led to increased efforts to immunize all eligible populations and has resulted in the recommendation that a series of two vaccine doses be used instead of the traditional single-dose protocol. The measles virus is so contagious that cases occur despite high levels of immunity in the population, and so the goal of prevention calls for vaccinating as many individuals in the population as possible. In the developing world measles is still a common childhood disease, and it has been estimated that measles cause 1 million to 2 million deaths annually worldwide. In the United States the mortality rate from measles is 3 in 1000 cases, primarily from respiratory and neurologic complications.

PATHOGENESIS

Measles is caused by a paramyxovirus that is spread by direct contact or by airborne droplets drawn into the host's respiratory tract. It and chickenpox are among the most easily transmitted infectious diseases. After inoculation the virus begins to replicate, and after 2 to 4 days it begins shedding and is communicable to other hosts. The acute infection is characterized by a marked depression of cellular immunity, which is probably a direct viral effect on B and T lymphocytes, and it is during this time that the prodromal symptoms start and progress. The depression of cellular immunity in the prodromal stage commonly produces leukopenia. A few days after upper respiratory symptoms have developed and progressed, the characteristic rash appears, produced by the reemergence of cellular immunity. Patients deficient in cellular immunity do not develop a rash but develop infections that result in death. Half the patients with an underlying malignancy or HIV who contact measles will die. The depression of cellular immunity in the prodromal stage sometimes results in the reactivation of tuberculosis or coccidioidomycosis and is the rationale for the recommendation not to perform skin testing after the administration of a measles vaccination or a case of measles.

In the absence of secondary complications, the appearance of the rash is soon followed by marked improvement in systemic symptoms such as fever, as the reinvigorated cellular immunity rapidly reduces the quantity of virus present in the host. The end result of a measles infection is a lifelong humeral immunity, which is passively transferred to a newborn. Newborns of immune mothers are protected by maternal antibody for the first few months of life.

The depression of cellular immunity also can contribute to the development of infections in other organ systems. Lower respiratory tract infections have been reported in up to 50 percent of measles cases. These infections include primary viral infections such as bronchitis and pneumonia in adults and croup and bronchiolitis in children as well as secondary bacterial infections such as pneumonia, sinusitis, and otitis media. Giant cell pneumonia may develop in immunocompromised patients without the presentation of the characteristic measles rash.

Measles often produces central nervous system symptoms, with a majority of uncomplicated cases exhibiting some transient EEG abnormalities. Between 0.05 and 0.1 percent of cases result in acute encephalitis, with these patients exhibiting fever, seizures, altered sensation, and occasional focal abnormalities. The mortality rate from measles encephalitis is 10 to 20 percent, with more than half these patients having residual neurologic effects. Encephalitis is thought to be due to an immune response directed at myelin structures. Subacute sclerosing panencephalitis (SSPE), a rare but fatal condition, can occur years after a measles infection. It is characterized by a progression of mental deterioration, seizures, and myoclonic jerks and is almost always fatal. It rarely occurs in patients whose immunity was conferred by immunization, and so the incidence of SSPE has decreased significantly in developed countries.

Acute measles infection can produce acute viral appendicitis and viral mesenteric adenitis, which can result in abdominal pain. An icteric hepatitis is present in up to 5 percent of adult measles cases. Viral keratitis is common and may progress to corneal ulcerations.

The measles virus poses problems in pregnant women in that maternal infection increases the risk of abortion and low birthweight infants. There is no evidence that measles causes birth defects; however, if maternal infection develops shortly before birth, the risk of the neonate developing measles is high. Neonates with measles bear some risk of death, especially if they are born preterm.

Individuals who received the inactivated measles vaccine before 1969 are susceptible to an often severe atypical form of measles. The inactivated vaccine of that era stimulated the production of antibody to only the viral hemagglutinin, not the fusion protein. A natural infection after vaccination with the inactivated vaccine often produced a severe illness with unusual and confusing features such as a noncharacteristic rash, pneumonitis, eosinophilia, coagulopathy, and an elevated erythrocyte sedimentation rate (ESR). The live-virus vaccines administered since 1969 stimulate antibody production to both the viral hemagglutinin and the fusion protein.

SIGNS AND SYMPTOMS

After infection and a 7- to 14-day incubation period, the patient begins to develop a fever, cough, coryza, and conjunctivitis. Fevers can be high and often are accompanied by anorexia, malaise, myalgia, and gastrointestinal symptoms. Within a day or two, an erythemetous maculopapular rash develops around and below the ears and quickly spreads downward to affect the trunk and extremities. A few days after the rash appears, the prodromal symptoms often begin to improve, and 5 to 6 days after appearing, the rash begins to turn a brownish color, starting with the earliest-appearing lesions. A generalized lymphadenopathy commonly appears in the prodromal phase and can persist for several weeks. The cough often persists after the resolution of the rest of the symptoms.

Two to 4 days after acute symptoms begin, Koplik's spots appear, which are diagnostic for measles. They present as small white to bluish white specks on a red base. They are typically present on the buccal or labial mucosa opposite the first and second molars.

SPECIAL CONSIDERATIONS

Bacterial infections are the most common complication, and pneumonia and otitis media are the most frequently found secondary infections, with pneumococci and group A streptococci being the most commonly responsible pathogens. Before the development of antibiotics, otitis media secondary to measles resulted in residual hearing loss in as many as 10 percent of cases. Bacterial infections should be suspected when fever recurs or persists and leukocytosis develops. Patients with a compromised immune system are at a much greater risk of secondary infection complications as well as a higher incidence of adverse outcomes from the primary measles virus infection.

DIFFERENTIAL DIAGNOSIS

The diagnosis of measles usually is made by recognition of the pattern of signs and symptoms and is particularly straightforward when Koplik's spots are present. The diagnosis can be difficult when the presentation is atypical, such as in individuals who were immunized with the inactivated measles vaccine, though suspicion should be enhanced if cases have been reported in the local area. Other diagnoses to consider include drug rashes, rubella, scarlet fever, secondary syphilis, Kawasaki disease, and infectious mononucleosis. Several of these diagnoses do not produce a prodrome; however, the diagnosis can be complicated if the patient had an upper respiratory infection before the development of a rash.

LABORATORY TESTS

The definitive diagnosis of measles is made by using acute and convalescent serum antibody titers. The obvious limitation of a diagnosis made by this method is that it is obtained after the patient has recovered and in the process has spread the highly contagious virus to many others. Isolation of the measles virus is difficult, and attempts at virus retrieval are advised only in unusual situations such as atypical measles, encephalitis after vaccination, and pneumonia without a rash in an immunocompromised patient. A complete blood count is helpful, since leukopenia is common in the prodrome phase and when the rash first presents; however, the interpretation may be compromised by the presence of a bacterial infection. A severe leukocytosis with less than 2000 cells/mm³ is correlated with a poor prognosis.

Measles has been known to produce elevations of liver function tests, and elevations of two to three times normal of serum aspartate aminotransferase (AST), lactic dehydrogenase, and creatine phosphokinase are not uncommon. As many as 5 percent of adults with measles exhibit an icteric hepatitis with hyperbilirubinemia. One-fifth of these patients have transient ECG changes, though measles-related cardiac complications are rare.

Because measles produces a transient depression of cellular immunity, skin tests that utilize the cellular immune system will be inaccurate. These include the purified protein derivative (PPD) and other skin tests for tuberculosis, the coccidiomycosis skin test, the candida control skin test, and skin testing for the identification of allergies. Suppression of immunity sufficient to invalidate these tests results from the measles live-virus vaccine as well as the natural infection, and it is advised that testing be delayed as long as 4 weeks after vaccination or infection.

TREATMENT

Treatment for active measles is generally supportive. Recently, interest in the use of antiviral therapy has increased, as the measles virus is susceptible in vitro to ribavirin. No controlled studies have demonstrated its effectiveness, and it is not currently U.S. Food and Drug Administration (FDA)-approved for use in measles.

The World Health Organization (WHO) and the United Nations International Children's Emergency Fund (UNICEF) advise the administration of vitamin A to certain populations of children with active measles. It is advised that vitamin A, which is available in the United States as an oral solution containing 50,000 IU/mL, be given to children 6 months to 2 years of age hospitalized with complications and also to patients older than 6 months with immunodeficiency, ophthalmologic evidence of vitamin A deficiency, impaired intestinal absorption, malnutrition including eating disorders, and recent emigration from an area with an over 1 percent measles mortality rate. Vitamin A therapy also is recommended for any population in which the measles mortality rate exceeds 1 percent. The recommended dosage is a single dose of 200,000 IU orally for children 1 year and older and 100,000 IU for children 6 months to 1 year. Children with ophthalmologic evidence of vitamin A deficiency should be retreated the next day and 4 weeks later.

The most effective treatment is prevention. Most developed countries have devoted resources to the control of measles by promoting mass immunization of the population. The currently available vaccine product is a live attenuated measles virus prepared in chick embryo cell culture. Approximately 95 percent of the recipients reach the desired level of immunity, though it is now known that antibody titers produced by vaccination tend to decrease over time in some individuals, in contrast to naturally acquired immunity, which is lifelong. The decrease in immunity over time in some vaccinated individuals was thought to contribute to the measles epidemics of the 1980s in the United States and led to the recommendation that all individuals born after 1957 receive two vaccinations. The vaccine is available as a single-disease product and in a combination product as measles-mumps-rubella (MMR) vaccine. It is generally advised that the MMR product be administered since vaccinated individuals are likely to be susceptible to mumps and rubella, unless the cost of the MMR compared to the cost of the measles-only vaccine is prohibitive.

The MMR should be given to susceptible individuals with measles exposure occurring no more than 72 h before vaccination. Vaccination within this time frame can prevent wild virus infection in some cases. This is the treatment most preferred in outbreaks in schools.

Immune globulin (IG) can be given to susceptible individuals up to 6 days after exposure. IG is utilized for the protection of household contacts, contacts 5 to 12 months of age, exposed infants less than 5 months of age if the mother is not immune, exposed immunocompromised individuals, exposed children and adolescents with HIV regardless of MMR status, and exposed pregnant women who are not immune. IG doses should be 0.25 mL/kg intramuscularly (0.5 mL/kg intramuscularly for immunocompromised children), with the maximum dose being 15 mL.

The preferred method of prevention is immunization of the population. All individuals born before 1957 are assumed to be immune from childhood infection from the wild virus; therefore, immunization of this population is unnecessary. MMR should be given to all children at 12 to 15 months of age, and a second dose should be given by 12 years of age. Some schools and public health jurisdictions now require that the second MMR be given for school entry, and this protocol is adequate provided that the first dose was not given before the first birthday. Individuals in the population born after 1956 who received only one MMR or received the inactivated vaccine (before 1969) should be reimmunized.

In areas with a low incidence of measles, the first MMR usually is given at age 15 months. In areas with a high incidence, the first MMR usually is administered at 12 months. During outbreaks, measles vaccine can be administered as early as 6 months; however, since many children immunized at this age do not become immune, those immunized before 12 months should be reimmunized at 12 to 15 months and then immunized again before 12 years of age. Immunizations given before the first birthday should not be considered part of the immunization series.

The measles vaccine has been known to produce fever in 5 to 15 percent of nonimmune recipients, usually beginning 7 to 12 days after vaccination and lasting 1 or 2 days but sometimes lasting up to 5 days. Rarely the vaccine will cause measles or complications of measles, and serious complications occur less frequently than 1 in 1 million. The vaccine is contraindicated during pregnancy, in individuals who have experienced anaphylaxis with egg antigens or neomycin, individuals with recent administration of IG, and immunocompromised individuals. Individuals with HIV should be immunized, as should those with inactive tuberculosis. After vaccination, PPD skin testing should be avoided for up to 6 weeks.

BIBLIOGRAPHY

Berkow R (ed): *Merck Manual of Diagnosis and Therapy,* 16th ed. Rahway, NJ, Merck Sharp & Dohme, 1992.

Brunell PA: *Cecil Textbook of Medicine,* 19th ed. Philadelphia, Saunders, 1992.

Cunningham GF, MacDonald PC, Gant NR, et al (eds): *William's Obstetrics,* 19th ed. Norwalk, CT, Appleton & Lange, 1993.

Hashmey R, Shandera WX: in Tierney LM Jr, McPhee SJ, Papadakis MA (eds): *Current Medical Diagnosis and Treatment,* 35th revision. Norwalk, CT, Appleton & Lange, 1996.

Hayden FG, Hayden GF: in Stein JH (ed): *Stein Internal Medicine,* 4th ed. Philadelphia, Saunders, 1994.

Levin MJ, Romero JR: in Hay WW Jr, Groothuis JR, Hayward AR, et al (eds): *Current Pediatric Diagnosis and Treatment,* 12th ed. Norwalk, CT, Appleton & Lange, 1995.

Mills J, Grossman M: in Stites DP, Terr AI, Parslow TP (eds): *Basic and Clinical Immunology,* 8th ed. Norwalk, CT, Appleton & Lange, 1994.

Peter G (ed): *1994 Red Book.* Elk Grove Village, IL, American Academy of Pediatrics, 1994.

Ray G: *Harrison's Textbook of Internal Medicine,* 12th ed. New York, McGraw-Hill, 1991.

Smith DS: in Rakel RE (ed): *Conn's Current Therapy, 1995.* Philadelphia, Saunders, 1995.

Chapter 9–17
MUMPS
Richard Dehn

DISCUSSION

Mumps is an acute generalized viral infection that characteristically causes painful enlargement of the parotid glands. In most cases, mumps is a benign self-limited illness, especially in the preadolescent age group. After puberty, the severity of the symptoms and complications increases significantly with age.

In nonvaccinated populations mumps is primarily a disease of childhood, and by age 15 over 90 percent of the population will have developed antibodies to mumps. As many as one-third of the cases are asymptomatic, and up to 90 percent of adults without a history of clinical mumps or mumps vaccination will have antibodies to mumps. In the United States the live attenuated virus vaccine was introduced in 1967, and this reduced the incidence of mumps by 98 percent. As a result of the immunization of school-age cohorts, the majority of nonimmune individuals are in the postpuberty age groups. This has contributed to the recent rise of mumps cases in older age groups, which have a higher frequency of complications and more severe symptomatology.

Most patients with clinical mumps have inflammation of the parotid glands. The parotitis of mumps has a characteristic "chipmunk" look, since the swelling lifts the earlobe outward and obscures the angle of the mandible. Often involvement is initially unilateral, followed 2 to 3 days later by contralateral involvement.

PATHOGENESIS

Mumps is caused by a paramyxovirus of which there is only one known serotype, though antigenic differences have been noted with different strains. Humans are the only known host of the mumps virus, although the virus can be introduced into several other mammals. The virus is spread to the host through saliva or secretions from the respiratory system, usually through direct contact or aerosol droplets. The virus is significantly less contagious than measles or chickenpox, though it is contagious enough that epidemics can occur in populations with a small proportion of susceptible individuals. The virus replicates in epithelial cells of the upper respiratory tract and spreads to the regional lymph nodes and then systemically. The virus has a high degree of affinity for glandular and nervous system structures; thus, the clinical manifestations are likely to occur in those organ systems. The incubation period is 7 to 25 days, usually averaging 16 to 18 days. The virus usually is communicable for an average of 7 days, starting 1 to 2 days before parotid involvement and lasting 5 days afterward; however, it has been reported to be communicable as early as 7 days before parotid involvement and to last as long as 9 days after the onset of parotitis. Up to 30 percent of mumps infections are subclinical. Among those which are symptomatic, the most commonly affected single organ is the parotid gland. Most patients with symptomatic mumps experience edema and tenderness of one or more salivary glands.

As many as 15 percent of patients with clinical mumps exhibit symptoms of meningitis, which usually is characterized by headache, lethargy, neck stiffness, and vomiting. The meningitis is thought to be caused by mumps virus replication in the ependymal cells of the choroid plexus, and virus can be found in the cerebrospinal fluid (CSF). Up to 50 percent of mumps patients symptomatic with parotitis and without meningitis have mild headache and mononuclear pleocytosis of the CSF. Severe encephalitis is rare (1 in 1000 cases) and has a relatively low mortality rate of 0.5 to 2.3 percent, seldom producing residual damage. The mumps virus is known to replicate in the testicles, producing orchitis. Orchitis is an unusual finding in prepubertal males but occurs in up to one-third of postpubertal males. Up to half the cases of mumps orchitis result in testicular atrophy, but sterility is uncommon. Mumps has been noted to cause oophoritis in postpubertal women, though the incidence is only about 5 percent. When the right ovary is involved, the clinical picture can resemble that of acute appendicitis. Premature menopause and infertility have been reported, though both are rare. Occasionally mumps produces mastitis. Several other glandular systems can be infiltrated by the mumps virus and produce clinical symptoms. Pancreatic inflammation can produce the symptoms of acute pancreatitis. Other uncommon presentations of mumps include thyroiditis, myocarditis, arthritis, prostatitis, lacrimal gland involvement, sensorineural deafness, renal function abnormalities, and thrombocytopenia.

Maternal mumps infection in the first trimester of pregnancy results in an increase in the frequency of spontaneous abortions and may be associated with a greater likelihood of low birth weight. No increases in birth defects have been noted in children born to mothers who had clinical mumps during the first trimester. There is no difference in the clinical course of mumps between pregnant patients and nonpregnant patients.

SIGNS AND SYMPTOMS

After the incubation period, the patient experiences a 12- to 24-h prodromal phase characterized by chills, low-grade fever, anorexia, and headache. It is not unusual for the prodrome to be absent. Parotitis then presents as an earache or jaw tenderness with mastication that worsens over the next 2 or 3 days until the gland reaches its maximum size. The patient usually experiences pain with chewing or swallowing and finds that the ingestion of acidic liquids causes severe parotid pain. The involved gland is swollen and tender, and the oral outlet ducts of the involved gland appear edematous and inflamed. The parotid gland is most commonly involved, though occasionally the submaxillary gland is involved, producing suprasternal edema. Often the parotid involvement is unilateral, only to be followed by contralateral involvement 2 to 3 days later. Parotid edema peaks on the second or third day and usually resolves within 7 days. Mumps has been known to produce a relapse of symptoms about 2 weeks after resolution, though the incidence of relapse is rare (Fig. 9-17-1).

Patients with symptomatic mumps commonly have headache and stiff neck. As many as half of these patients have a CSF pleocytosis, and up to 15 percent of all symptomatic measles cases progress to symptomatic meningitis. Males are two to three times more likely to have nervous system involvement than are

females. Meningitis usually presents 4 to 5 days after the onset of parotitis, though it is not unusual for it to present without parotid involvement. Meningitis symptoms usually resolve within a week but can persist up to 5 weeks.

Encephalitis is an uncommon complication of mumps. The symptoms may develop at the same time as parotid involvement or may present 1 to 2 weeks later. Findings include obtundation, seizures, and high fevers. A unilateral nerve deafness can occur, which is usually temporary. Mumps encephalitis has a low mortality rate, and residual damage is rare.

Orchitis is a common presentation in postpubertal males. The orchitis is usually unilateral, though it can be bilateral in up to one-third of cases. Orchitis typically presents within a week of the onset of parotitis, though it can develop as the only presenting symptom. Orchitis usually presents with severe testicular pain and swelling accompanied by fever, headache, nausea, and vomiting. The acute pain and swelling usually resolve within 7 to 10 days, but the symptoms can persist for several weeks. Up to 50 percent of involved testicles undergo some degree of atrophy after resolution of the infection. Sterility is rare even after bilateral involvement, and the subsequent development of testicular tumors is rare.

Postpubertal females can develop oophoritis and mastitis. Right-sided oophoritis can be confused with acute appendicitis. Pancreatic involvement can present as acute pancreatitis with a clinical picture of nausea, vomiting, severe epigastric pain, fever, and chills. Recovery usually occurs within a week.

Unusual complications include thyroiditis, myocarditis, arthritis, prostatitis, lacrimal gland involvement, sensorineural deafness, renal function abnormalities, and thrombocytopenia.

DIFFERENTIAL DIAGNOSIS

The parotitis of mumps is difficult to differentiate from other possible causes of tender neck masses. The presence of other mumps cases in the area or known exposure to mumps is helpful. Parotitis can be caused by several other viruses, such as influenza A virus, parainfluenza virus, coxsackievirus, and lymphocytic choriomeningitis virus. *Staphylococcus aureus* and streptococcal infections also can cause parotitis as well as diphtheria, typhoid, typhus fever, and infections resulting from poor oral hygiene. Care should be taken not to confuse parotitis with lymphadenopathy. Parotid duct obstruction and tumors should be considered.

Atypical presentations such as mumps meningitis and orchitis are difficult to diagnose. Other causes of orchitis, such as torsion, hematomas, hernias, tumors, epididymitis, and infection with other organisms, should be considered. The diagnosis in these cases probably will rely on laboratory testing.

LABORATORY TESTS

The diagnosis is easy to make from clinical signs in typical cases during an epidemic; however, mumps antibody titer from paired specimens of acute and convalescent serums is diagnostic if a fourfold increase is noted. Mumps virus can be isolated from samples obtained from saliva, urine, and cerebrospinal fluid for 4 to 6 days after the onset of parotitis.

The white blood cell count often is unaffected by mumps; however, elevated lymphocytes are not unusual. A white count higher than 20,000 with a polymorphonuclear predominance sometimes is found in patients with meningitis or orchitis. Parotid involvement often produces an elevated serum amylase, which complicates the diagnosis of pancreatitis. A normal serum lipase

Figure 9-17-1. Mumps in adult patient. *A.* Marked parotid swelling characteristic of mumps. *B.* Bilaterial parotid swelling in the same patient. (*Photos courtesy of Rodney L. Moser. Used with permission.*)

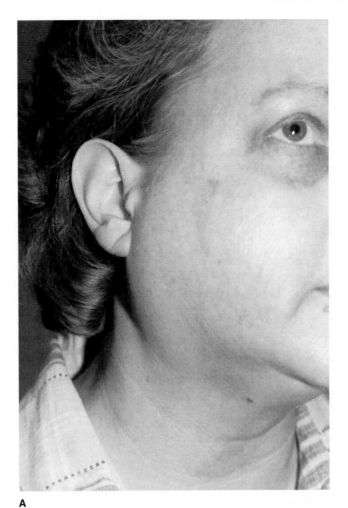

A

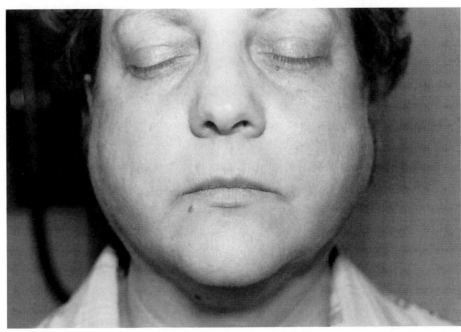

B

can indicate whether a patient also has pancreatic involvement. Patients with CNS involvement exhibit abnormalities of the CSF that are consistent with a viral infection.

TREATMENT

Treatment is supportive. Orchitis patients usually are advised to avoid activity, apply cold packs to the affected testicle, and wear appropriate support for the scrotum. Isolation from school, child care, and populations of susceptible individuals is appropriate for 9 days after the onset of parotitis. Serious complication such as meningitis, encephalitis, and pancreatitis may require hospitalization.

Mumps immune globulin has been found to be ineffective and has been withdrawn from the market. The administration of mumps live-virus vaccine after exposure is not effective in preventing infection but is not contraindicated.

The prevention of mumps cases through immunization is the preferred treatment. Mumps attenuated live-virus vaccine prepared in chick embryo cell culture was released in 1967 and has subsequently produced a 98 percent reduction in the number of cases reported. It produces immunity in 95 percent of those vaccinated, and serologic evidence suggests that immunity obtained from a single dose is long-lasting. It is available as a single-virus vaccine or combined with measles and rubella vaccines (MMR). Since it is known that mumps can transmit through a population containing only a small proportion of nonimmune individuals, the goal of immunization is the identification and vaccination of all susceptible individuals.

In the United States, all individuals born before 1957 are considered naturally immune and therefore do not need routine immunization. However, immunization in this age group is not contraindicated, as natural immunity will destroy the attenuated live virus of the immunization and such individuals therefore will not have any sort of immunization reaction. Any individual in that age group who is not naturally immune will have immunity conferred by the immunization.

It is recommended that children receive MMR after the first birthday. Generally this immunization is given at 15 months. A second MMR is recommended any time from school entry age (4 to 6 years) to the start of puberty. It is advised that the second MMR dose be given before the start of puberty so that any individual who does not receive immunity from the first vaccine will gain protection. Since mumps infection during puberty can involve the testes or ovaries and since the severity of cases increases with age, it is important that immunity be conferred before adolescence. The recent increase in adult mumps cases is indicative of the number of unvaccinated individuals in the population who were born after 1956 and did not receive the vaccine because MMR was not uniformly required for school entry in the 1970s.

Infants have mumps immunity for the first year of life if the mother was immune to mumps. It is this passive immunity that makes it impractical to give the attenuated live-virus vaccine in the first year of life. If an infant receives the mumps vaccine before the first birthday, it should be repeated at 15 months of age and again at school entry or before puberty.

All individuals in the population should be evaluated in regard to mumps immunity status. Individuals not immune by virtue of birth before 1957, not up to date with current immunization recommendations, or not shown by serology testing to be immune should be immunized.

Pregnancy is a contraindication to vaccination. Conception should be avoided for 3 months after vaccination. Inadvertent vaccination during pregnancy poses theoretical risks to the fetus, but there is no evidence that the fetus becomes infected with the virus.

Vaccination should be avoided in individuals who are immuno-compromised. The exception to this contraindication are patients with HIV, who should be immunized with MMR.

Patients who recently have received immune globulin or blood transfusions should avoid vaccination temporarily. The vaccine should be given at least 2 weeks before or 3 months after reception of the immune globulin or blood transfusion. The individual should be protected from mumps during that time by the antibodies in the blood products.

Since the mumps vaccine is derived from chick embryo cell cultures, it should be administered with caution in individuals who are allergic to eggs. Allergic reactions to the vaccine are rare.

The presence of fever is not a contraindication to vaccine administration. Individuals with upper respiratory infections and low-grade fever can be vaccinated; however, individuals who present with a fever suggestive of a more serious illness should have the vaccination withheld until after recovery. In recent studies, no differences were noted in immunity conferred by immunizations given to children with minor illnesses compared with those given to healthy children.

Adverse reactions to mumps vaccination are very rare. Most adverse reactions are time-limited and include neurologic deafness, rash, febrile seizures, parotitis, orchitis, meningitis, encephalitis, pruritus, and purpura. CNS reactions occur at a lower incidence than they do in unvaccinated populations.

BIBLIOGRAPHY

Berkow R (ed): *Merck Manual of Diagnosis and Therapy,* 16th ed. Rahway, NJ, Merck Sharp & Dohme, 1992.

Gnann JW: *Cecil Textbook of Medicine,* 19th ed. Philadelphia, Saunders, 1992.

Gordon RC: in Rakel RE (ed): *Conn's Current Therapy, 1995.* Philadelphia, Saunders, 1995.

Hashmey R, Shandera WX: in Tierney LM Jr, McPhee SJ, Papadakis MA (eds): *Current Medical Diagnosis and Treatment,* 35th revision. Norwalk, CT, Appleton & Lange, 1996.

Hayden FG, Hayden GF: in Stein JH (ed): *Stein Internal Medicine,* 4th ed. Philadelphia, Saunders, 1994.

Levin MJ, Romero JR: in Hay WW Jr, Groothuis JR, Hayward AR, et al (eds): *Current Pediatric Diagnosis and Treatment,* 12 ed. Norwalk, CT, Appleton & Lange, 1995.

Mills J, Grossman M: in Stites DP, Terr AI, Parslow TP (eds): *Basic and Clinical Immunology,* 8th ed. Norwalk, CT, Appleton & Lange, 1994.

Peter G (ed): *1994 Red Book.* Elk Grove Village, IL, American Academy of Pediatrics, 1994.

Chapter 9–18
PERTUSSIS
Richard Dehn

DISCUSSION

Pertussis, better known as whooping cough, is a highly communicable bacterial infectious disease with a significant morbidity rate in infants and young children. The illness presents in three distinct stages, the second of which is characterized by a severe paroxysmal cough with a unique inspiratory whoop. Uncomplicated pertussis usually has a 6- to 10-week course, though complications such as pneumonia are not uncommon.

Pertussis is highly contagious, infecting 70 to 100 percent of susceptible individuals. In unvaccinated populations pertussis is endemic, and in undeveloped regions of the world infant and childhood mortality rates are high. Improvements in supportive treatment in the United States at the beginning of the twentieth century and the subsequent development of antibiotics reduced mortality rates from pertussis; however, the incidence did not drop until the early 1950s, when the immunization of infants and children became prevalent. Before widespread immunization, the annual incidence in the United States was about 200,000 cases, compared with a recent annual incidence of about 4,000 cases. The mortality rate from pertussis has correspondingly dropped from 5,000 to 10,000 deaths per year in the prevaccination era to 4 to 11 deaths per year more recently. About three-fourths of the deaths occur in the first year of life. The fatality rate in children less than 6 months of age is 0.5 percent.

The reported incidence of pertussis in the United States increased from 0.54 to 0.95 case per 100,000 in 1978–1982 to 0.96 to 1.74 cases per 100,000 in 1983–1987. This has been thought to be due primarily to an increase in the proportion of unvaccinated individuals in the very young population. Factors contributing to the increase in the proportion of susceptible infants and young children include a significant number of parents withholding pertussis vaccine from their children because of the potential side effects, the existence of infant populations not receiving vaccinations, and the immigration of unvaccinated individuals to the United States.

PATHOGENESIS

Pertussis is caused by *Bordetella pertussis,* a nonmotile gram-negative coccobacillus first isolated by Bordet and Gengou in 1906. It usually is transmitted to the host by the inhalation of respiratory secretions from an infected individual. The organisms adhere to ciliated respiratory epithelial cells, where they replicate. *Bordetella pertussis* does not invade farther than the ciliated respiratory epithelial cells. The disease is produced by several bacterial toxins, including the pertussis toxin, which is responsible for lymphocytosis and many of the respiratory symptoms of pertussis. It is felt that the toxins cause tissue damage to specific organs in the respiratory system, since damage and symptoms persist long after the *B. pertussis* organism is no longer present. Further evidence supportive of pertussis being caused by toxins produced by *B. pertussis* is provided by the fact that treating individuals in the incubation period or the early catarrhal stage with antibiotics often ameliorates the disease. In these cases, the elimination of *B. pertussis* probably occurs before the production of toxins causes tissue damage. Infection with *B. pertussis* results in the production of antibody for about 5 years, while vaccination with killed whole virus produces about 3 years of immunity. Most older children, adolescents, and adults are susceptible to pertussis, and infections passed to young children by older members of the family are common. A natural infection and the prior completion of immunizations often result in milder subsequent infections. Infections in all but infants and young children rarely result in serious illness or complications but place susceptible youngsters at risk.

SIGNS AND SYMPTOMS

Pertussis presents in three distinct stages, with the first stage lasting 1 to 2 weeks and the second and third stages usually lasting 2 to 4 weeks. After infection of the host's respiratory tract with *B. pertussis* and a 7- to 10-day incubation period, the first stage, or catarrhal stage, begins. The catarrhal stage is characterized by mild nonspecific upper respiratory symptoms such as rhinorrhea, conjunctival injection, increased lacrimation, sneezing, and a troublesome hacking nocturnal cough that gradually becomes diurnal. Low-grade fever, listlessness, and anorexia are some-

times present; however, a fever higher than 38.3°C (101.0°F) is suggestive of a bacterial superinfection or a nonpertussis cause of the upper respiratory infection (URI). Pertussis in the catarrhal stage is difficult to distinguish from common URIs and thus often is not recognized at this stage. The host is most infectious to other susceptible individuals during this stage, and so the organism often is passed to others before it is clinically recognized. The catarrhal stage lasts about 2 weeks before the worsening cough becomes paroxysmal.

The second or paroxysmal, stage is characterized by bouts of 10 to 30 forceful coughs within a span of a few seconds, ending with an inspiratory whoop, though the whoop is not always exhibited in adults and infants. At the peak of the paroxysmal stage the host may experience as many as 25 paroxysms over a 24-h period, with more occurrences at night than during the day. Paroxysms can be accompanied by cyanosis, sweating, prostration, and exhaustion and often are followed by the expulsion of copious amounts of viscid mucus, which frequently results in vomiting. Cyanosis, neck vein congestion, bulging eyes, and protrusion of the tongue also can be present during attacks, as well as residual petechial hemorrhages, engorged conjunctivae, periorbital edema, and epistaxis. Attacks often are provoked by yawning, sneezing, or eating. Between attacks the patient appears normal. Except for a few scattered rhonchi, the chest examination is usually normal. The presence of fever in this stage is suggestive of a secondary infectious process.

After a paroxysmal stage lasting 2 to 4 weeks, the paroxysms gradually decrease in frequency and intensity. Vomiting and other symptoms produced by the intense paroxysms stop. Recovery progresses slowly, usually lasting an additional 3 to 4 weeks; however, this stage can last several months. The paroxysms evolve into a cough that resembles chronic bronchitis, though noxious stimuli and viral URIs can provoke a return of paroxysms.

DIFFERENTIAL DIAGNOSIS

At the onset pertussis is insidious, and in the catarrhal stage it is indistinguishable from a mild viral respiratory infection. Exposure to pertussis may provide a clue to the appropriate diagnosis during the catarrhal stage. The diagnosis of pertussis usually is entertained after the appearance of paroxysms; however, spasmodic coughing is not pathognomonic of pertussis. Bronchiolitis, cystic fibrosis, tuberculosis, foreign bodies, airway compression from lymphadenopathy or malignancy, and chlamydia and viral or mycoplasma pneumonia should be considered. Differentiation usually can be made by careful physical examination, laboratory findings, and the results of chest x-ray.

COMPLICATIONS

Up to 90 percent of the fatalities caused by pertussis are due to pneumonia, which is the most common serious complication. Interstitial and subcutaneous emphysema and pneumothorax are uncommon consequences of the increased intrathoracic pressure of the paroxysms. This can produce bronchiectasis in debilitated children, resulting in residual emphysema. Mucus plugs can cause atelectases. Severe paroxysms resulting in anoxia can cause hemorrhages into the brain, eyes, skin, and mucous membranes. Cerebral hemorrhage, cerebral edema, and toxic encephalitis may result in severe neurologic disorders. Paroxysms can produce frenulum ulcers as a result of abrasion with the lower incisors, and occasionally they result in rectal prolapse and umbilical herniation. It is not unusual to see convulsions in infants, but they are uncommon in older children. Otitis media is a common complication and should be treated with the appropriate antibiotic.

LABORATORY TESTS

The organism *B. pertussis* can be cultured from nasopharyngeal specimens in the catarrhal and early paroxysmal stages. Unfortunately, the likelihood of obtaining a positive culture starts to decrease at about the time in the course of the illness when the diagnosis of pertussis becomes obvious. A positive culture is considered diagnostic, and false-negative results are common, especially after the fourth week of the illness and in patients who have received antibiotics. Cultures are best plated at the bedside to freshly prepared Bordet-Gengou or charcoal agar medium, using small cotton swabs passed through the nose to the nasopharynx with 28-gauge zinc-coated wire. A direct immunofluorescent assay (DFA) of nasopharyngeal secretions is available at some laboratories but is less sensitive and specific than a culture, sometimes producing false-positive or false-negative results.

No single serologic test is specific or sensitive enough to confirm a diagnosis. Since each individual produces a different antibody response to pertussis infection or vaccination, serologic antibody results are difficult to interpret. Enzyme immunoassays for IgG antibody to pertussis toxin and IgA antibody to *B. pertussis* filamentous hemagglutinin are under investigation as diagnostic tests.

Pertussis often produces a lymphocytosis toward the end of the catarrhal stage. White blood cell counts are frequently in the range of 20,000 to 30,000/μL with 60 to 80 percent small lymphocytes, but the counts can be as high as 60,000/μL. The degree of lymphocytosis usually parallels the severity of the cough.

Bronchopneumonia and patchy atelectases often are seen on chest x-ray as thickened bronchi or a "shaggy" heart border.

TREATMENT

Treatment for pertussis once it has reached the paroxysmal stage is primarily supportive. Infants often require hospitalization, and occasionally older individuals may experience complications. Unnecessary manipulation and activity should be discouraged in the acute paroxysmal stage, since any form of stimulation can contribute to increased paroxysms.

Antibiotic therapy can stop the progression of the disease if it is given during the incubation period or the catarrhal stage. Antibiotics also are given to individuals beyond those stages to eradicate the *B. pertussis* organism even though this does not affect the course of the disease, thus preventing transmission of the disease to caretakers and family members. The antibiotic of choice is erythromycin 40 to 50 mg/kg/d in four divided doses, up to 2 g a day, for 14 days. The estolate form of erythromycin (Ilosone) is thought to be more active against *B. pertussis* and is preferred. An alternative to erythromycin is trimethoprim-sulfamethoxazole (Bactrim, Septra), 8 mg/kg/d trimethoprim and 40 mg/kg/d sulfamethoxazole in two divided doses; however, its efficacy has not been well studied. Antibiotic therapy also is recommended for all household contacts and other close contacts irrespective of vaccination status. The host and all contacts should be considered capable of shedding virus until 5 days after the start of antibiotic therapy.

Corticosteroids and albuterol have been used in the paroxysmal stage with variable results. Albuterol is commonly used in Europe, but its effectiveness has not been carefully evaluated. The use of corticosteroids can worsen a complicating infection, though in one study corticosteroid use significantly reduced the frequency of paroxysms. Pertussis immune globulin has been shown to be of no benefit.

Children under 7 years of age should be immunized with pertussis vaccine. A whole-cell killed-virus vaccine developed in the 1940s is available as a single-virus vaccine, as part of a combined vaccine with diphtheria and tetanus toxoids (DPT), and as a combined vaccine of DPT and *Haemophilus influenza* vaccine

(Tetramune). It should be given at 2, 4, and 6 months of age and again at 18 months and at school entry. The whole-virus component of the pertussis vaccine is associated with increased vaccination reactions with increased age, and so the pertussis vaccination is not recommended in individuals over 6 years of age. Recently acellular pertussis vaccines have been marketed that appear to produce milder vaccination side effects than do whole-cell vaccines. Acellular pertussis vaccines are currently recommended for the fourth and fifth doses of the vaccination schedule in children who previously were vaccinated with whole-cell vaccine. Three doses of whole-cell vaccine are effective in about 80 percent of recipients, and the immunity persists for about 3 years. The whole-cell pertussis vaccine generally has a higher incidence of adverse reactions than do other vaccines for childhood illnesses. In the United States media coverage of vaccination reactions has resulted in a significant number of parents refusing to vaccinate their children against pertussis. This population of unvaccinated infants and young children has contributed to the recent increase in pertussis incidence.

The most common reactions to the pertussis vaccine are inflammation at the site of injection and fever. As many as half the individuals receiving the whole-cell vaccine experience a local reaction or fever, though the incidence of these side effects is much lower when the acellular vaccine is used. Local reactions can be reduced by the administration of acetaminophen or another appropriate antipyretic at the time of injection and 4 and 8 h after the injection.

Allergic reactions are uncommon, with anaphylaxis occurring in approximately 2 cases per 100,000 injections, though death is extremely rare. The incidence of seizures within 48 h of vaccination with DPT is 1 in 1750 doses. Most of these seizures are thought to be fever-related and are not associated with residual neurologic symptoms or a greater risk of developing epilepsy. Inconsolable crying for more than 3 h occurs in 1 percent of individuals receiving the vaccine and can be seen as long as 48 h after the injection. A hypotonic-hyporesponsive episode presenting as a generalized collapse or shocklike state is seen in 1 in 1750 doses. There is no evidence of residual damage after these episodes. Generally, the incidence of all adverse reactions appears to be lower after the use of acellular vaccine, but large population studies have not been completed on the acellular vaccines.

Many severe reactions to the pertussis vaccine have been alleged but not proved. Severe adverse reactions, such as death, encephalopathy, the onset of seizure disorder, developmental delays, and learning disabilities, have been temporally related to the administration of the pertussis vaccine. In epidemiologic investigations, the incidence of pertussis vaccine–related severe acute neurologic illness has been estimated to be 1 in 140,000 DPT doses.

Contraindications to pertussis vaccine include an immediate anaphylactic reaction to a prior pertussis vaccination and encephalopathy within 7 days after a prior vaccination. Individuals experiencing a convulsion within 3 days of DPT vaccination, inconsolable crying with 3 days of DPT vaccination, a hypotonic-hyporesponsive episode within 48 h of DPT vaccination, or a fever of 40.5°C (104.9°F) or higher within 48 h of vaccination should consider the risks and benefits of additional vaccinations carefully.

BIBLIOGRAPHY

Berkow R (ed): *Merck Manual of Diagnosis and Therapy,* 16th ed. Rahway, NJ, Merck Sharp & Dohme, 1992.

Chambers HF: in Tierney LM Jr, McPhee SJ, Papadakis MA (eds): *Current Medical Diagnosis and Treatment,* 35th revision. Norwalk, CT, Appleton & Lange, 1996.

Edwards KM, Cattaneo LA: in Rakel RE (ed): *Conn's Current Therapy, 1995.* Philadelphia, Saunders, 1995.

Freij BJ, McCracken GH Jr. in *Harrison's Textbook of Internal Medicine,* 12th ed. New York, McGraw-Hill, 1991.

Hendley JO: in Stein JH (ed): *Stein Internal Medicine,* 4th ed. Philadelphia, Saunders, 1994.

Johnson RB Jr: in *Cecil Textbook of Medicine,* 19th ed. Philadelphia, Saunders, 1992.

Ogle JW: in Hay WW Jr, Groothuis JR, Hayward AR, et al (eds): *Current Pediatric Diagnosis and Treatment,* 12th ed. Norwalk, CT, Appleton & Lange, 1995.

Peter G (ed): *1994 Red Book.* Elk Grove Village, IL, American Academy of Pediatrics, 1994.

Ryan J, Grossman M: in Stites DP, Terr AI, Parslow TP (eds): *Basic and Clinical Immunology,* 8th ed. Norwalk, CT, Appleton & Lange, 1994.

Chapter 9–19
RABIES

Ralph Rice

DISCUSSION

Although rarely seen in the United States, rabies is perhaps the most feared potential consequence of animal bites. However, worldwide the incidence of rabies is much greater, with the World Health Organization reporting more than 20,000 deaths per year.[1,2] Although rabies was previously considered an endemic disease, mandatory vaccination of dogs and cats and animal control measures enacted in the 1940s and 1950s have resulted in a drop in human rabies in the United States from an average of 55 cases per year in the first half of the century to less than 1 case per year in 1980.[1,3] From 1980 until May 1996, a total of 26 cases of human rabies were reported by the Centers for Disease Control and Prevention.[4] The cost of rabies vaccination of pets and postexposure prophylaxis in the United States has been placed at $300 million annually.[1]

Wild animals are the main vector of rabies. The vast majority of rabies infections in humans and domestic animals come from skunks, raccoons, and bats, accounting for 83 percent of reported cases.[1] Other wildlife vectors include foxes, bobcats, coyotes, and wolves. Not commonly thought of as carriers of rabies, unvaccinated farm animals accounted for 11 percent of reported domestic animal cases in 1988.[1] Lagomorphs (rabbits and hares) and rodents are uncommon carriers of rabies. Amphibians, fishes, insects, and reptiles are noncarriers.

Rabies is present throughout the United States, with cases having been reported in every state. The prevalence of rabies shows the highest incidence in the following five geographic areas in the 48 contiguous states.[2,5,6]

1. The mid-Atlantic states of Pennsylvania, Maryland, New Jersey, Rhode Island, and West Virginia
2. The southeastern states of Florida, Georgia, Alabama, and South Carolina
3. The south-central states of Texas, Oklahoma, and Arkansas
4. The north-central states of Minnesota, Iowa, and the Dakotas
5. California

New England, the Pacific northwest, and some Rocky Mountain states, such as Utah, have an incidence of rabies in animals that is below the national average.

Table 9-19-1. Factors Influencing Susceptibility to Rabies

Host's genetic background and age
Infecting strain
Size of inoculum
Degree of innervation at site of injury
Proximity to CNS

SOURCE: From Baevsky and Bartfield;[1] Fishbein and Robinson.[6]

PATHOGENESIS

Transmission of the rabies virus most commonly occurs from inoculation with infected saliva. This may result from a bite, direct contact with mucous membranes, or a break in the skin. Transmission from inhalation has been reported four times, twice in workers in rabies research laboratories and twice after a spelunking exploration in caves inhabited by bats that carried the rabies virus.[3,6,7] Human-to-human transmission of rabies has occurred six times from corneal transplantation.[6]

Because of the nonspecific early signs and symptoms of rabies, it is important to obtain a history of an animal bite or bat exposure. The type of animal, its behavior, and the circumstances surrounding the injury, along with the location and ownership, if any, of the animal, are important items to obtain in the patient history. Bat bites may be small and go unnoticed, especially during the period of anxiety after an encounter with a bat. The Centers for Disease Control and Prevention (CDC) recommends that "in situations in which a bat is physically present and the person(s) cannot reasonably exclude the possibility of a bite exposure" and with inability to test the bat, exposure to the virus should be considered to have occurred.[4]

A number of variables determine the susceptibility of the host to infection. Table 9-19-1 lists those risk factors.

Initially, the virus replicates within the monocytes near the bite. The virus then enters the peripheral nervous system through unmyelinated terminal sensory and motor neurons. If the initial inoculum is large enough and is in direct contact with peripheral nerves, the virus may enter the nerve immediately. When transmission is acquired from inhalation, the virus invades the nervous system through the neuroepithelial cells on the mucosal surface. Once it is in nerve cells, the virus migrates through retrograde axoplasmic flow to the central nervous system (CNS). Symptoms of rabies arise when the virus reaches the CNS. This incubation period, before the onset of symptoms, averages 20 to 90 days[3] but may range from 4 days to 8 months or longer.[1,7] In the CNS, the virus replicates almost exclusively in the gray matter, with an ensuing encephalitis. The infection is disseminated through the body along the peripheral nerves and can infect other organs, including the salivary glands, the retinas and the corneas.

MICROBIOLOGY

The virus that causes rabies is a member of the Lyssavirus genus. It is bullet-shaped, measuring 75 by 180 nm and containing a single-stranded RNA genome.

SYMPTOMS AND OBJECTIVE FINDINGS

Rabies infection may be divided into four stages: incubation, prodrome, the neurologic period, and coma.

The *incubation stage,* described in "Pathogenesis," above, lasts from the time of viral inoculation until the onset of any symptoms. Like the other stages, it is highly variable. During this period the patient may remain asymptomatic. Most symptoms and signs usually are related to the bite and local wound healing, such as edema and erythema. If the incubation stage is prolonged, the initial injury site may be healed. A correct diagnosis during this period is not likely because of the paucity of symptoms.

Progression to the next stage—the prodrome—is associated with a poor outcome. This stage lasts 2 to 10 days. Most patients report pain, pruritus, or paresthesias at the site of the wound or in the entire limb. Itching may be severe to the point of causing significant excoriation. This sensation may be attributed to the proliferation of the virus in the sensory nerves. Fasciculations also may occur at the site of the bite. Other nonspecific constitutional symptoms may include fever, chills, malaise, fatigue, sore throat, headache, nausea, vomiting, anorexia, and a nonproductive cough.

Beginning with the onset of symptoms of CNS involvement and lasting 2 to 10 days, the neurologic period is marked by progressive deterioration of the patient's mental status. There may be, however, periods of normality during this stage. The hallmark symptoms of rabies infection—aerophobia and hydrophobia—usually are seen during this period. Aerophobia, or the fear of moving air, may be elicited by blowing air across a patient's face. This causes spasms of the muscles in the neck and pharynx. A combination of hypersalivation and difficulty swallowing may cause foaming at the mouth. Attempts to drink liquids cause violent, jerky spasms of the diaphragm and in other muscles of inspiration and deglutition, causing hydrophobia. Other nonspecific signs and symptoms during the neurologic stage are listed in Table 9-19-2.

Death during this "furious" phase may result from cardiovascular or respiratory collapse. If the patient does not die or become comatose, a "paralytic" phase may occur. This phase presents similarly to the Guillain-Barré syndrome, with an ascending symmetric or asymmetric paralysis, usually most pronounced in the bitten extremity. The paralytic phase is most commonly associated with bat bites.

The fourth stage is coma. Death from respiratory arrest, starvation, or dehydration normally occurs within 7 days. Intensive supportive care may prolong survival times, but rabies is almost uniformly fatal. According to the CDC, documented cases of survivors of human rabies in the United States have been limited to a total of four.

DIAGNOSTIC CONSIDERATIONS

During the incubation period rabies may be misdiagnosed as cellulitis because of lack of signs other than erythema and edema near the bite area. Presentation during the prodrome stage with nonspecific constitutional symptoms resembling an upper respiratory tract infection or gastroenteritis makes the correct diagnosis of rabies difficult.

More definitive signs and symptoms beginning in the neurologic stage should heighten the suspicion of rabies. The differential diagnosis (Table 9-19-3) remains extensive.

"Rabies hysteria" also should be considered in symptomatic patients. This occurs in a patient who is knowledgeable about the signs and symptoms of rabies and has a history of an animal bite, though the animal was not rabid.

Table 9-19-2. Nonspecific Findings During the Neurologic Stage of Rabies

Hyperactivity	Hyperreflexia
Hallucinations	Priapism
Muscle spasms	Anisocoria
Opisthotonia	Increased salivation
Lacrimation	Perspiration
Optic neuritis	Diplopia
Facial palsies	Fever to 40.6°C (105°F)

SOURCE: From Baevsky and Bartfield;[1] Doan-Wiggins;[5] Frenia et al.[7]

Table 9-19-3. Differential Diagnosis of Rabies During the Neurologic Period

Guillain-Barré syndrome	Tetanus
Brain tumor or abscess	Botulism
Metabolic encephalopathy	Polio
Cerebrovascular accident	Schizophrenia
Drug intoxication or withdrawal	Conversion reaction

SOURCE: From Baevsky and Bartfield;[1] Frenia et al.[7]

SPECIAL CONSIDERATIONS

People who are immunocompromised may not develop active immunity and may be predisposed to rabies. Immunosuppressive agents such as steroids should be given during the postexposure period only if they are needed to treat other medical conditions. Before immunosuppresive agents are given, vaccination to rabies should have been started and the serum should be tested for antibody production.

A low rabies antibody response has been reported with the administration of human diploid cell vaccine and chloroquine.[7] People traveling to countries with endemic malaria and rabies who are receiving prophylaxis for both should be aware of this interaction.

LABORATORY FINDINGS

A number of limited diagnostic tests are available to confirm rabies. The most common test in the United States is the rapid fluorescent focus inhibition test (RFFIT).[7] In this test, the patient's antibody titer to rabies is compared to a known standard. The results from this test are available within 24 h and have a specificity "approaching 100% with a sensitivity of approximately 90 percent."[1]

Immunofluorescent antibody staining for the viral antigen is another method of diagnosis. Specimens used for this include brain tissue, nerve tissue, neck skin, corneal impressions, serum, cerebrospinal fluid, and/or saliva.[5,7] The specimen is exposed to a fluorochrome-labeled antibody or antigen and then examined for fluorescence. Additional tests, often the RFFIT, are recommended to confirm negative results. Antibodies to the rabies virus usually are present in the serum and CSF within 1 week of the development of symptoms.

Mouse inoculation of infected tissue is a technique used to culture the rabies virus and confirm the fluorescent antibody test. If the mouse manifests symptoms of rabies, it is sacrificed and the brain is examined by direct fluorescent antibody testing. It should be noted that in cases of prolonged survival of the patient, mouse inoculation studies along with direct fluorescent antibody staining may be negative.[5,7] This autosterilization phenomenon is "thought to result from a large increase in antirabies antibody."[7]

Sections of brain tissue can be stained with Seller's stain and then examined by microscopy for Negri bodies, which are round or oval inclusion bodies seen in the cytoplasm and the nerve processes. This is the method most commonly used to examine an animal suspected of having rabies.

Standard laboratory tests for the diagnosis of rabies are nonspecific. Blood chemistry studies normally are unaffected by the infection.[1] White blood cell counts may be normal or elevated. A lumbar puncture may show an elevated opening pressure. The CSF may reveal an elevated protein level with a variable leukocytosis. Toxicologic screening of urine or blood is not useful in the diagnosis but can help rule out drug intoxication or withdrawal as a cause of the symptoms.

RADIOLOGIC STUDIES

Although not useful in the diagnosis, CT of the head may be useful in eliminating a brain tumor or abscess as a cause of the neurologic symptoms.

TREATMENT

As with any animal bite, the first step in proper treatment is cleaning the wound and the surrounding area. The incidence of developing rabies may be reduced by up to 90 percent by prompt washing of the area with soap or iodine solution.[1] Cleaning the wound with 1% to 2% benzalkonium chloride solution may have viricidal activity against localized rabies.

Pharmacologic Treatment

After Exposure

If a potential rabies exposure has occurred, postexposure prophylaxis should be administered. This consists of two components: passive immunization with immunoglobulin and active immunization with a vaccine.

One dose of human rabies immune globulin (HRIG) is given at the beginning of postexposure immunization, day 0. A dose of 20 IU/kg is given, with half the dose infiltrated around the site of the exposure (if anatomically possible) and the remaining portion given intramuscularly. Only the recommended dose of HRIG should be given, as passive immunization may partially suppress the active production of antibodies.[3,7] If it is not given with the vaccine, HRIG may be given within 7 or 8 days of the first dose of the vaccine. After this time an antibody response from the active immunization should have occurred. People who have been previously immunized do not receive HRIG.

Active immunization is obtained by administering 1.0 mL of human diploid cell vaccine (HDCV) or Rabies Vaccine Absorbed (RVA) intramuscularly into the deltoid or, in children, the anterolateral aspect of the thigh. The vaccine is given on days 0, 3, 7, 14, and 28.[1,6,7] The vaccine should not be mixed in the same syringe as the HRIG or administered at the same site, since neutralization may occur.[7] In cases where the patient has received a previous vaccination, the patient should receive 1.0 mL of the vaccine on days 0 and 3.[1,6]

Although there have been no treatment failures reported with the proper postexposure treatment with HRIG and HDCV or RVA in the United States, at least 18 people have contracted rabies outside the United States after receiving the vaccine.[3,6,8] These cases have been associated with improper wound care (inadequate cleaning, inappropriate timing of surgical closure), passive immunization not given or not given around the wound site, or reception of the vaccination in the gluteal region instead of the deltoid.

Treatment should begin as soon as possible after it has been determined that prophylaxis is necessary. Delays up to 5 days after exposure have not affected the success of treatment.[6]

The data involving treatment during pregnancy are limited. No fetal abnormalities have been associated with postexposure prophylaxis,[6,7] and pregnancy should not be considered a contraindication to treatment.

The patient's tetanus immunization status should be reviewed. If no booster has been received in the past 5 years or if the patient is unsure of his or her status, tetanus toxoid should be given.[9]

Many animal bites may require antimicrobial therapy (see Chap. 4-4).

Before Exposure

For persons with a high risk of rabies exposure, such as veterinarians, animal handlers, laboratory workers, spelunkers, and travelers to areas where rabies is endemic, prophylactic vaccination is recommended.[1,2,5,6] This series should begin at least 30 days before exposure or travel. HDCV or RVA 1.0 mL, should be given intramuscularly in the deltoid on days 0, 7, and 21 or 28. Booster vaccinations should be given to people who have a continued risk of exposure and a low antibody titer. Preexposure prophylaxis does not eliminate the need for postexposure treatment.

SUPPORTIVE MEASURES

When a case of rabies has progressed through the neurologic phase into the coma phase, intensive cardiovascular and respiratory support is required. As was noted earlier, starvation and dehydration are additional causes of death. All cases are most appropriately managed in an intensive care unit. In addition to supportive measures, some investigators have used antiviral drugs, interferon, and interferon inducers in the treatment of rabies.[10]

PATIENT EDUCATION

People, particularly children, should be warned to avoid contact with wild animals and unfamiliar domestic animals, especially animals that display bizzare, erratic behavior or hypersalivation. Wild animals should not be kept as pets. People with potential rabies exposure and bites of any kind should seek medical attention. People at high risk of exposure should receive prophylactic vaccination. Common sense is the key to prevention.

COMPLICATIONS AND RED FLAGS

Although it is recommended that prophylaxis be started as soon as rabies is suspected, regardless of the time elapsed after exposure, once the virus enters the peripheral nervous system, vaccination can no longer halt the infection.[1,6,7] The body starts to produce antibodies once clinical symptoms occur.

Adverse reactions to rabies prophylaxis are treated in the same manner as are reactions to other vaccines. Local or mild systemic reactions can be treated with anti-inflammatory medications and antipyretics. These minor reactions should not cause discontinuation of treatment. Antihistamines and epinephrine should be readily available in case an anaphylactic reaction occurs. The use of steroids during any reaction should be weighed against the consequence of inhibition of an immune response.

In incidences of anaphylaxis or serious systemic reaction, serious consideration must be given to the risk of developing rabies before the vaccination series is discontinued. Consultation with a local health department, the CDC, or other qualified experts may help in this decision.

OTHER NOTES AND PEARLS

Oral vaccines now being tested in an attempt to control rabies in wildlife.[1,6,7] In parts of Europe an orally absorbed vaccine distributed by aircraft and by hand has been used to control rabies in foxes. In late 1990, a recombinant rabies vaccine that had been effective in raccoons in the laboratory was distributed on a Virginia coastal island. The results of this and other studies involving skunks have been called "encouraging."[1,6]

Several countries have vaccination schedules that involve fewer doses and fewer clinic visits. One of these, recommended by the World Health Organization, has HDCV given bilaterally intramuscularly on day 0 (two doses) and then one dose given intramuscularly on day 7 and a final intramuscular dose given on day 21.[1,3] This dosing regimen has not been approved in the United States.

Also under investigation are interferon and interferon-inducing agents.[1,7] These agents may have antiviral and immunoregulatory activity, and the results of these studies have been promising.

REFERENCES

1. Baevsky RH, Bartfield JM: Human rabies: A review. *Am J Emerg Med* 11(3):279–286, 1993.
2. Warrell DA, Warrell MJ: Human rabies: A continuing challenge in the tropical world. *Schweiz Med Wochenschr* 125(18):879–885, 1995. (Abstract from MEDLINE Express computer search, May 15, 1996.)
3. Fishbein DB: Rabies. *Infect Dis Clin North Am* 5(1):53–71, 1991.
4. Center for Disease Control: Human rabies—Connecticut, 1995. *MMWR* 45(10):207–209, 1996.
5. Doan-Wiggins L: Animal bites and rabies, in Rosen P, Barkin RM, Braen GR, et al (eds): *Emergency Medicine: Concepts and Clinical Practice.* St Louis, Mosby Year Book, 1992, pp 868–875.
6. Fishbein DB, Robinson LE: Rabies. *New Engl J Med* 329(22):1632–1638, 1993.
7. Frenia ML, Lafin SM, Barone JA: Therapy review: Features and treatment of rabies. *Clin Pharm* 11:37–47, 1992.
8. Wilde H, Sirikawin S, Sabcharoen A, et al: Failure of postexposure treatment of rabies in children. *Clin Infect Dis* 22:228–232, 1992.
9. Sanford JP, Gilbert DN, Sande MA: Anti-tetanus prophylaxis, wound classification, immunization, in Sanford JP (ed): *The Sanford Guide to Antimicrobial Therapy.* Dallas, Antimicrobial Therapy, 1995, p 115.
10. Dutta JK, Dutta TK: Treatment of clinical rabies in man: Drug Therapy and other measures. *Clin Pharmacol Ther* 32(11):594–597, 1994.

Chapter 9–20
RESPIRATORY SYNCYTIAL VIRUS
Wayne J. van Deusen

DISCUSSION

Respiratory syncytial virus (RSV) is the most important and prevalent respiratory tract pathogen of early childhood. RSV is ubiquitous and causes a highly contagious and potentially devastating disease for the child and family. It primarily affects children in the first and second years of life. Younger children are more prone to contract the infection and more likely to develop severe symptoms. A longitudinal study in Houston found that 69 percent of children were infected in the first year of life and 83 percent were infected in the second. By age 2 years half these children had been reinfected. Reinfection is common, occurring at a rate of 10 to 20 percent, and may occur as early as a few weeks after recovery. Recurrences usually take place during subsequent annual outbreaks and are manifested as mild upper respiratory infections or tracheobronchitis in older children and adults. RSV is more common in boys than in girls (ratio, 1.5:5), and there is no difference between ethnic and racial groups; however, lower respiratory tract disease tends to occur earlier and have a higher incidence among lower socioeconomic groups and in crowded living conditions. The rate of admissions for RSV bronchiolitis and pneumonia in infants under 1 year is proportional to the number of RSV infections in the community. Estimates show that in urban settings at least half the susceptible infants undergo primary RSV infection during each epidemic. Infection is almost universal by the second birthday. The disease may last 3 to 7 days.

According to the American Academy of Pediatrics Committee on Infectious Disease, "approximately 300,000 US children are at risk for contracting RSV annually, with more than 90,000 hospitalizations and 4,500 deaths occurring each year."[1] In 1985,

in a report by the Institute of Medicine, it was estimated that the annual cost of RSV infection was $330 million. In 1991 the New England Medical Center calculated that the average cost of hospitalizing a child for RSV infection was $808, while later studies made an estimate of $5329 daily (ventilator therapy being one of the primary cost-enhancing factors). The cost is clearly dependent on the physician, the hospital, and the severity of the disease. The calculated mean cost of 15 days of treatment was $77,666, according to this study.[2]

The advent of RSV immune globulin is starting to offer a safe and cost-effective means of preventing the disease in high-risk children. In the past 5 years there have been new, effective drug treatments and improvements in drug regimens. There is promise for a vaccine in the foreseeable future.[3]

RSV is likely to be the cause of respiratory disease and should be suspected in the appropriate season of the year and in the presence of a typical outbreak in the community. RSV should be considered when the age of the child is under 2 years (but this is not always the case) and family epidemiology is consistent (siblings or parents with colds). It occurs in annual epidemics, typically in the winter and spring. Infections are sporadic and rare throughout the rest of the year. The virus is distributed worldwide, and in temperate locations yearly epidemics have occurred as early as December and as late as June but generally peak in January, February, or March. Most RSV infections are introduced by schoolchildren undergoing reinfection.

The high occurrence of RSV infection in the first months of life is unique among human viruses. Severe infections are uncommon in the first 4 to 6 weeks of life, and this may be attributed to the fact that placentally transmitted antibody provides some protection when it is in a high concentration. RSV is the only respiratory pathogen that causes severe illness at a time when maternal antibody is present and high antibody titers should modify or prevent infection. The incubation period from exposure to first symptoms is 4 days. Infants with lower respiratory tract illness tend to shed virus for 5 to 12 days after admission to the hospital. However, shedding has been reported for as long as 3 weeks. Infection is spread by close contact with large infected aerosolized droplets or fomites, typically by touching. The virus is transmitted by direct contact (fomite-skin-mucosa). RSV survives for hours on countertops, gloves, paper tissues, and cloth. It can also remain on skin for half an hour.[1] Nosocomial cross-infection in epidemics is also a concern. Due to the highly contagious nature of the virus, if hospitalization is imminent, infants at highest risk should be placed in "clean wards."[3]

Bronchiolitis, a clinical diagnosis, is an acute, common, often severe respiratory illness in children under age 2. Bronchiolitis is often indistinguishable from RSV pneumonia in infants, and the two conditions often coexist. RSV is the primary cause of bronchiolitis (about 45 to 75 percent of cases), childhood pneumonia (about 15 to 25 percent), croup (6 to 8 percent), and tracheobronchitis seen in the very young yearly. In an epidemic almost all cases of bronchiolitis are due to RSV. Mild bronchiolitis typically causes no long-term problems; however, it may cause 30 to 40 percent of hospitalized patients to wheeze in childhood. Viral agents such as RSV and parainfluenza virus are the most important primary infectious triggers of asthma early in life. The occurrence of chronic restrictive lung disease and bronchiolitis obliterans is rare.

A diagnosis of lower respiratory infection in infants may be made primarily by clinical and/or epidemiologic findings. In severe infections the prodromal rhinorrhea and cough are followed by dyspnea, poor feeding, listlessness, minimum wheezing, and hyperexpansion of the chest cavity. Apnea, a significant clinical concern, may be the principal presenting symptom in infants. What is of greatest concern in diagnosing and treating RSV is the question of possible bacterial involvement (e.g., *Chlamydia trachomatis*). However, other viruses must be considered as well to rule out the possibility of a mixed infection. This can be differentiated by x-rays (infiltrates present in bacterial infections), a history of conjunctivitis (positive chalmydial sign), and the prominence of cough (positive in bacterial infections) rather than wheezing. In bacterial infections, neutrophils typically increase and the white blood cell count can be elevated. However, the white count may be depressed in the presence of severe disease, high fever, and circulatory collapse. These parameters indicate the need for immediate adjunctive antibiotic therapy.

PATHOGENESIS

Inoculation typically occurs through the nose or in the conjunctiva of the eyes in susceptible subjects. In patients with bronchiolitis, proliferation and virus-induced necrosis of the bronchiolar epithelium, hypersecretion of mucus and round cell infiltration, and edema of the submucosa produce obstruction (mucus plug). This results in the obstruction of bronchioles, hyperinflation, and collapse of the distal lung tissue. Generalized infiltration of the lung ensues, epithelial necrosis may extend to both bronchi and alveoli, and the signs and symptoms of small-airway obstruction are evident. Some evidence suggests that immunologic injury is a factor in the pathogenesis of bronchiolitis resulting from RSV. Besides the destructive effect of the virus and the attendant host response, there appear to be injurious effects from superimposed bacterial infections (see Table 9-20-1).

RSV acts to initiate asthma through stimulation of afferent vagal receptors of the cholinergic system in the airways. In infants with RSV-associated wheezing, an IgE response to RSV can be initiated. This is not the case with RSV respiratory disease without associated wheezing. Wheezing with an RSV infection may unmask a predisposition to asthma.

MICROBIOLOGY

RSV belongs to the family Paramyxoviridae, the same family as the parainfluenza and mumps viruses, but is classified among the pneumoviruses. It is a medium-size membrane-bound RNA virus that develops in the cytoplasm of infected cells and matures by budding from the plasma membrane. It can grow in a number of types of tissue culture and shows the characteristic syncytial cytopathology.

SYMPTOMS AND OBJECTIVE FINDINGS

Rhinorrhea, which appears throughout the illness, and pharyngitis are the first signs of an infant infected with RSV. At the same time or within 1 to 3 days, a cough may appear with sneezing. A low-grade fever is common but is an inconsistent sign. Soon after the initial symptoms, an audible wheeze is often heard. Symptoms or secondary infections related to a mild upper respiratory tract infection appear, such as coryza, and otitis media is a common complication. The symptoms may get no worse than this in a mild infection.

In 10 to 40 percent of these patients, lower respiratory tract infection symptoms will occur. In premature infants in the first few months of life, apnea (a potentially life-threatening symptom) may be the presenting manifestation. There is no clear etiology, and apnea can occur in other respiratory infections. In RSV it typically resolves within the first 1 or 2 days of the illness. The more obvious signs of lower respiratory tract infection or bronchiolitis then appear, such as diffuse wheezing, variable fever, cough, rales, rhonchi, and decreased breath sounds. Intercostal or sub-

costal retractions, tachypnea with or without expiratory wheezes (up to 70 to 100 breaths per minute in the very young), and, if severe, central cyanosis, an indication of decreased gas exchange, are all indications of a potentially life-threatening situation. Typically present is the "barrel chest" appearance secondary to hyperinflation, which can be assessed by auscultation. Rash and conjunctivitis are unusual. The liver and spleen may be palpable and appear enlarged secondary to hyperinflation.

DIAGNOSTIC CONSIDERATIONS

Clinically, RSV may resemble *Chlamydia* pneumonitis, which may coexist. If fine rales are present but there is not a predominant fever or wheeze, *Chlamydia* pneumonitis should be considered. Cystic fibrosis (CF) and pertussis should be included in the list of differentials (see Chaps. 7-1 and 9-18). CF typically is associated with a family history, hyponatremia, or hypoalbuminemia. Pertussis is associated with a prominent cough.

LABORATORY TESTS

Immunofluorescent staining or enzyme immunoassay for viral antigen of nasal or pulmonary secretions or nasopharyngeal or throat swabbing for the RSV antigen is the most expeditious test and is 90 percent sensitive and specific. A tracheal aspirate is unnecessary. A routine culture takes 3 to 7 days to turn positive but remains the standard of diagnosis. When a respiratory sample is collected, it should be brought immediately on wet ice to the laboratory for testing, because the virus is heat-labile. Routine tests are nonspecific; the white cell count is normal or elevated, and the differential count can be shifted to the right or the left. Bacterial cultures usually grow normal flora. An elevated leukocyte count, lymphocytosis, and neutrophilia should suggest a bacterial superinfection or pertussis. Hypoxemia may give rise to hypercapnia. A sweat chloride test to rule out CF may be considered if there is evidence of hyponatremia or hypoalbuminemia. If Theophylline is instituted, levels for infants under age 1 should be performed to rule out drug toxicity.

RADIOLOGIC STUDIES

No consolidation or pleural effusions are seen in RSV. In about 10 percent of cases, air trapping is seen. Diffuse hyperinflation/expansion (50 percent) and peribronchial thickening (or interstitial pneumonia in 50 to 80 percent) are common. Segmental consolidation is seen in 10 to 25 percent of these patients. Atelectasis and patchy infiltrates occur in uncomplicated lower respiratory tract infections.

TREATMENT

Pharmacologic Management

The standard therapies include bronchodilators, terbutaline or epinephrine, theophylline, and the antiviral ribavirin. A bronchodilator therapy trial with albuterol or terbutaline (0.01 mg/kg up to 0.25 mg) or epinephrine (0.01 mL of 1:1000 solution per kilogram up to 0.3 mL) administered subcutaneously or by inhalation can be given to determine whether bronchospasm exists. If they help, nebulized treatments (every 2 to 6 h as needed) or intravenous or oral theophylline may be continued. Caution should be used in giving theophylline to infants less than 1 year of age (see "Laboratory Tests," above). Toxic levels can be reached quickly in this age group, and levels should be closely monitored. If there is no improvement with these therapies, treatment should be discontinued.

Antibiotics are of no value in the treatment of routine uncomplicated RSV infection because the risk of secondary infections is low for most infants with RSV. If chlamydia is suspected in an infant 1 to 4 months of age, erythromycin (40 mg/kg/d) may be beneficial. Otitis media is a secondary infection that often is associated with RSV, and standard oral antibiotics can be used to treat the infection. In older infants with interstitial pneumonia and when consolidation is found, parental antibiotics are indicated. Corticosteroids are not indicated except as a final effort in critical cases. Decongestants and expectorants are of no value in routine infections.

Ribavirin (hyperimmune RSV immunoglobulin G) is the only effective antiviral against RSV in humans that is both safe and effective.[4] It is very expensive (about $250 per daily dose estimated 1991 wholesale cost). It is administered early in the course of the infection by continuous aerosolization by a Small Particle Aerosol Generator (ICN Pharmaceuticals) for 12 to 18 h per day for 3 to 7 days. It affects viral shedding minimally but has a measurable modest effect on disease severity. It should be administered by a pediatric respiratory therapist in a well-ventilated negative-pressure room that contains additional respiratory equipment capable of preventing contamination of the room air. Anyone treating or caring for the child should wear a protective mask. Pregnant women should not care for patients receiving ribavirin. Bronchospasm can be exacerbated with this drug, and extreme caution should be used with ventilated patients.

Ribavirin's primary use should be reserved for premature infants and children with underlying cardiopulmonary conditions (underlying cyanotic congenital heart disease or bronchopulmonary dysplasia) and those (such as immunosuppressed transplant patients or patients with HIV infection) with immunologic anomalies that predispose them to severe or fatal infections.[5] The ones who would derive the most benefit from the use of ribavirin are unclear, as indicated in one study.[6] Also, there is no consistent dosing and administration of ribavirin between hospitals and specialty teams caring for these patients. In a report by the American Academy of Pediatrics Committee on Infectious Diseases, based on experience with more than 100,000 children treated with aerosolized ribavirin, the drug was proved to be safe and effective, with maximum benefit being derived from early intervention. The same report outlined the recommendations for the use of ribavirin based on the route of administration, cost, and need for hospitalization support. A recommendation for the strategy of selective use of ribavirin is also outlined in this report.[5]

Currently, safety and efficacy studies are investigating the roles of interferon α_{2A} and RSV-neutralizing antibody/respiratory syncytial immunoglobulin (RSIVIG) in the prevention of RSV disease in preterm babies and infants with and without bronchopulmonary dysplasia. In a controlled study of interferon α_{2A},[7] there was no statistically significant difference in the clinical course, duration of oxygen requirement, or physical assessment between treatment groups and control groups. Further studies evaluating various routes of delivery are under way. Prophylaxis of high-risk patients with RSIVIG appears to be safe and effective in high-risk children.[6] Recipients of high doses of RSIVIG showed a decreased incidence of moderate to severe RSV lower respiratory tract infection, fewer hospitalizations, fewer intensive care stays, and fewer days of ribavirin than low-dose or control subjects.[1] Maternal passive immunization is also being studied at this time.[8]

Despite serum antibody formation, there is no vaccine available. There is purified preparation of the fusion protein of RSV (PFP) that has undergone much of the required extensive vaccine testing, predominantly in adults.[9] It is now being tested in children, with studies using progressively younger age groups. It is being investigated for safety factors, immunogenicity, target population groups, dosing, and administration. However, the more compelling question under investigation involves whether a live-virus vaccine, attenuated-virus vaccine, or purified viral product would be best. Most likely, the 1 percent of the general population of 1-year-olds who acquire RSV in the first year of life would be good candidates for such a vaccine, although initiation in the neonatal period, while the immune system is changing and vulnerable, would be equally efficacious. Most importantly, high-risk children with bronchopulmonary dysplasia and cyanotic congenital heart disease would be excellent candidates for such a vaccine when it becomes available.[2,10]

SUPPORTIVE MEASURES

If a child is very hypoxic, unable to eat, or unable to maintain hydration because of respiratory distress, the child must be hospitalized and given humidified oxygen and tube feedings or intravenous nutrition. The child should be put in respiratory isolation. Sitting the child at an angle of 10 to 30° improves breathing. Many hospitals use preventive measures to stop the nosocomial spread of RSV by grouping patients with similar diagnoses (see "Discussion," above).

PATIENT EDUCATION

RSV is easily spread among all age groups and at home, but especially in high-exposure situations, e.g., day-care facilities, nurseries, pediatric wards, and institutions, where attack rates are higher (nearly 100 percent for young infants and 60 to 80 percent for older infants). Clean gowns and gloves and strict hand washing are mandatory for caretakers in or out of the hospital situation who work with patients with known severe respiratory conditions or established RSV infection.[3] During the RSV season, high-risk infants should be separated from other infants with respiratory symptoms. It is possible but has not been proved that breast milk contributes to a higher level of antibody against RSV and may offer some protection.[9]

DISPOSITION

The severity of RSV disease relates to the age of the patient and the patient's previous exposure to the virus. Older healthy children are typically less susceptible and less ill. Serious RSV infections can occur in elderly and immunocompromised adults. The prognosis is worse for young, premature infants and those with underlying neuromuscular, pulmonary, cardiovascular, and immunologic diseases. Outbreaks among bone marrow transplant and pediatric liver transplant patients have shown a high mortality rate. Infants with congenital heart disease are at risk for a severe or fatal RSV infection. Cardiac failure may occur secondary to pulmonary disease or myocarditis. The mortality of these hospitalized infants is about 2 percent.

COMPLICATIONS AND RED FLAGS

The most common complication is secondary bacterial infection of the middle ear or lung, most often by pneumococcus or *Haemophilus influenzae*. Mechanical ventilation may be required for respiratory failure or apnea. RSV may cause an acute exacerbation of asthma. In an interview by the American Academy of Pediatrics News, Dr. Kaufman was quoted as saying, "There's also a belief by many that RSV leads to respiratory complications later in life, such as asthma. That's not proven but there's anecdotal evidence. It's not just hospitalizations and mortality but complications in later life."[1] Table 9-20-1 provides an overview.

Table 9-20-1. Respiratory Syncytial Virus Overview (Bronchiolitis)

Recommended isolation period
  Infective period: during entire illness, particularly the first week
  Recommended isolation method: contact isolation for 14 days; staff may carry virus
Complications of severe RSV disease
  Short-term: apnea (most common complication in young infants)
  Long-term: recurrent wheezing, pulmonary function abnormalities
Risk factors for severe RSV disease
  Young age (especially less than 2 years old)
  Underlying medical problems: prematurity, lung disease (especially bronchopulmonary dysplasia), congenital heart disease, other major congenital anomalies
  Compromised immune function from chemotherapy or congenital immunodeficiency diseases
  Hospitalization during RSV season (nosocomial infection)
Clinical signs of RSV lower respiratory disease
  Fever usually is present early with upper respiratory tract signs but frequently disappears as disease progresses
  Retractions, tachypnea, crackles, wheezing, hypoxemia
  Cough (may persist for weeks)
  X-ray findings (do not always reflect severity of illness); bilateral interstitial pneumonitis or mild changes (peribronchial thickening and hyperinflation) with hyperinflation of lung (most common)
  Lobar, segmental, or subsegmental consolidation mimicking bacterial pneumonia (20 percent of children)

REFERENCES

1. Clark G: FDA OKs new RSV treatment. *AAP News,* February 1996, 12(2):1 and 20.
2. Meissner H: Economic impact of viral and respiratory disease in children. *J Pediatr* 124:2:S17–S21, 1994.
3. Hall CB: Respiratory syncytial virus: What we know now. *Contemp Pediatr,* 10(Suppl):S92–S110, 1993.
4. Groothius JR: Role of antibody and the use of respiratory syncytial virus immunoglobulin in the prevention of respiratory syncytial virus disease in preterm infants with and without bronchopulmonary dysplasia. *Pediatr Infect Dis J* 13(5):454–458, 1994; discussion, 13(5):457–458, 1994.
5. Committee on Infectious Diseases (American Academy of Pediatrics): Use of ribavirin in the treatment of respiratory syncytial virus. *Pediatrics* 92:501–504, 1993.
6. Moler FW, Steinhart M, Ohmit SE, et al: Effectiveness of ribavirin in otherwise well infants with respiratory syncytial virus–associated respiratory failure. *J Pediatr* 128:422–428, 1996.
7. Chipps BE, Sullivan WF: Alpha-2A-interferon for the treatment of bronchiolitis caused by respiratory syncytial virus. *Pediatr Infect Dis J* 12:653–658, 1993.
8. Englund JA: Passive protection against respiratory syncytial virus disease in infants: The role of maternal antibody. *Pediatr Infect Dis J* 13:449–453, 1994.
9. Tristram DA, Welliver RC: Respiratory syncytial virus: Can we improve our nature? *Pediatr Ann* 22(12):715–718, 1993.
10. Hall CB: Prospects for a respiratory syncytial virus vaccine. *Science* 265:1393–1394, 1994.

BIBLIOGRAPHY

Hashmey R, Shandera WX: Infectious diseases: Viral and richettsial, in Tierney LM Jr, McPhee SJ, Papadakis MA (eds): *Current Medical Diagnosis and Treatment,* 36th ed. Norwalk, CT, Appleton & Lange, 1997, p 1227.
Immunity, allergy and diseases of inflammation: Allergic disorders; Infectious diseases: Viral infections and those presumed to be call viruses; and The respiratory system; The upper respiratory tract, in Bralow L (ed): *Nelson Textbook of Pediatrics,* 14th ed. Philadelphia, Saunders, 1992, pp 589, 814–816, 1054, 1075.

Paisley JW, Levin MJ: Infectious diseases: Viral and rickettsial, in Hathaway WE Groothius jR, Hay WW Jr, Paisley JW, et al (eds): *Current Pediatric Medical Diagnosis and Treatment,* 10th ed. Norwalk, CT, Appleton & Lange, 1991, pp 819–820.
Stauffer JC: Lung, in Tierney LM Jr, McPhee SJ, Papadakis MA (eds): *Current Medical Diagnosis and Treatment,* 36th ed. Norwalk, CT, Appleton & Lange, 1997, pp 259.

Chapter 9–21
RUBELLA
Richard Dehn

DISCUSSION

Rubella, also known as German measles, is a viral illness that produces relatively mild symptoms. It is characterized by a discrete erythematous maculopapular rash that begins on the face and neck and rapidly spreads to the trunk and extremities. The rash sometimes is preceded by a low-grade fever and generalized lymphadenopathy, most notably in the suboccipital, postauricular, and posterior cervical nodes. This illness is often called the three-day measles, since the rash usually clears up within 3 to 4 days. Frequently children have subclinical cases or present with only one or two symptoms. Adults are more likely to experience a 1- to 5-day prodrome characterized by low-grade fever, headache, malaise, mild coryza, and conjunctivitis. Up to 50 percent of cases present with a rash, but leukopenia is common. Arthritis, especially in the small joints of the hands, is not an uncommon complication in adults, especially females. Encephalitis is a rare complication.

When rubella occurs in the mother during the first trimester of pregnancy, the fetus has an 80 percent chance of being infected with congenital rubella. Congenital rubella is known to produce a wide range of birth defects, the most common being a triad of malformations affecting the eyes, heart, and nervous system.

While rubella is a relatively benign viral illness in the postnatal population, its ability to produce serious birth defects when it is contracted by the mother in the first trimester of pregnancy provides justification for an immunization program to control the spread of rubella in the general population. In 1969 a live attenuated rubella virus vaccine was released both as a single-virus vaccine and in combination with the measles and mumps vaccines (MMR vaccine), and in the United States recommendations were made for a single-dose immunization of susceptible populations. This immunization campaign was directed primarily toward preschool and school-age children so that it would then reduce the exposure to pregnant women; it was successful in significantly reducing the incidence of congenital rubella syndrome from 20,000 cases during the 1964 epidemic to 175 cases in 1992. Recent serology studies have shown that up to 10 percent of the U.S. population is not immune to rubella, and so current immunization strategies have concentrated on immunizing subgroups that are likely to have low immunity, such as teenagers and young adults. Some studies have shown that up to 20 percent of 20-year-old females are not immune to rubella.

PATHOGENESIS

Rubella is caused by a rubavirus that resides only in human reservoirs. The postnatal form of rubella is transmitted by direct contact or aerosol droplets originating from nasopharyngeal secretions. After an incubation period of 14 to 21 days, symptoms may appear; however, in children infections are often subclinical and inapparent. It is thought that the virus invades the respiratory tract first and then disseminates to other organ systems. In postnatal cases the host will spread the virus beginning about a week before the appearance of symptoms and continuing for at least four days after the onset of the rash. The illness caused by postnatal rubella is generally benign but is of concern because of the possibility of passing congenital rubella to a first-trimester fetus.

Congenital rubella is a result of the passing of the rubella virus from an infected mother to her fetus. When a nonimmune mother is infected, the virus replicates in her respiratory system and then disseminates to other organ systems, including the placenta. If the infection presents early in gestation, it will establish a chronic intrauterine infection, which will produce endothelial damage to blood vessels, direct cytolysis of cells, and disruption of cellular mitosis. It has been shown that 80 percent of women with rubella infection and a rash during the first 12 gestational weeks have a fetus with congenital infection. At 13 to 14 weeks the incidence of congenital rubella drops to 54 percent, and by the second trimester it drops to 25 percent. The likelihood of congenital infection decreases even further as the pregnancy progresses. One study found birth defects in all infants infected before the eleventh gestational week, in only 35 percent of those infected at 13 to 16 gestational weeks, and in none of those infected after the sixteenth gestational week. These studies do not include several manifestations of congenital rubella that may not be apparent for several years or decades after birth, since the subjects were followed for only 2 years.

SIGNS AND SYMPTOMS

After a 14- to 21-day incubation period, up to 50 percent of these children have no signs or symptoms or just a fleeting light rash. A prodromal phase often precedes the appearance of an erythematous maculopapular rash that begins on the face and neck and quickly moves to the trunk and extremities. The prodromal phase often includes low-grade fever, minor upper respiratory symptoms, myalgias, transient polyarthralgias and polyarthritis, and lymphadenopathy that most commonly occurs in the suboccipital, postauricular, and posterior cervical nodes. The nodes are usually tender for only a few days but often remain palpable for up to a month. As the age of the host increases, the likelihood of a prodromal phase increases. Most young children do not experience a significant prodromal phase if they experience one at all, while most adults do. Arthralgias and arthritis are most common in adult women. Encephalitis is a rare complication and carries a 20 percent mortality risk; however, those who recover seldom exhibit permanent damage. Testicular pain is a common complaint in men and may indicate orchitis.

COMPLICATIONS

The major complication of rubella is congenital rubella. Congenital rubella has been associated with a wide range of birth defects. Its effects on the fetus cover a wide range of outcomes, from fetal death in utero to multiple anomalies to isolated hearing loss. Infants can appear normal at birth, only to have anomalies appear later. The most common abnormalities seen in congenital rubella include interuterine growth retardation, meningoencephalitis, cataracts, glaucoma, retinopathy, hearing loss, patent ductus arteriosus, pulmonary arterial hypoplasia, hepatosplenomagaly, and bone radiolucency. Less commonly seen are thrombocytopenia with purpura, dermal erythropoiesis resulting in bluish-red (blueberry muffin) skin lesions, adenopathy, chromosomal abnormalities, and interstitial pneumonia. Congenital rubella infants require close follow-up, since it is not unusual to

later find hearing loss, mental retardation, behavioral disorders, learning disabilities, endocrinopathies, and growth retardation. Infants with congenital rubella commonly continue to shed the virus for several months and sometimes up to a year, placing susceptible individuals at risk. An extended rubella syndrome with progressive panencephalitis and type 1 diabetes may not develop clinically until the second or third decade of life.

DIFFERENTIAL DIAGNOSIS

Because of the nonspecific nature of the signs and symptoms of postnatal rubella, it is difficult to differentiate it from several other common illnesses. Several common viruses, such as echoviruses, paraviruses, infectious monoucleosis virus, roseola virus, and even measles virus, can produce confusingly similar clinical pictures, as can some bacterial infections, such as streptococcal scarlet fever. It is generally accepted that the diagnosis of postnatal rubella cannot be made solely on the basis of clinical signs and symptoms and that only serologic evidence of infection is diagnostic.

LABORATORY TESTS

The diagnosis of rubella cannot be made reliably from the clinical signs and symptoms because of the nonspecific nature of the illness. The virus sometimes can be detected in throat, blood, and urine samples, but its isolation is time-consuming and expensive.

Most commonly the diagnosis of rubella infection is made by demonstrating at least a fourfold rise in rubella antibody titers, comparing serum samples from the acute and convalescent stages of the illness. Some laboratories can detect rubella-specific immunoglobin M (IgM) antibody, which is strongly suggestive of a recent infection. Other laboratory tests usually are not of much value in the management of postnatal rubella because of the mild nature of the illness.

TREATMENT

Treatment for rubella is supportive and usually is limited to symptomatic treatment for fevers, malaise, arthralgias, and arthritis. Prevention of rubella infections through immunization programs is generally considered the best treatment.

Since 1969 a live attenuated rubella virus vaccine has been available in the United States either as a single-virus vaccine or combined with measles and mumps vaccines. The current vaccine strain is grown in a human diploid cell line and confers immunity to about 98 percent of those immunized, with minimal side effects. It is thought that a single vaccination confers lifelong immunity to 90 percent of the recipients. Current recommendations call for the immunization of children after 12 months of age with the MMR and reimmunization at school entry or by 12 years of age. Individuals lacking a second immunization should be reimmunized or demonstrate serologic immunity to rubella. Postexposure immunization is not protective against rubella, but it is not contraindicated since the failure to contract rubella from the exposure will be followed by immunity from the vaccine. Contraindications to vaccination include pregnancy, recent administration of immune globulin (not including Rhogam), and patients with immunosuppression (not including those with HIV). The vaccine should not be given up to 3 months before conception; however, conception less than 3 months after vaccination does not justify terminating the pregnancy, since the maximum theoretical risk for congenital rubella from vaccination is 1.6 percent. Centers for Disease Control and Prevention (CDC) data show that among 226 rubella-susceptible women who accidentally received the rubella vaccine during the first trimester of pregnancy, none of the babies developed congenital defects although 2 percent had asymptomatic infection. It is also recommended that individuals receiving blood products or Rhogam before vaccine administration have rubella antibodies checked 8 or more weeks after vaccination to assess whether immunity was conferred.

Immune globulin (IG) sometimes is given to pregnant women after rubella exposure, though its use is not advised unless termination of the pregnancy is not an option. Data on this therapy are limited, though a dose of 0.55 mL/kg may prevent or modify the infection in an exposed individual. The data on the effect of IG on the fetus after exposure therapy are even more unclear. Several documented cases have demonstrated the presence of congenital rubella in infants born to mothers treated with IG shortly after exposure.

The most effective treatment for rubella a clinican can provide is to assure that all eligible individuals in the practice are appropriately immunized.

BIBLIOGRAPHY

Brunell PA: *Cecil Textbook of Medicine,* 19th ed. Philadelphia, Saunders, 1992.

Cunningham FG, MacDonald PC, Gant NF, et al (eds): *William's Obstetrics,* 19th ed. Norwalk, CT, Appleton & Lange, 1993, chap 58.

Georges P (ed): Rubella, in *1994 Red Book.* Elk Grove Village, IL, American Academy of Pediatrics, 1994, pp 406–412.

Hashmey R, Wayne X: Infectious diseases: Viral and rickettsial, in Tierney LM Jr, et al (eds); *Current Medical Diagnosis & Treatment,* 35th rev. Norwalk, CT, Appleton & Lange, 1996, pp 1172–1173.

Hayden FG, Hayden GF: *Stein Internal Medicine,* 4th ed. Philadelphia, Saunders, 1994, chap 246.

Levin MJ, Romero JP: *Current Pediatric Diagnosis and Treatment,* 12th ed. Norwalk, CT, Appleton & Lange, 1995, pp 1050–1051.

Morgan-Capneu P: Rubella and congenital rubella, in Rakel RE (ed): *Conn's Current Therapy, 1995.* Philadelphia, Saunders, 1995, pp 125–127.

Shehab ZM: Viral diseases: Rubella, Berkow R (ed): *Merck Manual of Diagnosis and Therapy,* 16th ed. Rahway, NJ, Merck, 1992.

Chapter 9–22
SYPHILIS

Meredith Hansen

DISCUSSION

Etiology

The etiologic agent of syphilis is *Treponema pallidum,* a spirochete. Humans are the only host for *T. pallidum.*

Epidemiology

The primary mode of transmission of syphilis is direct contact with infectious exudates from obvious or concealed lesions of the skin, mucous membranes, or body fluids and secretions (semen, saliva, blood, vaginal secretions). Syphilis also may be transmitted transplacentally from the mother to the fetus. Finally, intravenous needle sharing among drug users and blood transfusions can spread the infection. Risk factors known to increase the incidence of infection include multiple sexual partners, intravenous drug use, commercial sex work or sex with a commercial sex worker, young age, and incarceration. A causal relationship has been established between syphilis and the exchange of sex for "crack" cocaine. The syphilis epidemic peaked in 1990, when 51,060 cases

of primary and secondary syphilis and 55,132 cases of early latent syphilis were reported to the Centers for Disease Control and Prevention. A slight decrease in reported cases occurred from 1991 through 1996. The southern portion of the United States has the highest rates of occurrence. Reported incidence rates are disproportionately higher in blacks and Hispanics.

SIGNS AND SYMPTOMS AND OBJECTIVE FINDINGS

Because of the broad clinical spectrum and diverse treatment regimens, syphilis has been divided into five stages.

1. *Primary syphilis.* In primary syphilis, the most common clinical manifestation is a painless lesion (chancre), which appears 2 to 6 weeks after exposure. Initially, this lesion appears as a painless papule, but it quickly erodes into an indurated ulcer. Chancres usually are single lesions. The ulcer is generally well marginated. Localized, painless lymphadenopathy usually develops. Because chancres appear at the site of inoculation, they commonly present in the genital area. Chancres also may appear on the tongue, buccal mucosa, and lips. Healing of the chancre is spontaneous.

2. *Secondary syphilis.* Secondary syphilis typically appears 2 to 6 months after primary syphilis. Rarely, there is an overlap of symptoms. In secondary syphilis, the infection has progressed from a regional infection to a systemic one. The most common clinical manifestations in secondary syphilis are skin lesions. Syphilitic skin lesions may imitate a variety of dermatologic conditions (varicella, pityriasis rosea, tinea corporis, seborrheic dermatitis, acne vulgaris, tinea versicolor). These lesions may be transitory or may persist for months. Syphilis should be included in a differential diagnosis if any skin lesions present on the palms of the hands or the soles of the feet. Mucous membrane involvement is common with fused, hypertropic, painless papules in intertriginous areas of the body. The lesions present primarily in the genital and rectal areas and are called condylomata lata. Skin and mucous membrane lesions tend to be highly contagious, with the lesion borders teeming with spirochetes. Another common clinical manifestation of secondary syphilis is a generalized alopecia. Common constitutional symptoms include sore throat, fever, chills, headache, weight loss, anorexia, and generalized lymphadenopathy. Uncommon clinical manifestations include arthritis, osteitis, meningitis, iritis, uveitis, and hepatitis. With or without treatment, all the clinical manifestations of secondary syphilis resolve spontaneously.

3. *Latent syphilis.* In latent syphilis, the patient is asymptomatic but diagnostic testing is positive. Latency is divided into two phases. The early latent stage lasts up to 1 year. The late latent stage occurs after 1 year without symptoms. Theoretically, treatment for late latent syphilis requires therapy for a longer duration, because organisms are dividing more slowly; however, the validity of this division and timing is unproved. Latent syphilis often is found incidentally during a routine physical examination or prenatal visit. Unless the patient develops tertiary symptoms, the patient will remain in latent syphilis throughout his or her life.

4. *Tertiary syphilis.* Tertiary syphilis is a chronic inflammatory disease that can affect any organ system. Studies have shown that in patients with tertiary syphilis, cardiovascular syphilis presented in 10 percent, symptomatic neurosyphilis presented in 10 percent, and gummatous syphilis presented in 15 percent. In cardiovasular syphilis, aortitis with aortic insufficiency is the most common complication. Syphilitic aneurysms also may occur. In tertiary neurosyphilis, up to 40 percent of patients may be asymptomatic. In symptomatic neurosyphilis, the clinical manifestations include stroke, seizures, paresis, and tabes

Table 9-22-1. Manifestations of Neurosyphilis

Tabes dorsalis
    Ataxia
    Decreased vibratory sensation
    Decreased deep tendon reflexes
    Incontinence
    Cranial nerve palsies
    Argyll Robertson pupils
    Peripheral neuropathies
General paresis
    Tremors
    Personality changes
    Hyperactive reflexes
    Speech disorders
Stroke syndromes
Seizures

dorsalis, which involves destruction of the posterior column of the spinal cord. Neurosyphilis has a broad range of psychiatric and neurologic manifestations (Table 9-22-1). In gummatous syphilis, the development of gummas may occur on the skin, bone, and respiratory tract. Gummas are slowly enlarging, benign granulomatous lesions that are thought to result from a delayed hypersensitivity reaction.

5. *Congenital syphilis.* A dramatic rise in congenital syphilis has occurred in the 1990s, particularly in the inner cities. Syphilis in pregnancy causes infection in the fetus even if the mother is asymptomatic. Without treatment, 50 percent of the time the infant will die in utero or in the perinatal period. The most common clinical presentation of congenital syphilis is a child who appears healthy at birth but becomes ill weeks to months later. The symptoms include sneezing, rhinitis, and cutaneous lesions. Lymphadenopathy, hematologic abnormalities, and failure to thrive also may be present. Older children may present with interstitial keratitis, Hutchinson's teeth (sharp central incisors), or Clutton's joints (bilateral knee effusions). Making a diagnosis of congenital syphilis requires a high index of suspicion combined with accurate and appropriate testing. When an infant is born to a seropositive mother, the mother and child must be evaluated thoroughly and immediately. This is especially important if there is no record of treatment or if the birth mother was treated less than 1 month before delivery. No infant should leave the hospital without the serologic status of his or her mother having been documented at least once during pregnancy. Serologic testing should be performed at delivery in communities and populations at risk for congenital syphilis.

DIAGNOSTIC CONSIDERATIONS

Syphilis has been recognized as the "great masquerader." A plethora of illnesses mimic syphilis.

Primary Syphilis

Lymphogranuloma venereum, chancroid, herpes simplex, and labial, vaginal, or cervical cancer can mimic a syphilitic chancre. All genital lesions should be considered to be potential syphilis cases.

Secondary Syphilis

Mucocutaneous lesions may imitate a variety of dermatologic disorders. Syphilis should be considered in the diagnostic workup of most dermatologic lesions. Meningitis and hepatitis may be caused by other infectious agents. A patient with alopecia should be tested for syphilis before treatment. Condylomata lata may present as a verrucous lesion, imitating condyloma acuminata

(venereal warts). The initial treatment of venereal warts should include a serologic test for syphilis.

Tertiary Syphilis

Tertiary syphilis may affect any organ system. It must be differentiated from a primary neoplasm of the bone, skin, brain, liver, or lungs. Meningitis may be caused by a variety of infectious agents. Syphilis must be included in the differential diagnosis of any patient who presents with a focal neurologic presentation.

SPECIAL CONSIDERATIONS

Management of Sexual Partners

The sexual partners of infected patients must be evaluated and treated. Patients should be instructed to refrain from intercourse until the patient and his or her partners are cured. Persons exposed to a patient with syphilis in the prior 90 days should be treated regardless of the serologic findings.

HIV Infection

Serologic testing in HIV patients is considered highly accurate. With the exception of neurosyphilis, treatment regimens in HIV-infected patients are identical.

Pregnancy

Pregnant patients should receive the same treatment regimens. If a pregnant patient is allergic to penicillin, she should be hospitalized for desensitization and then treated with penicillin.

DIAGNOSTIC TESTING

Dark-field examination and direct fluorescent antibody testing remain the standard and only definitive methods of diagnosing early syphilis. Considerable skill is required in using this technique. Most hospitals are not equipped to provide these diagnostic tests.

Two types of antibodies are created in response to syphilis: a nontreponemal antibody and a treponemal antibody. Serologic testing has been developed around the two different antibody types. Nontreponemal tests are equally sensitive and are widely used for screening and diagnostic purposes. The two most common nontreponemal tests are the rapid plasma reagin (RPR) and the Venereal Disease Research Laboratories (VDRL). Nontreponemal titers usually correlate with disease activity and may be used as both quantitative and qualitative tests. While both tests are equally sensitive, titers between VDRL and RPR are not interchangeable. In the treatment of patients with primary syphilis, nontreponemal tests become seronegative within 1 year. In secondary syphilis, patients become seronegative within 2 or 3 years after treatment.

The most widely used treponemal test is the fluorescent treponemal antibody absorption (FTA-ABS) test. The two indications for ordering an FTA-ABS test are to confirm a diagnosis of syphilis based on the clinical presentation and to confirm a positive nontreponemal test result. The cost of this test discourages its use for screening purposes. A patient with a reactive treponemal test will have a positive test for a lifetime regardless of disease or treatment activity.

False-positive results are a consideration in performing nontreponemal tests for syphilis. The false-positive incidence rate for nontreponemal tests is 5 to 20 percent. Diseases that yield a false-positive result include infectious mononucleosis, herpes simplex, lupus, scleroderma, and various malignancies. False-negatives in nontreponemal tests are uncommon, and false-positive results in treponemal tests are rare. False-negative tests may occur in immunocompromised patients because of a reduced or absent antibody response. Patients tested in the incubating or early primary stages also may have a false-negative reaction, since nonspecific antibodies are not produced until 3 to 4 weeks after spirochete exposure.

No single test can be used for the diagnosis of neurosyphilis in all patients. The diagnosis can be based on various combinations of reactive serologic test results, abnormalities of the CSF cell count, or a reactive VDRL-CSF with or without clinical evidence of disease.

The diagnosis of congenital syphilis requires (1) a thorough physical examination, (2) a quantitative nontreponemal test of the infant's sera, not cord blood, (3) CSF analysis, (4) chest and extremity x-rays, (5) complete blood count (CBC), (6) liver function tests, and (7) a pathologic examination of the placenta and amniotic cord.

TREATMENT

Since the time of its initial use, penicillin has been the drug of choice for treating all stages of syphilis. There have been reports of rare cases of penicillin resistance.

Pharmacologic Management

For incubating, primary, secondary, and early latent syphilis, benzathine penicillin G is given at 2.4 million units intramuscularly as a single dose.

For late latent, gummatous, and cardiovascular syphilis, benzathine penicillin G is given at 2.4 million units intramuscularly weekly for 3 weeks. Patients should have a CSF exam to rule out neurosyphilis.

For neurosyphilis, 2 million to 4 million units of aqueous penicillin G is given intravenously every 4 h for 10 to 14 days. Penicillin G is the only documented treatment for neurosyphilis, congenital syphilis, and syphilis in pregnancy. Penicillin-allergic pregnant patients, infants, and patients with neurosyphilis should be treated with penicillin after desensitization. HIV-infected patients should be treated with the same regimens. Penicillin G is the drug of choice for the treatment of syphilis in HIV patients. Desensitization should occur before treatment if the patient is allergic to penicillin.

For congenital syphilis, the patient should receive, aqueous penicillin G 50,000 units/kg intravenously every 12 h (first 7 days of life) and then 50,000 units/kg every 8 h for 4 to 7 days or procaine penicillin G 50,000 units/kg intramuscularly daily for 10 to 14 days. Minimal clinical evidence exists regarding the efficacy of alternative treatment regimens.

Patient Education

Patients should be tested for HIV infection and advised to abstain from sexual activity until they and their partners are cured. Concurrent treatment of partners is essential even if they are asymptomatic. A history of a sexually transmitted disease (STD) places a patient at risk for subsequent STDs. When used consistently, condoms are effective in preventing STDs. Patient education in the proper use of condoms should occur during every patient visit for STDs.

DISPOSITION

Treatment failures with penicillin, though uncommon, may occur. Other than serologic retesting, definitive criteria for cure are not available. Patients with early syphilis (incubating, primary, secondary, and early latent) should undergo clinical reassessment and quantitative serologic testing 1, 3, 6, and 12 months after treatment. Patients with a prior history of syphilis will have their test titers decline more slowly than do those of other patients.

Patients with neurosyphilis should have follow-up serologic

testing along with CSF examination every 6 months for a minimum of 3 years.

Patients with HIV infection should be assessed clinically and serologically 1, 2, 3, 6, 9, and 12 months after treatment.

Patients who do not have declining serologic titers or remain symptomatic should be assessed for HIV infection, treatment failure, and possible reinfection. All states require notification of syphilis to public health agencies. Physician assistants should be knowledgeable about the reporting procedures for communicable diseases in their states.

COMPLICATIONS AND RED FLAGS

A complication of syphilis treatment is an intense, febrile reaction called a Jarisch-Herxheimer reaction; its etiology is unknown. This reaction occurs within 24 h after treatment, is self-limiting, and is common among early syphilis patients. Patients should be counseled about this reaction before treatment initiation. Pregnant women who develop a Jarisch-Herxheimer reaction are at increased risk for premature labor or fetal distress. The management of a Jarisch-Herxheimer reaction is limited to supportive care.

BIBLIOGRAPHY

Centers for Disease Control and Prevention: 1993 sexually transmitted diseases treatment guidelines. *MMWR* 42(No. RR-14):3–10, 27–46, 1993.
Hoffman I, Schmitz J: Genital ulcer disease: Management in the HIV era. *Postgrad Med* 98:67–80, 1995.
Isselbacher KJ, Braunwauld E, Wilson JD, et al (eds): *Harrison's Principles of Internal Medicine,* 13th ed. New York, McGraw-Hill, 1994, pp 726–736.
Preventive Services Task Force: *Guide to Clinical Preventive Services,* 2d ed. Alexandria, VA, International Medical Publishing, 1996.
Tierney LM Jr (ed): *Current Medical Diagnosis and Treatment,* 35th ed. Norwalk, CT, Appleton & Lange, 1996, pp 1227–1240.

Chapter 9–23
TETANUS
Richard Dehn

DISCUSSION

Tetanus, also known as lockjaw, is a neurologic disease that is caused by the exotoxin tetanospasmin elaborated by *Clostridium tetani,* a motile, gram-positive, anaerobic spore-forming bacillus. In most cases the organism is introduced into the host through a contaminated wound, though the suitability for infection is not necessarily related to the severity of the wound. The development of clinical tetanus is dependent on contamination of a wound by the organism, tissue characteristics in the area of the wound that are favorable for toxin production, and a susceptible host.

Clostridium tetani spores can be found in 20 to 65 percent of soil samples, with the highest population found in cultivated soil and the lowest in virgin soil. The organism is commonly found in human and animal wastes; thus, areas with poor hygienic practices have more organisms in the soil. As many as 10 percent of humans carry *C. tetani* in the colon. The organism also is found on inanimate objects such as nails and contaminated tools and in household dust. Another source of *C. tetani* is contaminated heroin. In undeveloped countries, the practice of applying contaminated soil or animal feces to an infant's umbilical stump and using contaminated instruments on the stump can cause neonatal tetanus in infants born to unvaccinated mothers.

The exotoxin tetanospasmin is one of the most potent known microbial toxins. The spores can remain viable in the soil for years and are difficult to eradicate. Eradication of the spore requires boiling for a minimum of 4 h or 12 min of autoclaving at 121°C (250°F). When the spores are subjected to an environment with a reduced oxidation-reduction potential, they revert to a vegetative form that produces tetanospasmin. The toxin is absorbed by the peripheral nerves and transported to the spinal neurons at a rate of about 250 mm/d. The toxin also can be carried to the nervous system by blood pathways. The toxin binds irreversibly to the ganglioside membranes of nerve synapses, blocking the release of inhibitory neurotransmitters in the motor neurons. Loss of the inhibitory function results in continuous motor firing, producing a generalized tonic spasticity that usually is superimposed on intermittent tonic convulsions.

Tetanus is not common in the developed world, where a large proportion of the population has been vaccinated. In the United States 53 cases were reported in 1988, including 1 case of neonatal tetanus. Almost all tetanus cases occur in unvaccinated or inadequately vaccinated individuals. Most cases occur in older adults, probably as a result of inadequate immunity in older populations. The overall fatality rate is 26 percent; however, 52 percent of patients with tetanus who are over 60 years old die. Although most cases in the United States occur as a result of wounds contaminated by soil, tetanus has occurred after surgery, injections, burns, skin ulcers, and tympanic membrane perforation. Drug addicts appear to be at risk, especially "skin poppers" (those who inject drugs subcutaneously). Heroin that is diluted with quinine lowers oxygen tension at the injection site, creating a favorable environment for the growth of *C. tetani*. Tetanus is common in the undeveloped world, especially in rural areas in warm climates where the soil is cultivated and conditions are unsanitary. It has been estimated that as many as 1 million infants die annually of neonatal tetanus.

PATHOGENESIS

Introduction of *C. tetani* spores into the host usually occurs through a contaminated wound; however, 20 percent of these patients present with no history of trauma or wound. If the wound is deep, contains necrotic tissue, or contains a foreign body, an anaerobic environment can be established that is favorable for the conversion of the spores to the vegetative form, which produces the exotoxin tetanospasmin. Although the growth of the organism usually is limited to the local wound site, the exotoxin is spread through peripheral nerves and the bloodstream. Eventually the toxin can be disseminated to motor end plates, spinal cord internuncial neurons, and some cranial ganglia, causing a generalized tonic spasticity that usually is superimposed on intermittent tonic convulsions. Peripherally, tetanospasmin can produce neuromuscular blockades, similar to the toxin of botulism, and can have a direct contraction-producing effect on muscles. Cinical symptoms also suggest that tetanospasmin disrupts the sympathetic nervous system. Once the toxin becomes fixed at a binding site, it cannot be reversed; however, patients who survive tetanus have no residual damage. Active infection with *C. tetani* does not produce immunity. Sometimes the effects of the toxin remain local.

SIGNS AND SYMPTOMS

After an incubation period that averages 7 days after the introduction of *C. tetani* spores, neurologic symptoms begin. The most common symptom is jaw stiffness, which often leads to the patient initially presenting to a dentist. Restlessness, irritability, dysphagia, headaches, fevers, sore throat, tonic spasms, and stiffness of the neck, arm, or legs sometimes are seen. Later in the illness, the patient complains of difficulty opening the mouth (trismus); this is why tetanus is commonly called lockjaw. Progression of the muscle spasms involving the facial muscles leads to a characteristic expression with a fixed smile and raised eyebrows called risus sardonicus. Spasms may progress to other muscle groups, including sphincteral spasms, which can cause urinary retention and constipation, and dysphagia, which can interfere with nutritional intake. The spasms can interfere with respiration, resulting in fatal asphyxia. The spasms often are precipitated by a minor stimulus such as a faint noise or a light touch.

The prognosis is related to the length of incubation and the speed with which the symptoms progress. Severe cases with a poor prognosis present after an incubation period of less than 7 days, with the symptoms evolving over 3 days or less. Moderately severe cases present after an incubation period of less than 10 days, with the symptoms progressing over 3 to 6 days, and mild cases present after 10 or more days, with the symptoms progressing over 4 to 7 days. Tetanus usually lasts 3 to 4 weeks regardless of the severity.

Neonatal tetanus presents in newborns within the first 10 days of life. An infant is susceptible if the mother was not vaccinated. The mortality rate of neonatal tetanus is higher than 70 percent.

DIFFERENTIAL DIAGNOSIS

A patient presenting with spasm or muscle weakness and a history of a wound suggests tetanus. Tetanus can mimic viral or bacterial meningitis or encephalitis, though in tetanus the CSF and the mental status examination are normal. Drugs in the phenothiazine class can produce a muscle rigidity similar to that of tetanus. Trismus can be mimicked by peritonsillar or retropharyngeal abscesses and other local infections and subluxation of the mandible. Strychnine poisoning also can present with similar symptoms.

LABORATORY TESTS

Clostridium tetani occasionally can be cultured from the wound; however, the absence of a positive culture does not exclude the diagnosis of tetanus. Laboratory analysis of blood and CSF usually is unaltered by tetanus until the disease produces complicating cardiopulmonary, fluid, and electrolyte problems. The absence of abnormal laboratory and radiologic studies should suggest a diagnosis of tetanus.

TREATMENT

Human tetanus immune globulin (TIG) (HyperTet) should be given as soon as possible at 3000 to 6000 units intramuscularly, avoiding injection in sites where previous tetanus toxoid vaccinations were administered. The purpose of TIG is to neutralize any free tetanospasmin; however, it is not known whether injection directly into the wound site is of any value. Equine tetanus antitoxin can be given if TIG is unavailable, but the patient should first be checked for hypersensitivity to horse serum. Animal serum is far less preferable than TIG because of more rapidly falling antitoxin levels and a considerable risk of serum sickness.

The wound should not be debrided until 3 to 4 h after the administration of immune globulin so that rising antitoxin levels will neutralize the tetanospasmin released during debridement. Thorough debridement is essential to stop the production of tetanospasmin. Metronidazole (Flagyl) is the drug of choice for eradication of the vegetative form of *C. tetani* after debridement. A loading dose of 15 mg/kg is given intravenously over 1 h, followed by 7.5 mg/kg intravenously given over 1 h every 6 h.

Procaine penicillin, penicillin G, and cephalosporins are also effective against *C. tetani*.

Additional treatment is supportive while one waits for the slow elimination of the tetanospasmin. Unnecessary stimulation should be avoided. Intravenous fluids and mechanical ventilation may be necessary. Muscle spasms can be controlled with benzodiazepines, chlorpromazine, or short-acting barbiturates. Diazepam (Valium) is the drug of choice, and for mild cases adults can be given 5 to 10 mg orally every 2 to 4 h, though severe cases may require 10 to 20 mg every 3 h by intravenous push. Effective respiration may require the use of a curariform agent.

Tetanus is preventable by vaccination. Under 1 percent of the recently reported tetanus cases in the United States have occurred in adequately vaccinated individuals. A 0.5-mL dose of tetanus toxoid vaccine stimulates active immunity to tetanus, and after completion of the primary series of vaccinations, antitoxin persists for at least 10 years. Additionally, individuals who have completed the primary series of vaccinations can boost their antitoxin levels for another 10 years by receiving an additional tetanus toxoid vaccination.

As a tetanus prevention strategy, it is recommended that all individuals in the population receive tetanus vaccination, preferably the absorbed tetanus toxoid formulation. The vaccination is available as a single agent or in several combinations with vaccines for pertussis [diphtheria-tetanus-pertussis (DTP) or diphtheria-acellular tetanus-pertussis (DTaP)], diphtheria [diphtheria-tetanus (DT) or adult diphtheria-tetanus (Td)], and *Haemophilus influenzae* (Tetramune).

Children beginning the initial vaccination series before age 7 should receive a total of five vaccinations. Usually a DTP is given at 2 months, 4 months, and 6 months of age, followed by a DTP or DTaP at 18 months and again before school entry at age 4 to 6 years. If the vaccination schedule is delayed, immunizations should continue with the first three doses given no less than 4 weeks apart, followed by a fourth dose at least 6 monts later and a fifth dose at school entry, unless the fourth dose was given after the fourth birthday.

Adults and children age 7 years or older beginning the initial vaccination series should receive a first and a second Td injection at least 4 weeks apart and a third Td at least 6 months after the second injection.

After the initial immunization series, a Td vaccination should be administered preventively every 10 years, except in individuals who are likely to incur contaminated wounds, who should be vaccinated every 5 years.

Because infection with *C. tetani* does not confer immunity, unvaccinated individuals surviving a case of tetanus who received immune globulin should begin the appropriate vaccination series after recovery from the illness. The vaccinations should be given at a site away from where the immune globulin was given. Individuals surviving a case of tetanus who did not receive immune globulin should begin the vaccination series during convalescence.

Appropriate treatment for individuals sustaining a wound is dependent on whether an individual completed at least three doses of the vaccination series and whether the wound characteristics are favorable for the growth of *C. tetani*. Clean and minor wounds in individuals who have received at least three doses of vaccine do not need revaccination unless the most recent dose was received more than 10 years previously, in which case a Td should be given. Individuals who received fewer than three doses of vaccine and present with a clean and minor wound should begin or continue the immunization series at that time. Individuals who received at least three doses of vaccine and who present with a wound that is not clean or minor should receive a Td if the most recent dose was received more than 5 years earlier. Individuals who had not received at least three doses of vaccine

and who present with a wound that is not clean or minor should receive 250 units of TIG intramuscularly or, after appropriate testing for sensitivity, equine tetanus antitoxin intramuscularly and begin or continue the immunization series at that time. The immunization series should always be administered at a site away from the site of the antitoxin injection. In HIV patients who present with a wound that is not clean or minor, TIG or equine tetanus antitoxin should be given regardless of the immunization history.

Neonatal tetanus can be prevented by immunizing the mother prenatally. Two doses of vaccine should be administered at least 4 weeks apart so that the second dose is received at least 2 weeks before delivery. Pregnancy is not a contraindication to the administration of a booster dose of tetanus toxoid.

Tetanus is most common in older adults, probably as a result of a lack of immunization compliance in that population. The immunization status of all individuals in the population, including elderly adults, should be assessed periodically and kept current.

The tetanus toxoid vaccination can produce local swelling, redness, and tenderness at the site of injection, especially if antitoxin is present. The administration of Td boosters at intervals shorter than 5 years can produce accentuated side effects. The side effects observed after the administration of combined vaccines often are due to the nontetanus components. Rarely, an individual is allergic to tetanus toxoid, and subsequent injections should be avoided in these individuals.

BIBLIOGRAPHY

Abrutyn E: Tetanus, in Fauci AS, Braunwald E, Isselbacher KJ, et al (eds): *Harrison's Principles of Internal Medicine,* 14th ed. New York, McGraw-Hill, 1998, pp 901–904.

Bartlett JG: *Cecil Textbook of Medicine,* 19th ed. Philadelphia, Saunders, 1992.

Berkow R: *Merck Manual of Diagnosis and Therapy,* 16th ed. Rahway, NJ, Merck Sharp & Dohme, 1992.

Chambers HF: Infectious diseases: Bacterial and chlamydial, in Tierney LM Jr et al (eds): *Current Medical Diagnosis and Treatment,* 35th revision. Norwalk, CT, Appleton & Lange, 1996, pp 1200–1201.

Georges P (ed): Tetanus, in *1994 Red Book.* Elk Grove Village, IL, American Academy of Pediatrics, 1994, pp 458–463.

Gilbert DN: *Stein Internal Medicine,* 4th ed. Philadelphia, Saunders, 1994.

Ogle JW: Infections: Bacterial and spirochetal, in Hay WW Jr et al (eds): *Current Pediatric Diagnosis and Treatment,* 12th ed. Norwalk, CT, Appleton & Lange, 1995, pp 1073–1074.

Rauscher LA: Tetanus, in Rakel RE (ed): *Conn's Current Therapy, 1995.* Philadelphia, Saunders, 1995, pp 128–131.

Chapter 9–24
TOXIC SHOCK SYNDROME
Jean M. Covino

DISCUSSION

Toxic shock syndrome (TSS), a multisystem illness caused by toxin-producing *Staphylococcus aureus,* was first described in 1978. In 1980 TSS was recognized as occurring in epidemic proportions in menstruating women who used tampons.[1] Subsequent research led to the elucidation of the pathophysiology and concentrated efforts targeted at disease control. Those efforts were to some degree successful. From 1980 to 1981, TSS occurred in

6 to 6.2 per 100,000 women. Currently the prevalence of this disease is 4 per 100,000 women.

PATHOGENESIS

A strong association was found between TSS and recovery of *S. aureus* from cervical or vaginal cultures obtained from affected women, and a distinct marker toxin, TSST-1, was isolated in up to 90 percent of strains.[2] Staphylococcal enterotoxins B and C1 also may play a role. The pathogenesis involves the establishment of a toxin-producing strain in a nonimmune individual under conditions conducive to toxin production. Presumably, the clinical manifestations of the syndrome are produced when the toxin is absorbed through mucous membranes or from a subcutaneous tissue site of colonization or infection.

EPIDEMIOLOGY

Epidemiologic studies showed a strong association of TSS with the use of tampons. The absorbency of tampons is directly related to the risk for TSS.[3] Public education to limit the duration of use of tampons and the removal of hyperabsorbent tampons from the market have resulted in a decrease in the number of reported cases. Currently, nonmenstrual TSS occurs as frequently as does menstrual TSS. Nonmenstrual TSS has been associated with cutaneous and subcutaneous abscesses, osteomyelitis, postsurgical wound infections, postpartum infection, and gynecologic procedures such as the loop electrosurgical excision procedure (LEEP). TSS also has been reported with the use of diaphragms.

SYMPTOMS AND OBJECTIVE FINDINGS

The onset of menstrual TSS typically occurs on the third or fourth day of menses. In 1980, the Centers for Disease Control and Prevention (CDC) compiled diagnostic criteria. The criteria are as follows:

- Temperature >38.9°C (102°F)
- Rash (diffuse, macular erythroderma that looks like sunburn)
- Hypotension
- Desquamation of palms and soles 1 to 2 weeks after onset of illness

The CDC criteria also include the involvement of three or more of the following organ systems:

- Gastrointestinal (vomiting or diarrhea)
- Muscular (myalgia or elevated creatine phosphokinase twice the upper limit of normal)
- Mucous membranes (hyperemia of vagina, oropharynx, or conjunctivae)
- Renal (blood urea nitrogen or creatinine over twice the upper limit of normal)
- Hematologic (platelet count <100,000/μL)
- Hepatic (total bilirubin, serum glutamic-oxaloacetic transaminase, and serum glutamate pyruvate transaminase over twice the upper limit of normal)
- Neurologic (disorientation or alteration in consciousness without focal neurologic signs)
- Negative tests for Rocky Mountain spotted fever, leptospirosis, and measles
- Negative throat, blood, and cerebrospinal fluid cultures

DIAGNOSTIC CONSIDERATIONS

The differential diagnosis includes any systemic illness associated with fever, rash, hypotension, and multiorgan system involvement, most commonly Kawasaki disease (see Chap. 10-6), Rocky Mountain spotted fever, streptococcal scarlet fever, and bacteremia.

SPECIAL CONSIDERATIONS

Most individuals develop antibodies to TSST-1 by the late teens. Toxic shock occurs predominantly in the population that lacks that antibody because of genetic factors or lack of exposure. It appears that adolescents are at increased risk for TSS.

LABORATORY TESTS

A complete blood count with differential, electrolytes, urinalysis, and renal and hepatic function tests should be done. Gram staining of the vaginal pool, cultures of body cavities (vagina, cervix, oropharynx, anterior nares, and throat), blood, urine, and any lesions and wounds should be done when applicable.

RADIOLOGIC AND OTHER DIAGNOSTIC STUDIES

No radiologic or other diagnostic studies are necessary.

TREATMENT

Therapy is both supportive and specific, with attention to aggressive fluid, electrolyte, and blood product replacement. Tampons and any other foreign bodies should be removed. Identification of the site of infection, drainage, and antibiotic therapy with a β-lactamase-resistant antistaphylococcal agent such as nafcillin or oxacillin (1 g intravenously every 4 h) should be given. If the patient is penicillin-allergic, vancomycin 500 mg every 6 h is indicated. Antibiotics do not change the course of the illness but may prevent relapses in tampon-associated cases.

Patients should be counseled to

1. Avoid tampon use for at least 8 months
2. Avoid superabsorbent tampons
3. Use tampons only intermittently and use sanitary pads at night
4. Remove the tampon and call a practitioner if vomiting, diarrhea, rash, or fever occurs

COMPLICATIONS

All suspected patients must be hospitalized. The case fatality ratio of TSS is approximately 3 percent. Up to 30 percent of menstruating women with TSS may have milder recurrences with subsequent menses. The recurrence rate drops to 5 percent if the patient receives β-lactamase-resistant antibiotics early in the disease process.

OTHER NOTES AND PEARLS

TSS may be present in a milder version, and so a high index of suspicion must be maintained. More severe cases most likely will present to the emergency room. Although TSS is not currently a common illness, the risk of TSS can be further reduced by counseling all menstruating female patients to use tampons intermittently, alternating with sanitary pads, and to use the least absorbent tampon that is necessary.

REFERENCES

1. Shands KN, Schmid GP, Dan BB: Toxic-shock syndrome in menstruating women: Association with tampon use and *Staphylococcus aureus* and clinical features in 52 cases. *New Engl J Med* 303:1436–1442, 1980.
2. Bohach GA, Fast DJ, Nelson RD: *Staphylococcal* and *Streptococcal* pyrogenic toxins involved in toxic shock syndrome and related illnesses. *Crit Rev Microbiol* 17:251–272, 1990.
3. Berkley SF, Hightower AW, Broome CV et al: The relationship of tampon characteristics to menstrual toxic syndrome. *JAMA* 258:917–920, 1987.

BIBLIOGRAPHY

DeCherney AH, Pernoll ML (eds): *Current Obstetric and Gynecology Diagnosis and Treatment,* 8th ed. Norwalk, CT, Appleton & Lange, 1994.

Ryan KJ, Berkowitz RS, Barbieri RL: *Kistner's Gynecology,* 6th ed. St. Louis, Mosby Year Book, 1995.

Chapter 9–25
TOXOPLASMOSIS
Dana Gallagher

DISCUSSION

Toxoplasmosis is a disease caused by the protozoan parasite *Toxoplasma gondii.* Transmission of the parasite can occur either congenitally or in adulthood.

Congenital acquisition occurs when nonimmune women are infected during pregnancy. Although maternal infection is typically mild, it can be devastating to the fetus. The severity of fetal sequelae is inversely proportional to gestational age at the time of the mother's infection.[1] Up to 50 percent of newly infected pregnant women pass the infection to their fetuses;[2] the risk of infection in the United States is about 1 per 1000 live births.[1]

Adult acquisition is usually a clinical "nonevent" in an immunocompetent adult, as these infections are asymptomatic. However, new or recrudescent infection with *T. gondii* can be a serious problem in immunosuppressed individuals, especially those with AIDS. In a pregnant AIDS patient, toxoplasmosis infection may reactivate and rarely cause congenital infection.[3,4]

PATHOGENESIS

With the exception of vertical transmission from an infected woman to her fetus, *T. gondii* is not transmitted from person to person. Cats are the definitive host of the parasite; oocysts pass through the feline gut lumen and out into the feces.[5] In children and adults, transmission can result from contact with litter boxes, sandboxes, and playgrounds in which cats have defecated.

Because the intermediate hosts of viable cysts include cattle, goats, and poultry, infections also may occur after the eating of raw or undercooked meat or the drinking of contaminated milk. *Toxoplasma gondii* also can be transmitted by transfusion or organ transplantation.

SYMPTOMS

Acquiring toxoplasmosis congenitally can result in microcephalus or hydrocephalus at birth and a variety of conditions later in childhood, including chorioretinitis, thrombocytopenia, mental retardation, hepatosplenomegaly, jaundice, cerebral calcifications, and abnormal findings in cerebrospinal fluid (elevated protein, pleocytosis).[6] Congenital toxoplasmosis also causes stillbirth.

In pregnant women, toxoplasmosis may be asymptomatic or may present with flulike symptoms of fever, malaise, and generalized lymphadenopathy.

The most common manifestation of toxoplasmosis in AIDS patients is encephalitis, presenting with focal neurologic findings such as altered mental status, seizures, and/or hemiparesis with or without headache and fever. However, *T. gondii* should be an etiologic suspect in pneumonitis and any unexplained disorder of the ocular, integumentary, cardiac, gastrointestinal, and/or genitourinary systems of AIDS patients.[7] Infection with *T. gondii* is asymptomatic in immunocompetent adults.

LABORATORY TESTS

Infection with *T. gondii* causes antibody reactions that are identifiable in blood; approximately 55 percent of all Americans[8] have been infected. However, it has been estimated that 80 percent of American women are uninfected and susceptible.[1] Therefore, prevention of congenital transmission is a critical issue.

A toxoplasmosis titer (the T in the TORCH obstetric panel) should be drawn at the first prenatal visit. The presence of IgM antibody indicates current infection.[9] Such a result should prompt a referral for genetics counseling.

A toxoplasmosis titer also is drawn at the initial evaluation of an HIV-positive patient. The purpose of the titer is to document the presence of IgG or IgM antibody and, if the titer is positive, to consider toxoplasmosis in any future presentation of neurologic symptoms. Toxoplasmosis does not typically reactivate until the CD count is $100/\mu L$. The prophylaxis for *Pneumocystis carinii* pneumonia (Bactrim DS 1 by mouth every day or three times a week), which is usually instituted when CD4 counts are $200/\mu L$, may prevent toxoplasmosis as well.

RADIOLOGIC STUDIES

If diagnosed with toxoplasmosis in the primary care setting, AIDS patients and those infected congenitally should be referred for specialty care. They probably will undergo CT brain scanning to ascertain the extent of infection and the response to treatment.

TREATMENT
Congenital Infection

Pharmacologic Management

Because of the potential for drug toxicity to the fetus, a specialist should be consulted to institute treatment during pregnancy. Similarly, chemoprophylaxis and treatment in newborns and young children should be managed by an infectious diseases specialist or another specialist.

Patient Education

To avoid infection, pregnant women should be advised not to clean cat litter boxes. They need not, however, avoid ordinary household contact with their pets.

An infected pregnant woman should be referred to a genetics counselor for a complete case-specific review of potential fetal effects and treatment options. Referrals for pregnancy termination should be made available at the patient's request.

AIDS

Pharmacologic Management

AIDS patients with toxoplasmosis are usually hospitalized acutely for a multidrug treatment regimen[10] and then take suppressive therapy for the rest of their lives. Ongoing management of AIDS patients should be handled in concert with an infectious diseases or AIDS specialist.

Patient Education

Patients with HIV should be advised not to clean cat litter boxes and, if it is necessary to do so, to be gloved and masked. Patients should not be advised to give away their cats, because the companionship of pets improves the quality of life.

COMPLICATIONS AND RED FLAGS

Immunocompromised individuals with toxoplasmosis need immediate referral to a specialist for further diagnostics and treatment.

NOTES AND PEARLS

Having received multiple complaints about test accuracy, the Centers for Disease Control and Prevention and the U.S. Food and Drug Administration are scrutinizing commercial serologic test kits for antitoxoplasma antibody.[11] One can expect both the accuracy and the labeling of commercial tests to improve.

With regard to treatment, national collaborative U.S. studies are continuing to determine the best therapeutic regimens for the treatment of congenital toxoplasmosis and toxoplasmosis in AIDS patients.

REFERENCES

1. Stamos JK, Rowley AH: Timely diagnosis of congenital infections. *Pediatr Clin North Am* 41:1020, 1994.
2. Holliman RE: Congenital toxoplasmosis: Prevention, screening and treatment. *J Hosp Infect* 30(Suppl):180, 1995.
3. Benenson AS (ed): Toxoplasmosis, congenital toxoplasmosis, in *Control of Communicable Diseases Manual,* 16th ed. Washington, DC, American Public Health Association, 1995, p 468.
4. Biedermann K, Flepp M, Fierz W, et al: Pregnancy, immunosuppression and reactivation of latent toxoplasmosis. *J Perinat Med* 23:191–203, 1995.
5. Cano RJ, Colome JS: *Diseases of the blood, lymph, muscle, and internal organs,* in *Essentials of Microbiology.* St. Paul, MN, West Publishing, 1994, p 534.
6. Hensyl WR (ed): *Stedman's Medical Dictionary,* 25th ed. Baltimore, Williams & Wilkins, 1991, p 1614.
7. Israelski DM, Remington JS: AIDS-associated toxoplasmosis, in *The Medical Management of AIDS,* 3d ed. Philadelphia, Saunders, 1992, pp 320–321.
8. Goldsmith RS: Toxoplasmosis, in Tierney LM Jr, McPhee SJ, Papadakis MA (eds), *Current Medical Diagnosis and Treatment,* 36th ed. Norwalk CT, Appleton & Lange, 1997, pp 1322–1325.
9. Jancin B: Toxoplasmosis testing urged before pregnancy. *Ob Gyn News,* April 1, 1996, p 12.
10. Sanford JP, Sande MA, Gilbert DN: *The Sanford Guide to HIV/AIDS Therapy. Vienna, VA, Antimicrobial Therapy,* 1995, p 81.
11. Brown SJ: Testing kits for toxoplasmosis are criticized. *Ob Gyn News,* April 1, 1996, p 12.

Chapter 9–26
VARICELLA
William H. Fenn

DISCUSSION

Varicella (chickenpox) is one of the most common exanthems of childhood. Over 90 percent of cases occur before age 10, with only 5 percent occurring in persons over 15 years of age. In the United States, acquisition of this disorder is almost universal, with more than 3 million cases annually. It is a major cause of lost time from school (morbidity) but in healthy children has a low mortality rate (2 to 3 deaths per 100,000 cases). The peak incidence occurs in late winter and spring.

PATHOPHYSIOLOGY

Varicella is caused by the varicella-zoster virus (VZV), a herpesvirus whose only known reservoir is humans. The disease is highly contagious (70 to 90 percent rate) via airborne droplets and direct transmission. Initial entry occurs in the nasopharynx, with a secondary viremia leading to the characteristic cutaneous eruption after an incubation period of 10 days to 2 weeks. Because colonization and initial replication in the nasopharynx occur before the rash, patients generally are contagious 1 to 4 days before the rash appears. Generally, the eruption lasts 4 to 5 days. As the lesions resolve, becoming noncontagious by crusting, VZV recedes to the secondary ganglia in a latent phase. One episode generally confers permanent immunity, although documented cases of second infections have occurred and subsequent reactivation of the virus is common (see Chap. 2-17).

SIGNS AND SYMPTOMS

Adult patients especially may complain of a mild prodrome of myalgias, fever, malaise, and headaches, but children frequently have no prodromal symptoms. The presentation is usually one of a pruritic vesicular rash that usually is accompanied by fever, malaise, anorexia, and a nonproductive cough. The rash generally starts on the face, with rapid spread to the trunk, where it predominates. The patient or parents may describe the rapid appearance of multiple "crops" of lesions over the course of a day.

OBJECTIVE FINDINGS

The characteristic varicella lesion is described as a "dewdrop on a rose petal" and occurs singly and in groups. The generalized exanthem starts as a rose-colored macule, evolving quickly into a papule, followed by the classic vesicles and pustules, which rapidly rupture and crust. At any given time, all lesion types occur simultaneously [Figs. 9-26-1 (Plate 22) and 9-26-2 (Plate 23)].

This was a clinical observation that in the past was useful in distinguishing VZV from smallpox infections. The lesions are more numerous on the trunk but occur on all areas of the skin and may involve the mucous membranes as well. A low-grade fever is usually present. Lymphadenopathy also may be present.

DIAGNOSTIC CONSIDERATIONS

A diagnosis of varicella is usually not difficult to establish. Disseminated herpes simplex virus (HSV) infection or disseminated vaccinia should be considered in immunocompromised populations.

SPECIAL CONSIDERATIONS

The course of the disease is generally more disabling in adults. Immunocompromised patients also have a more serious course, with a high potential for complications, and merit consideration for aggressive treatment.

LABORATORY TESTS

Although the diagnosis of varicella is usually obvious, Tzanck smears (see Chap. 2-16) occasionally may be useful. Viral cultures are possible, although the yield is low, and therefore they are of

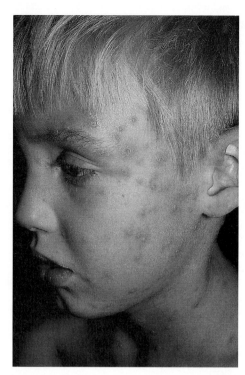

Figure 9-26-1 (Plate 22). Pediatric varicella with multiple vesicles and crusting. (*Photo courtesy of Rodney L. Moser. Used with permission.*)

little clinical use. Immunofluorescence staining of vesicle smears allows for direct identification when needed. Serologic studies are useful only retrospectively.

RADIOLOGIC AND OTHER DIAGNOSTIC STUDIES

No radiologic or diagnostic studies are necessary.

TREATMENT

Pharmacologic Management

Pharmacologic management remains somewhat controversial. Generally, systemic antihistamines are all that is necessary for symptom relief. Acyclovir (Zovirax), an antiviral agent, has been approved for the treatment of varicella, and reductions in lesion

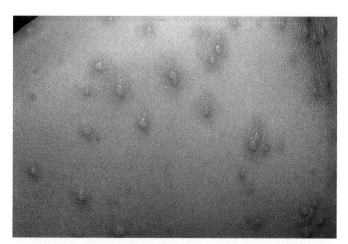

Figure 9-26-2 (Plate 23). Close-up of varicella vesicles showing the characteristic "dewdrop on a rose petal" appearance. (*Photo courtesy of Rodney L. Moser. Used with permission.*)

count and healing time have been documented when treatment is begun within the first 24 h of the disease. Acyclovir is clearly indicated in high-risk populations and adults, but whether its routine use in otherwise healthy children is indicated is a matter of considerable debate. Most authorities do not recommend the routine use of acyclovir. When acyclovir is used in varicella, a regimen of 80 mg/kg/d in four divided doses is used for children and 800 mg four times daily is used for adults. Treatment duration is 5 to 10 days. Antipyretics may be used; however, aspirin must be avoided because of its high degree of association with Reye's syndrome.

Supportive Measures

Measures to reduce scratching and thus reduce the well-known "pock" marking are helpful. Cool baths and compresses, oatmeal baths (Aveeno), and calamine lotion may be employed. Having children wear gloves or socks on their hands when they go to bed may reduce nocturnal scratching. Isolation of the patient while contagious is generally recommended, but as a result of the high rate of contagion and preclinical communicability, this is of limited practical effect. Most school districts require either a provider's statement of noncommunicability or the complete resolution of all lesions before readmitting a child to school after a varicella infection.

Patient Education

Patients and their parents should be educated about the expected course of the disease and the pros and cons of any treatment. One must ensure that the parents are well aware of the need to avoid aspirin. They should be advised that patients are no longer contagious when all lesions have crusted and no new lesions are appearing. The practitioner should inquire about nonimmune household contacts and advise the parents about the high degree of likelihood that those contacts will subsequently display symptoms.

Prevention

The introduction into the United States in 1995 of an approved VZV vaccine promises to reduce the morbidity rate of varicella greatly. Current recommendations of the Centers for Disease Control and Prevention's (CDC's) Advisory Committee on Immunization Practices call for children to receive a single vaccine dose between 12 and 18 months of age. Persons above this age who have not been vaccinated and lack a reliable history of varicella disease also should be vaccinated. Differing rates of efficacy have been reported in different study models, but the long-term results of mass immunizations are not yet evident.

High-risk nonimmune patients who have been exposed to varicella should receive varicella-zoster immune globulin (VZIG).

Disposition

Follow-up evaluation is not necessary in uncomplicated cases.

COMPLICATIONS AND RED FLAGS

Secondary bacterial infection of skin lesions is common and can lead to scarring. Progressive cough and fever, particularly in adults and very young children, should raise the suspicion of varicella pneumonia. Meningeal signs may suggest varicella encephalitis.

OTHER NOTES AND PEARLS

Many providers accept a parent's phone diagnosis and direct treatment without examining the patient. It is important to recognize the pitfalls of this practice in an era of risk management. However, it would be irresponsible to simply ask that a potentially infected child be brought into a crowded waiting room. Strategies such as bringing suspect patients in through an alternative entrance at the end of a clinical day can obviate these concerns.

BIBLIOGRAPHY

Fitzpatrick TB, Eisen AZ, Wolff K, et al (eds): *Dermatology in General Medicine,* 4th ed. New York, McGraw-Hill, 1993, pp 2543–2567.

Holmes SJ: Review of recommendations of the Advisory Committee on Immunization Practices, Centers for Disease Control and Prevention, on varicella vaccine. *J Infect Dis* 174(suppl 3): S342–S344, 1996.

Lookingbill DP, Marks JG: *Principles of Dermatology,* 2d ed. Philadelphia, Saunders, 1993, pp 167–168.

Chapter 9–27
LYMPHOGRANULOMA VENEREUM
Meredith Hansen

DISCUSSION

Etiology

The etiologic agent of lymphogranuloma venereum (LGV) is *Chlamydia trachomatis,* serotypes L1, L2, and L3. LGV is a sexually acquired chlamydial infection. These chlamydial serotypes are different from those that cause urethritis and cervicitis.

Epidemiology

While LGV is endemic in tropical regions, it is uncommon in the United States. Reported cases number less than 1000 per year. Risk factors include sexual contact with partners from endemic regions. The incubation period is 1 to 4 weeks after exposure. Occult infections are common.

SIGNS AND SYMPTOMS AND OBJECTIVE FINDINGS

Lymphogranuloma venereum can be divided into three clinical stages. Stage I presents as a painless papule that ulcerates; urethritis, or multiple lesions (usually pustules) that quickly ulcerate. These lesions resolve without treatment. Frequently, they go unnoticed by the patient.

In stage II, after the lesions disappear, the infection migrates to the pelvic and rectal lymphatic chains. The most common clinical presentation of LGV is tender, unilateral inguinal lymphadenopathy. The lymphadenopathy may progress to bubo formation, an accumulation of tender lymph nodes that may undergo suppuration. Buboes may become fluctuant and rupture. Sinus formation commonly results from spontaneous rupture. Anorectal presentations include proctitis and rectovaginal and perianal fistula formation. In women, inguinal nodes are less commonly affected and involvement is mainly of the pelvic nodes with extension into the rectum. Disseminated disease occurs infrequently, resulting in fever, nausea, arthritis, and meningismus.

Table 9-27-1. Differential Diagnosis of Genital Ulcers

Granuloma inguinale
Lymphogranuloma venereum
Haemophilus ducreyi (chancroid)
Herpes simplex virus
Syphilis

In stage III, regional lymphadenopathy resolves in 2 to 3 months with or without treatment. Scrotal and penile elephantiasis has been reported sporadically in endemic areas.

DIAGNOSTIC CONSIDERATIONS

Ideally, the sexually transmitted disease (STD) workup of a patient with genital ulcers includes serologic testing for syphilis, culture for *Haemophilus ducreyi* (chancroid), and viral culture for herpes simplex virus (HSV). In the United States, the most common causes of genital ulcers are HSV, primary syphilis, and chancroid. Studies have shown that coinfection with multiple diseases is present in 3 to 10 percent of patients with genital ulcers. A differential listing is given in Table 9-27-1.

SPECIAL CONSIDERATIONS

HIV Infection

Treatment of LGV infection in HIV-infected patients is identical to the treatment regimens listed under "Treatment," below.

Pregnancy

The treatment regimen for pregnant patients is the erythromycin regimen listed under "Treatment," below.

DIAGNOSTIC TESTS

The diagnosis is made by culture of the bubo aspirate or a serologic complement fixation test. These tests are expensive and not commonly available. A complement fixation test result higher than 1:32 is indicative of active disease. Occasionally, the diagnosis is made by excluding syphilis, chancroid, or HSV as the correct disease.

TREATMENT

Pharmacologic Management

The recommended regimen is doxycycline 100 mg orally two times a day for 21 days. Alternative regimens are erythromycin 500 mg orally four times a day for 21 days or sulfisoxazole 500 mg orally four times day for 21 days.

Azithromycin is currently used for uncomplicated genital chlamydial infections. At the present time, it is not recommended for LGV.

Surgical Management

Aspiration of fluctuant lymph nodes or buboes through intact tissue may prevent spontaneous rupture and subsequent fistula formation.

Patient Education

Genital lesions significantly increase the risk of acquiring HIV infection. HIV testing should be considered and offered to patients with genital ulcers. These patients must be advised to refrain from sexual activity until they and their partners are cured. Any sexual partner in the past 30 days should be examined and treated.

When used consistently, condoms are effective in the prevention of STDs. Patient education in the proper use of condoms should occur during every STD patient visit.

Disposition

A follow-up test to cure is not required. The disease course may be long and potentially disfiguring. The therapeutic response is monitored by resolution of the symptoms. Longer-term pharmacologic treatment than the regimen listed above may be indicated.

COMPLICATIONS AND RED FLAGS

Few states require partner contact tracing and notification for LGV infections. Physician assistants should be knowledgeable about the reporting procedures for communicable diseases in their states.

BIBLIOGRAPHY

Centers for Disease Control and Prevention: 1993 sexually transmitted diseases treatment guidelines. *MMWR* 42(No. RR-14):3–7, 47–56, 1993.

Goens JL, Schwartz R, DeWolf K: Mucocutaneous manifestations of chancroid, lymphogranuloma venereum and granuloma inguinale. *Am Fam Phys* 49:415–423, 1994.

Preventive Services Task Force: *Guide to Clinical Preventive Services*, 2d ed. Alexandria, VA, International Medical Publishing, 1996.

Tierney L, McPhee SJ, Papadakis MA: *Current Medical Diagnosis and Treatment*, 36th ed. Stamford, CT, Appleton & Lange, 1997, p 1272.

Chapter 9–28
MENINGITIS
Michaela O'Brien-Norton

DISCUSSION

Meningitis is an infection of the cerebrospinal fluid, including the ventricles of the brain, the subarachnoid space, and occasionally the optic nerve. The etilogy can be bacterial, viral, fungal, chemical, or neoplastic. In a matter of hours a person can have a fulminant case of bacterial meningitis; in milder cases, such as viral or fungal, a patient may have symptoms subacutely for several days.

Bacterial Etiologies

In a previously healthy adult, the three most prevalent causative organisms are *Streptococcus pneumoniae, Neisseria meningitides,* and *Haemophilus influenzae.* All three are commonly found in the nasopharynx. Over 15 other pathogens have caused meningitis. More than 2000 deaths occur annually in the United States from bacterial meningitis.

Viral Etiologies

Approximately 12,000 people in the United States are affected by viral, also referred to as aseptic, meningitis, in which bacterial cultures are negative. More than 90 percent of these people are under age 30. Over 40 different groups of viruses cause neurologic illness, and it tends to be a less severe illness than that caused by bacteria.

SIGNS AND SYMPTOMS

Fever is common in both forms: 38 to 40°C (100.4 to 104.0°F). Headaches are a prominent complaint, as is neck stiffness. Altered mental status consisting of lethargy, confusion, or even seizures is more common in bacterial meningitis but is seen in the aseptic form. Nausea and vomiting are common symptoms. A generalized petechial or purpuric rash can be present. Malaise is present in all cases, mimicking a flulike illness with an acute onset.

OBJECTIVE FINDINGS

It is important to review vital signs continuously, looking for elevated temperature, tachycardia, respiration (Cheyne-Stokes breathing seen in central tentorial herniation), and hypotension (systolic pressure less than 90 mmHg), which can signal impending shock. A rash can be present, either petechial or purpuric, over dependent areas of the body, but one must check the palms of the hands, the axillae, and the lower extremities. Nuchal rigidity ("stiff neck") is seen on forward flexion. This can further elicit a positive Kernig's sign, which involves pain on extension of the knees past 120° with the hips flexed. A positive Brudzinski's sign is flexion of the hips and knees produced by flexing the neck. It is important to check everywhere for sources of infection, especially HEENT, including the sinuses, ears, scalp, mouth, and throat. If papilledema or a fixed, dilated pupil (can indicate a tentorial herniation) is present, one should consider obtaining CT before doing a lumbar puncture. Both are ominous findings.

A neurologic exam is essential, checking cranial nerves II through XII and watching for subtle findings. It is important to discriminate between what a patient will not do and can not do. One must check the patient's mental status and perform sensory and motor examinations. If local neurologic deficits are found, CT is usually indicated before doing a lumbar puncture (LP). Increased intracranial pressure (ICP) can cause herniation of parts of the brain from the cranial vault into the tentorium. However, there must not be a delay in administering antibiotics.

DIAGNOSTIC CONSIDERATIONS

The following are the major diagnostic considerations:

- Brain abscess
- Fungi
- Malaria
- Subarachnoid hemorrhage
- Neoplasms
- *Rickettsia* spp.
- Toxic shock syndrome

SPECIAL CONSIDERATIONS

Infants under 3 months of age with a temperature of 38°C (100.4°F) or higher need a full sepsis workup. Since 1992, most pregnant women have been screened and treated before delivery for group B streptococci, a significant cause of neonatal sepsis. Infants and children may present with vague symptoms, such as poor feeding, irritability, respiratory distress, and lethargy. Fontanelles need to be checked for bulging, and a full blood and urine workup with cultures as well as an LP must be done.

The elderly may present only with lethargy. The presentation can be complicated by other underlying disorders that are common to this age group. Full workups often are indicated.

LABORATORY STUDIES

If there are no contraindications, an LP is performed in which four components of the cerebrospinal fluid are closely analyzed:

- Opening pressure
- Protein
- Glucose
- Cell count

Blood cultures, cultures of any focal infections, a complete blood count with differential, electrolytes, glucose, blood urea nitrogen, and creatinine also are ordered.

RADIOLOGIC STUDIES

Chest x-ray and sinus films are done to look for infection. Skull x-ray can rule out a fracture if CT is not done or is not available. CT is done to rule out skull fractures, paranasal sinusitis, osteomyelitis, epidural or brain abscess, obstructive hydrocephalus, and other lesions that may cause herniation.

TREATMENT

Bacterial Meningitis

Treatment consists of ampicillin 2 g intravenously every 6 h plus ceftriaxone 1 g bid or ampicillin 2 g intravenously every 6 h plus cefotaxime 1 g tid.

If there is a penicillin allergy, one should select an alternative, being aware that penicillin-allergic persons may cross-react with cephalosporins, as follows:

- Vancomycin for suspected gram-positive organisms
- Ceftriaxone 2 g intravenously once daily
- Cefotaxime 2 g intravenously every 4 h
- Chloramphenicol 4 to 6 g intravenously in a continuous infusion or divided doses

Neonates should receive ampicillin 100 to 200 mg/kg in a divided dose every 6 h plus either cefotaxime 50 to 100 mg/kg in a divided dose every 12 h or gentamycin 7.5 mg/kg in a divided dose every 8 hs.

Children should receive ampicillin and ceftriaxone or cefotaxime. First- and second-generation cephalosporins penetrate the blood-brain barrier poorly.

Viral Meningitis

There should be symptomatic treatment only: rest, fluids, pain relief and fever control. If the patient cannot tolerate oral fluids and medications because of nausea and vomiting, hospitalization for 24 to 48 h may be needed.

Supportive Measures

Hospitalization for bacterial meningitis is mandatory. Monitoring of vital signs, fluid intake and output, intravenous medications, and adequate caloric intake needs to be done. Repeat lumbar punctures are rarely needed.

Patient Education

Close contacts of patients who have bacterial meningitis may require vaccination and/or prophylactic treatment.

Children should have their hearing checked when they have recovered.

BIBLIOGRAPHY

Deresinski SC, Khan A, Koster F, et al: Emerging infections: Beyond the media hype. *Patient Care* 29(9):29–55, 1995.

Griffiss JM: Meningococcemia infections, in Issecbacher KJ, Braunwald E, Wilson JD, et al (eds): *Principles and Practice of Internal Medicine,* 13th ed. New York, McGraw-Hill, 1991, pp 641–644.

Chapter 9–29
MENINGOCOCCEMIA
Michaela O'Brien-Norton

DISCUSSION

Meningococcemia is a rapidly progressing systemic disease caused by *Neisseria meningitidis* that is carried in the nasopharynx in up to 40 percent of the population. A history of upper respiratory infection is common. Transmission is from person to person through inhaled droplets, usually from carriers, not from the patient. The carrier state is transient, and the organism usually disappears from the oropharynx within a few weeks to a few months. Healthy adults have specific antibodies that destroy the bacteria as they try to enter the bloodstream. Immune status is very important, and natural immunity usually develops by age 20. Approximately 15 to 20 percent of all teenagers are typically carriers of *N. meningitidis.* Antibodies of one strain of *N. meningitidis* usually induce antibodies to other strains, increasing natural immunity. The use of antibiotics has dramatically decreased the fatality of this disease. However, fulminant disease (overwhelming shock) receives much attention and is feared, as a previously healthy person can die in 24 to 48 h.

SIGNS AND SYMPTOMS

There is a prodromal period of cough, headache, sore throat, malaise, and then a sudden onset of high fever, chills (rigors, or shaking chills), and muscle aches, especially in the back, abdomen, and extremities, with nausea and vomiting. The patient looks quite ill. In seriously ill patients, confusion, delirium, seizures, and coma can develop.

OBJECTIVE FINDINGS

Fever and tachycardia are common findings. Hypotension can signal impending shock; it is defined as a systolic pressure less than 90 mmHg. Approximately 75 percent of all meningococcemia patients have a rash, either a spotty maculopapular rash (reminiscent of hives) or a petechial one. It can begin in the early stages and frequently is found in the axillae, flanks, wrists, and ankles. Petechiae can be mixed in with macular lesions. As the patient gets sicker, large ecchymotic areas can develop. Gram-negative diplococci can be obtained in scrapings of these lesions. The patient appears toxic. The degree of prostration may not coincide with the initial clinical findings, and the patient may inadvertently be sent home.

DIAGNOSTIC CONSIDERATIONS

The following are major diagnostic considerations:

- Toxic shock
- Malaria
- Echovirus
- Typhoid
- Brucellosis
- Meningitis, bacterial or viral
- Measles encephalitis
- Subacute bacterial endocarditis
- Subarachnoid hemorrhage
- Rickettsial infection: Rocky Mountain spotted fever

SPECIAL CONSIDERATIONS

Children can present with irritability (defined as a child who is inconsolable even by the closest caregiver), a mild rash, and low-grade fever. They also can present with a change in mental status (confusion), lethargy, or seizures.

LABORATORY TESTS

Blood cultures from multiple sites should be done 15 to 20 min apart on the theory that it then will be hard to miss anything. However, no studies to date have proved this. A complete blood count usually shows an elevated white count with a leftward shift, but it may be normal or even low, especially in immunosuppressed patients.

A platelet count will be decreased, and clotting times (prothrombin time and partial thromboplastin time) will be increased in the presence of disseminated intravascular coagulation (DIC). A lumbar puncture is done if meningitis is suspected. It can be negative or inconclusive early in the disease. A patient can have meningococcal meningitis or meningococcemia without meningitis.

A creatine phosphokinase can be done if a patient is extremely tender to light touch. In rare instances, complement testing is done in "chronic" neisserial infections. Hereditary defects in late complement components (C5 through C9) create a particular susceptibility to these infections.

TREATMENT

Aqueous penicillin is the drug of choice, administered at 4 million units every 4 h for 24 h until the patient is afebrile for 5 days. In a penicillin-allergic person, chloramphenicol is an effective alternative. The dose is usually 50 mg/kg daily in equally divided doses every 6 h intravenously until the patient is able to take oral medication.

Supportive Therapy

The patient is hospitalized, preferably in the intensive care unit, for 1 to 2 weeks. A patient this ill needs good nursing care, close monitoring of vital functions, proper nutrition and fluid maintenance, in addition to the intravenous antibiotics.

COMPLICATIONS AND RED FLAGS

Possible complications include the following:

- Waterhouse-Friderichsen syndrome, a condition in meningococcemia in which the adrenal glands hemorrhage

- Cranial nerve damage
- Arthritis
- Hydrocephalus
- Myocarditis
- Pericarditis
- Endocarditis
- Herpes labialis

An infectious disease specialist should be consulted to oversee the care of the patient.

BIBLIOGRAPHY

Deresinski SC, Khan A, Koster F, et al: Emerging infections: Beyond the media hype. *Patient Care* 29(9):29–55.

Griffiss JM: Meningococcemia infections, in Isselbacher KJ, Braunwald E, Wilson, JD, et al (eds): *Principles and Practice of Internal Medicine,* 13th ed. New York, McGraw-Hill, 1991, pp 641–644.

Chapter 9–30
FOOD-BORNE DISEASES
Rick Davis

INTRODUCTION

Food-borne illness is a significant health problem in the United States. The estimated incidence ranges from 6 million to 80 million cases per year. However, many cases are not reported or go unrecognized. Young children, the elderly, and immunocompromised patients are at increased risk of developing serious illness and death from food-borne disease. Transmission of the illness usually occurs by ingestion of contaminated food and person-to-person spread by a fecal-oral route. Several factors in recent years have contributed to the changing epidemiology of food-borne disease, including greater consumption of fresh fruits and vegetables, global trade, increased consumption of commercially prepared food, new methods of food production, and microbial adaptation.[1]

Food-borne disease can be categorized by the offending agents, such as viruses, bacteria, parasites, and chemical toxins, or by the predominant symptoms, incubation period, and duration of illness. This chapter covers two of the most common bacterial pathogens: *Salmonella* and *Shigella*. Other, emerging bacterial food-borne pathogens such as *Campylobacter jejuni* and *Escherichia coli* 0157:H7 are also covered (see also Chaps. 6-7 and 6-19).

Shigellosis
DISCUSSION

The "Shiga bacillus" was first described in 1898 by K. Shiga and later was called *Shiga dysenteriae*. The term *dysentery* refers to a diarrheal stool that contains pus (polymorphonuclear leukocytes) and blood.

Epidemiology

Over 15,000 cases of shigellosis are reported annually in the United States. *Shigella sonnei* and *Shigella flexneri* account for

90 percent of the reported cases. It is primarily a disease of children between 6 months and 5 years of age, especially children in day-care settings. *Shigella sonnei* is more common before age 15 years, and *S. flexneri* is more common in adults. Transmission is by a fecal-oral route with close personal contact or contaminated food or water. It is highly contagious, with an attack rate of 22 percent in healthy volunteers after the ingestion of only 180 organisms and a 57 percent attack rate after the ingestion of 5000 organisms. This is in comparison to *Salmonella,* which requires $>10^7$ organisms for a 50 percent attack rate. Shigellosis is endemic in Mexico, Central America, India, and southeast Asia.

Microbiology

Shigella spp. are aerobic, nonmotile gram-negative rods of which there are four major groups. Group A contains *Shigella dysenteriae* with 12 serotypes, group B contains *S. flexneri* with 14 serotypes and is common in tropical locales, group C contains *Shigella boydii* with 15 serotypes, and group D contains *S. sonnei* with 1 serotype and accounts for the majority of shigellosis cases in the United States and Europe. *Shigella* spp. produce intestinal damage by invading the colonic epithelium and producing an enterotoxin (Shiga toxin). Previous infection and the development of secretory IgA antibodies may provide some protection against reinfection.[2]

SIGNS AND SYMPTOMS

The classic clinical presentation of bacillary dysentery is cramping lower abdominal pain, fever, tenesmus (a painful urge to defecate with little or no evacuation), and multiple low-volume stools with bloody mucus. The symptoms usually begin within 24 to 72 h of ingestion and last for 5 to 7 days in adults and 2 to 3 days in children. The volume of diarrhea is usually less than 1 L per day. Malnourished children and debilitated adults are at risk of a more severe clinical course.

DIAGNOSTIC STUDIES

The clinical suspicion of shigellosis should be made in any patient with acute bloody diarrhea, abdominal cramps, and fever. Stool examination for fecal leukocytes and blood supports a diagnosis of dysentery. However, this cannot be differentiated from an acute presentation of ulcerative colitis (see Chap. 6-4) or other dysentery-producing pathogens, such as *Campylobacter* spp., *E. coli* 0157:H7, and *Salmonella* spp.

A stool culture should be performed to confirm the diagnosis and antibiotic sensitivity. Sigmoidoscopy is usually not necessary within the initial 4 or 5 days of symptoms. If the symptoms continue after treatment or last for more than 6 weeks, sigmoidoscopy with biopsy is indicated. If patients have been recently treated with antibiotics before the onset of diarrhea, a stool specimen for a *Clostridium difficile* assay should be obtained.

TREATMENT

Many patients with mild symptoms clear the infection without antibiotic therapy. A primary regimen for adults is a fluoroquinolone, such as ciprofloxacin 500 mg orally bid or norfloxacin 400 mg bid orally for 3 to 5 days. An alternative regimen is trimethoprim-sulfamethoxazole (TMP-SMX, Septra DS) bid orally for 3 to 5 days.[3] Resistance to trimethoprim-sulfamethoxazole is high, especially in the tropics. It has been suggested that shigellosis inadequately treated with trimethoprim-sulfamethoxazole may increase the risk of hemolytic-uremic syndrome.[4] Oral rehydration therapy is indicated for patients with mild disease. However, moderate to severe diarrhea may require intravenous fluid hydration. Traditionally, hypomotility agents are avoided in patients with dysentery to prevent the possible complication of toxic

mega-colon. However, some researchers are now advocating their use in mild disease.[3] Since shigellosis is a highly contagious disease, careful handwashing by the patient, family members, and the health care delivery team should be strongly encouraged. Shigellosis is reportable to the health department in some areas. One can refer to the local health department for reporting requirements.

Salmonellosis

DISCUSSION

Nontyphoidal Salmonellosis

Infections caused by any *Salmonella* spp. other than *Salmonella typhi* and *Salmonella paratyphi* are termed nontyphoidal salmonellosis. These species are the most common causes of bacterial food-borne illness in the United States. Five clinical syndromes, including typhoid fever, are commonly seen. Gastroenteritis with dysentery and dehydration occurs in approximately 75 percent of salmonella infections; bacteremia in 10 percent; localized infections that may involve the bones, joints, and meninges among others in 5 percent; and an asymptomatic carrier state in less than 1 percent of cases.

Microbiology

The genus *Salmonella* includes a large group of gram-negative bacilli with over 2000 serotypes. They are primarily intestinal parasites but may be found in contaminated water and sewage. *Salmonella enteritidis* has recently become the most common salmonella infection in the United States. It is found in undercooked eggs, homemade and unpasteurized ice cream, and poultry and livestock.[5] The bacteria invade the ileal mucosa and to a lesser extent the colonic epithelium after oral ingestion. They also may produce an enterotoxin that plays a role in the initial diarrhea. The development of infection is dependent on the number of organisms ingested (10^3 to 10^8) and the age and health of the human host.

Epidemiology

Salmonella may account for over 40 percent of reportable food-borne outbreaks. The most common serotypes are *S. enteritidis, Salmonella typhimurium, Salmonella heidelberg,* and *Salmonella newport.* The incidence of infection has been increasing over the past 20 years. Over 25,000 cases were reported each year in the 1970s, up to 45,000 cases were reported annually by the mid-1980s, and currently, although the disease is underreported, between 1 million and 4 million cases are suspected each year.[6]

SIGNS AND SYMPTOMS

Symptoms from salmonella gastroenteritis usually occur 6 to 48 h after ingestion but may be delayed for 7 to 12 days. The initial symptoms may be as mild as a few loose stools or as serious as severe watery diarrhea. A dysentery syndrome can occur, with colonic infection with frequent bloody mucoid stools of small volume, lower abdominal cramping, fever [usually $<38.9°C$ $(102°F)$], malaise, nausea, and vomiting that may last from 1 week to 2 to 3 months. The more common mild form of gastroenteritis usually lasts <5 days. Young children, the elderly, and immunocompromised patients are more likely to have a more severe course and a greater chance of complications.

Conditions that predispose patients to salmonella infection include hemolytic anemia, immunosuppression, achlorhydria, malignancy, and inflammatory bowel disease.[6]

DIAGNOSTIC STUDIES

The diagnosis is made by means of a strong clinical suspicion and a stool culture. Sigmoidoscopy and biopsy usually are not indicated unless the diarrhea becomes chronic (>6 weeks), and inflammatory bowel disease should be excluded.

TREATMENT

Supportive treatment with oral rehydration is indicated in mild to moderate disease. Antibiotic therapy should be avoided in this group because of the risk of prolonging a chronic carrier state (>1 year). However, severe disease and patients at risk for complications from salmonella infection (malignancy, immunosuppression, prosthetic valves, hemolytic anemias, and sepsis) should be judiciously treated.

The primary therapy in adults is ciprofloxacin 500 mg orally bid or norfloxacin 400 mg orally bid for 5 days.[3] Alternative therapies include ampicillin and trimethoprion-sulfamethoxazole, but there is a high incidence of resistance to these antibiotics.

Typhoid Fever
DISCUSSION

Typhoid, or enteric fever, can occur with any serotype of *Salmonella* but is most commonly associated with *S. typhi* and *S. paratyphi*. *Salmonella typhi* is found in chronic human carriers and in contaminated food and water systems. Flooding of a community sewage system with subsequent contamination of the drinking water supply is a common source.

SIGNS AND SYMPTOMS

Clinically, these patients gradually develop fevers to 40 to 41°C (104 to 105.8°F) during the first week. There is associated malaise, headache, and chills. Typically, the pulse rate is not elevated as it is with other febrile conditions. If untreated, the fever may last from 4 to 8 weeks. Splenomegaly may be seen, and during the first week of illness "rose spots" may be observed on the chest and abdomen; these are small raised erythematous macules that blanch. Constipation may occur early, followed by a mild diarrheal illness.

Complications are rare but carry a high mortality rate when they occur. Intestinal perforation and peritonitis are the most common, followed by biliary tract disease, septic shock, meningitis, and septic arthritis.

DIAGNOSTIC STUDIES

The diagnosis is made by isolation of the organism, usually by blood culture. Stool cultures may be positive by the second to third week of infection. Antibiotic sensitivity should be tested, as there is a high rate of drug resistance.[6]

TREATMENT

The recommended therapy is ciprofloxacin 500 mg orally bid for 10 days or ceftriaxone 2.0 g a day intravenously for 5 days. An alternative therapy is chloramphenicol 500 mg qid orally or intravenously for 14 days.[3]

Campylobacter Infections
DISCUSSION

Campylobacter spp. are present in several human infections, but *Camplyobacter jejuni* is a major cause of acute dysentery and an emerging food-borne pathogen. It is a motile gram-negative rod or spiral. Transmission occurs by the fecal-oral route and is associated with the ingestion of poultry, eggs, and raw milk and with sick pets (e.g., puppies). The pathophysiology is not well understood but may be via intestinal mucosal invasion and toxin production. It is commonly a disease of children under 5 years of age, especially those in day-care settings, and young adults. The incubation period is between 1 and 6 days, and the clinical symptoms usually last <1 week.

Complications of *Campylobacter* enteritis include toxic megacolon, Reiter's syndrome (see Chap. 10-9), and hemolytic-uremic syndrome (HUS).[2]

SIGNS AND SYMPTOMS

The clinical features include an initial fatigue and myalgia followed by nausea, anorexia, lower abdominal cramping pain, and watery or bloody diarrhea (commonly more than 10 stools per day). Stool examination is frequently positive for fecal leukocytes and blood.

DIAGNOSTIC STUDIES

The diagnosis is made by stool culture.

TREATMENT

The infection is usually self-limiting, but moderately severe cases may benefit from antibiotic therapy. The primary treatment regimen in adults consists of ciprofloxacin 500 mg orally every 12 h or norfloxacin 400 mg orally every 12 h for 5 days. There have been reports of quinolone-resistant strains in southeast Asia, Africa, and Mexico. An alternative therapy is azithromycin 500 mg orally daily for 3 days or erythromycin 500 mg orally bid for 5 days.[3]

Enterohemorrhagic *Escherichia coli*
DISCUSSION

Escherichia coli 0157:H7 is an emerging food-borne pathogen in the United States and is associated with significant morbidity and the HUS. Infection causes a bloody diarrhea that often is associated with the consumption of unpasteurized milk or contaminated beef, especially undercooked hamburger. The organism is present in the intestinal tract of approximately 1 percent of cattle. The beef often becomes contaminated during processing, at the time of slaughter. Grinding of hamburger transfers the pathogens to the interior of the meat, where they may survive inadequate cooking temperatures. The pathophysiology is incompletely understood, but the organism is believed to adhere to the intestinal mucosal surface and produce enterotoxins similar to Shiga toxin.

SIGNS AND SYMPTOMS

The clinical features vary from watery, nonbloody diarrhea and abdominal cramps to bloody diarrhea, fever, nausea, and vomiting. Children less than 5 years old and the elderly are susceptible to a more severe clinical course. Most cases of HUS occur in patients with bloody diarrhea.

DIAGNOSTIC STUDIES

Stools are usually positive for blood and fecal leukocytes. The organism can be cultured from the stool on a special agar from which the 0157 antigen can be assayed. It is recommended that all bloody stool specimens be cultured for *E. coli* 0157:H7.[4] Currently, no antibiotic treatment is recommended. It is suspected that treatment with trimethoprion-sulfamethoxazole may increase the likelihood of developing HUS. A retrospective study also associated HUS with patients treated with a hypomotility agent. One week after the onset of diarrhea, all patients should be monitored for the signs and symptoms of HUS, such as decreased urinary output and pallor. Management is supportive and includes maintenance of fluid and electrolyte balance and frequently dialysis.

PREVENTION

Changes in the production, processing, and marketing of the food supply have contributed to new food-borne pathogens and changes in the epidemiology of food-borne disease. Improved sanitation in food animal production, prevention of contamination, and education of food handlers and consumers (careful hand washing, cooking meat to the proper temperature, etc.) are necessary to reduce the risk of food-borne disease.

REFERENCES

1. Altekruse SF, Swerdlow DL: The changing epidemiology of food-borne diseases. *Am J Med Sci* 311:23–29, 1996.
2. LaMont T: Bacterial infections of the colon, in Yamada T (ed): *Textbook of Gastroenterology,* 2d ed. Philadelphia, Lippincott, 1995, pp 1891–1911.
3. Sanford JP, Gilbert DN, Moellering RC, Sande MA: *Guide to Antimicrobial Therapy,* 27th ed. Vienna, VA, Antimicrobial Therapy, 1997, pp 12–13, 42.
4. Boyce TG, Swerdlow DL, Griffin PM: Current concepts—*E. coli* 0157:H7 and the hemolytic-uremic syndrome. *New Engl J Med* 333:364–368, 1995.
5. Hennessy TW, Hedberg CW, Slutsker L, et al: A national outbreak of *Salmonella enteritidis* infections from ice cream. *New Engl J Med* 334:1281–1286, 1996.
6. Gorbach SL: Infectious diarrhea and bacterial food poisoning, in Sleisenger MH, Fordtran JS (eds): *Gastrointestinal Disease.* Philadelphia, Saunders, 1993, pp 1128–1173.

Chapter 9–31
TUBERCULOSIS
R. Scott Chavez

DISCUSSION

Tuberculosis (TB) is caused by an anaerobic tubercle bacillus of the genus *Mycobacterium.* Most mycobacteria can be isolated easily from environmental sources and are not pathogenic for humans. However, *Mycobacterium tuberculosis* is transmitted from person to person through the respiratory route and is highly communicable. If left unchecked, pulmonary tuberculosis has a morbidity rate of 33 percent and a mortality rate of 60 percent. On average, TB patients have a 22-year course of disease progression.

According to the World Health Organization (WHO), TB is the cause of more adult deaths worldwide than AIDS, malaria, and cholera combined. While current census tracking demonstrates that tuberculous infection may be declining worldwide, nations whose health care resources and social conditions are diminished continue to have a rise in TB rates. The highest TB death rates are experienced in Asia and the sub-Saharan African countries. Health authorities estimate that 30 million people will die from TB during the 1990s.

Before 1985, the United States experienced a 30-year downward trend in newly reported TB cases. However, the United States began tracking annual TB increases in 1985, with a 20.1 percent net gain that year. The three states that reported the largest increases were New York (84.4 percent), California (54.2 percent), and Texas (32.7 percent). The United States reported 26,673 cases in 1992 (approximately 10.5 cases per 100,000 population), a 1.5 percent increase from the previous year.

The states reporting the largest gains in 1992 were Virginia (20.6 percent), Illinois (6.5 percent), New York (3.3 percent), and California (2.1 percent). More recently, in 1994 and 1995, the United States recorded decreases in new TB cases. Public health experts postulate that the downturn in reported TB cases may be due to improved public and professional awareness, the implementation of Centers for Disease Control and Prevention (CDC) controls to prevent the spread of TB, and the Occupational Safety and Health Administration's (OSHA's) mandatory monitoring and controls.

However, TB continues to spread in indigent areas and is found primarily among AIDS patients, the elderly, minority group members, and the urban poor. TB is seen with equal prevalence in rural and urban settings, with the epidemic being focused in hospitals, nursing homes, homeless shelters, correctional institutions, and AIDS/HIV residential care facilities. The relationship between TB and HIV is serious worldwide. WHO estimates that by the year 2000, 14 percent of new TB cases will be associated with HIV. This is significant, since only 4 percent of all TB cases were associated with HIV in 1990.

Other risk groups are the young and the poor. They are more at risk to exposure to TB because of the fact that they live and work where the infection is most often found. Malnutrition, stress, and a compromised immune status are risk factors for promoting TB exposure. TB cases among nonwhites tend to be twice those among whites. Of special concern are blacks, Hispanics, Haitians, and southeast Asian minorities.

PATHOGENESIS

Tuberculosis, a chronic bacterial infection, is caused by *M. tuberculosis,* which can affect multiple organs but usually manifests in the lungs.

Mycobacterium tuberculosis is transmitted primarily through the respiratory route, although it can be transmitted through other routes. As an anaerobic tubercle bacilli, *M. tuberculosis* is carried in respiratory secretions by forming nuclei that are carried on liquid droplets, which are transported during sneezing, spitting, coughing, or even speaking.

What makes *M. tuberculosis* most troublesome is that it remains airborne for a considerable time after the liquid droplets have evaporated. Inhalation of just a few of the bacilli is needed for a person to become infected. The contagiousness of TB is dependent on the frequency and force of a host's cough, the number of bacilli in the expectorate, and the virulence of the infection. Patients who have extensive cavitary pulmonary TB, laryngeal tuberculosis, and endobronchial disease are highly contagious and should be handled with caution.

There are three encouraging factors. First, mycobacteria bacilli are susceptible to ultraviolet radiation. Second, most TB-infected patients do not excrete large amounts of *M. tuberculosis.* Third, most TB patients become noninfectious within 2 weeks after being placed on chemotherapy. A good TB intervention program is predicated on providing adequate ventilation, cough suppression, and appropriate antibiotic chemotherapy.

Microbiology

When the tiny (1 to 5 μm in diameter) airborne droplet nuclei of *M. tuberculosis* are inhaled, they become established in the pulmonary tissues and in some susceptible individuals may manifest throughout the body. In the initial 8 weeks of an *M. tuberculosis* infection, the tubercle bacilli multiply in an anaerobic intracellular environment. Lymphocytes and monocytes begin to interact with the bacilli and create a cell-mediated hypersensitivity. *Mycobacterium tuberculosis* affects monocytes and transforms them into specialized histiocytic cells, which form into granulomas. It is known that mycobacteria can remain dormant in microphages for many years, forming granulomas that become calcified and eventually are detectable on a chest radiograph.

Macrophages transport the bacilli to regional lymph nodes, which may calcify in the lymph node, providing access for systemic infection. A patient with both a calcified hilar lymph node and a calcified peripheral lung granuloma has a Ghon complex.

The initial TB infection may remain dormant for months, years, or even decades; however, it eventually progresses to full reactivation tubercular disease.

SYMPTOMS

Generally, patients with primary tuberculosis are asymptomatic. Usually, the onset of pulmonary tuberculosis is insidious and deteriorates the host through a chronic and progressive course. Primary tuberculosis may not progress to clinical symptomatology until long after the initial infection. Some patients may present with only an inferior or midlung pneumonia that is nonspecific and resolves without complications. However, primary tuberculosis may fulminate into full clinical tubercular disease shortly after the initial infection.

The point to remember about tuberculosis is that it is a chronic wasting disease that varies in its presentation. TB is known as the "great masquerader." There may be minimal infiltration that produces no clinical illness, or there may be extensive bacterial involvement that produces significant symptomatology. A patient can complain of fatigue, exhaustion, muscle weakness, weight loss, low-grade fever, and drenching night sweats as constitutional symptoms of reactivated pulmonary tuberculosis.

The primary respiratory symptom of TB is a chronic nonproductive cough. When sputum is produced, it is usually scanty and nonpurulent. If there is any hemoptysis, it usually is confined to blood streaking of the sputum. TB patients rarely have massive life-threatening hemoptysis.

OBJECTIVE FINDINGS

Generally, there are few physical examination findings in patients with pulmonary TB. Inspection of the chest cavity yields little information about the disease unless there is extensive wasting and the accessory respiratory muscles are pronounced as a result of the labored breathing or cough. Percussion along the isthmus and clavicles may reveal dullness, but only in extensive tubercular apical disease. Auscultation may also reveal little information except when there is apical disease (rales, wheezing) or extensive cavitation (amphoric breath sounds).

DIAGNOSTIC SCREENING

The tuberculin skin test is the standard method of screening for *M. tuberculosis* infection. The tuberculin purified protein derivative (PPD) is the preferred antigen. It should be applied in the intermediate-strength dose through the intracutaneous Mantoux test. Using a tuberculin disposable syringe, 0.1 mL of PPD tuberculin containing 5 tuberculin units (TU's), or intermediate-strength tuberculin, should be injected by the Mantoux method (intradermally into the volar surface of the forearm, approximately 1 to 2 in below the antecubital fossa). The Mantoux injection is made just under the surface of the skin with the needle bevel facing

Table 9-31-1. Population Group and PPD Reaction Size

Population Group	Positive PPD Reaction, mm
HIV-infected persons	Any reaction
Persons at risk or likely to be infected; particular caution with household contacts of tuberculous patients	5
Population groups at high risk of tuberculosis	10
Persons from low-risk general populations, especially in geographic areas known to have a high prevalence of nonspecific tuberculin reactivity	15

upward. A 6- to 10-mm-diameter wheal is formed from the injection.

Within 48 to 72 h the patient's sensitivity reaction to the PPD injection should be measured. The tuberculin skin test must be measured crosswise to the axis of the forearm. Measurement of the transverse diameter of the induration provides an assessment of current or past mycobacterial infection in the patient. Care should be taken to measure only the induration, not the erythema around the site.

The standard recording of a PPD measurement is made in millimeters, not in terms of one's observation of "positive" or "negative." A nonreactive PPD test is recorded as 00 mm when there is erythema with no induration. PPDs can be measured accurately up to 1 week after application. However, if the PPD reading is taken after 3 days beyond its implantation and the results appear negative, the standard of care requires a repeat Mantoux test.

What is the standard for determining a positive reaction for TB? For the past 30 years the definition of a positive reaction has been any induration of 10 mm. This figure was determined by accounting for false-positives caused by mycobacteria of the nontuberculosis type. The CDC and the American Thoracic Society (ATS) have revised the guidelines for Mantoux tuberculin skin test interpretation. A new definition of three cutoff values for significant reactions (or positive tests) has been established. Table 9-31-1 describes the method for interpreting positive skin reactions.

It is important to remember that the larger the tuberculin reaction, the more specific it is for *M. tuberculosis;* in general, a confidence level of 100 percent specificity is reached when PPD reactions of 15 mm are approached. However, caution should be exercised in interpreting PPD readings. The presence or absence of TB is not directly correlated to the size of the PPD skin reaction. Studies have demonstrated that noninfected, asymptomatic populations can have tuberculin skin reaction distributions identical to those of patients with known tuberculosis.

False-positives may result when a patient has been exposed to nonpathogenic environmental mycobacteria. The environmental climate greatly influences false-positives. For example, in northern climates false reactions to tuberculin reactivity are rather rare, while in the southeast costal area of the United States nonspecific tuberculin reactivity is commonly found. Generally, reactions smaller than 10 mm are read as cross reactions to environmental mycobacterial antigens and are not significant.

False-negatives can occur for a variety of reasons, such as acute infections, live-virus vaccines, poor nutritional status, metabolic derangements, immunosuppressive therapy, and lymphoid disease.

False-negatives often occur in the elderly. Elderly persons are well known to fail to react to initial testing. A repeat PPD test should be applied 7 to 10 days after the initial test. It is significant if a reaction occurs on the second PPD application in the elderly. False-negative results also may be obtained through technical errors such as the use of outdated materials or storage, dilution, contamination, and adsorption of tuberculin antigen material. Injecting subcutaneously, keeping PPD in syringes too long before use, and reading or recording errors by inexperienced readers are other causes of false-negatives.

Extreme tuberculin skin reactions are rare. However, if a patient complains of intense itching or a severe reaction 3 days after the administration of the PPD, relief can be sought through the application of a strong topical steroid (e.g., triamcinolone ointment 0.1%).

Of greatest concern in tuberculosis surveillance is anergy. Anergy is the absence of a tuberculin skin reaction in infected persons and should not be confused with false-negatives. Tuberculin skin testing fails in a number of cases: 15 percent of patients with newly acquired TB, approximately 50 percent of miliary TB patients and 33 percent of tuberculous pleurisy patients, and any individual who is immunosuppressed. Studies have demonstrated that 17 to 24 percent of hospitalized TB patients and 5 percent of ambulatory TB patients have a negative tuberculin skin test at the time of diagnosis. A study of men admitted to New York jails and detoxification centers demonstrated that poor nutritional status, weight loss, and needle sharing result in anergy. Generally, a positive skin test will occur 2 weeks after the initial therapy and some weight gain.

Caution should be followed in repeating PPD skin tests. In a person infected with *M. tuberculosis* as well as in an uninfected person, repeated PPD testing may cause hypersensitivity and result in a boosted reaction size. This reaction, whether it is due to nonspecific reactivity or to TB, should be read and judged with caution. Any small increase should be looked at with suspicion. It is best to think of the booster phenomenon as a "recall of waned immunity." The ATS and CDC define boosting as "an increase of more than 6 mm of induration from an initial negative test result to one that is positive." The concept of boosting is important in serial tuberculin testing because it may lead to an error in interpretation and unnecessary therapy. The boosting phenomenon, which was first observed in 1934, became more prevalent in the 1970s, when reports of TB conversion in hospital employees increased 10 percent. Boosting rarely occurs before 1 week after the initial testing. Boosting occurs in any age group but is more frequently encountered after 55 years of age. Pres-Stable and associates tested 2675 San Francisco nursing home residents (mean age, 72) and found boosting on a second test in almost 15 percent; when a third serial tuberculin test was given to 769 negatively tested residents, they found an additional 67 persons (8.7 percent) with positive tests.

To account for the boosting phenomenon, a two-step tuberculin skin testing protocol is recommended for persons with a high degree of suspicion for TB. The first test in a serial tuberculin skin test is read 7 days after application, and if there is less than 10 mm of induration, a second test is applied immediately and read 2 to 3 days later.

Patients can be classified into six categories. Table 9-31-2 lists the six classes of the standard international classification of tuberculosis. The classification is useful in maintaining a surveillance system for TB. Worldwide, the Mantoux tuberculin test remains the *sine qua non* surveillance tool for TB; however, sputum or tissue sampling is necessary to confirm the diagnosis.

SPECIAL CONSIDERATIONS

Special consideration must be given to children and pregnant women with TB. Aggressive and prompt treatment is required in infants suspected of having TB, because the risk of dissemination is far greater in infants than it is in adults.

Pregnancy is another special situation that requires prompt and effective treatment. Women who are pregnant and have

confirmed TB should be treated with isoniazid (INH), rifampin (RIF), and ethambutol(EMB) for a period of 9 months. Breast freeding can be encouraged, since very low levels of these anti-TB drugs have been found in breast milk and have been found to be nontoxic to a nursing newborn.

Streptomycin is the only licensed anti-TB drug that has been documented to have a deleterious effect on the fetus, causing congenital deafness. It should be avoided.

LABORATORY STUDIES

The diagnosis of TB is confirmed through bacteriologic examination of the sputum, urine, body fluids, or tissues of the patient. Patients with pulmonary TB most likely will have tubercle bacilli in their sputum. Most mycobacteria are acid-fast organisms that retain certain dyes after being washed in an acid solution. When a report indicates that acid-fast bacilli (AFB) are present on a stained sputum smear, one should suspect a diagnosis of TB. However, TB can be confirmed only after a culture has been grown and identified as *M. tuberculosis*. It takes approximately 4 to 8 weeks to obtain a primary isolation on classic media.

RADIOLOGIC STUDIES

The chest radiograph remains the essential tool for the diagnosis and evaluation of TB. The most typical lesion of pulmonary TB is multinodular infiltration in the apical posterior segments of the upper lobes and the superior segments of the lower lobes. Pulmonary TB patients frequently have cavitation with substantial amounts of infiltration in the same pulmonary segments. The standard views are posterior-anterior (PA) and lateral; however, on occasion lordotic views can obtain views of pulmonary tissue obscured by the intersection of the third and fourth posterior ribs, the second anterior rib, and the clavicle.

Serial films are important in judging the progression and activity of tuberculosis. In time, as the tuberculosis becomes inactive or heals, there will be fibrotic scarring. Healed primary lesions may calcify with the passing of years.

OTHER DIAGNOSTICS

Peripheral blood studies may demonstrate monocytosis in the range of 8 to 10 percent, an elevated erythrocyte sedimentation rate, and modest anemia. Otherwise, blood and chemical studies do not help in the diagnosis of TB.

TREATMENT
Pharmacologic Management

Tuberculosis patients generally are placed on a 6-month course of antituberculosis drugs. They are given isoniazid, rifampin, and pyrazinamide for 2 months, followed by isoniazid and rifampin for 4 months. Ethambutol or streptomycin is added in the first 2 months for patients with advanced disease. This regimen applies to both HIV-infected and uninfected persons.

With good patient compliance and in susceptible TB strains the success rate with the 6-month regimen in sputum conversion exceeds 90 percent. Patient compliance is the major detriment to a successful outcome of treatment. A new product developed to improve patient compliance, a triple-drug combination containing rifampin, isoniazid, and pyrazinamide (Rifater/Marion Merrell Dow), has been approved by the U.S. Food and Drug Administration (FDA). Rifater is given during the initial 2-month intensive treatment for the management of pulmonary tuberculosis (Table 9-31-3).

Table 9-31-2. International Classification of Tuberculosis Protocol

Class O	No history of tuberculosis exposure Not infected	An individual with no history of exposure whose reaction to the tuberculin skin test using 5 tuberculin units (TUs) PPD is <5 mm
Class I	Tuberculosis exposure No evidence of infection	An individual with a history of exposure (contact to a case of tuberculosis) whose reaction to the Mantoux tuberculin skin test using 5 TUs PPD is < 5 mm
Class II	Tuberculosis infection No disease	An individual who exhibits a significant reaction >5 mm if a close contact to a case of tuberculosis or if HIV-seropositive, >10 mm for all others) to the Mantoux tuberculin skin test using 5 TUs PPD but who has no radiographic evidence of tuberculosis and/or negative bacteriologic studies (if bacteriologic studies are done)
Class III	Tuberculosis Current disease	An individual with *M. tuberculosis* cultured or clinical and/or radiographic evidence of current disease
Class IV	Tuberculosis No current disease	An individual with history of previous episode(s) of tuberculosis or abnormal but stable roentgenographic findings, negative bacteriologic studies (if done), and no clinical evidence of current disease
Class V	Tuberculosis suspect	Diagnosis pending, awaiting results of culture or full clinical evaluation; an individual should not remain in this category more than 3 months

SOURCE: World Health Organization: Diagnostic Standards and Classification of Tuberculosis.

An antituberculosis regimen that has been highly effective in the United States consists of isoniazid 300 mg and rifampin 600 mg daily for 1 month, followed by isoniazid 900 mg and rifampin 600 mg twice weekly for 8 months.

If patients are compliant and take effective drugs, symptomatic improvement occurs within the first 2 to 3 weeks. Most patients will convert to negative AFB sputum occurs within the first 2 months. Radiographic evidence of clearing of infiltrates may occur within the first month but usually is recognized between the second and fourth months. Radiologic stability is demonstrated by serial chest films between 3 and 6 months. Drug therapy should be continued 6 months beyond the time when the patient reaches radiographic stability.

Nonpharmacologic Management

Patient noncompliance contributes to the emergence and transmission of drug-resistant organisms. Most patient defaults occur within the first 6 months of a treatment program. To counter this, short-course therapy and directly observed therapy (DOT) have been used to maintain patient compliance. The single most effective public health strategy against the emergence of drug-resistant TB is DOT.

In an on-site DOT program a comprehensive coordination of medical, nursing, and social services ensures that patients receive

and self-administer their antituberculosis medications. Patients on DOT receive daily or twice-weekly therapy. An appointment-based system keeps track of those reporting to the hospital or clinic, and outreach services are used to track patients who miss appointments.

The Bellevue, New York, DOT clinic reported that from November 1992 through July 1993, 113 patients were referred. These were HIV-infected patients, homeless individuals, illicit drug users, and alcoholics. This DOT program achieved a 90 percent (102 of 113 patients) bacteriologic cure rate, while 11 patients were lost to follow-up.[1] A comprehensive hospital-based tuberculosis DOT control program is capable of achieving a very high success rate; however, it is costly and time-consuming (Tables 9-31-4 and 9-31-5).

Supportive Measures

Patient activity and diet can be regular and as tolerated. TB patients are not contagious after a few days of treatment. Children, elderly patients, and pregnant patients require additional supportive measures. Bacillus Calmette-Guerin (BCG) should be given to uninfected children who are at high risk or when isoniazid is not feasible. Elderly patients generally experience more pronounced side effects of isoniazid. Pregnant patients should be given pyridoxine.

Table 9-31-3. Drugs Used to Treat Tuberculosis

Antituberculosis Drugs	Dose	Comments
Isoniazid (INH)	300 mg daily for 1 month, boosted to 900 mg twice weekly for 8 months	Causes a peripheral neuropathy that is preventable and reversible by the administration of pyridoxine; it is safe in pregnant patients
Rifampin (RIF)	600 mg daily for 1 month followed by 600 mg twice weekly for 8 months	Should always be used if the tuberculosis is disseminated or very extensive
Pyrazinamide (PZA)		Often added as the optimal third drug; in clinical trials, has been found to be particularly useful during the first 2 months of treatment
Rifater	120 mg rifampin, 50 mg isoniazid, 300 mg pyrazinamide	
Ethambutol (EMB)		Is bacteriostatic
Thioacetazone		Used in developing countries where drug costs are a limiting factor; combined with isoniazid, 12 to 18 months provides 80 to 90% cure rates
Streptomycin	15 mg/kg/d (IM)	Bactericidal against extracellular, metabolically active organisms; increased risk of fetal ototoxicity with use of streptomycin during pregnancy
Amikacin	15 mg/kg/d (IM or IV)	
Cycloscrine		
Ethionamide	500–1000 mg/d	
Ofloxacin	400 mg bid	
Ciprofloxacin	750 mg bid	

Table 9-31-4. Directly Observed Therapy Protocol Applies To

An individual who is a confirmed or suspected case of tuberculosis and is under the care of the New York City Department of Health Chest Clinics (NYCDOH), is to have medications given under a program of directly observed therapy (DOT)

DOT is a method where every dose of antituberculosis medications taken by the patient is directly observed and supervised by a health care worker or another responsible individual

If an individual is not being treated under a program of DOT, the physician must document the reason in the individual's clinic medical record. A contract should be signed by the patient, the clinic manager or clinic DOT provider (registered nurse, public health adviser), and the physician who is ordering DOT

An individual who is being cared for by a non-NYCDOH physician may also receive DOT at a NYCDOH Chest Clinic, in which case the physician in charge must review the individual's medical regimen

SOURCE: New York: New York City Department of Health. Bureau of Tuberculosis Control, Clinical Protocols. Internet address: www.ci.nyc.ny.us/nyclink/ntml/doh/html tb/cppcont.html

Patient Education

Patients should be instructed about the pathogenesis of their disease and the importance of completing the full course of prescribed therapy. They also should be instructed that rifampin colors tears, secretions, and urine orange. Patients with contact lens should be informed that rifampin may permanently stain their lenses. A well-educated patient and an alert provider are the principal safeguards against drug hepatitis.

Disposition

Generally, there are few complications, and if the patient is compliant with the medication regimen, full resolution of the disease can be expected. Patients should be followed every 2 to 3 months with chest radiographs. Children should be seen every 2 to 4 weeks.

COMPLICATIONS AND RED FLAGS

Multiple-drug-resistant tuberculosis (MDRTB) is defined as a TB infection that is resistant to at least two drugs. MDRTB is a growing problem in the treatment and management of TB. This

Table 9-31-5. Order of Priority for Inclusion in Directly Observed Therapy

If individuals with suspected or confirmed TB must be prioritized for DOT, the following conditions will have priority. If a choice must be made between AFB smear-positive persons who have the same level of resistance, those who are homeless, substance abusers, alcoholics, and those with a history of previous unsuccessful treatment for TB will have priority

AFB smear-positive TB resistant to at least isoniazid and rifampin

AFB smear-positive TB resistant to first-line anti-TB medications other than isoniazid and rifampin

AFB smear-positive TB susceptible to isoniazid and rifampin

AFB smear-negative, culture-positive TB resistant to at least isoniazid and rifampin

History of previous unsuccessful treatment for TB

AFB smear-negative, culture-positive TB resistant to first-line anti-TB medications other than isoniazid and rifampin

AFB smear-negative, culture-positive TB susceptible to isoniazid and rifampin

Culture-negative TB

Extrapulmonary TB

SOURCE: New York: New York City Department of Health. Bureau of Tuberculosis Control, Clinical Protocols, 1997. Internet address: www.ci.nyc.ny.us/nyclink/ntml/doh/html tb/cppcont.html

is especially true in New York City, where approximately 20 to 25 percent of newly diagnosed TB patients have organisms that are resistant to both isoniazid and rifampin.

At-risk populations for MDRTB include HIV-positive individuals; intravenous drug abusers; homeless people; people working or living in correctional institutions, nursing homes, and mental institutions; people exposed to patients with active TB; and health care workers. A high degree of suspicion for primary drug resistance should be raised when a patient has been exposed to noncompliant TB patients or MDRTB patients. Treatment, which must be individualized and based on susceptibility studies, should be initiated only in consultation with local experts or public health authorities. Some public health authorities add a fluoroquinolone to the initial protocol, with final decisions on therapy made when drug resistance studies have been completed. A fifth drug, such as streptomycin, cycloserine, or ethionamide, may be added.

Drug toxicity is always a concern in multiple drug therapy. Since there are multiple drug regimens for TB, toxicity becomes a factor in the choice of therapy. The toxicity of greatest concern is hepatitis. Approximately 3 to 5 percent of patients taking isoniazid and rifampin have a level of toxicity that requires a change in the regimen. Another 1.5 percent of patients taking isoniazid and ethambutol develop toxicities that require a regimen change. Approximately 30 percent of Asian groups and 2 to 5 percent of other populations have toxicity from isoniazid and thiacetazone. Generally, 25 percent of HIV-infected persons develop toxicity from antituberculosis drugs as well. To prevent toxicity side effects, the elderly, diabetic patients, alcoholic patients, and malnourished patients should be given pyridoxine (50 mg/d) concomitantly with isoniazid. Finally, there is little to gain from monitoring liver function serum enzymes, since normal values do not predict the absence or presence of toxicity, and isoniazid may cause transient rises three times the normal value.

In 1995 and 1996, the FDA approved three protease inhibitor drugs: saquinavir (Invirase), ritonavir (Norvir), and indinavir (Crixivan). Nelfinavir (Viracept) (Agouron Pharmaceuticals) was released in 1997. These drugs inhibit HIV protease and block HIV maturation and replication. To date they are the most potent antiretroviral agents available to treat seropositive HIV patients. However, these protease inhibitors interact with rifamycin derivatives, such as rifampin and rifabutin, and their use in HIV TB patients is done with caution.

NOTES AND PEARLS

What is in the future for the diagnosis and treatment of tuberculosis? As TB rates continue to grow worldwide, the need for additional research also grows. Current efforts in TB research have centered on epidemiology, diagnosis and susceptibility testing, treatment, and prevention. Current epidemiologic research focuses on the efficacy and efficiency of control measures to improve existing programs and determine how TB is increasing in developing and underdeveloped countries.

Diagnosis and susceptibility research is centered on rapid and faster techniques. A "third generation" of laboratory techniques soon will make testing not only more effective but also more efficient. These methods include direct testing of respiratory specimens through nonisotopic genetic probes, techniques utilizing the polymerase chain reaction (PCR), and other molecular procedures. These new procedures and protocols are expensive and time-consuming and require further research before they become widely available. Therapeutic research is working to improve the treatment and prevention of tuberculosis in HIV-infected patients and to develop new antimycobacterial agents. Additional research centers on the efficacy and duration of preventive regimens (e.g., the use of pyrazinamide and rifampin). Prevention of MDRTB transmission is also an important research area in which techniques of patient isolation, adequate and prolonged therapy, and better detection of resistant strains with gene amplification methods (PCR) are being conducted.

PATIENT RESOURCES

Facts about the TB Skin Test and Facts about Tuberculosis. American Lung Association, 1740 Broadway, New York, NY 10019-4373, (212) 315-8700.

TB: Get the Facts and Tuberculosis: Connection between TB and HIV. Centers for Disease Control and Prevention, Information Services Office, 1600 Clifton Road NE, Atlanta, GA 30333, (404) 639-1819.

PROVIDER RESOURCES

Core Curriculum on Tuberculosis. American Thoracic Society/Centers for Disease Control. Division of Tuberculosis Elimination, National Center for Prevention Services, Centers for Disease Control and Prevention, 1600 Clifton Road, Mailstop E-10, Atlanta, GA 30333, (404) 639-2508.

Initial Therapy for TB in the Era of Multiple Drug Resistance and Mantoux Tuberculin Skin Testing (videotape). Centers for Disease Control and Prevention, Information Services, 1600 Clifton Road NE, Atlanta, GA 30333, (404) 639-1819.

REFERENCES

1. Schluger N, Ciotoli C, Cohen D, et al: Comprehensive tuberculosis control for patients at high risk for noncompliance. *Am J Respir Crit Care Med* 151(5):1486–1490, 1995.

BIBLIOGRAPHY

American Academy of Family Physicians, Commission on Public Health and Scientific Affairs: *Age Charts for Periodic Health Examination.* Kansas City, American Academy of Family Physicians, 1993.

American College of Obstetricians and Gynecologists: *The Obstetrician-Gynecologist and Primary-Preventive Health Care.* Washington, DC, American College of Obstetricians and Gynecologists, 1993.

American Thoracic Society: Control of tuberculosis in the United States. *Am Rev Respir Dis* 146:1623–1633, 1992.

American Thoracic Society: Treatment of tuberculosis and tuberculosis infection in adults and children. *Am J Respir Crit Care Med* 149:1359–1374, 1994.

American Thoracic Society/Centers for Disease Control: Diagnostic standards and classification of tuberculosis. *Am Rev Respir Dis* 142:725–735, 1990.

Barnes PF, Barrows SA: Tuberculosis in the 1990s. *Ann Intern Med* 119:400–410, 1993.

Burk SA, Canales R, Rahr R, Ayachi S: The challenge of drug-resistant tuberculosis. *Phys Assist* 20:30–46, 1996.

Canadian Task Force on the Periodic Health Examination: The periodic health examination 1979. *Can Med Assoc J* 121:1194–1254, 1979.

Cavalieri SJ, Biehle JR, Sanders WE Jr: Synergistic activities of clarithromycin and antituberculous drugs against multidrug-resistant Mycobacterium tuberculosis. *Antimicrob Agents Chemother* 39(7):1542–1545, 1995.

CDC: Guidelines for preventing the transmission of tuberculosis in health-care settings with special focus on HIV-related issues. *MMWR* 39(No. RR-17):1–25, 1990.

CDC: *National Action Plan to Combat Multidrug-Resistant Tuberculosis.* Atlanta, U.S. Department of Health and Human Services Public Health Service, CDC, 1992.

Centers for Disease Control and Prevention (CDC): Guidelines for preventing the transmission of Mycobacterium tuberulosis in health care facilities. *MMWR* 43(No. RR-13):1–105, 1994.

Centers for Disease Control: *Control of Tuberculosis in Correctional Facilities—A Guide for Health Care Workers.* Atlanta, Centers for Disease Control, 1992.

Centers for Disease Control: Guidelines for preventing the transmission of tuberculosis in health-care settings, with special focus on HIV-related issues. *MMWR* 39(RR-17):1–29, 1990.

Centers for Disease Control: Prevention and control of tuberculosis in facilities providing long-term care to the elderly: Recommendations of the Advisory Committee for Elimination of Tuberculosis. *MMWR* 39(RR-10):7–20, 1990.

Centers for Disease Control: Prevention and control of tuberculosis in U.S. communities with at-risk minority populations and prevention and control of tuberculosis among homeless persons: Recommendations of the Advisory Council for Elimination of Tuberculosis: *MMWR* 41(RR-5):1–23, 1992.

Centers for Disease Control: Purified protein derivative (PPD) tuberculin anergy and HIV infection: Guidelines for anergy testing and management of anergic persons at risk of tuberculosis. *MMWR* 40(RR-5):27–33, 1991.

Centers for Disease Control: Screening for tuberculosis and tuberculous infection in high-risk populations: Recommendations of the Advisory Committee for Elimination of Tuberculosis. *MMWR* 39(RR-8):1–7, 1990.

Centers for Disease Control: The use of preventive therapy for tuberculous infection in the United States: Recommendations of the Advisory Committee for the Elimination of Tuberculosis. *MMWR* 39(RR-8):9–12, 1990.

Centers for Disease Control: Use of BCG vaccines in the control of tuberculosis: A joint statement by the Advisory Committee for Immunization Practices and the Advisory Committee for Elimination of Tuberculosis. *MMWR* 37:663–664, 669–675, 1988.

Cohn DL: Treatment and prevention of tuberculous in HIV-infected persons. *Infect Dis Clin North Am* 8(2):399–412, 1994.

Frieden TR, Sterling T, Pablos-Mendez A: The emergence of drug-resistant tuberculosis in New York City. *New Engl J Med.* 328:523–526, 1993.

Iseman MD, Cohn DL, Sbarbaro JA: Directly observed treatment of tuberculosis: We can't afford not to try it. *New Engl J Med* 328:576–578, 1993.

Lowrie DB, Tascon RE, Colston MJ, Silva CL: Towards a DNA vaccine against tuberculosis. *Vaccine* 12(16):1537–1540, 1994.

McGowan JE Jr, Metchock B, Nolte FS: Laboratory diagnosis of tuberculosis: Past, present, and future. *J Med Assoc Ga* 84(5):215–220, 1995.

Physicians' Desk Reference. Oradell, NJ, Medical Economics Company, 1993, pp 898–899, 1689–1692.

Pust RE: Tuberculosis in the 1990's: Resurgence, regimens, and resources. *South Med J* 85:584–593, 1992.

Chapter 9–32
HISTOPLASMOSIS
Kathryn Frake

DISCUSSION

Histoplasma capsulatum is a dimorphic fungus that is present in soil, particularly soil contaminated with the fecal material of blackbirds, pigeons, and chickens. Birds themselves are not carriers of *H. capsulatum;* however, the fungus grows well in soil that is nitrogen-enriched from bird droppings. Bats can be infected with the fungus, and *H. capsulatum* is excreted in their feces. Inhalation of spores from disturbed soil causes human infection and may result in a variety of clinical manifestations, depending on the amount of inoculum inhaled, the nature of the infecting aerosol, and the host's immunity.

Histoplasma capsulatum is present in temperate climates worldwide and is endemic in the United States along the Ohio and Mississippi river valleys. The endemic area also includes parts of Texas, Virginia, Delaware, and Maryland. Among individuals living in endemic areas, nearly 100 percent have positive histoplasma skin test reactivity. Isolated outbreaks have occurred in other areas. In New York City, for example, cases have been seen among people who have lived in Puerto Rico, the Dominican Republic, and Colombia. Other outbreaks have been described in San Francisco, Los Angeles, Minnesota, Iowa, and Florida, suggesting that there may be areas of *H. capsulatum*–contaminated soils outside the endemic region. Historically, most outbreaks result from massive exposure to *H. capsulatum* spores from large soil disturbances at the fringes of endemic areas, where the population lacks natural immunity, or in large cities where a proportion of the population is immunodeficient from HIV infection.

There are approximately 500,000 new *H. capsulatum* infections per year; however, in endemic areas very few individuals develop active disease. Among AIDS patients, the overall rate of histoplasmosis is 2 to 5 percent in the endemic areas of the United States and up to 25 percent in certain cities, such as Indianapolis, Kansas City, and Memphis.

PATHOGENESIS

After inhalation of *H. capsulatum* into the alveoli of the lungs, dissemination occurs via the blood and lymphatics. Circulating organisms are removed by the cells of the reticuloendothelial system (spleen, liver, bone marrow), but the fungus is not destroyed until 2 to 3 weeks later, when cell-mediated immunity develops. This immune response causes intense inflammation at sites of infection, and necrosis and calcification may occur. The results of this immune response may be noted as an incidental finding on a chest radiograph that demonstrates numerous small calcifications of uniform size.

In those with deficient cell-mediated immunity (AIDS patients, individuals receiving chronic glucocorticoids, patients on chemotherapy, and those with certain hematologic malignancies), a progressive form of primary infection may develop. Rarely, a progressive primary infection is seen in patients with normal immune systems. It is suspected that an unknown immune deficit exists in these so-called normal hosts. Additionally, a progressive primary infection of the lung that mimics tuberculosis can be seen in smokers with underlying chronic obstructive pulmonary disease (COPD).

SIGNS AND SYMPTOMS

Acute Primary Histoplasmosis

Sixty to ninety percent of primary histoplasmosis infections are asymptomatic. Clinically apparent infections are mild to moderate in severity with nonspecific presentations. Infants and young children are more likely to develop symptoms than are immunecompetent adults, and immune-deficient patients are more likely to progress to serious complications from primary infection.

The incubation period of primary infection is 3 to 21 days. In those who do have symptoms, fever, headache, malaise, a nonproductive cough, and substernal chest pain with inspiration are common. Pericarditis, which resolves in 1 to 3 months without treatment, may be present in up to 5 percent. Rarely, acute respiratory distress syndrome (ARDS) develops after extremely heavy exposures. Most ARDS patients improve after 2 to 6 weeks if they survive the initial critical care management. Females who are symptomatic are at greater risk of developing rheumatologic manifestations such as arthralgias, erythema multiforme, and erythema nodosum.

The lung examination is usually normal. Hepatosplenomegaly may be appreciated, particularly in children. Routine laboratory studies are nondiagnostic or may reveal mild anemia and elevated alkaline phosphatase in more severe cases. Chest radiography in asymptomatic patients is normal. In symptomatic patients, typical findings include patchy infiltrates with hilar and mediastinal adenopathy. Sputum may be cultured and is positive in 10 to 15 percent of patients with symptoms.

Influenza is the most common misdiagnosis; however, the sore throat and coryza typical of influenza are uncommon. Hilar adenopathy on chest radiography also may be seen in sarcoidosis and lymphoma patients, and the histopathology of sarcoidosis and histoplasmosis may be indistinguishable. Elevated serum angiotensin-converting enzyme (ACE) levels, which are often seen in sarcoidosis, may be seen in histoplasmosis as well, further confusing the diagnosis. Since most patients improve without treatment, the diagnosis is missed in the vast majority.

Chronic Pulmonary Histoplasmosis

Chronic pulmonary histoplasmosis (CPH) primarily affects males >50 years old with underlying COPD. CPH localizes to the apical regions of the lungs and causes chronic cough, weight loss, low-grade fever, and fatigue. Night sweats are not common. Twenty percent of these patients develop cavity lesions. The result of CPH is progressive worsening of the underlying COPD. If untreated, these cases sometimes resolve spontaneously. In most, however, insidious progression occurs.

Progressive Disseminated Histoplasmosis

Progressive disseminated histoplasmosis (PDH) occurs in 1 in 2000 healthy adults. It is more common in immunosuppressed patients, infants, and small children. Those with AIDS who reside in endemic areas are particularly susceptible. The clinical manifestations of PDH include

1. *Chronic PDH:* waxing and waning symptomatology
2. *Subacute PDH:* waxing and waning but relentless course
3. *Acute PDH:* fulminant, rapidly fatal course

Chronic PDH

Skin lesions are the most common clinically apparent manifestation of chronic PDH. Mouth ulcers are the cutaneous lesions that are most frequently seen. The ulcers are usually painful with heaped-up borders and may be mistaken for a malignancy. Hepatosplenomegaly is present in 30 percent. Chest radiography is negative, and laboratory studies are not usually helpful but may demonstrate mild anemia, leukopenia, and thrombocytopenia. Gradual weight loss, fatigue, and low-grade fevers occur in approximately 30 percent of these patients. The course is very protracted with asymptomatic periods, making the diagnosis extremely difficult.

Subacute PDH

Fever, weight loss, and malaise are consistent findings. Hepatosplenomegaly is more common, as are oral ulcers. Half these patients have anemia, leukopenia, and thrombocytopenia. The adrenal glands are commonly affected, and 5 to 10 percent of these patients develop adrenal insufficiency. Gastrointestinal masses and fistulations, endocarditis, chronic meningitis, and cerebral mass lesions may occur. Subacute PDH progresses to death in 2 to 24 months if left untreated.

Acute PDH

The incidence of acute PDH is rising along with the AIDS epidemic. Other susceptible individuals include the very young and those with lymphoblastic leukemia and Hodgkin's disease. In AIDS patients, acute PDH is often the AIDS-defining illness. CD4+ counts are usually <200 cells/μL. Fever, weight loss, fatigue, cough, and dyspnea are common. Hepatosplenomegaly and lymphadenopathy may be seen. The appearance of skin lesions varies considerably, with the most common presentation being a diffuse, erythematous maculopapular eruption. Purpuric lesions, skin ulcers, and vegetative lesions also may be seen. Mouth ulcers are less common, and the overall incidence of skin lesions (approximately 10 percent) is lower than that of chronic PDH. Anemia, thrombocytopenia, and leukopenia are very common. Chest radiography may demonstrate infiltrates or may be normal. CNS involvement is seen in 5 to 20 percent of cases. If untreated, acute PDH is always fatal, usually within a few weeks.

DIAGNOSTIC STUDIES

Culture and Tissue Staining

The diagnosis requires growth of the fungus from body tissues or fluid samples or staining for yeast forms in tissue sections. Cultures may require 4 to 6 weeks for growth; however, a DNA probe specific for histoplasma permits the identification of an isolate in 1 to 3 weeks. Success rates for culture vary from laboratory to laboratory, depending on experience. Sputum is positive in only 10 to 15 percent of those with acute pulmonary disease; however, sputum from patients with chronic histoplasmosis or cavitary lesions is more likely to be positive. In AIDS patients with acute PDH and abnormal chest radiographs, bronchial aspirates are positive in 80 to 90 percent. Blood and bone marrow are rarely positive in those with chronic PDH, but biopsy of oral lesions is usually diagnostic.

Serologic Tests

Tests for complement fixation antibodies are the most widely used. Two to twelve percent of the population in endemic areas will have chronically positive cultures. As a result, the lowest titer considered to be positive is 1:8. A single test of 1:32 or higher is more suggestive of histoplasmosis, while titers of 1:8 or 1:16 are less compelling but should be considered suspicious in the right clinical setting. Antibodies are detected in 5 to 15 percent of cases approximately 3 weeks after exposure and in 75 to 95 percent after 6 weeks. Thirty to fifty percent of immunodeficient hosts, however, fail to develop antibodies at sufficient titers for diagnosis.

Antigen Detection

The antigen detection technique is useful in patients who are immunodeficient when serologic titers are unreliable. Histoplasma antigen may be detected in the urine or serum by radioimmune assay (RIA). RIA can detect antigen in the serum of 50 percent of AIDS patients with acute PDH and in 90 percent of urine samples. It is less useful in those with self-limiting pulmonary histoplasmosis or cavitary disease.

The monitoring of urinary antigen may be used to determine the initial response to therapy and to detect relapses in AIDS patients who are on chronic suppressive therapy.

Skin Testing

Skin testing is of value only epidemiologically for mapping the distribution of the fungus. It is of little use for diagnosis.

TREATMENT

Acute Primary Histoplasmosis

No treatment is necessary unless the patient is severely ill. Ketoconazole 400 mg/d or itraconazole 200 mg/d for 4 to 6 weeks may be used. Amphotericin B may be used at 0.7 mg/kg/d for 2 to 3 weeks if an azole is contraindicated.

Chronic Pulmonary Histoplasmosis

Asymptomatic patients with thin-walled cavities and areas of interstitial pneumonitis may be followed radiographically over 2 to 4 months if they are not immunocompromised. Those with worsening or persistent radiographic pictures should be treated, along with symptomatic patients and those with thick-walled (>3 to 4 mm) cavities.

Amphotericin B may be used at 0.7 mg/kg/d to a total dose of at least 35 mg/kg. The relapse rate is high (20 percent), and surgical resection may be required in patients with relapse or progressive disease despite treatment. Ketoconazole and itraconazole may also be used at 400 mg/d and 200 mg/d, respectively, for 6 to 12 months. Efficacy is similar between the azoles and amphotericin B.

Chronic and Subacute Progressive Disseminated Histoplasmosis

Amphotericin B or the azoles at the same doses as those listed above may be used. Amphotericin B is the drug of choice if the patient is immunocompromised.

Acute Progressive Disseminated Histoplasmosis, Including Immune-Compromised Hosts

Emergent treatment with amphotericin B is needed. A 1-mg test dose is not advised, as this can cause a considerable delay in treatment. A dose of 25 to 30 mg given intravenously is administered immediately over several hours, followed by 0.7 to 1 mg/kg/d to a total dose of 35 mg/kg or 2.5 g.

Fifty percent or more of AIDS patients relapse after therapy; therefore, chronic suppression treatment is required with itraconazole at 200 mg/d. Urinary antigen should be monitored at the beginning and end of induction and every few months thereafter. Any increase in urinary antigen of at least 2 units should prompt additional studies, as this may indicate relapse.

BIBLIOGRAPHY

Bullock WE: Histuplasma capsulatum, in Mandell GL, Bennett JE, Dolin R (eds): *Principles and Practice of Infectious Diseases,* 4th ed. New York, Churchill Livingstone, 1995.

Johnson PC, Sarusi GA: Infections caused by dimorphic fungi, in Mandell GL, Bennett JE, Dolin R (eds): *Principles and Practice of Infectious Diseases,* 4th ed. New York, Churchill Livingstone, 1995.

Wheat J: Endemi mycosis in AIDS: A clinical review. *Clin Microbiol Rev* 8(1):146–159, 1995.

Wheat J, Hafner R, Korzun AH, et al: Itraconazole treatment of disseminated histoplasmosis in patients with the acquired immunodeficiency syndrome. AIDS Clinical Trial Group. *Am J Med* 98(4):336–342, 1995.

Chapter 10–1
COMMON COMPLAINTS OF THE WRIST, ELBOW, SHOULDER, AND ANKLE

Gloria M. Stewart

Many of the common complaints of the wrist, elbow, shoulder, and ankle that are seen in a primary care setting involve the diagnosis and treatment of tendinitis and bursitis. Therefore, a general discussion of tendinitis and bursitis precedes the sections on the various extremities.

Tendinitis

DISCUSSION

The tendon transfers the force of the muscle contraction to the bone, which in turn produces movement of the joint. Tendons are able to withstand large forces, with a breaking point that is said to be similar to steel. However, as a person ages, the strength of tendons is reduced and fibers shrink and stiffen, frequently resulting in tears from overuse.[1,2] Tendons appear white because they are relatively avascular, consisting of approximately 30 percent closely packed collagen fibers and 2 percent elastin and 68 percent water.[1,3]

Understanding of the anatomy of the muscle-tendon unit is helpful in the discussion of tendinitis or what is now called by some authors *tendinosis*. The muscle-tendon unit can be divided into three areas of concern. Region one is the insertion of the muscle into the tendon. An inflammatory response to injury located in this region would be referred to as *peritendinitis,* whereas an inflammatory response to injury in region three, at the insertion of the tendon into the bone, is referred to as *tendinitis* (tendinosis).[4] Tendinitis is considered to be an overuse syndrome, which involves a chronic inflammation process. The middle section, region two, of the muscle-tendon unit, is where an inflammatory response occurs in the synovial sheath surrounding the tendon. An inflammatory response in this region is referred to as *tenosynovitis.*[1,4,5,6,7] Tenosynovitis of the tendon sheath may be due to strain from overuse, a direct blow, or an infection.[1,4,6]

Trauma initiates an increase in blood supply, the invasion of inflammatory cells, oversecretion of synovial fluid, and an increase in fibronectin content, which cause adhesions between the tendon and its surroundings.[1,4,6] Usually, the sites of tendon injury are located where the muscle-tendon units cross more than one joint, where repetitive high-eccentric workloads generally occur. This process is time-dependent, characterized by tissue repair, regeneration, or scar formation from repeated microtraumas, or the destruction of a small number of cells.[2]

Inflammation is a necessary response to trauma. Macrotrauma, which is acute tissue destruction, is characterized by a defined time of onset, such as a sudden traumatic episode, like a spontaneous disruption of the tendon. Microtraumatic tendon injury is the chronic abusive load or overuse of the tendon, which results in an inflammatory response and is often found in patients who engage in repetitive overhand motions.[2]

As always, an accurate and complete history and physical check of the area of complaint should be explored for the various reasons that could cause tendinitis. Factors that lead to tendinitis may be best understood by grouping them as either intrinsic or extrinsic. Intrinsic factors include malalignment, excessive pronation, femoral neck anteversion, limb length discrepancy, muscular imbalance, and muscular insufficiency. Extrinsic factors include training errors, too much distance, excessive intensity, hill work, improper technique, fatigue, running on hard or uneven surfaces, environmental conditions, and inadequate footwear and equipment.[4,7]

SYMPTOMS

Typically the patient presents with a history of a gradual onset of localized pain and tenderness over the insertion of the tendon. The four cardinal signs of inflammatory response were defined by Celsus (1st century A.D.) as "rubor et tumor cum calore et dolore," redness and swelling with heat and pain, which can be reproduced as the patient moves the tendon.[1,2,4,6,8,9] Tenosynovitis in its acute state presents with pain on function, which progresses to pain at rest and diffuse swelling. Crepitation may also be felt by placing the fingers over the involved tendon while it slides up and down. In a patient with chronic tenosynovitis, the tendons may become thickened.[27]

DIAGNOSTIC TESTS

Conventional radiographs, ultrasound, and CT have a limited role in the diagnosis of injuries of tendons and muscles. Arthrography has been useful for evaluating injury to the rotator cuff, but the most useful diagnostic tool for the evaluation of an injured tendon is MRI.[3,9] The use of MRI with high intrinsic tissue contrast has the ability to separate normal from abnormal tendons. When looking at the MRI, normal tendons appear dark, whereas fat appears bright and muscle has an intermediate contrast.[9]

TREATMENT

Rest

The initial treatment of tendinitis should include rest. The practitioner should have the patient non-weight-bearing for the first 24 h and then slowly increase the motion and load to the area as tolerated by the patient. The key to any treatment is gradual progressive challenges in intensity and load. There is evidence that the repetitive motion may create positive signals for postinjury repair, and that a modified load has also been shown to be important to a successful return to prior performance levels.[2]

Cold Modalities

The use of cold as a modality produces an initial circulatory response of vasoconstriction resulting in reduced edema.[4,6,10,11,12] There is a secondary circulatory response that is called cold-induced vasodilation.[13] This secondary response occurs mainly in the periphery following cold immersion. Cold exposure blocks sensory transmission of the pain impulse, which in turn helps to decrease muscle spasm, thereby helping to control the pain of the patient. The use of cold exposure for an acute injury helps in the prevention of hemorrhage, inflammation, edema, muscle spasm, and pain.[12] The use of cold exposure for a chronic complaint helps the patient by preventing additional inflammation as a result of the rehabilitation process. Conventional cold therapy includes ice packs, ice-cup massage, or ice immersion baths. There are also commercially prepared products, including gel refrigerant packs, chemical packs, and coolant sprays. Commercially prepared products have a warning about potential package breakage, which could result in chemical burns and injuries.[12] Contraindications to using cold therapy are Raynaud's phenomenon, cardiovascular disease, cryoglobulinemia, and paroxysmal cold hemoglobinuria. Other problems with cold therapy are allergy, anesthetic skin, and arthritic conditions.[12]

Heat Modalities

Heat has always been an accepted method of treatment. The use of heat produces vascular changes by causing vasodilation, which produces an analgesic effect and also helps to move nutrients and oxygen into the affected area at the cellular level of metabolism and to remove waste products.[4,12] It has been suggested that for each 10°C (18°F) rise in temperature, the cell's chemical activity and the metabolic rate increases two to three times.[3] Various methods of heat modality include warm whirlpools, paraffin wax, moist heat packs, infrared heat, and therapeutic ultrasound. Each of these modalities helps to raise the temperature and, therefore, increase vasodilation.[12] Warm whirlpool baths are usually taken at a temperature of 39 to 41°C (102 to 106°F) for 15 to 20 min, depending on the body area.[10,12] During the treatment the patients can be actively moving the body part in the whirlpool within the pain tolerance level. Paraffin wax is used mainly for small joints such as fingers, hands, and wrists. This type of treatment is conducted for 20 to 30 min.[5,6,12] Although infrared heat results in a more rapid superficial temperature increase, it is not generally used in the primary setting.

Cold and Heat

The combination of cold and heat therapies, called contrast baths, is another modality for treatment of tendinitis. The heat therapy should be between 39 and 41°C (102 and 106°F) and the cold therapy between 10 and 15.5°C (50 and 60°F). Suggested times for each modality vary according to each practitioner. Some sources suggest 5 min for heat and 1 to 2 min for the cold, alternating for 30 min, whereas others suggest 1 min heat and 30 s cold or 30 s in heat with 1 min in cold. The treatment should always end with cold treatment. Theoretically, this method produces a maximum increase in blood flow to the involved area, which should increase the healing process.

PHARMACOLOGIC TREATMENT

The use of NSAIDs can be controversial. The suggested uses of NSAIDs are to control pain, to act as an anti-inflammatory agent that would presumably allow early activity, and to decrease inflammation, presumably resulting in faster healing.[14] However, it is necessary to remember that inflammation is a natural and necessary process for response to trauma. There have been studies that suggest that NSAIDs do not seriously delay the healing process and that the person can return to activity more quickly with NSAIDs being part of the treatment.[4] Another part of the controversy involves the adverse effects of GI upset, nausea, dyspepsia (one in three patients), ulcers (1 to 2 percent), and skin eruptions of pruritus and urticaria. It is said that approximately 50 percent of all patients all have an adverse reaction and that of this group 1 to 2 percent of these reactions could be serious.[14] The practitioner must remember the "triad syndrome": A patient with asthma, nasal polyps, and aspirin intolerance could have a fatal reaction.[14]

REHABILITATION

There are three phases of tendon healing: (1) the cellular reaction to injury, (2) fibrous protein and collagen synthesis, and (3) scar remodeling.[2,4,15] This inflammatory process lasts approximately from 5 to 7 days with the second phase of collagen synthesis starting 3 days after injury. When looking at this, it is necessary to consider the duration of injury vulnerability, always remembering that vulnerability to reinjury is proportional to the original severity of the tendon damage, the rate of healing of the person, and the demand on the tendon. Injured connective tissue may have only 70 to 80 percent of its original structural and biomechanical integrity up to and beyond 12 months after injury. It also must be remembered that immobilization is detrimental to the outcome strength of the repaired tendon, adding a longer recovery time once immobilization is discontinued.[2] Therefore, the practitioner must weigh the benefits versus the risks of each component of the treatment prescribed.

Most of the common complaints of tendinitis respond to a program of stretching and strenghtening. The program should be progressive both in intensity and the amount of load on the tendon. It is important that when a patient does any stretching the stretch be held for a minimum of 10 to 30 s and the patient does a minimum of three sets of 10 repetitions each day. It is important to remember that all rehabilitation programs should begin with a program of ice prior to stretching and strengthening and each session should conclude with the application of ice for an additional 20 min. An example of such a program would be as follows:

- Ice for 10 to 15 min.
- Warm up the area for 10 min.
- Do strengthening exercises in a progressive program.
- Ice for 20 min.

Bursitis

DISCUSSION

The bursa is the fluid-filled sac formed by two layers of synovial tissue; it contains a thin layer of joint fluid.[4,6] The bursa is located in places where friction would occur within the body tissues, such as between tendon and bone or between skin and bone.[4,5,6]

Acute bursitis occurs because of sudden direct trauma to areas, such as the prepatellar (between the patella and the skin) and the olecranon (between the olecranon process of the ulna and the skin). *Chronic* bursitis is caused by the overuse, or repetitive trauma, of muscles or tendons, a constant external compression, or trauma (healing). In both acute and chronic bursitis an inflammatory reaction occurs within the bursa.[1,4,8,11,16]

SYMPTOMS

Swelling, pain, some loss of function, and an increase in fluid in the bursa occurs.[4,6,8] Chronic bursitis may result in the walls of the bursa thickening, possibly leading to calcific deposits and degeneration of the internal lining of the bursa.[4,6,8,17]

TREATMENT

Use rest, compression, heat, and NSAIDs, and protect from further injury.

Painful Wrist

Common complaints of a painful wrist could include wrist tendinitis, DeQuervain tenosynovitis, carpometacarpal osteoarthritis, and ganglion cyst.

DeQuervain Tenosynovitis

DISCUSSION

DeQuervain tenosynovitis is an inflammation of the extensor pollicis brevis and abductor pollicis longus tendons of the thumb caused by overuse or repetitive gripping.[8,16,18] This leads to the irritation of the tendons and the sheath, resulting in a stenosing tenosynovitis.[4,6,8,16,19]

SYMPTOMS

The patient will complain of pain, sharp or aching, which may radiate into the hand or forearm, and the inability to grip. There is local point tenderness over the radial styloid process and weakness during thumb extension and abduction.[5,8,16] The pain is aggravated by isometric or resistive extension or abduction of the thumb.[5,8]

Patients may have a positive Finkelstein test. A Finkelstein test is performed by having the patient place a thumb into opposition and having the fingers cover the thumb, that is, make a fist with the thumb inside. The patient is then asked to put the wrist into ulnar deviation, causing a stretching of the tendon. A positive Finkelstein test results in pain of the thumb tendons: extensor pollicis longus, extensor pollicis brevis, and abductor pollicis longus.[6,8,9,16,20]

DIAGNOSTIC TESTS

X-rays of the wrist and thumb are usually normal, but would be appropriate to rule out other differential diagnoses. The standard views include anteroposterior (AP), lateral, pronation oblique, and axial.[10,20]

TREATMENT

The initial treatment consists of rest, ice, NSAIDs, and possibly phonophoresis.[6,8,18,19] After the acute signs have resolved, ice treatment before and after passive stretching will help prevent a recurrence. In patients who receive only rest and immobilization, it is effective in 25 to 75 percent.[19] If conservative treatment fails to work, then a local injection of steroids or surgical decompression should be considered.[5]

Carpometacarpal Osteoarthritis

DISCUSSION

The carpometacarpal (CMC) is one of the more common sites for osteoarthritis. Patients who do repetitive gripping and grasping or who work with machinery that involves excessive vibration often complain of pain at the base of the thumb.[4,8,21]

SYMPTOMS

The patient can experience some joint crepitation with circumduction. Generally, there is swelling, inflammation, pain when the joint is moved to its extremes, and local joint tenderness.[2,13] If this condition continues for several years, there is bone enlargement at the base of the thumb, which may cause a bony deformity (shelf sign), and loss of motion. The patient may also experience subluxation of the joint.[4,8,16]

DIAGNOSTIC TESTS

The x-ray of the thumb and wrist usually presents with joint narrowing, spur formation, and some varying degree of bony sclerosis.[8]

TREATMENT

Conservative treatment for this condition is initially rest and restriction of the gripping and grasping motion, and administration of NSAIDs. If the condition does not improve, referral of the patient to a hand surgeon is appropriate for possible local injection of steroid, implant arthroplasty, or tendon graft interposition.[4,16]

Wrist Ganglion

DISCUSSION

A wrist ganglion is the herniation of the joint capsule or of the synovial sheath of a tendon. The cyst, containing a mucinous colorless fluid and a benign palpable mobile mass with minimal tenderness usually appears slowly on the dorsum of the wrist.[4,5,6,8,9,18]

TREATMENT

The general procedure for treatment of a ganglion cyst is aspiration with chemical cauterization and application of a compression bandage. If the cyst returns, the next appropriate measure is to refer for surgical removal.[5,16,18] This does not mean a new cyst will not form.[8,16]

DIFFERENTIAL DIAGNOSIS

The differential diagnosis for wrist ganglion includes carpal scaphoid fracture, base of the second and third metacarpal fracture, hamate hook fractures, Colle's fracture, carpal tunnel syndrome, and dislocation of the lunate.

Painful Elbow

Lateral and Medial Epicondylitis

DISCUSSION

Lateral epicondylitis (tennis elbow) is an inflammatory response to overuse of the extensor-supinator muscles attached to the lateral epicondyle, from forced extension of the wrist, causing microtearing of the extensor carpi radialis and the extensor carpi ulnaris causing soft tissue failure.[5,8,22] Medial epicondylitis (Little League elbow, golfer's elbow) is the inflammatory response to overuse of the flexor-pronator muscles attached to the medial epicondyle of the humerus.[5,8]

SYMPTOMS

The patient experiences pain and weakness of the arm, with positive point tenderness over the lateral or medial epicondyle and with pain that may radiate down the forearm or up into the brachial radialis in the case of lateral epicondylitis. This localized area is usually between the radial head and the lateral epicondyle. Pain is aggravated by resistive wrist extension or flexion and a strong gripping motion.[4,5,8,16] Generally, there is full range of motion, but in some cases there is an inability to fully extend the elbow.[8,22] Swelling of the epicondyle may or may not always be present. To test the elbow, apply resistance to the patient's extended hand with the elbow flexed at 45°, while palpating either the lateral or medial epicondyle at the point of local tenderness. This maneuver results in moderate to severe pain over the epicondyle.[5,20]

DIAGNOSTIC TESTS

X-rays and laboratory tests are not necessary in the diagnosis of epicondylitis. However, x-rays would be used to distinguish a fracture or dislocation. The standard x-rays could include AP and lateral, and internal and external oblique; a reverse axial view may also be helpful.[3,10] MRI is now used to diagnose any change in the tendons and ligaments.[3]

TREATMENT

Treatment of either lateral or medial epicondylitis includes rest, ice, phonophoresis, curvilinear bend, NSAIDs, and strengthening and stretching exercises.[5,8] The key in treating epicondylitis is to have the patient begin a program of ice massage and stretching. The patient should stretch the arm so as to feel the stretch on either the lateral or medial epicondyle. The patient should hold the stretch position from 10 to 30 s for 10 repetitions, three times daily. Ideally, the patient would then progress to isotonic exercises that would strengthen the extensor or flexion mucles, always remembering to begin with low weight (1 lb) and increase only after experiencing no pain or discomfort after strengthening exercises.[5,8] If conservative measures do not result in recovery, then the use of steroid injections would be appropriate. After a steroid injection, the patient should rest the affected area for several weeks to ensure the healing process and to prevent any spontaneous rupture of the tendon.[4,8]

DIFFERENTIAL DIAGNOSIS

The differential diagnosis for epicondylitis includes sprain of the collateral ligaments of the elbow, strain of the musculotendinous units of the upper extremity, fractures of the ulnar or radius, osteochondritis dissecans, and dislocation of the radial head.[4] Dislocation of the radial head in association with an ulnar fracture is called a Monteggia fracture. Dislocation of the ulna with a fractured radius is called a Galeazzi fracture. Other problems to consider include dislocation of the olecranon process, referred pain of carpal tunnel syndrome, cervical radiculopathy, and rotator cuff tendinitis.

Olecranon Bursitis
DISCUSSION

Olecranon bursitis is the inflammation of the bursa located between the olecranon process of the ulna and the overlying skin.[6,8] This inflammation can be caused by multiple small blows (draftsman's elbow, student's elbow), a single traumatic blow, or repetitive flexion and extensions of the elbow.[4,5,8]

SYMPTOMS

The most common symptoms include stiffness and swelling posteriorly, and tenderness. If there is pain, malaise, fever, and erythema, then infectious bursitis must be considered.[4,5,6,16] If the bursitis becomes a chronic condition, there is the possibility of thickening of the bursal sac in 10 to 20 percent of patients.[8]

DIAGNOSTIC TESTS

X-rays are considered to be unnecessary for the diagnosis, unless there is a question of a possible fracture or dislocation. If it is being considered that this could be infectious bursitis, then the practitioner should aspirate the elbow and get the following laboratory values: cell count, gram stain, crystal analysis, and hematocrit to evaluate the fluid.[8]

TREATMENT

The conservative treatment includes rest, ice, aspiration, NSAIDs, or other analgesic for pain and compression. It is necessary to remember that with an elbow that has marked swelling, heat, and erythema, the fluid will have to be aspirated to rule out sepsis.[5,8,14,22] If conservative treatment does not produce results, then the practitioner can refer for steroid injections, and with chronic olecranon bursitis the patient should be referred for possible surgical excision.

DIFFERENTIAL DIAGNOSIS

The differential diagnosis for olecranon bursitis includes gout and infection.

Painful Shoulder

Common complaints of a painful shoulder could include acromioclavicular separations and sprains, bicipital tendinitis, rotator cuff tears, and adhesive capsulitis.

Acromioclavicular Joint: Separations or Sprains
DISCUSSION

The acromioclavicular (AC) joint and the ligaments are susceptible to injury from trauma and from overuse syndromes.[5,6,8] The joint comprises three important ligaments that hold the acromion, clavicle, and the coracoid process together. They are the acromioclavicular ligament, the coracoclavicular ligament, and the coracoacromial ligament.[4,6,16,23] During trauma the ligaments can experience varying degrees of tearing.

A first-degree sprain of any of the ligments is a stretching of the ligament. A second-degree sprain and/or separation is partial tearing of the superior and inferior acromioclavicular ligament. A third-degree sprain and/or separation is a complete tearing of the superior and inferior acromioclavicular and the coracoclavicular ligaments. Traumatic injury can result in a partial tear of the acromioclavicular ligament, which would then be called a first-degree separation or sprain. If the acromioclavicular ligament is completely torn, but the coracoclavicular ligament remains intact, this is often considered second degree. And when the acromioclavicular ligament and the coracoclavicular ligament are both completely torn, then this is often referred to as a third-degree sprain or separation.[4,5,6,16,24,25]

SYMPTOMS

The patient presents with the arm held close to the side and complains of pain and tenderness to palpation, and there may be swelling and deformity. Pain is also produced with downward traction or passive adduction across the chest. A second- or third-degree separation or sprain may include joint widening when traction is applied.[4,8,25]

A first-degree sprain presents with point tenderness, pain during range of motion, and no deformity. A second degree also has point tenderness, decreased range of motion (ROM) in abduction, and slight deformity. The third degree will have point tenderness, decreased ROM, and increased deformity.[4,5,6,8]

DIAGNOSTIC TESTS

Suggested x-ray views include AP, lateral, axillary, internal and external AP views.[3,4,9,10,25] The use of weighted x-ray views of the shoulder may show widening between the clavicle and the acromial process. If this demonstrates a >5-mm separation, then this is an indication of a separation.[8]

TREATMENT

The initial treatment is to limit the ROM of the arm. This can be accomplished by use of a shoulder immobilizer for 2 to 4 weeks or until patient does not experience pain.[4,5,8,16,25] The shoulder should be treated with ice for the first 48 to 72 h. The patient should not be allowed to lift objects that weigh more than 10 to 20 lb and may return to activity only after full ROM without pain is present.[4,5,6]

Bicipital Tendinitis

DISCUSSION

The tendon of the long head of the biceps can become inflamed as it passes through the bicipital (intertubercular) groove of the anterior head of the humerus. This tendon extends intraarticularly under the acromial process through the rotator cuff to its insertion at the top of the glenoid.[4,5,6,8] Repeated irritation of this tendon leads to microtearing and degenerative changes. This process could lead to spontaneous rupture and also subluxation of the tendon out of its groove, which generally occurs when the transverse ligament is ruptured.[8]

SYMPTOMS

Pain that can be aggravated by lifting or overhead pushing and pulling that is localized to the proximal humerus and anterior shoulder joint is diagnostic.[6,8,9] There will be localized tenderness approximately 1 in below the anterolateral tip of the acromion, when the practitioner palpates the passively moving arm during internal and external rotation.[5,6,8] Resistive supination of the forearm with elbow flexion aggravates the pain.[4,5,8,26] A positive Yergason test is used to measure instability and produces pain in the bicipital groove as the patient flexes the elbow at 90° with the wrist supinated against resistance.[4,24,25] A bicipital tendon that has ruptured presents as a bulge several inches above the antecubital fossa. The patient experiences a popping or snapping sensation as the tendon ruptures.[5,8]

DIAGNOSTIC TESTS

X-rays do not show tendinitis but help in the evaluation of possible calcification in the bicipital groove.[6,8]

TREATMENT

Rest, ice, phonophoresis, high-voltage electric stimulation, and NSAIDs are all appropriate modalities of treatment. After the first 24 to 48 h, the patient should begin with pendulum stretch exercises, progressing to isotonic exercises to help strengthen the tendon's internal and external rotators and avoiding horizontal abduction during the early stages of rehabilitation.[5,6,8,25,26] If after 6 months conservative treatment is unsuccessful, then the patient should be considered a candidate for surgical intervention.[25] Ten percent of cases progress to spontaneous rupture.[6,8] Surgical repair of a biceps tendon rupture is not usually suggested for noncompetitive participants.[5]

Rotator Cuff Tear

DISCUSSION

The rotator cuff muscles of the shoulder include the supraspinatus, infraspinatus, teres minor, and subscapularis (SITS).[4–6,8,24] The mechanism of injury (MOI) of rotator cuff injuries is the loss of normal integrity of the tendons, from repetitive overhead activities, such as pitching, swimming, and serving in tennis, all of which cause microtrauma.[4,5,6,9,24] The most likely tendon to be injured is that of the supraspinatus and then the infraspinatus.[5,6,8,25] As a patient engages in repetitive overuse activities, the rotator cuff may impinge on the acromion and the overlying coracoacromial ligament, causing microtrauma to the cuff, resulting in local inflammation, edema, cuff softening, pain, and poor function of the cuff. The poor blood supply to the tendon is suggested as one cause of early degeneration.[4] Other MOIs that cause rotator cuff tears would be those of an acute injury, such as a fall on an outstretched arm or directly onto the outer shoulder, which cause the humeral head to be impacted against the acromion, which could cause a tear to the cuff.[4,6,8]

SYMPTOMS

The patient experiences pain and weakness on external rotation and abduction. This position is commonly called the "empty-can" position, arm in 90° of horizontal abduction, 30° of forward flexion, and internally rotated.[4,6,7,8,16,20,24,25] The patient may also experience discomfort or dull aching deep pain at night and when the arm is passively taken into a position of horizontal adduction, flexion, and internal rotation.[4,5,9,24,25] When the patient has a partial tear, the motion of reaching overhead is not smooth. A patient who has a complete tear is unable to reach overhead, migrate anteriorly and superiorly, or, rarely, have the drop arm sign. The patient has decreased ROM, muscle atrophy, muscle weakness, and crepitus in the supraspinatus.[5,8,9] There may also be swelling of the subacromial bursa and the glenohumeral joint with large rotator cuff tears.

DIAGNOSTIC TESTS

The use of routine x-rays does not help in the diagnosis of rotator cuff tears, but may produce rotator cuff tendon calcification in approximately 30 percent of cases. The standard views for the shoulder are transaxillary lateral, AP internal, and AP external.[3,8,9,24,25] MRI is now used to show large transverse tears, but it may not be able to differentiate partial tears. MRI has been shown to be 95 to 100 percent accurate for full thickness tears and 84 percent accurate for partial thickness tears.[3,7] The use of arthrography has been beneficial to the diagnosis of tears of the rotator cuff.[3,8,24,25] Other diagnostic tests used for differential diagnoses could include erythrocyte sedimentation rate, a complete blood count, and a rheumatoid factor.[9]

TREATMENT

If the underlying problem of the patient is tendinitis, treatment is the same as for most tendinitis injuries. This includes rest, restriction of overhead motion, cold or heat, iontophoresis or phonophoresis, microelectrical nerve stimulation, NSAIDs, and stretching and strengthening programs (ice prior to and after exercise program).[5,8,24] A patient who does not respond to conservative treatments should be referred for possible steroid injection or surgery. Steroids must be used with caution because of the degeneration of the tendon and softening of the cuff during the early stages following injection.[4] Surgery should be a consideration after 6 months to 1 year of conservative treatment with the understanding that there is a 95 percent success rate with conservative treatment.[4,8,24,25]

Adhesive Capsulitis: Frozen Shoulder

DISCUSSION

When the patient complains of shoulder pain with significant loss of shoulder ROM, consider the diagnosis of adhesive capsulitis.[4] Whenever a patient experiences any type of inflammatory process, such as rotator cuff tendinitis, acute subacromial bursitis, or fractures that occur at the head or neck of the humerus, it could lead to progressive limitation in the ROM.[4,6,8] Adhesions often form between the joint capsule and the humeral head. This condition can also be caused by the lack of complete ROM over a long period of time. Commonly, this is associated with older adults who do not raise their arms over their head on a daily basis and is often referred to as a frozen shoulder.[4,6,8,9,25]

SYMPTOMS

The patient may complain of shoulder pain or discomfort, occurring primarily at night, with decreased ROM (external rotation and abduction).[8] As the condition progresses, the pain diminishes and the ROM becomes progressively less.[9] Common findings in a patient include an inability to raise the arms above the head and a decrease in passive ROM. Normal external rotation is 90°, and normal abduction is from 90 to 120°.[4,8] The patient is unable to perform the Apley scratch test, which requires patients to reach their midback at T8-T10 ventral level with their hand.[6,8,10]

DIAGNOSTIC TESTS

Routine shoulder x-rays can be used to help differentiate the diagnosis. Another radiology test that is used is arthrography, in which a normal glenohumeral joint fills with 7 or 8 mL of the contrast agent, as compared with a joint in an advanced case of adhesive capsulitis that will only accept 4 to 5 mL of contrast agent.[4,8]

TREATMENT

Conservative treatment involves the slow and tedious program of heat application prior to stretching with weighted pendulum exercises and passive stretch exercises.[4,8]

DIFFERENTIAL DIAGNOSIS

The differential diagnosis for adhesive capsulitis includes sternoclavicular dislocation, clavicular fractures, cervical disk disease, brachial plexus (thoracic outlet syndrome), and referred pain of spleen and gallbladder.

Painful Ankle

Common complaints of a painful ankle include lateral and medial ankle ligament sprains, peroneal tendon injury, and Achilles tendinitis.

Lateral Ankle Ligament Sprains

DISCUSSION

The ankle is one of the most commonly injured joints of patients involved in sports and everyday activities. The three bony structures that make up the ankle joint (hinge joint) are the talus, distal fibula, and distal tibia. There are also three ligamentous complexes that help to stabilize this joint: the lateral complex, medial complex, and interosseous complex (syndesmotic ligaments).[4,6,27] Lateral ankle sprains account for 85 to 95 percent of all ankle sprains and involve the lateral ligamentous complex of the anterior talofibular ligament, the calcaneofibular ligament, and the posterior talofibular ligament.[4,6,27] An ankle placed in a plantar flexed position has increased instability because of the position of the talus in the mortise. This position also causes the anterior talofibular ligament to be taut and at risk for injury, since the medial malleolus may act as a fulcrum, predisposing the ankle to lateral or inversion sprains.[4,6,16,27,28] The MOI is usually a cutting action or landing on an uneven surface, such as another person's foot.[4,6]

A lateral inversion sprain of the ankle most commonly occurs from the anterior ligament to the posterior ligament, with the most frequent being an anterior talofibular ligament sprain. Sprains are often classified as first, second, and third degree. First-degree sprain has minor tearing of the ligament, usually of the anterior talofibular ligament, with little or no instability of the ankle. A second-degree sprain is a partial tear of the anterior talofibular ligament with a minimal tear of the calcaneal fibular ligament, resulting in ankle instability. A third-degree lateral ankle sprain is a complete tear of the ligament with gross instability of the ankle joint.[4,6,28]

SYMPTOMS

The patient complains of pain and point tenderness over the injured ligament, localized swelling, decreased ROM, and ecchymosis, and may even have a palpable gap in the ligament.[4,6,27] To differentiate further the degree of injury: With a first-degree lateral ankle sprain there is point tenderness over the anterior talofibular ligament, with little or no instability, a negative anterior drawer sign, and negative stress x-ray; with a second-degree ankle sprain there is also a moderate anterior drawer sign, with normal stress x-rays or minimal talar tilt with moderate instability; and with a third-degree ankle sprain there is both a positive anterior drawer sign and positive stress films.[4,6,28]

To perform an anterior drawer test, grasp the patient's heel by cupping it firmly in one hand. While pulling the foot forward, push posteriorly on the anterior aspect of the distal tibia with the other hand.[4,6,27] To complete the evaluation of the ankle, a compression test and/or heel tap should be performed. A positive compression test and/or heel tap is usually associated with a fracture.[4,6,28]

DIAGNOSTIC TESTS

Routine x-rays of all ankle injuries include AP, lateral, mortise (AP with external rotation of 15 to 20 percent of the foot), oblique, and inversion stress. These help differentiate the type of ankle injury, for example, sprain, fracture.[4,10,27] If the x-ray indicates 15 to 30° of tilt of the talus within the mortise, then the anterior talofibular ligament and the calceneofibular ligament are torn.[4]

TREATMENT

The initial treatment for an acute ankle sprain includes rest, ice, compression, elevation (RICE) and the use of NSAIDs.[4,6,27] Rest requires non-weight-bearing for the first 24 h. Ice should be applied 20 min on and 20 min off while awake during the first 24 h. Compression can be accomplished by the use of an elastic wrap, with care given to proper circulation. A more successful procedure for compression is to apply an open-basket taping procedure or an Unna boot. All the procedures for compression should be applied with the ankle in neutral position, so that the ankle mortise is closed. This helps prevent further swelling within the mortise and reduce the recovery time of the patient. Finally, elevation of the ankle should be above the heart to help reduce the dependent swelling. A second-degree sprain requires more rehabilitation time, whereas a third-degree sprain treatment may include surgical repair of the ligament.[4–6,8,23]

The use of cold whirlpools [10 to 12.5°C (50 to 55°F)] for 15 to 20 min two to three times daily helps speed up the recovery. The use of cold helps to produce a local anesthesia, which decreases tissue metabolism and ultimately causes vasodilation, which assists in the reduction of swelling and removal of hematoma.[27] During the whirlpool treatment, the patient should be asked to move the ankle in flexion and extension because it has been shown that early progressive weight bearing and movement encourages early healing and return to normal function.[4,6,27] Refer back to the discussion on tendinitis for further explanation. Any rehabilitation program should begin with a cold whirlpool, progress to resistive exercises including heel cord stretching, continue with application of cold for 20 minutes, and conclude with taping or putting an air cast on the ankle until no pain occurs and stability returns. The patient should work on strengthening the ankle, with particular attention to restoring full strength to the peroneal muscles.[27,29]

Medial Ankle Ligament Sprain

DISCUSSION

The ligament of the medial complex of the ankle is called the *deltoid ligament*. It is made up of both superficial and deep fibers and serves as the primary resistance to foot eversion.[4,6,27] The medial ligament sprain or eversion sprain occurs less frequently and is often associated with a fracture of the lateral malleolus and/or rupture of the syndesmosis. The most common MOI is any action similar to stepping into a hole.[4,6,16]

SYMPTOMS

The patient complains of pain, point tenderness, swelling, decreased ROM, and ecchymosis with increased instability.[4,6]

DIAGNOSTIC TESTS

Routine x-rays of all ankle injuries include AP, lateral, and oblique. These help differentiate the type of ankle injury, that is, sprain or fracture.[4,10,27]

TREATMENT

The initial treatment should be RICE and NSAIDs. (See "Lateral Ankle Sprain.")

Peroneal Tendon Injuries

The peroneal tendons act as the primary lateral dynamic stabilizers of the ankle joint, and injury to these tendons occurs during forced plantar flexion and valgus of the foot. This occurs during maximal eccentric contraction when a load is applied.[4,30] Injuries to these tendons include tendinitis, subluxation, and rupture.[30]

Peroneal Tendinitis

Tendinitis occurs because of the placement of tendons around the lateral malleolus. Because of the pulley action around the tendon, the results can be decreased vascularity, inflammation, and degeneration change.[4,30]

SYMPTOMS

The patient complains of pain and point tenderness over the lateral malleolus, swelling, ecchymosis, and increased pain with active eversion.[4,30]

DIAGNOSTIC TESTS

Standard lower leg and ankle x-rays are appropriate, but the use of an MRI provides more information in determining the degree of injury to the tendon.[8] (See "Tendinitis" for further information about the use of MRI).

TREATMENT

The initial treatment should be RICE and NSAIDs. (See "Lateral Ankle Sprain.") It is important to remember that the inflammatory response lasts approximately 48 h and is vital to the healing phase. Since collagen protein is produced 3 to 4 days following injury, it is necessary to limit inflammation by the use of NSAIDs and cryotherapy.[30] (See "Tendinitis.")

Peroneal Subluxation

DISCUSSION

The MOI is a forceful dorsiflexion with inversion and contracture of the peroneal tendons, which causes the retinaculum of the joint to rupture and the tendons to sublux in front of the distal fibula.[6,30]

SYMPTOMS

The patient complains of swelling and point tenderness with possible subluxation (snapping) of the tendons.[6,30]

DIAGNOSTIC TESTS

Standard lower leg and ankle x-rays are appropriate, but the use of an MRI provides more information in determining the degree of injury to the tendon.[8] (See "Tendinitis" for further information about the use of MRI.)

TREATMENT

The initial treatment should be RICE and NSAIDs, and non-weight-bearing for 4 weeks in a cast or surgery.[30]

Peroneal Rupture

This is rare and would require surgery.

Achilles Tendinitis

DISCUSSION

The Achilles tendon is the largest tendon in the body. An inflammatory response to overload triggered by microscopic tearing of the collagen fibers is a complaint of the lower leg.[8,28,31] This could occur because of both intrinsic and extrinsic conditions. The intrinsic conditions include malalignment, tight hamstrings or calf muscles, cavus feet, heel or forefoot varus deformity, excessive supination and hyperpronation in midstance, and tight heel cord.[4,28–30] The extrinsic conditions are often the result of training errors, such as increased mileage, increased intensity of the sessions, repetitive hill running, progressing too quickly, running on uneven surfaces, and poor shoes.[4,30]

SYMPTOMS

The patient complains of pain, swelling, crepitation, heat, erythema, weakness secondary to pain, decreased motion, and tenderness to palpation.[4,6,8,28,30] Chronic symptoms include increased vascularity, thickening of tissue (tenosynovitis), and possibly nodules.[6,30]

DIAGNOSTIC TESTS

Standard lower leg and ankle x-rays are appropriate, but the MRI provides more information in determining the degree of injury to the tendon.[8] (See "Tendinitis" for further information about the use of MRI.)

TREATMENT

The initial treatment should be RICE, NSAIDs, gentle stretching, ultrasound, and orthotics, which may include the use of a heel lift (1/2 to 3/4 in).[4,6,28–30] The nodules can be surgically removed.[6] Steroid injections should be avoided because they weaken the tendon, which could result in rupture of the tendon.[29,30]

Achilles Rupture

Achilles rupture usually occurs as a result of a rapid push-off with the knee extended or landing with the foot in dorsiflexion. The rupture occurs more often 1 to 2 in above the insertion on the calcaneus, with patients decribing the injury as if someone had kicked them in the back of the leg.[4,6,28,30,32]

SYMPTOMS

Patients initially complain that they feel as if someone kicked the back of their leg. They present with pain, swelling, possibly a palpable gap, weak or absent plantar flexion of the foot, inability to walk on the toes, and possibly a positive Thompson test. The Thompson test is performed by squeezing the muscle belly of the gastrocnemius-soleus muscle while the patient is either in the prone position or on the knees in a chair. Squeezing the muscle will normally cause the ankle to plantar flex.[4,6,28,30,32]

DIAGNOSTIC TESTS

Standard lower leg and ankle x-rays are appropriate, but the use of an MRI provides more information in determining the degree of injury to the tendon.[8] (See "Tendinitis" for further information about the use of MRI.)

TREATMENT

The initial treatment should be RICE and NSAIDs. Following this, conservative treatment includes casting the lower leg in slight plantar flexion for 3 to 6 weeks. This is the procedure often followed for the older or nonactive patient and for partial tears of the Achilles tendon. For a complete tear of the tendon, and for athletes, the surgical approach is preferred. Surgery restores 75 to 90 percent of original function and requires an aggressive rehabilitation program of 3 to 4 months.[4,6,28,32]

DIFFERENTIAL DIAGNOSES OF COMMON ANKLE PAIN

The differential diagnosis should include undisplaced spiral fracture of fibula, avulsion fracture of the distal tip of the fibula, fracture of the fifth metatarsal, posterior tibial tendinitis, and stress fracture.

REFERENCES

1. O'Brien M: Functional anatomy and physiology of tendons, *Tendinitis I: Basic Concepts.* Philadelphia, Saunders, *Clin Sports Med* 11:505–520, 1992.
2. Leadbetter W: Cell-matrix response in tendon injury, *Tendinitis I: Basic Concepts.* Philadelphia, Saunders, *Clin Sports Med* 11:533–578, 1992.
3. Pope C: Radiologic evaluation of tendon injuries, *Tendinitis I: Basic Concepts.* Philadelphia, Saunders, *Clin Sports Med* 11:579–600, 1992.
4. *Athletic Training and Sports Medicine.* Park Ridge, IL, American Academy of Orthopaedic Surgeons, 1991.
5. Anderson M, Hall S: *Sports Injury Management.* Baltimore, Williams & Wilkins, 1995.
6. Arnheim D, Prentice W: *Principles of Athletic Training,* 8th ed. St Louis, Mosby, 1993.
7. Jarvinen M: Epidemiology of tendon injuries in sports. *Tendinitis I: Basic Concepts.* Philadelphia, Saunders, *Clin Sports Med* 11:493–504, 1992.
8. Anderson B: *Office Orthopedics for Primary Care Diagnosis and Treatment.* Philadelphia, Saunders, 1995.
9. Greene H (ed): *Clinical Medicine,* 2d ed. St Louis, Mosby, 1991.
10. Belhobek G, Richmond B, Piraino D, et al: Special diagnostic procedures in sports medicine, *Office Practice of Sports Medicine.* Philadelphia, Saunders, *Clin Sports Med* 8:517–537, 1989.
11. Kibler W, Chandler J, Pace B: Principles of rehabilitation after chronic tendon injuries, *Tendinitis I: Basic Concepts.* Philadelphia, Saunders, *Clin Sports Med* 11:661–672, 1992.
12. Rivenburgh D: Physical modalities in the treatment of tendon injuries, *Tendinitis I: Basic Concepts.* Philadelphia, Saunders, *Clin Sports Med* 11:645–660, 1992.
13. Kulund D: *The Injured Athlete.* Philadelphia, Lippincott, 1982.
14. Weller J: Medical modifiers of sports injury: The use of nonsteroidal antiinflammatory drugs (NSAIDs) in sports soft-tissue injury, *Tendinitis I: Basic Concepts.* Philadelphia, Saunders, *Clin Sports Med* 11:625–644, 1992.
15. Fyfe I, Stanish W: The use of eccentric training and stretching in the treatment and prevention of tendon injuries, *Tendinitis I: Basic Concepts.* Philadelphia, Saunders, *Clin Sports Med* 11:601–622, 1992.
16. O'Donogue D: *Treatment of Injuries to Athletes,* 4th ed. Philadelphia, Saunders, 1984.
17. Dambro M: *The 5 Minute Clinical Consult.* Baltimore, Williams & Wilkins, 1995.

18. Mirabello S, Loeb P, Andrews J: The wrist: Field evaluation and treatment, *Injuries of the Hand and Wrist.* Phildelphia, Saunders, *Clin Sports Med* 11:1–26, 1992.
19. Kiefhaber T, Stern P: Upper extremity tendinitis and overuse syndromes in the athlete, *Injuries of the Hand and Wrist.* Philadelphia, Saunders, *Clin Sports Med* 11:39–56, 1992.
20. Magee D: *Orthopedic Physical Assessment,* 2d ed. Philadelphia, Saunders, 1992.
21. Kahler D, McCue III F: Metacarpophalangeal and proximal interphalangeal joint injuries of the hand, including the thumb, *Injuries of the Hand and Wrist.* Philadelphia, Saunders, *Clin Sports Med* 11:57–76, 1992.
22. Yocum L: The diagnosis and nonoperative treatment of elbow problems in athletes, *Office Practice of Sports Medicine.* Philadelphia, Saunders, *Clin Sports Med* 8:439–454, 1989.
23. Booher J, Thibodeau G: *Athletic Injury Assessment.* St Louis, Times Mirror/Mosby, 1985.
24. Collins L: Shoulder pain in the overhand athlete. *J Am Acad Physician Assist* 7:415–423, 1994.
25. Jobe F, Bradley J: The diagnosis and nonoperative treatment of shoulder injuries in athletes, *Office Practice of Sports Medicine.* Philadelphia, Saunders, *Clin Sports Med* 8:419–439, 1989.
26. Ellenbecker T, Derscheid G: Rehabilitation of overuse injuries of the shoulder, *Office Practice of Sports Medicine.* Philadelphia, Saunders, *Clin Sports Med* 8:583–604, 1989.
27. Ryan J, Hopkinson W, Wheeler J, et al: Office management of the acute ankle sprain, *Office Practice of Sports Medicine.* Philadelphia, Saunders, *Clin Sports Med* 8:477–497, 1989.
28. Hamilton W: Foot and ankle injuries in dancers, *Foot and Ankle Injuries.* Philadelphia, Saunders, *Clin Sports Med* 7:143–173, 1988.
29. Mattalino A, Deese J Jr, Campbell E, et al: Office evaluation and treatment of lower extremity injuries in the runner, *Office Practice of Sports Medicine.* Philadelphia, Saunders, *Clin Sports Med* 8:461–476, 1989.
30. Frey C, Sherett M: Tendon injuries of the ankle in athletes, *Foot and Ankle Injuries.* Philadelphia, Saunders, *Clin Sports Med* 7:103–118, 1988.
31. Komi P, Fukashiro S, Jarvinen M: Biomechanical loading of Achilles tendon during normal location, *Tendinitis I: Basic Concepts.* Philadelphia, Saunders, *Clin Sports Med* 11:521–532, 1992.
32. Donnelly R: Recognizing and managing Achilles tendon rupture. *J Am Acad Physician Assist* 7:406–414, 1994.

Chapter 10–2
COMMON FRACTURES AND DISLOCATIONS
Karen A. Newell

The intent of this chapter is to review pertinent anatomy and basic orthopedic principles involved in the identification, management, and treatment of common fractures and dislocations.

TYPES OF FRACTURES AND DISLOCATIONS

Open or compound fracture Fracture communicates with the outside environment through skin that is broken (may be subtle).
Closed or simple fracture Fracture has no potential for communication with the outside environment. Skin is intact.
Complete fracture Both cortices are broken.

Incomplete fracture One cortex is broken. Example: greenstick/ buckle or torus (common in children), where force applied bows the bone in such a way that only one side fractures.
Transverse fracture Fracture line is perpendicular to the long axis of the bone.
Oblique fracture Fracture line runs oblique to the long axis of the bone.
Spiral fracture Fracture associated with rotational forces that spiral down the long axis of the bone.
Comminuted fractures Fracture produces two or more fragments.
Segmental fracture Comminuted fracture which involves a free central fragment between two main sections of bone.
Articular fracture Fracture extends into or involves the articulating surface of a joint.
Pathologic fracture Fracture occurs secondary to diseased or abnormal bone.
Stress fracture Repetitive forces can weaken bone.
Avulsion fracture Bony fragment ("chip") has been pulled off by ligaments or tendons attached to it.
Depressed fracture Fracture fragment is depressed below the bone surface.
Impaction Compression of bone. This crush injury occurs when bone is forced into bone.
Dislocation The articular surfaces of bones that usually form a joint are completely out of contact with one another, usually associated with damage to joint capsule and surrounding soft tissue structures.
Subluxation Incomplete dislocation in which the articular surfaces of bones that usually form a joint are partially out of contact with one another.

OTHER DEFINITIONS

Closed reduction Correction of the fracture from external manipulation, considered conservative management.
Open reduction internal fixation (*ORIF*) Correction of the fracture by surgical repair usually requiring placement of hardware (e.g., plates, screws).
Delayed union Slow bone healing (not healed in expected time).
Nonunion Failure of fragments of bone to heal together.

DESCRIPTIVE TERMS

It is imperative that accurate terminology and description be used when discussing specific fractures. Fractures are always discussed with location of distal fragments in relation to the proximal fragment.

Displacement Refers to amount of lateral location of distal fragment with relationship to the more proximal fragment while maintaining alignment with the long axis of the bone (e.g., 50 percent displaced means half the bone width is displaced laterally between the distal and proximal fragments).
Nondisplaced Fracture without lateral movement of distal fragment maintaining alignment with long axis of the bone on both anteroposterior and lateral x-ray views.
Separation Distance in millimeters that two fragments are from each other.
Angulation The distal fragment long axis and the proximal fragment long axis are at an angle which can be measured in degrees and described with distal fragment location with respect to the proximal fragment.

RED FLAGS

Any open fracture or joint requires immediate consultation with the orthopedic service and typically is surgically irrigated in the operating room. On initial presentation give consideration to obtaining wound cultures, keeping the patient NPO, initiating IV prophylactic antibiotics such as 1 g cefazolin or 1 g ceftriaxone, and tetanus prophylaxis. The wound should be dressed with a sterile gauze soaked in normal saline covering any exposed bone.

It is important to note whether the fracture extends into the joint line or articulating surface (intraarticular). These often require special consideration by the orthopedic service.

Fractures in children that involve the epiphysis (physis), which is the location for bone growth, are particularly important and should include consultation with the orthopedic service, particularly if they are displaced.

SALTER-HARRIS CLASSIFICATION

Class I Fracture through the growth plate.
Class II Fracture through the growth plate and metaphysis.
Class III Fracture through the growth plate and epiphysis.
Class IV Fracture through the metaphysis, growth plate, and epiphysis.
Class V Growth plate crushed, may not be evident on x-rays.

HISTORY

A detailed mechanism of injury is invaluable information obtained from the patient or any witnesses in orthopedic trauma. Specific areas of pain or what motions exacerbate or relieve the pain is also helpful information. Check for any areas of anesthesia or paresthesia. Get previous medical and surgical history, including current medications and allergies. Knowledge of dominant hand, occupation, and serious hobbies are important for clinical decision making.

PHYSICAL EXAMINATION

Carefully inspect skin for associated laceration, abrasion, or communication with the underlying fracture or joint. Note any swelling, discoloration, or deformity of the site. Thoroughly palpate, including all bones and joints, especially the joint above and the joint below. Give a meticulous neurovascular examination, including range of motion, motor, sensory and all pulses, and capillary refill distal to affected extremity. It may be helpful to compare with the contralateral side. Do not administer local anesthetics until after the sensory examination. Carefully document, including any previous musculoskeletal injury and baseline status prior to new injury. All jewelry on the affected extremity should be removed. A ring cutter may be necessary in some cases.

RADIOLOGIC STUDIES

Consider obtaining films of the joint above and the joint below. Possible films of uninvolved side for comparison are especially helpful in children with physis injury.

SOME OF THE MORE COMMON FRACTURES AND DISLOCATIONS

Upper Extremity

Anterior Dislocations

Incidence 90 to 95 percent are anterior, the most common major joint dislocation.
Mechanism Abduction and external rotation of the arm.

Presentation Severe pain and immobility of the shoulder, visible deformity of normal rounded shoulder as prominent acromion with "squared off" appearance at the shoulder; usually patient is holding affected arm with contralateral hand in slight abduction.
Physical examination Particular attention to sensation of lateral shoulder, since axillary nerve damage may be associated.
X-ray Look for associated fracture of humeral tuberosities, often note Hill-Sachs lesion (compression divot on humeral head).
Reduction Successful in the emergency department after ruling out coexistence with other upper extremity fractures, passive reduction with the Stimson technique: 10 to 15 lb of weight secured to the affected wrist with patient lying prone on a stretcher for 20 to 30 min, analgesia (morphine, 3 to 5 mg IV every 10 to 15 min, naloxone, 0.4 to 2 mg IV every few minutes as needed for reversal if necessary) may be necessary to help relax musculature; occasionally slight internal and external rotation by the clinician while in this position may be enough to reduce; Milch technique: clinician slowly abducts and externally rotates the arm to an overhead position, once fully extended gentle traction can be applied; postreduction films should confirm reduction; sling and swathe, analgesics, orthopedic follow-up in 3 to 5 days.

Posterior Dislocations

Incidence Rare.
Mechanism Occurs with direct trauma to the front of the shoulder as from landing on an outstretched hand during a fall. Can occur during seizure as the posterior muscles are stronger than the anterior, resulting in forceful muscle contraction that pulls the humeral head out of the glenoid fossa.
Presentation Severe discomfort; visible prominence may be noted posteriorly with relative shallow anterior shoulder appearance, held adducted against chest and internally rotated.
Physical examination Patient resists movement, especially abduction, and is unable to externally rotate past neutral.
X-ray Often missed on x-rays (estimated up to 50 percent); therefore, always order anteroposterior *and* lateral views. Axillary views (scapular Y) may be helpful in those read as negative with a high clinical index of suspicion; however, they may be difficult to obtain secondary to patient's inability to abduct.
Reduction May require sedation or general anesthesia for reduction. Reassess axillary nerve and neurovascular state postreduction.

Clavicle Fractures

Incidence The most common fracture in children.
Mechanism Blow to the shoulder or fall onto an outstretched hand.
Presentation Localized tenderness, edema, deformity.
Physical examination Consideration of great vessel injury.
X-ray Plain views may miss it. May require CT.
Treatment Figure eight dressing, sling.

Proximal Humeral Fractures

Incidence Usually in the elderly, secondary to a fall on an outstretched hand.
Presentation Pain, tenderness, deformity, edema, ecchymosis.

Physical examination Assess axillary nerve by testing lateral shoulder sensation, as well as other nerves and arteries.

X-ray Anteroposterior, lateral, and axillary views.

Treatment Uncomplicated minimally displaced fractures require sling and swathe, analgesia, orthopedic referral.

Complication "Frozen shoulder"; prevent with early rehabilitation.

Humeral Shaft Fractures

Incidence Healthy active adults; occurs in middle third of humerus.

Mechanism Blow to the shoulder or fall onto an outstretched hand.

Presentation Pain, tenderness, deformity, edema, ecchymosis.

Physical examination Careful assessment of radial nerve, as often an associated injury (assess wrist extension).

X-ray Obtain anteroposterior, tangential scapular lateral views of the humerus.

Treatment If uncomplicated, coaptation U splint/sugar tong splint of the upper arm, sling and swathe, appropriate analgesics, orthopedic referral in 3 to 5 days.

Radial Head Subluxation (Nursemaid's Elbow)

Incidence Common in children from 1 to 4 years of age since the radial head is the same size as the neck; after age 7 occurrence is rare since the radial head enlarges and is more difficult to sublux.

Mechanism Sudden jerk of the hand while the forearm is extended and pronated.

Presentation Child avoids use of the affected arm but does not appear in great distress; forearm is held in slight flexion and pronation; resists supination; usually no edema.

X-ray Not indicated unless history warrants it.

Reduction Clinician places thumb over the radial head, while the other hand placed at the wrist initiates full supination; a palpable "click" should be felt; if not, fully flex at the elbow or fully extend; may require repeated attempts, no immobilization is required unless multiple episodes occur, which warrant a sling or long arm cast and orthopedic follow-up.

Radial Head and Neck Fractures

Mechanism Trivial trauma.

Presentation Vague discomfort noted over the proximal forearm.

X-ray Often normal despite fracture; occasionally will note a positive fat pad sign (radiolucent area noted on lateral view just posterior to distal humerus suggestive of intraarticular bleeding).

Physical examination Exacerbation of pain during rotation of the forearm and hyperflexion and hyperextension at the elbow.

Treatment for uncomplicated cases Sling (remove several times during the day for gentle range of motion if tolerated), analgesics, application of ice, orthopedic follow-up in 10 to 12 days (films repeated at this time may show fracture line).

Elbow Dislocation

Incidence Most elbow dislocations are posterior.

Mechanism Fall onto an outstretched hand.

Presentation Elbow held at 45° of flexion; may develop marked edema.

Physical examination Careful neurovascular assessment with attention to brachial artery; ulnar, radial, and median nerves.

X-ray Lateral view demonstrates posterior displacement of both radius and ulna; anteroposterior view may show displacement either medial or lateral with radius and ulna normally aligned with relationship to each other; may be associated with other injuries.

Reduction After appropriate sedation: while gentle wrist and forearm traction is applied by one clinician, the other clinician provides countertraction on the upper arm. Next, downward pressure is applied to the proximal forearm to disengage the coronoid process, and the elbow is flexed. A palpable "clunk" can be felt: full range of motion should be possible. If not, entrapment might have occurred: splint the patient in 90° flexion from axilla to base of the digits.

Nightstick Fracture

Mechanism Trauma to ulna resulting while trying to protect oneself by blocking blows during an altercation.

Presentation Pain, edema over ulnar aspect of the forearm.

Reduction Long-arm splint; ORIF if conservative reduction fails.

Colles' Fracture

Fracture just proximal to the distal radius with dorsal displacement (Smith's fracture, reverse Colles' fracture); same fracture with volar displacement.

Incidence The most common fracture of the distal radius.

Mechanism Fall onto an outstretched hand.

Presentation Pain, swelling, tenderness, "dinner fork" deformity, limited range of motion.

Physical examination Attention to the radioulnar joint.

Treatment Volar wrist splint, elevation, analgesics, orthopedic follow-up in 3 to 5 days.

Monteggia's Fracture or Dislocation

Ulna fracture usually in the proximal third, and radial head dislocation.

Ulna fracture usually in the proximal third, and radial heal dislocation.

Mechanism Forced pronation of the forearm or direct blow over the posterior aspect of the ulna.

Presentation Pain at elbow, resists flexion and extension; shortened forearm with palpable radial head in antecubital fossa.

Treatment Orthopedic referral, often operative.

Galeazzi's Fracture

Radius fracture usually located at the junction of the middle and distal thirds; subluxation of inferior radioulnar joint.

Mechanism Direct blow on the dorsilateral wrist or from a fall.

Presentation Ulna head may be prominent.

X-ray Often a widened space between the distal radius and ulna on anteroposterior films.

Reduction ORIF.

Scaphoid and Navicular Fractures

Mechanism Fall on outstretched hand.
Presentation Point tenderness localized to the anatomical snuff-box, may have swelling but many look normal; x-rays are often read as negative since the fracture may not show initially (repeat films at 10 to 14 days may demonstrate the fracture line). If the patient has pain with snuffbox pressure despite normal films (including a scaphoid view), treat in a thumb spica splint for 4 to 6 weeks. These fractures are often missed and because of the blood supply, which may be interrupted, may subject a patient to avascular necrosis.

Bennett's Fracture

Fracture of the base of the first metacarpal.

Mechanism Axial loading to the thumb.
Treatment Often requires surgical repair.

Rolando's Fracture

Fracture of the base of the first metacarpal.

Mechanism Axial loading to the thumb.
Treatment Often requires surgical repair.

Metacarpal Shaft Fracture

Treatment Nondisplaced fractures can be treated in a gutter splint with orthopedic follow-up; those with any angulation, rotation require prompt orthopedic referral.

Metacarpal Neck Fractures

Incidence Commonly seen in the fourth and fifth digits.
Mechanism Fifth digit referred as Boxer's fracture; results from striking an object with the closed fist. Usually the distal fracture fragment appears volarly angulated on x-ray.
Presentation Localized tenderness and edema, may have loss of knuckle prominence on making a fist.
X-ray Obtain anteroposterior, lateral, and oblique views.
Reduction The fourth digit can accept up to 20° of volar angulation and the fifth up to 40° of volar angulation to be considered acceptable, provided no rotational component is present. (Have patient make a fist; look at fingertips for rotation). If greater than the accepted angles are noted, a hematoma block (aspiration of dark blood confirms location, place 3 to 5 mL of 1% plain lidocaine into the fracture site by an experienced clinician) can be given and closed reduction done to a more acceptable angle, spliting in an ulnar gutter splint (fourth and fifth metacarpophalangeal at 90°, fourth and fifth interphalangeal joints fully extended, wrist in 15° of extention), analgesics (e.g., ibuprofen, 400 mg PO every 6 h), elevation; orthopedic follow-up in 5 to 7 days.
Pitfalls Careful examination of the skin overlying the metacarpophalangeal joint is imperative if history suggests striking another person in the mouth (clench fist injury in which human oral contaminants may be introduced into the joint space as these are treated aggressively as a human bite to prevent severe infection; often present with severe soft tissue hand infection 3 to 5 days after injury with little external sign of laceration from tooth and no recollection of previous trauma). Second and third metacarpal neck fractures require almost perfect reduction to maintain normal hand function and are best referred for orthopedic consultation.

Proximal and Middle Phalanx Fracture

Treatment Often referred to orthopedic service for operative repair since they often involve articular surfaces, displacement, or rotation.

Interphalangeal Dislocation

Incidence Very common, may be associated with ligamentous injury.
Physical examination Neurovascular documentation.
X-ray To rule out associated fracture.
Reduction 1% plain digital block may be useful but is not mandatory. While stabilizing the proximal segment, the distal segment can be pulled longitudinally, then dislocation reduced. Confirm postreduction assessment of intact collateral ligaments and full restoration of motor function. Discharge with a volar splint with the proximal interphalangeal joint segment flexed at 15 to 20° and early orthopedic follow-up in 3 to 5 days. If reduction is not easy, then refer to an orthopedic specialist, since it may require open reduction secondary to soft tissue.

Mallet Avulsion Fracture

Mechanism Extensor tendon pulls off segment of bone.
Treatment If segment is greater than 25 percent of the articular surface, it may require operative pinning. If less, it may be treated in a extension splint. It can result in a mallet finger deformity.

Distal Phalanx Fracture: Tuft Fracture

Mechanism Smashing fingertip in door, dropped objects.
Physical examination Careful to rule out open fracture; often associated with nail bed injury, which may require careful repair.
Treatment May require evacuation of subungual hematoma (portable electrocautery).

Lower Extremity

Pelvic Fractures

Mechanism High-energy trauma (motor vehicle accident, fall from height); second most common cause of death associated with trauma—head injury is first; 50 percent have other fractures or major injuries; commonly associated with bladder rupture, urethral tear, sacral root damage.
Presentation Usually associated with multiple life-threatening injuries and hemorrhagic shock, pelvic or perineal edema, ecchymosis, hematoma.
Physical examination After attention to head, thoracic, abdominal, and genitourinary injuries, do urethral, pelvic, and rectal examination (high riding prostate or decreased/absent sphincter tone). Do a neurovascular assessment. Attempt to rock the pelvis by exerting bimedial pressure and anterior to posterior pressure to each anterior superior iliac spine and anterior to posterior pressure over the pubic rami.
X-ray May include a variety of views such as anteroposterior, lateral, internal and external oblique, inlet and outlet plain films. Look for widened sacroiliac joint or symphysis pubis, disruption of pelvic ring; often requires CT scans or other special studies.
Treatment Close cardiovascular monitoring for hemorrhagic shock, orthopedic consultation, and admission.

Hip Dislocation

Incidence Most occur posteriorly.
Presentation With severe discomfort of the hip and inability to ambulate.
Physical examination Reveals a shortened, slightly flexed, adducted, and internally rotated lower extremity. Can coexist with associated fractures.
Reduction Prompt reduction by the orthopedic service within several hours minimizes chances of avascular necrosis from interrupted blood supply to the femoral head.

Slipped Capital Femoral Epiphysis

Incidence Children or adolescents, minor or unrecalled trauma.
Presentation Hip or knee pain, limp.
Physical examination Pain exacerbated with internal rotation of the hip.
X-ray Anteroposterior, lateral, and frog leg (hips flexed to 90° and abducted 45°) demonstrate posterior and inferior displaced femoral epiphysis.
Treatment Crutches, orthopedic consultation; late complications include avascular necrosis of the femoral head and premature closure of the epiphyseal plate.

Femoral Shaft Fractures

Mechanism Direct blow, twisting of the leg, gunshot wounds.
Presentation Usually associated with high-energy trauma. May have multiple injuries and significant blood loss. Limb may appear shortened or angulated. Often associated with pelvis and knee injuries.
Physical examination Careful skin and neurovascular examination to rule out open fracture and involvement of the femoral artery or sciatic nerve.
Treatment Intravenous fluids, monitor for hemorrhagic shock, traction splint, orthopedic referral, admission.

Patellar Dislocation

Mechanism Twisting force on an extended knee; often recurrences because medial joint capsule damaged.
Presentation Patella may be found laterally; severe pain and deformity noted; often already reduced.
Reduction Hyperextension of the knee, flexion at the hip, with manual manipulation of patella back into place.
X-ray Postreduction to rule out associated fracture.
Treatment Immobilization in Jones splint or straight leg knee immobilizer, does not incorporate the ankle.

Tibial Shaft Fractures

Incidence The most frequently fractured long bone; often open fracture; often associated with a fibular fracture.
Mechanism Direct blow, twisting forces, gunshot wound.
Physical examination Careful skin assessment because the anterior bone surface is very close to skin; careful and frequent neurovascular assessment necessary.
Pearls Be suspicious of compartment syndrome; beware as skin color and pulses may appear normal.
Treatment Elevate, analgesics, traction splint, orthopedic referral, admission.

Maisonneuve Fracture

Incidence Ruptured deltoid ligament with a high fibular fracture.
Presentation Pain over lateral proximal leg over proximal fibula.
X-ray Wide mortise despite negative leg and ankle films.
Treatment Usually operative to restore joint and syndesmosis.

Fifth Metatarsal Fracture: Avulsion (Ballerina Fracture) versus Jones Fracture (Transverse)

Mechanism Plantar flexion, inversion injury "twist ankle" versus forceful planting of foot as in motor vehicle accident or dropped object on foot.
Presentation Point tender over base of the fifth metatarsal; may have edema, ecchymosis.
Reduction Hard-soled shoe versus short leg splint.
Pearls In all ankle injuries be sure to also assess the base of the fifth metatarsal because it is often missed. X-ray views should be based on where point tenderness exists. Many patients with fifth metatarsal fractures have had ankle films but no radiologic assessment of the foot. Jones fractures are notorious for developing nonunion or delayed union.

BIBLIOGRAPHY

Jenkins JL, Loscalzo J: *Manual of Emergency Medicine.* Boston, Little Brown, 1995, chap 6, pp 57–86.
Posen RB, Barkin: *Emergency Medicine Concepts and Clinical Practice.* 1992, chaps 29–37, pp 522–777.
Saunders CE, Ho MT: *Current Emergency Diagnosis and Treatment.* Norwalk, CT, Appleton & Lange, 1992, chap 22, pp 316–355.
Tintinalli JE, Ruiz E, Krome RL (eds): *Emergency Medicine: A Comprehensive Study Guide,* 4th ed. New York, McGraw-Hill, 1996, Sect. 21, pp 1205–1276.

Chapter 10–3
RHEUMATOID ARTHRITIS
Pamela Moyers Scott

DISCUSSION

Rheumatoid arthritis (RA) is a chronic, systemic disease characterized by symmetric synovial inflammation of the peripheral joints, especially the proximal interphalangeal and metacarpophalangeal joints of the hands, wrists, elbows, knees, ankles, and subtalar joints of the feet. Its etiology is unknown.

Rheumatoid arthritis affects approximately 1 percent of the U.S. population.[1] It is more common in women than men. There appears to be a genetic predisposition to developing RA. Onset of symptoms is generally in the fourth or fifth decade of life. Advancing age is a risk factor for developing RA. Symptoms can vary from intermittent arthralgias to severe, debilitating deformities and extraarticular manifestations.

SIGNS AND SYMPTOMS

Generally the presenting complaint in a patient with RA is pain, swelling, and stiffness of the aforementioned joints. The pain is usually bilateral and aggravated by movement. Morning stiffness, or that occurring after periods of inactivity, often lasts more than 1 h.

Table 10-3-1. Criteria for the Diagnosis of Rheumatoid
Arthritis

At least four of the following criteria must be present to establish the
diagnosis of RA:
1. Morning stiffness of ≥ 1 h for at least 6 weeks
2. Arthritis (diagnosed by a health care provider) simultaneously present in ≥ 3 peripheral joints, for a minimum of 6 weeks duration
3. Arthritis of the wrists or metacarpophalangeal or proximal interphalangeal joints of the hands, diagnosed by a health care provider, and present for at least 6 weeks
4. Peripheral joint arthritis that is symmetric, observed by a health care provider, and present for a minimum of 6 weeks
5. Rheumatoid nodules diagnosed by a health care provider
6. Positive serum rheumatoid factor (RF) done by a method that has a false-positive rate in $\leq 5\%$ of the unaffected control subjects
7. Radiographic changes that are characteristic for RA—hand x-rays revealing erosions or unequivocal bony decalcification

SOURCE: Modified from Lipsky PE: Rheumatoid arthritis, in Fauci AS, Braunwald E, Isselbacher KJ, et al (eds): *Harrison's Principles of Internal Medicine*, 14th ed. New York, McGraw-Hill, 1998, pp 1880–1888.

Constitutional symptoms are also common. They include low-grade fever, early afternoon fatigue, malaise, weakness, anorexia, and weight loss.

OBJECTIVE FINDINGS

On physical examination, the affected joints reveal swelling, tenderness, decreased range of motion, and warmth secondary to the synovial inflammation. Erythema is generally not present.

If the inflammation is not controlled, several characteristic deformities can occur. They are the *Z deformity,* caused by radial deviation at the wrist and ulnar deviation of the fingers; *swan-neck deformity,* due to the hyperextension of the proximal interphalangeal joints (PIPs) and flexion of the distal interphalangeal joints (DIPs); and *boutonniere deformity,* defined as a flexion deformity of the PIPs with extension of the DIPs.

Extraarticular manifestations consist of dermatologic complications such as vasculitis and rheumatoid nodules. Rheumatoid nodules are subcutaneous nodules of varying sizes that occur on the extensor surfaces of periarticular structures, especially the elbows, sacrum, and occiput. The presence of rheumatoid nodules or vasculitis indicate a more aggressive form of RA.

Cardiac and pulmonary manifestations are also seen. Most cardiac disease is asymptomatic; it can consist of pericarditis and inflammatory lesions similar to rheumatoid nodules forming in the myocardium and heart valves.[2] Cardiac tamponade and death are possible, but rare.

Pulmonary complications can be asymptomatic, such as rheumatoid pleural disease, or life-threatening when pleural nodule-like lesions become infected and cavitate or rupture into the pleural space causing a pneumothorax.[2] Chronic obstructive pulmonary disease can occur, consisting of dyspnea, chronic cough, interstitial fibrosis, and/or bronchiectasis.

Central nervous system involvement is rare; however, rheumatoid vasculitis and rheumatoid nodule-like granulomas occasionally develop in the meninges.[2] Extracranial rheumatoid vasculitis is rarely associated with a mononeuritis multiplex syndrome, and the proliferating synovium can compress nerve roots producing neurologic symptoms.

Ophthalmologic complications can include Sjögren's syndrome, episcleritis, scleritis, and scleromalacia perforans.[2]

DIAGNOSTIC CONSIDERATIONS

The diagnostic criteria for RA appear in Table 10-3-1. Other collagen vascular diseases (e.g., lupus, polyarteritis, and progres-

sive systemic sclerosis) must be considered in the differential for RA. Systemic diseases with joint manifestations, such as acute rheumatic fever, sarcoidosis, and amyloidosis, must be considered. Infectious joint disease (e.g., gonococcal arthritis and Lyme disease) must be excluded. Finally, other forms of arthritis must be considered, including osteoarthritis, ankylosing spondylitis, gouty arthritis, and psoriatic arthritis.

SPECIAL CONSIDERATIONS

Juvenile rheumatoid arthritis (JRA) is estimated to affect approximately 200,000 children in the United States.[3] It is characterized by the objective findings of chronic inflammation in one or more joints for at least 6 weeks duration in someone less than 16 years old. As with RA, there are no specific diagnostic tests and the etiology remains unknown.

LABORATORY TESTS

There are no specific tests to establish or exclude the diagnosis of RA. The rheumatoid factor (RF) is present in approximately 90 percent of all patients with RA.[4] However, it is also present in approximately 5 percent of the general population and 10 to 20 percent of individuals ≥ 65 years old.[1] RF can also be seen with connective tissue diseases and various infectious processes (e.g., syphilis, hepatitis, rubella, influenza, mononucleosis, and malaria). Although the RF factor is nondiagnostic, it has some prognostic value for patients with RA. Higher titers are associated with more severe forms of the disease and more extraarticular manifestations.

The erythrocyte sedimentation rate (ESR) is generally elevated. However, there is a small subset of patients with RA who have normal ESRs.[4] C-reactive protein, if tested, is almost always elevated. A normocytic, normochromic anemia can also be present in patients with RA.

RADIOLOGIC STUDIES

There are no specific x-ray changes indicating RA, except those listed in Table 10-3-1.

OTHER DIAGNOSTICS

Synovial fluid analysis will confirm the presence of an inflammatory arthritis; however, it is not specific for RA.[1]

TREATMENT

The goals of treatment of rheumatoid arthritis are to reduce pain, relieve inflammation, prevent deformity and disability, and educate the patient regarding the disease process.

Pharmacologic Management

Because of the aggressive nature of RA, the length of time for the disease-modifying antirheumatic drugs (DMARDs) to be effective, and the toxicities associated with nonsteroidal anti-inflammatory drug (NSAID) usage, accepted pharmacologic therapy for RA is changing from the traditional pyramid approach to more rapid administration of DMARDs.[5–7]

Unless significant joint pathology and/or extraarticular manifestations are already present, NSAIDS are still the first-line agents. When choosing a NSAID, it is important to consider the impact of side effects, costs, dosing convenience, and compliance for each patient.

The risk of GI toxicity, especially hemorrhage, is a serious complication of NSAID therapy. Cytoprotective agents, like misoprostol (Cytotec), should be considered in all patients receiving an NSAID. Risk factors that increase the likelihood of an adverse GI complication include a previous GI bleed, history of peptic ulcer disease, advancing age, smoking, and oral corticosteroid therapy. Misoprostol is currently the only agent with FDA approval for this. However, omeprazole (Prilosec) and famotidine (Pepcid) have been successfully used for this purpose.[8]

NSAIDs are also associated with renal and hepatotoxicity. The greatest risk for renal complications occurs in the elderly, diabetics, hypertensives, individuals with preexisting renal disease, and patients on diuretic therapy. Patients who consume large amounts of alcohol are probably at the greatest risk of hepatic complications.

Before instituting NSAID therapy, obtain baseline liver functions, renal functions, potassium, and a complete blood cell count (CBC). A CBC, creatinine, and potassium should be repeated in 1 month and again every 6 months thereafter.[8] If the initial liver function testing is normal, then additional testing is usually unnecessary.[8]

It is also necessary to advise the patient of these potential complications and their signs and symptoms, and to report them immediately if they do occur. Patients should also be informed of the importance of the laboratory studies.

If NSAIDs alone fail to alleviate symptoms in 1 to 2 months, then a DMARD should be instituted. Because of its safety profile and cost, the antimalarial, hydroxychloroquine (Plaquenil), is probably the best first-line agent for primary care providers to prescribe.[5,6] The dose is 200 mg twice a day.[5,6]

No additional laboratory monitoring is required with treatment with hydroxychloroquine. However, patients taking this agent should have regular, complete ophthalmologic examinations to detect the presence of the side effect of retinal toxicity.

If the patient is still symptomatic after 3 to 4 months of the above two agents, most rheumatologists would now recommend proceeding directly to methotrexate [(MTX); Rheumatrex].[5] MTX is generally given in doses of 7.5 to 15 mg 1 day per week.[5,6] It is contraindicated in individuals with renal insufficiency, hepatic impairment, alcohol abuse, significant lung disease, diabetes, and morbid obesity.

Before MTX therapy is instituted, the clinicians should obtain a baseline CBC, hepatic panel, creatinine, hepatitis B and C antibodies, and chest x-ray.[5] The CBC, creatinine, and liver function studies should be repeated every 1 to 2 months on therapy; individuals taking MTX continuously for longer than 3 to 5 years, should have a liver biopsy performed.[5]

Low-dose oral corticosteroids (less than 10 mg/day) have a disease modifying effect in addition to the weak anti-inflammatory properties seen at this dose. Although they are effective in reducing symptoms, they are associated with many systemic complications. These include adrenal suppression, diabetes, peptic ulcer disease, osteoporosis, hypertension, glaucoma, increased susceptibility to infection, and mood disturbances. Therefore, they should be used only under the supervision of a rheumatologist.

Intraarticular corticosteroids are useful in controlling acute flares involving only one or two joints. They should not be given more frequently than at 3- to 4-month intervals.

Other DMARDs include sulfasalazine (Azulfidine), injectable gold salts (Solganal), oral gold (Auranofin), cyclosporine (Sandimmune), azathioprine (Imuran), and penicillamine (Cuprimine). Unless the practitioner is very familiar with these agents, they should be used only in conjunction with a rheumatology consult. Combinations of these drugs are now being used with increased effectiveness but no increased toxicity.[9]

Surgical Management

Surgery is only indicated in RA when all other treatment modalities have failed and the patient has significant structural joint damage. The most successful surgeries for RA include carpal tunnel release, resection of the metatarsal heads, and total knee and hip arthroplasties.[6]

Supportive Measures

Daily exercise with the goal of maintaining or increasing joint mobility and muscle strength is an important component of the treatment plan. Adequate rest, including naps, is essential. Splints, orthotic devices, and physical therapy are also useful modalities.

PATIENT EDUCATION

The patient and family have to be educated on the disease process itself, the purpose of each intervention (including physical therapy, medications, laboratory monitoring, and exercise), and potential complications from medications. They can obtain more information by contacting the Arthritis Foundation at 1-800-283-7800 or at http://www.arthritis.org.

DISPOSITION

The severity of the symptoms and the medications used to treat the patient determine the frequency for follow-up. Individuals in remission should be seen at least semiannually.[6]

At each visit, the activity level of the disease should be assessed. At a minimum this should consist of an ESR; questions regarding pain status, presence of swelling, changes in morning stiffness, and amount of fatigue; and a physical examination of the affected joints.

COMPLICATIONS

The patient should be referred to a rheumatologist if not responding to therapy, if significant disease is present, or if extraarticular complications are identified.

OTHER NOTES AND PEARLS

A new medication is currently being investigated for RA, tenidap (Enable). Its mechanism of action is to interfere with the cytokines, thus decreasing inflammation and blocking pain.

REFERENCES

1. Lipsky PE: Rheumatoid arthritis, in Fauci AS, Braunwald E, Isselbacher KJ, et al (eds): *Harrison's Principles of Internal Medicine,* 14th ed. New York, McGraw-Hill, 1998, pp 1880–1888.
2. Hess E: Rheumatoid arthritis—epidemiology, etiology, rheumatoid factor, pathology, pathogenesis, in Schumacher RH (ed): *Primer on the Rheumatic Diseases,* 9th ed. Atlanta, Arthritis Foundation, 1988, pp 83–96.
3. Lindsley C: Juvenile rheumatoid arthritis, in Rakel RE (ed): *Conn's Current Therapy,* 1996. Philadelphia, Saunders, 1996, pp 941–945.
4. Peterson LS, Cohen MD: Rheumatic disease: How to use the laboratory in the workup. *Consultant* 6:1329–1337, 1996.
5. McGuire J, Lambert E: Rheumatoid arthritis, in Rakel RE (ed): *Conn's Current Therapy,* 1996. Philadelphia, Saunders, 1996, pp 938–941.
6. Primary care update: Guidelines for managing rheumatoid arthritis. *Consultant* 9:1859–1867, 1996.
7. Kremer JM: Disease-modifying drugs for RA: Current patterns of clinical use. *J Musculoskelet Med* 9:11–19, 1996.

8. Clough J, Lambert T, Miller D: The new thinking on osteoarthritis. *Patient Care* Sept 15:110–137, 1996.

9. O'Dell JR, Hair CE, Erikson N, et al: Treatment of rheumatoid arthritis with methotrexate alone, sulfasalazine and hydroxychloroquine, or a combination of all three medications. *New Engl J Med* 334:1287–1291, 1996.

Chapter 10–4
ANKYLOSING SPONDYLITIS

Pamela Moyers Scott

DISCUSSION

Ankylosing spondylitis (AS), also known as Marie-Strümpell disease and Bechterew's disease, is an inflammatory arthritis that primarily affects the axial skeleton and occasionally the large peripheral joints. Although AS is considered a rheumatoid disease, its main pathologic changes are concentrated around the enthesis, not the synovium as seen in rheumatoid arthritis. For purposes of classification, it is considered to be one of the seronegative spondyloarthropathies. The pathogenesis is uncertain; most consider it to be an immune-mediated disease.

Patients begin noticing symptoms in late adolescence or their early twenties. Onset of symptoms after the age of 40 years is rare. There appears to be familial clustering of the disease. AS affects more men than women. The course of the disease ranges from mild stiffness to a completely fused spine with severe peripheral joint arthritis and extraarticular complications.

SIGNS AND SYMPTOMS

The presenting symptom of AS is generally aching low back pain. It is associated with morning stiffness and stiffness following inactivity that can last up to several hours; however, these symptoms decrease with exercise and activity. Nocturnal exacerbations of pain can occur. In later stages of the disease, the pain can be constant. However, most patients have episodes of pain-free periods followed by acute exacerbations.

Occasionally, other structures are the site of the presenting symptom of AS. Most commonly these sites include the costosternal junctions, spinous processes, iliac crests, greater trochanters, ischial tuberosities, tibial tubercles, and heels.[1]

Constitutional symptoms (e.g., low-grade fever, fatigue, weight loss, anorexia, and night sweats) are sometimes the presenting complaint. This is especially true in adolescents.[1]

Extraarticular involvement is rarely the presenting symptom. These extraarticular diseases can include neurogenic conditions, such as sciatica, cauda equina syndrome, and complications resulting from spinal fractures; cardiac conditions, including aortic insufficiency, conduction defects, and cardiomegaly; and pulmonary conditions, manifesting as pulmonary fibrosis, cyst formation, and *Aspergillus* infections.[1]

OBJECTIVE FINDINGS

Limited spinal motion is always present in AS. The Schober test is probably the simplest and quickest method to obtain an

Table 10-4-1. Diagnostic Criteria for Ankylosing Spondylitis

According to the modified New York criteria, the presence of radiographic confirmed sacroiliitis, plus one of the following criteria is diagnostic for ankylosing spondylitis:

1. History of inflammatory back pain consisting of an insidious onset before 40 years of age, morning stiffness with resolution by exercise or activity, and present for greater than 3 months before seeking treatment.
2. Decreased range of motion of the lumbar spine as defined by the Schober test.
3. Limited chest expansion.

SOURCE: Adapted from Taurog and Lipsky.[1]

objective assessment. To perform this maneuver, find the patient's iliac crests, visually make a line connecting the two, and mark where this line intersects with the spine. Then make an X 5 cm above and 10 cm below this mark. Have the patient forward flex as much as possible, then remeasure the distance between the two marks. Most authorities agree that an increase of >5 cm between the two measurements is normal.[1] Some authors, however, believe the distraction is age-dependent and should be greater than this in younger individuals.[2]

Limited chest expansion is also a characteristic finding. It is quantitatively evaluated by measuring the difference between maximum inspiration and maximum forced expiration around the chest at the nipple line in men and just below the breasts in women. Normal chest expansion is considered to be ≥5 cm.

Bony tenderness and/or muscle spasms may or may not be present. Loss of lumbar lordosis, accentuation of thoracic kyphosis, and cervical forward flexion are sometimes evident on physical examination. In severe disease, flexure contractures of the hip and knee are evident.

If involved, physical findings relating to the aforementioned extraarticular complications are present.

DIAGNOSTIC CONSIDERATIONS

The modified New York criteria for diagnosing ankylosing spondylitis are outlined in Table 10-4-1. AS must be distinguished from the other seronegative spondyloarthropathies such as Reiter's syndrome (characterized by a more sudden onset, mucous membrane involvement, conjunctivitis, and urethritis), psoriatic arthropathy (characterized by dermatologic involvement), intestinal arthropathy (characterized by gastrointestinal involvement and sudden onset of affecting peripheral joints), and reactive arthropathy (a nonspecific form of seronegative spondyloarthropathy with a sudden onset).

Other conditions in the differential include rheumatoid arthritis, osteoarthritis, herniated intervertebral disk, and DISH syndrome (diffuse idiopathic skeletal hyperostosis).

SPECIAL CONSIDERATIONS

Onset of AS during adolescence is generally associated with a more severe form of the disease and a poorer prognosis. AS in women tends to progress less frequently to total ankylosis; however, women often have more peripheral arthritis and incidence of isolated cervical ankylosis.[1]

LABORATORY TESTS

There are no laboratory tests specific for AS. The HLA-B27 antigen is present in approximately 90 percent of patients with AS of most ethnic groups; however, it is only present in approximately 50 percent of African Americans with AS.[1] Additionally, this antigen occurs in 4 to 8 percent of all Caucasians and 2 to 4 percent of all African Americans.[2] Therefore, a negative result is more useful in excluding the diagnosis than a positive result is in confirming the diagnosis.

The erythrocyte sedimentation rate (ESR) is mildly elevated in individuals with active disease. C-reactive protein and IgA levels are often elevated. Rheumatoid factors and antinuclear antibodies are negative unless AS is accompanied by another rheumatoid disease. Occasionally, a mild normocytic, normochromic anemia may be seen. The alkaline phosphatase is increased in severe disease.

RADIOGRAPHIC STUDIES

Lumbar spine x-rays initially reveal findings consistent with bilateral sacroiliitis (blurring of the cortical margins of the sacroiliac joints, followed by erosions, sclerosis, and pseudowidening of the joint space). Early changes seen in the spine itself consist of diffuse vertebral squaring, osteoporosis, spotty ligament calcifications, and early syndesmophytes (a bony formation that occurs as the outer annular fibers erode). As the syndesmophytes continue to grow and the ligamentous calcifications become diffuse, the vertebral bodies become fused. This represents the classic bamboo spine of AS; however, this finding is seen only in a minority of the patients with severe disease.

OTHER DIAGNOSTICS

Other diagnostic procedures are unnecessary unless the patient is experiencing extraarticular symptoms.

TREATMENT

The goals of treatment are to alleviate pain and prevent, delay, or correct deformities.

Pharmacologic Management

Nonsteroidal anti-inflammatory drugs (NSAIDs) are currently the drugs of choice. Indomethacin (Indocin) is often considered by many authorities to be the most effective NSAID for the treatment of AS.[1,2] However, it would probably be best to reserve it for individuals who do not respond to other NSAIDs because it is associated with a much greater incidence of agranulocytosis and aplastic anemia. When choosing an NSAID, consider the impact of side effects, costs, dosing convenience, and compliance for each patient.

The risk of GI toxicity, especially hemorrhage, is a serious complication of NSAID therapy. Cytoprotective agents, like misoprostol (Cytotec), should be considered in all patients receiving an NSAID. Risk factors that increase the likelihood of an adverse GI complication include a previous GI bleed, history of peptic ulcer disease, advancing age, smoking, and oral corticosteroid therapy. Misoprostol is currently the only agent with FDA approval for this. However, omeprazole (Prilosec) and famotidine (Pepcid) have been successfully used for this purpose.[3]

NSAIDS are also associated with renal and hepatotoxicity. The greatest risk for renal complications occur in the elderly, diabetics, hypertensives, individuals with preexisting renal disease, and patients on diuretic therapy. Patients who consume large amounts of alcohol are probably at the greatest risk of hepatic complications.

Before instituting NSAID therapy, obtain baseline liver functions, renal functions, potassium, and a complete blood cell count (CBC). A CBC, creatinine, and potassium should be repeated in 1 month and again every 6 months thereafter.[3] If the initial liver function testing is normal, then additional testing is usually unnecessary.[3]

Sulfasalazine (Azulfidine), which is indicated for the treatment of ulcerative colitis, has been proved to be effective in reducing the pain and inflammation associated with AS.[1,4] The dosage is 2 to 3 g/day.[1]

Narcotics and muscle relaxants should be used only for limited periods of time for acute exacerbations. Oral corticosteroids do not have a role in the treatment of AS. Intraarticular corticosteroids may be beneficial when peripheral joint pain is the main concern. They should not be given any more frequently than once every 3 to 4 months.

Surgical Management

Total hip arthroplasty is indicated in a patient with severe hip joint arthritis. Other surgical procedures that may benefit patients with AS are correction of extreme flexion of the spine or of atlantoaxial subluxation.[1]

SUPPORTIVE MEASURES

Daily exercise is essential in the treatment of the patient with AS. Stretching and strengthening exercises have to be an integral component of these programs to maintain and/or improve range of motion and to prevent contractures and deformities. Postural training, including sleep positions, is also required. A competent physical therapist, with experience in treating AS patients, is able to assist in devising individualized exercise programs.

PATIENT EDUCATION

Patient and family education regarding AS and its potential complications is essential. The expectations of therapy, including the importance of regular exercise, regular follow-up, and potential adverse reactions from medications, also need to be discussed.

Additionally, patients need to be informed that there is a 10 to 20 percent risk of their children having the disease.[5]

DISPOSITION

At a minimum, the patient should be seen at 3- to 6-month intervals. Each visit should include measurements of the patient's height, chest expansion, lumbar flexion (Schober test), and occiput-to-wall distance with thoracic spine held against the wall. The patient should be monitored for problems and potential adverse reactions to medications.

Obviously, if the patient has a more severe form of the disease or extraarticular complications, more frequent follow-up will probably be required.

COMPLICATIONS

Patients should be referred to as rheumatologist if they are not responding to therapy or have complex extraarticular manifestations.

OTHER NOTES OR PEARLS

There are some theories that exist that implicate infective agents as the precipitating factor for acute flares; the two most implicated organisms are *Klebsiella* and *Mycoplasma*.[5]

REFERENCES

1. Taurog JD, Lipsky PE: Ankylosing spondylitis, reactive arthritis, and undifferentiated spondyloarthropathy, in Fauci AS, Braunwald E, Isselbacher JK, et al (eds): *Harrison's Principles of Internal Medicine*, 14th ed. New York, McGraw-Hill, 1998, pp 1904–1909.

2. Hellmann DB: Ankylosing spondylitis: Why the morning stiffness in a younger patient? *Consultant* 10:2169–2172, 1996.
3. Clough J, Lambert T, Miller D: The new thinking on osteoarthritis. *Patient Care* Sept 15:110–137, 1996.
4. Dougados M, vam der Linden S, Leirosalo-Repo M, et al: Sulfasalazine in the treatment of spondyloarthropathy: A randomized, multicenter, double-blind, placebo-controlled study. *Arthritis Rheum* 38:618–627, 1995.
5. Calin A: Ankylosing spondylitis and the spondyloarthropathies, in Schumacher HR (ed): *Primer on the Rheumatic Diseases,* 9th ed. Atlanta, Arthritis Foundation, 1988, pp 142–147.

Chapter 10–5
GOUT

Richard Dehn

DISCUSSION

Gout is a unique form of recurrent acute arthritis caused by the precipitation of monosodium urate crystals into the synovial fluid of the joints. It is most often characterized by the abrupt onset of a monoarticular arthritis that starts as an agonizing, pulsating pain followed by a quick progression of excruciatingly tender erythematous edema, known as pseudocellulitis.

Gout most frequently presents in middle-aged males, with a peak age of onset of 45. The overall incidence of gout is 1 percent, though prevalence increases with age, approaching 5 percent in males over 65. The initial arthritic attack is almost always in the lower extremity, most often affects a single joint, and over half the time is in the metatarsophalangeal joint of the great toe. Other joints are less frequently involved in early attacks, and include the joints of the foot, ankle, and knee. The first attack often occurs at night, with the patient reporting no symptoms or a slight tingling sensation upon retiring. The attack rapidly progresses to where the joint is so inflamed and tender that the patient cannot tolerate the weight of the bed covers on it. On examination the joint inflammation may be so intense as to suggest a septic joint or cellulitis.

Attacks will often follow a minor trauma, an emotionally stressful experience, surgery, the stress of a medical illness, fatigue, or an overindulgence of food or alcohol. The first attack may be quite short, and a second attack may not occur for several years. Without treatment, attacks become more frequent and last longer, and continued progression leads to the development of destructive tophi and renal involvement.

PATHOGENESIS

Gout is caused by the deposit of urates in various locations in the body, producing secondary problems. The urates are deposited as a result of chronically high concentrations of serum uric acid. The urate precipitants are found as urate crystals in the joint synovial fluid, as encapsulated lesions containing urate crystals known as tophi usually located near joints, as urate crystals deposited interstitially in the kidney, and as uric acid stones in the urinary system. The presence of urate crystals in body structures initiates an inflammatory response that leads to the symptoms. When the urate crystals in the synovial fluid elicit an inflammatory response, the presentation is that of acute gouty arthritis. The

tophaceous urate crystal deposits stimulate a chronic low-grade inflammatory response, with the chemical mediators of the inflammation producing the destruction of nearby tissues, usually bone or cartilage. Likewise, urate crystal deposits in the kidney stimulate an inflammatory response that over time decreases renal function. Additionally, uric acid urolithiasis can cause obstructive renal disease.

The extravascular deposit of urate crystals is a response to chronically high concentrations of uric acid in the serum. If uric acid concentrations in the serum are lowered, the extravascular deposits dissolve and the urates return to the serum. If serum concentrations are kept low over a long period of time, extravascular deposits disappear.

High serum levels of uric acid are caused by a metabolic overproduction of uric acid, urinary underexcretion of uric acid, or a combination of both mechanisms. It is believed that most cases of gout are caused by decreased renal clearance of urate. This may be a primary idiopathic abnormality, it may be secondary to pharmacologic agents, or it may be secondary to renal disease. Overproduction is most often caused by a genetically transmitted mechanism; however, it can also be secondary to any condition that exhibits increased rates of cell proliferation and cell death, such as leukemia or psoriasis.

Gout is associated with increased body mass, hypertension, and hypertriglyceridemia. Although diet is a factor in the overproduction of urates, restrictions in consumption of high-purine foods is only of marginal value, with the possible exception of organ meats and beer.

Many commonly used pharmacologic agents reduce renal uric acid excretion. Thiazide diuretics, furosemide, pyrazinamide, ethambutol, and cyclosporine can all increase serum uric acid concentrations by this mechanism. Aspirin also decreases renal urate excretion, and therefore should be avoided by patients predisposed to gout.

LABORATORY TESTING

Virtually all patients with gout have above-average serum uric acid levels, and a majority of gout patients have elevated levels. A normal serum uric acid level at the time of an acute attack is probably due to a stress-induced uricosuric process; however, most patients present with an elevated or high-normal level.

The gold standard in the diagnosis of gout is identification of urate crystals in synovial fluid from the inflamed joint. The crystals are visible inside polymorphonuclear leukocytes. Aspirating the joint for evidence of urate crystals is essential to differentiate gout from pseudogout, which is usually caused by deposition of calcium pyrophosphate dihydrate crystals. Joint aspiration also rules out a septic joint process.

A measurement of uric acid renal clearance can be calculated by a 24-h urine collection. In the typical middle-aged male patient, this is not particularly useful, but in identifying the patient where gout is secondary to overproduction from a disease state or where underexcretion is secondary to renal failure, 24-h urine studies are valuable. A spot estimate can be calculated to make a rough estimate as to whether the patient's hyperuricemia is a result of overproduction or underexcretion by obtaining a random urine uric acid and multiplying the value by the serum creatinine value. This product should then be divided by the random urine creatinine. A result of <0.6 is likely to point to underexcretion; if it is >0.6, overproduction should be suspected, and if it is approximately 0.6, a mixed cause should be considered.

DIAGNOSTIC CONSIDERATIONS

In acute attacks of arthritis, despite the characteristic history and physical findings suggestive of gout, several other diagnoses should be considered. Pseudogout can easily be confused with gout; however, pseudogout is usually found in larger joints. Both gout and pseudogout respond to anti-inflammatory acute treatments; however, pseudogout does not respond to uric acid reduction therapies. The only definitive diagnostic test for accurately discriminating gout from pseudogout is the synovial fluid aspiration analysis. A septic joint process should also be entertained and ruled out.

In an acute gouty arthritis patient, consider the possibility that the urate hyperproduction could be secondary to a malignancy or hyperthryroidism, or the possibility that the urate underexcretion could be secondary to renal disease. Additionally, patients with gout should be evaluated for treatable associated signs and symptoms such as obesity, hypertension, hyperlipidemias, and diabetes mellitus.

TREATMENT

Pharmacologic Management

Treatment of gout is determined by whether the patient is in the acute stage or the asymptomatic stage. In the acute stage, treatment is aimed at stopping the inflammatory process in the affected joint. This is usually done by giving high doses of a short-half-life NSAID such as ibuprofen, 800 mg four times daily, or indomethacin, 100 mg then 50 mg four times daily. These regimens are continued until the joint improves dramatically, usually a few days, and then are reduced to 600 mg three times daily and 50 mg three times daily, respectively.

Colchicine can also be used, one tablet (0.6 mg) every 1 to 2 h until the symptoms improve, GI toxicity occurs, or a maximum of 7 gm has been taken in 48 h. If the symptoms improve, the dose should be reduced to 0.6 mg two times daily. The use of colchicine should be carefully monitored owing to its potential toxicity.

Corticosteroids can be used in either parenteral or oral formulations. A course of oral prednisone, 40 to 60 mg daily for 1 week with a tapered withdrawal or a single intramuscular injection of a sustained-released corticosteroid such as triamcinolone (Kenalog) 40 to 60 mg can be used if NSAIDs are contraindicated. Injection of corticosteroids into the joint is also effective; however, it is important that the volume injected by kept to a minimum since large volumes increase the symptoms. Injection of the joint requires starting an additional anti-inflammatory agent to prevent resumption of the gout symptoms in a few days.

Adrenocorticotrophic hormone (ACTH) is effective and is appropriate in patients unable to use NSAIDS or corticosteroids. It has a faster onset of action than other agents, but must be given intramuscularly, intravenously, or subcutaneously. It also has a rebound effect, requiring the addition of another agent after the symptoms have improved.

Additionally, patients with acute gout should be advised to avoid dehydration to enhance uric acid renal clearance and to prevent the accumulation of urate crystals in the kidneys.

Supportive Measures

The goal of the treatment of symptomatic gout is the prevention of future attacks. Overweight patients should be advised to reduce their body mass to reduce uric acid production, and excesses of food and alcohol consumption should be avoided. A significant number of first-attack patients will not experience another attack, and many others will not have the second attack for several years, so it is not unreasonable to stop treating these asymptomatic gout patients after 2 weeks of anti-inflammatory medications. Patients experiencing more than two attacks a year are candidates for prophylactic NSAID or colchicine therapy, or may elect to use an agent to lower serum uric acid. Patients exhibiting tophi

or renal involvement also should be placed on a serum uric acid lowering agent.

Serum uric acid can be reduced by pharmacologic agents that reduce uric acid synthesis or increase renal excretion of uric acid. Allopurinol is effective in inhibiting the production of uric acid, and once-a-day dosing makes it convenient to take. It should be started at 100 mg daily and increased until serum uric acid levels off at the 5- to 6-mg/dL range. Serious toxic side effects such as rashes, interstitial nephritis, liver damage, fever, leukocytosis, and bone marrow suppression will usually present early in treatment, so it is important to begin with a low dose.

Uricosuric agents can also be used to increase the renal excretion of uric acid. Probenecid (Benemid), 250 mg twice daily, can be given and titrated up to 2 g daily in divided doses until serum uric acid levels off at the 5- to 6-mg/dL range. Sulfinpyrazone (Anturane) can be started at 100 mg twice daily and titrated up to 800 mg/day until the desired serum uric acid level is attained.

Because allopurinol is more convenient to take and has fewer interactions with other medications, it is used most commonly for serum acid reduction despite the fact that most gout patients are underexcreters, it is more expensive than uricosuric agents, and it can produce more serious side effects than the uricosuric agents.

One must remember when starting a uric acid lowering agent that sudden changes in serum uric acid levels are likely to trigger an acute gout attack. When starting a patient on allopurinol or a uricosuric agent an anti-inflammatory agent should also be started, such as an NSAID or low-dose colchicine, 0.6 mg twice daily. This should be continued until the serum uric acid levels have reached the desired therapeutic range.

BIBLIOGRAPHY

Berkow R (ed): *The Merck Manual of Diagnosis and Therapy,* 16th ed. Rahway, NJ, Merck, 1992.

Fauci AS, Braunwald E, Isselbacher KJ, et al (eds): *Harrison's Principles of Internal Medicine,* 14th ed. New York, McGraw-Hill, 1998.

Gaarden W, Smith JB, Bennett LH Jr, Claude J: *Cecil Textbook of Medicine,* 19th ed. Philadelphia, Saunders, 1992.

Hellmann DB: *Current Medical Diagnosis and Treatment,* 35th rev. Appleton, WI, Appleton & Lang, 1996.

Howe S, Edwards NL *Conn's Current Therapy.* Philadelphia, Saunders, 1995.

Terkeltaub RA: *Stein's Internal Medicine,* 4th ed. Philadelphia, Saunders, 1994.

Chapter 10–6
KAWASAKI DISEASE
Wayne J. van Deusen

DISCUSSION

Kawasaki disease (KD), Kawasaki syndrome, or mucocutaneous lymph node syndrome was previously described as, and cannot be easily distinguished from, infantile polyarteritis. It was first noted in Japan after World War II and was described further in 1967. It is now known to exist in other parts of the world, in a number of races, and appears to be increasing in frequency, sporadically and in epidemics. By the end of 1994, 125,000 cases

Table 10-6-1. Overview of Kawasaki Disease

Sex	No predilection
Age at onset	Usually before age 5
Pathogenesis	Unknown
Prodromal signs and symptoms	Fever, adenopathy, conjunctivitis, rash
Nature of eruption	Cracked lips, "strawberry tongue," maculopapular polymorphous rash, peeling skin on fingers and toes
Clinical characteristics	Fever, conjunctivitis, oral changes, swelling and peeling of hands and feet (extremities), rash, cervical and/or generalized adenopathy, coronary vasculitis
Other diagnostic features (criteria)	Angitis of coronary arteries
Laboratory tests and characteristics	Thrombocytosis, elevation of sedimenation rate, abnormal cardiac vessels on echocardiogram
Diagnosis	Clinical
Therapy	Intravenous gammaglobulin, aspirin
Natural history	Self-limited, fatal in 1–2%, long-term coronary and large-vessel damage

had been reported in Japan and it has replaced acute rheumatic fever in the United States and abroad as the leading cause of acquired heart disease in children.[1] It is a febrile multisystem disease predominantly of children 5 years of age or younger. There is no evidence of person-to-person transmission, and the etiology is unknown. Although KD can occasionally affect adults, as of 1994 there have been only 39 documented cases of adult KD, and many of these were diagnosed prior to the very similar toxic shock syndrome (TSS).[1,2]

Cardiac involvement is the predominant manifestation of the disease. Vasculitis of the large coronary blood vessels occurs, which leads to dilation, aneurysm formation and rupture, thrombosis, myocardial ischemia, myocarditis, pericarditis, acute myocardial infarction, and stenosis. Within the first 2 weeks of the disease process, evidence of coronary vasculitis can be detected by two-dimensional echocardiography. During the healing period, alternating areas of coronary dilation and stenosis occur, which may lead to myocardial infarction and death. Rapid diagnosis by characteristic clinical signs, followed by long-term follow-up of these patients, is critical to avoid these cardiovascular complications. Echocardiography should be performed on any child with known or suspected KD at presentation and again within the first 2 to 3 weeks of the course of the disease[1] (see Table 10-6-1).

Disease manifestations and diagnosis depend on the stage in which the disease presents. Recovery is generally complete in patients where vasculitis is not detectable, and second attacks are rare. Early studies in Japan indicated that 1 to 2 percent of the children died of cardiac complications within 1 to 2 months after onset. New data have indicated a drop to 0.14 percent mortality.[1] Children with cardiac involvement generally do well, although long-term prognosis is unknown. Likewise, coronary vascular changes and their relation to the incidence and severity of atherosclerotic coronary disease later in life are not known. Reports now indicate a later occurrence of large-vessel aneurysms other than coronaries.

PATHOGENESIS

Current theories describing the pathogenesis of KD are inconclusive or have not been substantiated. Because of the similarities between streptococcal scarlet fever and KD, some investigators have often considered *Streptococcus pyogenes* as an etiologic agent in the illness.[3] Others implicate the presence of a staphylo-

coccal toxin that acts as a superantigen and interacts with the body's T cells. Other infectious agents such as *Rickettsia*, retrovirus, and environmental toxins, have been implicated but not proved.[4] There are epidemiologic and clinical features of the disease that implicate an immune-mediated syndrome. However, no agents have been identified, and there is no evidence that immune aberrations have any central role in the disorder.[1]

SYMPTOMS AND OBJECTIVE FINDINGS

KD is characterized by three phases. In the first, or acute phase, patients have onset of fever from the first day, which may last 10 to 14 days. During this phase, other characteristic physical findings are noted and systemic complaints are prominent. On auscultation, signs of myocarditis-induced congestive heart failure are present. Tachycardia and a gallop rhythm are more prominent than expected from fever or anemia.[5] In the second, or subacute phase (onset days 10 to 14, lasting 21 to 25 days), symptoms occurring in the acute phase resolve and distal to proximal periungual desquamation of the fingers and toes begins. It is at this time that most structural cardiac involvement is noticed; however, the development of coronary aneurysms has been detected by electrocardiography as early as day 7. Lastly, in the convalescent stage (about day 25 to as long as 8 weeks after onset), the physical symptoms resolve and systemic problems and laboratory values gradually return to normal[6] (see Table 10-6-2).

The disease is characterized by prolonged fever [generally higher than 40°C (104°F)] lasting for more than 5 days (usually one to several weeks) that is unresponsive to antibiotics. Almost all affected children are irritable and may have altered mental status.

At least four of the following five areas of involvement will be noted on physical examination:

1. Adenopathy is generally cervical. Less often there is generalized lymphadenopathy from one to several (1.5 cm or greater) *non*suppurative, nontender, large nodes.

Table 10-6-2. Diagnostic Criteria and Noncardiac Symptoms

Diagnostic criteria
  Fever of at least 5 days duration
  Presence of 4 of the 5 following conditions:
  1. Bilateral *non*exudative conjunctival injection
  2. Changes of the mucosa of the oropharynx (including injected pharynx; injected, dried, or fissured lips; "strawberry tongue" or inflammation)
  3. Changes of the peripheral extremities (edema or erythema of the hands and feet, desquamation usually beginning periungually)
  4. Rash primarily truncal, polymorphous but nonvesicular
  5. Cervical lymphadenopathy—Illness not explained by other known disease process

Noncardiac features
  Extreme irritability (especially infants), altered mental status
  Arthralgia, arthritis
  Aseptic meningitis
  Hepatic dysfunction and hepatosplenomegaly
  Hydrops of the gallbladder
  Diarrhea, vomiting, abdominal pain
  Sterile pyuria from the meatus (urethritis)
  Ulcerative stomatitis
  Cough (possibly associated with infiltrates)
  Pneumonitis, mild radiologically but not clinically apparent
  Otitis media
  Uveitis, iridocyclitis (by slit lamp)
  Cranial nerve palsies
  Erythema and induration at site of Bacille Calmette-Guérin (BCG) inoculation (rare in the United States but common in Japan)
  Peripheral gangrene

2. Bilateral *non*exudative conjunctivitis.
3. Dry, erythematous, cracked and fissured lips; injected oral and pharyngeal mucous membranes; these may include an infected pharyx or "strawberry tongue."
4. A polymorphous rash, which may be an erythematous skin eruption, a maculopapular, morbilliform, or erythema multiforme. There may be desquamation of the rash, especially in the perineum.
5. Edematous and painful hands and feet with erythema of the palms and soles, which may be followed by peeling under the fingernails and toenails.

Transient arthritis can occur, particularly in older children; it is identified as symmetric painful joint swelling affecting large and small joints.

Other common acute manifestations may include diarrhea, vomiting, abdominal pain, hydrops of the gallbladder, sterile pyuria from the meatus (urethritis), tympanitis, ulcerative stomatitis, cough (possibly associated with infiltrates), rhinorrhea, aseptic meningitis, seizures or cranial nerve palsies, and hepatosplenomegaly. Uveitis or iridocyclitis is frequently found in children by slit lamp, even in the absence of overt conjunctivitis. Peripheral large arterial aneurysms (axillary, popliteal) and evidence of distal vascular compromise may be noted on physical examination.

"Case reports suggest that infants with KD have atypical presentations and a high complication rate, likely related to delayed diagnosis and treatment," according to Joffe and colleagues.[7] Atypical cases may manifest only fever, rash, conjunctival infection, and pharyngeal signs, with characteristic coronary lesions appearing later. These patients are typically 1 year of age or younger, often have an incorrect admitting diagnosis (e.g., gastroenteritis, viral syndrome, or sepsis), and have high morbidity.[7]

DIAGNOSTIC CONSIDERATIONS

Before a diagnosis of KD is made a broad range of multisystem diseases that might mimic the disease should be considered. Alternative clinical diagnoses should be carefully considered and rapidly excluded because of the urgency of a quick and accurate diagnosis.

The differential diagnosis includes

- *Septic or severe scarlet fever* Distinguished from KD by age of onset, absence of conjunctival involvement, and recovery of group A steptococci.
- *Toxic shock syndrome* Closely resembles KD; both have fever and are unresponsive to antibiotics. Hyperemia of mucous membranes and erythematous rash with subsequent desquamation are seen in both as well; however, typically absent or very rare in KD are diffuse myalgia, vomiting, and shock.
- *Carbamazepine hypersensitivity* It was described by Hicks and coworkers that carbamazepine hypersensitivity mimicked KD.[8]

Other potential differential diagnoses include drug reactions, toxic epidermal necrolysis, leptospirosis, Epstein-Barr virus, juvenile rheumaoid arthritis, infection, measles, Rocky Mountain spotted fever, acrodynia, Stevens-Johnson syndrome, other vasculitis syndromes, and sepsis.[1,2]

LABORATORY TESTS

Although there are no specific diagnostic laboratory tests, thrombocytosis and increased sedimentation rate in the second or third week can be striking. Anemia is also common. Factors associated with increased risk of coronary artery aneurysms include impressive leukocytosis with a predominance of immature forms as well

as a greatly elevated C-reactive protein. Hemolytic complement levels are high. Tests for autoantibodies such as antinuclear antibodies (ANA) and rheumatoid factors are negative. Mild proteinuria, pyuria, and cerebrospinal fluid pleocytosis may be present. Serum hepatic transaminases and bilirubin levels may be slightly elevated.

RADIOLOGIC AND SPECIALIZED DIAGNOSTIC STUDIES

There are no direct diagnostic tests for KD, although the demonstration of coronary artery involvement is highly suggestive of KD. Cardiac-oriented chest x-rays, electrocardiograms, and echocardiograms are vital to the initial evaluation of the patient. Two-dimensional echocardiography is most useful for the diagnosis of coronary vascular disease and coronary vascular dilation or aneurysm formation. (*Remember:* These should be done initially and within a 2- to 3-week follow-up.) Arteriography of the coronary vessels and larger central vessels to reveal lesions may be warranted by physical examination; however, they are invasive and are not routinely needed.

Histologic changes noted at autopsy of fatal lesions include intense inflammatory cell infiltrates of the media and intima of the large coronary vessels and other central vessels. Arterial obstruction by platelet thrombi resembles the rare condition indistinguishable from KD, previously called infantile periarteritis nodosa.

TREATMENT

Pharmacologic Management

Primary management involves adjunct high-dose aspirin and intravenous immunoglobulin.[9] Aspirin should be given starting with 80 to 100 mg/kg/day in four to six divided doses; once fever resolves and after the first few days, the aspirin can be reduced to 3 to 5 mg/kg/day in a single daily dose with or without dipyridamole. Aspirin should be given for at least 6 weeks and up to 3 months, until the sedimentation rate normalizes.

Aspirin is used initially for its antithrombotic (antiplatelet) effect if the echocardiogram is normal. If coronary abnormalities are present, aspirin therapy may be continued indefinitely. Therapeutic serum concentrations of salicylates may be difficult to achieve even at doses up to 100 mg/kg/day. Chronic therapeutic salicylate administration is relatively safe, even in small children. Medical providers, patients, and parents must be aware of the potential toxic side effects. Overdose can be avoided if the dose is calculated with care and parents watch their children for side effects of salicylism, such as rapid heavy breathing, drowsiness, or other central nervous system changes. Dose-related tinnitus, common in adults, is rarely noted in children. Gastrointestinal complications may be avoided by eating prior to taking the medication. Some specialists advocate the use of adjunct heparin or warfarin (Coumadin) for patients with persistent, large, or multiple, nonobstructive or obstructive aneurysms.

Administration of intravenous immune globulin (IVIG) in a single high dose during the acute febrile phase of the disease elicits a dramatic response in the prevention of coronary artery aneurysm formation. Immunoglobulins are proteins that are produced by B lymphocytes. During production, IVIG, a commercial product, is well preserved both structurally and functionally to native immunoglobulin G (IgG), with a half-life of 18 to 23 days. It acts to reduce the inflammatory response of KD. A single large dose of IVIG (2 g/kg) over 10 to 12 h, within 10 days of onset, has been shown to be as efficacious as a regimen of 400 mg/kg daily for 4 days, which was previously considered to be the standard of care.

When administered early, IVIG decreases the incidence of coronary vascular damage and coronary artery aneurysm formation. Once aneurysms have formed, however, IVIG has no curative effect.[9] Fever and other attendant systemic manifestations often resolve within 24 h of initiating therapy. If given to symptomatic patients [febrile, high erythrocyte sedimentation rate (ESR)] 10 days after onset of symptoms, it may provide symptomatic relief. Side effects of IVIG, although rare, may include anaphylaxis, chills, fever, headache, and myalgia. *Note:* Use of corticosteroids should be avoided and is contraindicated because it may increase the likelihood of coronary aneurysms.

Thrombolysis with streptokinase is recommended for the active phase of coronary artery thrombosis. Peripheral artery ischemia may be treated with thrombolytic drugs and prostaglandin E (PGE$_1$) infusion.[9] Careful repeated follow-up examinations by stress testing, echocardiography, and at times angiography should be performed to assess coronary vascular changes.

Surgical Management

Aortocoronary bypass surgery with internal mammary artery or saphenous vein grafts is rarely indicated. It has been proved useful in symptomatic patients if tests reveal signs of severe stenotic lesions (>75 percent occlusion) and myocardial ischemia, or infarction with obstruction.

DISPOSITION

During the acute illness, and for 2 to 3 months thereafter (usually at weeks 2, 4, and 8), patients should be monitored closely by a pediatric cardiologist with serial electrocardiography, chest x-rays, and M-mode and two-dimensional echocardiography.[10] If abnormalities are detected on electrocardiography, selective coronary angiography should be performed. If myocardial ischemia with obstruction or infarction exists, and is detected early, cardiac catheterization and bypass surgery are warranted.

COMPLICATIONS AND RED FLAGS

If left untreated, 20 percent of patients with KD develop cardiovascular complications in the acute stage of the illness: primarily, myocarditis, pericarditis, and arteritis of the coronary vessels, which predisposes them to aneurysm formation. These typically occur between 7 and 45 days after the onset of the acute illness. Myocardial infarction may occur secondary to thrombosis at this stage.[10] Death, which presumably results from arteritis, occurs in 1 to 2 percent of these patients. Other reports cite development of arteritis of extremity vessels and peripheral gangrene with KD. The etiology of these complications is unknown.[1]

REFERENCES

1. Shulman ST, De Inocencio J, Hirsch R: Kawasaki disease. *Pediatr Clin North Am* 42(5):1205–1220, 1995.
2. Jackson JL, Kunkel MR, Libow L, et al: Adult Kawasaki disease: Report of two cases treated with intravenous gamma globulin. *Arch Intern Med* 154:1398–1405, 1994.
3. Akiyama T, Yashiro K: The probable role of *Streptococcus pyogenes* in Kawasaki disease. *Eur J Pediatr* 152:82–92, 1993.
4. Nadel S, Levin M: Kawasaki disease. *Curr Opin Pediatr* 5:29–34, 1993.
5. Sundel RP, Newburger JW: Kawasaki disease and its cardiac sequelae. *Hosp Practice* 28(11):51–54, 57–60, 64–66, 1993.
6. Appelgate BL: Kawasaki syndrome: An important consideration in the febrile child. *Postgrad Med* 97(2):121–126, 1995.
7. Joffe A, Kabani A, Jadavji T: Atypical and complicated Kawasaki disease in infants: Do we need criteria? *West J Med* 162:322–327, 1995.
8. Parha S, Garoufi A, Yiallouros P, et al: Carbamazepine hypersensitivity and rickettsiosis mimicking Kawasaki disease. *Eur J Pediatr* 152:1040–1041, 1993.
9. Von Planta M, Fasnacht M, Holm C, et al: Atypical Kawasaki disease with peripheral gangrene and myocardial infarction: Therapeutic implications. *Eur J Pediatr* 154:830–834, 1995.
10. Yamamoto LG, Martin JE: Kawasaki syndrome in the ED. *Am J Emerg Med* 12(2):178–182, 1994.

BIBLIOGRAPHY

Paisley JW, Levin MJ: Infectious diseases: Viral and rickettsial, in Hathaway WE, Groothius JR, Hay WW Jr, et al (eds): *Current Pediatric Medical Diagnosis and Treatment,* 10th ed. East Norwalk, CT, Appleton Lange, 1991, pp 463–464.
Groothuis JR: Infectious diseases: Viral and rickettsial, and Anti-infective chemotherapy, in Tierney LM Jr, McPhee SJ, Papadakis MA (eds): *Current Medical Diagnosis and Treatment,* 34th ed. Norwalk, CT, Appleton & Lange, 1995, chaps 30 and 36, pp 1153, 1159, 1329.
Hay WW Jr et al: Immunity, allergy and diseases of inflammation *and* Infectious diseases: Viral infections and those presumed to be caused by viruses, in Bralow L (ed): *Nelson Textbook of Pediatrics,* 14th ed. Philadelphia, Saunders, 1992, Chap. 11, Sec. 11.58, pp 629–631 *and* Chap. 12, Sec. 12.18, 12.20, pp 700, 708.

Chapter 10–7
LOW BACK PAIN
Howell J. Smith III

DISCUSSION

Low back pain (LBP) produces a short-term impairment in at least 80 percent of the U.S. population at some time in each person's life. Causes for LBP are numerous. Mechanical pain resulting from injuries to muscles, tendons, ligaments, deep fascia, disks, or bones accounts for most cases of back pain. The remaining sources include cauda equina syndrome, infection, aortic aneurysm, and neoplasms. These conditions require immediate intervention to prevent further neurologic deficits, massive blood loss, shock, or subsequent death. Low back problems are one of the most common reasons patients seek medical care. It is essential that health care providers obtain a careful medical history and then perform a thorough physical examination that is guided by the symptoms. Using the history and physical examination, a treatment plan is then developed using the flow chart shown in Fig. 10-7-1. Referral to appropriate specialists should occur when primary care providers believe the condition exceeds their expertise. Additionally, consultation is indicated when the patient's condition deteriorates, if the neurologic deficit progresses, or if a secondary cause of back pain is identified that requires skills beyond those of a primary care provider.

Mechanical Low Back Pain

This condition most commonly occurs during the productive years, between ages 30 and 60. Even though this is by far the most common cause of LBP, it should be a diagnosis of exclusion after other causes have been ruled out. At increased risk for LBP are individuals with poor conditioning, poor abdominal musculature, poor posture, or poor body mechanics, or who are pregnant or obese. Additionally, those working in occupations with heavy exertional activities or those who are exposed to vibrations by vehicles or heavy machinery are more prone to LBP. Underlying

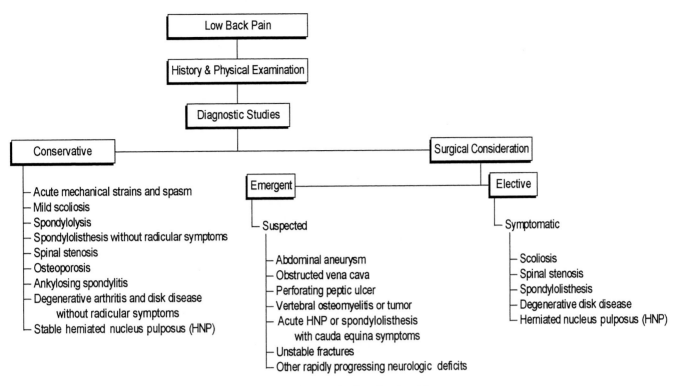

Figure 10-7-1. Low back pain algorithm.

psychological etiologies are common and may include manipulation, boredom, dissatisfaction with jobs or personal lives, drug and alcohol addiction, and clinical depression. Secondary gain, whether it be workers' compensation, a settlement from a lawsuit, or attention is frequently associated with chronic LBP patients.

SYMPTOMS

The symptom that is most indicative of mechanical low back is intermittent pain that correlates with certain body postures or positions. The pain and discomfort are apt to be acute in onset. Many may be able to relate an identifiable cause for their pain, like moving or unusual weekend athletic activity. Symptoms are usually aggravated with activities and are improved with rest. Between 30 and 60 percent of patients report a prior history of back pain. The natural progression of those presenting with mechanical LBP has been demonstrated to be that 50 percent of patients will recover within 2 weeks and 90 percent recover by 4 weeks. Acute exacerbations generally last less than 3 months, and chronic exacerbations last 3 months or longer. Fortunately, less than 5 percent of patients will develop a chronic low back syndrome.

OBJECTIVE FINDINGS

Most patients who present with lumbosacral strain have a diffuse area of tenderness on the affected side. Range of motion of the spine, hips, or lower extremities may be restricted by pain. The examination is unremarkable for neurologic findings. Motor strength, sensation, and deep tendon reflexes are intact. The Babinski test is negative. Rectal tone is good. The straight-leg raising (SLR) test is negative. Although not very specific, the SLR test is a sensitive indicator for disk herniations at the L4-L5 and L5-S1 levels. Leg length discrepancy as well as hamstring tightness are commonly overlooked as sources for LBP.

RADIOLOGIC STUDIES

Anteroposterior and lateral x-rays are standard views.

TREATMENT

Pharmacologic Management

Acetaminophen can be used for mild to moderate cases. Unless contraindicated, nonsteroidal anti-inflammatory drugs (NSAIDs) are prescribed for moderate to severe cases. Patients who have self-medicated with over-the-counter NSAIDs prior to presentation are usually not taking full therapeutic dosages. If a patient's response to the first prescribed NSAID is inadequate, then changing medications is often helpful. Muscle relaxants should be reserved for those patients with muscle spasm, since most cause sedation. This may interfere with the patient returning to work and mobilizing early. Narcotic agents should be used only if the previous treatment fails. If prescribed at all, they should be for no longer than 3 weeks to avoid addiction. Narcotic use should be carefully monitored in patients with chronic pain syndromes. Tricyclic antidepressants may be an appropriate adjunct for patients with chronic LBP.

Supportive Measures

Modalities such as ice, heat, and ultrasound are often helpful. Traction and lumbosacral corsets have not proved effective in the treatment of acute low back symptoms. During the past 5 years, the treatment strategy has changed from prolonged bed rest to encouraging early mobility. New studies indicate that no bed rest and performing normal activities as pain allows is superior to placing the patient on bed rest. Bed rest is utilized for patients with severe acute LBP and should be kept to a minimum. Two days have been shown to be as effective as 7 days. Patients placed on bed rest should be instructed to avoid sitting while in bed.

PATIENT EDUCATION

Patients should be instructed on use of proper body mechanics when lifting and advised to use good postural positions. Enrollment in "low back school" or a referral to physical therapy has proved beneficial to reduce recurrence of symptoms. Abdominal strengthening exercises can begin when pain subsides.

Herniated Lumbar Disk

Lumbar disk herniation is found most commonly in individuals between the ages of 20 and 50. Disks can protrude, extrude, or be free fragments in the canal. Individuals at increased risk are those in occupations that require prolonged sitting and repetitive lifting. Disk herniations most commonly occur at the L4-L5 and L5-S1 levels. Most herniations are posterolateral because the posterior longitudinal ligament is the weakest. In acute injuries, the pain is usually severe and is commonly associated with a flexion strain or other traumatic event.

Sciatica and radicular symptoms may be present, and the patient may report pain relief with rest. Cauda equina compression syndrome involves an acute massive central disk prolapse and presents with paresthesias and pain in the posterior thighs and legs. There are varying degrees of motor function loss in the legs and feet, and possible bowel and bladder dysfunction. This is truly an orthopedic emergency that requires immediate referral to an orthopedic spine surgeon or neurosurgeon. An immediate MRI and surgery (as directed by MRI findings) are necessary to arrest progression of neurologic loss.

Individuals with chronic disk herniation report a wide range of symptoms. With aging, degenerative disk change includes loss of water content and annular tears, which predisposes to herniation of nuclear material. Most individuals with this condition have symptoms that progress gradually and intensify. The pain may be dull to severe and may not necessarily be present in the back. The hallmark complaint is lower extremity pain that radiates from the buttocks to the posterolateral thigh and calf and frequently into the foot. Valsalva and other straining maneuvers that may further compress the involved neurologic structure frequently intensify the symptoms. Clinically, on physical examination, the amount of sensory and motor changes directly correlates with the degree of compression. Conservative treatment methods previously mentioned are generally attempted for mild and transient conditions. Unresolved conditions and those that progressively worsen are considered surgical candidates, based on MRI, electromyogram (EMG), and nerve conduction velocity (NCV) studies.

Vertebral Etiologies

SCOLIOSIS

Most severe cases of scoliosis are identified in adolescence. Surgical intervention is indicated for severe and unstable cases. Mild scoliosis, which is often detected when evaluating adults with LBP, is generally treated like mechanical LBP.

SPONDYLOLYSIS

A defect in the pars interarticularis is the most common cause of LBP in children and adolescents. The defect is thought to be a fatigue fracture from repetitive hyperextension stresses. It is commonly found in gymnasts, divers, football linemen, and weightlifters.

Although spondylolysis can be seen on some lateral studies, an oblique view best visualizes the defect. When present, the pars defect appears as a defect or break in the "Scottie dog's

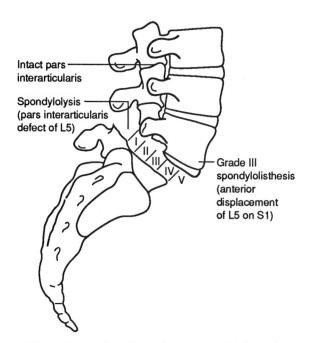

Figure 10-7-2. Spondylolysis and spondylolisthesis.

neck." Defining acute-versus-chronic etiologies can become an issue, especially in workers' compensation cases. A nuclear scan with an increased uptake is consistent with an active lesion or fracture. Treatment of acute injuries should include avoidance of heavy lifting and hyperextension activities. Symptomatic relief measures should include rest and NSAIDs.

SPONDYLOLISTHESIS

Spondylolisthesis is the anterior displacement of one vertebra on another. It most commonly occurs at L4-L5 or L5-S1. The slippage is usually due to a pars interarticularis defect. The severity of the slip is based on the amount of displacement or degree of the spinal column compared with S1 on the lateral x-ray: Grade I = 0 to 25 percent; II = 25 to 50 percent; III = 50 to 75 percent; IV = 75 to 100 percent; V = >100 percent. More than 100 percent displacement is called *spondyloptosis* (see Fig. 10-7-2).

Patients with less than 50 percent displacement (grades I and II) usually can be asymptomatic or have minimal mechanical LBP symptoms. Patients with slippages of greater than 50 percent (grades III, IV, and V) usually experience moderate to severe pain and sciatica, and may complain of a variety of lower extremity neurologic symptoms. The degree of neurologic involvement runs from rare to the possibility of a full-blown cauda equina syndrome in high-degree slips. The treatment for asymptomatic spondylolysis and a minimal spondylolisthesis is observation with no restrictions. There is a 60 percent success rate of treating symptomatic grades I and II spondylolisthesis patients with conservative treatment. Spinal fusion is often necessary to stabilize patients with grades III, IV, and V slippages. Most neurologic deficits are L5 radiculopathy associated with L5-S1 spondylolisthesis. Cauda equina symptoms are associated with grades III, IV, or V slips. Fortunately, this amount of neurologic loss is rare. Suspicion of cauda equina involvement is an orthopedic emergency that needs immediate attention by either an orthopedic spine surgeon or a neurosurgeon.

SPINAL STENOSIS

Spinal stenosis is a three-joint complex (disk and facet joints) condition that narrows the neural foramen, creating compression on the spinal cord. Most cases of stenosis are from the degenera-

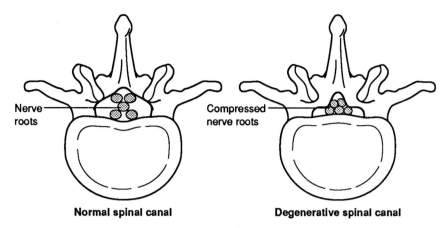

Figure 10-7-3. Spinal stenosis.

tive changes of a collapsing disk and subsequent facet arthritis. The average age of a patient with stenosis is 60 years. Stenosis is the most common cause for neurologic leg pain in the elderly. Patients with stenosis have a narrowing of the central canal and the lateral recesses where the nerve roots are contained (see Fig. 10-7-3). This can create a lumbosacral radiculopathy and neurogenic claudication. Most patients complain that the pain worsens during the day. A common description is low back and bilateral extremity pain in the buttocks, legs, and thighs after ambulating or standing. Patients also relate that downhill walking makes the pain worse. Neurogenic claudication pain is relieved by 15 to 30 min in a supine position with a pillow under the knees. Patients also report relief of their symptoms by leaning forward while standing, which has been termed the "shopping cart" position. The physical examination may be normal. Increased discomfort with spinal extension suggests stenosis. Neurologic findings vary, and, when present, impairment at several spinal levels is often noted.

Radiographs usually demonstrate extensive vertebral osteophytes and degenerative disk disease. MRI and CT studies are used to evaluate the severity of the condition and for preoperative planning. Conservative treatment consists of NSAIDs and avoidance of aggravating activities such as walking. Bicycling may be recommended as an alternative aerobic activity. Epidural steroid injections may provide short-term relief. Surgical decompression is needed for long-term resolution for those with significant discomfort and neurologic compression.

OSTEOPOROSIS

(See Chap. 5-2, "Osteoporosis.") This is the most common cause of metabolic bone disease in the United States. This age-related decrease in bone mass, most commonly seen in postmenopausal women, is usually associated with the loss of estrogen. Osteoporosis is a contributing cause of 1 million fractures per year. This process primarily affects the cancellous bone. The spine, hip, and pelvis are the most commonly affected areas. Most vertebral fractures secondary to osteoporosis occur between T11 and L1. Individuals affected may be completely asymptomatic or may suffer from severe back pain.

ANKYLOSING SPONDYLITIS

(See Chap. 10-4, "Ankylosing Spondylitis.") This chronic systemic inflammatory disease of the joints and the axial skeleton commonly has an onset in the late teens or early 20s and usually occurs before age 40. This disorder affects three times more men than women. The onset is gradual with intermittent exacerbations and back pain radiating down the leg(s) posteriorly. Complaints

of progressive morning stiffness over several months that is relieved with exercise are common. Physical examination findings may include painful sacroiliac joints, reduced mobility of the spine, and possible uveitis. Studies indicate that 85 percent of patients with ankylosing spondylitis (AS) have an elevated erythrocyte sedimentation rate (ESR), the rheumatoid factor is generally negative, and HLA-B27 antigen is present in 90 percent. The earliest x-ray changes are widening and sclerosis of both sacroiliac joints, which are best visualized on the anteroposterior pelvis view. As the disease progresses, x-ray changes may include what has been labeled the "bamboo" spine. This appearance is a combination of calcification of the anterior spinal ligament and bony bridging of the vertebral bodies. Treatment consists of stressing the importance of postural breathing, NSAIDs, and physical therapy.

SPINAL TUMORS

Primary spinal tumors are rare, accounting for less than 10 percent of all bone tumors. Tumors in individuals younger than 21 years old are usually benign. More than 70 percent of primary spinal tumors in individuals older than 21 years of age are malignant. Multiple myeloma (see Chap. 13-12, "Multiple Myeloma") is the most common primary bone tumor. Metastatic tumors are common. Between 50 and 70 percent of individuals with terminal cancer have vertebral metastasis. More than 75 percent of tumors in the vertebral body are malignant. Known malignancy and a tender spinous process, with or without back pain, is extremely suspicious for a vertebral or epidural metabolic disease. Night pain that is slow, progressive, persistent, dull, and made worse by recumbency should also be aggressively investigated. Neurologic deficits are common at the time of presentation. X-rays may identify only as little as 30 percent of spine lesions associated with pain. Nuclear imaging demonstrates increased uptake in areas of activity. CT scan is utilized to evaluate the extent of the tumor. Treatment consists of a biopsy, radiation therapy and chemotherapy, or, in selected cases, surgical excision with spine stabilization.

SPINAL INFECTIONS

Infections of the vertebrae (osteomyelitis) and of the soft tissues surrounding the spine are rare and are commonly associated with a postoperative surgical procedure or injection. Other causes may include tuberculosis, primary or metastatic tumors of the spine and spinal cord, or infections secondary to myelograms. The most common organisms cultured are *Staphylococcus aureus, Pseudomonas,* and *Escherichia coli.* Individuals with increased risks include drug abusers, those with diabetes mellitus, and those who are immunologically suppressed. Back pain, malaise, fever, sepsis, wound drainage, and an elevated ESR are classic at presentation. The neurologic examination may be normal to a complete cauda equina compression, which is a frequent presentation with spinal tumors. Conditions with acute neurologic changes that are progressing to cauda equina compression need immediate surgical intervention. Other infectious processes require a combination of wound management techniques that include incision and drainage and intravenous antibiotics.

REFERRED PAIN

The causes for referred pain to the back are numerous, many of which can be life-threatening. Etiologies may include herpes zoster renal calculi, urinary tract infection, peptic ulcer disease, carcinoma of the pancreas, prostatitis, prostatic carcinoma, inferior vena cava obstruction, and abdominal aortic aneurysm. Pain may be intermittent or acute and excruciating. Patients will normally present with the expected signs and symptoms for the particular condition. Treatment is directed by the severity of the condition at time the patient presents.

DIAGNOSTIC STUDIES

It is important to carefully choose the diagnostic studies ordered and then place them into a proper perspective when evaluating LBP. Some studies are costly, and all can be misleading, which can confuse the treatment plan.

Radiologic Studies

Anteroposterior and lateral x-rays are baseline studies. Additional views may include a "coned down" (spot) view of the lumbar and sacral spine. Oblique, flexion, and extension views are taken to more clearly define and evaluate specific etiologic pathologies. Lumbosacral x-rays in general have a very low specificity. Degenerative changes in patients older than 40 years old are not uncommon. For this reason, some clinicians may not order x-rays while initially evaluating apparent simple mechanical strains. X-rays should be obtained when a fracture, metastatic bone disease, infection, chronic inflammatory disease, or a congenital or developmental anomaly is suspected. Spinal radiographs may be required for medicolegal documentation by workers' compensation protocols to assess for preexisting conditions.

Specialized Studies

Specialized studies may be required to assess for a more definitive diagnosis. MRI is best utilized to evaluate soft tissue structures and neural compression. Research investigation conducted on asymptomatic individuals demonstrated that more than 33 percent had a substantial abnormality. CT is best utilized to evaluate osseous structures. It should be noted that CT imaging, like MRI, is expensive and has shown a large number of asymptomatic individuals with abnormalities. EMG and NCV are usually reserved for individuals with neurologic changes to assess the physiologic integrity and level of nerve root involvement. Nuclear imaging is helpful to diagnose acute subtle fractures, as well as neoplastic and infectious lesions.

Serum Tests

A complete blood cell count (CBC) and ESR are relatively inexpensive and should be performed when assessing the patient for possible infection, inflammatory processes, and blood loss. A decreased hemoglobin and hematocrit are diagnostic for anemias with various pathologies. The white blood cell count is generally elevated in infectious processes, and the ESR is the most sensitive and early indicator for an inflammatory response. Additional serum tests may be ordered as appropriate, including serum calcium, alkaline phosphatase, serum protein electrophoresis, rheumatoid factor, antinuclear antibodies, and HLA-B27.

RED FLAGS

Individuals with recent trauma, as from a motor vehicle accident, fall, or strenuous lifting activity, are at an increased risk for fracture, disk herniation, and spinal cord compression. Patients older than 50 years of age are at an increased risk for carcinomas and infections. The history, physical examination, and diagnostic studies should be ordered with these considerations in mind.

CONCLUSIONS AND OUTLOOK

Back and spine disorders are the most frequent and most costly musculoskeletal conditions causing limited activity during the working years. Back impairment is the most common chronic impairment for individuals under the age of 45 and ranks third behind arthritis and heart disease for individuals in the 45- to 64-year-old age group. Low back pain is a major cause of time and productivity loss at work. More than 400,000 U.S. workers are disabled annually by back pain. Medical care costs for LBP are more than $13 billion annually. Primary care providers must be comfortable in evaluating and treating patients with LBP. Recently there has been an acute interest and awareness in fitness and health that will hopefully decrease the morbidity associated with chronic lower back disability. Many large corporations have already installed fitness gyms and other incentives in an attempt to reduce stress and improve employee fitness and health, thus reducing time lost from the workplace.

BIBLIOGRAPHY

Frymoyer JW: Lumbar spine, in *Orthopaedic Knowledge Update 4.* Rosemont, IL, American Academy of Orthopaedic Surgeons, 1993, pp 491–498.
Hellmann DB: Arthritis and musculoskeletal disorders, in Tierney LM Jr, McPhee SJ, Papadakis MA (eds): *Current Medical Diagnosis and Treatment.* Norwalk, CT, Appleton & Lange, 1996, pp 755–756.
Miller MD: Spine, in *Review of Orthopaedics.* Philadelphia, Saunders, 1992, pp 147–164.
Way LW: Orthopedics, in *Current Surgical Diagnosis and Treatment.* East Norwalk, CT, Appleton & Lange, 1994, pp 1101–1104.
Winter RB: Tumors and infections of the spine. American Academy of Orthopaedic Surgeons, Eleventh Annual Comprehensive Review Course, Chicago, IL, 1995.
U.S. Department of Health and Human and Human Services: Acute Low Back Problems in Adults: Assessment and Treatment, AHCPR Publication no 95-06343, 1994.

Chapter 10–8
OSTEOARTHRITIS
Pamela Moyers Scott

DISCUSSION

Osteoarthritis (OA), or degenerative joint disease (DJD), is the most common form of arthritis. It is estimated that it affects approximately 16 million Americans.[1] OA is characterized by a progressive loss of articular cartilage and new bone formation consisting of osteophytes (at the joint margins) and sclerosis (subchondral).

Risk factors for OA include increasing age, obesity, female gender, repetitive joint usage (either occupational or recreational), major joint trauma, and a genetic predisposition. Racial differences also exist; however, it is unclear if they are genetic or life-style related.[2]

Risk factors for increased symptomatology, in terms of pain and disability associated with OA, include being female, divorced, unemployed, and on Medicaid.[2]

SIGNS AND SYMPTOMS

The predominant symptom of osteoarthritis is pain. It is generally aggravated by activity and alleviated by rest. In the more advanced stages of the disease, the pain can be constant. It is most often defined as a deep ache and confined to one or a few joints. It is generally unilateral, although bilateral disease involvement is possible. Onset is usually insidious. The most commonly affected joints are the knees, hips, spine, thumb bases, and distal interphalangeal joints of the hands.

It may be associated with stiffness following a period of inactivity, including sleeping at night. However, the stiffness is usually completely resolved within 30 min. Unless another condition is associated with OA, systemic symptoms and inflammation are generally absent.

OBJECTIVE FINDINGS

On physical examination, the affected joint or joints usually reveal tenderness to palpation, decreased range of motion, instability, bony enlargement, and crepitus. As the disease progresses, these findings become more prominent and can lead to gross deformity. Synovial effusions and synovitis may be present.

The presence of bony enlargement of the distal interphalangeal joints (Heberden's nodes) and the proximal interphalangeal joints (Bouchard's nodes) are pathognomonic for OA.

DIAGNOSTIC CONSIDERATIONS

The diagnosis of osteoarthritis can usually be made on the basis of history and physical alone. However, other forms of arthritis should be considered in the differential, including rheumatoid, gouty, psoriatic, erosive inflammatory, and spondyloarthropathic. Bursitis and tendonitis can sometimes mimic OA.

SPECIAL CONSIDERATIONS

OA frequently occurs as a result of an associated disease state and/or causative factor. These conditions include acute and repetitive trauma; inflammatory arthritis; bone diseases, such as Paget's and osteoporosis; metabolic and endocrine disorders including diabetes mellitus, hypothyroidism, hyperparathyroidism, acromegaly, hemochromatosis, gout, and ochronosis; congenital and developmental disease, like Legg-Calve-Perthes, slipped epiphysis, and bone dysplasias; Charcot's joints; and frostbite.[2]

When this occurs, it is classified as secondary osteoarthritis. OA without a causative factor or associated disease state is termed primary (or idiopathic).

LABORATORY TESTS

Laboratory studies in the evaluation of osteoarthritis are indicated only to rule out other etiologies or secondary causes. In OA, the erythrocyte sedimentation rate (ESR) is normal to slightly elevated.

RADIOGRAPHIC STUDIES

Plain films of the affected joint may confirm the diagnosis. Very early in the course of the disease, however, the x-ray may be normal. Typical radiographic findings of OA include joint space narrowing, osteophytes, sclerosis, and possibly bony cyst formation. When interpreting these radiographic results in the evaluation of a patient with joint pain, it is important to remember that severity of disease on x-ray does not necessarily correlate with severity of symptoms.

OTHER DIAGNOSTICS

Other diagnostic studies are not necessary to make the diagnosis of osteoarthritis. However, they may be required to determine the etiology of secondary osteoarthritis.

TREATMENT

Since osteoarthritis cannot be cured, therapy is aimed at reducing pain and minimizing disability.

Pharmacologic Management

First-line medication of OA is now acetaminophen in fixed or as-needed doses up to a maximum of 4 g/day. Although long-term acetaminophen usage has been associated with liver toxicity, it most often occurs in association with heavy alcohol consumption.[3] Patients should be counseled accordingly. Long-term acetaminophen usage has also been associated with renal failure; however, the incidence appears to be less than seen with long-term nonsteroidal anti-inflammatory drug (NSAID) usage.[1]

In patients who do not respond to maximum acetaminophen therapy and nonpharmacologic approaches, an NSAID is then the drug of choice. None of the currently available NSAIDs appears to be superior to the others in the treatment of all patients with OA.[3] When choosing an NSAID, the impact of side effects, costs, dosing convenience, and compliance for each individual patient must be considered.

The risk of GI toxicity, especially hemorrhage, is a serious complication of NSAID therapy. Cytoprotective agents, like misoprostol (Cytotec), should be considered in all patients receiving an NSAID. Risk factors that increase the likelihood of an adverse GI complication include a previous GI bleed, history of peptic ulcer disease, advancing age, smoking, and oral corticosteroid therapy. Misoprostol is currently the only agent with FDA approval for this. However, omeprazole (Prilosec) and famotidine (Pepcid) have been successfully used for this purpose.[3]

NSAIDs are also associated with renal and hepatotoxicity. The greatest risk for renal complications occurs in the elderly, diabetics, hypertensives, individuals with preexisting renal disease, and patients on diuretic therapy. Patients who consume large amounts of alcohol are probably at the greatest risk of hepatic complications.

Before instituting NSAID therapy, obtain baseline liver functions, renal functions, potassium, and complete blood cell count (CBC). CBC, creatinine, and potassium tests should be repeated in 1 month and again every 6 months thereafter.[3]

If the initial liver function testing is normal, then additional testing is usually unnecessary.[3]

It is also necessary to advise the patient of these potential complications and the signs and symptoms of such. Patients should be told to report them immediately if they do occur and told about the importance of the laboratory studies.

If NSAIDs alone do not control the patient's symptoms, consider adding acetaminophen (up to the maximum dose of 4 g/day) on an as-needed basis to the regime.

If the patient is intolerant of NSAIDs or has a severe aspirin allergy, the nonacetylated salicylates such as salsalate (Salflex, Disalcid) and choline magnesium trisalicylate (Trilisate) may be effective. These drugs are associated with less renal and GI toxicity than the NSAIDs; however, they are usually not as effective of an analgesic.

Other oral medications for pain relief include the opioids. Their primary role is in providing immediate relief in acute flares of OA. Occasionally, they are used long term in the management of osteoarthritis in individuals who are poor surgical candidates and in whom other treatments fail to provide relief, in patients who cannot tolerate any of the other oral regimes, and in individuals where the risk of NSAID complications outweigh the hazards of long-term opioid therapy (i.e., addiction and impairment).

If oral medications are ineffective or poorly tolerated in the management of osteoarthritis, intra- or periarticular injections of corticosteroid may provide the patient with relief. They should not be used in anyone contemplating arthroplasty since they could cause a residual infection of the joint leading to an infected prosthesis. They should not be given any more frequently than every 3 to 4 months because they might increase the rate of cartilage breakdown. Injectable and oral corticosteroids have no role in the treatment of OA.

Nonpharmacologic Management

Because of the potential of adverse drug reactions, nonpharmacologic approaches must be incorporated into the initial treatment plan for patients with osteoarthritis. These consist of exercise, weight reduction, and topical applications.

Low-impact, non-weight-bearing exercise is recommended to reduce pain and increase joint stability via improved muscle tone. Examples of these activities include swimming, water aerobics, low-impact aerobics, and bicycling. Any activity that causes pain that persists for greater than 2 h should be avoided. Additionally, if the joint becomes painful during exercise, the patient must take a break.

Because obesity can cause an accelerated rate of destruction of the weight-bearing joints, especially the knees, weight reduction in these individuals is essential. Studies indicate that even a modest weight loss can result in a significant reduction of symptoms in OA.[3]

Some patients respond to the topical application of heat, some cold, and others alternating heat and cold (known as contrast baths). Another topical therapy that many patients respond to is capsaicin cream (Zostrix), 0.025 to 0.25% several times per day. Rubefacients containing methyl salicylate (e.g., Thera-Gesic) and various sports creams have been effective in reducing pain in some patients.

Surgical Management

Total joint arthroplasty (TJA) is the ultimate solution in the treatment of osteoporosis. Because of the risks of mechanical failure and need of repeat procedures, TJA should only be considered if all other treatment options have been unsuccessful. Other surgical options include arthroscopic joint washout, tidal lavage, osteotomy, chondroplasty, and laminectomy.

SUPPORTIVE MEASURES

In addition to the nonpharmacologic approaches previously mentioned, physical therapy often increases function and decreases pain in osteoarthritic joints.

PATIENT EDUCATION

The patient must be made aware that treatment will control, but not cure the disease. Advise the patient that OA is usually a progressive disease process that often requires increased medical management, including the possibility of surgery. The importance of the nonpharmacologic modalities must be stressed. Finally, the patient needs to be aware of potential complications of the drug therapies. Patients may obtain additional information and resources by contacting the Arthritis Foundation at 1-800-283-7800 or http://www.arthritis.org.

FUTURE MANAGEMENT

Preliminary research is being done on disease-modifying medications. The most promising at this point are the chondroprotective agents such as polysulfate glycosaminoglycans.[2,3] Research is also being conducted on techniques to diagnose OA based on serology testing for the macromolecules being released from degenerating bone and cartilage (e.g., glycosaminoglycans).[2]

COMPLICATIONS AND RED FLAGS

Patients who are not adequately responding to conservative therapy should be referred to an orthopedic surgeon.

OTHER NOTES AND PEARLS

Articular cartilage is essentially aneural. Therefore, the pain associated with OA has an etiology in other intra- and/or periarticular structures.

REFERENCES

1. Primary care update. New management guidelines in osteoarthritis of the hip. *Consultant* (2):341–343, 1996.
2. Brandt K: Osteoarthritis, in Isselbacher K, Braunwald E, Wilson J, et al (eds): *Harrison's Principles of Internal Medicine,* 13th ed. New York, McGraw-Hill, 1994, pp 1692–1698.
3. Clough JD, Lambert T, Miller DR: The new thinking on osteoarthritis. *Patient Care* Sept 15:110–137, 1996.

Chapter 10–9
REITER'S SYNDROME
Jean M. Covino

DISCUSSION

Reiter's syndrome is a form of reactive arthritis (ReA) that refers to an acute, nonsuppurative sterile inflammatory condition that occurs in response to an infectious process (usually enteric or urogenital) elsewhere in the body. Reiter's syndrome is the most common form of ReA and consists of mucocutaneous, urogenital, and ocular manifestations.

PATHOGENESIS

Reiter's syndrome occurs predominantly in individuals with the histocompatibility locus A B27 (HLA-B27) haplotype. The pathogenesis of Reiter's syndrome is poorly understood and an area of ongoing research. Most investigators postulate that a preceding infection serves as a trigger in a genetically predisposed host and that the disease may then persist or recur despite eradication of the infection.[1] The mechanism by which inflammation or infection of a mucosal surface might initiate a sustained systemic illness or how the organisms reach the affected joints is unknown. What is known is that initial manifestations of Reiter's syndrome tend to be more severe and the natural course more aggressive in persons with the HLA-B27 haplotype than in those without it.[1] The HLA-B27 haplotype is found in 70 to 80 percent of white patients, compared with 6 to 8 percent of whites in the general population; in blacks with Reiter's syndrome, the reported prevalence of HLA-B27 has varied from 15 to 75 percent, compared with about 2 percent in blacks in the general population.[2]

Incidence and Epidemiology

Although cases of Reiter's syndrome have been reported worldwide, the incidence and prevalence of this disease are uncertain and may vary geographically.[1] Epidemiologically, it is characterized by both an endemic, or venereal form, usually sexually acquired, and a less common epidemic or dysenteric form, most often associated with enteric infections. Although postdysenteric Reiter's syndrome occurs in children, most patients are adults. Peak onset of Reiter's syndrome is during the third decade of life.[1] Postvenereal Reiter's syndrome affects men more than women; male-female ratios ranging from 9:1 to 5:1 have been reported.[2] The ratio was once thought to be 20:1, but this was most likely the result of underreporting of cases in women, who often have less severe disease. The dysenteric form of Reiter's syndrome affects equal numbers of both sexes.[2]

Microbiology

Chlamydia trachomatis (serotypes D through K) is the most common infectious organism found in patients with Reiter's syndrome. It has been documented in approximately 50 percent of men with sexually acquired Reiter's syndrome.[1,2] At least 50 percent of all patients with Reiter's syndrome have high antichlamydial antibodies suggestive of a recent infection.[2,3] *Ureaplasma urealyticum* is another possible candidate. Enteric pathogens implicated in Reiter's syndrome include *Campylobacter, Shigella, Salmonella, Yersinia,* and possibly *Cryptosporidium* and *Giardia* species.

SIGNS AND SYMPTOMS

The diagnosis is straightforward in patients with arthritis, conjunctivitis, and urethritis. However, fewer than one-third of patients with Reiter's syndrome present with all three clinical findings.[2]

Urogenital findings include urethritis, dysuria, or prostatitis in males. Urethritis is an early symptom and can occur 2 to 4 weeks after sexual exposure or cessation of a gastrointestinal illness. Women may present with cervicitis or vaginitis. However, a clear spectrum of urogenital symptoms in women with Reiter's syndrome still needs to be described.

Ocular manifestations occur in up to 50 percent of patients with the sexually acquired form of the disease and up to 90 percent of the cases following the epidemic form of the disease. As with other symptoms, the ocular manifestations may be recurrent. Conjunctivitis, often mild enough to go unnoticed, is the most common ocular manifestation. Although uncommon at initial presentation, keratitis, iritis, and uveitis are other possible symptoms.

Arthritic manifestation is the last clinical feature of the triad to occur. Asymmetric polyarticular synovitis-tendinitis can be seen initially, followed by persistence in one or two joints. Any joint can be involved, but knees, ankles, and toes are most commonly affected. Later involvement may include the fingers and the wrists. Tendon insertion sites (entheses) are common points of inflammation, and areas include insertion of the Achilles tendon and the plantar fascia. A classic enthesitic feature is dactylitis, which causes "sausage-shaped" fingers or toes. This clinical finding occurs only in Reiter's syndrome and psoriatic arthritis. Sacroiliitis is also a common finding, occurring in up to 10 percent

of cases acutely and more commonly in those with chronic Reiter's syndrome.

Dermatologic manifestations often include mucocutaneous lesions and occur in about 50 percent of patients. Circinate balanitis is the most common cutaneous manifestation, occurring in approximately 20 to 40 percent and up to 85 percent of men with the sexually acquired form of the syndrome. These lesions start as vesicles that quickly rupture to form painless superficial erosions, which in circumcised individuals can form crusts similar to the lesions of keratodermia blennorrhagica. Lesions of keratoderma blennorrhagica begin as erythematous macules that gradually enlarge to form hyperkeratotic papules, sometimes with red halos and occasionally with central clearing. The lesions most commonly appear on the plantar surfaces of the feet, but may occur anywhere. They resemble psoriasis both grossly and histologically. In as many as 20 percent of patients with Reiter's syndrome, especially those with the sexually acquired form, painless shallow ulcers can occur on the tongue, palate, buccal mucosa, tonsillar pillars, or pharynx. Nail involvement occurs in as many as 19 percent of patients, manifested by thickening and brown-yellow discoloration.

Other systemic manifestations are common and include malaise, fever, anorexia, and weight loss. Transient and usually benign electrocardiographic abnormalities, including atrioventricular conduction disturbances, ST-segment elevation or depression, and nonspecific T-wave changes, can occur.

DIAGNOSTIC CONSIDERATIONS

Other arthritic conditions that should be considered in the differential diagnosis of Reiter's syndrome include ankylosing spondylitis, colitic arthritis, gonococcal arthritis, systemic lupus erythematosus, Lyme disease, psoriatic arthritis, rheumatic fever, and rheumatoid arthritis. (See corresponding chapters.)

SPECIAL CONSIDERATIONS

A correlation between Reiter's syndrome and HIV infection was reported in the late 1980s.[4,5] However, more recent studies have failed to show a link between the two diseases.[6] This remains an area of debate with some investigators.

LABORATORY TESTS

Laboratory findings are nonspecific and do not help establish a diagnosis. The erythrocyte sedimentation rate (ESR) and C-reactive protein levels are usually elevated but do not correlate with disease activity. Mild anemia and leukocytosis with a shift to the left may occur.

RADIOLOGIC STUDIES

In early disease, there are usually absent radiographic findings or evidence of soft tissue swelling. With persistent disease, there may be radiographic evidence of joint space erosion, periostitis with reactive new bone formation, or spurs at the insertion of the plantar fascia. About 50 percent of patients have evidence of sacroiliitis.

OTHER DIAGNOSTICS

Synovial fluid analysis is rarely specific and resembles septic arthritis. It may show a white blood cell count of 500 to 50,000 cells/μL, predominantly neutrophils, elevated protein and complement levels, and normal glucose levels. A Gram stain should be negative for any organisms. Microbiologic identification of specific organisms is helpful but is usually not successful. Attempts to culture the infectious agent from the urethra, cervix, or stool should be made, if possible. Antichlamydia antibody tests for IgG and IgM may prove the presence of infection, but are not necessary for the diagnosis and are lengthy and costly.

TREATMENT

Although there is no cure for Reiter's syndrome, antibiotic therapy is indicated. Recent data suggest that recurrent arthritis was much lower in patients treated with antibiotics for chlamydial urethritis.[7] Most authorities currently recommend doxycycline, 100 mg two times daily, for an extended period of time based on the patient's clinical response. Whether antibiotics are indicated for patients with postdysenteric Reiter's syndrome is unknown because few clinical studies are available in this subgroup.

Treatment with nonsteroidal anti-inflammatory drugs (NSAIDs) such as indomethacin (Indocin) (75 to 150 mg/day in divided doses) may help alleviate some of the arthritic symptoms. Other NSAIDs may also be effective. Corticosteroid therapy given orally or by intraarticular injection is not effective. Sulfasalazine (Azulfidine), methotrexate (Rheumatrex), azathioprine (Imuran), and bromocriptine mesylate (Parlodel) may help patients with persistent debilitating disease that is refractory to NSAIDs.

Physical therapy may also help alleviate some symptoms.

COMPLICATIONS AND RED FLAGS

Most patients are symptom-free 2 months to 1 year after the diagnosis is made, so overall prognosis is good. The acute syndrome may recur in about 15 percent of patients and may manifest as back pain, heel pain, arthritis, or any of the initial symptoms. Twenty percent of patients may develop chronic arthritic symptoms with the potential for degenerative changes. Other documented long-term sequelae, especially in sexually acquired cases, include complete heart block, myocarditis, pericarditis, acute aortitis with aortic valve incompetence, and congestive heart failure. Death from Reiter's syndrome is rare.

NOTES AND PEARLS

Since Reiter's syndrome is a clinical diagnosis with no definitive laboratory test, a high index of suspicion must be maintained. Always consider this diagnosis in a patient with asymmetric inflammatory arthritis or tendinitis. A careful history may elicit genitourinary or ocular symptoms 1 to 4 weeks prior to the reactive disease. Careful inspection of the glans penis, including retraction of the foreskin, and the oral mucosa in all male patients presenting with acute arthritic symptoms is essential.

REFERENCES

1. Keat A: Reiter's syndrome and reactive arthritis in perspective. *New Engl J Med* 309:1606, 1983.
2. Cush JJ, Lipsky PE: Reiter's syndrome and reactive arthritis, in McCarty DJ, Koopman WJ (eds): *Arthritis and Allied Conditions,* 12th ed. Philadelphia, Lea & Febiger, 1993.
3. Handsfield HH, Pollock PS: Arthritis associated with sexually transmitted diseases, in Holmes KK, Mardh PA (eds): *Sexually Transmitted Diseases,* 2d ed. New York, McGraw-Hill, 1990.
4. Winchester R, Bernstein DH, Fisher HD, et al: The co-occurrence of Reiter's syndrome and acquired immunodeficiency. *Ann Intern Med* 106(1):19–26, 1987.
5. Berman A, Espinoza LR, Diaz JD, et al: Rheumatic manifestations of human immunodeficiency virus infection. *Am J Med* 85(1):59–64, 1988.
6. Clark MR, Solinger AM, Hochberg MC: Human immunodeficiency virus infection is not associated with Reiter's syndrome: Data from three large cohort studies. *Rheum Dis Clin North Am* 128(1):267–276, 1992.
7. Bardin T, Enel C, Cornelis F, et al: Antibiotic treatment of veneral disease and Reiter's syndrome in a Greenland population. *Arthritis Rheum* 35(2):190–194, 1992.

Chapter 10–10
SYSTEMIC LUPUS ERYTHEMATOSUS
William A. Mosier

DISCUSSION

Systemic lupus erythematosus (SLE) is a chronic multisystemic inflammatory disease. Its chief characteristic is the development of abnormal immune system products that the body fails to suppress. SLE is named for the erythematous rash that appears on the face in about 50 percent of cases. In fact, the term *lupus* (Latin for "wolf") was first applied to the disease in 1230 A.D. because of the rash resembling the mask appearance over the malar eminence of a wolf's face. SLE can vary greatly in its presenting symptoms, clinical manifestation, and course.

A hallmark of SLE is the presence of antibodies to nuclear components found in the blood. The typical case of SLE progresses in a chronic, irregular manner. Episodes of active disease state are interspersed with long periods of seemingly complete or nearly complete remission. SLE may present in a mild form. Although it is not typical, SLE can have a fulminating presentation and be rapidly fatal. Infection is a major cause of morbidity and mortality rates in patients with SLE. Some patients die from vascular lesions affecting the central nervous system, the heart, or the kidneys, whereas others die from the complications of secondary infection. There is no known cure.

Ninety percent of all cases occur in women. In fact, SLE affects women eight times more often than it does men. At age 30, the ratio of women to men is 10:1. The ratio in juveniles is closer to 2:1 and in persons over age 65 the ratio appears to be about 3:1. The prevalence rate among women between ages 15 and 64 is 1 in 700 women. Symptoms usually appear between the ages of 15 and 25 years. The prevalence in the general population is about 1 in 1000.

Although SLE affects all ethnic groups, in the United States the prevalence is three times higher among African Americans than Caucasians. It may be slightly more common in the native American population than in Caucasians. Data are unclear as to its actual prevalence in the Asian population.

PATHOGENESIS

SLE is a disease of unknown etiology. It may actually represent several different disease entities that manifest a clinical expression through a common pathway. It is a disease of immunologic malfunctioning. This malfunctioning results in autoimmune reactions against host antigens that lead to inflammation and tissue damage resulting in cellular and organ dysfunction. Both environmental and genetic factors play an important role in the cause and pathogenesis of SLE. The serum of patients with SLE contains antibodies to nuclear antigens. (See "Laboratory Tests," below.) The apparent diversity of antibodies in SLE may be explained by the common chemical features among the antigens, rather than by any diversity of antibody specificities. The antibodies to nuclear antigens (ANA) participate in the pathogenesis of SLE by forming antigen-antibody complexes with their specific antigens. SLE may be triggered by bacterial, chemical, or viral antigens in genetically predisposed individuals. Drugs, such as hydralazine and procainamide, can induce a disease state that appears identi-

Table 10-10-1. Medications That Can Induce Symptoms
of SLE

Acebutolol	Ethosuximide
Atenolol	Hydralazine
Carbamazepine	Isoniazid
Chlorpromazine	Labetalol
Clonidine	Methyldopa
D-penicillamine	Procainamide

cal with SLE (see Table 10-10-1). A genetic predisposition for
SLE is suggested by the increased rate of subclinical abnormalities discovered in relatives of patients with SLE and by the increased occurrence of SLE in the second twin in monozygotic
twins.

SYMPTOMS

A young female patient presenting with a fever, rash, and arthritic
pain should be evaluated for SLE. About 90 percent of all patients
with SLE experience nondeforming arthritis. Morning stiffness,
usually due to arthralgia, with swelling and effusion is common.
About 50 percent of patients with SLE are photosensitive. Those
with photosensitivity may experience a worsening of symptoms
after sun exposure.

Alopecia may often occur, however it is usually reversible.
Ulcerations of the mouth and lips may also occur. The two principal affective symptoms encountered in SLE are anxiety and depressed mood. Headaches are also a common complaint (see
Table 10-10-2).

OBJECTIVE FINDINGS

Because the severity of symptoms can vary so greatly and because
they may occur spread out over many years, diagnosis may also
be delayed for many years. The three most common clinical
findings are fever, rash, and arthritic pain. Other findings may
include cardiac abnormalities, hemolytic anemia, neurologic abnormalities, polyarthralgia, polyserositis (such as pleurisy and
pericarditis), renal abnormalities, and thrombocytopenia
purpura.

After an acute attack of SLE, remission usually occurs. There
can typically be an interval of several symptom-free years. However, an eventual reoccurrence is likely. In any case the course

Table 10-10-2. American College of Rheumatology (ACR)
Criteria for the Classification of SLE

Malar rash
Discoid rash
Photosensitivity
Oral or nasopharyngeal ulcers
Nonerosive arthritis
Pleuritis
Pericarditis
Proteinuria (>500 mg/dL)
Cast cells
Psychosis
Seizures
Hemolytic anemia
Leukopenia (<4000/mL)
Lymphopenia (<1500/mL)
Thrombocytopenia ($<100,000$/mL)
Antinuclear antibodies (ANA)
Anti-dsDNA
Anti-Smith antigen
False-positive Veneral Disease Research Laboratories (VDRL) test
Positive lupus erythematosis cell preparation

is unpredictable and may recur without apparent cause. Factors
that can precipitate exacerbation are certain medications, emotional or physical stress, infection, sunlight, and the trauma of
surgery.

Fever Involvement

A low-grade fever occurs in the majority of patients with SLE.
Less frequently, a high-grade fever may manifest in isolation
or may accompany multisystemic involvement. Caution must be
taken to differentiate a fever caused by SLE versus one caused
by a secondary infection.

Musculoskeletal Involvement

An acute attack of SLE may consist of symmetric and polyarticular arthritis. The hands, wrists, elbows, knees, and ankles are
commonly involved. The inflammatory appearance of the joints
may or may not be notable. Myalgia and muscle weakness are
common. Symptoms of fibromyalgia are also common in SLE.

Skin Involvement

Skin lesions can be an important diagnostic clue to SLE. A patient
with SLE may present with subacute, acute, or chronic skin
involvement. Although acute cutaneous lupus typically presents
as an erythematous (butterfly appearing) rash extending from
the bridge of the nose to the malar areas; it may occur in other sun-
exposed areas. The subacute cutaneous lupus typically consists of
an erythematous, papulosquamous eruption. The eruptions may
appear annular. These discoid lesions may be found on the face,
neck, or scalp. In chronic cutaneous lupus, there are patches of
atrophic skin, depigmented at the center with increasing degrees
of pigmentation toward the edges. Telangiectasia, scaling, periungual erythema, and palmar erythema may also be present. Alopecia is a typical finding. However, this plugging of hair follicles
often resolves during periods of remission.

Renal Involvement

Lupus nephritis may be present in most cases of SLE. It is a benign
focal proliferative lesion that usually resolves spontaneously. A
remitting and relapsing membranous glomerulonephritis may
produce a nephrotic syndrome. A progressive renal failure may
develop. Renal insufficiency and renal hypertension may result
from a diffuse proliferative glomerulonephritis. In more than 50
percent of lupus patients with renal disease, the pathology
changes over time.

Nervous System Involvement

CNS involvement occurs in about 50 percent of patients with SLE.
Reactive depression is the most common presentation. About 20
percent of patients with SLE have an organic brain syndrome
involving varying degrees of disorientation, intellectual deterioration, and memory impairment. Approximately, 10 percent of
patients with SLE may manifest psychosis. Patients who develop
psychosis may show evidence of seizure activity. The cranial
nerves may be affected, causing facial weakness, ptosis, or diplopia. The CNS manifestations are usually transient. Even the psychosis may be episodic and will often clear dramatically. Cranial
or peripheral neuropathies, headaches, chorea, ataxia, impaired
work capacity, and impaired social functioning may also be
present.

Cardiac Involvement

The most common cardiac manifestation is pericarditis. Pericardial effusion may be present. A friction rub is often identifiable
on auscultation. Raynaud's phenomenon (cold- or stress-induced

vasospasms of the hands and feet) can be observed in 30 percent of SLE patients. About 15 percent of patients with SLE may have cardiac valvular disease. Atherosclerotic coronary artery disease may account for as many as 30 percent of SLE deaths.

Pulmonary Involvement

A possible cause of an audible friction rub could be pleural effusion. Acute or chronic parenchymal pulmonary involvement may be present in SLE. Acute lupus pneumonitis may be present. It is characterized by a sudden onset of fever and dyspnea with pulmonary infiltrates. Alveolar hemorrhage is the second most prevalent syndrome. It manifests, as the name implies, with bleeding in the lungs and an inevitable decrease in hematocrit. If not treated promptly, both syndromes can quickly progress to respiratory failure. An interstitial lung disease may develop and manifest as either inflammatory alveolitis or interstitial fibrosis. Inflammatory alveolitis responds to immunosuppressive therapy, whereas interstitial fibrosis does not. The pulmonary hypertension that can manifest in SLE presents with dyspnea on exertion. The pulmonary involvement can resemble primary pulmonary hypertension.

DIAGNOSTIC CONSIDERATIONS

The differential diagnosis includes rheumatoid arthritis, scleroderma, mixed connective tissue disease, thyroid disease, primary fibromyalgia, and Lyme disease.

SPECIAL CONSIDERATIONS

It is imperative to remember that patients with active SLE are predisposed to opportunistic infections. Another important consideration is the emotional state of patients with SLE because their psychological condition will influence their perception of pain, physical function, the successfulness of rehabilitation, and their quality of life.

Fertility is not affected by SLE, and pregnancy is not necessarily contraindicated. A patient with active SLE may experience flare-ups during pregnancy. However, there is no increased risk of flare-ups as a result of pregnancy.

LABORATORY TESTS

The diagnosis of SLE is confirmed by the finding of abnormal ANA levels (titers of 1:80 or higher). The most specific finding in active SLE is a high titer of double-stranded deoxyribonucleic acid antibodies (anti-dsDNA). Other antigen specificities that may be found in SLE are anti-DNP (deoxyribonucleoprotein), anti-RNA (ribonucleic acid), antihistones, anti-Sm (Smith), anti-nRNP (non-histone ribonucleoprotein), anti-PCNA (proliferating cell nuclear antigen), antinuclear matrix, anti-Golgi, and/or antiribosomes.

Elevated serum levels of auto antibodies to ribosomal P proteins are specific for SLE when psychiatric symptoms are present. Antineuronal antibodies are found in as many as three-fourths of patients with neuropsychiatric symptoms of SLE. High titers to anti-dsDNA are encountered in roughly 50 percent of patients with SLE. Anti-Sm antibodies are highly specific for SLE. However, they only occur in 50 percent of cases.

Antibodies to DNA can be determined by indirect immunofluorescence, immunodiffusion, counterimmunoelectrophoresis (CIE), hemagglutination, radioimmunoassay (RIA), and enzyme-linked immunoassay (ELISA).

LE cells (live neutrophils that engulf the nucleus of dead, fragmented neutrophils after being bound by ANA and comple-

ment) are found in the joint fluid, bone marrow, and pleural and pericardial effusion of more than 85 percent of patients with SLE.

Humoral immune phenomena may be uncovered by studying the immunoglobulins. Serum protein electrophoresis may demonstrate elevated gamma globulin. Lupus anticoagulants, that are sometimes seen in SLE are immunoglobulins of IgG or IgM class that bind to phospholipids. They are present in 10 percent of patients with SLE. Both congenital and acquired IgA deficiency have been associated with SLE.

Cellular immune phenomena may be demonstrated with major histocompatibility complex (MHC) of the DR3 type in more than 50 percent of cases. Complement components C3, C4, and CH_{50} (hemolytic complement) may demonstrate an alternate pattern in SLE. C3 may be normal in acute SLE, but low in active or chronic SLE. C4 may appear normal in chronic SLE but low in the acute, active state. Low CH_{50} can be associated with active SLE whether acute or chronic. Measurement of static and functional complement levels may be a useful guide to the activity of SLE in a specific patient.

The lupus band test is a skin biopsy that may be positive for IgG or IgM in more than 90 percent of specimens taken from patients with SLE. Biopsies from sun-exposed skin of the dorsum of the forearm are positive more than 80 percent of the time. However, a positive test is not specific only to SLE.

Hematologic findings may demonstrate a hemolytic anemia, leukopenia (<4000/mL), lymphopenia (<1500/mL), or thrombocytopenia (platelets <100,000/mm³). A false-positive result on the serologic test for syphilis (VDRL) is a common finding in patients with SLE.

Urinalysis may uncover proteinuria (>500 mg/day), pyuria, hematuria, and granular or red cell casts.

RADIOLOGIC STUDIES

When pulmonary involvement is suspected, a chest radiograph may indicate patchy alveolar infiltrates which can be indicative of acute lupus pneumonitis.

OTHER DIAGNOSTICS

Analysis of synovial fluid may evidence only mild inflammation. Leukocytes are typically lower than the count found in rheumatoid arthritis. Histologic synovial tissue study may reveal significantly less inflammatory response than is seen in rheumatoid arthritis. A limited joint infiltration of lymphocytes and plasma cells with marginal evidence of edema and some fibrinoid necrosis are often the only histologic synovial findings.

Magnetic resonance imaging (MRI) may be useful for revealing abnormalities associated with the neuropsychiatric manifestations of SLE. Symmetrically distributed areas of increased signal intensity in the subcortical white matter may be present in patients with cognitive dysfunction, generalized seizures, or psychosis. These abnormalities are not present when the patient is in remission.

TREATMENT

Treatment for the various presentations of SLE is controversial. Response to treatment is difficult to evaluate because the symptom patterns and course vary so greatly from patient to patient.

Pharmacologic Management

The usual treatment is with immunosuppressive drugs, such as prednisone (5 to 15 mg daily). In the majority of patients, the cutaneous lesions of SLE respond to antimalarial drugs such as chloroquine and hydroxychloroquine. In some instances arthritis and arthralgia also respond to these drugs. Maintenance therapy with hydroxychloroquine may even reduce the frequency of flare-ups. Patients found to be resistant to antimalarial medication may respond to azathioprine, dapsone, or the retinoids. Nonsteroidal anti-inflammatory medications can be useful for many patients suffering from active SLE. However, care must be taken to avoid the typical gastrointestinal side effects as well as an aspirin-induced hepatitis that may present in patients with active SLE. Salicylates must be avoided in cases of severe thrombocytopenia and when renal disease is present. The treatment of depression and fibromyalgia secondary to SLE may respond to tricyclic antidepressants and selective serotonin re-uptake inhibitors.

Supportive Measures

Bed rest is indicated for patients with active SLE. Because emotional and physical stress can have a negative impact on the immune system, patients should be encouraged to avoid high-pressure situations.

PATIENT EDUCATION

Because all SLE-related skin lesions are either precipitated or exacerbated by sun exposure, patients should be cautioned against exposure without sun block. Patients must be taught that sunlight exposure can also cause flare-ups in other organ systems, not only the skin. When exposure to sunlight cannot be avoided, patients should be instructed to use sunscreens that contain aminobenzoic acid (PABA) and also have a high protective factor (PF) rating of at least 30. Patients should also be taught relaxation techniques to use during periods of stress. Patient and family education are critical. Many symptoms of SLE improve with the proper balance of exercise, rest, and adequate stress management.

DISPOSITION

Follow-up and management depend on whether the patient is in a period of remission or exacerbation of symptoms. The prognosis for patients with SLE is difficult to determine. The most frequent cause of death is active renal disease often accompanied by complications in other organ systems as well as a superimposed infection. Any follow-up activity must be planned so as to ensure a timely intervention of management that will assist the patient in maintaining a satisfactory quality of life.

COMPLICATIONS AND RED FLAGS

Because the toxicity from corticosteroids is predictable and cumulative over time, extreme care must be taken when treating with these preparations. The incidence of herpes zoster occurring because a patient is being treated with immunosuppressive drugs can be as high as 20 percent. Steroid-induced psychosis is also a serious complication to guard against. Controversy exists over the use of postmenopausal estrogen replacement therapy in women diagnosed with SLE. There is evidence that postmenopausal estrogen is associated with an increased risk of developing SLE.

OTHER NOTES OR PEARLS

Elevated serum levels of autoantibodies to ribosomal P proteins are not associated with nonpsychiatric manifestations of SLE. They are a useful measure because they are specific for SLE only when there is severe depression or psychosis. To assist patients in understanding their condition better refer them to the Lupus Foundation of America (1-800-558-0121 or 1-301-670-9292).

BIBLIOGRAPHY

Boumpas DT, Fessler BJ, Austin HA: Systemic lupus erythematosus: Emerging concepts. I: Renal, neuro psychiatric, cardiovascular, pulmonary, and hematologic disease. *Ann Intern Med* 122:940, 1995.

Boumpas DT, Austin HA, Fessler BJ: Systemic lupus erythematosus: Emerging concepts. II: Dermatologic and joint disease, the antiphospholipid antibody syndrome, pregnancy and hormonal therapy, morbidity and mortality, and pathogenesis. *Ann Intern Med* 123:42, 1995.

Gladman DD, Urowitr MB: Systemic lupus erythematosus, in Klippel JH, Dieppe PA (eds): *Rheumatology.* London, Mosby-Year Book Europe, 1994.

McGuire JL, Lambert RE: Systemic lupus erythematosus and overlap syndromes, in Kelley WN, Dupont HL, Glick JH, (eds): *Textbook of Internal Medicine,* 3d ed. Philadelphia, Lippincott-Raven, 1997.

Mills JA: Systemic lupus erythematosus. *New Engl J Med* 330:1871, 1994.

Robinson DR: Systemic lupus erythematosus. Rheumatology, in Dare DC, Federman DD (eds): *Scientific American Medicine.* New York, Scientific American, 1996.

Rothfield NF: Systemic lupus erythematosus: Clinical aspects and treatment. Arthritis and allied conditions, in McCarty DJ, Koopman WJ (eds): *A Textbook of Rheumatology,* 12th ed. Philadelphia, Lea & Febiger, 1993.

Sanchet-Guerrero J, Liang MH, Karlson EW, et al: Post menopausal estrogen therapy and the risk for developing systemic lupus erythematosus. *Ann Intern Med* 122:430, 1995.

Schur PH: Clinical features of SLE, in Kelley WN, Harris ED, Ruddy S, (eds): *Textbook of Rheumatology,* 4th ed. Philadelphia, Saunders, 1993.

Tan EM: Auto antibodies in systemic lupus erythematosus, in McCarty DJ, Koopman WJ (eds): *Arthritis and Allied Conditions: A Textbook of Rheumatology,* 12th ed. Philadelphia, Lea & Febiger, 1993.

Wallace DJ, Hahn BH, Quismorio FP Jr, (eds): *Dubois' Lupus Erythematosus,* 4th ed. Philadelphia, Lea & Febiger, 1993.

Chapter 10–11
CARPAL TUNNEL SYNDROME
David Zinsmeister

DISCUSSION

Carpal tunnel syndrome is the most common peripheral nerve entrapment. The anatomy of the wrist causes the median nerve to be subject to compression and perhaps ischemia in the confined space formed by the carpal bones and transverse carpal ligament. The syndrome commonly occurs alone as the result of repetitive overuse; however, it may be present in association with local or systemic conditions that alter the space of the carpal tunnel. The disorder is three times more common in women than in men and occurs most often in middle age. The dominant hand is usually the first to be involved, but symptoms are frequently bilateral by the time the patient presents. Numerous studies have linked carpal tunnel syndrome to the workplace with some reporting as high as 56 percent of all cases directly attributed to occupational activities.

PATHOGENESIS

The carpal tunnel is formed by the bones of the carpus on the dorsal aspect of the wrist and the transverse carpal ligament (flexor retinaculum) on the volar aspect. Within the tunnel lies

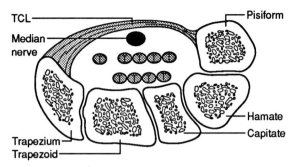

Figure 10-11-1. The carpal tunnel and its contents. TCL = transverse carpal ligament; trapezium; trapezoid; capitate; hamate; pisiform; median nerve; T = tendons.

the median nerve, the flexor digitorum superficialis and profundus tendons, the flexor pollicis longus tendon, and synovial sheaths (Fig. 10-11-1). Compression of the median nerve within this fibro-osseous canal can arise from any condition that causes an alteration in the volume of the tunnel.

Repetitive overuse is the most common cause of median nerve compression at the wrist. Actions performed repetitively in the workplace or during leisure activities may result in swelling of the synovium or thickening of the transverse carpal ligament, causing compression of the nerve. Other common local causes include osseous changes from fractures, dislocations, or arthritic changes in the bone that compromise the space within the tunnel. A variety of systemic conditions can cause the syndrome, and a complete listing can be found in Table 10-11-1. Rarely, carpal tunnel syndrome can be of familial origin.

Regardless of the causes of reduced space within the tunnel, the median nerve, which can be likened to the consistency of overcooked spaghetti, is compressed by the unyielding fibrous and osseous structures that form the tunnel or occupy it with the nerve. At the microscopic level, compression impedes the venous return of the nerve, which impairs the intrafunicular circulation. This results in increased pressure that leads to ischemia, anoxia, and impaired nutrition of the nerve. Edema occurs and protein leakage into the surrounding tissue promotes the proliferation of fibroblasts that form constrictive endoneural tissue. Finally,

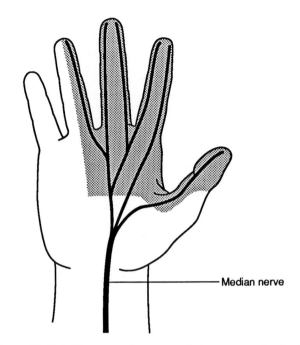

Figure 10-11-2. The normal pattern of the sensory distribution of the median nerve in the hand.

wallerian degeneration occurs with loss of axons, and the few surviving nerve fibers become encased in a dense, avascular epineurium.

Variations in the sensory and motor distribution of the median nerve must be kept in mind when evaluating a patient with suspected carpal tunnel syndrome. The palmar cutaneous branch that supplies the proximal palm exits the median nerve radially before entering the carpal tunnel. Owing to overlapping innervation from the ulnar, radial, and lateral cutaneous nerves, compression of this branch rarely causes a discernible loss of sensation in the proximal palm in the syndrome.

As the median nerve exits the carpal tunnel, its sensory fibers divide into common digital nerves, which supply the distal palm and further subdivide into the proper digital nerves near the web space, which supply the thumb and fingers. The typical sensory innervation pattern of the thumb and fingers by the median nerve includes the palmar aspect of the thumb, index finger, long finger, and the radial aspect of the ring finger. The nerves continue to supply the tips of the digits and extend dorsally to the distal interphalangeal joint of the fingers and interphalangeal joint of the thumb (Fig. 10-11-2). Common variations of this pattern include innervation of the ulnar side of the ring finger by the median nerve and ulnar nerve innervation that extends to the ulnar aspect of the long finger. Cadaver studies have shown that in 80 percent of the specimens dissected, the ulnar aspect of the ring finger was innervated by both the radial and ulnar nerves.

Distal to the transverse carpal ligament, the recurrent motor branch supplies the muscles of the thenar eminence. The typical pattern includes the abductor pollicis brevis, opponens pollicis, and flexor pollicis brevis. This pattern, however, is present in only one-third of the population. Variations include ulnar innervation to one or all of the thenar muscles or combinations of innervation by both median and ulnar nerves to the individual muscles. The terminal motor branches of the median nerve usually supply the lumbricals of the index and long fingers. The most common variation of this pattern is partial innervation of the long finger lumbrical by the median nerve.

The median nerve also carries sympathetic fibers that supply the skin, blood vessels, and sweat glands. When compression

Table 10-11-1. Causes of Carpal Tunnel Syndrome

Local	Connective tissue disorders
Repetitive overuse	Rheumatoid arthritis
Flexor tenosynovitis	Scleroderma
Wrist fractures and dislocations	Polymyalgia rheumatica
Hematomas	Systemic lupus erythematosis
Infections	Gout
Carpal tunnel stenosis	Chondrocalcinosis (pseudogout)
Exostosis/osteophytes	Amyloidosis
Ganglion cyst	
Anomalous muscles and tendons	
Endocrine disorders	Other
Diabetes mellitus	Pregnancy
Hypothyroidism	Long-term renal failure
Hyperthyroidism	Multiple myeloma
Acromegaly	Familial carpal tunnel syndrome
Calcium abnormalities	Other polyneuropathies
	Estrogen and/or progesterone
	Snake bite
	Vitamin B_6 deficiency (?)
	Idiopathic

affects the sudomotor and vasomotor fibers in carpal tunnel syndrome, trophic changes in the skin and coolness and dryness of the palm and digits occur.

SYMPTOMS

When evaluating a patient with suspected carpal tunnel syndrome, it is necessary to keep in mind the seemingly endless variety of terms that a patient may use to describe the symptoms. Although terms such as paresthesia (tingling), dysesthesia (an unpleasant perception to a normal stimulus), and hypesthesia (an elevated threshold to stimulus perception) have very specific implications, patients speak in terms of "numbness, crawling bugs, and burning pain." Further affecting the patients' inability to communicate their experience is the anatomic and physiologic differences between the A-delta and C fibers that are responsible for nociception.

A-delta fibers are responsible for the ability to sense acute pain. They are dense and myelinated, and have the ability to transmit rapidly via direct pathways to specific areas of the cortex. C fibers, which are responsible for sensation in chronic conditions, are sparse and unmyelinated but transmit slowly and are integrated with several other pathways before they reach a wide area of the cortex. Since carpal tunnel syndrome is a chronic compression neuropathy, transmission of the patient's sensations occurs primarily through C-fiber pathways. This results in the inability to describe precisely the sensation felt or define its exact location.

At the onset, the symptoms of carpal tunnel syndrome are usually preceded by activities such as typing, use of vibrating tools, or doing fine detail work that requires the wrist to be flexed. Early in the course of the process, the pain is intermittent and is described as a dull ache at the wrist during or shortly after use. As time progresses, the patient classically complains of burning pain, numbness, and tingling in the areas of the hand supplied by the median nerve. As compression of the nerve continues, the symptoms become constant and more severe. The pain may begin to radiate up the arm and can be felt as high as the shoulder. The pattern may develop where the patient wakes up 2 to 3 h after retiring because of pain and numbness in the hand. This is due to the loss of conscious control of the wrist extensors while sleeping, which causes the wrist to flex, thus narrowing the carpal tunnel.

Clumsiness and weakness are common complaints with the syndrome and can be attributed to both altered sensation and muscle weakness. Patients may report dropping objects and the inability to perform fine motor skills that require the use of the thumb and index finger. These symptoms suggest involvement of the recurrent motor branch of the median nerve that innervates the muscles of the thenar eminence and the terminal motor branch that supplies the lumbricals.

When asked to demonstrate what is done to relieve their symptoms, most patients shake their wrist. This is known as the *flick sign* and is common in patients with carpal tunnel syndrome.

OBJECTIVE FINDINGS

When inspecting the hand and wrist, the examiner should make note of the color, temperature, and texture of the skin and the presence or absence of thenar muscle atrophy. With the exception of advanced cases of carpal tunnel syndrome with severe compression of the median nerve, the inspection portion of the examination should be normal. At the end stages of long-standing compression, the tips of the thumb, index finger, long finger, and ring finger become smooth, cool, and dry, which represents trophic changes of sensory and autonomic impairment. Atrophy of the thenar muscles is a late finding and when present indicates that sensory involvement and weakness are advanced.

The sensory examination should begin by asking the patient to outline the area of sensory abnormality. Once this is defined, testing by light touch is frequently all that is required to confirm the involved area. If results are negative, a gentle pin prick is useful to reveal the deficit. Two-point discrimination is often a late finding and, if affected, typically is 1 cm or greater. In the normal, uncalloused hand two-point discrimination is 5 to 6 mm. To obtain a baseline, the unaffected hand and the ulnar distribution of the affected hand should be tested first, since a 1- to 2-mm variance in two-point discrimination can be expected. Testing of vibratory sense with a tuning fork is useful when evaluating polyneuropathies but is of limited value in compression neuropathies such as carpal tunnel syndrome.

Phalen's test is a provocative method of eliciting symptoms in patients without objective neurologic deficits and has been found to be positive in 76 percent of the patients with carpal tunnel syndrome. This test can easily reproduce the symptoms by having the patient markedly flex the wrist for 1 min. After 1 min has elapsed, paresthesias or numbness in the distribution of the median nerve occur if compression is present. Even if paresthesias do not develop, sensory examination will typically reveal areas of hypesthesias within the sensory distribution of the median nerve. It must be noted that paresthesias will develop in normal persons if wrist flexion is sustained long enough and will result in a false-positive Phalen's sign.

Tinel's sign can be elicited by tapping along the course of the nerve as it passes under the transverse carpal ligament. A positive Tinel's is present when paresthesias are reproduced by the tapping. Pain at the wrist without paresthesias should be considered percussion tenderness and does not constitute a positive Tinel's sign. The symptoms produced by Phalen's and Tinel's tests may not be present equally in the sensory distribution of the median nerve. This is due to the arrangement of the nerve fibers with those supplying the long finger being closest to the transverse carpal ligament.

The motor examination is usually normal except in advanced cases of the syndrome. When motor deficits are noted, severe compression of the median nerve is present. Motor testing is normally limited to the abductor pollicis brevis since it is the least likely of the thenar muscles to receive innervation from the ulnar nerve and is the easiest to isolate. The abductor pollicis brevis is tested for strength by having the patient abduct the thumb away from the palm against resistance. It is important to ensure that the thumb is in a plane perpendicular to the palm when conducting this test; otherwise, the extensor muscles will assist with the movement.

DIAGNOSTIC CONSIDERATIONS

A listing of local and systemic conditions that are associated with the syndrome can be found in Table 10-11-1. These processes can be eliminated by the absence of other symptoms and signs noted during the general history and physical examination. It is of prime importance to exclude entrapment of the median nerve at other levels or nerve root involvement (Fig. 10-11-3).

Entrapment of C6 or C7 spinal nerve roots can also cause pain and paresthesias in the fingers innervated by the median nerve along with pain in the forearm and shoulder. Nerve root involvement, however, is usually accompanied by pain and stiffness in the neck and is rarely bilateral or develops the pattern of night pain. In addition, nerve root entrapment at these levels will cause pain and paresthesias in the dorsal aspect of the hand and involves the reflexes and motor strength at higher levels in the upper extremity.

Thoracic outlet syndrome may mimic carpal tunnel syndrome in that thenar atrophy may present. The sensory abnormalities

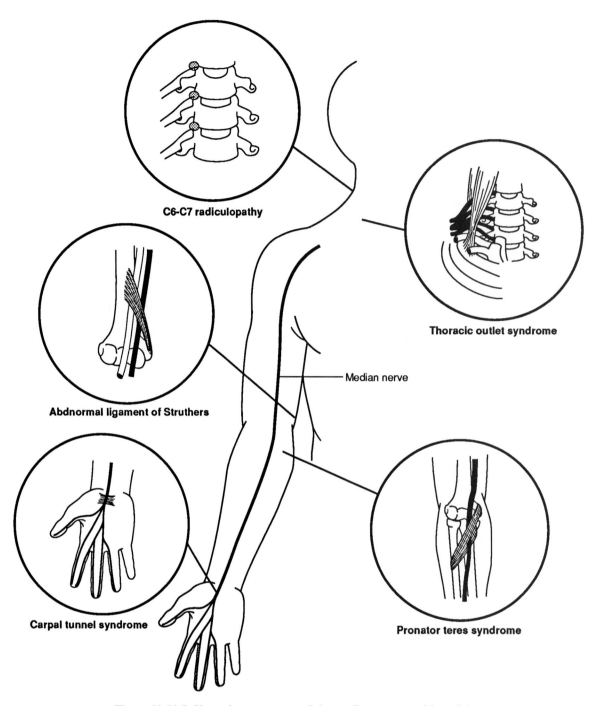

C6-C7 radiculopathy

Thoracic outlet syndrome

Abdnormal ligament of Struthers

Median nerve

Carpal tunnel syndrome

Pronator teres syndrome

Figure 10-11-3. Sites of entrapments of the median nerve and its origins.

in thoracic outlet syndrome differ and present in the dermatomes of C8 and T1 and involve the ring and little fingers and the medial aspect of the forearm.

In 2 percent of the population a spur occurs at the medial supracondylar region of the distal humerus. When the spur is present, the ligament of Struthers may be abnormally attached to it and form a canal through which the median nerve and brachial artery pass. Compression may occur with repetitive flexion of the elbow and resemble carpal tunnel syndrome. In addition to the picture of median nerve compression, the classic presentation of pain, pallor, pulselessness, paresthesias, and paralysis that indicates arterial occlusion occurs in the regions distal to the elbow that are supplied by the brachial artery.

Compression of the median nerve can occur at the proximal forearm where the nerve passes between the two heads of the pronator teres. The symptoms associated with pronator teres syndrome are an aching pain in the anterior aspect of the forearm that is worsened by activities that involve repeated pronation and pain and paresthesias in the median nerve distribution in the hand. Physical examination findings include a hard, tender pronator teres and a Tinel's sign over the muscle.

A small number of patients may have carpal tunnel syndrome and another coexisting neuropathy that contributes to their symptoms. Most commonly a cervical radiculopathy is the other process involved. When this occurs, the term *double crush syndrome* is applied. Although no evidence exists to establish whether there is a pathologic connection or the conditions coexist purely by chance, double crush syndrome should be suspected in the patient with profound symptoms or an atypical presentation of carpal tunnel syndrome.

DIAGNOSTIC STUDIES (NERVE TESTING)

Nerve conduction velocity (NCV) and electromyogram (EMG) are valuable studies that can be readily obtained to aid in the diagnosis of carpal tunnel syndrome. NCVs can be performed on both motor and sensory nerves. To test the motor portion of the median nerve in carpal tunnel syndrome, electrodes are placed at various points along the nerve to stimulate the abductor pollicis brevis. The latency, which is the time from the onset of the stimulus until the muscle responds, is then measured. From this conduction velocity, amplitude and duration can be obtained. If a sensory portion of the median nerve is being tested, an electrode is placed proximal to the transverse carpal ligament and a recording of the potential is obtained distally. As with motor testing, sensory responses are calculated and reported in terms of conduction velocity, amplitude, and duration.

Conduction velocity is a direct measurement of latency and records the time from stimulus to response. In carpal tunnel syndrome, conduction velocity is delayed owing to the demyelination of median nerve fibers. Amplitude represents the number of functioning myelinated fibers that can carry the stimuli and is reduced in carpal tunnel syndrome. Duration indicates the uniformity of the conduction velocity of the axons and is increased (dispersed) if carpal tunnel syndrome is present.

EMG examination of suspected carpal tunnel syndrome consists of inserting a needle electrode into the abductor pollicis brevis and measuring the electrical activity when the muscle is relaxed and again when it is fully contracted. During full relaxation the electrical activity of the abductor pollicis brevis is silent if the muscle is normal. If carpal tunnel syndrome is present and wallerian degeneration has occurred and the axons are disrupted, the denervated muscle spontaneously fires during relaxation and produces fibrillation potentials and positive sharp waves. Fibrillation potentials on the EMG resemble the pattern of atrial fibrillation on electrocardiography (ECG), and positive sharp waves look very similar to a pathologic Q wave found in myocardial infarction. Fibrillation potentials and positive sharp waves can be found in a variety of muscle disorders and should therefore not be considered diagnostic of carpal tunnel syndrome.

RADIOLOGIC (IMAGING) STUDIES

Radiographs of the wrist may reveal an osseous cause for median nerve compression at the wrist. Malunion of old fractures of the radius, ulna, and carpal bones along with arthritic spurs may extend into the tunnel and reduce its space. Posteroanterior lateral, oblique, and carpal tunnel views are routinely used to evaluate the wrist. Computed tomography has been used to evaluate the size of the carpal tunnel in research but has yet to provide a direct correlation to the clinical syndrome and is not routinely used. Magnetic resonance imaging has provided a means to view the median nerve, tendons, sheaths, and transverse carpal ligament, but as with computed tomography, the clinical relevance of MRI findings is lacking.

TREATMENT

Conservative treatment of carpal tunnel syndrome consists of splinting the wrist in the neutral position and avoiding repetitive activities of the hand and wrist. Anti-inflammatory agents are prescribed to reduce the inflammation and swelling of the synovial tissues. Corticosteroid injections into the carpal tunnel are useful adjuncts in treatment. If injections are utilized, the median nerve should be avoided. The purpose of the steroid is not to treat the nerve directly but to reduce the inflammation and swelling of the surrounding synovium. Referral to a therapist for tendon gliding exercises and custom splinting is also helpful in the conservative management. These modalities reduce or eliminate the symptoms in about two-thirds of the patients with mild to moderate compression neuropathy.

Patients who fail to respond to conservative therapy or who have marked symptoms such as sensory loss, weakness, or atrophy at the time of presentation are candidates for surgery. In most cases the procedure simply consists of releasing the transverse carpal ligament through an incision in the palm. If indicated, some patients may require a synovectomy or neurolysis. Endoscopic release is frequently employed and facilitates early hand mobilization. Compression dressing and splinting are continued for several weeks postoperatively, followed by supervised therapy. Most patients report resolution of pain, paresthesias, and nocturnal symptoms once the incisional pain has dissipated. Return of full sensation and strength may take several months after the surgery. If thenar atrophy is present preoperatively, the recovery period can be prolonged.

COMPLICATIONS AND RED FLAGS

Complications most commonly reported include wound infection, incomplete relief of symptoms, prolonged scar pain, and return of the syndrome after initial surgical success. In rare instances reflex sympathetic dystrophy, bow-stringing of the flexor tendons, and joint contractures occur.

BIBLIOGRAPHY

Goldner RD, Goldner JL: Compression neuropathies of the hand and forearm, in Sabiston DC (ed): *Textbook of Surgery,* 15th ed. Philadelphia, Saunders, 1997, pp 1479–1486.

Griffin JW, Peripheral neuropathies, in Stobo JD, (ed): *The Principles and Practice of Medicine,* 23rd ed., Stamford, CT, Appleton & Lange, 1996, pp 881–889.

McCue FC, Alexander EJ, Baumgarten TE: Median nerve entrapment at the elbow in athletes. *Operative Techniques Sports Med* 4(1):21–27, 1996.

Palmar D: Carpal tunnel syndrome in athletes. *Operative Techniques Sports Med* 4(1):33–39 (1996).

Stewart JD: *Focal Peripheral Neuropathies,* 2d ed. New York, Raven, 1993.

Venna N: Peripheral neuropathies, in Noble J (ed): *Textbook of Primary Care Medicine,* 2d ed. St Louis, Mosby, 1996, pp 1408–1431.

Chapter 10–12
CERVICAL STRAIN AND SPRAIN
Stephen M. Cohen

DISCUSSION

The neck injury termed *whiplash* was first described by an American orthopedist in 1928. Cervical strain (muscle-tendon injury) and/or sprain (ligamentous injury) primarily involves damage to the soft tissues of both the anterior and posterior neck. Although most episodes are the result of hyperextension forces, hyperflexion and rotational forces may also cause injury to soft tissue. This injury primarily affects adults. Motor vehicle collisions, diving accidents, and falls account for the primary mechanisms in this injury.

The damage to soft tissue is directly proportional to the forces applied and creates a continuous scale of injury from minimal to severe. Any structure in the neck can be damaged by the forces of extreme or rapid flexion, extension, or rotation. Muscle, tendons, ligaments (such as anterior longitudinal), the esophagus, trachea, nerve roots, sympathetic chain, and fascia may all be damaged. Resulting tissue swelling and inflammation can compound the initial damage.

Often overlooked in neck injury is the risk of cerebral concussion and contusion. When the head is thrown forward, rapid deceleration occurs as the neck flexes to the full forward position. However, the brain continues its forward movement (as a result of inertia) and strikes the frontal cranial vault. Similar injury can occur posteriorly as the head decelerates when the neck goes into full extension. This phenomenon may explain much of the brain damage noted in "shaken baby syndrome." As a result of the brain injury, many patients experiencing cervical strain or sprain injury have abnormal electroencephalograms (EEGs) and associated complaints. This underappreciated phenomenon may account for many of the psychiatric and cognitive symptoms in patients with chronic complaints after neck injury.

SIGNS AND SYMPTOMS

The most common symptoms reported at presentation are acute, delayed, or chronic headache; dizziness; hearing loss; visual disturbances; alterations in smell or taste; and difficulty in cognitive function (primarily word differentiation, concentration, and short-term memory).

Symptoms are extremely variable depending on forces applied, mechanism and degree of injury, and chronology of presentation. Headache is often described as tension-like, starting at the base of the skull near the suboccipital triangle or occiput, shoulders, or midback. The common complaint of muscle spasm can affect thoracic back, neck, shoulders, and facial muscles.

Aggravation or acute onset of temporal mandibular joint dysfunction and pain have been reported. In a delayed or chronic presentation the pain of the original injury can be recreated by triggers such as posture and stress days, weeks, or months after the injury.

OBJECTIVE FINDINGS

Often there are delayed symptoms with cervical strain or sprain. As soft tissue swelling progresses, neck musculature becomes stiff and may progress to painful spasm. Neck range of motion often becomes decreased. Pain often centers around neck and suboccipital region, although symptoms may include upper back and shoulder pain if spasm persists and spreads caudally.

The mechanics of neck injury may cause symptoms to begin from any previous injured disk herniation or musculoskeletal condition. Underlying and preexisting disease processes in the neck that may precipitate pain in flexion or extension injuries include arthritis, disk annulus fracture, microtears and herniation, and spondylosis. The pain from underlying neck entities is often of a magnitude that exceeds what might be expected with a given mechanism of injury. Additionally, the mechanics of injury may facilitate new fracturing of the disk annulus or facet joint surfaces.

Neurologic examinations are most often normal or without significant findings. Severe mechanical injury may stretch nerve roots and the sympathetic nerve chain, causing symptoms of blurred vision, tinnitus, nausea, vomiting, and occasional dizziness. Pronounced neck and upper back spasm can present with numbness and tingling sensations superficially, but rarely will be confused with peripheral nerve or radicular injury. If unilateral sternocleidomastoid muscle damage and swelling occurs, torticollis of varying degrees may also occur acutely.

DIAGNOSTIC CONSIDERATIONS

Diagnosis and proper evaluation begin with a complete history and physical examination with concentration on the musculoskeletal and neurologic component of the head, neck, upper torso, and extremities. Careful examination should focus on discovery of underlying and preexisting conditions separate from the often obvious soft tissue injury.

SPECIAL CONSIDERATIONS

Many cervical injuries, especially from motor vehicle accidents, present "packaged" by emergency medical personnel to the emergency department. The use of rigid collar and backboard in these cases demands attention to neurologic evaluation and consideration of more severe injury. Proper evaluation and judgment is necessary to guide the removal of these appliances. At a minimum, a full lateral roentgenogram (visualizing completely to the C7-T1 disk space) should be accomplished prior to removal of any prehospital applied collars.

LABORATORY STUDIES

With injury secondary to forceful trauma of unknown cause, a blood alcohol, drug screen, glucose, and complete blood cell count (CBC) may be warranted. Laboratory examination to evaluate extent of cervical soft tissue injury is not necessary or helpful separate from determining the medical cause of the injury, or contributing factors leading to the mechanism of the injury.

RADIOLOGIC STUDIES

Radiographic evaluation in sprain or strain injury most often is normal. Progression of symptoms, muscle spasm, and increased chronicity can cause reversal of the normal curvature on lateral neck films. This presentation is often noted by chiropractic examination, but is insignificant on initial presentation unless accompanied by degenerative changes or segmental collapse. Correlation with long-term structural changes has not been shown.

Although only 80 to 85 percent accurate at detecting abnormality, the anterior-posterior (AP) and the lateral plain roentgenogram of the cervical spine are considered the minimal examination to rule out structural abnormality. Serious bony injuries have been detected in "minor" presentations of neck pain and stiffness after low-velocity events. Although uncommon, a high index of suspicion should be present in the evaluation of all neck injury.

The essence of radiologic examination is to rule out subluxation or fracture associated with soft tissue injury. A concerted effort must be made to clearly visualize C1-C7 with preference for seeing the top of T1 if possible. A "swimmer's" view of C7 may be necessary if this cannot be accomplished. Lateral examinations can often be utilized to assess the severity of prevertebral, soft tissue swelling. Attention must be directed to the alignment of spinous processes on AP views of the cervical spine to detect malrotation defects and ligamentous rupture in the rotational plane.

In addition to AP and lateral radiographs, flexion and extension views can be very helpful, some say essential, in delineating and defining ligamentous injury in whiplash. The practitioner should remember the significant part the ligamentous structures play in stabilization. The degrees of "kinking," or kyphosis, and "fanning," or spread of spinous processes, are useful observations to separate minor soft tissue injury from more significant ligamentous tears. Wide-spaced spinous processes on lateral radiographs may indicate complete disruption of ligamentous structures.

OTHER DIAGNOSTICS

CT and MRI may be indicated to evaluate extent of swelling and damage. These examinations may also be utilized to delineate

Table 10-12-1. Muscle Relaxant Medications

Metaxalone, 400 mg (Skelexin)	800 mg 3–4 times daily for 7–10 days	For muscle spasm pain, not in renal or hepatic deficiency. Watch for drug-induced anemia. Must take regularly to gain blood levels.
Cyclobezaprine, 10 mg tabs (Flexeril)	10 mg, 3 tid for muscle spasm; 60 mg maximum; no longer than 3 weeks	Danger in cardiac disease, thyroid disease, or with MAOIs. May cause drowsiness, dizziness, GI upset, HA = headache.
Orphenadrin citrate, 100 mg (Norflex), sustained release	100 mg bid for painful muscle spasm	Contains sulfites. Precautions: coronary disease, arrythmia, asthma. Interacts with anticholinergic, ETOH and CNS depressants. May cause tachycardia, dizziness GI upset, urinary retention.
Chlorzoxazone (Parafon Forte)	500 mg qid; 750 mg max qid	Potentiation hazard with CNS depressants and alchol. GI upset not uncommon. Heptacellular toxicity (rare).
Methocarbamal (Robaxin)	1.5 g 4 times daily for 48–72 h, then 4 g daily (divided)	May potentiate CNS depressants. Drowsiness, dizziness, GI disturbance, blurred vision, HA reported.
Carisoprodol (Soma)	350 mg 4 times daily	Contraindicated in prophyria. Potentiates CNS depressants; May cause orthostatic hypotension, rash, tachycardia, epigastric distress.

NOTE: MAOI = monoamine oxidase inhibitor; HA = headache; ETOH = ethyl alcohol.

small or occult fractures associated with the injury. Bone scans are generally not indicated, since most will be "hot" throughout the area due to acute inflammation and swelling. Tomograms may also assist in the visualization of occult or suspected fractures but are not helpful in acute presentations.

TREATMENT

Pharmacologic Management

Nonsteroidal anti-inflammatory medications (NSAIDs) in combination with analgesics given in amounts necessary to relieve pain in the acute phases are essential. Muscle relaxant medication, such as metaxalone or methocarbamol, in combination with salicylate or anti-inflammatory medication for acute spasm is also well tolerated and assists in the most common cause of acute pain.

Rarely is diazepam (Valium) or narcotic necessary in either the acute or chronic stages, and both should be avoided if possible. Regardless of the medication, care must be taken to ensure proper instruction, patient use, and follow-up. None is intended for use in children, and caution must be used in adolescents. The most common musculoskeletal pain and spasm medications are noted (see Table 10-12-1).

Vitamin C in dosages of 500 to 1500 mg orally per day may assist in the healing of soft tissue and is a useful adjunct in the treatment of suspected soft tissue damage in the cervical spine region. Commercially available OTC preparations are sufficient and cost effective for this purpose.

In severe cases with suspected transient cord compression, methylprednisolone given within 8 h of injury may be helpful in preventing more permanent cellular changes in the soft tissue zone of injury, especially if nerve tissue is involved centrally or peripherally. These patients require hospitalization and MRI or CT evaluation of spinal cord and column.

Supportive Measures

Aggressive application of conservative treatment modalities are essential in whiplash injury. Rest with 48 to 72 h (primary inflammatory period) of cold-pack therapy is beneficial in reducing inflammation and acute pain. Treatment in the acute injury should then be followed by physical examination to reassess symptoms. Moist hot packs, manual muscle therapy, trigger point manual therapy, electrical stimulation, and other modalities can relive the pain and spasm associated with injury once the primary inflammatory period has passed.

Although many clinicians recommend a soft foam collar for support in the early phases of injury, there is no proven stabilization with their use. Soft collars appear not to alter the degree of persistent pain in those patients who develop chronic syndromes. The use of soft collars may lead the patient to long-term, psychological dependency on such appliances and is not recommended.

Once the acute inflammatory phase has passed, range-of-motion (ROM) must be preserved with slow and controlled movement. Once motion becomes stiff and reduced from full range, it may be difficult to recover full motion as time progresses. Gentle ROM exercise in a warm shower twice daily is very beneficial to facilitate early motion of a stiff neck. This may be begun as early as 4 to 7 days after injury, depending on severity and results of follow-up examination.

Aerobic exercise is also recommended to ensure circulatory enhancement in the area of injury. Walking, bike riding, swimming, and easy jogging are best to decrease jarring of high-impact exercise. Recommend a program of three to four sessions of exercise per week for 20 to 40 min/day. The usual precautions in prescribing aerobic exercise to any patient should be employed, including evaluation of other anatomic and physiologic subsystems.

PATIENT EDUCATION

Patient education and support are vital in the acute injury and chronic syndrome. The emotional impact of this injury can be disabling and severe. Many patients describe not being "believed" and being treated indifferently by practitioners, which causes great anxiety in the patient with chronic or reoccurring symptoms. Depression is also an extremely common diagnosis in chronic pain syndromes of the neck. Support and complete patient education throughout the process of therapy, which may be months or years, is vital to a positive outcome. "Learn to live with it" instruction is often unjustified, since improvement is possible with attention and persistent conservative treatment.

The regularly prescribed use of muscle relaxant and anti-inflammatory medication cannot be stressed enough in the acute phase of this injury (24 to 72 h). The patient must clearly understand that waiting until symptoms begin or get worse is often "too late." PRN (as needed) instruction has no place in the treatment of the acute phase of whiplash injury.

DISPOSITION

Most patients recuperate from this type of injury in 30 to 60 days with conservative care. The remaining 35 percent continue to have varying degrees of symptoms from months to years. Approximately 18 percent have persistent symptoms that they attribute to the primary traumatic event after 2 years. Most of this group have identifiable preexisting conditions prior to injury. Relapse and setback in treatment commonly cause the patient to become frustrated with therapy. This is to be expected and is a normal course for strain or sprain injury to the cervical spine. The practitioner should be patient and attentive to these concerns.

As the patient begins to heal, triggering events may cause setback, pain, and spasm. Posture (work, sleep, and recreation), stress, recreational activity, and other environmental factors can stimulate muscle spasm and acute pain attacks. Psychological support and therapy modalities should be utilized to break spasm cycles, gain patient confidence, and facilitate long-term healing and dealing with the injury. This may involve months or years.

Permanent laxity of supporting structures may be identified after the conversion to a chronic pain syndrome. Chronic pain presentations after injury demand regular evaluation for instability and structural changes. This is especially true in any new or progressive radiculopathy after strain or sprain injury.

COMPLICATIONS AND RED FLAGS

Immediate attention should be directed at any neurologic deficit (paresthesia, muscle weakness, loss of reflexes, sensory loss, or radiculopathy) or radiographic evidence of more severe bony injury. Any deficit in the acute presentation should be considered for additional studies such as MRI and immediate stabilization with rigid collar system and neurologic consultation.

Any difficulty swallowing or talking should alert the evaluator to the possibility of significant soft tissue swelling in the neck. Airway support may be indicated in severe injuries and should be available. Facial or chest injury alerts the examiner to the strong possibility of more severe underlying bony injury in head, face and/or spine.

The examiner should remain alert to signs and symptoms that indicate more severe injury or complications. Epidural hematoma, internal carotid artery occlusion, abducens nerve palsy, and retropharyngeal hematoma have been reported in whiplash injury. Additionally, any transient ischemic attacks, dizziness, or similar events within 3 months of a whiplash injury should alert the practitioner to the possibility of circulatory injury, especially in the posterior cerebral system.

NOTES AND PEARLS

Any acute strain or sprain injury of the cervical spine can aggravate preexisting cervical inflammatory or degenerative processes. Old radiographic studies should be obtained for comparison, when possible, because vital information can be helpful in evaluating pain syndromes. Additionally, facet arthritides cannot be ignored. Degenerative facet joint surfaces, when aggravated by acute strain or sprain injuries, can manifest with severe spasm and a chronic course.

Those patients with small vertebral canal architecture (congenital small diameter) appear to have a more chronic course and worse prognosis. In such cases, the stretch and microtears of superficial neural structures adjacent to and including the cord may inhibit expeditious recovery.

Patient support and rigorous patient education as to the use of medication, modalities, range of motion, heat or cold therapy, and support systems is often the difference between patient satisfaction and treatment failure. Rapid and aggressive management of the acute trauma may avoid or substantially reduce the chronic pain syndromes after neck injury.

BIBLIOGRAPHY

Griffiths HJ, Olson PN, Everson LI, et al: Hyperextension strain or "whiplash" injuries to the cervical spine. *Skelet Radiol* 24(4):263–266, 1995.

Helliwell PS, Evans PF, Wright V: The straight cervical spine: Does it indicate muscle spasm? *J Bone Jt Surg Ser B* 76:103–106, 1994.

Mercier LR: *Practical Orthopedics.* St Louis, Mosby, 1995.

Pennie BH, Agambar LJ: Whiplash injuries. *J Bone Jt Surg Ser B* 72:277, 1990.

Praemer A, Furner S: *Musculoskeletal Conditions in the United States.* Park Ridge, IL, American Academy of Orthopedic Surgeons, 1992.

Radanov BP, Sturenegger M, DiStefano G: Long-term outcome after whiplash injury. A 2-year follow-up considering features of injury mechanism and somatic, radiologic, and psychosocial findings. *Medicine* 74(5):281–297, 1995.

Viktrup L, Knudsen GM, Hansen SH: Delayed onset of fatal basilar thrombotic embolus after whiplash. *Stroke* 26(11):2194–2196, 1995.

Chapter 10–13
HIP FRACTURES
David Zinsmeister

DISCUSSION

The term *hip fracture* applies to fractures of the proximal femur. Common locations for fracture are the femoral neck, intertrochanteric region, and subtrochanteric region, with isolated fractures of the greater and lesser trochanter occurring less frequently. Stress fractures of the hip are becoming more prevalent, and the hip is a relatively common site of pathologic fracture. Fractures of the femoral head occur with dislocation of the hip and fracture of the acetabulum and are not generally considered to be hip fractures.

Femoral neck fractures occur at the subcapital, neck, and basicervical regions. Intertrochanteric fractures are defined as having the primary fracture line extending between the greater and lesser trochanter, and subtrochanteric fractures are those with the primary fracture between the lesser trochanter and a point 5 cm distal. Each type of fracture has variants that significantly alter treatment and prognosis based on the anatomic and biomechanical influences at the fracture site (see Boxes 10-13-1 and 10-13-2).

PATHOGENESIS

As the average age of the population has increased, the incidence of hip fractures has climbed dramatically. Between 1965 and 1981, the number of hip fractures tripled. Currently, more than 275,000 hip fractures occur each year in the United States, with the estimated cost of treatment exceeding $6 billion. By the year 2040, the incidence of hip fracture is projected to be 500,000 per year. Among medicare patients, the rate of fracture was highest in the South and lowest in the Northeast.

Age, sex, and race place certain individuals at a higher risk for hip fracture. About 85 percent of all hip fractures occur in individuals over 65 years old. By age 80, 93 percent of all women will have sustained at least one fracture, 33 percent of which will be a hip fracture. White women are at twice the risk for hip fractures as are blacks and Hispanics and at 2.7 times the risk as white men.

BOX 10-13-1

SKELETAL AND VASCULAR ANATOMY

Cortical bone is thinnest at the femoral neck and contributes to the higher incidence of fractures in this area. The metaphyseal region is largely trabecular bone and contains the calcar femorale, a dense plate of cortical bone that serves as a posteromedial buttress. Intertrochanteric and subtrochanteric fractures involving this buttress create instability in this region and increase the risk of malunion and nonunion. The proximal femoral diaphysis consists largely of cortical bone, and when subtrochanteric fractures occur, there is less surface area for healing, and this may lead to delayed union, nonunion, and malunion.

The proximal femur receives its blood supply from branches of the femoral artery and the foveal artery (Fig. 10-13-A). The retinacular arteries supply the neck and most of the femoral head. Although the foveal artery provides blood to the femoral head, its contribution alone is not sufficient to sustain viability. Therefore, disruption of the retinacular vessels in femoral neck fractures increases the likelihood of osteonecrosis of the head and nonunion.

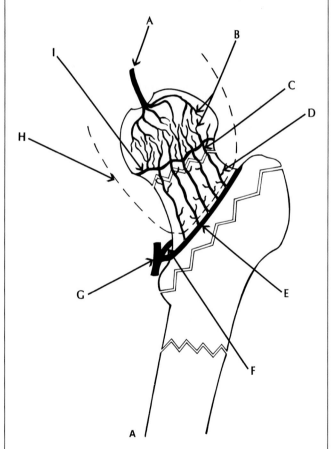

Figure 10-13-A. Vascular anatomy of the proximal femur. *A.* Foveal artery. *B.* Epiphyseal arteries. *C.* Retinacular arteries. *D.* Metaphyseal arteries; extracapsular arterial ring. *E.* Lateral femoral circumflex. *F.* Medial femoral circumflex. *G.* Femoral artery. *H.* Capsule. *I.* Intracapsular arterial ring.

BOX 10-13-2

BIOMECHANICS

Forces applied across the hip from body weight and muscle can amount to three times body weight in a single-limb stance. In the early 1900s, James Koch,[1] using theoretical analysis, calculated that compression stress at the medial cortex of the subtrochanteric region exceeds 1200 lb/in^2. This was confirmed more than 50 years later using strain gauge measurements.

Franklin Ward in 1838 was the first to describe the trabecular orientation of the proximal femur that represents the bone's response to stress, known as Wolff's law. He identified five trabecular groups that result from bone formation in response to compression, tension, and muscle counterbalance.

In 1976, M. Singh[2] devised a grading system for osteoporosis that is based on the disappearance pattern of these trabecular groups, as determined by x-ray films. The trabeculae in Ward's triangle are the first to disappear, followed by the secondary compressive, secondary tensile, primary tensile, and eventually the primary compressive groups. The disappearance pattern is a useful guide to estimate the degree of osteopenia present (Fig. 10-13-B).

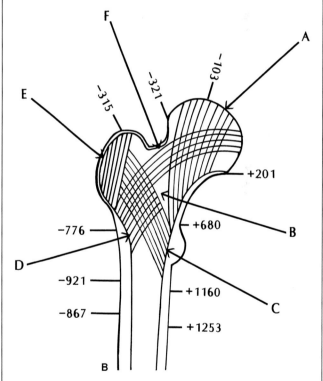

Figure 10-13-B. The bone's response to forces across the hip. Trabecular group patterns as described by Ward. *A.* Primary compressive. *B.* Ward's triangle. *C.* Secondary compressive. *D.* Secondary tensile. *E.* Greater trochanter. *F.* Primary tensile. Numbers on periphery indicate pounds per square inch as calculated by Koch. Positive numbers represent compressive stress; negative numbers indicate tension stress.

The relationship of osteoporosis and osteomalacia to hip fracture has been studied extensively. Although they are not causes of hip fracture, they are contributing factors. Osteoporosis (decreased density with normal mineralization) and osteomalacia (decreased mineralization) result in a density or mineralization level below what is required for mechanical support. It has been reported that by age 65, 50 percent of all women will have a bone density or mineral content below the threshold required for fracture and that by age 85, 100 percent of women are below this threshold (see Chap. 5-2).

Radiographically, osteoporosis and osteomalacia are indistinguishable. Clinical manifestations, laboratory studies, and noninvasive methods to determine bone density help differentiate between the two processes, but bone biopsy is required for definitive diagnosis.

Other risk factors include the use of psychotropic drugs, Alzheimer's disease, excessive alcohol intake, and a prior history of hip fracture.

Mortality rates within the first year after injury vary from 14 to 21 percent. Patients with significant medical problems (American Society of Anesthesiologists III/IV) had a 1-year mortality rate of 49.4 percent as compared with 8.0 percent for healthier patients. Patients are at the greatest risk of death within the first year after injury, and the mortality rate 1 year after fracture is comparable to that of the age and sex-matched population that has not sustained hip fracture.

HISTORY

Hip fractures in the young adult usually result from high-energy trauma, such as motor vehicle accidents or falls from great heights. In the absence of a history of either of these injuries, inquiry should be made concerning alcohol use, current medications, and medical conditions that may have predisposed the patient to fracture from a simple fall. A history of insidious groin pain that occurs with increased activity in a young, active adult may indicate stress fracture.

In the elderly, hip fracture occurs with minor trauma such as falls in the home, missteps, and twisting injuries. Preexisting medical conditions such as diabetes mellitus, cardiac arrhythmias, disorders of equilibrium, cancer, arthritis, and neurologic conditions that result in muscular paresis, weakness, and instability are common and may initiate the fall. Current medications should also be assessed as possible contributing factors. In patients older than age 75, the fall is more likely to be caused by organ failure than accident.

OBJECTIVE FINDINGS

In young adults with a hip fracture, concomitant injuries resulting from high-velocity trauma are common and should be aggressively sought. Common coexisting injuries include those of the chest, abdomen, spine, and head of a life-threatening nature that require emergency treatment. Once life-threatening injuries are stabilized, obvious injuries of the extremity should not become the total focus of attention and preclude a complete orthopedic examination. Subtle hip fractures are occasionally missed because of a more dramatic fracture of the ipsilateral femoral shaft (Fig. 10-13-1). In contrast, hip fractures in the elderly are usually isolated injuries. The physical examination should be complete and ensure both that medical conditions are stabilized before surgery and that previously unrecognized conditions are identified and treated.

Physical findings on examination of the hip vary, depending on the location of the fracture and degree of displacement. In a

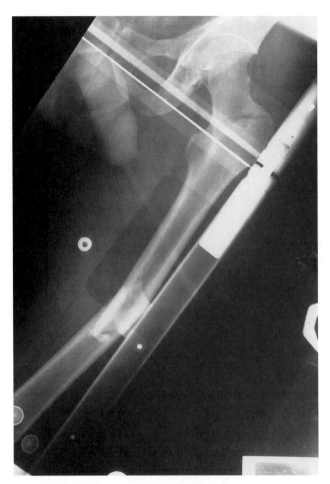

Figure 10-13-1. Fracture of the femoral shaft and ipsilateral basicervical fracture of the proximal femur in a polytrauma patient.

stress fracture of the femoral neck the patient may be ambulatory with an antalgic gait. Range of motion usually is normal, and tenderness may be elicited over Scarpa's triangle. Displaced femoral neck fractures present with the classic findings of shortening, abduction, and external rotation of the injured extremity. Any attempt at motion elicits extreme pain. In the case of an impacted or nondisplaced femoral neck fracture, the patient may remain ambulatory for several days before presentation with physical findings similar to a femoral neck stress fracture.

Intertrochanteric fractures have the features of the displaced femoral neck fracture except that a greater degree of external rotation and generalized hip tenderness with swelling exists. Subtrochanteric fractures result in varus angulation distal to the greater trochanter. This physical finding is caused by the pull of the hip abductors and flexors on the proximal fragment and adductors on the distal fragment. Hip examination findings vary with pathologic fractures, depending on the type of tumor, its location, and the extent of cortical involvement.

RADIOLOGIC AND IMAGING STUDIES

Good quality anteroposterior (AP) radiographs of the pelvis and AP and true lateral films of the hip are the mainstays in the diagnosis of hip fracture. If hemiarthroplasty or total hip arthroplasty is being considered, a low AP view of the pelvis should be obtained for component measurement. Tomograms are helpful in detecting discrete, nondisplaced femoral neck fractures.

FEMORAL NECK FRACTURES

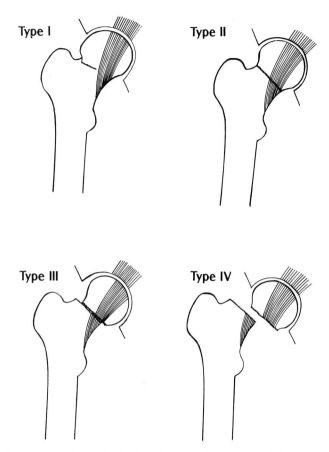

Figure 10-13-2. Garden's classification of femoral neck fractures. *(From Garden[3] with permission.)*

Technetium 99m scanning assists in the diagnosis of nondisplaced and stress fractures of the femoral neck and aids in tumor evaluation. Currently, computed tomography and magnetic resonance imaging have a limited role in traumatic fractures of the hip but help in the evaluation of the cortex and medullary canal in pathologic fractures.

TREATMENT

Femoral Neck Fractures

Femoral neck fractures are classified by Garden[3] into four types based on the amount of displacement shown on prereduction radiographs (Fig. 10-13-2). Type I is an incomplete or complete fracture, impacted with valgus angulation of the head; type II is a complete fracture without displacement; type III is a complete fracture with partial displacement; and type IV is a complete fracture with total displacement.

Type I and type II fractures are considered stable because of preservation of the retinacular vessels and carry the best prognosis. The displaced type III and type IV fractures are comminuted posteriorly, which renders the fracture unstable and results in a higher incidence of nonunion and osteonecrosis resulting from vascular insufficiency to the femoral head.

General agreement exists that in the young, active adult the femoral head should be preserved and the fracture internally

fixed with multiple pins or screws. When treating the elderly patient, most authors advocate pin or screw fixation in type I (Fig. 10-13-3) and type II fractures and hemiarthroplasty or total hip arthroplasty for type III and type IV (Fig. 10-13-4) fractures under certain conditions. Relative indications for selecting arthroplasty over internal fixation include physiologic age over 70, failure to achieve adquate reduction, advanced arthritis, osteogenic bone stock, Parkinson's disease, spastic hemiplegia, and pathologic fracture. Both internal fixation and arthroplasty have been reported as acceptable forms of treatment for displaced femoral neck fracture in the elderly, but a consensus on optimal treatment has not been reached.

Intertrochanteric Fractures

The integrity of the posteromedial buttress is of prime importance in intertrochanteric fractures. Posteromedial comminution and fracture extension result in loss of stability and varus collapse. Kyle and Gustilo's modification[4] of Boyd's classification of intertrochanteric fractures recognizes four basic types of fractures based on the location and degree of comminution that affects stability (Fig. 10-13-5). Type I is a stable, nondisplaced intertrochanteric fracture; type II is a stable, displaced intertrochanteric fracture with fracture of the lesser trochanter and varus deformity; type III is an unstable, displaced intertrochanteric fracture with fracture of the greater trochanter, posteromedial comminution, and varus deformity; and type IV is an unstable, displaced intertrochanteric fracture with subtrochanteric extension, pos-

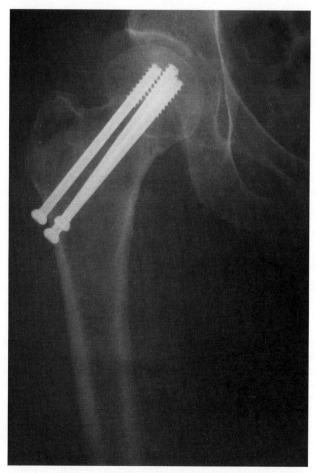

Figure 10-13-3. Type I femoral neck fracture in an elderly woman. The fracture is internally fixed with cannulated screws.

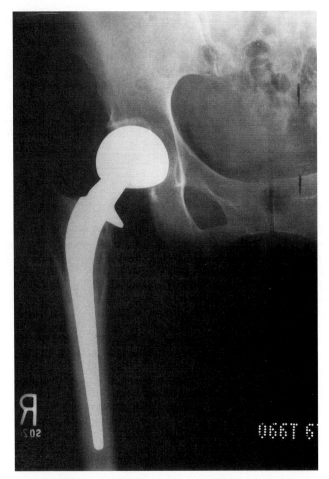

Figure 10-13-4. Postoperative radiograph of a patient with a type IV femoral neck fracture treated with cemented bipolar hemiarthroplasty.

teromedial comminution, fracture of the greater trochanter, and varus deformity.

Internal fixation of intertrochanteric fractures centers around correcting the varus deformity and regaining and maintaining stability. The sliding compression screw and side plate device is usually used to treat stable and unstable fractures. It allows controlled impaction of the fracture and resists deforming forces (Fig. 10-13-6).

Subtrochanteric Fractures

Russell and Taylor's classification system[5] for subtrochanteric fractures incorporates extension of the fracture into the piriformis fossa and posteromedial cortex, a process that alters treatment and prognosis (Fig. 10-13-7). Within this classification system, a type I fracture does not extend into the piriformis fossa, type II involves the fossa, A indicates sparing of the posteromedial cortex, and B indicates comminution and inadequate posteromedial support. This combination results in four fracture types: IA, IB, IIA, and IIB, with IA having the best prognosis and IIB the worst.

With the piriformis fossa and lesser trochanter intact, type IA fractures are treated with standard intramedullary nailing that locks into the calcar femorale. Type IB fractures that are comminuted posteromedially, thus preventing locking in this region, are internally fixed with a reconstruction nail that locks in the femoral head (Fig. 10-13-8). Type II fractures that involve the fossa and prevent nail introduction are treated with a compression screw

and side plate device that stabilizes the fracture. Indirect reduction techniques and bone grafting are helpful adjunctive methods in these difficult cases.

Stress Fractures of the Femoral Neck

A recent prospective study of 1049 stress fractures identified 54 femoral neck stress fractures in 49 patients. Numerous classification systems for this type of fracture exist, and all center around the involvement of the compression and tension cortices. If only the compression side is involved (Fig. 10-13-9), treatment consists of rest and restricted weight bearing. In the case of tension side fracture, disruption of both cortices, or displacement, the fracture is internally fixed with multiple parallel pins or screws. Callus, sclerosis, and fracture may not be apparent radiographically for several weeks after the onset of pain, and scintigraphy is required for early diagnosis and assessment of the tension side.

Pathologic Fractures

Metastatic neoplasms are the most common malignant bone tumor, with the femur being fourth in frequency of osseous sites for metastasis. Primary tumors that frequently metastasize to bone are breast, lung, thyroid, kidney, and prostate, with hematogenous spread being the usual route. Radiation therapy is the principal treatment modality for bony metastasis, and the goals of internal fixation are pain relief, restoration of function, and early mobilization, thus enhancing quality of life and facilitating provision of care.

Indications for internal fixation of impending pathologic fractures are a painful lesion more than 2.5 cm in diameter or destruc-

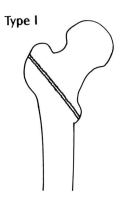
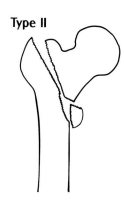
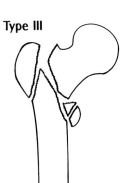
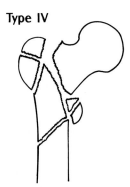

Figure 10-13-5. Kyle and Gustilo's modification of Boyd's classification of intertrochanteric fractures. *(From Kyle[4] et al with permission.)*

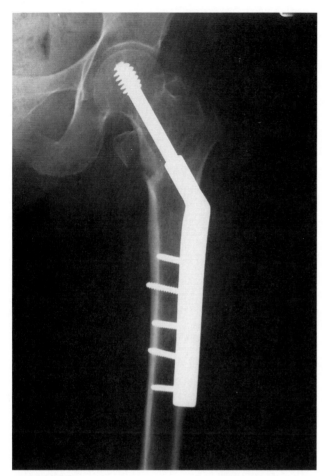

Figure 10-13-6. Type III intertrochanteric fracture after internal fixation with a sliding compression screw and side plate device.

tion of more than 50 percent of the cortex. In addition to sparing the patient the painful experience of acute fracture, fixation of impending pathologic fractures results in lower surgical mortality and fewer complications.

SPECIAL CONSIDERATIONS

Indications for the nonoperative treatment of hip fractures are rare. Operative fixation is generally considered the conservative option with relative contradications limited to nonambulatory, severely demented patients in little pain and those with life-threatening conditions who are at a high risk of death from anesthesia. However, patients with severe traumatic brain injury can experience spontaneous and often dramatic recovery. Therefore, if otherwise indicated, operative fixation of the fracture should be accomplished under the optimistic assumption that the patient will achieve normal ambulatory status.

AFTERCARE

The principal goals of aftercare of all hip fractures are early mobilization and prevention of complications. The patient should sit upright within the first 24 h after surgery and begin assisted touchdown weight bearing as soon as tolerated. Progression to full weight bearing with cane or walker is advanced during the next 6 to 12 weeks, depending on fracture type. Hip and knee range-of-motion exercises are initiated and advanced during the process of fracture healing.

Various methods exist for using prophylactic anticoagulants in hip fracture patients. The goals of therapy are to provide adequate

protection against thromboembolic disease and decrease the risk of bleeding. Support stockings, foot pumps, and elevation of the extremity also help venous return. Prophylactic cephalosporin antibiotics are used and continued for 24 to 72 h postoperatively. Discharge planning for the elderly should include an evaluation of the home environment and often requires the assistance of social service and home nursing agencies.

COMPLICATIONS AND RED FLAGS

Early significant complications are wound infection and thromboembolic disease. Elderly patients are more susceptible to cardiac failure, pulmonary insufficiency, and genitourinary infections, especially if immobilization is prolonged. The polytrauma patient is at an increased risk for adult respiratory distress syndrome, shock, and disseminated intravascular coagulation.

Osteonecrosis and nonunion continue to be the main complications of displaced femoral neck fractures in young adults treated with pins or screws. The incidence of nonunion and osteonecrosis ranges from 5.5 to 14 percent and 19 to 33 percent, respectively. Complications for elderly patients treated with arthroplasty include component loosening, acetabular erosion, and heterotopic ossification. Reoperation rates for component loosening and acetabular erosion have been reported as 13.7 percent for fixed femoral head devices and 7.2 percent for cemented bipolar prosthesis. Heterotopic bone formation of significance occurs in 1 to 2 percent of arthroplasty patients.

Complications of intertrochanteric and subtrochanteric fractures treated with a sliding compression screw and side plate device are penetration of the femoral head and neck and device failure resulting in nonunion and malunion. Failure rates vary, depending on fracture stability, from 4.8 to 11.5 percent in inter-

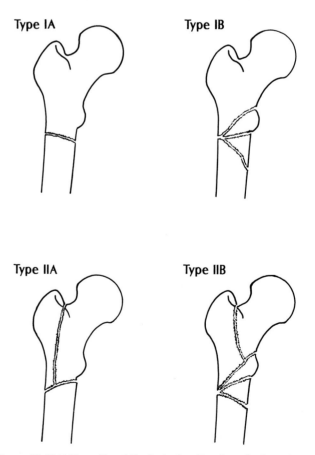

Figure 10-13-7. Russell and Taylor's classification of subtrochanteric fractures. *(From Russell[5] with permission.)*

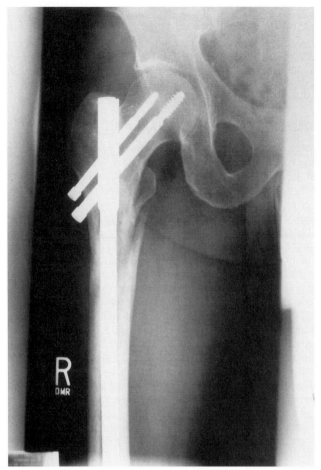

Figure 10-13-8. Type IB subtrochanteric fracture after fixation with an interlocking reconstruction nail introduced into the piriformis fossa.

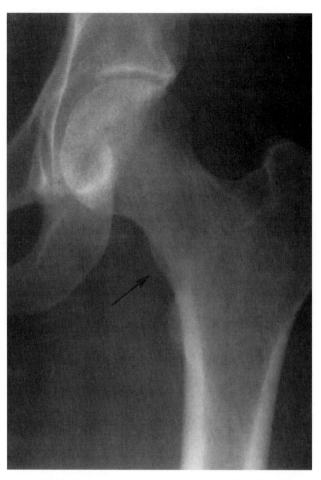

Figure 10-13-9. Callus formation *(arrow)* indicating stress fracture of the compression cortex.

trochanteric fractures and a reported nonunion rate of 5 percent in a variety of subtrochanteric fractures. In subtrochanteric fractures treated with interlocking medullary nailing, delayed union, and nonunion are occasionally reported.

NOTES AND PEARLS

The incidence of hip fracture can be expected to increase as the average life expectancy for Americans becomes longer. In the elderly population, white women with type I osteoporosis are at the greatest risk for hip fracture from minor trauma. High-energy trauma is the predominant cause for hip fracture in young adults, who frequently sustain concomitant life-threatening injuries.

The primary diagnostic tool in the evaluation of hip fractures is fracture classification based on plain radiographs. To be usesful, a classification system must guide appropriate treatment and indicate prognosis. Numerous classifications exist, and the practitioner should consider the strengths and weaknesses of each when selecting a classification system.

Surgery is the treatment of choice for fracture of the hip with few contraindications. Femoral neck, intertrochanteric, and subtrochanteric fracture are the types usually encountered, each with its own variants that alter treatment and prognosis. Aftercare of the patient with fracture of the hip is individualized on the basis of the patient's needs, with early mobilization and the prevention of complications being common goals in the treatment of all hip fractures.

REFERENCES

1. Koch JC: The laws of bone architecture. *Am J Anat* 21:177, 1917.
2. Singh M, Nagrath AR, Manini PS: Changes in the trabecular pattern of the upper end of the femur as an index of osteoporosis. *J Bone Jt Surg* 52A:457–467, 1976.
3. Garden RS: Low angle fixation in fractures of the femoral neck. *J Bone Jt Surg* 438:647, 1961.
4. Kyle RF, Gustilo RB, Premer RF: Analysis of 622 intertrochanteric hip fractures: A retrospective and prospective study. *J Bone Jt Surg* 61A:216–221, 1979.
5. Russell TA: Fractures of the hip and pelvis, in Crenshaw AH (ed): *Campbell's Operative Orthopaedics,* 8th ed. St Louis, Mosby Year Book, 1992, vol 2, pp 895–987.

BIBLIOGRAPHY

DeLee JC: Fractures and dislocation of the hip, in Rockwood CA, Green DP (eds): *Fractures in Adults,* 3d ed. Philadelphia, Lippincott, 1996, vol 2, pp 1659–1826.

Laros GS: Intertrochanteric fractures, in Evarts CM (ed): *Surgery of the Musculoskeletal System,* 2d ed. New York, Churchill Livingstone, 1990, vol 3, pp 2613–2639.

Lhowe DW: Intracapsular fractures of the femoral neck, in Evarts CM (ed): *Surgery of the Musculoskeletal System,* 2d ed. New York, Churchill Livingstone, 1990, vol 3, pp 2549–2592.

Michelson JD, Cowen EL, Morris MT: Epidemiology of hip fractures among the elderly. *Clin Orthopaed Rel Res* 311:129–135, 1995.

Zinsmeister DE: The diagnosis and treatment of hip fractures. *J Am Acad Physician Assist* 8(6):542–551, 1993.

Chapter 10–14
EVALUATING TRAUMATIC KNEE PAIN

David Zinsmeister
Howell J. Smith III

DISCUSSION

History

Pain, to a greater or lesser extent, is a feature of any traumatic process involving the knee. When eliciting a history of traumatic knee pain, it is useful to develop a systematic approach that is all-inclusive so as to avoid the pitfall of focusing on the pain rather than the associated symptoms and signs that are of significance in establishing the diagnosis.

Pain related to trauma is rapid in onset, and the patient is evaluated at an early point in the process, usually within hours or days. A key feature in evaluating pain due to trauma is the mechanism of injury. With an understanding of the anatomy of the knee and the biomechanical forces that act on the knee, the clinician can, in the interview process, identify the structures involved, question the patient on related symptoms, and confirm the diagnosis with an equally systematic approach to the physical examination (Fig. 10-14-1).

Mechanism of Injury

A sudden twisting of the knee with the foot planted, knee flexed, and tibia internally rotated may tear the anterior cruciate ligament (ACL), medial collateral ligament (MCL), or medial meniscus. With the knee in this position, the anterior cruciate ligament is taut. If enough force is applied either by forward momentum or a force applied from behind (a clipping injury), the ligament is stretched beyond its elastic limits and is torn. As the ligament tears, the tibia translates anteromedially and can shear the medial meniscus. If enough valgus stress is applied during a clipping-type injury, fibers of the MCL may also be torn.

When a pure varus or valgus stress is applied to the knee, the primary and secondary stabilizers can be involved. The primary stablizer for the medial aspect of the knee is the medial collateral ligament, with the secondary stabilizers being the anterior and posterior cruciate ligaments. The lateral aspect of the knee is stabilized primarily by the lateral collateral ligament, and the anterior and posterior cruciate ligaments provide secondary support.

A history of a major force applied just below the knee joint, which forces the tibia posteriorly, or a sudden stop such as stepping in a shallow hole can cause an isolated tear of the posterior cruciate ligament (PCL) or posteriorly dislocate the knee and damage the popliteal artery.

A direct fall on the knee will involve the anterior structures of the knee. Commonly injured are the bursae, patella, and the articular surface of the femur. Fracture of the patella may result, as well as osteochondral fracture of the articular cartilage of the patella or femur. Because of its unprotected location, the prepatellar bursa is usually involved to some degree in any injury, however minor, to the anterior surface of the knee from blunt trauma.

Knee pain originating from trauma of the extensor mechanism requires violent contraction of the quadriceps against resistance. This is commonly seen in basketball players during a rebound play when an attempt is made to extend the weight-bearing leg against the downward force of the body. When this occurs, the extensor mechanism can sustain four types of injury:

1. A tear of the quadriceps tendon
2. A transverse fracture of the patella
3. A tear of the patellar tendon
4. An avulsion of the tibial tubercle

Patella dislocation can occur as a result of virtually any rotational force on the knee. Because of the alignment of the proximal and distal tendinous attachments, and the pull of the vastus lateralis, the patella dislocates laterally and in the process tears the medial retinaculum. The patient usually gives a history of a twisting injury to the knee and a deformity that followed. Since most patella dislocations spontaneously reduce, the deformity is not present when the patient presents.

Effusion

Effusion is the presence of free fluid within the joint. The two primary types of effusion in the acutely injured knee are blood and synovial fluid. The onset of the effusion in relationship to the injury is a key differentiating point in establishing clinically whether the effusion is secondary to bleeding or from the accumulation of synovial fluid. Bleeding within the knee can come from four sources:

1. A torn ligament
2. A torn tendon
3. A fracture
4. A torn meniscus

The tibial intracondylar artery lies on the anterior surface of the anterior cruciate ligament and is covered by the ligamentum mucosa. When the ACL is stretched or torn, the artery is damaged and the joint fills with blood. Since this is arterial bleeding, the effusion is rapid and the artery continues to bleed until enough blood accumulates within the knee to tamponade the bleeding. The typical history obtained when an anterior cruciate ligament is torn is that of an inversion injury to the knee followed by a massive, rapid effusion that is present within 5 to 10 min following the injury.

The vascular supply to the meniscus is limited to the outer one-third, with the central two-thirds being avascular. This had led to the terminology of the *red zone* (vascular) and the *white zone* (avascular) being applied to meniscal tears. The terms are more than descriptive since treatment and prognosis are also dependent on the zone of injury. When a meniscus is torn within the red zone, bleeding occurs but at a much slower rate than when the ACL is torn. The pattern of the effusion in a meniscal tear is what appears to be minor swelling at the time of injury but is noted to be a pronounced effusion when arising the next day. This is due not only to the accumulation of blood within the knee but also to inflammation of the synovium secondary to bleeding, which causes the production of synovial fluid within 6 to 8 h. If a meniscal tear occurs within the white zone, fluid forms, but usually at a slower rate.

Locking

True locking occurs when the knee is unable to be fully extended because of a mechanical obstruction. When trying to elicit this symptom during the history, it is important to be careful in questioning the patient. When carefully questioned, most patients who feel locking is present actually describe stiffness. When true locking occurs, it is usually unexpected and the patient is unable to extend the knee past a given point. The end point of extension is usually the point of maximum pain, and to fully extend the knee past the obstructed end point, some type of manipulation

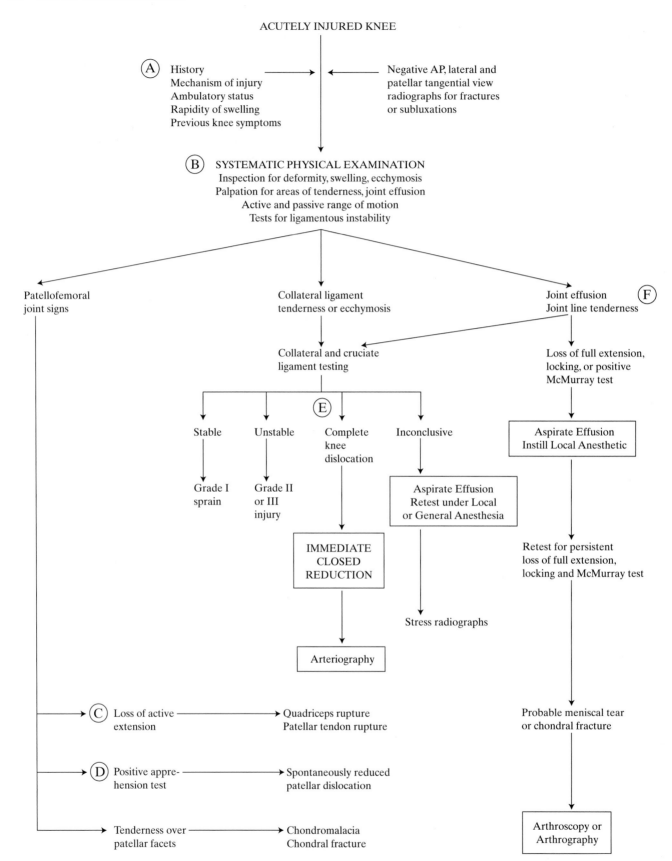

Figure 10-14-1. Algorithm for the evaluation of traumatic knee pain. *(Published with permission from RW Buchholz, FG Lippert, DR Wenger (eds): Orthopaedic Decision Making. Toronto, Decker, 1984, pp 46–47.)*

on the behalf of the patient is required, a pop is felt, and the knee will freely move again.

The most common cause of knee locking is a torn meniscus. Locking, however, will occur only if the torn portion is detached from the central body of the meniscus to the point where it will freely extend into the joint and impinge between the femur and tibia. Other causes of locking include an osteochondral fracture that is detached and free to migrate within the joint (joint mouse) and a large tibial remnant of a torn anterior cruciate ligament.

Instability

Patients usually describe instability as "giving way" and, when present, it indicates injury to the primary or secondary ligamentous stabilizers of the knee. Isolated tears of the MCL and lateral collateral ligament (LCL) rarely produce symptoms of instability. In contrast, tears of the ACL and PCL typically cause pronounced symptoms. ACL tears are noted by most patients to be symptomatic when pivoting is attempted; however, some may experience marked "giving way" in straight-line walking.

PHYSICAL EXAMINATION

General

The patient should be dressed to allow full exposure of both lower extremities from the feet to the upper thighs. For ambulatory patients, the knee examination begins by assessing gait. A gross assessment can be performed by observing the patient as he or she walks into the examination room. Both lower extremities should be inspected for symmetry (quadriceps atrophy, gross effusion), general condition of the skin (erythema, ecchymosis, abrasions, wounds), and range of motion. The examiner should then carefully palpate the bony structures, joint lines, muscles, ligaments, tendons, bursae, and popliteal area, noting areas of tenderness or edema. Generally, range of motion and other specialized tests are performed on the uninjured knee first. This gives the examiner a baseline for comparison as well as demonstrates to the patient the maneuvers that will be performed on the injured knee.

Palpation

A careful and systematic palpation of the bony and soft tissue structures of the knee can provide the examiner with a considerable amount of information as to what structures may be involved in the injured knee. Palpable tenderness in the acutely injured knee is typically pinpoint and is a key diagnostic indicator as compared with the generalized tenderness found in chronic knee pain. Since many of the knee's contours disappear when the knee is fully extended, more accurate information can be obtained when the knee is palpated in a flexed position. One of the easiest positions for both the patient and examiner is to have the patient sit on an examination table with the examiner sitting on a stool facing the patient. An alternative position is to place the patient supine and flex the knee. Either of these two non-weight-bearing positions relaxes the muscles, tendons, and ligaments surrounding the knee joint.

Palpation of the anterior aspect of the knee should begin with the extensor mechanism and proceed from proximal to distal to include the quadriceps tendon, patella, patellar tendon, and tibia tubercle. Any tenderness or defects in these structures can indicate injury to the mechanism. The medial retinaculum should also be examined. Tenderness along the medial retinaculum, with or without a palpable defect, may be the only indication of a patella dislocation that has spontaneously reduced. The examination should then proceed to the femoral condyles. Tenderness along the condyles may indicate the presence of an osteochondral fracture.

There are four bursae located around the anterior aspect of the knee that can be a cause of pain in the traumatized knee:

1. The prepatellar bursa
2. Superficial infrapatellar bursa
3. Deep infrapatellar bursa
4. The pes anserine bursa

The prepatellar bursa overlies the patella, the superficial and deep infrapatellar bursae are anterior and posterior to the patellar tendon, and the pes anserine bursa is located at the flare of the medial tibial plateau, just medial to the tibia tubercle. When palpating the bursae, swelling, crepitus, and tenderness are key signs that indicate traumatic inflammation that may be the source of pain.

The medial and lateral joint lines should then be palpated for defects and tenderness. Since several overlying structures are present at the joint lines, palpation must continue beyond the joint lines to isolate the structures involved. When palpating for the medial meniscus, the tibia should be internally rotated. In this position the medial meniscus becomes more prominent along the upper medial tibial plateau both anteriorly and posteriorly. The lateral joint line should be examined in a similar manner to detect any tenderness that may indicate a lateral meniscal tear. Palpation of the joint lines should extend to the posterior aspect of the knee since the posterior horn of the meniscus is a common location for tears. Tenderness in this region may be the only finding to indicate meniscal pathology.

In addition to meniscal tears, central joint line tenderness may indicate damage to the MCL or LCL. When central tenderness is noted at the medial joint line, palpation should continue proximally to the medial epicondyle of the femur and distally to the medial tibial plateau. If central tenderness is noted at the lateral joint line, the central area should be palpated from the lateral epicondyle of the femur to the head of the fibula. Any tenderness extending into the regions described above helps the examiner to differentiate a ligament injury from meniscal pathology.

The posterior area of the knee should be palpated for the pulse of the popliteal artery, which lies deep to the fascia, posterior tibial nerve, and popliteal vein. Since the artery is well protected, it is rarely injured except in posterior dislocations of the knee. However, the artery should be palpated in all cases of traumatic knee pain to exclude vascular compromise due to swelling.

Measuring Range of Motion

Range of motion is measured with the patient lying supine. The patient is then instructed to raise the entire lower extremity with the knee fully extended as high as possible off the table and hold it at the end point. Flexion of the thigh is actually due to contraction of the iliopsoas muscle but is critical to ensure that the leg has adequate clearance off the table. The patient is then instructed to flex the knee as far as possible (try to touch the posterior thigh with the heel of the foot) and a measurement of flexion is taken with a goniometer. The patient is then asked to extend the knee as far as possible, and a measurement of extension is recorded. In the normal knee, the range of motion arc is from 0° of extension to 135° of flexion.

In the event of a disruption of the extensor mechanism, the leg cannot be extended actively despite the patient's best efforts, and must be supported against gravity. If a large tear of a meniscus is present and displaced into the joint, the patient is able to fully flex the knee; however, extension blocks at a given point (locked knee). This can be confirmed by the examiner attempting to passively extend the knee. If the examiner cannot passively extend the knee past the same point, then mechanical obstruction of extension is confirmed. Comparison of active and passive knee extension is also useful to help differentiate extension lag from flexion contracture in the patient with chronic knee pain.

Measuring Quadriceps Atrophy

Appreciable quadriceps atrophy is most commonly the result of a chronic knee problem and typically involves the vastus medialis. This muscle is responsible for the last 30° of extension and is the first to atrophy if a condition is present that prevents the patient from achieving full extension. An acute injury may present with atrophy but should prompt the examiner to inquire about previous injuries. Quadriceps atrophy, if noted visually, should be confirmed and quantified by measuring the circumference of both quadriceps muscle groups at a specified point proximal to the superior pole of the patella and comparing the measurements. The measurements should then be documented comparing the right and left circumferences in centimeters and the distance from the superior pole of the patella at which the measurement was obtained. An example of documenting the finding would be

Circumferential quadriceps measurements obtained 10 cm proximal to the superior pole of the patella: right 45 cm, left 43 cm.

Tests for Joint Effusion

Two tests commonly used to detect the presence of an effusion are the bulge test and patella ballottement test.

- The *bulge test* is performed with the patient in the supine position with the knees fully extended and relaxed. The suprapatellar pouch is then massaged or "milked" distally while the examiner inspects for a bulge at the medial sulcus, which, if present, indicates the presence of an effusion.
- The *patella ballottement test* is performed with the knee in the same position as described above. When performing this test, the examiner applies downward pressure to the patella, compressing it against the femoral condyle. If an effusion is present, the examiner will appreciate a click when the downward pressure is applied.

Tests for Meniscal Pathology

Two tests are used to test for meniscal pathology: the McMurray test and the Apley compression/distraction test.

- The *McMurray test* is the maneuver most commonly used to detect tears in either the medial or lateral meniscus. To perform the test, the patient is placed in the supine position and the knee is passively flexed. To test the medial meniscus, the leg is internally rotated by grasping the ankle with one hand and applying a slight valgus stress to the knee with the other and then slowly bringing the knee to full extension. To test the lateral meniscus, the leg is externally rotated and varus stress is applied. A palpable or audible click that occurs at the joint line when the knee approaches full extension suggests a meniscal tear. To determine that the click originates from the joint line, the examiner should place the palm of the hand used to apply the varus or valgus stress over the patella and the thumb and index finger at the joint lines since clicks and clunks can come from other structures within the knee. It is important to keep in mind that a meniscal tear may be present even if the McMurray test fails to elicit a click at the joint line. The stress and rotation maneuvers applied to the knee while performing the test force the femoral condyle to glide over the torn portion of the meniscus and to displace it; the click is produced when the femoral condyle slips off the torn portion. If the tear is too small for the condyle to displace, no click will occur, but the patient will usually still experience pain or discomfort.

- The *Apley compression/distraction test* is another method used for detection of meniscal pathology and is helpful in differentiating the source of medial and lateral joint line pain. The test is performed with the patient in the prone position with the knee flexed to 90°. The examiner then exerts downward pressure on the foot. By applying downward pressure, the menisci are compressed between the femoral condyles and the tibial plateau and, if a tear is present, pain can be elicited at either the medial or lateral joint lines. If the patient does not experience pain on compression, the examiner then stabilizes the thigh with one hand and pulls upward on the leg with the other. If the joint line pain is due to an injury of the medial or lateral collateral ligaments, pain will be elicited upon distraction.

Tests for Ligamentous Stability

Due to the wide variation of ligamentous laxity among individuals, the uninjured knee should be examined first to establish a baseline. Some patients have extremely "tight" knees, whereas others have "loose" knees. The variance is so great that the uninjured knee in a patient with a significant degree of ligamentous laxity will resemble a complete ligament tear in the patient with normally tight knees.

The MCL and LCL are tested by applying varus and valgus stress to the knee. To perform these tests, the patient is placed in the supine or sitting position and the examiner supports the lower extremity with the knee fully extended to facilitate complete relaxation of the quadriceps and hamstring muscles. To test the MCL, valgus stress is applied by pressing on the lateral aspect of the knee while at the same time distracting the leg laterally. To test the LCL, varus stress is applied by pressing on the medial aspect of the knee and simultaneously distracting the leg medially.

The knee should be examined for joint laxity by applying valgus and varus stress with the knee in full extension and flexed to 30°. With the knee in full extension, the ACL and PCL act as secondary stabilizers and may prevent the examiner from appreciating the full extent of injury sustained by the MCL or LCL. With the knee flexed to 30°, the ACL and PCL are relaxed and the joint line opens significantly if a complete disruption (third-degree sprain) of the ligament has occurred. If a first-degree sprain (stretching) or second-degree sprain (partial disruption) is present, the patient experiences pain when the MCL or LCL is stressed, but the joint line does not open.

The integrity of the ACL is best assessed by the *Lachman test*, which is well tolerated, if performed correctly, by patients with acute ACL tears. To perform the test, the patient is placed in the supine position on the examination table and the examiner stands next to the injured knee. The patient is then instructed to relax all muscles and to remain supine during the examination. Most patients attempt to partially sit up to view the test; however, this causes the quadriceps and hamstrings to contract, which produces a false-negative test. The examiner then stabilizes the distal femur just above the knee with one hand and passively flexes the knee to 15° with slight external rotation. The tibia is then grasped with the other hand just below the knee, and a downward motion is applied to the femur while an upward motion is applied to the tibia. If the ACL is intact, the degree of tibial translation in relationship to the femur should be equal to that of the uninjured knee. If the extent of tibial translation is greater, but has a soft end point, the ACL is partially torn. If the tibia freely translates anteriorly from the femur, the ACL is completely torn.

The integrity of the ACL can also be determined by the *anterior drawer test*. This test is also performed in the supine position, but the hip and knee are flexed and the patient's foot is flat on the table. The examiner stabilizes the extremity by lightly sitting on the foot from the side of the examination table. The hands of the examiner are then "cupped" around the proximal tibia into the popliteal fossa, and the examiner gently pulls the proximal tibia forward to assess the amount of anterior tibial translation in relationship to the femoral condyles. To perform the posterior drawer test to assess the integrity of the PCL, the examiner simply pushes the proximal tibia posteriorly to determine the amount of posterior tibial translation in relationship to the femoral condyles.

NOTES AND PEARLS

The acutely injured knee should be examined as soon as possible since edema, point tenderness, and discoloration are initially localized over the injured structures. Over time, as the edema, ecchymosis, and tenderness become more diffuse, isolating the specifically injured structures becomes more difficult. A careful neurovascular examination should be performed, especially with an edematous knee, since the popliteal vessels are frequently injured with posterior knee dislocations. The inability to bear weight, guarding to prevent movement of the knee joint, and marked edema or ecchymosis are signs that are highly suggestive of a severe injury.

BIBLIOGRAPHY

Bradford DS, Pashman RS, Hu SS: Orthopedics, in Way LW (ed): *Current Surgical Diagnosis & Treatment,* 19th ed, Norwalk, CT, Appleton & Lange, 1994, pp 1011–1129.

Caldwell GL, Allen AA, Fu FH: Functional anatomy and biomechanics of the meniscus, in Drez D, DeLee JC (eds): *Operative Techniques in Sports Medicine.* Philadelphia, Saunders, 1994, vol 2, no 3.

DeHaven KE: Acute ligament injuries and dislocations, in Evarts CM (ed): *Surgery of the Musculoskeletal System,* 2d ed. New York: Churchill Livingstone, 1990, vol 4, pp 3255–3282.

Giles RS, Scott N, Insall JN: Injuries of the knee, in Rockwood CA, Green DP (eds): *Fractures in Adults,* 4th ed. Philadelphia, Lippincott, 1996, vol 2, pp 2001–2126.

Greenleaf JE: Physical diagnosis of collateral ligament and combined ligament injuries, in Drez D, DeLee JC (eds): *Operative Techniques in Sports Medicine.* Philadelphia, Saunders, 1996, vol 4, no 3, pp 148–157.

Seidel HM, Ball JW, Dains JE (eds): *Mosby's Guide to Physical Examination,* 3d ed. St Louis, Mosby, 1995, pp 644–711.

Chapter 10–15
OSGOOD-SCHLATTER DISEASE
Patti Pagels

DISCUSSION

Osgood-Schlatter disease is an overuse syndrome that occurs exclusively in young people (ages 8–18) causing pain, swelling,

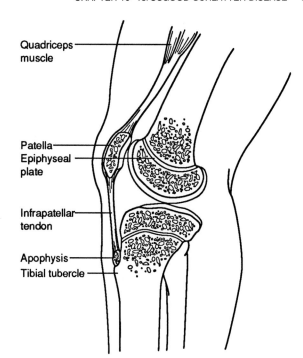

Figure 10-15-1. Lateral view of tibial tubercle, apophysis, and quadriceps muscle.

and erythema of the anterior tibial tubercle (see Fig. 10-15-1). It is commonly referred to as *traction apophysitis.* The apophysis (unique to the immature skeleton) is a growing layer of bone that attaches the infrapatellar tendon of the quadriceps to the anterior tibial tubercle. During the growth spurt, an imbalance develops between the apophysis and the quadriceps. Traction is placed on the loosely attached apophysis by the somewhat inflexible quadriceps, making it susceptible to injury. Forceful, repetitive contraction of the quadriceps during activities involving running, jumping, and pivoting can avulse the apophysis completely or partially from the tibial tubercle. Continued activity following apophyseal injury leads to inflammation. If athletic activities are not modified, swelling and erythema may result from a painful non-union between the apophysis and the tibial tubercle.[1] Since the apophysis is not contiguous with the physis (growth plate), this condition is rarely serious. Conservative measures and skeletal maturity bring resolution to the vast majority of cases. The prevalence and incidence of traction apophysitis is unknown. Approximately 20 to 25 percent of patients present with a bilateral condition.[2] Subsets of patients at greatest risk for developing this condition are ages 11 to 15, males more than females, those at the peak of the growth spurt, and especially young athletes who participate in a single sport year-round.[1]

SIGNS AND SYMPTOMS

Pain, swelling, and erythema of the anterior tibial tubercle, resulting in a painful limp, are the most common presenting symptoms in the adolescent patient.

Examination of an adolescent with painful limp should focus initially on the musculoskeletal system. It is important to exclude systemic condition that could manifest themselves as joint or bone pain. Since hip pain is often referred to the knee, a thorough examination of both hips and knees is indicated. Osgood-Schlatter disease is a diagnosis made by history and direct physical examination of the knee. It is considered good practice to followup the physical assessment with a radiograph of the knee to rule out other more serious conditions (see "Radiologic Studies," below).

Table 10-15-1. Physical Examination Findings in
Osgood-Schlatter Disease

Typical findings
  Localized pain, swelling, and erythema over the anterior tibial tubercle
  Increased knee pain with squatting, crouching, or jumping
  Pain increases with resisted extension of the knee at 90°
  No pain with straight leg raise
  Condition may be bilateral
Atypical findings
  Acute onset
  Medial or lateral knee tenderness
  Ballottable patella or effusion
  Cruciate or collateral ligament laxity
  Joint warmth
  Popping, clicking, or crepitus
  Hip pain
  Fever or multiple joints with tenderness, erythema, or swelling

Typical and atypical physical examination findings are found in Table 10-15-1. Atypical findings warrant a search for other causes.

DIAGNOSTIC CONSIDERATIONS

A painful limp in the adolescent can be the result of other causes. In evaluating suspected Osgood-Schlatter disease, it is important to consider both common and uncommon differentials (see Table 10-15-2).

SPECIAL CONSIDERATIONS

Sports notorious for producing this overuse syndrome are long-distance running, jumping, basketball, and soccer. Adolescents may experience pain and discomfort at the knee for up to 2 years, particularly if they remain physically active. The swelling at the anterior tibial tuberosity may persist into adulthood.

LABORATORY STUDIES

Laboratory testing is not required unless a systemic condition or a septic joint is suspected. Tests to rule out these conditions may be appropriate in the primary care setting.

RADIOLOGIC STUDIES

A simple AP and lateral view of the proximal tibia and knee can rule out other lesions. Expected findings in Osgood-Schlatter disease are tissue swelling, thickened patellar ligament, and an

Table 10-15-2. Differential Diagnosis of Osgood-Schlatter
Disease

Common differentials
  Sindig-Larsen-Johansson syndrome
  Trauma
  Tibial stress or plateau fractures
  Patellofemoral stress syndrome
  Patellar tendinitis
  Shin splints
Uncommon differentials
  Slipped capital femoral epiphysis
  Juvenile rheumatoid arthritis
  Neoplasia
  Sickle cell pain crisis
  Legg-Calve-Perthes disease
  Septic arthritis or osteomyelitis

irregular tibial tuberosity.[3] Small spicules of bone within the patellar tendon are sometimes seen. These avulsions usually reunite in time. A very small number of patients complain of persistent pain and may require surgical excision of the unattached fragment(s).

TREATMENT

Treatment is conservative and focuses on pain control. A trial of NSAIDs,[1] taken with meals, may bring relief. A short course of analgesics may be considered when pain is severe. Activity should be restricted during analgesic use.

Local steroid injections are not recommended since they weaken tendons.

SUPPORTIVE MEASURES

The mainstays of treatment are rest, ice, compression, and elevation (RICE) and modified activity. If pain is pronounced, a trial of crutches or a knee immobilizer in extension for 2 to 3 weeks may bring relief.[1] Plaster casting is no longer recommended.

PATIENT EDUCATION

Education should include parents in an effort to reduce the number of visits for the same problem and costly trips to specialists. To prevent symptom flare-ups, the following are recommended:

1. Immediately ice the affected knee after activity. Frozen bags of peas work nicely.
2. Have the patient do quadriceps strengthening and stretching[1] with 30 daily repetitions of straight leg raises for 2 to 3 weeks, followed by another 2 to 3 weeks with 5- or 10-lb weights added to the ankles.
3. Activity should be stopped at the onset of pain to prevent extension of the inflammatory cycle.
4. Use protective padding against direct trauma to the tubercle during athletic activities.
5. Activities that aggravate the symptoms may have to be eliminated until skeletal maturity has been achieved.

DISPOSITION

Conservative measures can safely be employed for up to 2 years or until skeletal maturity is complete.

COMPLICATIONS

Seek consultation for prolonged disability not responding to conservative measures or symptoms that persist beyond the age 18 or longer than 2 years. In rare cases surgical excision of ossicles embedded in the infrapatellar tendon may be indicated to relieve pain.

PEARLS

Osgood-Schlatter disease sounds ominous. Take the time to educate and assure the child's family that this is a self-limited condition with very low risk for surgery or permanent disability.

The American Academy of Family Physicians provides a patient information sheet on Osgood-Schlatter disease. It is an excellent resource for patients and families that may be reproduced for nonprofit educational purposes.

REFERENCES

1. Peck DM: Apophyseal injuries in the young athlete. *Am Fam Phys* 51(8):1891–1895, 1897–1898, 1995.
2. Behrman RE, Kleigman RM, Nelson WE, Vaughan VC III: *Nelson Textbook of Pediatrics,* 14th ed. Philadelphia, Saunders, 1992, p 1705.
3. Dandy DJ: *Essential Orthopaedics and Trauma,* 2d ed. Edinburgh, Churchill Livingstone, 1993, pp 324–325.

Chapter 10–16
POLYMYALGIA RHEUMATICA AND TEMPORAL ARTERITIS

Daniel P. Radawski
Laura M. Capozzi

DISCUSSION

Polymyalgia rheumatica (PMR) is a disease characterized by aching and stiffness primarily in the proximal muscles and synovial joints of the shoulder and hip girdle. The chief pathologic finding in PMR is lymphocytic synovitis in these joints. The etiology of PMR is poorly understood, but genetic and immunologic factors are thought to play a role. The prevalence of PMR is approximately 1 in 200 persons older than 50 years with an incidence rate of 50 per 100,000 persons over age 50. PMR tends to be self-limited with symptoms of several months' to several years' duration.

Temporal arteritis (TA) is also known as giant cell, cranial, or granulomatous arteritis. TA is a vasculitis that most often affects the temporal artery but may affect any branch of the cranial arteries originating from the arch of the aorta. A subtle, more generalized vasculitis may accompany TA. Biopsies of an affected artery demonstrate granulomatous inflammatory infiltrates. The inflammation is often segmental or patchy with histiocytes, monocytes, lymphocytes, and giant and other cells infiltrating the vessel walls. The etiology of TA is unknown, but environmental factors such as infectious agents, exposure to sunlight, and contact with birds may be involved. Human parvovirus B19 has recently been identified in temporal artery tissues in TA patients. The recent observation in Minnesota of a regular cyclic pattern in incidence rates over time may also support the hypothesis of an infectious cause for TA. The prevalence of TA is about 1 in 500 persons older than 50 years with an average annual incidence of approximately 20 per 100,000 persons over age 50. TA may lead to irreversible blindness or stroke if untreated.

Both PMR and TA occur more frequently in patients of central and northern European ethnic backgrounds. The incidence is less frequent in Asian and African-American groups and southern Europeans. They occur in women twice as frequently as in men. Fifty percent of patients who have PMR are also found to have TA. Patients with TA are also found to have PMR in a range from 18 to 78 percent.

SIGNS AND SYMPTOMS

PMR is characterized by aching and stiffness of the shoulder and pelvic girdle muscles and may be of abrupt or gradual onset. These symptoms most often occur in the morning on arising and should, for diagnostic consideration, last for at least 1 h or more and be present for 1 month or longer. Aching and stiffness also follow other periods of inactivity. This pain and stiffness may begin in one location but soon becomes symmetric and may involve other areas including the buttocks and neck. The distal upper and lower extremities may also be involved. The discomfort may become severe enough to interfere with usual activities and may be associated with systematic constitutional symptoms such as fatigue, loss of sleep and/or weight, or low-grade fever. The symptoms are generally unremitting.

Headache is the most common symptom of TA. The headache may be mild or severe and, as mentioned, is most often present in the region of a temporal artery but infrequently may present in other areas of the head including frontal and occipital areas, depending on the cranial artery affected. Jaw claudication is the next most frequently encountered symptom, occurring in approximately 50 percent of patients. Jaw claudication is more likely to occur with increased use of the muscles of mastication during prolonged chewing of foods such as meat. Visual disturbances occur in approximately 30 percent of patients and may include diplopia, blurred vision, transient visual loss (amaurosis fugax), and partial or complete blindness. Mononeuritis multiplex or polyneuropathy may also be present. Patients with TA may have transient ischemic attacks or strokes that are preventable or treatable with prompt parenteral corticosteroid administration. Constitutional symptoms such as fever, malaise, or fatigue may be present.

OBJECTIVE FINDINGS

Objective findings in PMR are minimal. PMR is a diagnosis of exclusion with objective findings often being related to other diseases. Muscle tenderness may be present, but in objective testing muscle weakness is most often nonexistent or minimal and must be differentiated from hesitancy to perform strength testing because of pain and/or tenderness. Painful areas are less tender to examination than would be expected by the history of disability and pain. Synovial thickening may occur and is most often present in the wrist or knees but is usually mild. Swelling has been noted in the hands and feet in some instances along with pitting edema.

The objective findings in TA may be enlargement, tenderness, and/or erythema over the affected temporal, occipital, or other scalp artery. Bruits or pulse deficits may be present over the carotid, subclavian, or brachial arteries. Large artery and aortic arch involvement may be present initially or later as part of the disease. Funduscopic examination in patients with visual symptoms may include papilledema, and hemorrhage and/or exudates. Optic nerve atrophy may appear later.

DIAGNOSTIC CONSIDERATIONS

Because of the overlap of PMR and TA, signs and/or symptoms and objective findings of PMR may be present in TA. Conversely, history and physical examination of patients with PMR necessitates evaluation for possible symptoms and signs of TA. At present, temporal artery biopsy is not generally recommended in patients with PMR who are asymptomatic for TA. The diagnosis of PMR to a significant degree is a diagnosis of clinical exclusion of other diseases. The differential diagnosis for PMR includes late-onset rheumatoid arthritis (RA) and other rheumatic diseases, including polymyositis, systemic lupus erythematosus, and granulomatous vasculitis. Fibromyalgia, bacterial endocarditis, amyloidosis, and paraneoplastic syndromes secondary to malignant neoplasms may also be considered. It may be difficult to distinguish PMR from RA. The absence of rheumatoid factor, a more benign course, constitutional symptoms, and large joint involvement with abrupt onset indicate PMR. Polymyositis and systemic lupus erythematosus can be identified with associated symptoms and signs and by screening with creatine kinase and antinuclear-antibody testing, respectively. Patients with fibromyalgia should meet the criteria of 11 of 18 specific tender points on digital palpation as determined by the American College of Rheumatology.* These patients should also have a history of widespread pain and other associated symptoms. Patients with bacterial endocarditis include a subset of patients whose bacterial endocarditis is accompanied by prominent musculoskeletal symptoms early in the course of the disease. These patients also display various stigmata of bacterial endocarditis. Patients with hypothyroid myopathy should have other stigmata of hypothyroidism with concomitant abnormalities in thyroid testing. Patients with muscle tenderness from paraneoplastic PMR syndrome are usually identified by associated symptoms, signs, and tests that indicate malignancy. The malignant neoplasms associated with paraneoplastic PMR syndrome include many hematopoietic and nonhemopoietic cancer.

The differential diagnostic considerations for TA may include the following: tension vascular headaches, temporal mandibular joint dysfunction, systemic infections, amyloidosis with prominent vascular involvement, neoplasms, and atherosclerotic vascular disease. Tension vascular headaches may be similar in location to TA with tenderness of the muscles. However, there should be no enlargement of vessels or unexplained erythema. Temporal mandibular joint dysfunction should be discernible on history and physical examination. The other conditions should be differentiated on the basis of associated findings.

LABORATORY STUDIES

In both PMR and TA the erythrocyte sedimentation rate (ESR) as determined by the Westergren method is usually elevated. With PMR, the average ESR is 40 to 50 mm/h as minimal criterion for the diagnosis. With TA, the average ESR is 80 to 100 mm/h. The ESR may occasionally be normal in PMR or TA. Elevated C-reactive proteins; normochromic, normocytic anemia; leukocytosis; thrombocytosis; a mild elevation in hepatic enzymes; and an inflammatory response pattern of serum protein electrophoresis may be seen in both PMR and TA. Radiologic studies are not usually performed in PMR and are infrequently performed in TA. PMR does not usually require other diagnostic tests. A biopsy on a 3- to 5-cm segment of clinically abnormal artery should be performed in TA. This biopsy should be obtained prior to initiating therapy when possible, since corticosteroids rapidly suppress the inflammatory findings. However, histologic features remain normal up to 2 weeks or more after the initiation of corticosteroid therapy in TA. Multiple sections of biopsy specimens should be examined after appropriate staining. The specimens should be examined for the stigmata of chronic vasculitis.

TREATMENT

The treatment of choice for both PMR and TA is usually corticosteroid therapy. With PMR, 10 to 20 mg of prednisone is given in a single or divided daily dose. This should bring prompt relief of the symptoms within 24 to 48 h. Rapid resolution of pain and stiffness suggests the diagnosis of PMR. Slow tapering of the corticosteroids over months to minimize symptomatic flare-ups is usually indicated. From 15 to 70 percent of patients still require corticosteroids after 2 years, and 25 to 50 percent experience relapse after termination of corticosteroid. The route of cortico-

steroid treatment in TA is determined by symptomatology. If visual or strokelike symptoms are imminent or present, aggressive and immediate therapy with intravenous steroids is indicated. Otherwise, TA is treated with 40 to 60 mg of prednisone daily given in a single or divided dose. Once the clinical symptoms and laboratory tests have normalized, the steroid dose can be decreased by approximately 10 percent of the total dose per week. At levels below 10 mg/day, the reduction should be spaced at wider intervals. The other drugs that have been found to be helpful are nonsteroidal anti-inflammatory drugs in low-grade PMR and methotrexate in some cases of TA.

In both PMR and TA, patients should be followed at regular intervals. In PMR, the improvement or defervescence of muscle aching and stiffness should be monitored with appropriate adjustment of steroids. In TA the patient should be seen on a more frequent basis not only to assess the course of the disease but also to determine any potential vision or other central nervous system involvement.

SPECIAL CONSIDERATIONS

Thoracic arch aneurysm may be a late manifestation of TA occurring 5 to 7 years after the initial diagnosis. These aneurysms may rupture. Evaluation for this complication should be considered.

PATIENT EDUCATION

Patients with PMR and TA should be educated regarding the course and potential complications of their illness. Teach patients with PMR the signs and symptoms of TA, and also teach patients with TA the signs and symptoms of PMR. Patients should also be educated about the side effects of nonsteroidal anti-inflammatory and corticosteroid drugs. These patients should understand the course of their illness and central nervous system complications including diplopia, blindness, blurring, partial vision loss, transient ischemic attacks, and stroke.

OTHER NOTES AND PEARLS

PMR should be considered in patients 50 years or older with persistent proximal shoulder and hip girdle pain and stiffness of greater than 1 month duration lasting for greater than 1 h following periods of inactivity. Consider the diagnosis of TA in patients who are 50 years old or older with new-onset headaches that involve the region of the superficial temporal artery. Observe the temporal artery for signs of disease, including enlargement, erythema, or tenderness. In older patients who have new-onset frontal or occipital headaches, include TA in the differential diagnosis.

BIBLIOGRAPHY

Bennett J, Plum F: *Cecil Textbook of Medicine,* 20th ed. Philadelphia, Saunders, 1996.

Brooks RC, McGee SR: Diagnostic dilemmas in polymyalgia rheumatica. *Arch Intern Med* 157: 162–168, 1997.

Fauci AS, Braunwald E, Isselbacher KJ, et al (eds): *Harrison's Principles of Internal Medicine,* 14th ed. New York, McGraw-Hill, 1998.

Hunder G: Polymyalgia rheumatica/giant cell arteritis. *Mayo Clinic,* 18th Annual Practice of Internal Medicine. Rochester, MN, May 1997.

Hurst J: *Medicine for the Practicing Physician,* 4th ed, Stamford, CT, Appleton & Lange, 1996.

Marsh C, Mazzaferri E: *Internal Medicine Pearls.* Philadelphia, FA Davis, 1993, pp 187–189.

Salvarani C, Gabriel S, O'Fallon W, et al: The incidence of giant cell arteritis in Olmstead County, Minnesota: Apparent fluctuations in a cyclic pattern. *Ann Intern Med* 123(3): 192–194, 1995.

---

*The locations of these specific tender points are diagrammed in many textbooks, including *The Arthritis Foundation Primer on the Rheumatic Diseases,* Chap. 41.

Chapter 10–17
OSTEOMYELITIS

Stephen M. Cohen

DISCUSSION

Osteomyelitis customarily describes an inflammatory process of the bone and attached structures, including joint and muscle attachments. The term most often suggests an acute or chronic inflammation caused by a microorganism. The terminology is most commonly applied to bacterial infection, but any microorganism can cause the inflammatory reaction. Fungal and viral infections have also been found to be as causative agents in osteomyelitis.

Generally osteomyelitis is categorized by pathway of infection and host vascularity. Hematogenous osteomyelitis occurs when spread of infection occurs through the bloodstream from distant infection foci. Contiguous osteomyelitis, the most common type, occurs secondary to infection of tissue close to the bone, resulting in direct spread of the contaminant. Where vascular insufficiency is present, as in diabetes and aging, infection is most often contiguous, and the diminished vascular status can accelerate local effects of the infection. Whether hematogenous, or contiguous with or without vascular insufficiency, bone infection requires prompt and deliberate attention to limit morbidity rate, structural damage, and deformity.

SIGNS AND SYMPTOMS

Osteomyelitis may present with local and/or systemic signs of infection. Systemically, the patient may present with malaise, fever, chills, night sweats, anorexia, and/or irritability as in any generalized infective process. Local signs and symptoms may help to identify anatomic involvement. Local signs and symptoms may include limitations of motion around the infection, erythema, drainage through sinus tracts, nonhealing wounds or ulcers, local swelling, pain, warmth, and discomfort. Joint dysfunction, pain, and limited motion may occur if the joint is involved or in close proximity to the bone infection. Presenting features may be chronic or acute, depending on duration and onset.

DIAGNOSTIC CONSIDERATIONS

Diagnosis and proper evaluation begin with a complete history and physical examination with a keen focus on history of present illness. The chronology of symptoms related to causative events is often the key to proper diagnosis. Risk factors should be noted and may include neuropathies, fractures, intravenous drug use and abuse, renal failure and hemodialysis, internal fixation devices, and vascular insufficiency, as in peripheral vascular disease or diabetes. Other history should include inquiry about recent pharyngitis, cellulitis, abscesses, respiratory infection, animal bites, diabetes, and puncture wounds. Detailed history should also include prior antibiotic treatment and use for the bone presentation and other subsystems. Host immunologic status must always be considered, especially in vertebral bone infection.

Etiologic Considerations

Most often hematogenous osteomyelitis is of bacterial origin, most commonly *Staphylococcus aureus*. After *S. aureus,* the common etiologic bacteria vary with age of presentation. In the neonate group B streptococci and *Escherichia coli* are most common after *S. aureus*. In the age group from 1 month to 16 years, *Haemophilus influenzae* and group A streptococci are common along with *S. aureus.*

In the adult over the age of 16 years, the clinician must consider gram-negative bacilli and the anaerobes in addition to streptococci and *S. aureus*. The gram-negative bacteria, such as *Pseudomonas* and *Klebsiella,* are common in immunosuppression, nosocomial infection, and intravenous drug abuse. *Escherichia coli* is usually the cause of spinal osteomyelitis following urinary tract infection or instrumentation. In patients with sickle cell, infections with *S. aureus* and *Salmonella* are not infrequent.

Differential Diagnosis

Other disease states that may present concurrently or in a similar manner to osteomyelitis include osteoarthritis, rheumatoid and crystalline arthritis, stress fractures, neuropathic joint syndromes, bone and joint tumors, aseptic bone infarction, and other systemic infections.

LABORATORY STUDIES

Optimally, a sample of fluid or tissue sample from the infected area is required for accurate and precise diagnosis. Culture and antibiotic sensitivity of these samples or histologic examination is the best demonstration of diagnostic features. Blood cultures are unpredictable and may show as much as 50 percent false-negative in hematogenous osteomyelitis.

White blood cell (WBC) count can be variable in chronic osteomyelitis, but often is elevated in acute disease. Erythrocyte sedimentation rate (ESR) is nonspecific and often elevated. Caution must be applied to the evaluation of patients who have had prior treatment with surgery or antibiotics, since presentation features may make diagnosis difficult. This is especially true in the chronic presentation.

RADIOLOGIC STUDIES

Although findings may not appear until later in the infection course, plain radiographs of painful or locally inflamed areas can be diagnostic. On plain film, acute osteomyelitis may produce soft tissue swelling, periosteal reaction, cortical irregularities, and/or demineralization. Fewer than one-third of cases have plain film evidence of osteomyelitis at 7 to 10 days. Most cases do not manifest radiographic evidence of infection until 3 to 4 weeks.

CT scan may show increased density within the marrow, but this may be difficult to visualize early in the disease course.

MRI may show replacement of marrow fat with edema (water) and exudate resulting in a decreased signal on T1, and an increased signal on T2 images. This finding is not specific for osteomyelitis, however, and can also be found in tumor, acute infarction, or fracture. The sensitivity and specificity of MRI for the detection of acute osteomyelitis is about 95 percent each. MRI may be particularly useful in evaluation of the spine osteomyelitis, showing a characteristic pattern of confluent vertebral body and disk involvement.

Indium 111 white blood cell imaging has shown promise in the imaging of adult osteomyelitis. In this technique, 60 mL of the patient's blood is removed, spun down to obtain WBCs for labeling, and then reinjected. Images are performed 24 h following injection. Uptake occurs at the site of any infection or inflammation with WBC aggregation. Infections that do not generate a significant leukocyte response tie (chronic, parasitic, or fungal infection) may best be evaluated with other techniques. Indium 111 WBC imaging is not commonly performed in children because of the high radiation exposure and the potential for more mutagenic effects on lymphocytes given the expected longer life span of the child.

Technetium-99m-methylene diphosphonate (MDP) bone scan is highly sensitive, but not very specific for osteomyelitis. Any insult to bone may produce an abnormality. The three-phase bone scan has a reported sensitivity of 95 percent and a specificity of 78 percent for identification of osteomyelitis in nontraumatized bone. Specificity drops to about 35 percent in patients with complicating bone conditions such as recent surgery or hardware. In an adult, a negative bone scan essentially rules out infection. Bone scans may remain positive on delayed images for up to 1 to 2 years following successful treatment of osteomyelitis due to continued remodeling. Gallium imaging is better when assessing response to treatment.

Gallium 67 Imaging: The addition of gallium 67 imaging to conventional radiologic studies of bone is also reported to increase specificity and to provide a slight improvement in sensitivity. The gallium scan can be positive as early as 4 h after the onset of infection, and it is usually positive by 24 h. Gallium imaging is hindered by the same lack of specificity as conventional bone scintigraphy because gallium localizes to bone as a calcium-like material. In osteomyelitis, gallium uptake should be either equal to or greater in intensity than the uptake on the bone scan. The normal limb is used to determine the degree of intensity of the abnormality. A normal gallium scan virtually excludes the diagnosis of acute osteomyelitis with a high degree of certainty.

Gallium is also effective for identifying osteomyelitis in neonates and children owing to better identification of lesions adjacent to the growth plates. In this setting, a gallium examination should be used when the bone scan is inconclusive or shows a cold defect. Following treatment, uptake of gallium should decrease even if the bone scan remains abnormal. Gallium activity frequently does not completely return to normal, but this should not be considered indicative of chronic osteomyelitis. If the gallium scan does return to normal, a cure can be predicted with high reliability.

Bone marrow scintigraphy in acute osteomyelitis may show a marrow defect in approximately 5 days. This can be useful in the differentiation of bone infarction from infection in sickle cell patients who present with acute symptoms.

OTHER DIAGNOSTICS

When fluid aspiration is not possible or unobtainable, a needle biopsy (open or closed) may be necessary to obtain tissue suitable for histologic study and culture.

CLASSIFICATION

The Cierny (University of Texas) classification system uses the following categories for osteomyelitis:

1. *Medullary (Type I)* The primary lesion is endosteal, the etiology is variable, the nidus is constant, there is an ischemic scan, chronic granulations are present, and the trabeculae are sequestered.
2. *Superficial (Type II)* The outer surface of bone is affected, and there is a compromised soft tissue envelope surrounding the bone.
3. *Localized (Type III)* There is full-thickness cortical involvement, and infection usually begins after trauma. The entire lesion can be completely excised and covered with a cuff made of viable tissue while preserving bone.
4. *Diffuse (Type IV)* There is circumferential, complete bone involvement where an intercalary segment of skeleton must be removed to effect treatment and cure. There may be an infected non-union and/or an end-stage septic joint present with obvious destruction.

Table 10-17-1. Empirical Intravenous Therapy Guidelines

Organism or Circumstances	Medication and Dosing
Staphylococcus aureus and coagulase negative *Staphylococcus*	Nafcillin* or cloxacillin, 2 g IV q4–6h
Penicillin allergy	Clindamycin,† 600 mg IV q8h
Methicillin-resistant *Staphylococcus* or empirical when infection involves prosthetic joint	Vancomycin,‡ 1 g IV q12h
Coagulase negative *Staphylococcus*	Nafcillin, 2 g IV q4–6h
Streptococcus	Penicillin G, 2–4 million units IV q4h, or cefazolin, 1 g IV q8h
Enteric gram-negative bacilli or *Pseudomonas*	Piperacillin, 4 g IV q4–6h plus aminoglycoside
Mixed aerobic and anaerobic organisms (diabetes or animal or human bite wound)	Beta-lactamase inhibitor combination therapy (e.g., ticarcillin = clavulanate 3.1 g q6h IV)
Mixed gram-positive and anaerobic organisms	Clindamycin, 600 mg IV q8h
High-risk patient (e.g., IV drug abuse or hemodialysis patients)	Cloxacillin or nafcillin with gentamicin (gentamicin = 1.5 mg/kg IV q8h)
High-risk patient with penicillin allergy (when aminoglycoside is contraindicated)	Clindamycin with gentamicin or clindamycin with ceftriaxone or cefotaxime or ciprofloxacin

* Adding metronidazole to either nafcillin or cloxacillin has the same spectrum of activity as clindamycin alone.

† Watch for diarrhea with and without *Clostridium difficile* infection with clindamycin.

‡ Watch for ototoxicity with extended therapy.

The Time Element Classification has the following types:

1. *Acute* Acute inflammation, inflammation of periosteum
2. *Chronic* Long term with soft and bone tissue changes
3. *Subacute* Without signs and symptoms; silent infection

TREATMENT

Successful treatment is proportional to virulence of disease, suitable antibiotic use, the bone involved, status of blood supply, duration of antibiotic therapy, and treatment duration. The overall goals of therapy are to stop continued infection and spread, stop sepsis and death, reduce signs and symptoms, and prevent the complications of infection, including bone and tissue loss and disability. With prudent and timely treatment, morbidity rate can be reduced and limb salvage accomplished. Beginning treatment immediately in adult, chronic osteomyelitis is less important than in acute or subacute processes.

Pharmacologic Management

As in all infectious disease therapy, antimicrobial agent therapy should be based on susceptibility testing (sensitivity) and organism identification by a sample of fluid or tissue taken prior the start of therapy. Initial therapy begins immediately with intravenous antimicrobial agents on diagnosis and continues for 2 to 3 days (Table 10-17-1).

Further treatment of acute osteomyelitis is based on reassessment of the patient, but it should continue for 4 to 6 weeks minimum on an outpatient basis. Chronic osteomyelitis may require longer therapy. Oral antibiotics are used only after intravenous therapy is complete, an organism is identified, and patient compliance is assured (Table 10-17-2).

Table 10-17-2. Commonly Used Oral Therapy in Osteomyelitis (After Intravenous Therapy)

Medication	Dose
Cloxacillin	1 g PO q6h
Ciprofloxacin	750 mg PO bid
Clindamycin	300 mg PO q6h

Antimicrobial therapy may also be administered locally in the form of antimicrobial-impregnated polymethylmethacrylate (PMMA) beads implanted at the time of surgery.

Surgery

Most cases of chronic osteomyelitis require debridement surgery in addition to any antibiotic therapy. Surgery is the treatment of choice in chronic osteomyelitis and should be strongly considered in initial, acute infection. Infective tissue has the ability to lie dormant, and wide surgical excision of all subacute infected tissue is mandatory for cure. Current understanding of osteomyelitis requires clinicians to understand that incomplete excision is wasted effort. The principles of surgery include adequate drainage; thorough debridement of granulation, scar, and dead bone; obliteration of dead space; and directed, specific antibiotic therapy. This surgical process often entails creating wide margins of excision with large tissue defects. Defect management is accomplished with cancellus bone graft, simple approximation, transposition of local tissues, and vascularized tissue flaps. Secondary intent healing is not recommended because it leaves an avascular scar.

The surgeon may consider the temporary implantation of antibiotic-impregnated PMMA (bone cement) beads into the surgical wound. Methylmethacrylate beads impregnated with antibiotic have been utilized by some to increase the level of antibiosis at the wound site in chronic osteomyelitis. There is a risk that the presence of these beads may inhibit the obliteration of dead space after surgery. Positive results with beads appear to be directly related to extent and success of debridement and adequacy of wound coverage.

Surgical intervention is accomplished for debridement, to remove inflammatory tissue, to reduce the bacterial load factor, and to establish an environment where antibiotics work more efficiently. Free tissue transfer flaps and bone grafting to fill tissue voids left by surgical excision currently appear to offer the best chance for successful treatment of osteomyelitis by assisting in increasing circulation to the area.

PATIENT EDUCATION

Patient must be included in all decisions of treatment so they may understand the potential chronic nature of this disease. Cure of osteomyelitis with medical treatment alone or inadequate surgical debridement is unpredictable and uncertain. Most patients underestimate the commitment to the treatment course once begun. Additionally, weight-bearing or mechanical stress on the infected bone can reduce healing potential and potentiate infection. Patients must be instructed to remain non-weight-bearing.

DISPOSITION

Medical treatment is extremely unpredictable when utilized without surgical debridement. Because cure rates are low in the long bones without surgery, recurrence can be assumed with antibiotic treatment only. If hematogenous spread can be verified, cure with antibiotic alone increases. Antibiotic compliance and correct dosing for 6 weeks or longer is mandatory for cure. The patient may be monitored in the treatment period with antimicrobial blood levels, antibacterial titer, and erythrocyte sedimentation rate (ESR).

COMPLICATIONS AND RED FLAGS

Complications of acute osteomyelitis include death, chronic osteomyelitis, growth disturbance, physeal damage, involvement of adjacent joint, local extension into soft tissues and abscess formation, pathologic fracture, bacteremia, and prosthetic loosening (if involved).

Chronic recurrent multifocal osteomyelitis (CRMO) is a complication that was first described 1972. It is a subacute form of osteomyelitis characterized by symmetric bone lesions and associated with palmoplantar pustulosis. The etiology of CRMO has been hypothesized to be immune or viral in origin. CRMO occurs most in older children, and blood cultures are often negative. Slow resolution followed by recurrence months to years later is the course.

PEDIATRIC CONSIDERATIONS

Any child who has sustained minor trauma and not recovered appropriately should be considered for osteomyelitis. In children osteomyelitis develops mostly in male children between 8 and 12 years. Pediatric bone infection most commonly occurs in the metaphyseal region of the long bones where turbulent, slowed blood flow near the growth plate and decreased phagocytic activity may favor bacterial deposition. Transient bacteremia, considered a probable cause, is common in pediatrics and may be initiated by tooth brushing, pharyngitis, ear infection, or similar minor events. Recent varicella infection may predispose to streptococcal osteomyelitis. *Salmonella* osteomyelitis has been noted in pediatric patients with sickle cell disease.

Epiphyseal and joint involvement is common in children under 18 months of age due to the presence of transphyseal vessels. In older children the growth plate prevents the spread of infection into the epiphysis. In neonates with osteomyelitis, systemic disturbances may be mild or absent. Detection is therefore frequently delayed, and involvement can be multicentric. Differential diagnosis must include juvenile rheumatoid arthritis and tumor such as Ewing's sarcoma. Radiographic signs may take 7 to 10 days to become evident. Culture of aspirate material is most reliable compared with Gram stain or blood cultures.

OTHER NOTES AND PEARLS

Hematogenous vertebral osteomyelitis is almost always a monomicrobial infection affecting the older population. *Staphylococcus aureus* is the most common microorganism isolated in this group. Gram-negative bacilli may be seen in elderly males with urinary tract infections. Hematogenous vertebral osteomyelitis is treated primarily by conservative care in the form of immobilization and parenteral antibiotics. Indications for surgery are rare and should be reserved for patients resistant to treatment or with septic course, abscess formation, or neurologic deficits.

BIBLIOGRAPHY

Anthony JP, Mathes SJ: Update on chronic osteomyelitis. *Clin Plast Surg* 18:515–523, 1991.

Anthony JP, Mathes SJ, Alpert BS: The muscle flap in the treatment of chronic lower extremity osteomyelitis: Results in patients over 5 years after treatment. *Plast Reconstr Surg* 88:311–318, 1991.

Dirschl DR, Almekinder LC: Osteomyelitis—Common causes and treatment recommendations. *Drugs* 45:29–43, 1993.

Job ML, Matthews HW: Bone and joint infection, in Herfindal E, Gourley D (eds): *Textbook of Therapeutics.* Baltimore, Williams & Wilkins, 1996.

MacDougall CA, McCormack J: Drug therapy in osteomyelitis, in McCormack J, Brown G, Levine M, et al (eds): *Drug Therapy Decision Making Guide.* Philadelphia, Saunders, 1996.

Mandell GL, Douglas RG Jr, Bennett JE (eds): *Principles and Practice of Infectious Diseases,* 3d ed. Toronto, Little, Brown, 1991.

Mercier LR: *Practical Orthopedics.* St Louis, Mosby, 1995.

Steffanovski N, Van Voris LP: Pyogenic vertebral osteomyelitis. *Contemp Orthop* 31:159–164, 1995.

Vibhagool A, Calhoun J, Mader J, et al: Therapy of bone and joint infection. *Hosp Form* 28:63–85, 1993.

Wladvogel FA: Osteomyelitis, in Gorbach S, Bartlett J, Blacklow N (eds): *Infectious Diseases.* Philadelphia, Saunders, 1992.

Chapter 11–1
SEIZURE DISORDERS (EPILEPSY)
William A. Mosier

DISCUSSION

A seizure disorder (epilepsy) is best described as a symptom of brain dysfunction involving a paroxysmal and disorganized depolarization of neurons in the brain and the spread of the resulting discharge. The word *epilepsy* is derived from the Greek *epilepsia*, "a seizing." It refers to the many varying types of recurrent seizures produced by sudden, excessive neuronal discharges in the brain. A seizure is an uncontrolled synchronous firing of a group of cerebral neurons. The spread of a seizure involves the progression of surges of disorganized electrical impulses in the brain to surrounding or closely interconnected groups of neurons, engaging them in similar activity. Many abnormal depolarizations have no clinical manifestations; however, when manifestations are present, the result is seizure activity. The term *epilepsy* encompasses convulsive "disorders" with loss of consciousness as well as nonconvulsive seizures with only a slight change in conscious awareness. Generally, the term *epilepsy* is reserved for patients who have experienced at least two and usually three recurrent seizures without clear precipitating factors. Seizures produced by cerebral ischemia, hypoxia, hypoglycemia, cocaine abuse, and withdrawal from alcohol, barbiturates, or benzodiazepines should not be referred to as epilepsy.

The prevalence of seizure disorders is roughly 6 in 1000 in the general population. In the United States, about 1 percent of the population, approximately 2 million people, has active epilepsy. Another 7 million persons have had at least one seizure at some point during their lifetimes. This represents 1 in every 11 persons. It has been estimated that 200,000 persons experience seizures more than once a month.

It also has been estimated that one-fourth of all patients with seizure disorders continue to suffer seizure activity despite receiving treatment. Although seizures can develop at any time of life, 75 percent of new cases present in childhood. Seizure disorders are slightly more prevalent in males and in lower socioeconomic groups.

The two most widely accepted ways of classifying seizures are the International Classification of Epileptic Seizures (ICES) and the International Classification of Epilepsies (ICE). In these systems, seizures are divided into two broad categories:

1. Generalized seizures
2. Localization-related (partial, focal) seizures

Generalized seizures are most often genetic in origin and begin from both sides of the brain simultaneously. Localization-related seizures usually are restricted to specific regions of the brain and most often are acquired. These so called local seizures can be separated further into simple and complex seizures. The most common idiopathic localization-related seizure disorder is benign childhood epilepsy with centrotemporal spikes (benign rolandic epilepsy). It occurs most frequently between ages 3 and 13. It presents with simple partial seizures manifesting sensorimotor symptoms that affect predominantly the face and particularly the mouth.

Seizures also can be divided into two types: convulsive and nonconvulsive. The most familiar expression of convulsive seizures is the generalized tonic-clonic form often referred to as grand mal seizures. They commonly begin in late adolescence. The most familiar expression of nonconvulsive seizures is called an absence seizure (petit mal). These seizures usually begin in early childhood (Table 11-1-1).

PATHOGENESIS

The causes of seizures are as varied as the possible clinical manifestations. Seizures may result from idiopathic factors or may be produced by disease processes or brain trauma. Given the appropriate chemical and electrical stimuli, seizure activity can occur even in a "normal" brain. Certain regions of the brain are particularly sensitive to seizure activity, especially the motor cortex and the limbic system. The temporal lobe, the amygdala, and the hippocampus are all especially susceptible to biochemical disturbances. Age and developmental factors are significant influences in the genesis of seizure disorders (Table 11-1-2).

SIGNS AND SYMPTOMS

One of every five individuals diagnosed with a seizure disorder (epilepsy) may not actually have epilepsy. The most important consideration in seeking a diagnosis is taking a thorough history of the initial seizure and any subsequent presumed seizures as well as a detailed family history. The history frequently uncovers the seizure type. The interview must include questioning about a history of early morning seizure activity or jerking behavior and establishing whether the patient felt tired after a seizure. Evidence of feeling fatigue during the postictal state can rule out absence seizures, which are marked by a rapid return to feeling normal.

Seizure disorders are classified according to their presenting clinical features and the patterns that are observed on the electroencephalogram. Because an accurate diagnosis of a seizure disorder involves so many factors, the following diagnostic considerations should apply in assessing a patient. A determination must be made as to

1. Whether seizure activity actually occurred
2. Whether the seizures are localized or generalized in nature
3. Whether consciousness was impaired
4. Whether convulsions occurred

Generalized seizures of the tonic-clonic type are characterized by an aura (a rising or sinking sensation) followed by a sudden loss of consciousness. During the period of unconsciousness, the body develops a tonic (stiffening) response that usually lasts less than a minute. Then the body undergoes a series of muscle contractions that represent the clonic phase. The entire seizure may typically last 3 min.

Generalized absence seizures usually present as brief, mild episodes lasting only 5 to 30 s. They tend to cause no dramatic physical changes and may go unnoticed. An absence seizure is characterized by a sudden stop in activity and a blank, vacant stare lasting only seconds. The individual may then immediately resume activity, completely unaware that he or she just experienced a seizure.

Partial seizures can be classified as complex or simple. A partial seizure with impaired consciousness is referred to as a complex partial seizure. A partial seizure without compromised conscious-

Table 11-1-1. Classification of the More Common Seizures

Type	Characteristics	Location
LOCALIZATION-RELATED SEIZURES (FOCAL, LOCAL, PARTIAL)		
Motor	Aura	Cortical foci of spikes and slow waves seen on EEG
Sensory Somatosensory	Tingling, numbness	Parietal lobe
Visual	Flashing lights and color	Occipital lobe
Temporal lobe Complex partial (psychomotor)	Lip smacking, chewing	Anterior temporal lobe foci
GENERALIZED SEIZURES		
Tonic-clonic (grand mal)	Aura, unconsciousness, tonic-clonic movements, postictal drowsiness	Single or multiple cortical foci of spikes seen on EEG; can be in any area of cortex
Absence (petit mal)	Staring, speech arrest (brief spells)	Synchronous, symmetric, 3-per-second spike and wave discharges with no cortical localization seen on EEG
Myoclonic	Quick repetitive jerks	Multifocal spikes seen on EEG

ness is called a simple partial seizure. When a seizure persists for an extended period, more than 30 min, or occurs so frequently that there is no recovery between attacks, this is referred to as status epilepticus (see "Complications and Red Flags," below).

OBJECTIVE FINDINGS

The clinical features of a seizure disorder depend largely on the regions of the brain initially involved and the rate and pattern of spread of the abnormal discharge. The neurologic examination may uncover evidence of a localized brain lesion or an organic disorder. In children, the examination must include looking for developmental delays, adenoma sebaceum (a sign of tuberous sclerosis), and organomegaly (which could indicate a storage disease).

Table 11-1-2. Causes of Seizure Activity

Cause	Result
Birth trauma	Anoxia, contusion
Congenital	Abnormal development
Metabolic	Disorders of amino acid or vitamin metabolism, lipidoses, hypoglycemia, hypocalcemia, hyponatremia, uremia
Infection	Encephalitis, meningitis, brain abscess
Perinatal injury	Temporal lobe sclerosis, cerebral palsy
Neoplastic	Primary and metastatic tumors
Vascular	Arteriovenous malformation, arteritis, hematoma, sickle cell disease, postinfarction, hypertension
Postnatal trauma	Anoxia, contusion, penetrating head wound
Toxins or withdrawal	Alcohol, barbiturates, cocaine, lead, organic phosphates, steroids, abrupt medication changes, Reye's syndrome

Table 11-1-3. Diagnostic Tools for Screening Seizure Disorders

Electroencephalogram
Computerized tomography and/or magnetic resonance imaging
Fasting blood glucose
Serum urea nitrogen, calcium, and phosphorus
Sedimentation rate
Urinalysis
Positron emission tomography with fluorodeoxyglucose (in surgical candidates)

DIAGNOSTIC CONSIDERATIONS

A diagnosis of seizure disorder can have profound medical and psychological implications for a patient. Consequently, careful attention should be given to exploring the nonepileptic disturbances that produce abnormalities of neurologic function similar to those of the seizure disorders. The differential diagnosis should include conversion hysteria (psychogenic origin) as well as cerebrovascular insufficiency (drop attacks) and syncope.

SPECIAL CONSIDERATIONS

The chief issues in managing seizure disorders in children are accurate diagnosis, appropriate selection of an antiepileptic drug, and supportive management to minimize the adverse effects of seizures on maturation. Many children have self-limiting seizures. An accurate diagnosis can prevent the overprescribing of antiepileptics that may have a negative impact on a child's cognitive functioning and academic achievement. Children with seizure disorders have a higher incidence of learning disabilities and other neurologic handicaps than do their peers. Antiepileptic drugs also can contribute to learning problems. Because these problems are so common among children treated for seizure disorders, testing and remedial help for the child should be recommended to the parents.

DIAGNOSTIC TESTS

The use of the EEG is indispensable in considering a diagnosis of seizure disorder. An EEG can provide a precise definition of the nature of the abnormal neural discharge and often can be used to establish the seizure type. It is best performed on the patient in both awake and sleeping states, utilizing hyperventilation and phobic stimulation. EEG can detect focal and diffuse brain dysfunction. The two typical patterns to look for are a slowing and the classic epileptiform activity, which is brief and starts and stops abruptly. The number of epileptiform discharges between seizures, referred to as interictal discharges, does not correlate with frequency of seizures. In fact, the interictal EEG of an awake patient with a seizure disorder may be totally normal. EEG patterns of partial and generalized seizures are typically quite distinct. Partial seizures can produce a focal slowing of the background rhythm, focal spikes, or even sharp waves.

With generalized seizures, EEG tracings may demonstrate a bilateral or widespread spiking and slow wave pattern or a polyspiking and slow wave pattern over the entire frontal and central regions of the brain. Because many epileptiform patterns are confusing and may lead to a misdiagnosis, interpretation of EEG results requires caution and expertise (Table 11-1-3).

TREATMENT

The management of seizures is based primarily on empirical observations of how certain types of seizures present in relation to the age of the patient and the response of seizure activity to therapeutic intervention. The question of whether to treat with medication is complicated by the fact that the recurrence rate after a single seizure varies from 15 to 60 percent. However, after two seizures, the risk of eventually experiencing a third seizure rises to 85 percent. Therefore, treatment decisions must be individualized to the needs of each patient because the consequences and recurrence rates of seizures are so varied. The aim of treatment is to control seizure activity without drug toxicity. Single-drug therapy is effective in about 50 percent of patients.

Pharmacologic Management

The initial drug management of seizure disorders is generally as follows:

- *Partial seizures:* valproate, phenytoin, or carbamazepine
- *Generalized seizures with convulsions (tonic-clonic or myoclonic):* valproate
- *Generalized seizures without convulsions (absence):* valproate or ethosuximide

There are many anticonvulsant drugs, but those listed above are the mainstay of drug therapy. The safest first-line drug is valproate. When this therapy alone is not effective, phenytoin, cabamazepine, or ethosuximide therapy should be attempted.

Before the initiation of monotherapy with valproic acid or divalproex sodium, a blood count that includes platelets, bleeding time, and liver function should be ordered. This should be repeated after 10 days of therapy and then monthly for the first 6 months of treatment. The dose should be increased gradually from 250 mg/d to 750 mg or even 1500 mg daily, often in divided doses. Nausea and vomiting usually are a problem only if the dose is increased too rapidly. Gastrointestinal (GI) side effects can be minimized if the medication is taken with meals. Occasional complaints include hair loss, tremors, and weight gain. It is important to avoid abrupt cessation of the medication.

Supportive Measures

Even with adequate seizure control utilizing anticonvulsive therapy, many patients require concomitant psychological support services, such as individual or group counseling.

Patient Education

Patient education should emphasize helping the patient recognize seizure triggers. Although there may be no special triggers in some patients, others find that flickering lights (even sunlight), stress, lack of sleep, and lack of food may be associated with a greater likelihood of seizure activity.

The most common cause of an unexpected seizure is failure to take the medication as prescribed. Therefore, an individualized educational plan of care should provide the patient and the patient's family members with informational tools that will enhance their understanding of the patient's seizure disorder. The significance of reminding the patient about the importance of taking all medications appropriately cannot be overemphasized. The risks of driving an automobile and work-related issues also must be reviewed in counseling the patient about his or her seizure risk. Parents of children with seizure disorders must be cautioned against overprotectiveness.

DISPOSITION

Most genetically predisposed seizure disorders are well controlled with the proper medication management, as are most acquired partial seizure disorders. In both children and adults, early initiation of treatment produces the most favorable prognosis as long as there is no underlying progressive structural disease.

COMPLICATIONS AND RED FLAGS

Status epilepticus refers to

1. Seizure activity that is so frequent or prolonged that it persists for at least 30 min
2. Seizure activity occurring with impaired consciousness and without a return of consciousness between seizures

The most frequently occurring type of status epilepticus is generalized convulsive status epilepticus (GCSE). It constitutes a medical emergency that necessitates prompt treatment to avoid neurologic damage. Intravenous diazepam or lorazepam and phenytoin are the first-line therapies for GCSE. Most patients respond to the initial treatment. However, refractory status epilepticus may require pentobarbital, phenobarbital, or inhalational anesthetic agents.

Surgical intervention is appropriate for selected patients who remain intractable after intensive medical therapy. About 10 percent benefit from anterior temporal lobectomy, amygdalohippocampectomy, or corticotomy.

OTHER NOTES AND PEARLS

Refractory complex partial seizures may be due to inadequate dosing of the anticonvulsant medication, an inappropriate choice of medication, or the presence of aggravating factors such as stress, sleep deprivation, menses, and alcohol. Patient noncompliance with taking medication must always be considered if refractory seizures persist.

Research is being conducted using biofeedback as a treatment for seizures. In theory, the patient learns how to reproduce the brain waves that seem to prevent seizures. However, some studies indicate that the ability to control seizure activity fades once the biofeedback training is discontinued. For a patient who is a nonresponder to medication, researchers at Johns Hopkins Medical School have developed a diet, called the ketogenic diet, that is being studied in children with severe seizures. This is a high-fat, low-carbohydrate, low-protein diet that must be followed with exactness to control seizure activity. It is not recommended without close medical supervision. For information on the ketogenic diet, contact Johns Hopkins Pediatric Epilepsy Center, 600 North Wolfe Street, Baltimore, MD 21287.

BIBLIOGRAPHY

Annegers JF, Rocca WA, Hauser WA: Causes of epilepsy: Contributions of the Rochester Epidemiology Project. *Mayo Clin Proc* 71:570–575, 1996.
Britton JW, So EL: Selection of antiepileptic drugs: A practical approach. *Mayo Clin Proc* 71:778–786, 1996.
Cascino, GD: Generalized convulsive status epilepticus. *Mayo Clin Proc* 71:787–792, 1996.
Chabbolla DR, Krahn LE, So EL, et al: Psychogenic nonepileptic seizures. *Mayo Clin Proc* 71:493–500, 1996.
Hauser WA, Annegers JF, Rocca WA: Descriptive epidemiology of epilepsy: Contributions of population-based studies from Rochester, Minnesota. *Mayo Clin Proc* 71:576–586, 1996.
Jack CR: Magnetic resonance imaging in epilepsy. *Mayo Clin Proc* 71:695–711, 1996.
Krahn LE, Rummans TA, Peterson GC: Psychiatric implications of surgical treatment of epilepsy. *Mayo Clin Proc* 71:1201–1204, 1996.
Mosewich RK, So EL: A clinical approach to the classification of seizures and epileptic syndromes. *Mayo Clin Proc* 71:405–414, 1996.
Trenerry MR: Neuropsychologic assessment in surgical treatment of epilepsy. *Mayo Clin Proc* 71:1196–1200, 1996.

Wass CT, Rajala MM, Hughes JM et al: Long-term follow-up of patients treated surgically for medically intractable epilepsy: Results in 291 patients treated at Mayo Clinic Rochester between July 1972 and March 1985. *Mayo Clin Proc* 71:1105–1113, 1996.

Westmoreland BF: Epileptiform electroencephalographic patterns. *Mayo Clin Proc* 71:501–511, 1996.

Zupanc ML: Update on epilepsy in pediatric patients. *Mayo Clin Proc* 71:899–916, 1996.

Table 11-2-1. Neurologic Signs Associated with MS

Abnormal pupillary responses
Abnormal speech patterns
Altered eye movements
Circumscribed sensory disturbances
Limb spasticity
Localized weakness
Overactive tendon reflexes
Paleness of the optic discs
Visual field disturbances

Chapter 11–2
MULTIPLE SCLEROSIS
William A. Mosier

DISCUSSION

Multiple sclerosis (MS) is a slowly progressive demyelinating disease of the central nervous system (CNS). It results in varied neurologic symptoms with periods of alternating remission and exacerbation. The cause is unknown, and current therapy is only marginally effective. The disease generally begins in early adult life. The onset of symptoms rarely occurs before age 15 and after age 40. The name *multiple sclerosis* refers to two features of the disease:

1. *Multiple* indicates that many areas of the brain, spinal cord, and optic nerve are affected.
2. *Sclerosis* suggests that there are hardened plaques in the involved areas.

The course is highly unpredictable. Remissions may last months or years. However, over the course of the disease the intervals between remissions become shorter.

PATHOGENESIS

The pathologic focus of MS is the fatty myelin coating on nerve fibers in the CNS. MS attacks the myelin, forming plaque in varying locations in the brain, spinal cord, and closely related structures. The prevalence of MS varies from region to region. It appears to be more common in temperate zones. There are an estimated 250,000 cases of diagnosed MS in the United States. The factors that determine susceptibility to MS appear to be acquired before age 15. The incidence of MS is higher in urban settings than in rural areas. It also manifests more frequently among affluent socioeconomic groups. Blood relatives of patients with MS are eight times more likely to develop the disease than is the general population. These epidemiologic factors suggest a viral or altered immune response in a genetically susceptible individual as the probable etiology. MS is the most common demyelinating disease of the CNS.

MICROBIOLOGY

MS attacks the myelin that covers nerve fibers. The damaged myelin cells cause plaques of demyelination with destruction of oligodendroglia, primarily in the white matter of the cervical and dorsal region of the lateral and posterior columns, the optic nerves, and the periventricular areas. Tracts in the midbrain, pons, and cerebellum and gray matter in the cerebrum and spinal cord also may be invaded. Chemical changes in the lipid and protein constituents of myelin have been identified in and around the plaques associated with MS.

SYMPTOMS

The onset of MS is usually insidious. Symptoms often develop over the course of a few days, remain stable for several weeks, and then recede. The most frequently presenting symptoms include

1. Paresthesias in one or more extremities, on one side of the face, or in the trunk
2. A feeling of clumsiness in or weakness of a hand or leg
3. Visual disturbances (e.g., retrobulbar optic neuritis, diplopia, foggy vision, scotomas, partial blindness)

Other symptoms include transient weakness of one or more extremities, minor gait disturbance, limb fatigue, bladder control problems, ocular palsy, dizziness, male impotency, and psychological changes such as mood swings, apathy, and depression. Exposure to excessively warm temperatures tends to exacerbate the symptoms. The symptoms may present months to years before the disease is diagnosed.

OBJECTIVE FINDINGS

Most neurologic findings are nonspecific, but certain signs are suggestive of MS:

1. *Internuclear ophthalmoplegia.* Paresis of the medial rectus muscle on lateral conjugate gaze but not on convergence can be noted. Nystagmus can be seen in the abducting eye.
2. *Lhermitte's sign.* Neck flexion produces a sensation of an electrical charge that runs down the back and into the legs.
3. *Optic neuritis.* Decreased visual acuity, a defective pupillary reaction to light (Marcus Gunn pupil), edema of the optic discs, and hyperemia can all be early signs of MS. Noted pallor of the temporal half of the disc develops as a later sign of MS (Tables 11-2-1 and 11-2-2).

Table 11-2-2. Typical Findings on Eye Examination in MS

Centrocecal scotomas
Impaired color vision
Impaired visual acuity
Marcus Gunn pupils
Nystagmus
Optic nerve atrophy

Table 11-2-3. Findings on Laboratory Tests and Radiologic Studies in MS

Test	Findings
Cerebrospinal fluid	Abnormal protein composition >55% of time
Computed tomography	White patches notable with high contrast
Magnetic resonance imaging	Areas of abnormal nerve tissue
Evoked potential studies	Pattern shift of brainstem auditory, somatosensory, or visual evoked potentials may appear abnormal in early stages of MS

DIAGNOSTIC CONSIDERATIONS

Multifocal and recrudescent CNS diseases, such as systemic lupus erythematosus (SLE) and Behçet's disease, can mimic MS. Additional considerations in the differential must include amyotrophic lateral sclerosis (ALS), arthritis of the cervical spine, cerebral infarction, CNS abscess or tumor, hereditary ataxia, pernicious anemia, ruptured intervertebral disk, meningovascular syphilis, cryptococcosis, toxoplasmosis, sarcoidosis, syringomyelia, and vascular malformations of the brain and spinal cord. When the presenting complaints are vague and there are minimal findings, a diagnosis of conversion disorder (hysteria) may be considered.

SPECIAL CONSIDERATIONS

In the early stages, MS often is inaccurately mislabeled as hysteria. It is important to avoid this mistake. No blood test, x-ray study, or other type of objective examination can determine with total certainty that a patient's presenting complaints are caused by MS. MS is diagnosed from clinical findings. Laboratory procedures can only lend support for the diagnosis.

LABORATORY STUDIES

The only useful laboratory test for MS is an examination of the cerebrospinal fluid (CSF). However, all the abnormalities induced by MS are not unique to this disease alone. The characteristic changes in the CSF that occur in MS also may be seen with some infections, other demyelinating diseases, and other CNS diseases of unknown etiology. In MS, proteins associated with the myelin of the CNS—myelin basic proteins—often are found in higher than normal concentrations. They represent a crude measure of the extent of myelin damage in the CNS. The most characteristic CSF finding in MS is elevated immunoglobulin G (IgG). An elevated kappa chain content of the CSF may be a better indicator of MS than is IgG (Table 11-2-3).

RADIOLOGIC STUDIES

Computed tomography (CT) with contrast and magnetic resonance imaging (MRI), especially nuclear magnetic resonance (NMR), can provide assistance in the investigation of MS. Determining that an area of damage is afflicted by demyelination rather than a tumor or damaged blood vessels is better achieved with MRI than with CT. The plaques of demyelination seen in MS show up as white patches on both CT with contrast and MRI.

OTHER DIAGNOSTICS

Evoked potential studies are a noninvasive tool to assess nerve fiber conduction in the visual, auditory, and somatosensory path-

ways. Test results may uncover unsuspected problems in parts of the nervous system that are still asymptomatic.

TREATMENT

There is no cure for MS. Although spontaneous remissions make treatment efficacy difficult to evaluate, treatments to manage acute exacerbations and complications are utilized. Treatment is currently aimed at relief of symptoms and prevention of relapse.

Pharmacologic Management

Interferon β_{lb} (Betaseron) is an agent that has been approved for use in ambulatory patients with relapsing-remitting multiple sclerosis (RRMS). It tends to reduce the frequency and severity of exacerbations. The recommended dose is 0.25 mg (8 million IU) administered subcutaneously every other day. It is supplied as a lyophilized powder in a single-use vial with a separate vial of sodium chloride to be used as a diluent; it should be stored under refrigeration. The side effect profile includes "flulike" symptoms such as fever, chills, and myalgia. Other side effects, such as palpitations, dyspnea, menstrual disorders, possible abnormal liver function, decreased white blood cell count, and depression, also are seen.

Adrenocorticotropic hormone (ACTH) and corticosteroids have been widely used to treat MS since 1970. However, optic neuritis may be the first sign of MS or may occur during an exacerbation. Since optic neuritis can be worsened by corticosteroids such as prednisone, treatment with prednisone during a flare-up of MS is potentially dangerous. Other risks include steroid-induced hypertension and diabetes mellitus.

Muscle relaxants may be helpful in the treatment of the spasticity and muscle stiffness that often develop with MS. The benzodiazepines are used frequently for this purpose. Clonazepam (Klonopin) is usually adequate to improve mobility. It should be noted, however, that after taking a benzodiazepine for several months, a patient will notice withdrawal effects if the drug is discontinued. Insomnia and restlessness are commonly noticed. Therefore, when a patient is in a period of remission, benzodiazepine discontinuation should be done in a tapered manner.

Supportive Measures

Massage and passive range-of-motion exercise of weak limbs can make patients more comfortable. Physical therapy can help preserve as much muscle function as possible and should be emphasized. Most treatment is aimed at relieving symptoms. Wearing braces or using a cane, walker, wheelchair, or battery-powered vehicle may become necessary. Adequate rest and a healthy, well-balanced diet are important. Providing the patient with encouragement and reassurance is essential.

Patient Education

Because living with MS can be difficult, these patients should be encouraged to join an MS support group. They also should be counseled about avoiding emotionally and physically stressful situations in an attempt to control symptoms. These patients must be reminded to consult their health care providers as soon as the symptoms become apparent in an attempt to shorten any exacerbation of the disease.

DISPOSITION

In some patients, especially those who develop MS in middle age, there can be a rapid downhill course with recurrent urinary tract infections that can pose a risk of kidney failure. Therefore, a neurology consultation should be sought immediately after the onset of symptoms.

COMPLICATIONS AND RED FLAGS

A common complication of MS and of the medications used to treat the associated symptoms is depression. It may result from the stress of the condition, the demyelination process, steroid withdrawal, or a drug reaction. Regardless of the cause, the treatment of choice is antidepressant therapy. Although psychotherapy may be beneficial, an antidepressant drug alone is often sufficient. Fluoxetine (Prozac) is particularly useful because of its benign side effects profile. A single 20-mg capsule taken each morning with breakfast is often adequate. Widely prescribed alternatives include imipramine (Tofranil) 100 mg at bedtime and amitriptyline (Elavil) 10 to 25 mg tid. However, both imipramine and amitriptyline can interfere with bladder emptying and may contribute to urinary retention if the patient already has bladder problems. As a result of already disturbed functioning of the CNS, an MS patient on an antidepressant must be monitored for abnormal body temperatures or blood pressure problems. A neurological consultation is always advisable at the onset of an exacerbation of symptoms.

OTHER NOTES AND PEARLS

Many types of treatment have been applied to the management of MS, but few have demonstrated efficacy in clinical studies. Tried and failed therapies include acupuncture, chiropractic, cyclosporine, evening primrose oil, fatty acid supplements, hyperbaric oxygen, megavitamins, and vitamin E. No totally adequate treatment for acute or chronic MS is currently available. However, research continues in an attempt to find the cause and effective treatments to control, prevent, and reverse this disease. Treatments currently under study include antiviral agents, bee-sting venom, ciliary neurotrophic factor, copolymer-1, cytokines, immunosuppressant drugs, lymphocytapheresis, monoclonal antibodies, oral bovine myeline, prostaglandins, thymectomy, total lymphoid irradiation, 3,4-diaminopyridine, and 4-aminopyridine. The future management of MS may result from research into the molecular genetics of demyelinating diseases. The only certainty at present is that the eventual eradication of MS is expected sooner rather than later.

BIBLIOGRAPHY

Beck RW, Cleary, PA, Anderson MM Jr, et al: A randomized controlled trial of corticosteroids in the treatment of acute optic neuritis. *New Engl J Med* 326:581, 1992.

Cutler RWP: Demyelinating disease. *Scientific American*–Medicine. 11 Neurology, IX:1–5, 1993.

Fowler CJ, van Kerrebroeck PEV, Nordenbo A, et al: Treatment of lower urinary tract dysfunction in patients with multiple sclerosis. *J Neurol Neurosurg Psychiatry* 55:986, 1992.

Lechtenberg R: *Multiple Sclerosis Fact Book,* 2d ed. Philadelphia, Davis, 1995.

Likosky WH, Fireman KB, Elmore R, et al: Intense immunosuppression in chronic progressive multiple sclerosis: The Kaiser study. *J Neurol Neurosurg Psychiatry* 54:1055, 1991.

Lublin FD, Whitaker JN, Eidelman BH, et al: Management of patients receiving interferon β-lb for multiple sclerosis: Report of a consensus conference. *Neurology* 46:12–18, 1996.

McDonald WI: Multiple sclerosis: Diagnostic optimism. *Br Med J* 304:1259, 1992.

Paty DW, Li DKB, et al: Interferon β-lb is effective in relapsing-remitting multiple sclerosis: II. MRI analysis results of the multi-center, randomized, double-blind, placebo-controlled trail. *Neurology* 43:662–667, 1993.

Ron MA, Feinstein A: Multiple sclerosis and the mind [editorial]. *J Neurol Neurosurg Psychiatry* 55:1, 1992.

Chapter 11–3
HEADACHES
Andrea G. Weiss

Organic Headache (Secondary)
DISCUSSION

Secondary headache represents symptoms of organic disease as classified by the Headache Classification Committee of the International Headache Society in 1988. There are multiple causes of organic headaches (Table 11-3-1).

PATHOPHYSIOLOGY

The pain from headache can originate extracranially from skin, fat, muscle, blood vessels, periosteum, and fascial regions of the neck. Head pain also can originate intracranially from the great venous sinuses, the dura at the base of the skull, the dural arteries, and the large arteries at the base of the brain. All these regions have pain fibers. The fifth cranial nerve serves most of the facial area and is responsible for pain arising above the tentorium. Actual brain parenchyma, most of the dura, the arachnoid, and the pia mater are incapable of producing pain arising above the tentorium. The ninth, tenth, and eleventh cranial nerves and the upper cervical spinal nerves serve the region below the tentorium; pain often is referred to the neck and the occipital region of the

Table 11-3-1. Causes of Headache

Acute-onset headache
Meningitis
Intracranial hemorrhage (stroke or ruptured aneurysm)
Stroke
Increased intracranial pressure (cerebral edema, hypertensive encephalopathy, hemorrhage)
Viral illness
Sinusitis
Glaucoma
Metabolic imbalances (hypoglycemia, carbon monoxide poisoning)
Acute presentation of recurrent headache
Persistent or recurrent headache
Migraine with or without aura
Tension-type headache
Cluster-type headache
Postconcussion syndrome
Intracranial mass or lesion (abscess, neoplasm, arteriovenous malformation, subdural hematoma)
Cervical muscle strain or spasm
Temporal arteritis
Post-lumbar puncture–type headache

head. The pain-sensitive structures of the head and neck are affected by the following pain-producing mechanisms: distention, dilation, inflammation, tension, and traction.

HISTORY TAKING

An accurate, detailed history is the most important part of the evaluation in distinguishing acute from chronic from recurrent headache. The six principal areas covered in the headache history are

1. Location
2. Character
3. Typical location and character
4. Duration
5. Precipitating and/or aggravating factors
6. Ameliorating factors
7. Medication history

Location

Asking about the location of the head pain is occasionally but not always useful in making a diagnosis. Unilateral headache suggests a migraine, whereas a headache that begins unilaterally and then progresses to a bilateral distribution can be a sign of elevated intracranial pressure (ICP).

Character

Most patients describe their headaches as intense. Asking a patient to provide a description of the pain may be more useful in determining whether it is sharp, piercing, or exploding pain. One should ask if it is made worse by bending forward, having a bowel movement, or coughing. This may be suggestive of an intracranial source. Is the headache occurring in a location typical of prior headaches, and is it usual in character? This information helps differentiate between chronic headaches and those of new onset suggestive of a possible intracranial bleed.

Precipitating, Aggravating, and Ameliorating Factors

Any history suggesting head trauma (recent or in the past) is a "red flag" and warrants methodical investigation. Therefore, one should inquire about associated head trauma or injuries. A history of lethargy, confusion, vomiting, and/or dizziness concomitant with head trauma raises the possibility of a subacute or chronic subdural hematoma. If the headache improves where the patient lies down, this also suggests an intracranial process.

A physician assistant must use a systematic approach to headache assessment to prevent the pitfalls of overdiagnosis and underdiagnosis, which can have life-threatening consequences. As determined from a careful history, the basic critical distinctions between acute versus chronic, episodic versus continuous, and spontaneous versus traumatic headache can aid the clinician in demonstrating rational approaches to the use of further diagnostic tests, appropriate consultation, and ultimately the proper medical management.

PHYSICAL EXAMINATION

The physical examination is an essential part of the evaluation of headache to search for a serious underlying pathology. Despite the advent of sophisticated imaging techniques, the history and physical examination remain indispensable. The blood pressure and temperature should be checked for elevations. The scalp needs to be thoroughly inspected and palpated for any signs of swelling, discolorations, and tenderness. Also, one should palpate

for tenderness over the temporal arteries; it is necessary to palpate directly over the temporomandibular joint ligaments to elicit tenderness or an audible "pop or click." A sterile gloved finger should be used to probe any scalp lacerations to assess their depth and possible penetration of the skull. Pupils should be assessed for loss of reactivity; a fixed, dilated pupil warrants further investigation into a possible brain abscess or malignancy. Ocular disc margins are examined for clarity; papilledema indicates elevated ICP. One should determine nuchal rigidity on anterior flexion; when present, it is consistent with meningeal irritation. Finally, one should conduct a thorough neurologic examination, looking for ataxia, alterations in mental status (lethargy, confusion, alterations in speech and behavior), focal deficits (positive Babinski's sign), and meningeal signs (Brudzinski's and Kernig's signs).

DIAGNOSTIC CONSIDERATIONS

In evaluating a patient with headaches, the issue of the need for an imaging study of the head commonly arises. Mitchell and colleagues[1] studied the utility of head computed tomography (CT) in patients with headaches, particularly those with abnormal physical examinations or unusual headache characteristics. Only 1 percent of patients with normal physical examinations had an abnormal CT scan, whereas 10 percent of patients with abnormal examinations and 12 percent with unusual histories had abnormal scans. None of the patients with normal examinations and unusual histories had abnormal scans.

Therefore, with the acute onset of headache or a history of a worsening chronic or recurrent headache, emergency CT is the test of choice for prompt detection of potentially life threatening lesions (an intracranial mass or hemorrhage). If the headache is accompanied by meningeal signs of irritation or evidence of increased ICP, a lumber puncture and culture should be performed as well as a complete blood cell count and chemistry profile. Examination of the cerebrospinal fluid should follow a CT to rule out an infectious etiology as long as there is no evidence of markedly increased ICP.

A new onset of headache in an elderly patient may represent the onset of temporal arteritis, especially if it is accompanied by palpable tenderness over a temporal artery. An elevated sedimentation rate helps confirm giant cell arteritis. Finally a neurologic or neurosurgical consultation is recommended in patients with severe headache in whom a definitive diagnosis cannot be established. A consultation also is useful with infection and/or trauma when CT is abnormal and in the presence of altered mental status.

Organic Headaches Resulting from Mass Lessions

DISCUSSION

Mass lesions can cause headache by displacing pain-sensitive structures. Approximately one-third of patients with a mass lesion have headache as an early symptom of the disease. The pain often is reported as being localized to the side of the lesion; however, there are a variety of other presentations, none of which are precisely diagnostic. The headache may be described as mild or severe, persistent or intermittent, sharp or achy, throbbing or pressure-like. Characteristically, the headache remains in one location and becomes progressively worse, lasting for several months. In particular, patients may report that the headache is worse upon awakening. Generally, there are progressive changes in mental status and/or the development of neurologic deficits such as diplopia. Initially these headaches are aggravated by a cough, straining at the stool, lying down, and bending over. However, as ICP increases, the headache becomes more generalized and is associated with nocturnal awakening, dizziness, and vomiting (with or without preceding nausea) and can include generalized convulsions. In patients with a brain tumor, headache may be the sole initial complaint, unaccompanied by focal neurologic deficits. However, as the condition progresses, neurologic deficits usually arise.

The following tumors tend to produce general cerebral symptoms or seizures: metastatic carcinoma, glioblastoma multiforme, astrocytoma, oligodendroglioma, meningioma, and primary reticulocell sarcoma of the cerebrum.

The tumors that tend to elevate ICP without conspicuous localizing signs include medulloblastomas, ependymomas of the fourth ventricle, hemangioblastomas, pinealomas, colloid cysts of the third ventricle, gliomas of the tegmentum of the midbrain with blocking of the aqueduct, and craniopharyngiomas.

TREATMENT

Pharmacologic Management

Steroid therapy is initiated before tissue diagnosis in symptomatic patients with a CT or MRI that reveals edema surrounding an intracranial mass lesion. Although the information regarding the optimal steroid dose is mostly anecdotal, several guidelines have been established. There is a clear dose-related clinical response to corticosteroids. The majority of these patients respond favorably to dexamethasone 4 to 6 mg given by mouth or parenterally four times daily. In critically ill patients and patients who do not exhibit a favorable response to the initial therapy, one should consider massive doses such as 25 mg four times a day. The benefit for patients receiving this dose is that it allows time for more definitive therapies such as life-saving surgical decompression. Other interventions, such as radiation, chemotherapy, and surgical intervention, should be sought whenever appropriate.

Organic Headaches Resulting from Brain Abscesses

DISCUSSION

A headache caused by a brain abscess may present as a mass lesion causing headache, particularly during the latent stages of abscess growth. The formation of a brain abscess involves two stages. Initially a diffuse, poorly marginated area of infection is associated with edema and destruction of brain tissue. Over 4 to 9 days the center of the infection turns into semiliquid pus and necrotic brain tissue. Once this stage is reached, the infection may not be curable by medical therapy (e.g., antibiotics) alone. Encapsulation by gliotic tissue occurs gradually, and a free abscess forms. Lung abscesses, parenteral drug abuse, and parameningeal infections may serve as the source or reservoir for this type of brain infection. The symptoms of a brain abscess manifest as a subacute progression of focal neurologic signs of headache and altered mental status. Seizures occur in 20 to 25 percent of these patients.

DIAGNOSTIC STUDIES

The definitive diagnosis of brain abscess is made during surgery, although characteristic findings may be seen on MRI or CT.

Arteriography is relatively ineffective in localizing a brain abscess.

A patient with a suspected brain abscess is advised to undergo a search for a parameningeal infection. Adequate views of the mastoids and sinuses are critical, since a brain abscess caused by sinusitis usually occurs adjacent to an infected sinus cavity.

TREATMENT

Treatment consists of surgery with drainage of the abscess cavity by needle aspiration or total excision of the affected region. The best surgical treatment remains controversial: There are advocates of aspiration and defenders of total surgical excision. CT-guided stereotactic biopsy and intraoperative ultrasound make most areas of the brain relatively safe for aspiration. There is good evidence that complete excision of superficial lesions eliminates the risk of recurrence. Antibiotics are used both preoperatively and postoperatively. Antibiotic therapy alone is recommended in patients with multiple or surgically inaccesible lesions and patients who are poor candidates for surgery.

Organic Headaches Resulting from Subdural Hematoma

DISCUSSION

Headache caused by a subdural hematoma is another type of mass lesion: a collection of blood between the dura and the underlying brain tissue. It is present in 10 to 15 percent of patients with severe head injuries. Acute subdural hematomas frequently result from high-speed impact accidents and are associated with severe primary brain damage.

A subacute subdural hematoma is suspected when, after several days of headache or diminished alertness, deterioration of consciousness develops. Chronic subdural hematomas, in contrast to other forms of hematomas, may follow a trivial trauma that may go unnoticed by the patient and the patient's family members. Commonly, a gradual drift into stupor or coma is preceded by a headache.

DIAGNOSTIC STUDIES

Subdural Hematoma

CT is the test of choice for a subdural hematoma to demonstrate a mass effect and a midline shift beyond the thickness of a hematoma associated with brain injury.

Subacute and Chronic Subdural Hematomas

The CT density of a hematoma changes from hyperdense to isodense to hypodense (relative to brain tissue) as time progresses after a head trauma. In the isodense stages, a sizable hematoma may not be detectable by CT unless intravenous contrast is administered to enhance the vascular membranes. MRI has replaced CT as the study of choice for distinguishing subacute from chronic subdural hematomas. If MRI is not available, contrast CT, nuclear brain scanning, or arteriography can aid in this diagnosis. In the presence of cerebral edema, ICP monitoring is usually necessary during both the intraoperative and the postoperative phases.

Subarachnoid Hemorrhage from Aneurysmal Rupture

Acute rupture of a brain aneurysm produces the sudden onset of a headache that reaches its maximum intensity immediately. It often is accompanied by meningeal irritation and occasionally by an abrupt loss of consciousness. Subarachnoid hemorrhage (SAH) is one of the most common causes of death in apparently healthy young adults. However, SAH also occurs later in life, with the average age being 50. While a majority of these cases are caused by the rupture of an intracranial source, SAH also may result from head trauma, venous thrombosis, blood dyscrasias, and a variety of metabolic causes.

In the absence of any rupture, 10 to 15 percent of patients with an arteriovenous malformation (AVM) may experience chronic headaches characterized by unilateral throbbing-type pain. An acute onset of intense head pain indicates an AVM rupture. Unlike migraine, there are no prodromal or associated symptoms.

TREATMENT

Because even the lastest-generation CT scanners are not sensitive enough to detect all SAHs, lumbar puncture remains an essential second step in ruling out SAH. CT is not infallible in detecting blood in the CSF. Lumbar puncture seems to be more sensitive and specific with regard to positive findings. Finally, it should be noted that MRI is no more accurate than CT in ruling out SAH. Angiography may be used, since early surgery (24 to 48 h) has been demonstrated to be the treatment of choice for accessible ruptured aneurysms with minor neurologic impairment. Surgery is also the treatment of choice for any aneurysm that is surgically accessible. AVMs, however, may or may not be amenable to surgery, since there is a risk of recurrent hemorrhaging from AVMs.

Organic Headaches Resulting from Stroke

DISCUSSION

Head pain is frequently a presenting feature of an ischemic (embolic or thrombotic) and hemorrhagic stroke such as primary intracerebral hemorrhage and SAH. Many patients report other neurologic deficits before complaining of a headache because these symptoms (inability to talk or feel an arm or leg) seem more compelling and frightening. Headache may precede, exist concomitantly with, or follow a cerebrovascular accident (CVA) (see Chap. 1-3).

On occasion headache may present sooner than the actual signaling of a stroke in evolution. Patients suffering from a stroke involving a large arterial occlusion may surprisingly present with head pain as the sole (initial) symptom. Patients with cortical lesions on CT have been found to have a headache more often than do individuals with deeper infarcts (e.g., SAH versus an ischemic stroke). Headache is more common with posterior circulatory infarcts than it is with anterior circulatory infarcts.

Ischemic strokes present as a primary thrombotic occlusion of a vessel or occlusion of a vessel by fragments from a distant source (embolism). The neurologic deficit associated with an embolism characteristically begins suddenly, with a maximum deficit occurring at the onset. Preceding transient ischemic attacks (TIAs) may occur but are less common than is primary thrombosis. Preceding TIAs are common with thrombotic strokes. This type of stroke also progresses over hours or days, with the neurologic deficit fluctuating or changing in a stepwise fashion, the so-called stroke in evolution. The treatment for stroke is covered in Chap. 1-3.

Organic Headaches Resulting from Bacterial Meningitis

DISCUSSION

Bacterial meningitis from infection or hemorrhage produces pain that is severe, acute in onset, generalized in location, and constant. The headache produced by this condition may be defined as inflammatory. The symptoms may include a severe headache, vomiting, drowsiness, and stupor and have been known to cause coma in extreme cases (see Chap. 9-28).

The causes of bacterial meningitis that vary with age are as follows:

1. *Streptococcus pneumoniae* causes 30 to 50 percent of cases in adults, 10 to 20 percent of cases in children, and up to 5 percent of cases in infants.
2. *Neisseria meningitidis* causes 10 to 30 percent of cases in adults and 30 to 40 percent in children up to age 15. It is rare in infants.
3. *Haemophilus influenzae* type B is responsible for 35 to 45 percent of cases in children but only 1 to 3 percent in adults. It is rare in infants.

Other pathogens may include *Staphylococcus aureus, Staphylococcus epidermidis*, group B streptococci, *Escherichia coli*, and other Enterobacteriaceae, such as *Klebsiella, Enterobacter, Proteus*, and *Citrobacter* spp. Other sources of meningitis include *Treponema pallidum*, Borrelia burgoferi, and *Leptospira interrogans*. Patients with lowered cell-mediated immunity, including transplant recipients, are especially susceptible to intracellular parasites such as *Listeria* spp.

DIAGNOSTIC STUDIES

The following are considered routine tests in all patients with presumptive bacterial meningitis: a complete blood count with differential including a peripheral blood smear, blood cultures, blood urea nitrogen and serum creatinine, serum glucose, electrolytes, and urinalysis. If nephrotoxic drugs are to be used, a baseline serum creatinine clearance is advised. One should obtain a chest x-ray and CT of the head to seek a possible parameningeal focus of infection. After a CT scan, a lumbar puncture needs to be performed to obtain a culture and sensitivities of the organisms in cerebrospinal fluid.

TREATMENT

Once the presumptive diagnosis of bacterial meningitis has been made, antibiotic treatment must be initiated immediately. The initial therapy for bacterial meningitis usually includes intravenous ampicillin 12 g a day divided into four doses. If ampicillin-resistant strains of *H. influenzae* are common in a particular geographic area, it is reasonable to add ceftriaxone 4 to 6 g a day divided into two doses. The alternative treatment is chloramphenicol 4 g a day intravenously divided into four doses and erythromycin 4 g a day intravenously divided into four doses. Pediatric treatments and medication doses are beyond the scope of this chapter. Once antibiotic sensitivities are known through lumbar puncture or blood cultures, a more specific antibiotic selection can be made to provide optimum antibiotic availability for the identified pathogen.

Other Headache Syndromes

CERVICAL ARTHRITIS

Occipital headache associated with pain on movement of the neck may be due to problems in the cervical spine. Arthritic changes can be confirmed by plain x-ray examination of the cervical spine to aid in the diagnosis of cervical arthritis. A trial of aspirin in combination with diazepam can give some relief to these patients. Many patients may also benefit from anti-inflammatory drugs. A cervical collar can be worn during the acute phase, combined with topical therapy such as cold and/or heat applications, in conjunction with physical therapy and cervical traction.

LUMBAR PUNCTURE HEADACHE

The headache that occurs after a lumbar puncture is exacerbated by standing and relieved by lying down. These headaches appear to be caused by persistent leakage of CSF from the subarachnoid space. Management consists of bed rest, analgesics, and hydration. When conservative treatment fails, an epidural blood patch is 90 to 100 percent effective. In this procedure, autologous blood is injected epidurally at or around the site of the previous lumbar puncture site, effectively tamponading the dural leak. Since the blood spreads both circumferentially and longitudinally along as many as nine spinal segments, the precision of the second puncture is not critical so long as the epidural space is injected.

SINUSITIS

Acute sinusitis is accompanied by a recent history of nasal stuffiness or discharge associated with pain on percussion over the sinuses. These patients often describe frontal headache and increased facial pressure when leaning forward and sometimes note upper tooth pain (see Chap. 3-1).

ACUTE CLOSED-ANGLE GLAUCOMA

The headache associated with a red, painful eye can be produced by acute closed-angle glaucoma. Open-angle glaucoma, which is more common, does not produce headache (see Chap. 14-1).

TEMPOROMANDIBULAR JOINT SYNDROME

Head pain caused by the temporomandibular joint syndrome is characterized by pain on chewing or jaw use with radiation into the ear. These patients may describe joint clicking when yawning as well as jaw restriction.

COLD STIMULUS HEADACHE

A cold stimulus headache results from external exposure to cold or the ingestion of a cold substance ("ice cream headache"). The pain is nonpulsatile and reaches a peak intensity about 25 to 60 s after exposure. The great majority of patients with migraine also experience ice cream headache. No treatment is necessary; the headache usually can be avoided by stirring ice cream to a semisolid consistency.

TOXIC HEADACHE

Headaches that are secondary to drugs or environmental exposure are extremely common and often go undiagnosed. Such exposure may aggravate a migraine or tension headache or an unspecified variety of headache. Generally speaking, these headaches tend to be generalized, persistent, and throbbing in nature. Their intensity increases with further exposure to ingestion of the offending agent. Drugs commonly associated with headache include atenolol, nifedipine, cimetidine, ranitidine, and various estrogens. Other implicated substances are nitrates and nitrites, monosodium glutamate, and carbon monoxide.

Nonorganic Benign Headache

DISCUSSION

In 1988, the Headache Classification Committee of the International Headache Society (IHS) classified headaches into organic and nonorganic disorders. The three primary benign types are tension-type headaches (TTHs), cluster headaches, and migraine headaches with and without an aura.

Headaches do not represent a single disease but instead reflect a diverse set of clinical syndromes that may be interrelated. Therefore, primary (benign nonorganic) headaches cannot be "cured." Many patients seem perplexed at medical providers' inability to stop their head pain. The exact etiology of primary benign headache is unknown.

SYMPTOMS

Depending on the type of nonorganic benign headache, the severity and nature of the pain as well as the degree of incapacity vary from person to person. The onset, frequency, location, character, and duration of the pain are very important to determine and may offer important diagnostic clues. The pain may have patterns that disturb sleep, worsen with straining or lifting, or are accompanied by other symptoms, such as dizziness, nausea, vomiting, photophobia, phonophobia, strange smells, and scintillating scotomas. Patients may mention certain triggers or patterns of timing that aggravate or ameliorate the head pain.

OBJECTIVE FINDINGS

Most patients with an active headache appear to be uncomfortable and show various signs of being in pain. The presence of high blood pressure and/or fever should alert the clinician to the possibility of an intracranial bleed or infection, such as meningitis. One should note the patient's vital signs and examine for nuchal rigidity. It is necessary to check the patient's pupils and optic discs for irregularities, such as papilledema. One should look for visual field defects, assess facial asymmetry, test the proximal and distal muscles in the upper and lower extremities, and check all deep tendon reflexes, gait, finger-to-nose movements, and rapid rhythmic movements to differentiate between organic and nonorganic disease.

DIAGNOSTIC CONSIDERATIONS

In evaluating a patient with headaches, the issue of the need for an imaging study of the head commonly arises. Mitchell and colleagues[1] studied the utility of head CT in patients with headaches, particularly those with abnormal physical examinations or unusual headache characteristics. Only 1 percent of patients with normal examinations had an abnormal CT, whereas 10 percent of patients with abnormal examinations and 12 percent with unusual histories had abnormal CT. None of the patients with normal examinations and unusual histories had abnormal head CT scans.

Tension-Type Headache (Muscle Contraction)

PATHOPHYSIOLOGY

Stressful events produce a biochemical change in the brain by which serotonin levels are generally reduced. Theoretically, this biochemical change manifests in a depressive state, although the precise biochemical counterpart of depression is not known. In endogenous depression, endorphin levels decrease, facilitating the transmission of pain impulses that can leave the patient more susceptible to pain. Muscles become tonic and contracted. Vasoconstriction occurs, causing an ischemic-type muscle pain with focal tenderness.

SYMPTOMS

Two varieties of TTHs have been identified: episodic and recurrent TTHs. The constant bilateral pain form of episodic or acute TTHs typically occurs in the late afternoon, lasting from 30 min to several days. It is accompanied by pain that is typically described as constricting in character and bilateral in location and often is associated with anorexia. Physical activity does not exacerbate this type of head pain. Chronic TTHs by definition occur more than 15 days a month for more than 6 months. Unlike the acute form of TTH, chronic TTHs may cause occasional nausea but no vomiting. This type of pain seldom awakens the patient from sleep. TTHs can be precipitated by stress and lack of sleep. Muscle tenderness in the neck and shoulder regions is common. The pain is described as pressure-like, squeezing, or tightening and accumulates throughout the day. Generally, TTHs begin in early adulthood while migraines usually begin in childhood.

OBJECTIVE FINDINGS

Physical examination generally reveals no abnormal findings, with the exception of tenderness and/or palpable muscle spasms at the base of the head, and neck, and/or shoulder region. Also, the patient may complain of pain when asked to perform active range-of-motion exercises of the neck.

TREATMENT

For patients who experience TTHs, pharmacologic treatment considerations include nonsteroidal anti-inflammatory drugs (NSAIDS) alone or in combination with a muscle relaxant. When headaches are not relieved with these agents, consideration of a narcotic is appropriate, to be used on an "as needed" basis alone or with an NSAID. Antidepressants also should be considered appropriate treatment; tricyclics tend to work better than the selective serotonin reuptake inhibitors (SSRIs). The side effects of tricyclics, however, may make these agents less appealing for patients to use (see Table 11-3-4).

Cluster Headaches

PATHOPHYSIOLOGY

The etiology of cluster headaches is not well understood. Popular theories include a vascular headache disorder and a disturbance of the serotoninergic mechanism. This type of headache occurs more commonly in middle-aged men than in women and has no familial predisposition.

SYMPTOMS

The pain is a severe unilateral pain that intensifies around one eye or the temple region. The character of the pain usually is described as sharp and piercing through the affected eye. Episodes last 15 min to 3 h and may recur as many as eight times a day. Headaches often occur 1 or 2 h after the patient falls asleep, thus awakening the patient from sleep. Associated symptoms may include increased eye lacrimation, rhinorrhea, ipsilateral nasal congestion, redness of the affected eye, and Horner's syndrome (seen in approximately 25 percent of cluster headache patients). Spontaneous remission may occur, with the patient remaining symptom-free for several weeks before the next recurrence.

TREATMENT

For abortive treatment one should give oxygen 2L via a mask. Injectable medications such as sumatriptan (Imitrex) and dihydroergotamine (DHE) can be administered intramuscularly, intravenously, or subcutaneously, with oral and self-injectable forms being available. The contraindications to these medications are discussed below in the section on migraine treatment. Oral ergotamines also may be used. Prophylactic regimens include calcium channel blockers and lithium. Verapamil and lithium carbonate are the preferred treatments for chronic cluster headaches.

Migraine Headache

DISCUSSION

Migraine headache is a familial disorder with autosomal dominant inheritance. These patients tend to be young to middle-aged; 80 percent have a history of the first attack before the age 30. About 75 percent of migraine headaches occur without auras, while 20 percent occur with auras. Less than 5 percent are so-called migraine variants, which include hemiplegia with ophthalmologic varieties of ocular dysfunction such as scotomas.

PATHOPHYSIOLOGY

There is a process within both the intracranial and the extracranial vascular structures with phases of vasoconstriction, vasodilation, and inflammation. Vasoconstriction produces anoxia and acidosis and a systemic drop in serum serotonin levels. During this phase a patient may experience neurologic changes called an *aura* that may include several physiologic dysfunctions, such as facial paresthesias and/or partial defects in the visual fields. Anoxia and acidosis cause a local metabolic change and a reaction potentiated by a drop in serotonin that increases cerebral blood flow and causes marked dilation of intracranial and extracranial arteries. Treatment is designed to alter the serotonin receptor reaction in the brain.

SYMPTOMS

Migraine with Aura

Auras are characterized by sensory changes, most often visual symptoms, which range from haziness, to shimmering light waves (scintillating scotomas), to bright or dark holes in the visual field and frank hemianopia. Sensory symptoms also may include tingling paresthesias of the face or upper body, with the legs and trunk seldom involved. No aura symptom lasts longer than 60 min, and several may occur at once. These symptoms precede a

Table 11-3-2. Acute Abortive Treatment Medications for Migraine

Drug	Route	Dose, mg	Comment
Sumatriptan	SC	6	May repeat once after 1 h; up to 24 h; do not use concommitantly with ergot alkaloids; contraindicated in presence of uncontrolled HTN, hx of AMI, peripheral vascular disease, pregnancy
	PO	25, 50, 100	As above; response rates somewhat lower than parenteral routes; start with 25–50 mg; if ineffective, increase to 100 mg;
Dihydroergotamine	IV, IM, SC		often coadministered with metoclopramide or any other antiemetic; individualize dose to patient, usually in range of 0.5–1.5 mg IV, IM administered in office; SC useful in home
Ergotamine tartrate	SL	2	May repeat twice;
(with or without caffeine)	PO	1	with caffeine, 100 mg; oral dose two tablets at onset of headache, may repeat one every 30 min to 6 max;
Isometheptene mucate	PO	65/100/325	maximum of 5 capsules in 24 h or 2 stat, repeat 2 caps in 1h, then stop
Dichloralphenazone			
Acetaminophen			
High-dose nonsteroidal anti-inflammatory drugs			See Table 11-3-2; rebound can occur
Adjunctive therapy			
Phenothiazines	IV	10–12.5	Chlorpromazine
	PR	25	Chlorpromazine

headache by 30 to 60 min. Most cases of ophthalmoplegia resolve without residual deficits. Repeated episodes of vasospasm-induced ischemia, however, may produce infarction, thus causing permanent neurologic deficits in the brain. The head pain itself is paroxysmal, unilateral in location, and associated with nausea, vomiting, photophobia, and phonophobia. The medical history and physical examination, including a complete neurologic examination, often do not suggest other disorders.

Migraine without Aura

Attacks of migraine with an aura last 4 to 70 hs and include at least two of the following characteristics: unilateral location, pulsating quality, moderate to severe intensity, inhibition of daily activities, aggravation by physical activities, and association with at least one of the following signs: nausea, vomiting, phonophobia, and photophobia. The history and neurologic examination do not suggest another secondary, organic headache disorder.

TREATMENT

Nonpharmacologic Therapy

Nondrug therapy is essential in a motivated patient. Nearly all primary benign headaches are associated with a component of stress of anxiety. Without exploration of these underlying issues, clinicians provide a disservice to patients by often prescribing unnecessary medications. Helpful nonpharamcologic techniques may include pscyhotherapy, relaxation techniques, massage, relaxation exercises, and biofeedback.

Abortive Therapy

Abortive therapy (Table 11-3-2) involves both oral and injectable deliveries of pharmacologic medications. The oral forms include ergotamines (tablets and suppositories), isometheptene mucate, NSAIDS, phenothiazines, ketorolac, and transnasal butorphanol.

Dihydroergofamine (DHE-45) given intramuscularly or intravenously in combination with an antiemetic [prochlorperazine Compazine) or droperidol (Inapsine)] is another choice for abortive therapy. Side effects may include nausea, vomiting, chest pain, and transient myalgias and arthralgias. This regimen is contraindicated in patients with cardiovascular disease, peripheral vascular disease, and significant liver or renal disease.

When used subcutaneously, sumatriptan, works quickly. Side effects may include flushing, chest tightness, chest pain, and transient paresthesias. This is contraindicated in patients on monoamine oxidase (MAO) inhibitors, patients with poorly controlled hypertension, and pregnant or nursing women. One should avoid using this drug if ergotamines have been used within the past 24 h. Sometimes a second injection of sumatriptan has been shown to be effective if the patient's symptoms are partially reduced after the initial injection.

Table 11-3-3. Nonsteroidal Anti-Inflammatory Drugs

Drug	Route	Dose, mg/d
Naproxen	PO	250–500 bid
Fenoprofen	PO	600 tid
Flurbiprofen	PO	100 bid
Ketoprofen	PO	75 tid

NOTE: Prophylactic doses for daily use in migraine and chronic tension-type headaches.

Table 11-3-4. Beta Blockers

Drug	Route	Dose, mg/d
Propanolol	PO	60–160
Nadolol	PO	20–120
Timolol	PO	10–20
Metoprolol	PO	100–200
Atenolol	PO	25–100

NOTE: Prophylactic doses for migraine and tension-type headaches. Side effects may include fatigue, depression, diarrhea, and slow heart rate; may exacerbate underlying asthma and congestive heart failure. One approach recommends beginning at the lowest dose and progressing to the highest dose tolerated before including or switching to additional therapy.

Table 11-3-5. Antidepressants

Drug	Route	Dose, mg/d
Tricyclic Antidepressants*		
Nonsedating types		
Desipramine	PO	5–30
Protriptyline	PO	25–150
Sedating types		
Amitriptyline	PO	10–150
Doxepin	PO	10–150
Imipramine	PO	10–150
Nortriptyline	PO	10–150
Serotonin Reuptake Inhibitors†		
Fluoxetine	PO	10–80
Sertraline	PO	50–200
Paroxetine	PO	20–60

* Side effects may include drowsiness, dryness of mouth, weight gain, constipation, and urinary retention.
† Side effects may include drowsiness, nausea, sweating, and irritability, but these drugs seem better tolerated than tricyclics.
NOTE: Used in prophylactic doses for migraine and chronic tension-type headaches, particularly but not exclusively those with a depression component.

PREVENTION

Preventive therapy is indicated for patients who suffer from debilitating headaches at least 2 to 3 days per month. Pharmacologic interventions may include calcium channel blockers (verapamil and diltiazem), which take 4 to 6 weeks to work. In contrast, beta blockers (propanolol) have an onset of only 2 to 3 days, but not all patients receive relief from this category of drugs. Tricyclic antidepressants are more effective than SSRIs and work well in patients in whom there is a component of depression and/or anxiety (Tables 11-3-3 through 11-3-6).

NOTES AND PEARLS

The following points should be noted:

- Changing headaches can be a predictor of more serious consequences.
- Any headaches that occur after age 50 are more of a concern than are headaches that begin at an earlier age.
- A headache after age 40 that is abrupt in onset should raise the possibility of an organic cause such as an intracranial hemorrhage.
- A headache that radiates all over the head is usually more innocuous than a headache that remains unilateral and stays in the same location.
- Narcotic medications should be used with caution in patients with chronic headaches. One must be aware of drug-seeking behaviors and other signs of drug dependency.

Table 11-3-6. Calcium Channel Blockers

Drug	Route	Dose, mg/d
Verapamil	PO	120–480
Flunarizine	PO	10
Diltiazem	PO	90–360
Nifedipine	PO	10–30

NOTE: Verapamil and flunarizine seem to be the most effective for migraine. Constipation is the most common side effect.

REFERENCE

1. Mitchell CS, Osborn RE, Grosskreutz SR: Computed tomography in the headache patient: Is routine evaluation really necessary? *Headache* 33:82–86, 1993.

BIBLIOGRAPHY

Asmark HH, Lundberg P: Drug-related headache. *Headache* 29:441, 1989.
Caesar R, Kramer DA, Gavin LJ: Acute headache management: The challenge of deciphering etiologies to guide assessment and treatment. *Emerg Med Rep* 16:117–128, 1995.
Dalesso DJ: Diagnosing the severe headache. *Neurology* 44:S6–S12, 1994.
Forsyth PA, Posner JB: Headaches in patients with brain tumors: A study of 111 patients. *Neurology* 43:1678, 1993.
Gorelick PB: Ischemic stroke and intracranial hematoma, in Olesoen J (ed): *The Headaches*. New York, Raven Press, 1993, p. 642.
Koudstaal PJ: Headache in transient or permanent cerebral ischemia. *Stroke* 22:754–759, 1991.
Kumar KL: Recent advances in management of migraine and cluster headaches. *J Gen Intern Med* 9:339–348, 1994.
LeBlanc R: The minor leak preceding subarachnoid hemorrhage: *J Neurosurg* 66:35–39, 1987.
Morgenlander JC: Lumbar puncture and CSF examination. *Postgrad Med* 95:125–131, 1994.
Moskowitz MA, Macfarlane R: Neurovascular and molecular mechanisms in migraine headaches. *Cerebrovasc Brain Metab Rev* 5:159, 1993.
Olsen KS: Epidural blood patch in the treatment of post lumbar puncture headache. *Pain* 30:293–301, 1987.
Pearce JMS: Cluster headache and its variants. *Postgrad Med J* 68:517, 1992.
Pearce JMS: Headache. *J. Neurol Neurosurg Psychiatry* 57:134–143, 1994.
Rapoport AM: Update on severe headache. *Neurology* S5, 1994.
Sames TA et al: Sensitivity of new-generation computed tomography in subarachnoid hemorrhage. *Acad Emerg Med* 3:16, 1996.
Silberstein SD: Tension-type and chronic daily headache. *Neurology* 26:469–471, 1993.
Weir BK: Headaches form aneurysms. *Cephalgia* 14:79–87, 1994.
Welch KMA: Drug therapy of migraine. *New Engl J Med* 329:1476, 1993.

Chapter 11–4
ALZHEIMER'S DISEASE
Freddi Segal-Gidan

DISCUSSION

Alzheimer's disease (AD) affects an estimated 4 million Americans. It is considered to be the fourth leading cause of death among adults, accounting for approximately 120,000 deaths per year. It is a degenerative disorder of the brain involving changes in the number, structure, and function of neurons in the cerebral cortex, producing loss of memory and intellectual function (see Chap. 11-5) along with changes in personality and behavior. The illness lasts on average 8 years, but this varies widely and can reach 15 or more years. There is no known cause or cure, but new therapies to delay the course of the disease are rapidly entering the market. Treatment is aimed at early diagnosis and supportive services for the patient and family.

Table 11-4-1. Prevalence of Alzheimer's Disease with Increasing Age

Age, years	Prevalence, %
60–64	1
65–69	2
70–74	4
75–79	8
80–84	16
>85	30

Advancing age remains the primary risk factor. The incidence of AD is 1 in 100,000 at age 50 and 1 in 1000 at age 70 (Table 11-4-1). AD occurring before age 65 is classified as presenile or early-onset AD. When the disease manifests after age 65, it is called senile or late-onset AD. AD affects women almost twice as often as men, though this may be partially due to the longer life span of women. Other risk factors include lower level of education, a family history of AD, and a history of head trauma. AD in persons with a first-degree relative (parent or sibling) with the disease is often referred to as familial AD, while in those without a family history it is termed sporadic AD, although these are somewhat arbitrary classifications.

PATHOGENESIS

The primary feature of AD is loss of neurons in the cerebral cortex. In 1911 Dr. Alois Alzheimer first described the presence of tangled bundles of fibers within the nerve cell (neurofibrillary tangles) and deposits (plaques) over the cortex in the brain of a 59-year-old woman who had died after a 5-year course of progressive dementia. The presence of neurofibrillary tangles and senile plaques in certain regions of the brain remains the basis for a definitive diagnosis of AD. The deposition of amyloid in the cerebral and meningeal blood vessels (cerebral angiopathy) also is commonly seen pathologically in AD.

SYMPTOMS

The hallmark of AD is the presence of a progressive dementia of no known etiology. In early AD there are recent memory problems (forgetfulness), impaired problem solving, and often difficulty making decisions. Social demeanor is usually preserved. In this stage patients may be aware of their deficits and try to compensate or may withdraw from interactions. They tend to become fearful and anxious and often are depressed.

As the disease progresses, language problems are common, with word-finding difficulty (e.g., "that thing" or "thing you write with" for a pen or pencil) and paraphasic errors ("clock" for "watch," "spoon" for "fork"). Visual-spatial difficulties increase the risk of the patient getting lost, and functional problems require increasing outside supervision. Behavioral problems and personality changes become more common in the middle stages of AD. Wandering, pacing, agitation, and paranoia are more characteristic of AD than of other dementias.

In the later stages cognitive and functional impairment is profound, requiring supervision and assistance in most activities. Severe language problems (aphasia), motor planning (apraxia), and incontinence are common. Individuals with AD die with the disease not from it. Death associated with end-stage dementia and immobility usually results from accompanying infection (pneumonia, urinary, sepsis).

OBJECTIVE FINDINGS

In the history, the key element is the course of the disease, which is insidious and slowly deteriorating. AD patients typically (though not always) are physically quite healthy, have a sparse past medical history, and take no or very few medications. Mental status testing is essential for documenting the presence of a dementia and decline over time. The physical examination is typically normal in AD patients. Increased tone and certain frontal release signs (suck, grasp) are common in the latter stages of the disease.

DIAGNOSTIC CONSIDERATIONS

The clinical accuracy of diagnosis is about 85 percent. The diagnostic criteria for AD were established in 1984 and are accepted worldwide (Table 11-4-2). A definitive diagnosis of AD can be made only on brain autopsy and requires a preexisting clinical diagnosis of probable AD.

SPECIAL CONSIDERATIONS

The primary population affected by AD is over age 65, although about 10 to 15 percent of cases occur before that age. Although the diagnostic criteria set 40 to 90 as the age limits, rare cases have been diagnosed before age 40, and with the aging of the population, AD is increasingly being diagnosed in those in the tenth decade and beyond.

LABORATORY TESTS

There is to date no definitive laboratory test for AD. A laboratory evaluation for dementia is essential (see Chap. 11-5) and should be negative. If laboratory abnormalities are identified, they must be addressed and corrected before a clinical diagnosis of AD can be made with any certainty. For instance, previously undiagnosed hypothyroidism must be treated appropriately, thyroid levels must be normalized for several months, and then repeat cognitive testing must be done to establish a persistent and progressive dementia before a clinical diagnosis of AD should be made.

RADIOLOGIC STUDIES

There are no definitive radiologic studies. Serial computer tomography (CT) or magnetic resonance imaging (MRI) of the brain over several years may show evidence of increasing generalized cortical atrophy (ventriculomegaly and enlargement of the sulci). Single-photon-emission computer tomography (SPECT) and

Table 11-4-2. Criteria for the Diagnosis of Alzheimer's Disease

Clinical diagnosis of definitive Alzheimer's disease
  Presence of a dementia by clinical examination and documented by mental status testing
  Deficits in two or more areas of cognition
  Progressive worsening of memory and other cognitive functions
  No disturbance of consciousness
  Onset between ages 40 and 90, most often after age 65
  Absence of systemic disorder or other brain diseases that could account for the progressive deficits in memory and cognition
Clinical diagnosis of definitive Alzheimer's disease
  Dementia syndrome in the absence of another neurologic, psychiatric, or systemic disorder sufficient to cause dementia and in the presence of variations in onset, presentation, or clinical course
  Presence of a second systemic or brain disorder sufficient to produce dementia that is not considered to be the cause of the dementia
  A single, gradually progressive severe cognitive deficit in the absence of another identifiable cause
Definitive Alzheimer's disease
  Clinical criteria for definitive Alzheimer's disease
  Histopathologic evidence obtained from a biopsy or autopsy of the brain

SOURCE: Adapted from McKahnn et al.

positron-emission tomography (PET) typically show reduced blood flow and metabolism in the temporal and parietal lobes of the brain. It remains uncertain whether these findings are sensitive and specific for AD.

OTHER DIAGNOSTICS

Comprehensive neuropsychological testing may be helpful, especially in the early stages. It can identify specific areas of cognitive decline and their severity. Most AD patients show reduced short-term memory, although there may be considerable variation in test results between patients.

TREATMENT

There is no curative or preventive treatment for AD. Intervention is aimed at improving function and maintaining maximum independence for as long as possible.

Pharmacotherapy

There are currently two medications approved specifically for the treatment of AD, tacrine, (Cognex) and donepezil (Aricept). Both are cholinesterase inhibitors and have been shown to slow the rate of decline in 15 to 40 percent of individuals in the early to moderate stages of AD. Tacrine requires more frequent dosing and has some risk of hepatotoxicity. Aricept has few side-effects and is dosed once daily making it easier for patients and their caregivers to manage. A number of other drugs that may slow the rate of cognitive decline or stop further progression of the disease are in large-scale trials to assess their efficacy and safety but will not be available for 3 to 5 years.

Estrogen and nonsteroidal anti-inflammatory drugs (NSAIDs) have recently been shown to have a protective effect on AD (see Chap. 11-5 for a discussion of pharmacologic therapy for behavioral problems associated with dementia).

Supportive Measures

Individuals with AD should be encouraged to remain as independent as is safely possible. A regular schedule should be maintained to minimize confusion and new learning for a person with AD.

Wandering behavior is seen frequently in patients with AD, although it also may occur with other dementia syndromes. Wandering itself is not a problem, but it presents challenges to the caregiver in regard to the safety of the patient. The goal should be not to stop the wandering (or pacing) but to ensure the safety of the wanderer. Regular physical activity, such as walking and riding a stationary bicycle, may help dissipate excess energy and thus diminish the frequency of wandering. Identification bracelets are an important preventive measure in case the individual becomes lost. Physical and chemical restraints, while frequently used in the past, are not considered appropriate except in extreme cases.

Patient Education

Patients in the early stages should be told about the diagnosis so that they can make appropriate future plans. It is important that the family know what level of care the patient wants. The execution of a durable power of attorney for health care (DPAHC) if not previously done should be encouraged among those who are cognitively able.

One of the most difficult problems with AD, as with other dementias, is driving (see Chap. 11-5). One should be aware of one's state's laws regarding reporting requirements. Individuals with early AD may still retain the capacity to operate a motor vehicle safely, but those in the middle to later stages are a danger to themselves and others on the road.

Table 11-4-3. Resources for Information and Assistance

National Alzheimer's Association 70 E. Lake Street Suite 600 Chicago, IL 60601 Tel: 800-621-0379
ADEAR (Alzheimer's Disease Education and Referral) Center PO Box 8250 Silver Spring, MD 20907-8250 Tel: 301-495-3311

The bulk of care for individuals with AD falls on their families. Caregivers need accurate information, emotional support, anticipatory guidance, and respite. Placement out of the home in a supportive housing environment or nursing home may have to be considered, depending on the patient and family's abilities, resources, and desires. Some AD patients remain at home until death, while others require out-of-home placement early in the course of the disease. The Alzheimer's Association and the National Institute on Aging's Alzheimer's Disease Education and Referral Center (ADEAR) are important national resources for families and professionals (Table 11-4-3). Local chapters can provide literature, support groups, and referral to day-care programs, paid in-home aides, and nursing homes.

DISPOSITION

A diagnosis of AD represents the beginning of an ongoing need for reevaluation and monitoring. Cognitive status should be reassessed at least annually to document a progressive decline consistent with AD. Changes in function should be assessed, and caregivers should be assisted in appropriate ongoing management. The physician assistant may need to suggest out-of-home placement or provide referrals for increased in-home assistance. Intercurrent medical problems should be treated in accordance with the patient's stated wishes.

COMPLICATIONS AND RED FLAGS

AD is a slowly progressive disease of neurodegeneration. Individuals without objective decline over a 1- to 2-year period may be incorrectly diagnosed. Any marked change over a short period (hours or days) in cognition or function may signal a delirium and warrants a complete evaluation for the underlying cause (Table 11-4-4). Seizures or falls in the early stages are extremely rare in AD, although they are common in the late stages of the disease.

AD is a terminal disease, but with good supportive care individuals may live for many years. In the latter stages of the disease the patient requires total care, including feeding and turning in bed regularly to avoid pressure sores (see Chap. 2-11). When a patient loses the ability to swallow, the family and the provider face the difficult decision of whether to initiate tube feeding in

Table 11-4-4. Common Causes of Delirium

Medications (prescribed, over-the-counter, illicit)
Infectious (pneumonia, urinary, decubitus)
Cardiovascular (congestive heart failure, myocardial infarction)
Cerebrovascular (cerebrovascular accident, trauma, tumor)
Metabolic (hypo- or hyperthyroid, hypo- or hyperglycemia)
Thermoregulatory (hypo- or hyperthermia)
Psychiatric (bipolar, grief and/or loss, depression)
Environmental (relocation, institutionalization)

this terminal stage of AD. The use of nasogastric feeding tubes is only temporary (1 to 2 weeks), and then placement of a gastric feeding tube must be considered.

NOTES AND PEARLS

A genetic link to an increasing incidence of AD has been detected in recent years. Currently markers on four chromosomes (1, 14, 19, and 21) have been shown to be associated with the development of AD. A strong association has been demonstrated between the apolipoprotein E (apo E) E^4 allele and the development of late-onset AD. The apo E genetic test is widely available, and its results indicate which allele combination a person has inherited. Higher susceptibility to AD is indicated if the person has one or two E^4 alleles. The apo E genotype is only one risk factor and should not be used as a clinical predictor of AD. In the presence of a late-onset dementia, genetic testing for apo E may help confirm a diagnosis of AD, but in the absence of a dementia, the test is not predictive.

BIBLIOGRAPHY

Alzheimer's Association: The use of APOE testing in Alzheimer's disease. *Res Pract* 5, 1996.

Davis KL, Thal LJ, Gamzu E, et al: A double-blind placebo-controlled multicenter study of tacrine for Alzheimer's disease. *New Engl J Med* 327:1253–1259, 1992.

Growdon J: Treatment of Alzheimer's disease. *New Engl J Med* 328:1306–1308, 1992.

McKahnn G, Drachman D, Folstein M, et al: Clinical diagnosis of Alzheimer's disease: Report of the NINCDS-ADRDA Work Group. Department of Health and Human Services Task Force on Alzheimer's Disease. *Neurology* 34:939–944, 1984.

Morris JC: Differential diagnosis of Alzheimer's disease. *Clin Geriatr Med* 10(2):257–275, 1994.

Whitehouse PJ, Geldmacher DS: Pharmacotherapy for Alzheimer's disease. *Clin Geriatr Med* 10(2):339–350, 1994.

Chapter 11–5
DEMENTIA
Freddi Segal-Gidan

DISCUSSION

Dementia, from the Latin *de mens,* literally means "out of one's mind." It refers to a clinical condition in which there is impairment of memory and other cognitive abilities, resulting in a loss of function. Diagnostic criteria according to the *Diagnostic and Statistical Manual of Mental Disorders,* 4th ed (DSM-IV) include memory impairment, at least one other area of cognitive decline, and associated functional problems (see Table 11-5-1).[1] Dementia is a syndrome that represents the final common clinical expression of a variety of diseases that damage the brain (Table 11-5-2). Most dementias are irreversible, but there are many conditions with symptoms that may mimic a dementia, especially in the elderly.

Table 11-5-1. DSM-IV Criteria for Dementia

A. The development of multiple cognitive deficits manifested by both
  (1) memory impairment (impaired ability to learn new information or to recall previously learned information)
  (2) one (or more) of the following cognitive disturbances:
    (a) aphasia (language disturbance)
    (b) apraxia (impaired ability to carry out motor activities despite intact motor function)
    (c) agnosia (failure to recognize or identify objects despite intact sensory function)
    (d) disturbance in executive functioning (i.e., planning, organizing, sequencing, abstracting)
B. The cognitive deficits in Criteria A1 and A2 each cause significant impairment in social or occupational functioning and represent a significant decline from a previous level of functioning

SOURCE: Diagnostic and Statistical Manual of Mental Disorders, 4th ed (DSM-IV). Washington, DC, American Psychiatric Association, 1994.

Dementias occur at all ages but increase in incidence with increasing age. The aging of the population means that there will be a growing prevalence of dementing illnesses with associated increasing costs, direct and indirect, for the care of individuals with these conditions. Early recognition of a dementia is important to prevent excessive morbidity and premature mortality and to give the patient time to make plans for future needs and care.

SYMPTOMS

It may be difficult at times to differentiate the cognitive changes associated with normal aging from those of early dementia. The

Table 11-5-2. Causes of Dementia in Adults

Primary degenerative diseases
  Alzheimer's disease
  Pick's disease
Cardiovascular disorders
  Vascular disease (multi-infarct)
  Vasculitis
Neurologic diseases with dementia
  Huntington's disease
  Parkinson's disease
  Progressive supranuclear palsy (PSP)
  Amyotrophic lateral sclerosis (ALS)
  Multiple sclerosis (MS)
  Intracranial structural lesions
  Normal-pressure hydrocephalus (NPH)
  Tumors
  Subdural hematomas
Metabolic or systemic conditions
  Hypo- or hyperthyroidism
  Hypo- or hyperglycemia
  Sarcoidosis
  Nutritional deficiencies
Infections
  Syphilis
  HIV-AIDS
  Meningitis
  Encephalitis
  Creutzfeld-Jakob disease
  Brain abscess
Sensory deprivation
Depression
Intoxication
  Drugs
  Alcohol
  Heavy metals
  Carbon monoxide
  Industrial agents (organophosphates)

Table 11-5-3. Differentiating Delirium from Dementia

Characteristic	Delirium	Dementia
Onset	Abrupt	Gradual
Course	Fluctuating, days to hours	Stable over days to weeks
Duration	Hours to weeks	Years
Alertness	Abnormal: increased or decreased	Usually normal
Attention	Impaired	Usually normal
Orientation	Impaired for time Mistakes unfamiliar for familiar	Impaired
Memory	Immediate and recent memory impaired	Recent impaired; remote intact until late
Thinking	Disorganized	Impoverished
Perception	Illusions, hallucinations	Usually normal
Speech	Abnormal: slow or rapid	Word finding
Sleep-awake cycle	Disrupted	Fragmented sleep
Physical illness	Present	Often absent

earliest symptoms of dementia often go unrecognized by patients, their families, and health care providers. Routine mental status testing among the elderly may help uncover an early dementia months or years sooner than it would otherwise be detected. When symptoms appear suddenly, it is important to differentiate delirium from dementia (Table 11-5-3) in order to initiate appropriate treatment promptly.

The history in a suspected dementia patient should always be confirmed by a collateral source. An individual may have little or no insight into his or her cognitive decline. Often it is the family, the employer, or a close relative who notices a change in intellect, behavior, or function and brings the patient to the attention of the health care system. It is important to document the onset of cognitive problems and functional decline: Was there a gradual onset, or did things change over a short period? What activities can the person no longer perform? Most dementias, regardless of etiology, manifest progressive decline in a number of areas that can be monitored over time (Table 11-5-4).

In the early stages there are often difficulties with judgment and complex problem solving, resulting in problems with tasks such as balancing a checkbook, paying taxes, and cooking. The patient may be apathetic and withdraw from the usual activities and social gatherings. As a dementia progresses, memory problems become more apparent, the ability to function outside one's own home declines, and personal care and hygiene may be neglected and require supervision. In the late stages of dementia individuals require increasing assistance for most basic tasks, such as dressing and bathing; they become incontinent (usually of urine first) and need 24-h supervision for safety because of their severely impaired memory and judgment. In the terminal stages a dementia patient is bed-bound, requires total care, and may have to be fed.

OBJECTIVE FINDINGS

A comprehensive physical examination, including mental status testing to document cognitive ability, is essential in the diagnosis of dementia. A number of validated, brief screening instruments can easily be mastered and any one of them can be used routinely in the context of a standard history and physical examination (Table 11-5-5). Each instrument tests a variety of cognitive domains and can be used to screen for dementia, but none is diagnostic in and of itself. Referral for definitive neuropsychological testing should be considered for those in the very early stages of

a suspected dementia (clinical dementia rating of 0.5), those who score within normal limits but remain suspicious for a dementia, and those with an unusual pattern of decline.

A thorough neurologic examination is required to detect findings of neurodegenerative diseases in which dementia is a component and other conditions that can exacerbate or contribute to an existing dementia.

DIAGNOSTIC CONSIDERATIONS

There are over 60 conditions that can manifest themselves as a dementia or in which a dementia is a primary symptom. The acronym DEMENTIA provides a helpful tool for remembering the causes of dementia that can be reversed or arrested (Table 11-5-6).

Numerous medications, as well as over-the-counter and illicit drugs, can alter cognition and produce an apparent dementia (Table 11-5-7).

Depression is not an uncommon occurrence concurrently with a dementia but also may produce symptoms of cognitive and functional decline that present as a dementia (pseudodementia). Metabolic conditions such as hypo- and hyperthyroidism and hypo- and hyperglycemia can produce alterations in cognition. Common eye and ear disorders, such as cataract and ceruminosis, often come on gradually, are asymptomatic, and may disturb cognition and function.

Nutritional problems, especially malnourishment and vitamin B_{12} deficiency, are known to impair cognition. Thyroid disease (hypo- and hyperthyroidism) and thermoregulatory problems also can produce a dementia syndrome. Trauma, especially subdural hematomas and intracranial masses, can affect cognition and appear insidiously or abruptly as confusion. Infectious diseases such as pneumonia, urinary tract infections, and syphilis present in the elderly subtly and can produce a delirium that often is mistaken for dementia. In younger individuals HIV-AIDS is increasing as a primary cause of dementia. Alcohol use and arteriosclerotic disease (cardiac and cerebral) may be the underlying reason for a decline in cognitive and other functional abilities.

Cerebrovascular disease (vascular or multi-infarct dementia) accounts for about 15 percent of all dementias in the United States and a considerably higher percentage in other countries (e.g., Japan). These patients usually have a stepwise pattern of decline with periods of stability. They frequently have hypertension, diabetes, peripheral vascular disease, and cardiac problems (arrhythmia, angina, congestive heart failure). In patients with large-vessel disease, cognitive deficits are associated with hemiplegia or aphasia. Small-vessel disease is more difficult to detect, as there may be no or only very subtle neurologic abnormalities on physical examination.

Normal-pressure hydrocephalus (NPH) is the most common structural abnormality associated with dementia. It is one of the few surgically correctable causes of dementia. Classically, the patient presents with the triad of early dementia, urinary incontinence, and gait ataxia. Surgical shunting of CSF can produce a significant improvement in cognition and function, especially when it is done early in the course.

There are a number of neurodegenerative diseases in which dementia can be a prominent symptom. The most common are Parkinson's disease (see Chap. 11-7), Huntington's disease, and multiple sclerosis (see Chap. 11-2).

SPECIAL CONSIDERATIONS

Undiagnosed or misdiagnosed dementia is a costly illness in terms of both dollars and lives. Not all dementia is Alzheimer's, even in those over age 65. Forty percent of dementias in persons over

Table 11-5-4. Clinical Dementia Rating Scale

Process	Healthy CDR 0*	Questionable Dementia CDR 0.5	Mild Dementia CDR 1	Moderate Dementia CDR 2	Severe Dementia CDR 3
Memory	No memory loss or slight inconsistent forgetfulness	Mild consistent forgetfulness; partial recollection of events; "benign" forgetfulness	Moderate memory loss, more marked for recent events; defect interferes with everyday activities	Severe memory loss; only highly learned material retained; new material rapidly lost	Severe memory loss; only fragments remain
Orientation	Fully oriented	Fully oriented	Some difficulty with time relationships; oriented for place and person at examination but may have geographic disorientation	Usually disoriented for time, often for place	Orientation to person only
Judgment, problem solving	Solves everyday problems well; judgment good in relation to past performance	Only doubtful impairment in solving problems, similarities, differences	Moderate difficulty in handling complex problems; social judgment usually maintained	Severely impaired in handling problems, similarities, differences; social judgment usually impaired	Unable to make judgments or solve problems
Community affairs	Independent function at usual level in job, shopping, business and financial affairs, volunteer and social groups	Only doubtful or mild impairment, if any, in these activities	Unable to function independently in these activities though may still be engaged in some; may still appear normal on casual inspection	No pretense of independent function outside home	No pretense of independent function outside home
Home and hobbies	Life at home, hobbies, intellectual interests well maintained	Life at home, hobbies, intellectual interests well maintained or only slightly impaired	Mild but definite impairment of function at home; more difficult chores abandoned; more complicated hobbies and interests abandoned	Only simple chores preserved; very restricted interests, poorly sustained	No significant function in home outside of own room
Personal care	Fully capable of self-care		Needs occasional prompting	Requires assistance in dressing, hygiene, keeping of personal effects	Requires much help with personal care; often incontinent

Clinical Dementia Rating Scale for More Severe Stages of Dementia (Usually Institutionalized)

Process	Profound CDR 4	Terminal CDR 5
Speech and language	Speech usually unintelligible or irrelevant; unable to follow simple instructions or comprehend commands	No response; no comprehension
Recognition	Occasionally recognizes spouse or caregiver	No recognition
Feeding	Uses fingers more than utensils; requires much assistance	Needs to be fed; may have nasogastric tube; may have swallowing difficulties
Continence	Frequently incontinent despite assistance or training	Total incontinence
Mobility	Able to walk a few steps with help; usually chair-bound; rarely out of home or residence; purposeless movements often present	Bedridden; unable to sit or stand; contractures

* CDR = clinical dementia rating. Score as 0.5, 1, 2, 3 only if impairment is due to cognitive loss.

SOURCE: Adapted with permission from Hughes CP, Berg L, Danziger WL, et al: A new clinical scale for the staging of dementia. *Br J Psychiatry* 140:566, 1982.

age 65 are due to other causes. Among younger individuals, HIV-AIDS is the fastest growing cause of dementia.

LABORATORY TESTS

No single test or laboratory formula for detecting and diagnosing a dementia exists. A comprehensive hematologic workup is required to look for possible underlying causes or contributing factors (Table 11-5-8). HIV testing should be done in individuals with dementia and a history of high-risk behavior recently or in the past 5 to 10 years.

An electrocardiogram is important to rule out an underlying myocardial infarction and serve as a baseline for current or future pharmacologic treatment of associated behavioral problems.

RADIOLOGIC STUDIES

The use of brain imaging remains controversial. The American Academy of Neurology has suggested that a neuroimage be obtained at least once in all cases of dementia.[2] Neither computed tomography (CT) nor magnetic resonance imaging (MRI) of the brain is diagnostic unless an underlying intracranial structural process is involved. Such imaging is definitely warranted if one suspects a stroke, tumor, or subdural hematoma.

OTHER DIAGNOSTICS

An electroencephalogram (EEG) should be considered if there is the possibility of an underlying seizure disorder but is not

Table 11-5-5. Mental Status Screening Instruments

Folstein Mini-Mental State Exam (MMSE)
Blessed Memory-Information-Concentration Test
Short Portable Mental Status Questionnaire (SPMSQ)
Cognitive Capacity Screening Exam
Mental Health Questionnaire
Kokman Short Test of Mental Status

Table 11-5-7. Drugs That Affect Cognition

Antianxiety agents (benzodiazepines)
Antidepressants (lithium, amitriptyline)
Antihistamines (diphenhydramine, hyroxyzine)
Antihypertensives (clonidine, hydralazine, methyldopa, propranalol, reserpine)
Antimicrobials (isoniazid)
Antiparkinsonian drugs (amantadine, bromocriptine, carbidopa)
Antipsychotics (haloperidol, thiothixene, thoridazine, chlorpromazine)
Cardiovascular (atropine, digitalis, diuretics, lidocaine)
H_2 blockers (cimetidine)
Hypnotics (barbiturates, benzodiazepines, chloral hydrate)
Narcotics (codeine, meperidine, morphine, propoxyphene)
Steroids

routinely recommended. Lumbar puncture is indicated when there is suspicion of a CNS infection, a reactive (positive) serum syphilis serology, and hydrocephalus and when there is a rapidly progressive or unusual dementia. Positron-emission tomography and single-photon-emission computed tomography scans remain experimental in the diagnostic workup of dementia.

Referral to a psychologist for comprehensive neuropsychological testing may be necessary in the very early stages and for individuals with cognitive deficits that are difficult to assess with screening tests. Psychological referral for assessment and therapy for individuals with depression should be considered. A psychiatric consultation may be required for the associated behavioral problems.

TREATMENT

The appropriate treatment depends on an accurate diagnosis of the underlying cause of the dementia. If delirium is suspected as the cause or as a contributing factor, treatment of the delirium should be undertaken aggressively.

Pharmacologic Management

All medications, prescription and nonprescription, that are not absolutely essential should be discontinued. Some medications cannot be stopped abruptly but must be reduced in dose gradually. Alcohol and any illicit drug use must cease for several months before an accurate assessment of cognitive status can be obtained.

Depression, either as the primary underlying diagnosis or as a contributing factor, warrants pharmacologic therapy along with counseling, psychotherapy, and other appropriate activities. Antidepressants with minimal anticholinergic activity should be started at a low dose, with gradual increases every 1 or 2 weeks. If the depressive symptoms include insomnia, nortriptyline and trazodone, which have sedating qualities, can be tried. When there is agitated depression, the selective serotonin reuptake inhibitor (SSRI) agents [fluoxetine (Prozac), paroxetine (Paxil)] may be more appropriate. A practitioner unfamiliar with these medications should consult with or refer to a geriatric psychiatrist for assistance.

Many dementia patients experience disruptive behaviors of agitation, anxiety, aggression, and delusions or hallucinations during the course of illness. These behaviors are very frightening to caregivers and often precipitate institutionalization. It is important to assess whether these behaviors are part of a delirium

caused by an underlying acute illness and, if so, to treat the intercurrent illness appropriately. Behavioral problems are best managed by environmental manipulation such as taking the individual for a drive or a walk, playing soothing music, and engaging the patient in a distracting activity (puzzles, painting, etc.). When psychotic behaviors persist and present a potential danger, antipsychotics should be considered (Table 11-5-9). The difficulty is that most of these agents can cause increased confusion and agitation or severe lethargy.

Supportive Measures

Many community resources can provide ongoing assistance for an individual with dementia. Senior centers with structured activities may be appropriate for an individual with an early or mild dementia. Adult day-care programs are appropriate for community-dwelling individuals in the mild to moderate stages of a dementia. They provide structured daily activities, socialization, and supervision as well as a respite for caregivers. In-home assistance or out-of-home placement in a supervised living situation may be necessary for a person with a dementia who lives alone. Referral to a hospice for dementia in the terminal stages is appropriate.

Patient Education

Patients and families need accurate diagnostic information to understand the etiology of the dementia. Referral to national associations and their local chapters such as the Alzheimer's

Table 11-5-8. Laboratory Workup for Dementia

Essential
  Complete blood count with differential
  Electrolytes
  Blood urea nitrogen and creatinine
  Glucose
  Liver function tests
  Calcium, magnesium
  Protein, albumin
  Thyroid-stimulating hormone
  Vitamin B_{12}, folate
  Syphilis serology
  Urinalysis
  Chest x-ray
  Electrocardiogram
Selective/optional
  Neuroimage of brain (CT or MRI)
  Electroencephalogram (EEG)
  Lumbar puncture
Experimental
  Single-photon-emission computed tomography
  Positron-emission tomography
  Genetic testing (apolipoprotein E)

Table 11-5-6. Reversible Causes of Dementia

D: drugs
E: emotional and endocrine disorders
M: metabolic disorders
E: eye and ear dysfunctions
N: nutritional deficiencies
T: tumor or trauma
I: infections
A: alcohol, anemia, atherosclerosis

Table 11-5-9. Pharmacologic Agents for Behavioral Management in Dementia

Agent	Usual Daily Dose	Indicative Behavior
Haloperiodol	0.5 mg (0.5–3 mg)	Agitation, delusions
Thioridazine	75 mg (10–75 mg)	Agitation, delusions,
	25 mg (10–75 mg)	insomnia
Buspirone	15 mg (5–40 mg)	Agitation, anxiety
Trazadone	100 mg (50–400 mg)	Agitation, insomnia
Oxazepam	10 mg (20–60 mg)	Anxiety
Lorazepam	1 mg (0.5–6 mg)	Anxiety
Temazepam	15 mg (15–30 mg)	Insomnia
Nortriptyline	50 mg(50–100 mg)	Depression
Fluoxetine	20 mg (5–40 mg)	Depression
Paroxitine	20 mg (20–50 mg)	Depression
Venlafaxine	75 mg (75–200 mg)	Depression
Carbamazepine	600 mg (800–1200 mg)	Agitation
Propranolol	20 mg (60–240 mg)	Agitation

Association, Parkinson's Foundation, and Multiple Sclerosis Society is appropriate for individuals with specific dementia diagnoses. Libraries and local bookstores have many books on dementias written for the consumer that can help the family understand the illness better. There are even books that help children deal with a family member with dementia. The American Association of Retired Persons (AARP) and the National Institutes of Aging publish free pamphlets about memory loss, aging, and dementia.

Those in the early stages of a dementia who maintain the ability to communicate their needs should be encouraged to discuss their wishes for future care and to complete an advanced directive (preferably a durable power of attorney for health care). The issue of driving is among the most difficult for these patients, their families, and providers. Individuals with many conditions, including most dementias, that impair the ability to operate a motor vehicle should not drive, as they may be a danger to themselves and others. In many states, such as California, dementia is included in the list of "reportable diseases" to the department of motor vehicles. Families are often relieved and patients are angered when they are informed that a patient should no longer be driving. Referral to a driver's assessment program (such as 55 Alive, sponsored by the AARP) or for testing by the state's department of motor vehicles may be necessary to demonstrate the inability of a patient with dementia to operate a car safely.

DISPOSITION

Follow-up depends on the underlying etiology of the dementia. If a structural lesion is found, appropriate referral to a neurosurgeon is required. When a delirium or an intercurrent acute problem is found, it should be treated and followed appropriately. Cognitive status should be reassessed several months after the correction of any underlying problem.

COMPLICATIONS AND RED FLAGS

Regardless of the age of the patient, changes in cognition and function should not be ignored or considered "normal." When cognitive and functional status deteriorate abruptly, hospitalization may be required. When the behavioral problems associated with a dementia are severe, the patient may require psychiatric intervention and hospitalization.

NOTES AND PEARLS

The initial diagnosis of dementia cannot be made in an individual who is comatose, in the postoperative state, or in an emergency room. Serial examinations over a period of time are the best way to make an accurate clinical diagnosis of dementia. Dementia

assessment centers in many metropolitan areas, often affiliated with medical schools, can provide comprehensive assessment and family education and assist in the management of patients with behavioral problems or unusual findings.

REFERENCES

1. American Psychiatric Association: *Diagnostic and Statistical Manual of Mental Disorders,* 4th ed. Washington, DC, American Psychiatric Association, 1994.
2. Corey-Bloom J, Thal LJ, Galasko D, et al: Diagnosis and evaluation of dementia. *Neurology* 45:211–218, 1995.

BIBLIOGRAPHY

Emergy VA, Oxman TE (eds): *Dementia Presentations, Differential Diagnosis and Nosology.* Baltimore, Johns Hopkins University Press, 1994.
Maletta GJ: Treatment considerations for Alzheimer's disease and related dementing illnesses. *Clin Geriatr Med* 4(4):699–702, 1988.
Schmitt FA, Ranseen JD, DeKosky ST: Cognitive mental status examinations. *Clin Geriatr Med* 5(3):545–581, 1989.

Chapter 11–6
MYASTHENIA GRAVIS
Christopher C. Stephanoff

DISCUSSION

Myasthenia gravis (MG) is one of three disorders that affect the myoneural junction. Each of these disorders presents with varying symptoms of weakness, fatigue, and delayed recovery time, with the characteristic symptoms being a result of transmission abnormalities.[1] As an autoimmune disease, MG manifests when circulating antibodies attack and destroy acetylcholine receptors on the postganglionic membrane of the neuromuscular junction, which is the interface between the nerve and muscle fibers. It functions as a chemical pathway through which an action potential is conducted from the presynaptic to the postsynaptic nerve element. Loss of these receptor sites greatly reduces a neurotransmitter's effectiveness.[2]

Individual nerves originating in the spinal cord and brainstem branch extensively, each interfacing with and innervating as many as 2000 skeletal muscle fibers at a point termed the synapse (Fig. 11-6-1). The three basic components of the synapse are the presynaptic membrane, the synaptic cleft, and the postsynaptic membrane. Acetylcholine, a neurotransmitter, is synthesized and stored in vesicles on the presynaptic membrane. If an arriving stimulus possesses sufficient intensity, acetylcholine molecules are released and traverse the synaptic cleft to bind with receptor sites on the postsynaptic membrane. Depolarization takes place at the postsynaptic membrane, causing an influx of sodium and an efflux of potassium ions. The resulting action potential is reproduced along the sarcolemma, producing contraction of the innervated muscle fiber or fibers. Relaxation—cessation of myofibril contraction—takes place when the enzyme acetylcholinesterase destroys acetylcholine molecules. Research has shown that in the synapse, myasthenic patients produce yields and concentrations of acetylcholine that are comparable to those of nonmyasthenic patients. However, in a myasthenic patient, circulating acetylcholine receptor antibodies (AChR-ab) reduces the num-

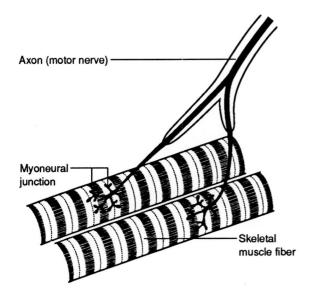

Figure 11-6-1. Motor unit. Motor neuron and muscle fibers innervated by that neuron.

ber of receptor sites on the postsynaptic membrane and bind themselves to those which remain. Depolarization thresholds are achieved less frequently, reducing propagated action potentials (Fig. 11-6-2).

Early muscular weakness and fatigue ensue because fewer muscle fibers are recruited for contraction. Thus, MG patients often describe their symptoms as being more pronounced at the day's end.[3] Although acetylcholine antibodies are known to cause their motor deficiency, their mechanism of action is poorly understood. Also, no direct correlation exists between the number of circulating antibodies and the severity of the disease.

Two pieces of credible evidence support the theory of acetylcholine receptor antibodies. First, children born to myasthenic mothers have only temporary symptoms of the disease that resolve shortly after birth. Second, plasmapheresis, which is included among treatment regimens, provides temporary symptomatic relief.[1] Histologically, no changes in muscle parenchyma are seen.

Although MG may manifest at any age and in both sexes, two incidence peaks are seen: young adult females and elderly males. The incidence of the disease ranges anywhere from 1 in 10,000 to 1 in 20,000 people. Also, no apparent racial or geographic predilections exist. In older patients, it is more common to find an increase in thymus gland masses, whether they are malignant or benign. The significance of this finding lies in the potential for remission or a decrease in symptoms after excision of the tumor.[2,4]

SIGNS AND SYMPTOMS

Muscle weakness, fatigue, and delayed recovery, which increase with exercise and decrease with rest, are the symptoms that most frequently prompt affected individuals to seek medical attention. In most patients, the disease has an insidious course, manifested initially as impaired ocular movement and eyelid droop (ptosis). For the remainder of patients, the onset is abrupt. In less than 20 percent of MG patients, ocular involvement is the sole manifestation, but most patients have additional striated muscular involvement.

Motor weakness in striated muscles may be exacerbated by stressors such as illness and, in the case of females, menses. Other regions of the body with a high incidence of involvement include the muscles of mastication and swallowing, the muscles of respiration, and the proximal skeletal muscles. Paresthesia, or sensory loss, is not evident in a myasthenic patient. The course of the disease is variable in that it may be remitting, static, or progressive.

DIAGNOSTIC STUDIES

Diagnosing MG, as with other disease entities, begins with a detailed medical history and careful physical examination. Too often, MG is a diagnosis of exclusion. Patients presenting with "weakness" as the chief complaint often are thought to be malingering, not taken seriously, and believed to have an underlying psychiatric problem.[4] Eliciting a history of extreme end-of-day muscle weakness, diplopia, ptosis, and weakness and fatigue improved by rest provides the clinician with the "keys" to an accurate diagnosis.

Physical diagnostic confirmation should include repetitive exercises directed at reproducing the symptoms stated in the chief complaint. For example, the patient is instructed to maintain an upward gaze for several minutes, and as the levator oculi becomes fatigued, the practitioner looks for the eyelids to begin closing over the eyes. Diplopia or ocular divergence may be reproduced by examining the "cardinal fields of gaze and confrontation."[5] In patients with difficulty eating and/or drinking, swallowing small sips of water may reproduce the symptoms of drooling and/or choking.[1] Clinicians may employ a variety of tests to achieve an accurate diagnosis.

The infusion of 2 mg of edrophonium chloride (Tensilon) is often used. Tensilon, an anticholinesterase agent with rapid onset and short duration, quickly resolves clinical symptoms and temporarily restores normal muscle function. If the first infusion fails to alleviate or at least improve the symptoms, a second infusion with 8 mg is recommended. Two infusions rather than one of 10 mg are used to prevent potential side effects such as nausea, diarrhea, salivation, and syncope. Repetitive nerve stimulation (RNS), evaluation of action potentials, and serum analysis of anti-AChR antibodies may be necessary when the results of Tensilon injections are inconclusive.[4]

Electric shocks delivered to a myasthenic patient at a rate of two to three per second will evoke a decreased amplitude in action potentials of approximately 10 to 15 percent.[6] Repeating the RNS while dosing the patient with edrophonium will inhibit this reaction. Serum antibodies are present in approximately 80 percent of those affected and are considered pathognomonic.[4] In a patient in whom a thymoma is under consideration as the cause, a thoracic CT or MRI is suggested.[7]

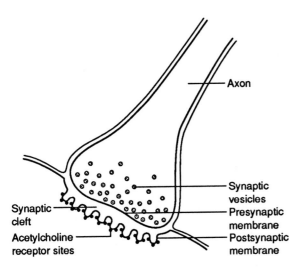

Figure 11-6-2. Synapse demonstrating relationship between neural and muscular structures.

TREATMENT

Definitive evaluation and care of patients who are thought to be affected with MG should be undertaken by a neurologist. Follow-up depends on the extent of involvement, the course of the disease, and the treatment regimen necessary. In the past, the diagnosis of MG meant almost certain death, usually as a result of respiratory failure.[2]

Today, medical and surgical treatment modalities enable most patients to resume fully productive lives. Treatments include anticholinergic medications, thymectomy, immunosuppression, and plasmapheresis. Anticholinergic medications such as oral pyridostigmine improve all the symptoms in some but not all MG patients.

Pyridostigmine is prescribed at a starting dose of 60 mg three to five times daily. The onset of action is 15 to 30 min, with a duration of 3 to 4 h. The dosing schedule of the medication should coincide with the times of greatest need.

Surgery may be necessary in patients who are found to have a thymoma, especially those with malignant tumors. Up to 85 percent of myasthenic patients who undergo thymectomy improve, and approximately 35 percent can discontinue oral therapy entirely. Recommendations for thymectomy are questionable in pediatric and geriatric patients, yet it remains the mainstay of treatment in teenagers and middle-aged patients.

Therapy with immunosuppressive agents such as corticosteroids demonstrates a spectrum of symptom remission in nearly all MG patients. Dosing of glucocorticoids should begin between 15 and 25 mg per day, increasing slowly (usually 5 mg every 3 days). Dose increases should continue until an improvement of symptoms or a maximum dose of 50 mg per day is reached. Some authors recommend maintaining the effective level for 1 to 3 months and then modifying the regimen so that patients ultimately receive 100 mg on alternate days. Any patient receiving prolonged glucocorticoid therapy should receive serial follow-up to monitor and treat possible side effects.

Since the circulating antibodies are found in a myasthenic patient's plasma, short-term plasmapheresis may be used in the event of medical procedures or for the prevention of a respiratory crisis. This process involves removing several liters of the patient's blood, centrifuging it to remove plasma that contains the receptor antibodies, and then reinfusing red blood cells with artificial plasma.[4]

Supportive Measures

With a myasthenic patient, prevention of symptoms is critical. Avoidance of offending stimuli, ample physical rest, and a healthy diet should be emphasized in counseling sessions.

Patient Education

Educating patients empowers them. Their active participation provides them with a sense of control in managing their disease. Tailoring a "self-help" protocol to fit their individual needs can be a powerful adjunct to "prescribed" therapies. For example, rest periods during the day give affected skeletal muscle groups recoupment time. Fatigue induced by stress may be alleviated by stress management classes. Dietitians may be consulted to discuss proper diets, including those high in potassium. Finally, support groups can lend an ear to patients and their caregivers and families.

COMPLICATIONS

Myasthenic or cholinergic crises are conditions requiring emergency treatment. A myasthenic crisis results from too little medication and/or too many stressors. Stressors, as was previously mentioned, can include infection, injury, and medication changes. A cholinergic crisis, by contrast, is directly related to increased anticholinergic activity, often as a result of overmedication. In both cases, patients frequently present to emergency rooms in varying levels of respiratory failure. Immediate treatment must include airway, breathing, and circulation (ABC) protocols because respiratory failure is the myasthenic complication that is most responsible for death. Urgent management includes instituting the therapy necessary to correct the underlying cause. Possibilities include reducing or stopping anticholinergic medication, infection treatment with appropriate antibiotics, pulmonary therapy, and, as was mentioned earlier, plasmapheresis.

REFERENCES

1. Andreoli TE, Bennett JC, Carpenter CC, Plum F: Disorders of myoneural junction and skeletal muscle, in *Cecil Essentials of Medicine*, 4th ed. Philadelphia, Saunders, 1997, pp 921–922.
2. Seybold ME: Diseases of the neuromuscular junction, in Stein JH: *Internal Medicine*, 4th ed. St. Louis, Mosby, 1994, pp 1104–1106.
3. Hartung MS: Neurologic disorders with generalized symptomatology. Myaesthenia gravis, in Price SA, Wilson LM: *Pathophysiology: Clinical Concepts of Disease Processes*, 4th ed. St. Louis, Mosby, 1992.
5. Bates B: The nervous system, in *A Guide to Physical Examination and History Taking*, 6th ed. Philadelphia, Lippincott, 1995, pp 491–554.
6. Devinsky O, Feldman E, Weinreb H, Wilterdink J: Neuromuscular junction disease. Postsynaptic disease, in *The Resident's Neurology Book*. Philadelphia, Davis, 1997, pp 177–178.
7. Myers AR: Disorders of the neuromuscular junction. Myasthenia gravis, in *National Medical Series for Independent Study*, 3d ed. Baltimore, Williams & Wilkins, 1997, pp 641–642.

Chapter 11–7
PARKINSON'S DISEASE
Kimberly Brown Paterson

DISCUSSION

In 1817, Dr. James Parkinson, a London physician, published his famous "Essay on the Shaking Palsy," in which he described the important and singular condition now known as Parkinson's disease.[1]

Isolated symptoms and features of Parkinson's disease—the characteristic shaking or tremor and the hurrying festination of gait and speech—have been described by physicians back to the time of Galen. However, it was Parkinson who first saw every feature and aspect of the illness as a whole.[2]

Parkinson's disease is a degenerative disorder of the basal ganglia of unknown etiology. It is a relatively common disorder that occurs in all ethnic groups, with an approximately equal sex distribution. The most common variety, idiopathic Parkinson's disease (paralysis agitans; Latin for "shaking palsy"), begins most often between 45 and 65 years of age. Twenty percent of people older than 65 and more than 50 percent of those older than 85 have signs of parkinsonism, according to a recent study. A positive family history is present in about 5 percent of these patients, but genetic factors are not thought to be important determinants of the disease.[3]

PATHOGENESIS

The principal pathologic feature of Parkinson's disease is degeneration of the substantia nigra, particularly the zona compacta. Degenerative changes also are found in other brainstem nuclei, especially the locus coeruleus and the dorsal metanucleus of the vagus. The Lewy body (the pathologic hallmark of Parkinson's disease) is found in degenerating neurons in most cases of idiopathic Parkinson's disease. Pathologic changes occur less predictably in the globus pallidus, striatum, and cortex.

Neurons of the substantia nigra project to the corpus striatum (caudate nucleus and putamen), where they release the neurotransmitter dopamine. Loss of striatal dopamine is the principal biochemical defect in Parkinson's disease. An imbalance of dopaminergic and cholinergic activity has been proposed to explain clinical phenomena in diseases of the basal ganglia. A relative excess of dopaminergic activity produces involuntary movements; a relative excess of cholinergic activity produces akinesia and rigidity.[3]

Symptoms and Signs

Diagnosis early in the disease, when the symptoms are mild and may be confined to one side of the body, can pose a problem. However, fully developed Parkinson's disease is unmistakable. Tremor, rigidity, bradykinesia, and postural instability are the cardinal features of the disease and may be present in any combination. The tremor of Parkinson's disease occurs most commonly with the patient at rest. It involves the face, tongue, and limbs and is often asymmetric. Characteristically, it is usually slower in frequency than essential tremor and has a "pill rolling" motion in the hands at about four to six cycles per second.

Rigidity, defined as an increase in resistance to passive movement, is responsible for the characteristically flexed posture seen in Parkinson's disease patients. Cogwheel rigidity refers to the combined rigidity and tremor elicited by extending the flexed forearm or by pronation-supination movements. Bradykinesia (slow movement) and postural instability are also disabling symptoms associated with the disease. Patients also describe nightmares, depression, excessive salivation, difficulty turning in bed and buttoning clothes or cutting food, and problems walking. Orthostatic hypotension, constipation, cognitive impairment, micrographia, hypophonia, urinary incontinence, and impotence are symptoms of the more advanced stages of Parkinson's disease. The diagnosis is based on history and clinical findings. CT, MRI, EEG, and cerebrospinal fluid are typically normal.

CLINICAL DIAGNOSES

Neuropsychological testing may help define intellectual impairment. Critical evaluation of a patient who is suspected of having Parkinson's disease should include the following checklist:

- Relatively immobile face with widened palpebral fissures
- Variable resting tremor
- Meyerson's sign (repetitive tapping over the bridge of the nose produces a sustained blink response)
- Infrequent blinking
- Rigidity in some or all limbs
- Fixed facial expression
- Slowness of voluntary movements
- Seborrhea of face and scalp
- Mild blepharoclonus
- Circumoral tremor

Table 11-7-1. Pharmacologic Preparations Used to Treat Parkinson's Disease

Medication	Dose	Indications
Carbidopa-levodopa immediate-release (IR) (Sinemet)	25 mg/100 mg 2–8 tabs/d	Early to advanced disease
	25 mg/250 mg 2–8 tabs/d	Moderate to advanced disease
	10 mg/100 mg prn	Added to above preparations to even response in advanced disease
Carbidopa-levodopa controlled-release (CR) (Sinemet CR)	25 mg/100 mg 2–8 tabs/d	For early to advanced disease
Selegiline (Eldepryl)	5 mg bid	Administered to patients receiving Sinemet; believed to slow disease progression
Trihexyphenidyl (Artane)	1–5 mg tid	Anticholinergic used to suppress resting tremor
Amantadine (Symmetrel)	100 mg bid	Anticholinergic used to suppress resting tremor
Benatropine (Cogentin)	0.5–2 mg tid	Anticholinergic used to suppress resting tremor
Procyclidine (Kemadrine)	2.5–5 mg tid	Anticholinergic used to suppress resting tremor
Propranolol	40–80 mg tid	Beta blocker useful for action tremor
Bromocriptine (Parlodel)	2.5–30 mg qd	Beta blocker useful for action tremor
Pergolide (Permax)	0.75–3 mg qd	Beta blocker useful for action tremor

Other findings may include drooling resulting from impairment of swallowing, soft and/or poorly modulated voice, impairment of fine or rapid movements, micrographia (difficulty walking where the gait is characterized by small shuffling steps), and difficulty turning and stopping. No alternation in the tendon reflexes or plantar responses is typically noted. Dementia may be present in 15 to 30 percent of Parkinson's disease patients (notably, it is more prominent in patients who are not severely affected by tremor).[1]

TREATMENT

To treat Parkinson's disease it is necessary to restore the dopaminergic function lost with degeneration of the substantia nigra in the extrapyramidal pathway. Therefore, the principal pharmacologic agent for treating Parkinson's disease is levodopa, which usually is administered in combination with carbidopa to prevent enzymatic conversion of levodopa to dopamine in peripheral tissues (Table 11-7-1).

The levodopa-carbidopa combination should be taken without food because amino acids from ingested proteins interfere with its intestinal absorption. An acceptable response to this formulation can be seen by severely limiting protein intake until dinner. The daily allowance of protein (0.8 g/kg of body weight) can then be provided by dinner and an evening snack.

Physical therapy or speech therapy helps many patients. Home additions of aids to daily living, such as rails or banisters placed around the home, special table cutlery with large handles, and nonslip rubber mats, often can improve the quality of life.[3]

Table 11-7-2. Information Sources for Parkinson's Disease

American Parkinson's Disease Association, Inc.
1250 Hylan Boulevard, Suite 4B
Staten Island, NY 10305
1-800-223-2732

National Parkinson's Foundation
1501 NW Ninth Avenue, Bob Hope Road
Miami, FL 33136-1494
1-800-327-4545

Parkinson's Disease Foundation
710 W. 168th Street
New York, NY 10032
1-800-457-6676

Patient information and resources concerning Parkinson's disease are readily available (Table 11-7-2).

DIAGNOSTIC CONSIDERATIONS

As was noted above, early-onset Parkinson's disease is difficult to diagnose, particularly if the tremor is minimal or absent. This makes the differential exceedingly extensive (Table 11-7-3).

NOTES AND PEARLS

Various other therapeutic approaches are being studied. Transplanting substantia nigra tissues from human fetuses into the brains of patients with Parkinson's disease has scientific appeal. However, the technique raises many medical ethical questions and continues to be experimental.

Medical treatment of Parkinson's disease patients can be most rewarding because of the noticeable improvement in their ability to perform daily living activities. However, if the initial treatment becomes less effective, evaluation by a neurologist may be necessary.

Table 11-7-3. Differential Diagnoses of Parkinson's Disease

Differential Diagnosis	Symptoms
Advanced age	Mild hypokinesia
	Slight tremor
Depression	Expressionless face
	Poorly modulated voice
	Reduction in voluntary activity
Wilson's disease	Early age at onset
	Presence of abnormal movements
	Kayser-Fleischer rings
	Chronic hepatitis
Huntington's disease	Rigidity
	Bradykinesia
	Family history
	Accompanying dementia
Shy-Drager syndrome	Postural hypotension
	Anhidrosis
	Decreased sphincter control
	Cerebellar neurologic deficits
Steele-Richardson-Olszewski syndrome (supranuclear palsy)	Bradykinesia and rigidity
	Pseudobulbar palsy
	Axial dystonia
Creutzfeldt-Jakob disease	Dementia
	Myoclonic jerking
	Ataxia
	ECG markings that may mimic atrial flutter

REFERENCES

1. Olanow CW: A 61 year old man with Parkinson's disease. *JAMA* 275:716–722, 1996.
2. Sacks OW: *Awakenings.* Garden City, NY, Doubleday, 1973.
3. Aurinoff MJ: Parkinson's disease and other extrapyramidal disorders, in Fauci AS, Braunwald E, Isselbacher KJ, et al (eds): *Harrison's Principles of Internal Medicine,* 14th ed, New York, McGraw-Hill, 1998, pp 2356–2363.

Chapter 11–8
BELL'S PALSY
R. Scott Chavez

DISCUSSION

Approximately 25 of every 100,000 people annually in the United States are diagnosed with Bell's palsy, a paralysis of the muscles innervated by the facial nerve. Bell's palsy, also known as idiopathic facial paralysis, generally is unilateral and occurs equally in males and females but predominantly in individuals over 30 years of age.

PATHOGENESIS

Bell's palsy is idiopathic with some degree of genetic predisposition. The facial nerve becomes inflamed within the facial canal, causing total or partial paralysis of the facial muscles. Exposure to cold has been known to precipitate an attack. Some theorists hypothesize that a vasoconstrictor, such as endothelin, may play a role in the mechanism of the onset of facial nerve paralysis. It is highly unusual to have bilateral paralysis, and other causes should be investigated.

Microbiology

No known microbiologic cause has been associated with Bell's palsy. Viral factors have been assumed to cause Bell's palsy. However, the etiology is still a maze of unknowns.

SYMPTOMS

A Bell's palsy patient commonly presents with a sudden onset of paralysis of the facial muscles. The patient may complain of tingling or numbness on the affected side. Drooling is often present. The patient's ability to blink is affected, and subsequently a loss of tear production is common. On occasion the patient complains of excessive tear production. In addition, the patient may complain of an earache on the affected side.

OBJECTIVE FINDINGS

Clinically, the diagnosis is made from the patient's presentation of paralyzed facial muscles. Inability to smile, wrinkle the forehead, or express taste on the affected side is a clinical sign of Bell's palsy.

DIAGNOSTIC CONSIDERATIONS

When a patient presents with vesicles along the outer ear canal or behind the ear, the condition is due to herpes simplex and is called the Ramsay Hunt syndrome. Bilateral facial paralysis can be due to Guillain-Barré syndrome or meningitis. Other causes of facial paralysis include multiple sclerosis, sarcoidosis, temporal bone fracture, meningitis, otitis media, parotid gland tumor, osteoma of the skull, and leukemic or carcinomatous meningitis.

SPECIAL CONSIDERATIONS

The clinician should be especially sensitive to underlying subclinical infections such as tuberculosis and systemic mycoses.

LABORATORY STUDIES

There are no routine laboratory tests for Bell's palsy. If it is clinically warranted, a spinal tap may be performed to rule out other causes. The cerebrospinal fluid will be mildly elevated 33 percent of the time. Patients should undergo electromyography within the first 3 weeks of onset. Serial electromyography will determine the extent of recovery of facial motor function.

RADIOLOGIC STUDIES

Magnetic resonance imaging (MRI) may be ordered to rule out posterior fossa lesions or tumors; however, a high level of clinical suspicion should dictate its use. There are no routine radiologic studies.

TREATMENT

Pharmacologic Management

Bell's palsy patients are initially treated with a 14-day steroid dose pack. Prednisone 80 mg once daily for 3 days, then 60 mg once daily for 3 days, then 40 mg once daily for 3 days, and then 20 mg once daily for 3 days is the usual dosing regimen. Corticosteroid therapy should begin soon after the onset of the initial symptoms of Bell's palsy. Treatment beyond 4 days after the onset is usually ineffective.

Supportive Measures

The patient should be instructed to close and patch the eye on the affected side. This guards against corneal abrasion and ulcerations. Artificial tears and ophthalmic lubricants also may be used.

Patient Education

The patient should be given a lot of reassurance and a detailed explanation of the viral disease. The patient's concern about disfigurement and loss of function should be addressed directly with the patient. Often patients think they have had a "stroke."

DISPOSITION

Patients are monitored on an outpatient basis and should be checked monthly for 6 to 12 months. Generally, complete recovery can be expected and full function of the facial muscles will be restored. However, each patient is different, and recovery may be slow. In a study conducted by the Department of Otolaryngology, Head and Neck Surgery at Louisiana State University Medical Center in Shreveport, electroneurographic and facial grading functions were performed on 32 patients with Bell's palsy. The authors found that the period between 10 and 14 days after onset was the most valuable for predicting recovery. According to the study's findings, serial electroneurograhic recordings provide reliable prognostic information on recovery from Bell's palsy.

COMPLICATIONS AND RED FLAGS

The single most important complication of Bell's palsy is corneal abrasion or ulceration. Appropriate monitoring and eye protection are critical. The use of methylcellulose eye drops may be helpful. As with the use of any corticosteroids, caution should be taken in administering such medications to patients with diabetes or peptic ulcer disease, pregnant patients, and patients on live vaccines (e.g., measles, mumps, rubella and live oral polio vaccine).

BIBLIOGRAPHY

Ikeda M, Iijima M, Kukimoto N, Kuga M: Plasma endothelin level in the acute stage of Bell's palsy. *Arch Otolaryngol Head Neck Surg* 122(8):849–852, 1996.

Qiu WW, Yin SS, Stucker FJ, et al: Time course of Bell's palsy. *Arch Otolaryngol Head Neck Surg* 122(9):967–972, 1996.

Chapter 11–9
INTRACRANIAL ANEURYSM/ INTRACRANIAL ANEURYSMAL HEMORRHAGE
Laura M. Capozzi

DISCUSSION

Intracranial aneurysm is seen in 1 to 6 percent of adults as a fairly incidental finding at autopsy. However, a feared complication of aneurysm is a rupture resulting in an intracranial subarachnoid hemorrhage. Aneurysms are commonly located at the branching points of the major arteries, traveling through the subarachnoid space at or near the circle of Willis. Cerebral angiography reveals 0.5 to 1 percent occurrence of small asymptomatic aneurysms among adults. It has been estimated from autopsy and angiography results that 1 million to 12 million Americans have intracranial aneurysms. The most common type of aneurysm is the saccular, or berry, aneurysm, followed by the fusiform aneurysm. A saccular aneurysm is characterized by a distinct neck and dome within the aneurysm. A fusiform aneurysm presents as a diffuse enlargement of an artery without an identifiable neck; these aneurysms are caused by atherosclerosis, trauma, infection, or tumor. Aneurysms typically rupture at the dome.

Aneurysms are classified by cause, size, site, and shape. These factors in combination are important in determining the treatment.

The majority of intracranial aneurysms are unruptured at autopsy. With the widespread use of diagnostic imaging techniques such as MRI and CT, many unruptured and asymptomatic aneurysms can be diagnosed. The rate of rupture increases with the size of the aneurysm (usually 10 mm or larger) and with advancing age up to the eighth decade; these ruptures occur more often in women than in men.

Epidemiology

The majority of intracranial aneurysms are located in the anterior circulation, usually at the junction of the internal carotid and posterior communicating arteries, in the anterior communicating artery complex, or at the trifurcation of the middle cerebral artery. Aneurysms of the posterior circulation are most commonly found at the bifurcation of the basilar artery or at the junction of a vertebral artery and an ipsilateral posterior inferior cerebellar artery. Interestingly, multiple aneurysms, usually two or three, are found in 20 to 30 percent of people with an aneurysm.

Subarachnoid hemorrhage is a common problem associated with intracranial aneurysm. The yearly incidence is about 1 per 10,000 people, and it is associated with high rates of morbidity and mortality. Approximately 12 percent of these patients die before receiving medical care, and 40 percent die within 1 month of hospitalization. Among those who survive, 30 percent have major neurologic deficits. Despite advances in diagnosis and medical or surgical intervention strategies, the fatality rate for aneurysmal subarachnoid hemorrhage has not changed over the past few decades.

Among patients with an aneurysmal subarachnoid hemorrhage, 2 percent develop a new aneurysm each year. In this patient group, the incidence of aneurysmal rupture is about 6 per 10,000 persons per year. This is substantially higher than the incidence of aneurysmal subarachnoid hemorrhage in the general population.

PATHOGENESIS

Evidence supports the role of genetic factors in the pathogenesis of intracranial aneurysms. These patients are thought to have developmental defects in the arterial wall. Many inherited connective tissue disorders have been associated with intracranial aneurysms, most notably autosomal dominant polycystic kidney disease, Ehlers-Danlos syndrome type IV, neurofibromatosis type I, and Marfan syndrome. Seven to twenty percent of patients with an intracranial aneurysm have a first- or second-degree relative with a confirmed intracranial aneurysm.

Environmental Risk Factors

Acquired factors also may play an important role in the pathogenesis of intracranial aneurysms. Among the environmental risk factors that may predispose a person to an aneurysmal subarachnoid hemorrhage, cigarette smoking is the only one that has been consistently identified in all the populations studied and is easily the most preventable. The risk of an intracranial aneurysmal hemorrhage is 3 to 10 times higher among smokers than among nonsmokers. The risk rises with increases in cigarette pack-years. Cigarette smoking decreases the effectiveness of proteolytic enzymes (proteases) such as elastase. The imbalance in these proteases may result in the degradation of connective tissues, including the arterial wall.

Other Factors

Hypertension is frequently studied in relation to the development and rupture of intracranial aneurysms. Although many studies support the relationship between hypertension and intracranial aneurysm, some do not support an increased risk of intracranial aneurysm in patients with hypertension. Although the incidence of aneurysmal subarachnoid hemorrhage is generally higher in women, before age 50 men are more likely to have an aneurysmal subarachnoid hemorrhage than are women. The use of low-dose oral contraceptives in premenopausal women is thought to decrease the risk of an aneurysmal subarachnoid hemorrhage. Additionally, the risk is lower among women who receive hormone replacement therapy postmenopausally.

Alcohol can lower the risk of an aneurysmal subarachnoid hemorrhage when it is consumed at low levels. However, heavy drinking, especially binge drinking, appears to increase that risk.

Data on hypercholesterolemia as a risk factor for aneurysmal subarachnoid hemorrhage are inconsistent. Pregnancy carries some risk for rupture of aneurysms that is related to the hemodynamic and endocrine changes that occur. The highest incidence of rupture occurs during the second trimester.

SIGNS AND SYMPTOMS

Although most intracranial aneurysms are asymptomatic until they rupture, the typical presentation is that of a severe headache of acute onset. The headache is often unusual and acute and may precede the rupture by several days or weeks in one-third to one-half of patients. This prodromal headache often is accompanied by nausea and vomiting, with loss of consciousness at times. This headache may be referred to as a "warning leak" of blood into the wall of the aneurysm or into the subarachnoid space.

Rupture is most common during times of exertion or stress but may occur at any time. Global or focal neurologic abnormalities may be found on physical examination. Meningismus and intraocular subhyaloid hemorrhages are two signs that are helpful in diagnosing a subarachnoid hemorrhage.

The signs of meningeal irritation are secondary to blood byproducts in the subarachnoid space. Neck stiffness therefore may not be noted until several hours after the hemorrhage. Circulation of bloody cerebrospinal fluid down the spinal axis may cause severe low back pain and even bilateral radicular leg pain.

When an intracranial aneurysm becomes large, it may cause a mass effect. The most common symptom associated with a mass effect is headache, and the most common sign is palsy of the third nerve, usually involving the pupillary fibers. This palsy is caused by an aneurysm at the junction of the carotid artery and the posterior communicating artery or an aneurysm of the upper end of the basilar artery. Other signs and symptoms that depend on the location of the aneurysm include brainstem dysfunction, visual field defects, trigeminal neuralgia, cavernous sinus syndrome, seizures, and hypothalamic-pituitary dysfunction.

DIAGNOSTIC CONSIDERATIONS

Intracranial aneurysms are typically asymptomatic unless they cause a mass effect by means of their size or location. However, headaches caused by "leaking" intracranial aneurysms must be differentiated from migraines and other types of headaches. The onset of the prodromal headache associated with an intracranial subarachnoid hemorrhage usually does not last longer than 2 weeks. Acute, severe headache in a patient warrants CT scanning in persons who have a family history of intracranial aneurysm or autosomal dominant polycystic kidney disease. In this patient group, the incidence of ruptured intracranial aneurysms is four times higher than that of the general population.

SPECIAL CONSIDERATIONS

The most important predictor of outcome is the clinical condition the patient exhibits on arrival at the hospital. The scale developed by the World Federation of Neurological Surgeons is the most widely used (Table 11-9-1). It is based in part on the Glascow Coma Scale (Table 11-9-2).

LABORATORY STUDIES

If the symptomatology and signs indicate the likelihood of an intracranial aneurysm with bleeding and if CT is negative, a

Table 11-9-1. World Federation of Neurological Surgeons Grading Scale for Subarachnoid Hemorrhage

Grade	Score	Motor Deficit
I	15	Absent
II	13 or 14	Absent
III	13 or 14	Present
IV	7–12	Absent or present
V	3–6	Absent or present

lumbar puncture should be performed to confirm the presence or absence of xanthochromia or blood. Electrolytes should be monitored to prevent hyponatremia, which can lead to neurologic deterioration.

RADIOLOGIC STUDIES

CT scanning should be the first diagnostic study performed to evaluate the possibility of subarachnoid hemorrhage. Within the first 24 h, scanning detects up to 95 percent of hemorrhages; its sensitivity decreases to 50 percent within 1 week. MRI is not sensitive enough in detecting early hemorrhage but may be helpful in detecting subacute or chronic hemorrhage of more than a 2-week duration.

In patients at high risk for aneurysm with subsequent rupture, conventional angiography should be the first diagnostic study performed. The most commonly used imaging techniques are angiography, MRI angiography (MRA), and helical CT angiography. Helical CT angiography is similar in sensitivity to MRA. They vary in terms of the ability to be a useful diagnostic tool. MRA is the most convenient diagnostic study since it is noninvasive, but it may not be able to detect aneurysms smaller than

Table 11-9-2. Glasgow Coma Scale

Eye opening (E)
  4: opens eyes spontaneously
  3: opens eyes to voice
  2: opens eyes to pain
  1: no eye opening
Best motor response (M)
  6: obeys commands
  5: localizes to pain
  4: withdraws to pain
  3: abnormal flexor response
  2: abnormal extensor response
  1: no movement
Best verbal response (V)
  5: appropriate and oriented
  4: confused conversation
  3: inappropriate words
  2: incomprehensible sounds
  1: no sounds

Scores from the three categories are summed to determine the severity of injury:

$$E + M + V = 9 \text{ (comatose)}$$
$$E + M + V = 9\text{–}12 \text{ (moderate head injury)}$$
$$E + M + V = 13\text{–}15 \text{ (minor head injury)}$$

Generally, patients with World Federation of Neurological Surgeons (WFNS) grades of IV or V have a poor outcome and prognosis despite medical and surgical intervention. Patients with WFNS grades of I and II have a better prognosis, although 30 percent do not survive until surgery.

mm. MRA is the best method for detecting a thrombus (uncommon) within an aneurysm, while CT scanning is preferred to detect calcification within the aneurysmal wall. Helical CT scanning is useful in the presurgical evalution of patients, since it can show relationships between the aneurysm and structures of the skull.

OTHER DIAGNOSTICS

Lumbar puncture should be performed if an intracranial hemorrhage is suspsected but is not revealed by CT. Xanthochromia (yellow discoloration) of the supernatant after centrifuging of the cerebrospinal fluid is diagnostic of a subarachnoid hemorrhage. Xanthochromia is caused by the breakdown of blood products in the cerebrospinal fluid several hours after the initial hemorrhage. Xanthochromia is present in all patients between 12 h and 2 weeks after a hemorrhage and is detectable for several weeks afterward.

TREATMENT

The goal of treatment is to remove the aneurysm from the intracranial circulation while preserving the parent artery. Removal usually is achieved by surgical resection or endovascular occlusion techniques. Medical treatment includes control of blood pressure and keeping the patient quiet. Pharmacologic treatment includes the use of mannitol to control cerebral edema and calcium channel blockers (e.g., nimodipine) to control arterial vasospasm.

Surgical resection involves the placement of a clip across the neck of an aneurysm. Its proven efficacy makes it the most desirable and definitive treatment. The timing of surgery after an intracranial hemorrhage is controversial. Early surgery within 48 to 72 h seems preferable, since the incidence of another intracranial subarachnoid hemorrhage is highest during this period. The rate of recurrent hemorrhage varies from 4 to 20 percent within 24 h. Additionally, arterial vasospasm occurs after an intracranial subarachnoid hemorrhage, resulting in arterial narrowing, a primary cause of cerebral ischemia. Early surgery can prevent this complication. Although the exact cause of the vasospasm is not known, it is related to the amount of blood present in the brain after a hemorrhage. Late surgery performed between day 10 and day 14 after an intracranial subarachnoid hemorrhage can be more difficult than early surgery because of secondary brain edema and a tenacious clot around the aneurysm.

Hydrocephalus also may occur during both the early course and the late course in 10 to 30 percent of these patients. Its presence usually indicates a poor prognosis. Ventricular drainage should be performed to prevent further neurologic deterioration.

Endovascular therapy is becoming a useful treatment modality involving the insertion of soft metallic coils within the lumen of the aneurysm. Obliteration occurs through thrombus formation within the entire aneurysm. This technique is most useful for saccular aneurysms.

Patient Education

Screening is suggested in patients who have two or more family members who have had an intracranial aneurysm and those with autosomal dominant polycystic kidney disease. Smoking cessation is an absolute necessity for patients who have been diagnosed with an intracranial aneurysm, particularly patients who have had an intracranial subarachnoid hemorrhage. As was mentioned previously, the rate of hemorrhage is directly related to the number of cigarettes smoked, with heavy smokers having a greater incidence of hemorrhage than light smokers.

COMPLICATIONS AND RED FLAGS

The following complications may be seen:

- Acute onset of a severe, often unusual headache, usually with activity
- Family history of intracranial aneurysms or autosomal dominant polycystic kidney disease
- Third nerve palsy involving pupillary fibers and visual field defects

OTHER NOTES AND PEARLS

Physical examination reveals a subhyaloid hemorrhage. These vitreous ocular hemorrhages occur between the retina and the vitreous membrane and are gravity-dependent. As a result, they appear convex at the bottom and flat at the top.

BIBLIOGRAPHY

Fauci AS, Braunwald E, Isselbacher KJ, et al (eds): *Harrison's Principles of Internal Medicine*, 14th ed. New York, McGraw-Hill, 1998.

Meyer FB, Morita A, Puumala M, Nichols D: Subject review: Medical and surgical management of intracranial aneurysms. *Mayo Clin Proc* 70(2):153–172, 1995.

Schievink W: Medical progress: Intracranial aneurysms. *New Engl J Med* 336(1):28–40, 1997.

Chapter 12–1
DYSMENORRHEA
Cheryl Gregorio

DISCUSSION

The normal menstrual cycle is almost always accompanied by perimenstrual symptoms, which usually resolve spontaneously and are minimally disruptive. Menstrual cramps begin within approximately 1 to 2 h of bleeding and subside within 24 to 48 h. The intensity of symptoms varies widely among women. Dysmenorrhea represents the severe end of the clinical spectrum; however, there are no definitive diagnostic criteria. When the symptoms become incapacitating or the patient seeks treatment, the clinical diagnosis is established.

Dysmenorrhea occurs with ovulatory cycles, and is categorized as primary, secondary, or membranous.[1] Primary dysmenorrhea is frequently distinguished by the absence of pelvic pathology and is the center of this discussion. Secondary dysmenorrhea is discussed elsewhere in association with specific disorders and diseases (e.g., endometriosis). Since the membranous type is rare, it is only mentioned. In membranous dysmenorrhea the pain is due to passage of a cast of the endometrium through the cervical os.

EPIDEMIOLOGY

Dysmenorrhea is the most common gynecologic complaint and usually begins within 4 years of menarche. Prevalence estimates vary, but surveys conducted between 1980 and 1990 reported 60 to 80 percent of respondents with some menstrual pain.[2] Daily impairment rates vary more widely. Surveys found approximately 50 percent reported some disability of daily life. School absenteeism for adolescent females ranged from 10 percent frequently missing school to 50 percent missing school occasionally. Disability of adult women between the ages of 21 to 45 is common. There are no available studies to document the disability, actual interference of daily life, or absenteeism for these adult women.

Factors consistently shown to be associated with increased incidence of dysmenorrhea are early menarche, heavy menstrual flow, and family history of dysmenorrhea in mother or sister. Specifically, family tendency to have severe symptoms has been reported in several studies. It is unclear whether this is primarily due to the "modeling" of attitudes from mother to daughter, information and education of the young female before menarche, or emotional anxiety. However, studies are underway linking a genetic contribution to the likelihood of dysmenorrhea.[3]

PATHOGENESIS

Synthesis of a number of biochemical agents in the endometrium is accelerated by the rapid decline of progesterone that occurs in the luteal phase, just preceding menstruation. Prostaglandins $F_{2\alpha}$ and E_2, leukotrienes, and possibly prostacyclin have been identified as important, contributing biochemical agents. Prosta-glandin production increases during the first 2 to 3 days of the menstrual cycle. Prostaglandins act directly on the myometrium (uterine musculature), increasing the intensity and frequency of uterine contractions. They cause constriction of the uterine arteries, leading to uterine ischemia, tissue trauma, necrosis, and finally the endometrial shedding of menstruation. The most recent hypothesis reveals that prostaglandin E_2 may increase the sensitivity of peripheral pain fibers. Psychological factors were long thought to be a primary cause of dysmenorrhea, until the discovery of the current biologic causes. These factors, including attitudes passed from mothers to daughters mentioned previously, may play a role in women with unresponsive dysmenorrhea and should be considered.

SIGNS AND SYMPTOMS

The diagnosis of primary dysmenorrhea should be a diagnosis of exclusion. History includes onset of problems months to years after menarche; midline cramping (with or without systemic symptoms), symptoms within the first 24 to 48 h of menses, duration 1 to 3 days, moderate menstrual flow; and no pain any other time. Constitutional symptoms may include nausea, vomiting, headache, malaise, fatigue, and/or low back pain. Symptoms are individualized and vary in intensity.

The physical examination does not reveal any anatomic abnormality or significant pelvic disease.

DIAGNOSTIC TESTS

In patients with a suggestive history and normal pelvic examination, no diagnostic testing is required. A reasonable approach is to proceed with either single or combined therapy through several cycles.

If the patient is unresponsive, further diagnostic testing may be required, including ultrasound and/or laparoscopy. As a final assessment, if laparoscopy is negative and treatment is ineffectual, psychological evaluation should be considered.

DIAGNOSTIC CONSIDERATIONS

The most common misdiagnosis for primary dysmenorrhea is secondary dysmenorrhea due to endometriosis. These symptoms occur 1 to 2 weeks prior to menses, and resolve with the onset of menstruation or shortly thereafter. Women with endometriosis often report dyspareunia; by contrast women with primary dysmenorrhea rarely report this symptom.

TREATMENT

Medical management is the mainstay of treatment. For most women prostaglandin synthetase inhibitors (nonsteroidal anti-inflammatory medications) and/or oral contraceptives are effective therapy. Surgical therapy is reserved for a small number with severe, unresponsive pain.

Prostaglandin Synthetase Inhibitor (Antiprostaglandins)

The antiprostaglandins mechanism of action is to block the synthesis and release of prostaglandins. Antiprostaglandins are most

Table 12-1-1. Prostaglandin Synthetase Inhibitors*

Drug	Dosage
Ibuprofen (Motrin)	400–600 mg every 4–6 h
Naproxen (Naprosyn)	500 mg stat, 250 mg every 6–8 h
Ketoprofen (Orudis)	25–50 mg every 6–8 h
Fenoprofen (Nalfon)	200 mg every 4–6 h
Meclofenamate (Meclomen)	100 mg twice daily
Mefenamic acid (Ponstel)	500 mg stat, 250 mg every 6 h
Naproxen sodium (Anaprox)	550 mg stat, 275 mg every 6–8 h

* Individual patients may respond differently to each medication. It would be appropriate to use a loading dose on the first day and to experiment for effect.

effective when taken before the initiation of pain. Generally these medications are interchangeable with respect to overall effectiveness. The initial choice is best made on the basis of cost, with subsequent modifications based on experience with side effects and effectiveness. Ibuprofen is a good initial choice, because it is available in generic form without a prescription, is the least expensive, and is safe. Experience has shown some women do poorly with one medication in this class but respond positively to another. For this reason it is acceptable and reasonable to experiment. The major side effects are gastrointestinal (nausea, vomiting, diarrhea), renal (fluid retention, decreased renal function in persons with renal vascular disease), and central nervous system (syncope, sedation). Women with known allergy to aspirin should not use antiprostaglandins. Table 12-1-1 shows a list of antiprostaglandins and the recommended dosage.

Oral Contraceptives

The mechanism of action is probably related to the absence of ovulation and an altered endometrium inhibiting prostaglandin release. Oral contraceptives are the treatment of choice for women who fail treatment on antiprostaglandins. Cyclic administration of any low-dose formulation is acceptable. It is preferable to begin with a monophasic one, since these are anecdotally more efficacious than the newer triphasic preparations. If there are other reasons to prefer a triphasic one, a reasonable approach is to try it for a few cycles, then switch to a monophasic one if there is no response. If neither oral contraceptives nor antiprostaglandins are 100 percent effective, a combined therapy is an appropriate alternative.

Alternative Therapies

The mainstays of treatment are antiprostaglandins and oral contraceptives; however, alternative therapies are available. These are effective at varying degrees. A discussion of dysmenorrhea would not be complete without mentioning these options:

1. *TEN (transcutaneous electrical nerve stimulation)* This technique works by blocking efferent pain stimuli and reducing central awareness of pain. It has been used for many types of musculoskeletal pain. This has limited practical application. It can be expensive, units may not be readily available, and it is inconvenient to carry around a unit for 1 to 3 days. There are no significant side effects with TENS.
2. *Ovulation suppression* Suppressing ovulation by using means other than oral contraceptives may be an option for women who are not surgical candidates or in whom other therapies failed. The practical choice would be depomedroxyprogesterone acetate IM. It is relatively inexpensive, provides contraception, and has few side effects, and the effect is completely reversible. Ovulation, however, may not resume for several months.

3. *Surgical therapy* In a few women, medication does not control dysmenorrhea and surgical therapies should be considered. Laparoscopic presacral neurectomy and resection of the uterosacral ligament may likely become more popular for unresponsive patients. In rare instances, hysterectomy may be considered for those cases in which child-bearing is no longer desired.

REFERENCES

1. Gerbie MV: Complications of menstruation; Abnormal uterine bleeding, in *Current Obstetrics and Gynecology,* 8th ed. East Norwalk, CT, Appleton & Lange, 1994.
2. Johnson SR: Dysmenorrhea and premenstrual syndrome, in *Gynecology and Obstetrics: A Longitudinal Approach.* New York, Churchill Livingstone, 1993.
3. Kendler KS, Silberg JL, Neal MC, et al: Genetic and environmental factors in the etiology of menstrual, premenstrual and neurotic symptoms: A population based twin study. *Psychol Med* 22:85, 1992.

Chapter 12–2
VULVOVAGINAL CANDIDIASIS
Peggy Valentine

DISCUSSION

Approximately 75 percent of women experience at least one episode of vulvovaginal candidiasis in their lifetime. The majority of cases (80 to 90 percent) are caused by *Candida albicans.* The remaining 10 percent are caused by *Candida glabrata* or *Candida tropicalis.* The typical complaint includes vulvar pruritus (of varied intensity) and vaginal discharge. The consistency of the discharge may vary from thin and watery to thick and lumpy ("cottage cheese"). Predisposing factors include pregnancy, oral contraceptives, diabetes mellitus, and recent antibiotic use. During pregnancy and while women are taking oral contraceptives, the high levels of hormones are thought to promote *Candida* growth in the vagina. Vaginal colonization is frequently observed in diabetic women, and antibiotics are thought to eliminate the protective vaginal flora. Wearing poorly ventilated underwear or tight-fitting clothing that increases perineal moisture and temperature are other predisposing factors. It is estimated that 10 to 20 percent of women normally harbor *Candida* species and yeasts without being symptomatic.

SIGNS AND SYMPTOMS

The most common symptom, vulvar pruritus, is present in nearly all symptomatic individuals. Vaginal discharge may vary in quantity and appearance. Other complaints include vaginal soreness, irritation, vulvar burning, dyspareunia, and external dysuria due to contact of urine with inflamed labia. The symptoms may be exacerbated just prior to the menstrual period with some relief at the onset of menstrual flow. Vulvovaginal candidiasis is usually not sexually transmitted, but male partners of affected women may develop balanoposthitis. More frequently, a transient rash, erythema, and pruritus may develop shortly after unprotected sexual intercourse. Same sex partners can transmit candidiasis by sharing unwashed clothing or sex toys. The symptoms are self-limiting and respond well to topical antifungal agents.

OBJECTIVE FINDINGS

Findings include vulvar erythema and vaginal discharge, which may be watery or thick with clumps like cottage cheese. The discharge often adheres to vaginal mucosa.

DIAGNOSTIC CONSIDERATIONS

Diagnosis can be made when the patient has signs and symptoms of vaginitis, when the wet mount demonstrates yeast, and when the vaginal yeast culture is positive.

SPECIAL CONSIDERATIONS

Acute vulvovaginal candidiasis occurs frequently among women infected with HIV, but insufficient information exists to determine the optimal management. The current recommended treatment is the same. Vulvovaginal candidiasis is common during pregnancy. Only topical "azole" therapies should be used (for 7 days) in pregnant women.

LABORATORY TESTS

A wet mount or saline preparation should be done to identify yeast cells or mycelia microscopically. The clinician should also observe for the presence of clue cells and motile trichomonads on the same slide. The use of 10% KOH (potassium hydroxide preparation) is important for revealing the presence of germinating yeast. Vaginal pH is usually normal (4.0 to 4.5); if the pH is higher than 5.0, consider bacterial vaginosis, trichomoniasis, or a mixed infection. A vaginal culture should be performed if microscopic findings are negative or inconclusive and vulvovaginal candidiasis is suspected based on signs or symptoms. A positive culture, however, does not necessarily mean that *Candida* is responsible for vaginal symptoms.

TREATMENT

Oral or topical azole preparations provide more effective treatment than simple nystatin preparations. Approximately 80 to 90 percent of patients completing azole therapy experience relief of symptoms and have negative cultures.

Recommended regimens are either butoconazole 2% cream, 5 g intravaginally for 3 days, or clotrimazole, 1% cream, 5 g intravaginally for 7 to 14 days. *Caution:* These vaginal preparations are oil-based and may weaken latex condoms and diaphragms.

Other therapy includes clotrimazole, 500 mg vaginal tablet; one tablet in a single application. Single-dose therapy should be reserved for uncomplicated mild-to-moderate vulvovaginal candidiasis. Multiday regimens (3 and 7 days) are the preferred treatment for severe or complicated cases. An example is miconazole, 200 mg vaginal suppository; one suppository for 3 days.

Alternative regimens include oral azole agents such as fluconazole (Diflucan), which may be as effective as topical agents and have a high patient acceptance. Use fluconazole, 150 mg as a single oral dose. Ketoconazole (Nizoral), 100 mg daily, or fluconazole, once weekly, for up to 6 months are thought to reduce the frequency of recurrent infections.

PATIENT EDUCATION

Now that self-medication with OTC preparations is available, patients should be advised that if symptoms persist or recur within 2 months, they should seek medical care.

COMPLICATIONS AND RED FLAGS

Women who experience three or more recurrent episodes of vulvovaginal candidiasis per year should be evaluated carefully. Diabetes mellitus, immunosuppression, broad-spectrum antibiotic use, corticosteroid use, and HIV infection may present as recurrent vulvovaginal candidiasis.

BIBLIOGRAPHY

Centers for Disease Control and Prevention: 1993 sexually-transmitted diseases treatment guidelines. *MMWR* 42(No. RR-14):70–72, 1993.

Mou SM: Gynecologic infections, in Seltzer VL, Pearse WH (eds): *Women's Primary Health Care-Office Procedures and Practice.* New York, McGraw-Hill, 1995.

Solbel JD: Vulvovaginal candidiasis, in Holmes KK, Mardh P-A, Sparling PF, et al (eds): *Sexually Transmitted Diseases,* 2d ed. New York, McGraw-Hill, 1990.

Chapter 12–3
BACTERIAL VAGINOSIS
Peggy Valentine

DISCUSSION

Bacterial vaginosis is the most common cause of malodorous (fishy smelling) discharge in sexually active women. Vaginal irritation and pain are uncommon, and if present, one should rule out coexisting conditions such as trichomoniasis, and vulvovaginal candidiasis. No single pathogen is responsible for bacterial vaginosis. An overgrowth of anaerobic bacteria (e.g., *Bacteroides* spp., *Mobiluncus* spp.), *Gardnerella vaginalis*, and *Mycoplasma hominis* replace the normal lactobacillus vaginal flora. The cause of this vaginal overgrowth is unknown. It remains unclear whether bacterial vaginosis is sexually transmitted, although some studies have demonstrated an increased prevalence among women with multiple sex partners. Treating the male partner has not proven beneficial in preventing recurrence of the disease, and further research is needed to understand the disease course. Bacterial vaginosis has been associated with endometritis, pelvic inflammatory disease (PID), and vaginal cuff cellulitis following invasive genitourinary procedures. There may be a risk of prematurity and chorioamnionitis among pregnant women with this infection.

SIGNS AND SYMPTOMS

The most common symptom is genital malodor, described as "fishy smelling," and the second most common symptom is increased vaginal discharge. Over half of all women have no symptoms at all. Abdominal pain and pruritus are rarely reported.

OBJECTIVE FINDINGS

Inspection reveals a nonviscous, homogeneous white noninflammatory discharge that adheres to the vaginal walls, often visible on the labia and fourchette. Usually no signs of inflammation are noted. The vaginal pH is usually greater than 4.5.

DIAGNOSTIC CONSIDERATIONS

Diagnosis is made by using clinical or Gram stain criteria. Clinical criteria should include three of the following signs and symptoms:

1. Homogeneous, white, noninflammatory discharge that adheres to the vaginal walls
2. Presence of clue cells on wet mount by microscopic examination
3. pH of vaginal fluid greater than 4.5
4. Fishy odor of vaginal discharge before or after addition of 10% KOH (whiff test)

SPECIAL CONSIDERATIONS

• Women of childbearing age who are sexually active.

LABORATORY TESTS

The pH of vaginal secretions is normally less than 4.4. Vaginal pH is best determined by swabbing the lateral and posterior fornices of vagina and placing sample directly on pH paper, look for pH greater than 4.5. One should avoid cervical mucus since the pH is approximately 7.0. Place a drop of vaginal fluid on a glass slide and add a drop of 10% KOH, a fishy smelling odor will be released (whiff test). *Saline wet mount* is done to detect clue cells, usually without polymorphonuclear neutrophils. Take a sample of vaginal fluid with a swab, and mix on a glass slide with a drop of normal saline. Microscopic examination should reveal squamous vaginal epithelial cells covered with many bacteria, giving them a stippled or granular appearance. *Cultures for Gardnerella vaginalis* are not recommended since it can be isolated from vaginal cultures in half of normal women; therefore, it is not very useful in diagnosing bacterial vaginosis.

TREATMENT

The primary goal is to relieve vaginal signs and symptoms. Treatment of sexual partners is not recommended, since this does not prevent recurrent infection in women. However, some clinicians empirically treat partners of patients with frequently recurring bacterial vaginosis. Commercially available lactobacillus preparations have not been shown to be effective.

The treatment of choice is metronidazole (Flagyl) 500 mg PO twice daily for 7 days. Patients should be advised to avoid alcohol during treatment with metronidazole and for 24 hours thereafter. Metronidazole is contraindicated in pregnancy.

Alternative Regimens (somewhat less efficacious) include metronidazole 2 g orally in a single dose or metronidazole gel, 0.75%, one full applicator (5g) intravaginally twice daily for 5 days or Clindamycin cream, 2%, one full applicator (5g) intravaginally HS for 7 days (still under investigation). Clindamycin cream is oil-based and may therefore weaken latex condoms or diaphragms, or Clindamycin 300 mg PO twice daily for 7 days may be given.

PATIENT EDUCATION

The patient should be informed of her diagnosis and the importance of complying with treatment in preventing recurrence. Since bacterial vaginosis is associated with sexual activity, abstinence or condom use are recommended.

DISPOSITION

If the symptoms resolve, follow-up visits are not necessary. Since recurrence of bacterial vaginosis is common, alternative treatment regimens should be used in such cases.

BIBLIOGRAPHY

Centers for Disease Control and Prevention: 1993 sexually-transmitted diseases treatment guidelines. *MMWR* 42(No. RR-14):68–70, 1993.
Hillier S, Holmes KK: Bacterial vaginosis, in Holmes KK, Mardh P-A, Sparling PF, et al (eds): *Sexually Transmitted Diseases,* 2d ed. New York, McGraw-Hill, 1990.
Mou SM: Gynecologic infections, in Seltzer VL, Pearse WH (eds): *Women's Primary Health Care: Office Practice and Procedures.* New York, McGraw-Hill, 1995.

Chapter 12–4
PREMENSTRUAL SYNDROME
Dana M. Gallagher

DISCUSSION

Premenstrual syndrome (PMS) is a common condition, affecting up to 90 percent of women at some time before menopause. PMS is a constellation of physical and/or affective symptoms that recurs cyclically between ovulation and onset of the menses. Premenstrual symptoms abate after menses begins.

In some women, physical symptoms predominate, for example, bloating, tender breasts, and fatigue, whereas others are more bothered by emotional lability and depression. Symptoms may be mild or moderate, and may vary in both type and intensity from cycle to cycle. Less than 10 percent of women suffer severe premenstrual symptoms.[1] Women whose chief complaints are affective are much more likely to have severe PMS than women whose complaints are primarily physical.[2]

PATHOGENESIS

The cause of PMS is unknown, although the patient may recall childbirth or tubal ligation as the event that precipitated her premenstrual symptoms. A variety of possible etiologies have been proposed, including estrogen-progesterone imbalance, vitamin and/or mineral deficiency, neurotransmitter dysfunction, prolactin excess, and psychiatric disorders. To date, none of these theories (either individually or in combination) have been proved.

Since the etiology is unknown and symptom presentation is variable, the treatment is, understandably, individualized.

SYMPTOMS

Physical symptoms can include (but are not limited to) bloating and weight gain, tender breasts, bowel changes, food cravings, headache, and acne. Affective changes can include (but are not limited to) agitation, irritability, rage, crying "for no reason," depression, and homicidal and/or suicidal ideation. Although patients may experience a combination of these, medical intervention is typically sought for relief of one or two particularly disagreeable symptoms.

OBJECTIVE FINDINGS

If the examination takes place during the premenstruum, it may be possible to document physical findings (e.g., to observe a fine tremor, or chart a weight gain or a tender breast examination). Or, the patient may be unusually tearful, agitated, or testy during the office visit. Most often, however, there are no objective findings.

DIAGNOSTIC CONSIDERATIONS

Diagnosing PMS requires a minimum of 2 to 3 months of daily symptom charting by the patient. She must note not only her symptoms but also their cyclicity and severity. It is not uncommon for women to learn during symptom charting that their symptoms are not cyclic. When cyclicity is not verified, another cause should be sought. Since symptom charts make the diagnosis, this documentation is critical, even for the woman who is certain she has PMS. (One of the author's patients documented weekday symptoms that disappeared after she quit her job.)

LABORATORY TESTS

There are no laboratory tests to diagnose PMS. However, laboratory tests may be ordered depending on the patient's presenting complaint. For example:

- A 49-year-old with PMS symptoms should have follicle-stimulating hormone (FSH) levels drawn to screen for menopause.
- A patient complaining of intense premenstrual fatigue should be screened for anemia.
- A patient complaining of depression and sluggishness should be screened for hypothyroidism.

RADIOLOGIC AND OTHER DIAGNOSTIC STUDIES

There are no diagnostic studies for PMS.

TREATMENT

Pharmacologic Management

The selective serotonin reuptake inhibitor fluoxetine (Prozac), has proved helpful in 50 percent of women with premenstrual affective symptomatology.[3] Dosage is 20 mg orally taken in the morning.

In women with severe affective symptomatology, alprazolam, 0.25 mg qid, is helpful[3] when used from day 18 of the cycle until menses, with a gradual taper to day 1 and 2 menses. Taking the drug only during the luteal phase decreases the risk of dependence. Still, alprazolam use should be reserved for those with severe symptoms who do not respond to other regimens.

For women with fluid retention, anecdotal reports support the use of spironolactone, 25 mg qid, at onset of symptoms.[4]

Although both micronized progesterone, 300 mg qid, and oral contraceptives have been widely touted for PMS treatment, there is no scientific evidence to support their use.

Supportive Measures

Avoidance of sugar and alcohol may ameliorate premenstrual symptoms of hypoglycemia. Caffeine should be avoided to decrease breast tenderness and irritability. Salt intake can be restricted to decrease bloating and fluid retention. Regular aerobic exercise helps fight depression and fluid retention. Although vitamin and mineral regimens have been recommended for treatment of PMS, none has shown conclusive effectiveness. If the patient requests vitamin supplementation, a good multivitamin with a full B complex and 1000 mg of calcium can be suggested. For reducing breast tenderness, anecdotal reports support the use of 250 mg gamma-linoleic acid (Evening Primrose Oil) daily.

PATIENT EDUCATION

Self-help books, support groups, and individual, couples, or family therapy may be useful. Offer the patient the option of bringing her spouse or partner to office visits so you can answer questions. Partners frequently have helpful insights about the patient's symptoms and the success of the treatment program. Inform the patient that improvements brought on by diet, exercise, and vitamin supplementation may be subtle over time, not immediate and dramatic. Life-style changes may also be more helpful if observed throughout the cycle rather than in the premenstruum alone.

NOTES AND PEARLS

Once PMS is treated and diagnosed, be sure to evaluate the progress of the patient at intervals. Because of the chronic and somewhat unpredictable nature of the syndrome, the patient continues to be at risk for depression. Should there be a flare-up of symptoms after the patient has responded to treatment, reevaluate the current treatment regimen and look for potential new problems.

REFERENCES

1. Tierney LM Jr, McPhee SJ, Papadakis MA (eds): *Current Medical Diagnosis and Treatment,* 37th ed. Stanford, CT, Appleton & Lange, 1998, pp 693–694.
2. Barnhart KT, Freeman EW, Sondheimer SJ: A clinician's guide to the premenstrual syndrome. *Med Clin North Am* 79(6):1458, 1995.
3. More help for severe PMS. *Mod Med* 63:8–10, 1995.
4. Griffith CJ: Premenstrual syndrome: An update. *J Am Acad Phys Assist* April 1995, p 35.

Chapter 12–5
CYSTOCELE AND RECTOCELE
William A. Mosier

DISCUSSION

A *cystocele* is a downward displacement of the bladder that forms a herniation of the anterior vaginal wall below the floor of the bladder. It bulges into the anterior aspect of the vagina, anteriorly. The urinary bladder becomes displaced from weakening of the anterior vaginal wall. Cystoceles can range from mild to severe in their presentation. However, as a rule, they progress slowly.

A *rectocele* is a bulging of the posterior vaginal wall resulting from a herniation of the anterior rectal wall through a relaxed or ruptured vaginal fascia and the rectovaginal septum. In essence it is a rectovaginal sacculation that results from a trauma to the levator muscles and stretching or tearing of the supporting fascia.

PATHOGENESIS

A cystocele results from a loss of support by the structures that are normally responsible for maintaining it. This commonly occurs after childbearing. These structures are typically the pubocervical or paravaginal fascia and the permanent stretching of the oblique tunnel of the levator sling through which the vagina passes.

A rectocele results from weakened or torn support structures status after childbirth and further weakening produced by repeated straining during defecation. A rectocele cannot occur without a definite fascial defect. When not due to the trauma of childbirth, it is due to a congenital or inherent weakness in fascial and muscle supports. No matter what the cause, once the herniation starts, the weakened fascial supports gradually give way.

SYMPTOMS

The severity of complaints varies widely with cystocele. Patients may complain of a sensation of fullness or bulging in their vagina, a bearing down sensation, a urinary stress incontinence, or a vaginal protrusion. The severity of complaints also depends on the degree of prolapse present. A bearing down discomfort is often aggravated by physical exercise or prolonged standing. If descent of the bladder is extreme, discomfort may be aggravated even by walking or prolonged sitting. Urinary symptoms are common in patients with a cystocele because of the difficulty in voiding completely. Due to sepsis, the patient may experience frequent urinary tract infections. The descent of the bladder can drop its anterior portion below the level of the bladder neck. This creates a mechanical problem that results in difficulty evacuating. This often leads to irritability of the bladder and urinary frequency.

The symptoms related to having a rectocele are usually few and considerably less severe than those of a cystocele. A slight, or even moderate, rectocele is generally asymptomatic. A patient may have a minimal discomfort during the Valsalva maneuver or may be aware of a bulge in the vaginal vault. Some patients may complain that defecation can be accomplished only with digital pressure applied vaginally against the sacculation. However, symptoms are rarely ever severe enough to require surgical intervention or even a pessary. It is usually an associated cystocele and uterine descent that produce discomfort.

OBJECTIVE FINDINGS

When the vaginal vault is inspected, it is important to distinguish between a cystocele and a rectocele. The distinction between the two is quite obvious.

In the case of a cystocele, a weakness of the anterior vaginal wall causes a visible bulging and is readily palpable. The bulging is usually spherical and often fills the vaginal orifice. On palpation, the mass has soft consistency and an elastic feel to the touch. A cystocele may be so small that it is not obvious when the patient is in a supine position. Asking the patient to perform a Valsalva maneuver can often make the cystocele more readily palpable.

The diagnosis of a rectocele can also be made via visualization and palpation. A finger placed on the anal canal and pressure exerted toward the upper part of the vagina will make a defect in the posterior vaginal wall obvious. If the patient is asked to perform a Valsalva maneuver, the protrusion of the posterior vaginal wall expands. The defect is usually noted above the anal sphincter.

DIAGNOSTIC CONSIDERATIONS

There are very few pathologic entities that can be confused with a cystocele or rectocele. However, the differential should include (1) enterocele, (2) urethrocele, and (3) vaginal cysts. Gartner's duct cysts, on rare occasion, have been found to dissect beneath the anterior vaginal wall epithelium and assume a cystocele-like position.

TREATMENT

Nonsurgical Management

Nonsurgical intervention should include an attempt to use muscle strengthening exercises to improve the muscle tone of the levator ani muscles. In the postnatal patient, a pessary may be useful immediately after delivery, especially if the uterus is retroverted and produces strain on the supporting ligaments. A pessary used to elevate the uterus may facilitate the muscles to regain adequate tone. A pessary, however, will not cure a prolapse. It can only prevent it from becoming worse.

For the older patient who is not planning any more children and who is an unsuitable candidate for surgical repair, a supporting pessary can be effective if a cystocele is accompanied by a prolapsed uterus. If there is so much relaxation of the support tissue that a prolapse is precipitated by coughing or defecation, a pessary will have no practical usefulness. Pelvic muscle exercises (Kegel exercises) are used to strengthen the muscles surrounding the opening of the urethra, vagina, and rectum. Hormone replacement therapy (HRT) may be useful, especially for postmenopausal women.

Surgical Management

Cystocele and rectocele repairs are considered a regular step in performing vaginal hysterectomies and pelvic floor repairs.

There is usually no urgency for repair of a cystocele. Surgery is indicated if the patient is having the following symptoms:

1. Repeated bouts of cystitis or other chronic urinary tract infections
2. Painful symptoms or a feeling of pressure
3. A cystocele that is growing

When surgery is indicated, the repair is usually done along with other procedures such as a vaginal hysterectomy or pelvic floor repair in conjunction with a urethrocele repair.

The basic surgical technique for cystocele is as follows:

1. A midline incision is made through the anterior vaginal mucosa. The incision should extend from the external urinary meatus to the cervix.
2. At the cervix, a transverse incision, through the mucosa over the anterior cervix, is performed that joins with the midline incision to form an inverted T.
3. Dissection is then performed laterally to the margin of the defect.
4. The bladder should be detached from the anterior cervix and elevated with interrupted sutures.
5. Any excess vaginal mucosa should also be excised.
6. Interrupted stitches, using absorbable suture, are then used to approximate the cut edges of the vaginal mucosa to carry out a full-thickness repair.
7. If a layered repair is being carried out, then the fascia and mucosa should be approximated separately.

Since a small rectocele usually causes a patient minimal problems, surgical repair is typically done only when there is prolapse of other pelvic viscera. It is usually recommended that a rectocele be repaired only if there is significant problem with perineal relaxation. However, a large rectocele should be repaired surgically if the patient has difficulty with fecal elimination specifically caused by the rectocele.

When an abdominal hysterectomy is performed, even an asymptomatic rectocele should be corrected, because it is quite common for patients to complain of rectocele symptoms after the removal of the uterus even if they were previously unaware of the presence of a rectocele. When surgical repair of a rectocele is indicated, it is usually done in conjunction with repair of the perineum.

The basic surgical technique for rectocele is as follows:

1. A midline incision is usually initiated unless there are lacerations. If lacerations are present, a diamond-shaped area of mucosa is first excised. The incision continues through the vaginal mucosa, stopping posterior to the cervix.
2. A transverse incision is then made, just posterior to the cervix, to meet with the midline incision.
3. Dissection of the vaginal mucosa is then performed laterally until reaching the margin of the defect.
4. Beginning posteriorly, the repair is performed by bringing the diverging fibers of paravaginal fascia to the midline, using absorbable suture.
5. When reaching the perineum, the suturing must accommodate the inclusion of the medial margins of the puborectalis fibers of the levator ani muscles.
6. It is important to remember to restore the triangular shape of the perineum.

SUPPORTIVE MEASURES

No specialized postoperative care is necessary for the patient who undergoes a cystocele or rectocele repair. However, adequate fluids and analgesics should be given, and a low-residue diet and stool softener should be utilized during the initial postoperative period to ensure that no solid material comes through the anus while the tissue is healing. The perineum should be washed (sitz baths) to avoid secondary infection.

PATIENT EDUCATION

Patient education must include a discussion with the patient about family planning. Usually patients should postpone any cystocele or rectocele repair until after they have completed all plans for having any more children. This is due to the probability that subsequent deliveries will destroy surgical repair of a cystocele or rectocele.

Patients should be taught how to perform Kegel exercises. They should be told to contract the pelvic muscles for about 10 s, 20 times in a row, at least six times per day.

If a pessary is inserted, patients must be advised that they should not be experiencing any pain or bleeding. They should be instructed to contact the provider if they encounter pain from the use of a pessary.

DISPOSITION

If a patient using a pessary is unable to remove it herself nightly, at bedtime and reinsert it each morning, she must be examined at least every 3 months for vaginal irritation. Postmenopausal patients prescribed a pessary should be managed with estrogen therapy in an attempt to improve the resistance and tone of the vaginal epithelium.

COMPLICATIONS AND RED FLAGS

If urinary stress incontinence is present with cystocele, this may be a sign of a coexisting urethrocele or other serious problem. Because of the exposed position and thin overlying vaginal epithelium, a cystocele may ulcerate and cause bleeding or a discharge. Urinary retention caused by bladder descent can easily bring on infection. Therefore, checking for cystitis is most important.

When the upper part of the posterior wall rolls out over the perineal body, this is usually not a rectocele but rather an enterocele.

OTHER NOTES OR PEARLS

Always check for a urethrocele. Stree incontinence is the chief symptom of a urethrocele. A rectocele is the least common type of prolapse. When there is a prolapse of the rectum, it is usually associated with a cystocele in uterine descent and a lacerated perineum.

BIBLIOGRAPHY

Baker VV, Deppe G: *Management of Perioperative Complications in Gynecology.* Philadelphia, Saunders, 1997.
Droegemueller W, Sciarra JJ (eds): *Gynecology and Obstetrics.* Philadelphia, Lippincott, 1991, vol 1, pp 61–63.
Lee RA: *Atlas of Gynecologic Surgery.* Philadelphia, Saunders, 1992.
Nichols DH: *Gynecology and Obstetric Surgery.* St Louis, Mosby-Year Book, 1993, chaps 21, 22.

Chapter 12–6
ECTOPIC PREGNANCY
Cheryl Gregorio

DISCUSSION

Ectopic (extrauterine) pregnancy accounts for approximately 2 percent of all pregnancies and remains the most common cause of maternal death in the first 20 weeks of pregnancy. It is responsible for more than 15 percent of all obstetrical maternal deaths in the United States. The risk for ectopic pregnancy increases with age: women 35 to 44 years of age are three to four times more likely than those 15 to 25 years of age to be at risk. Overall the risk of maternal death from ectopic pregnancy is 10 times greater than term childbirth and 50 times greater than abortion.

The Centers for Disease Control and Prevention (CDC) began keeping statistics on ectopic pregnancies in 1970, and since that time the incidence has increased four- to fivefold. However, the incidence for the maternal mortality rate has decreased sevenfold.[1] Unfortunately, references and investigators rarely agree on many aspects of the descriptions of the women most likely to experience ectopic pregnancies. Pernoll and Garmel report increases in the lower socioeconomic groups without regard to race, whereas Hickok and Patton report race as a factor, not income.[2,3]

The primary causes of ectopic pregnancy include conditions that impede or prevent passage of the fertilized ovum through the fallopian tube. Chronic salpingitis and pelvic inflammatory disease (PID) have been implicated. However, the rate for PID and salpingitis have remained stable over the past several years, and tubal histology has been reported as normal in as many as 70 percent of pathologic specimens. Increasing rates of tubal surgeries and assisted reproductive technologies have been suggested as possibilities.

Management has been influenced by the availability of quick and sensitive tests for human chorionic gonadotropin (hCG), technical advancement in ultrasonography, and early diagnostic laparoscopy. It is estimated that early detection is responsible for a 20 percent reduction of rupture prior to intervention, and the diagnosis is being made prior to rupture in 80 percent of cases.[3] Early detection now allows greater flexibility in management, including extensive use of linear salpingotomy or segmental resection, and nonoperative management.

PATHOGENESIS

Ectopic pregnancy appears to be a process seen almost exclusively in humans. The symptoms occur later in the pregnancy, including rupture of the tube and intraperitoneal hemorrhage. The mechanism of pain involves the distention of the fallopian tube due to the growing fetus. Although implantation and pregnancy can occur at any point along the reproductive path, approximately 95 percent implant within the fallopian tube. One important aspect of *all* ectopic pregnancy is the lack of resistance of the endosalpinx to invasion by the trophoblast. The trophoblast implants beneath the endosalpinx in the muscle and connective tissue. Then the trophoblast invades the blood vessels to cause local hemorrhage. A hematoma in the subserosal space enlarges as the pregnancy progresses, with possible bleeding in the distal end of the tube but not out the lumen. Distention, thinness of the tube, and the trophoblast predispose to rupture.[4] Rupture occurs when the ovum erodes through the tubal wall, and the serosa ruptures when stretched to the breaking point. Other implantation sites, in descending order, are ovary, abdomen, compound (heterotrophic), and cervix. The tube itself has statistical differences. The closer to the ovary, the more likely the implantation will occur, resulting in the highest statistical rate at the ampulla (78 percent). The highest morbidity rate results from the cervical pregnancy. It has statistically the lowest implantation rate. Each of the implantation sites may present with its own pathology.

ETIOLOGY

Conditions that impede the passage of the fertilized ovum through the tube are tubal factors, zygote abnormalities, ovarian factors, and exogenous hormones.

Tubal Factors

Fifty percent of tubal specimens reveal chronic salpingitis histologically. Other tubal factors include adherent folds of tissue due to developmental abnormalities (atresia, congenital diverticula, lengthy or tortuous tubes), abnormal tubal anatomy due to maternal use of diethylstilbestrol (DES) in utero, previous tubal or pelvic organ microsurgery, tubal ligation, and conservative treatment of unruptured ectopic pregnancy. These conditions are consistent with intrinsic adhesions. Extrinsic adhesions, like peritonitis, transplants, pelvic tumors, and endometriosis, have been implicated.

Zygote Abnormalities

Chromosomal defects, gross malformations, and neural tube defects have been reported. An increased incidence of zygote abnormalities has been reported with abnormal sperm counts and spermatozoa.

Ovarian Factors

There is evidence of ectopic development with the fertilization of an unextruded ovum, transmigrated ovum, post-mid-cycle fertilization, and ovarian enlargement due to fertility medications.

Exogenous Hormones

The administration of exogenous hormones may play a role in ectopic pregnancies. Increasing incidence of ectopic gestation, varying from 4 to 16 percent, has been reported with progestin-only contraceptives, progesterone secreting IUDs, and "morning after pills"[4] (see Fig. 12-6-1).

SIGNS AND SYMPTOMS

There are no pathognomonic signs or symptoms of ectopic pregnancy, but a combination of findings should be suggestive. A sexually active woman in the reproductive age group presenting with abdominal pain, amenorrhea, and/or vaginal bleeding must be evaluated for ectopic pregnancy.

Symptoms

Of the following symptoms, one or all may be present. The more of them present, the higher the index of suspicion. Abdominal or pelvic pain (99 percent)[4] may be generalized, diffuse, or localized. It has been described as colicky, intermittent, and sharp, also as crampy and constant. The pain may begin as early as 1 week past a missed menses or as late as the 16th week of gestation. Abnormal uterine bleeding (75 percent) results from the sloughing of the decidua of the endometrium. Bleeding may range from spotting to heavier than normal menstrual-like flow. A history of missed menses (amenorrhea—68 percent) is usually not given, though typically patients have missed their last normal menses. By the time symptoms have developed, it is usually 6 weeks past the last period. Faintness and syncope (37 percent) may present late in the course of development and may be associated with hypovolemic shock due to rupture or impending rupture.

Signs

Physical examination findings range from totally normal in cases of early ectopic pregnancy to hypovolemic shock and an acute abdomen in ruptured ectopic pregnancy. Diffuse or localized abdominal tenderness, with or without rebound, rigidity, or decreased bowel sounds may be present. With adnexal tenderness, pain may be exquisite on palpation or slight cervical or uterine motion. A unilateral or cul-de-sac (adnexal mass) mass may be present, which is usually boggy and poorly delineated. Uterine changes of pregnancy do not correlate to the duration of the ectopic pregnancy. The uterus may range from normal size to 12 weeks' gestational size.

DIAGNOSTIC TESTS

Routine and special examinations are necessary for the timely and ultimately lifesaving diagnosis of extrauterine pregnancy. A pregnancy test must be of primary importance. With the sensitive assays available today, a negative test excludes the possibility of ectopic pregnancy. A positive test focuses on complications of pregnancy. Quantitative serum β-hCG levels should be followed at 2-day intervals. The levels should increase more than 60 percent within 48 h. The pregnancy is not progressing appropriately if this criterion is not met.

Other hematology tests are usually *not* helpful in diagnosis, but may indicate other complications. Occasionally, the hematocrit may be low, and the complete blood count may identify a

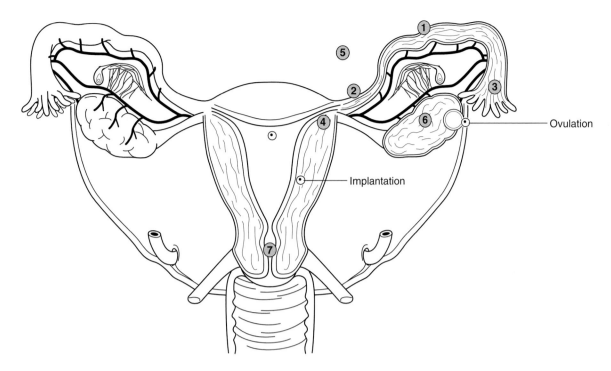

Figure 12-6-1. From ovulation to normal implantation the journey for an ovum can be arduous. At any of these sites the ovum may implant. The most common ectopic sites to the least common in descending order are: (1) ampullary, 78%; (2) isthmus, 12%; (3) fimbrial, 5%; (4) interstitial, 2 to 3%; (5) abdominal, 1 to 2%; (6) ovary, ≈ 1%; (7) cervix, .5%. (*From Bates et al.*[5])

blood loss anemia and leukocytosis. The white blood cell count, if elevated, would be an indication of infection, not ectopic pregnancy. Serum progesterone has been reported to assist diagnosis of an abnormal pregnancy.[5] A progesterone less than 5.0 ng/mL indicates a nonviable pregnancy. The test identifies only the pregnancy, not the location of the pregnancy.

Pelvic ultrasonography is an excellent adjunct to quantitative hCG. It can image a pregnancy within the uterine cavity reliably, but not outside. Transabdominal ultrasound should identify an intrauterine pregnancy with a serum level 6000 mIU/mL hCG; however, transvaginal ultrasound is more sensitive and reveals an intrauterine pregnancy with 2000 mIU/mL hCG.

Culdocentesis is a procedure to determine *ruptured* ectopic pregnancy. It can identify a hemoperitoneum. An 18-gauge needle is inserted into the posterior fornix between the uterosacral ligaments, through the cul-de-sac, into the peritoneal cavity. A negative aspirate (clear peritoneal fluid) indicates no hemorrhage, but does not rule out an *unruptured* ectopic pregnancy. A positive aspirate (nonclotting blood) indicates hemorrhage into the abdominal cavity that has undergone fibrinolysis. Clotting blood indicates penetration of a main vessel or rapid blood loss into the abdomen. An empty aspiration is nondiagnostic or equivocal. It simply means no information was obtained. Unfortunately, "no findings" does not rule in or out ectopic pregnancy. It must be remembered that culdocentesis is an invasive procedure and, as such, carries its own inherent risks. It may be argued that equivocal or negative findings do not negate the necessity of doing a laparoscopy.

The most accurate method of diagnosis is direct visualization through either laparoscopy or laparotomy, and these carry a combined misdiagnosis rate of 2 to 5 percent.

TREATMENT

Traditional therapy is surgical removal of the tube. The advent of conservative surgeries has helped to maximize preservation of the reproductive organs. Laparoscopic surgery allows for diagnosis and definitive treatment at the same time, with minimal inconvenience with respect to morbidity, cost, hospitalization, and lost work time.

Linear salpingotomy involves opening the tube at the implantation site, removing the pregnancy, and allowing the incision to heal by secondary intention. "Segmental resection" removes the portion of the tube containing the pregnancy.

In selected cases nonsurgical (expectant) management is advocated. This allows the pregnancy to spontaneously regress. Regression is documented with serial hCG levels. If trophoblastic function continues, surgery or methotrexate therapy is considered.

Rarely, abdominal pregnancy continues to viable fetal age. The fetus survival is approximately 10 to 20 percent, and greater than half of the survivors have significant deformities.[5] The patient is given the option of continuing an abdominal pregnancy or terminating. Regardless of the choice the patient makes, the placenta is retained in the abdomen to prevent possible hemorrhage. Later the placental remains are resolved (dissolved) with methoxtrexate. Ovarian pregnancy is dealt with at the time of diagnosis. Cervical pregnancy may be confused with incomplete abortion and may present with uncontrollable bleeding. Hysterectomy may be required for maternal survival.

REFERENCES

1. Ectopic pregnancy. *MMWR* 44(3):46–48, 1995.
2. Pernoll ML, Garmel SH: Early pregnancy risks, in *Current Obstetrics and Gynecology, Diagnosis and Treatment,* 8th ed. East Norwalk, CT, Appleton & Lange, 1994, pp 314–320.
3. Hickok LR, Patton PE: Ectopic pregnancy, in *Obstetrics and Gynecology: A Longitudinal Approach.* New York, Churchill Livingstone, 1993, pp 263–272.
4. Pernoll ML, Garmel SH: Early pregnancy risks, in *Current Obstetrics and Gynecology, Diagnosis and Treatment,* 8th ed. East Norwalk, CT, Appleton & Lange, 1994, p 315.

5. Bates GW, Barzansky BM, Beckman CRB, et al (eds): Ectopic pregnancy, in *Obstetrics and Gynecology for Medical Students.* Baltimore, Williams & Wilkins, 1992, pp 290–291, 293.

Chapter 12–7
MASTITIS
Dana M. Gallagher

DISCUSSION

Mastitis (breast infection) is characterized by unilateral breast tenderness, with localized warmth, swelling, and redness. Mastitis typically occurs after, but is not confined to, the onset of breastfeeding in a first pregnancy. If not promptly treated with antibiotics, mastitis can progress to abscess, which necessitates surgical drainage.

PATHOGENESIS

Factors inducing mastitis include poor drainage of a breast duct, the presence of a microorganism, and susceptibility to infection brought on by exhaustion and stress. Rare causes of mastitis include tuberculosis[1] and lupus erythematosus.[2]

Plugged ducts and mastitis must be understood on a continuum and differentiated. Plugged ducts occur when the milk flow is obstructed (for example, by tight bras or baby carriers), or following a missed or short feeding. Dried secretions on the nipple can cause backup of the milk flow as well. It is incumbent on the mother to watch for the tender lumps that signal plugged ducts and to remove the cause immediately. Mastitis is the end result of plugged ducts.

The most common microbial cause of mastitis is *Staphylococcus aureus; Escherichia coli* is a frequent culprit as well.[1] Common culprits in mastitis-associated abscesses include *S. aureus* and the anaerobes *Bacteroides* and *Peptostreptococcus.*[3]

SYMPTOMS

A localized area of erythema, heat, swelling, and tenderness is present. Fever [38°C (101°F)], along with intense breast pain and an overall feeling of malaise, is typical.

In contrast to symptoms of mastitis, plugged ducts are characterized by minor unilateral breast pain without heat or redness. There is no fever, and the woman feels well.

LABORATORY TESTS

The diagnosis of mastitis is made clinically. However, when mastitis does not improve after treatment, cultures of breast milk may be helpful. Prior to obtaining a culture, the breast and hands should be thoroughly washed; then a midstream clean catch should be manually expressed.

The placement of a purified protein derivative (PPD) may be useful in ruling out tuberculosis as an etiology. Though currently rare, as the incidence of tuberculosis rises, this cause of mastitis may become more prominent.

RADIOLOGIC STUDIES

Radiologic studies are not done, unless there is no clinical improvement with appropriate antibiotic treatment. If etiology of an inflamed breast is uncertain, an ultrasound and/or mammogram may be ordered to rule out inflammatory breast cancer.

TREATMENT

Pharmacologic management, dicloxacillin, 500 mg orally qid for 10 days, should be started immediately. If allergic, PCE, 333 mg orally tid for 10 days, is recommended. Response should be dramatic. The patient should be seen in follow-up within 72 h.

PATIENT EDUCATION[4,5]

Antibiotics pass through the breast milk, but do not harm the baby. Even though symptoms are likely to improve almost immediately, an entire 10-day course of treatment should be completed. Stopping antibiotic treatment too soon predisposes the woman to recurrent mastitis.

Since exhaustion compromises the immune system, rest (especially early in the infection) is important. If the nursing bra is uncomfortable or tight, remove it. Nurse frequently, at least every 2 h. Weaning at this time can slow healing and promote breast abscess. Hot moist heat should be applied locally prior to nursing. Nursing should start on the unaffected side, while the affected side "lets down." If the baby refuses to nurse from the affected side, a breast pump should be used, since drainage is a critical part of treatment. If the baby nurses only casually from the affected breast, drainage should be completed by breast pump. Acetaminophen can be used to ease pain. The woman should drink plenty of water.

COMPLICATIONS AND RED FLAGS

In the case of an inflamed breast that does not respond to antibiotics within 72 h, the diagnosis should be reviewed. The differential diagnosis includes resistant or atypical microorganisms, breast abscess, and inflammatory breast cancer.

REFERENCES

1. Lawrence RA: *Breastfeeding, A Guide for the Medical Profession,* 4th ed. Chicago, Mosby-Year Book, 1994, p 261.
2. Cernea SS, Kihara SM, Sotto MN, Vilela MAC: Lupus mastitis. *J Am Acad Dermatol* 29(2-2):343–346, 1993.
3. Dahlbeck SW, Donnelly JF, Theriault RL: Differentiating inflammatory breast cancer from acute mastitis. *Am Fam Phys* 52(3):930, 1995.
4. Huggins K: *The Nursing Mother's Companion.* Cambridge, MA, Harvard Common, 1986, p 95.
5. Jolley S: *Breastfeeding Triage Tool.* Seattle–King County Department of Public Health, 1996, p 43.

Chapter 12–8
PELVIC INFLAMMATORY DISEASE
Jean M. Covino

DISCUSSION

Pelvic inflammatory disease (PID) is defined as the acute clinical syndrome associated with the ascending spread of microorganisms (unrelated to pregnancy or surgery) from the vagina or cervix to the endometrium, fallopian tubes, and/or contiguous structures.[1] Infections are usually primary and are sexually transmitted. A smaller percentage of cases can be secondary to invasive uterine procedures or to parturition.

Incidence

More than 1.4 million women are diagnosed with PID every year in the United States.[2] Since PID is not a reportable disease in the United States, these numbers may be an underestimate. Recent data concluded that a strategy of identifying, testing, and treating women at risk for cervical *Chlamydia* infection was associated with a reduced incidence of PID.[3]

Pathogenesis

The pathogenesis of PID is poorly understood. Mechanisms cited as possibly contributing to the canalicular upward spread of microorganisms include changes in cervical mucus, adherence and ascent of spermatozoa, presence of cervical ectopy, IUD insertion, menstruation, and vaginal douching.

Microbiology

PID is a polymicrobial infection. Sexually transmitted organisms such as *Neisseria gonorrhoeae* and *Chlamydia trachomatis* account for roughly 80 percent and 51 percent of cases, respectively.[2] Other microorganisms implicated in PID include *Mycoplasma hominis, Peptococcus* species, *Mobiluncus* species, *Bacteroides* species, *Haemophilus influenzae, Streptococcus* species, *Gardnerella vaginalis, Ureaplasma urealyticum,* and possibly viruses.

Risk Factors

Certain risk factors have been associated with PID and should be sought while taking a history from any women with lower abdominal pain. These risk factors include age <25 years old, multiple sexual partners, presence of an IUD, and recent invasive gynecologic procedure. Also recent data from epidemiologic studies suggests that smoking and use of vaginal douches are associated risk factors.[4,5]

SYMPTOMS

There is no single historical, physical, or laboratory test that is pathognomonic in diagnosing PID. PID is a clinical diagnosis. Symptoms associated with PID include bilateral lower abdominal pain, irregular uterine bleeding, dysuria, and increased or changed vaginal discharge.

OBJECTIVE FINDINGS

Clinical findings associated with PID include temperature >38.0°C, palpable adnexal swelling and/or tenderness, cervical motion tenderness, and an abnormal cervical and vaginal discharge.

LABORATORY FINDINGS

Laboratory studies do not generally add to the accuracy of diagnosing PID. White blood cell (WBC) count and the erythrocyte sedimentation rate (ESR) may or may not be elevated in an acute case of PID. C-reactive protein may be elevated. Vaginal and cervical discharges should be checked by a wet mount examination for the presence of WBCs, since their absence makes the diagnosis of PID less likely. Cervical Gram stain should be done and checked for >5 WBCs/high-power field and for intracellular gram-negative diplococci. A sensitive urine pregnancy test should be done to rule out ectopic pregnancy. Syphilis serology should be ordered, and HIV testing and counseling should be encouraged since a diagnosis of PID suggests high-risk behavior. Pelvic ultrasound is not useful in diagnosing PID, but can help evaluate any pelvic masses.

INVASIVE TECHNIQUES

Invasive procedures are usually not indicated. Culdocentesis, if performed on a woman with PID, shows elevated concentrations of WBCs. Culture of the material is rarely helpful because of contamination by vaginal organisms. If an endometrial biopsy is done, it may suggest histopathologic evidence of endometritis, which correlates well with the presence of salpingitis. Results, however, can take several days. Laparoscopy is the specific means for diagnosing acute salpingitis and is considered the gold standard for confirming the diagnosis. However, the expense and the risk of the procedure must be considered. In most cases PID can be reasonably diagnosed without using the invasive procedures that tend to be reserved for cases where the diagnosis is imperative but remains uncertain (e.g., differentiation of acute appendicitis from PID).

DIAGNOSTIC CONSIDERATIONS

The two most important differential diagnoses that must be considered are ectopic pregnancy and acute appendicitis. Failure to recognize and treat either of these two can have devastating consequences. Other possible differentials include ovarian torsion, ruptured or hemorrhagic ovarian cyst, endometriosis, irritable bowel syndrome, and somatization disorder.

SPECIAL CONSIDERATIONS

Women ages 15 to 24 years who smoke, have multiple sexual partners, and admit to using vaginal douches are at the greatest risk for developing PID. PID in adolescents is more likely to result in infertility and ectopic pregnancy. PID is rare during pregnancy. Patients who are pregnant or HIV-positive with the diagnosis of PID should be hospitalized and treated with parenteral antibiotics.

TREATMENT

All patients with peritoneal signs or abscess formation should be admitted to the hospital and placed on parenteral antibiotics. Criteria for inpatient treatment of PID include:

1. Adolescence
2. Pregnancy
3. Unreliable patient
4. Patient who cannot tolerate oral medications
5. HIV-positive patient
6. No response to outpatient treatment after 72 h
7. Uncertain diagnosis

No single therapeutic regimen has been established for persons with PID. When selecting a treatment regimen, health care providers should consider availability, cost, patient acceptance, and geographic differences in antimicrobial susceptibility. Recent studies have demonstrated the presence of bacterial vaginosis–associated bacteria in addition to sexually transmitted organisms and suggest that treatment of acute PID must be broad spectrum in nature and effective against anaerobic bacteria as well as *N. gonorrhoeae* and *C. trachomatis.*[6]

Outpatient Therapy

The 1993 recommendations of the Centers for Disease Control and Prevention for treatment of PID are two types.[7] Regimen A calls for ceftriaxone (Rocephin), 250 mg IM (or any other third-generation cephalosporin), *or* cefoxitin (Mefoxin), 2g IM + 1 g of probenecid concurrently, *plus* doxycycline, 100 mg bid for 14 days. Regimen B consists of ofloxacin (Floxin), 400 mg PO bid for 14 days, *plus* clindamycin (Cleocin), 450 mg PO qid, *or* metronidazole (Flagyl, Protostat), 500 mg PO bid for 14 days. *Note:* Azithromycin is an approved single-dose therapy for cervical *Chlamydia* infection but costs roughly four times as much as doxycycline.

Inpatient Regimen

Regimen A consists of cefoxitin, 2g IV every 6 h *or* cefotetan, 2g IV every 12 h, *plus* doxycycline, 100 mg IV or PO every 12 h. Regimen B calls for clindamycin, 900 mg IV every 8 h, *plus* gentamicin, loading dose IV or IM (2 mg/kg of body weight), followed by a maintenance dose (1.5 mg/kg) every 8 h. Inpatient regimens should be continued for at least 48 h after clinical improvement, then followed with doxycycline, 100 mg PO bid or clindamycin, 450 mg PO qid, to complete a total of 14 days of therapy. Evaluation and treatment of sex partners of women who have PID is vital to reduce the chance of reinfection.

COMPLICATIONS AND RED FLAGS

The majority of women with acute PID recover completely. However, there are some long-term consequences of this disease. These sequelae include:

1. Risk of repeated episodes
2. Chronic pelvic pain, usually due to adhesion formation
3. Increased risk of ectopic pregnancy due to scarring of fallopian tubes
4. Infertility due to scarring of the fallopian tubes

About 11 percent of women are infertile after a single episode of PID, 23 percent after two episodes, and 50 percent after three or more episodes. The increased risk of infertility and ectopic pregnancy is directly related to duration of symptoms before treatment.

OTHER NOTES OR PEARLS

Symptoms associated with PID usually occur within 7 days of the beginning of menses. This is probably due to the opening of the cervix at that time. Always do a pregnancy test on any menstruating female patients who present with lower abdominal pain in spite of when they say their last menses took place. The clinical presentation of PID may help reveal which pathogen is responsible. For example, patients with gonococcal PID often present with an acute onset with temperatures 38.0°C or higher, palpable adnexal mass, and peritoneal signs. Therapeutic response is rapid. Patients with *Chlamydia* PID often have an insidious onset, complain of irregular bleeding, and have ESR >30 mm/h. *Chlamydia trachomatis* and *N. gonorrhoeae* are often found together in cases of PID, so treatment to cover both organisms is standard procedure. It has recently been suggested that before performing a surgical abortion, treatment of bacterial vaginosis (symptomatic or asymptomatic) should be considered to prevent PID.[8]

REFERENCES

1. Centers for Disease Control: Antibiotics-resistant strains of *Neisseria gonorrhoeae*. Policy Guidelines for detection, management, and control. *MMWR* 36:55, 1987.
2. Quan M: Pelvic inflammatory disease: Diagnosis and management. *J Am Board Fam Phys* 7:110–123, 1994.
3. Scholes D, Stergachis A, Heidrich FE, et al: Prevention of pelvic inflammatory disease by screening for cervical chlamydial infection. *New Engl J Med* 334:1362–1366, 1996.
4. Marchbanks PA, Lee NC, Peterson HB: Cigarette smoking as a risk factor for pelvic inflammatory disease. *Am J Obstet Gynecol* 162:639–644, 1990.
5. Scholes D, Dailing JR, Stergachis AS: Current cigarette smoking and risks of acute pelvic inflammatory disease. *Am J Public Health* 82:1352–1355, 1992.
6. Sweet RL: Role of bacterial vaginosis in pelvic inflammatory disease. *Clin Infect Dis* 20 (suppl 2):S271–275, 1995.
7. Centers for Disease Control and Prevention: 1993 sexually transmitted disease treatment guidelines. *MMWR* 42 (RR-14):75–81, 1993.
8. Joesoef MR, Schmid GP: Bacterial vaginosis: Review of treatment options and potential clinical indications for therapy. *Clin Infect Dis* 20 (suppl 1):S72–79, 1995.

Chapter 12–9
POLYCYSTIC OVARY SYNDROME
Dana M. Gallagher

DISCUSSION

Polycystic ovary syndrome (PCOS) is a common endocrine disorder characterized by hyperandrogenism and chronic anovulation. Hyperandrogenism manifests clinically as hirsutism, acne, and male-pattern alopecia, whereas anovulation encompasses a variety of possible menstrual disruptions, including amenorrhea, oligomenorrhea, dysfunctional uterine bleeding, and infertility. Although some have considered obesity to be essential to the diagnosis of PCOS, approximately one-half of women with PCOS are of normal weight.

Polycystic ovary syndrome is also associated with insulin resistance[1] and dyslipidemia.[2,3] In the obese patient, weight loss may improve the entire clinical picture by normalizing insulin and lipid levels, and stabilizing menstrual cycling.

PATHOGENESIS

The cause of PCOS is unknown. Historically, PCOS was attributed to a disorder of the hypothalamic-pituitary axis resulting in ovarian hyperandrogenism. More recently, it has been postulated that hyperinsulinism is an important precursor to hyperandrogenism. Although hyperandrogenism and hyperinsulinemia are features of PCOS, their mechanism of pathogenicity is unclear.

There have also been data to support the notion that PCOS is inherited. However, the responsible gene has not yet been pinpointed.[4]

SYMPTOMS

The patient presents with a history of menstrual irregularity, often since menarche. She may also be quite concerned about (and perhaps ashamed of) hirsutism, alopecia, and acne.

OBJECTIVE FINDINGS

Weight should be recorded. Examination of the skin may reveal excessive hair on the face, chin, chest, abdomen, and thighs. Identifying hirsutism should be achieved by both visual examination and palpation, since women typically remove excess hair to appear in public comfortably. Acne and seborrhea may be present; alopecia should be documented. Since these symptoms may be (wrongly) perceived as a lack of cleanliness or womanliness by the patient, care should be taken during the interview and examination not to shame her with tactless questioning or comments.

The presence of acanthosis nigricans (thick, brown skin in body folds) indicates hyperinsulinemia and should also be charted.

DIAGNOSTIC CONSIDERATIONS

The differential diagnosis includes hyperprolactinemia, acromegaly, and congenital adrenal hyperplasia. These can be ruled out through clinical examination, laboratory testing, and imaging studies (prolactin levels, serum growth hormone, CT and/or MRI).

LABORATORY TESTS

It is unclear what (combination of) laboratory tests clinch the diagnosis of PCOS. However, depending on history and clinical presentation, the following may be useful:

- *Luteinizing hormone (LH) levels* Hypersecretion is typical but normal levels do not rule PCOS.
- *Serum testosterone and androstenedione levels* Again, hypersecretion is typical but there may be individual variation.
- *Fasting lipid panel and glucose tolerance testing*

RADIOLOGIC STUDIES

Increasingly, pelvic sonogram is the gold standard for diagnosing PCOS. However, clinical and biochemical markers taken together are highly correlated with ultrasound findings.[5]

TREATMENT

Pharmacologic Management

Depending on the severity of the hirsutism, patients may opt to treat with spironolactone, 25 mg tid-qid,[6] or with low-dose oral contraceptives (containing 30 to 35 μg of ethinyl estradiol).[7] Patients with acne may respond well to oral contraceptives or can be treated with topical preparations or antibiotics (see Chap. 2-29). Alopecia may improve after treatment with oral contraceptives. Anovulation (menstrual irregularities) can be cycled with low-dose oral contraceptives.

Supportive Measures

For hirsutism, patients may pluck excess hair or use depilatories. For more permanent hair removal, referral to a skilled electrologist should be made. With regard to alopecia, changes in hairstyling may camouflage hair loss.

PATIENT EDUCATION

Patients should be informed that acne, hirsutism, and alopecia are slowly changing conditions, and that at least 6 months of treatment should be allowed to achieve noticeable improvement. Inform the patient that treatment for PCOS should continue for at least 1 year prior to tapering treatment. Many women will relapse when treatment is discontinued; treatment over a period of several years may be necessary to maintain beneficial response. Patients desiring pregnancy should be referred to an infertility specialist for evaluation and treatment. The use of spironolactone for hirsutism and dermatologic agents like isotretinoin (Accutane) must be discontinued because of potential teratogenicity. Overweight patients should be encouraged to start a regular program of exercise and weight reduction.

DISPOSITION

Patients should be evaluated at least yearly with a routine gynecologic examination. Patients with hyperinsulinemia and dyslipidemias should be followed at intervals congruent with office protocol.

NOTES AND PEARLS

It is likely that increased emphasis will be placed on treating hyperinsulinemia, since it appears to underlie the hyperandrogenism, chronic anovulation, and long-term cardiovascular risks associated with PCOS.

REFERENCES

1. Davidson MB: Clinical implications of insulin resistance syndromes. *Am J Med* 99(Oct):420–426, 1995.
2. Wild RA: Obesity, lipids, cardiovascular risk, and androgen excess. *Am J Med* 98(Suppl 1A):1A-27S to 1A-32S, 1995.
3. Bates B: Many young women with PCOS have lipid abnormalities. *Ob Gyn News* August 15, 1996, p 14.
4. Jacobs HS: Polycystic ovary syndrome: Etiology and management. *Curr Opin Obstet Gynecol* 7:203–208, 1995.
5. Franks S: Polycystic ovary syndrome. *New Engl J Med* 333(13):853, 1995.
6. MacKay HT: Gynecology, in Tierney LM Jr, McPhee SJ, Papadakis MA (eds): *Current Medical Diagnosis and Treatment*, 35th ed. Stanford, CT, Appleton & Lange, 1996, p 656.
7. Redmond GP: Androgenic disorders of women: Diagnostic and therapeutic decision making. *Am J Med* 98(Suppl 1A):1A-127S, 1995.

Chapter 12–10
SEXUAL ASSAULT
Jean M. Covino

DISCUSSION

Sexual assault (rape) is a violent crime directed mostly against women. It is defined as act(s) of sexual intimacy performed without the consent of the victim through the use or threat of force or when the victim is unable to give consent because of physical or mental disability.

Incidence

Rape is the most underreported violent crime in the United States. It is estimated that at least 20 percent of adult women have experienced sexual assault during their lifetimes. Approximately 100,000 cases of rape are reported annually in the United States, and this most likely represents only a small fraction of the actual cases. According to the U.S. Department of Justice, this accounts for approximately 6 percent of all violent crimes.[1] Note that statistics collected by law enforcement agencies are low estimates since many victims are especially reluctant to report this crime.

Incidence of Sexually Transmitted Infections

The types of sexually transmitted diseases associated with sexual assault are gonorrhea (up to 12 percent); trichomonas vaginalis, monilial vaginitis, and bacterial vaginosis (more than 6 percent each); *Chlamydia* (more than 4 percent); herpes (less than 2 percent); and syphilis (less than 4 percent). (See associated chapters.) Studies have shown that HIV infections are not likely to be contracted during an assault.[2]

Epidemiology

Although sexual assault does occur in any age group, victims are more likely to be young, single, female members of minority groups with a low socioeconomic status. Rape is more prevalent in urban areas. More sexual assaults occur during the summer months, whereas the fewest occur during the winter months.

HISTORY AND PHYSICAL EXAMINATION

The history should include a detailed account of the assault and a complete gynecologic history, including the use of any contraceptives. The victim must be asked if consciousness was lost at any time or if she or he has defecated, voided, douched, bathed, or showered since the incident. The victim must be questioned regarding the orifice(s) of penetration and whether ejaculation took place.

The physical examination should include general appearance and assessment of psychological and emotional status. The entire body must be checked for signs of trauma, the condition of the external genitalia documented, and a speculum examination performed. Pubic hair is combed and cut and fingernail scrapings are collected with standard rape kits. Photographs should be taken if appropriate. Counseling services should be provided and follow-up appointments arranged.

In many areas, usually through emergency departments, specially trained sexual assault medical examiners are available to collect acute forensic evidence. Whenever possible, victims should be referred to these individuals.

SPECIAL CONSIDERATIONS

The very young, very old, and handicapped are particularly vulnerable to sexual assaults. Every state has laws that require the reporting of child abuse. Health care providers should contact their state or local child protective service agency about child abuse reporting requirements in their areas.

LABORATORY TESTS

Initial diagnostic tests for sexually transmitted diseases (STDs) after sexual assault recommended by the Centers for Disease Control and Prevention (CDC) include cultures for *Neisseria gonorrhoeae* and *Chlamydia trachomatis* from any potentially infected sites and wet mount and culture of vaginal swab specimen for *Trichomonas vaginalis* infection. The wet mount can also check for evidence of bacterial vaginosis or yeast. Collect a serum sample to be preserved for subsequent analysis if follow-up serologic tests are positive (see 12 week follow-up), and perform HIV testing (optional, see 12 week follow-up).

Follow-up examination 2 weeks after assault should include cultures and wet mount tests should repeated unless prophylactic treatment has already been provided.

Follow-up examination 12 weeks after assault should include serologic tests for syphilis and HIV infection. If positive, testing of the serum collected at the initial examination will assist in determining whether the infection antedated the assault.

RADIOGRAPHIC AND OTHER DIAGNOSTIC STUDIES

There are no appropriate studies.

TREATMENT

Although not all experts agree, most patients probably benefit from STD prophylaxis because follow-up of patients may be difficult. Patients may be reassured if offered treatment or prophylaxis for possible infection.[3] The regimen recommended by the CDC includes ceftriaxone (Rocephin), 125 mg IM stat, plus metronidazole (Flagyl), 2g PO in a single dose, plus doxycycline, 100 mg bid for 7 days.[3] Postcoital contraceptive therapy should be offered to postpubertal adolescents and adult women of childbearing age who were raped less than 72 h ago.

COMPLICATIONS

Aside from obvious physical complications that may occur during a violent attack, health care providers must be aware of the psychological and emotional stress a rape victim undergoes. Eventual psychological manifestations are related to posttraumatic stress disorder. More than half of rape victims experience difficulty in reestablishing sexual or emotional relationships with spouses or other sexual partners. It is very important to offer psychiatric follow-up and counseling to all sexual assault victims.

NOTES AND PEARLS

The majority of rape victims who come to the emergency room do not openly admit to having been sexually assaulted. They may complain of being mugged or may voice concern about HIV or other STDs. Recent data have supported an association of sexual assault history with eating disorder symptoms.[4] Unless the health care provider is thorough in obtaining a sexual history, assault victims will remain unidentified.

REFERENCES

1. Federal Bureau of Investigation: *Uniform Crime Reports for the United States.* Washington, DC: US Department of Justice, 1991.
2. Holmes KK, Mardh P-A, Sparling PF, et al (eds): Sexual assault and sexually transmitted diseases, in *Sexually Transmitted Diseases,* 2d ed. New York, McGraw-Hill, 1990.
3. Centers for Disease Control and Prevention: 1993 sexually transmitted diseases treatment guidelines. *MMWR* 42(14):97–102, 1993.
4. Laws A, Golding JM: Sexual assault history and eating disorder symptoms among white, hispanic, and African-American women and men. *Am J Public Health* 86(4):579–582, 1996.

Chapter 12–11
TRICHOMONIASIS
Peggy Valentine

DISCUSSION

Trichomoniasis is a common sexually transmitted infection, caused by a flagellated protozoan, *Trichomonas vaginalis.* Some infected individuals have no symptoms, but women usually present with a diffuse, malodorous yellow-green vaginal discharge that may be frothy. Vulvar irritation is a common complaint. A "strawberry cervix" is observed in 1 to 2 percent of women on speculum examination and 50 percent on colposcopy. Women who use barrier methods such as diaphragms and condoms are least likely to acquire this infection. The majority of men are asymptomatic. Coexistent gonorrhea and other sexually transmitted diseases (STDs) are not uncommon in persons infected with *Trichomonas.* It is therefore important for the clinician to carefully evaluate patients with STDs for other pathogens.

SIGNS AND SYMPTOMS

The infection elicits an acute inflammatory response of the vagina, resulting in a vaginal discharge with polymorphonuclear neutrophils (PMNs). Vaginal discharge, the most common symptom, may be malodorous. Nearly half of affected women will complain of pruritus and dyspareunia. Many note worsening of symptoms following the menstrual period. Lower abdominal pain and tenderness of the adnexa and uterine fundus are uncommon symptoms. The majority of men have no symptoms. Those presenting with symptoms may complain of purulent, mucopurulent, or mucoid discharge, occasionally with mild urethral irritation.

OBJECTIVE FINDINGS

Homogeneous discharge varies in amount, is usually green-yellow in color, and is sometimes foamy or frothy. The vaginal mucosa is often erythematous, and occasionally petechiae are noted on the cervix, giving it a strawberry appearance.

DIAGNOSTIC CONSIDERATIONS

Diagnosis is made by observing the motile parasites on wet mount examination. Trichomonads are ovoid and slightly larger than PMNs. It is unfortunate that wet mount does not always reveal trichomonads, and a vaginal culture may be necessary for confirmation of the diagnosis.

LABORATORY TESTS

Using the wet mount, sweep the anterior and posterior fornices with a cotton swab, place a drop of the secretions on a microscopic slide, mix with one drop of slightly warm saline. Cover with a cover slip and examine under low then medium magnification. Motile trichomonads confirm the diagnosis; increased numbers of PMNs are usually present. Culture for *T. vaginalis* only if the wet mount is negative and clinical suspicion of trichomoniasis is high.

TREATMENT

Treatment for patient and partner is recommended. Metronidazole (Flagyl), 2 g orally in a single dose, is the recommended regimen. Adverse reactions of metronidazole include the following:

- Many patients complain of a metallic taste while taking metronidazole.
- Alcohol should be avoided. Metronidazole produces a disulfiram-like (Antabuse) effect, causing nausea and flushing in some individuals.
- The prothrombin time may be prolonged in patients taking warfarin and metronidazole.

As an alternative treatment, use metronidazole, 500 mg twice daily for 7 days. Metronidazole gel has not been studied for trichomoniasis treatment. There are no effective alternatives to metronidazole therapy. Use of metronidazole is contraindicated in the first trimester of pregnancy, but may be considered after the first trimester with a 2-g single dose.

DISPOSITION

Follow-up is unnecessary for men and women who become asymptomatic after treatment.

PATIENT EDUCATION

Sexual partners should be treated. Coitus should be avoided until therapy has been completed by patient and partner and both are without symptoms. To limit the possibility of recurrence, the patient should be given information on the benefits of a mutually monogamous sexual relationship and the recommendation of using barrier methods.

BIBLIOGRAPHY

Centers for Disease Control and Prevention: 1993 sexually-transmitted diseases treatment guidelines. *MMWR* 42(RR-14):70–72, 1993.

Mou SM: Gynecologic infections, in Seltzer VL, Pearse WH (eds): New York, *Women's Primary Health Care: Office Practices and Procedures.* McGraw-Hill, 1995.

Rein MF, Muller M: Trichomonas vaginalis and trichomoniasis, in Holmes KK, Mardh P-A, Sparling PF, et al (eds): *Sexually Transmitted Diseases,* 2d ed. New York, McGraw-Hill, 1990.

Chapter 12–12
BREAST MASS
Noel J. Genova

DISCUSSION

Evaluation of a breast mass implies separating very common, normal "lumps" in women's breasts from cancerous lesions (see Chap. 13-4). Unfortunately, there is no simple method. In many cases, biopsy is the only way to distinguish whether a breast mass is malignant. The information in this chapter is intended to help the clinician decide if, when, and where to refer a woman who presents with a breast mass. Heavy emphasis on the need for referral and biopsy of breast masses may appear to many primary care clinicians as "overkill."

Consider the following:

- Mammography has an overall false-negative rate of 10 to 15 percent. Because of the technical limitations of mammography, the false-negative rate in women younger than 50 years old who present with a breast mass is higher than the rate for women older than 50.[1]
- Mammography cannot be used at all in pregnant women or women younger than 20 years of age, and it is difficult to interpret for women younger than 30 to 35. Sonography, which could be used in these women, is of little value in diagnosing breast cancer, but can be useful in distinguishing cysts from solid masses.[2,3]
- Failure to diagnose breast cancer is a common and costly cause of malpractice claims.[2] Reassurance regarding a lump, thereby avoiding a biopsy, is not helpful to a woman who ultimately learns that the lump was malignant, especially if her prognosis is poor by the time her cancer is diagnosed and treated.

DIAGNOSTIC CONSIDERATIONS

Worrisome breast masses are generally described as dominant, firm, and discrete, and they may or may not be mobile. Bilateral, tender masses that resolve spontaneously within a few weeks or months are not generally clinically suspicious. Benign masses that are the most difficult to distinguish from cancerous lesions are cysts and fibroadenomas. Both occur very commonly in premenopausal women. Typically, fibroadenomas are firm, have discrete borders, and are freely movable. Cysts are also most common in premenopausal women, but are soft, are often fluid-filled, and may come and go, particularly with relation to the menstrual cycle. Cysts may be both resolved and proved benign if needle aspiration yields clear fluid and renders the cyst nonpalpable. Bloody aspirates must be submitted for cytology. Fibroadenomas are solid masses and do not yield fluid with needle aspiration.

Other causes of breast mass are more readily distinguished from breast cancer on history, but still must be referred to a surgeon. Breast abscesses, like other abscesses, are red, hot, and tender and may be draining purulent fluid. Lactating women with persistent, painful masses should be referred to a surgeon to rule out galactocele. Breast trauma may result in fat necrosis.[1]

Although the physical examination has limitations in establishing a diagnosis of breast cancer, having a slightly lower sensitivity than mammography alone, it should be performed by a clinician for all women who present with breast mass. Breast self-examination should be taught to all women, allowing them to separate normal supportive tissue, ribs, and general premenstrual swelling from discrete masses. Suspicious clinical findings (including nonspontaneous nipple discharge, especially if bloody), whether discovered by the woman or the clinician, should *never* be disregarded because of a normal mammogram. Cancer cannot be ruled out unless the mass resolves with needle aspiration or is negative on biopsy.

Mammography, therefore, is helpful as a diagnostic tool (as opposed to a screening tool), only in conjunction with history, physical examination, and needle aspiration or biopsy. Its greatest diagnostic use is to rule out occult cancers, especially those occurring bilaterally, which occur in 3 percent of patients who present with newly diagnosed breast cancer.[2]

Although evaluation of risk factors is important from a public health and epidemiologic point of view, it is of little diagnostic value in determining whether an individual has breast cancer. With the important exception of increasing age as a risk factor, 75 percent of women with breast cancer do not appear to be at high risk.[1] Although women ages 30 to 50 account for many tragic cases of early death from breast cancer, the rate of diagnosed disease climbs rapidly in each decade after age 50 [see Figs. 12-12-1 (Plate 24), 12-12-2 (Plate 25), 12-12-3 (Plate 26)].[1]

SPECIAL CONSIDERATIONS: TEAM APPROACH AND PATIENT INVOLVEMENT

Because biopsy is the only truly accurate method for diagnosis of a breast mass, a primary care clinician must have ready referral resources and should be familiar with their preferences. For example, does the surgeon want the patient to bring her mammogram films with her or delay any diagnostic workup until after personally evaluating the patient? Which mammography facilities in town prefer to work with surgeons to perform directed-needle biopsy, as opposed to those who specialize in screening procedures? How far does the patient have to travel to see a surgeon who is familiar with diagnosing breast conditions?

Patients should be offered all alternatives, with explanations of the risks and benefits of observation, needle biopsy, and exci-

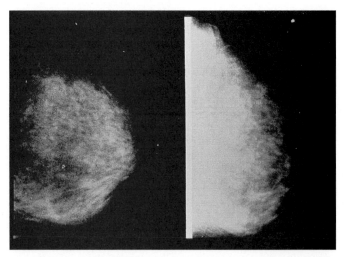

Figure 12-12-1 (Plate 24). Quality assurance for mammography is critical. These images are of the same breast. The image on the left shows a breast that is not properly compressed. It could have mistakenly been read as a dense, glandular breast with no abnormality visualized. The image on the right shows the same breast with proper compression. It is much easier to find a white density indicative of cancer on the right image than on the left image. *(From the American Medical Women's Association for the Breast and Cervical Cancer Education Project for Primary Care Providers, under a cooperative agreement with the Centers for Disease Control and Prevention.)*

sional biopsy. Considering that there is often no clear-cut "best" time for biospy, it is helpful if the woman herself has some input into all decisions made regarding her diagnosis and treatment, if applicable.

Centers specializing in diagnosis and treatment of breast conditions may have resources that are helpful to both patients and

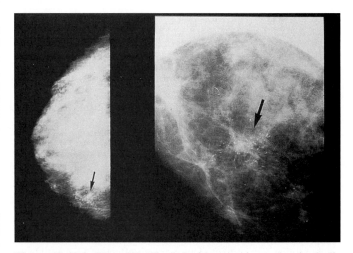

Figure 12-12-2 (Plate 25). The left side contains a density indicated by the black arrow. The cone-compression view on the right reveals a finding even more ominous than the original film, illustrating how useful cone-compression mammography can be. This finding represented carcinoma. *(From the American Medical Women's Association for the Breast and Cervical Cancer Education Project for Primary Care Providers, under a cooperative agreement with the Centers for Disease Control and Prevention.)*

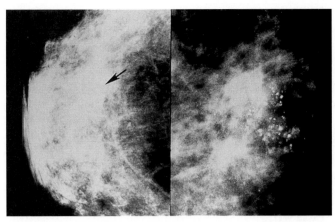

Figure 12-12-3 (Plate 26). On the left side, the radiologist has noted some white specks. These represent microcalcifications in the breast. Imaging these with a magnification view as shown on the right helps identify the sizes and shapes of the calcifications. These are highly suggestive of carcinoma because they are pleomorphic, that is, of different sizes and shapes. In general, cone compression mammography is used to evaluate densities further, and magnification views are done to identify and discern calcifications. *(From the American Medical Women's Association for the Breast and Cervical Cancer Education Project for Primary Care Providers, under a cooperative agreement with the Centers for Disease Control and Prevention.)*

primary care clinicians. Identification of patient education materials, self-help groups, and educators specializing in breast cancer (for example) may ultimately be important to women who are referred for evaluation of a breast mass.

FUTURE TRENDS AND CONTROVERSIES

Breast cancer remains a significant cause of death for American women (nearly 45,000 deaths estimated for 1996).[4] It appears that mortality rates from breast cancer are declining among white women, although the cause for this decline is unclear.[4] Genetic testing, which might help to identify those very young women who are at risk of developing breast cancer, is not yet ready for use in the general population.[5]

Evaluation of any clinically suspicious breast mass must be done by the primary care clinician in consultation with a surgeon and a radiologist. Many masses, even in the presence of a normal mammogram, require biopsy, either by fine-needle aspiration, stereotactic biopsy, or open surgical biopsy. Choice of biopsy method depends on the patient's age, type of mass, mammographic findings, and preference of the consulting surgeon.[3]

REFERENCES

1. Carlson KJ, Eisenstat SA, Frigoletto FD, et al: *Primary Care of Women.* Chicago, Mosby, 1995, pp 221, 222, 400, 401.
2. Donegan WL: Evaluation of a palpable breast mass. *New Engl J Med* 327(13):937–939, 1992.
3. Evaluation of Common Breast Problems: A Primer for Primary Care Providers, prepared by The Society of Surgical Oncology and The Commission on Cancer of the American College of Surgeons for The Centers for Disease Control and Prevention, 1995.
4. American Cancer Society: Cancer Facts and Figures, 1996.
5. Langston AA, Malone KE, Thompson JD, et al: BRCA1 mutations in a population-based sample of young women with breast cancer. *New Engl J Med* 334(3):137–142, 1996.

Chapter 12–13
CANCER OF THE CERVIX/ THE ABNORMAL PAP SMEAR
Amelia Naccarto-Coleman

DISCUSSION

Epidemiology

Since the introduction of the Pap (Papanicolau) smear in 1943, the incidence and mortality rate of invasive cervical cancer in the United States has declined more than 50 percent as the result of regular periodic screening. Carcinoma of the cervix accounts for approximately 16,000 new cases (6 percent of all cancers) and 5000 cancer deaths in the United States each year. However, in other countries, the prevalence of this disease is highly variable. Worldwide, it continues to be the second most common malignancy in women. These differences are attributed to low socioeconomic status, nonparticipation in screening programs, and several epidemiologic cofactors that have influenced the development of the human papillomavirus (HPV) infection.

Concurrent with the declining mortality rates for invasive carcinoma is the appearance of increasing incidence rates for carcinoma in situ (CIS). This shift has been linked to the efficacy of screening and a trend toward cigarette smoking and earlier sexual activity. Rates for CIS reach a peak during the reproductive years in both African American and white women. After the age of 25, however, the rates for invasive disease are different. Incidence rates for African-American women dramatically increase with age but stabilize over time for white women.

Overall, more than 25 percent of invasive cervical cancer occurs in women older than 65, and about 50 percent of all women who die from cervical cancer are older than 65 years of age. These patterns demonstrate the need to reach out to older women, ethnic minorities, poor women, and the uninsured who have not had the benefit of regular screening.

Pathogenesis and Natural History

Unique to cervical cancer is the etiologic relationship between the infectious HPV agent and development of preinvasive and invasive cervical lesions. According to the 1996 National Institutes of Health Consensus Statment on Cervical Cancer, HPV DNA is present in more than 93 percent of all cervical cancer and precursor lesions. More than 70 types of HPV have been identified. However, only 23 of these types actually infect the cervix, and out of these approximatley 10 are associated with invasive disease. These 10 are further divided into low- and high-risk categories. Both low-risk (types 6 and 11) and high-risk types (16, 18, 31, and 45) account for more than 80 percent of all cervical intraepithelial neoplasias (CIN). In highly invasive carcinomas, the high-risk types predominate, with HPV-16 in 50 percent of cases and HPV-18 in 20 percent. Approximately 70 to 80 percent of all cervical cancers are squamous cell (epidermoid). The remaining 20 to 30 percent are either adenocarcinoma, mixed epithelial carcinomas, or undifferentiated carcinomas.

Understanding the pathophysiology of the disease is the key to reducing the morbidity and mortality rates of invasive carcinoma. Cytologic screening assists the practitioner in identifying the precursor lesions that eventually progress to frank carcinoma. This preinvasive stage, detected by Pap smear screening, provides a unique opportunity to control any further progression of the disease. The entire spectrum of this cellular disorder is manifested by progressive atypical changes in growth and maturation. These

Table 12-13-1. Risk Factors for Cancer of the Cervix

Cigarette smoking
Early age at first intercourse
Low socioeconomic status
Infrequent Pap smears
History of genital warts
Multiple sex partners
Immunosuppression
DES (diethylstilbestrol) daughters

morphologic changes are responsible for initiating CIN, defined as the preinvasive phase of cervical cancer. Cervical epithelium is composed of two different cell types, columnar and squamous. Columnar epithelial cells that are exposed to the vaginal environment are continually replaced or repaired by stratified squamous epithelial cells. This benign regenerative process, called *metaplasia,* is a normal occurrence during a female's neonatal period, adolescence, and first pregnancy. However, certain environmental and hormonal conditions (see Table 12-13-1) can alter this benign process which results in cellular abnormalities known as *dysplasia.*

These conditions, or risk factors, include early age of first intercourse, early first pregnancy, multiple sex partners, herpesvirus type 2 infections, HPV, and intrauterine exposure to exogenous estrogen (diethylstilbestrol, DES). Anatomically, the area most vulnerable to these carcinogenic stimuli is located between the old and the new squamocolumnar, epithelial junction called the *transformation zone.* Approximately 95 percent of all squamous intraepithelial neoplasia develops within this zone. In most cases, the preinvasive stage either regresses entirely or remains static for several years before any further progression occurs. However, when progression does occur, the malignant cells push their way through the basement membrane and gradually invade the cervical stroma. Initially, this process results in microinvasive carcinoma but can evolve into frankly invasive carcinoma over time. Despite negative cytology or cervical biopsy results, a cone biopsy is needed to determine the presence or absence of invasion.

Although cervical cancer is primarily a disease of local infiltration, the tendency for lymphatic dissemination is the hallmark. In more extensive disease, infiltration of the underlying tissue extends beyond the pelvic floor to the bladder and the rectum. The more advanced the local disease, the greater the likelihood of lymphatic spread and distant metastases. The FIGO staging method is used by the health care provider to estimate the extent of disease and aid in planning treatment. This clinical staging method is based on physical examination and noninvasive testing. The International Classification System adopted by the Federation of Gynecology and Obstetrics (FIGO) is the most widely used system.

SIGNS AND SYMPTOMS

Preinvasive stages, such as CIN or CIS, are generally asymptomatic and detected by cytologic findings on routine Pap smears. The most common symptom of invasive carcinoma is abnormal or irregular vaginal bleeding. This can include intermenstrual bleeding, postcoital bleeding, or heavy menstrual bleeding (menorrhagia) (see Table 12-13-2).

Table 12-13-2. Most Common Signs and Symptoms of Carcinoma in Situ

Bleeding
Discharge
Cervical appearance

Vaginal discharge is the second most common symptom. Preinvasive cervical neoplasia rarely produces any physical findings, especially if the lesion is endocervical. Cervical lesions and epithelium that appear suspicious, white (leukoplakia), or bloody should be considered for immediate biopsy. Pelvic pain, hematuria, or urinary frequency are usually seen only in advanced stages of the disease.

As the disease progresses, infiltrative cancer can produce cervical enlargement, firmness, and irregularity. Three growth patterns that are clinically seen include exophytic, endophytic, and ulcerative. Exophytic lesions can appear cauliflower-like and bleed easily with palpation. Earlier stages of invasive disease often present with superficial changes that can mistakenly be interpreted as cervicitis or ectropion. Often, there is an associated vaginal discharge that can be either bloody, serous, or purulent. Rectovaginal examination is crucial in determining the extent of the involvement. Advanced disease with extensive parametrial involvement may reveal a nodular thickening of the uterosacral ligaments with loss of mobility and fixation of the cervix. Signs of metastasis can include (1) enlarged supraclavicular and inguinal nodes, (2) unilateral, pitting edema of a lower extremity, (3) evidence of disease in the vagina, (5) anemia, and (4) weight loss.

SCREENING RECOMMENDATIONS

The Pap smear is the clinician's primary tool in the detection of cervical dysplasia and preinvasive neoplasia. The cervical-vaginal Pap smear examines exfoliated cells from the cervix and the uterus to detect pathologic abnormalities and cellular alterations of the uterine cervix in asymptomatic women. It is never used diagnostically. It has been estimated that with regular screening the incidence of invasive cervical cancer has decreased as much as 70 percent. Despite this decline, there is still a large number of women who do not have regular Pap smears, especially elderly African American and middle-aged poor women. Some areas report that 75 percent of women ages 65 or older have not had a Pap smear within the previous 5 years. Since 20 percent of the total number of invasive cervical carcinoma cases occur in women aged 65 or older, and 40 to 50 percent of all women who die from cervical cancer are older than 65, an extra effort targeted at this population is important.

Currently, the screening recommendations of the American College of Obstetricians and Gynecologists, American Cancer Society, and the National Cancer Institute are as follows:

- Initiate annual Pap testing at the onset of sexual activity or age 18, whichever comes first.
- After three or more consecutive, satisfactory, and normal examinations, the Pap smear can be performed less frequently at the discretion of the patient and the clinician.
- There is no established upper limit of age for testing.

THE PAP TEST

The sensitivity and specificity of the Pap smear largely depends on the clinician's technique and/or the laboratory's interpretation. In spite of the best collection technique, specimen handling, or screening procedure, a 10 to 20 percent false-negative (missed lesion) rate is still reported. Efficacy is also limited by poor patient compliance, failure to identify high-risk patients, inaccurate or incomplete laboratory reports, and inadequate follow-up. Regardless of the explanation, Pap smear results are reliable only for screening purposes. All abnormal Pap smears require follow-up evaluations and histologic confirmation to make a diagnosis. It is important to note that cytology does not equal histology.

COLLECTION TECHNIQUES

Inspection

Visually inspect the cervix before collecting a sample. Locate the transformation zone. In postmenopausal and pregnant women, the transformation zone is often difficult to locate.

Instruction

Idealistically, patients should be scheduled for routine Pap smears during the proliferative phase of their menstrual cycle, which is the week immediately following their period. Ask the patient if she has noticed an abnormal vaginal discharge, evidence of infection, or expects to have her menses during the time of her visit. Avoid sampling if she is menstruating or complaining of a heavy discharge attributable to infection. Instruct the patient to avoid intercourse or use any intravaginal products for at least 24 to 48 h prior to the examination.

Identifying Information

Label the patient's slide prior to collection. Provide the laboratory with a clinical history and any abnormal findings. Alert the cyto-pathologist to patients who present with a history of intermenstrual, postcoital or postmenopausal bleeding, high risk for cervical pathology, or any visible lesions on examination. Include the last menstrual period (LMP), obstetrical history, sexual history, hormonal use, and history of previous Pap smears.

Cellular Composition

Avoid using lubricants of any kind. Moisten the speculum with water or saline if necessary. Reliable smears must include adequate numbers of squamous epithelial cells sampled from the endocervical canal and the transformation zone. Avoid preparing slides with epithelial cells that are obscured by blood, inflammatory cells, or foreign material. Sample both the endocervix and ectocervix with a spatula and a cytobrush. Gently cleanse the cervix with a cotton swab to remove any blood, mucus, or discharge. Insert the cytobrush into the cervical canal and rotate it no more than 360°. Spread the material evenly onto a glass slide. Rotate a wooden Ayres spatula around the external os (portio) and then roll either onto the same slide or a second slide. Immediately spray the slide with fixative.

Quality Control

Use an experienced, certified, and reputable laboratory that has been endorsed by either the American Society of Cytologists or the College of American Pathologists, or both. Inquire about the quality control process, including communication and reporting methods, technical equipment, and adequate staffing.

CYTOLOGIC CLASSIFICATION: THE BETHESDA SYSTEM

The National Cancer Institute changed the nomenclature for dysplasia in 1988 and developed the current reporting method known as the Bethesda System. Updated in 1991 and 1992, this system has replaced the earlier interpretations and reflects the current understanding of the development and progression of cervical neoplasia. The Bethesda System relies on the pathologist for a diagnosis and appropriate follow-up recommendations. The format of this reporting system includes the components listed in the following paragraphs.

Statement of Specimen Adequacy

Satisfactory versus unsatisfactory is determined by the presence or absence of both endocervical and metaplastic ectocervical cells. Satisfactory smears can be limited by the following four factors:

1. Lack of metaplastic or endocervical cells
2. Partially obscuring inflammation, blood, or debris
3. Drying artifact
4. Lack of patient information

Unsatisfactory implies that either more than 75 percent of the cells were obscured by blood, inflammation, or debris, or that the slide was broken in transit.

General Categorization

Within the system, two new classification terms are introduced: statement of general categorization and descriptive diagnosis of the general categorization.

Squamous intraepithelial lesion (SIL) encompasses CIN I, II, and III and describes two categories: low-grade squamous intraepithelial lesions and high-grade squamous intraepithelial lesions. Low-grade SIL (LGSIL) includes cellular changes associated with HPV infection and mild dysplasia or CIN I. High-grade SIL (HGSIL) includes moderate to severe dysplasia or (CIN II) and carcinoma in situ or (CIN III).

DIAGNOSTIC CONSIDERATIONS

The uterine cervix can present with a number of pathologic conditions, including each of the following:

- *Infections* Commonly associated with acute and/or chronic cervicitis, symptoms usually include a vaginal discharge. Clinicians may choose to perform a KOH preparation or wet mount to diagnose *Trichomonas, Candida,* or bacterial vaginosis. Microbiology cultures are useful for diagnosing bacterial infections, and serologic methods aid in the diagnosis of syphilis, herpes, and *Chlamydia.* Microscopic features of *Trichomonas, Candida,* and herpes can also be found on Pap smears.
- *Preinvasive Lesions or CIN* Cervical lesions that are visualized on speculum examination need to be differentiated between early invasive cancer or secondary carcinoma of the cervix and benign conditions such as eversion, polyps, and papillary endocervicitis. Multiple biopsies may be necessary before a final diagnosis can be made. Occasionally, metastatic ovarian, bladder, and breast carcinoma have spread to the cervix by direct extension from the uterine corpus or vagina. Lymphomas will also rarely present as a cervical tumor.
- *Dysplasia and/or atypia* Dysplasia and/or atypia detected on Pap smears need to be thoroughly evaluated to rule out invasive carcinoma, infectious processes (other than HPV), cellular reparation, and hormonally induced changes in the postmenopausal patient. The infectious processes that can produce atypical changes include bacterial vaginosis, *Candida, Trichomonas, Chlamydia trachomatis,* and *Neisseria gonorrhoeae.*
- *Invasive carcinoma* Microinvasive squamous carcinoma is the earliest invasive form of lesion, defined as less than 3 mm beyond the basement membrane but without invading the lymphatic system. Further extension is staged on the FIGO system and based on the degree and location of invasion.
- *Miscellaneous* Microglandular endocervical hyperplasia can present with a polypoid mass appearing within the endocervical canal. These lesions are often observed in pregnancy or in women who take oral contraceptives. Endocervical polyps are occasionally seen in women and may present with a history of abnormal bleeding or vaginal discharge. Flat condyloma are seen as a result of an infection with the human papilloma virus.

DIAGNOSTIC STUDIES

Whenever a clinician receives an abnormal Pap smear report that is suggestive of dysplasia, preinvasive disease (CIS), or invasive carcinoma, the patient is required to undergo a thorough investi-

Table 12-13-3. Indications to Perform a Cone Biopsy or
Conization

Two-step discrepancy between cytology and histology
Suspicion of microinvasive carcinoma
Poor cervical visualization

gation, using the simplest procedure, to ensure an accurate diagnosis. Patients who require further evaluation can be sorted into several distinct groups: (1) those with unsuspected invasive cancer, (2) those with observable lesions that are amenable to office or outpatient treatment, and (3) those who require diagnostic (and often therapeutic) conization. This process of selecting patients for further studies begins with an analysis of the Pap smear, which is used as a screening test for dysplasia and cancer. Colposcopy is the diagnostic test that is used to evaluate any abnormalities that are discovered on the Pap smear or observed on the cervix. Additionally, the diagnostic evaluation of cervical cancer also includes obtaining biopsies of representative areas of the cervix. Several modalities can be used for this procedure, including (1) endocervical curettage, (2) directed biopsies, (3) conization or cone biopsies, and (4) Schiller's test.

Colposcopy

Colposcopic examination uses a vaginal speculum, binocular magnification, and an intense light source to view the uterine cervix. After staining the cervix with a 3 to 5% solution of acetic acid (Schiller's test), a satisfactory examination will identify any lesions or abnormalities and allow the entire transformation zone of the cervical epithelium to be visualized. Abnormal findings that indicate dysplasia and CIS are (1) white epithelium and (2) a mosaic pattern of the surface capillaries. Early stromal invasion is suspected when bizarre capillary configurations are seen. With the exception of pregnancy, whenever these abnormalities are seen, a directed biopsy with evaluation of the endocervical canal by curettage should always be performed. Both specimens need to be submitted separately for pathologic assessment. Indications for colposcopy include the following:

1. Pap smears consistent with dysplasia or carcinoma
2. Pap smears consistent with evidence of HPV infection
3. Pap smears reported as atypical squamous cells of undetermined significance (ASCUS) or repeated ASCUS
4. Pap smears with repeated inflammation
5. Abnormal appearance of the cervix
6. Patients with a history of DES exposure

ECC and Biopsy

An endocervical curettage (ECC) is a general scraping of the interior wall of the cervix and best performed before taking any biopsies. Do not perform ECCs on pregnant patients. Specimens are submitted separately and labeled as such. In females who present with a dysplastic smear, an estimated 5 to 10 percent of the results are positive for dysplasia. Cervical biopsies of defined or well demarcated lesions are then obtained. Concern is warranted if a significant discrepancy is found between the colposcopic impression, the Pap cytology, and the biopsy histology. Generally, 10 percent of colposcopies with directed biopsies and ECC have a discrepancy between the screening Pap and the histologic data from the biopsy and ECC. A difference of one grade is common and acceptable. However, when a two-grade discrepancy occurs, a cone biopsy or conization is needed for further tissue diagnosis (see Table 12-13-3).

Cervical conization is the most commonly employed modality for diagnostic evaluation if the endocervical curettage reveals dysplasia. It can be performed by using either the cold-knife

technique, a laser, or a heated wire loop known as the LEEP procedure. Risks include infection, blood loss, anesthesia, and, in women who are considering pregnancy, cervical incompetence. The LEEP method claims less marginal tissue destruction, which provides for a more reliable pathologic assessment, less postoperative bleeding, better visualization of the squamous columnar junction, and greater ease to perform.

Schiller Test

The Schiller test is nonspecific for cancer but can reveal the presence of immature metaplastic epithelium if nonstaining of the cervix is seen after its application.

MANAGEMENT OF ABNORMAL PAP SMEARS

All abnormal Pap smears require further evaluaton. Management is individualized and dependent on the interpretation of the cytologic characteristics of the reporting classification system. Unfortunately, this process is a continuing source of confusion. The Bethesda System has gained widespread acceptance in laboratory and clinical practice today, replacing the outdated CIN grading system and class system. The responsibility of the treating practitioner, therefore, is to thoroughly understand the cytopathologist's report and translate the results to ensure optimal patient care. Comparison of the nomenclature for each of the classification systems is demonstrated in Table 12-13-4.

Evaluating abnormal Pap smears is a challenging task. It requires a broad knowledge of the disease process, different nomenclature for multiple classification systems, controversial treatment guidelines for low-grade lesions, competing modalities for diagnostic evaluation, financial restrictions in managed care environments, continuing education on current technologies, sampling techniques and screening methods, educating patients on disease prevention, and communicating test results effectively and reassuringly. However, whenever an abnormal Pap smear is suggestive of cervical neoplasia, the patient should be referred for diagnostic evaluation and histologic correlation.

Statement of Specimen Adequacy

Initial review of all Pap smears should begin with the statement of specimen adequacy. The presence of endocervical cells has traditionally been the gold standard for the adequacy of the specimen because it indicates that the transformation zone has been adequately sampled. This is confirmed in the reported findings by the cytopathologist as "satisfactory for evaluation." The absence of these cells is interpreted as "unsatisfactory for evaluation" and requires another sampling. "Satisfactory for evaluation but limited by" indicates that the interpretation may be compromised by either inadequate information, insufficient cellular material, or inability to interpret because of obscuring material. In

Table 12-13-4. Comparison of Classification Systems

Class	CIN	Bethesda	Description
I	Normal	Normal	Normal
II	HPV	ASCUS	HPV
II	Atypia	ASCUS	Atypia
III	CIN I	LGSIL	Mild dysplasia
III	CIN II	HGSIL	Moderate dysplasia
III	CIN III	HGSIL	Severe dysplasia
IV	CIS	HGSIL	CIS
V	Invasive carcinoma	Invasive carcinoma	Invasive carcinoma

NOTE: HPV = human papillomavirus; CIN = cervical intraepithelial neoplasia; CIS = carcinoma in situ; ASCUS = atypical squamous cells of undetermined significance; LGSIL = low-grade squamous intraepithelial lesions; HGSIL = high-grade squamous intraepithelial lesions.

this situation, the decision making is based on the history and the provider's clinical knowledge of the patient. Either close monitoring or repeating the Pap smear is acceptable if no cellular abnormality is reported.

General Categorization

The next area to assess is the general categorization of the specimen. Here, the pathologist states if the smear is within normal limits or if it possesses any cellular abnormalities. Abnormalities are elaborated and categorized as descriptive diagnoses under the headings of benign cellular changes or epithelial cellular abnormalities.

Benign Cellular Changes

Included under this description are the following:

1. Infection
2. Nonspecific inflammation associated with atrophy
3. Radiation-induced cellular disturbances and changes associated with certain chemotherapeutic agents
4. Benign reactive alterations from chronic irritation caused by intrauterine devices

A short course of therapy with vaginal estrogen cream may reverse the abnormalities associated with atrophy. In every case, though, the PA should rely on the clinical history to interpret the cellular changes that are reported. Frequently, the abnormalities can be better defined after a short observation period. If the second examination after treatment or observation shows that the cellular changes have resolved, routine follow-up is considered to be sufficient. If the changes persist and their cause undetermined, colposcopy and probable biopsy are necessary for a definitive diagnosis.

Epithelial Cell Abnormalities

Epithelial cell abnormalities are either of squamous cell origin or glandular origin. This classification introduces the term squamous intraepithelial lesion to encompass all grades of CIN. SIL is further subdivided into low grade, high grade, atypical, and invasive as follows:

1. ASCUS
2. LGSIL
3. HGSIL
4. SCC, or squamous cell carcinoma

LGSIL includes cellular changes that are associated with HPV infection and CIN I. HGSIL is associated with CIN II and III. The presence of CIN is strongly suggestive of a history of human papillomavirus infection. Some studies demonstrate that lesions reported with mild dysplasia or CIN I/LGSIL will spontaneously regress without any further intervention. However, because there is no way to predict which lesions will progress, it has become common practice in the United States for all dysplastic Pap smears (CIN) to be followed up with colposcopy and directed biopsy to histologically define and diagnose the level of dysplasia or carcinoma present.

Most of the controversy revolves around the classification of ASCUS. The presence of ASCUS in young women generally indicates the presence of HPV infection. Older women may have a variety of abnormalities. The challenge for the cytopathologist and the clinician lies in the interpretation of the results which can either be a florid benign reactive process or a preneoplastic one. The major dilemma revolves around the issue of whether a "wait and see" approach is appropriate for women with ASCUS or LGSIL diagnoses. An upcoming new clinical trial will be testing three different ways to manage these mild cervical lesions as listed below:

Table 12-13-5. Clinical Guidelines

Obtain pertinent information from health history.
Ask the question, "Who is at Risk?"
  Family history of DES, reproductive cancers
  Past medical history of abnormal Pap smears, STDs, or prior treatment
  Surgical history (pelvic)
  Symptoms of abnormal bleeding, vaginal discharge, or dyspareunia
    Risk factors (nutrition, smoking, HPV)
    Sexual activity (birth control method, age at first intercourse, multiple partners and male factors)
Evaluate risk.
Follow recommended NIH guidelines for follow-up Pap smears.
Obtain proper specimen to ensure accuracy.
Educate patient in preparation, scheduling, and significance of examination.
Follow correct procedure (unlubricated speculum and immediate fixative).
Sample correct area (transformation zone).
Select reputable laboratory.
Learn reporting systems, nomenclature, and interpretation.
Understand treatment options, limitations, and criteria for referral.
Schedule appropriate follow-up and implement tracking system.
Use every visit as an opportunity to educate and screen.
Practice good interpersonal and communication skills.

1. Observation and follow-up Pap smears every 6 months
2. Immediate colposcopy and biopsy
3. HPV DNA testing to distinguish between high- and low-risk lesions

Currently, however, an acceptable plan in managing ASCUS is to repeat the Pap smear every 3 months for 1 year. Colposcopy is indicated, however, if a second Pap smear is reported abnormal consecutively within that time frame.

SUMMARY

Appropriate guidelines to follow in the evaluation of abnormal Pap smears are listed in Table 12-13-5. The role of the physician assistant is extremely important in the screening and evaluation of all Pap smears, regardless of results. Communication is a key element in both preventive education and diagnostic evaluation. Patients should be easily referred for any malignancy and treatment decisions dependent on specific protocols. As a physician assistant, the provision of compassionate care and understanding, availability for counseling, reassurance, and explanations, and meticulous follow-up or tracking is absolutely imperative for meeting the criteria of optimal patient care.

PATIENT EDUCATION MATERIALS

"Should I have a Pap Smear?" (free brochure). Send a self-addressed stamped envelope to Pap Smear, American Society of American Pathologists, Box MT, 2100 West Harrison Street, Chicago, IL 60612.
Questions and Answers about the Pap smear. Write to Office of Cancer Communications, National Cancer Institute, Bldg. 31, Rm 10A24, Bethsda, MD 20892 or call 1-800-4-CANCER.

BIBLIOGRAPHY

Beckman CR, Ling FW, Barzansky BM, et al: *Obstetrics and Gynecology,* 2d ed. Baltimore, Williams & Wilkins, 1995.
Brotzman GL, Apgar BS: Cervical intraepithelial neoplasia: Current management options. *J Fam Pract* 39:271–278, 1994.
Consensus Development Conference Statement Cervical Cancer, NIH 1996, April 1-3 (cited November 11, 1996).
DeCherney AH, Pernoll ML (eds): *Current Obstetric and Gynecologic Diagnosis and Treatment,* 8th ed. East Norwalk, CT, Appleton and Lange, 1994.

Fauci AS, Braunwald E, Isselbacher KJ, et al (eds): *Harrison's Principles of Internal Medicine,* 14th ed. New York, McGraw-Hill, 1998.

Hacker NF, Moore JG: *Essentials of Obstetrics and Gynecology,* 2d ed. Philadelphia, Saunders, 1992.

Jacobs AJ, Gast MJ: *Practical Gynecology.* East Norwalk, CT, Appleton and Lange, 1994.

Kurman RJ, Solomon D: *The Bethesda System for Reporting Cervical/ Vaginal Cytologic Diagnoses: Definition, Criteria and Explanatory Notes for Terminology and Specimen Adequacy.* New York, Springer-Verlag, 1994.

Matsuura Y, Kawagoe T, Toki N, et al: Early cervical neoplasia confirmed by conization: Diagnostic accuracy of cytology, colposcopy and punch biopsy. *Acta Cytol* 40:241–246, 1996.

Mayeaux EJ Jr, Harper MB, Abreo F, et al: A comparison of the reliability of repeat cervical smears and colposcopy in patients with abnormal cervical cytology. *J Fam Pract* 40:57–62, 1995.

Rubin SC, Hoskins WJ: *Cervical Cancer and Preinvasive Neoplasia.* Philadelphia, Lippincott-Raven, 1996.

Swinker M, Cutlip AC, Ogle D: A comparison of uterine cervical cytology and biopsy results: Indications and outcomes for colposcopy. *J Fam Pract* 38:40–44, 1994.

Chapter 12–14
CONTRACEPTION
Noel J. Genova

DISCUSSION

Providing contraception is a task performed in partnership with the patient. The patient requires and expects the clinician's expertise and understanding of prescription methods and skill at performing an invasive procedure. However, any skill is useless, and possibly harmful, if the particular life-style, religious, and comfort requirements of each patient are not elicited, heard, understood, and taken into consideration as the chosen method is provided.

For sexually active patients who do not desire pregnancy or who wish to delay pregnancy for medical reasons, effective contraception is not optional, nor is it a treatment for any disorder. In this sense, it presents a unique challenge in medicine, that is, preventing potentially serious side effects of an elective intervention, thereby avoiding iatrogenic injury, while achieving a high rate of effectiveness in prevention of unplanned pregnancy without compromising future fertility.

METHODS OF CONTRACEPTION

Barrier Methods

Barrier methods include male and female condoms, vaginal spermicides, cervical cap, and diaphragm. Except for the cervical cap and diaphragm, which require prescriptions, instruction for use, and fitting by a clinician, barrier methods are available over the counter at fairly reasonable cost. With the important exception of allergy to their components, latex and the spermicide nonoxynol-9, these methods are virtually free of side effects. The failure rate of the most effective of these methods (the male condom plus spermicide), when used consistently and properly, approaches that of the combined oral contraceptive. There is less than 1 pregnancy per 100 couples annually.[1]

Diaphragms are relatively easy to fit and are popular among couples who wish to avoid the side effects of more effective methods. They are especially appropriate for highly motivated couples who are willing to accept the possibility of an unplanned pregnancy (often referred to as delay of pregnancy rather than prevention of pregnancy).

Cervical caps require special training and approval for fitting for clinicians who wish to offer them to their patients. They may be left in place before intercourse longer than a diaphragm, but are more difficult for the woman to insert.

The female condom is less effective, more expensive, and more difficult to use correctly than the male condom. Its only advantages are that it has greater anatomic area of coverage, which inhibits transmission of viruses that live on the skin, such as herpes simplex virus (see Chap. 2-16) and human papillomavirus (see Chap. 2-18), and that it does not cause latex allergy.

Special Considerations

Because barrier methods are primarily obtained over the counter, there is no need, and in fact potentially no opportunity, for clinicians to perform, or even suggest, screening for reproductive system diseases. Individuals using barrier methods for contraception may seek the services of a health care provider only when a more effective method is desired, a method fails, or a woman suspects pregnancy.

Patient Education

Education regarding use of barrier methods for contraception and as a way to reduce the chance of becoming infected with a sexually transmitted disease is being done by the public health and education communities, rather than by medical professionals in the individual clinical setting. Certainly, if the need for instruction or increasing awareness of the availability of the methods arises, it should be addressed by any clinician providing services of any type.

Future Trends

Because of their usefulness in preventing the spread of sexually transmitted diseases, barrier methods will remain popular, used with or without additional, more effective methods.

To address the major problem of latex allergy, several companies have developed polyurethane male condoms. (The only female condom currently marketed in the United States is made of polyurethane.) One brand, currently available mainly in western states, has been approved by U.S. Food and Drug Administration (FDA), and several others are being studied and considered. Breakage and slippage remain problems with all condoms. New products are being developed and studied to improve condom effectiveness.[2]

Hormonal Methods

Hormonal methods include combined oral contraceptives and the progesterone-only oral contraceptives, including the "mini-pill," injectable medroxyprogesterone acetate (DMPA, Depo-Provera), and levonorgestreal subdermal implants (Norplant). For overall balance of effectiveness, ease of use, cost, and side-effect profile, hormonal methods appear to be the most popular contraceptive methods currently used in the United States.[3] All these methods require prescriptions and monitoring and have significant potential side effects, including death. However, rates of serious complications must be compared with those associated with pregnancy and childbirth, since users of these methods are at risk for pregnancy. Although these methods require clinician visits for use, increasing their cost and decreasing their convenience to the patient, there is a built-in opportunity for reproductive health and cardiovascular screenings, which may be of great benefit to women using these methods.

Combined Oral Contraceptives

Using combined oral contraceptives (birth control pills, the pill) is a popular method that has been available for contraceptive use in the United States since 1960. At this point, risks, benefits, and failure rates have been well studied, and statements concerning their use may be made to women with a high degree of certainty. Detailed patient information is provided by the manufacturer with every package of pills sold. Clinicians prescribing oral contraceptives should be familiar with their product labeling, which includes absolute contraindications, warnings, death rates per 100,000 users per year broken down by age group, benefits, and instructions for use.

All combined oral contraceptives include an estrogen, usually ethynyl estradiol, and a progesterone, which varies by product. Dosage of the estrogen component and strength as well as dosage of the progesterone differ from one pill to another. All types of pills utilize 21 "active" pills. Some may contain seven "inactive" pills for improved daily compliance. Exposure to hormones for 3 weeks followed by a 1-week hiatus suppresses ovulation while stimulating the endometrium sufficiently to cause a withdrawal flow or "period" every 4 weeks. Triphasic pills vary the dosage of progesterone within each cycle (increasing the dose incrementally throughout the cycle, mimicking the natural hormonal cycle), whereas monophasic pills contain a consistent dose of progesterone throughout the cycle.

Most women can safely use oral contraceptives. It is the clinician's responsibility to select those women who cannot safely use this method. Education on use and how to manage side effects is vitally important. This includes adjusting the dosages of estrogen and progesterone in a way that minimizes "nuisance" side effects such as weight gain, headaches, irregular vaginal bleeding, and moodiness.

Absolute contraindications[4] to use of oral contraceptives are the following:

- History of cardiovascular disease, including non-pregnancy-related hypertension
- Any type of thrombophlebitis, including pulmonary embolism
- History or suspicion of reproductive organ cancer, including breast cancer
- Liver disease, including current abnormal liver function tests
- Pregnancy
- Smoking beyond age 35

Relative contraindications[4] include the following:

- History of migraine headache
- Gallbladder disease
- Family history of cardiovascular disease
- Diabetes
- Smoking before age 35
- Hypercholesterolemia
- Depression

Many common major illnesses are not contraindications to pill use, including asthma, congenital cardiac abnormalities, diabetes, and seizure disorders (see "Special Considerations," below). In these cases, specialist consultation may be helpful if the clinician who is caring for the woman's reproductive health needs is not the primary provider for the significant illness, as is frequently the case. Bear in mind that these women are frequently advised to avoid pregnancy, at least until their illness is under good control and/or teratogenic medications can be discontinued or changed. Risks of birth control pills must be weighed against the physical and psychological harm that could result from an ill-timed pregnancy.

Adjusting the dosage of estrogen and progesterone to mitigate side effects can be either rational, as in controlling breakthrough bleeding, or trial and error, as in alleviating decreased libido, moodiness, or mild depression. In general, beginning with 20, 30 or 35 μg estrogen is advisable, with an increase in the event of early-cycle (first-week) breakthrough bleeding or a decrease in the event of mild headaches, breast enlargement or tenderness, or weight gain.

Progesterone deficiency, especially in triphasic pills, leads to late-cycle breakthrough bleeding, uterine cramping, and heavy, prolonged periods. Changing to a monophasic pill often improves both symptoms and compliance. Mood changes are best handled by changing the type of progesterone used and adding vitamin B_6 (pyridoxine), 50 to 100 mg orally per day.[5]

Some patients may require several pill changes during their first year using this method, which may be frustrating to both the patient and the clinician. If side effects are not serious and the patient desires to continue oral contraceptives, the clinician can work with the patient to arrive at a dosage that minimizes any undesired effects.

Some Special Considerations

Women who have difficulty taking the pill consistently should use an alternative method. This group of women are often thought of as unreliable, but also include women who travel frequently for business, or work rotating shift schedules.

Antibiotics and anticonvulsant medications may decrease the effectiveness of oral contraceptives. A backup method, usually condoms and spermicide, should be recommended during antibiotic use and for 7 days after antibiotics are discontinued. Concomitant use with anticonvulsants is controversial, with some references advising discontinuation of the pills and others advising use of a pill containing 50 μg of ethynyl estradiol. The latter approach has the advantage of offering a highly effective method for women who must chronically use teratogenic medications. Consultation with a neurologist is wise in these cases.

Potentially serious conditions are possible. These include borderline hypertension, mild dyslipidemias, and migraine headaches. Women must be informed of the risks of continuing oral contraceptive use and closely monitored. Choose an alternative contraceptive method if a preexisting condition is exacerbated. The clinician must offer detailed information and follow-up regarding reasonable alternatives such as an intrauterine device (IUD), subdermal implant (Norplant), or elective surgical sterilization.

Patient Education

All patients presenting for contraceptive services should have access to appropriate patient education materials. This includes instruction on natural family planning for those couples who desire nonmechanical fertility control methods. Use of oral contraceptive pills must be an informed choice, and the role of patient education in making that choice cannot be overstated.

Future Trends

Oral contraceptives may become even more popular if they are sold over the counter in the United States, as they are in many other countries.

Although not approved by the FDA, the "morning after" approach uses high doses of birth control pills taken within 72 h of unprotected intercourse as emergency contraception.[6] Although the effectiveness of postcoital contraception is difficult to study in controlled trials, this intervention may be approximately 75 percent effective in preventing pregnancy when used correctly.[7] This method is frequently used after a sexual assault.

Finally, as a result of information published in the *Lancet* and the *British Medical Journal* in 1995 and 1996,[8,9] it appears that oral contraceptives with the progestin desogestrel have an increased chance of causing deep vein thrombosis as compared with other low-dose oral contraceptive pills. Although there is no current plan to remove these pills from the market, patients using desogestrel-containing pills should be informed of the potential increased risk.

Progesterone-Only Methods

With the exception of the mini-pill, which is slightly less effective than combined oral contraceptives, these methods have two advantages over estrogen-containing pills. First, they have fewer absolute contraindications, and second, their delivery systems do not depend on daily use.

These methods, in contrast with combined oral contraceptives, may be used by lactating women, women with a history of cardiovascular disease including hypertension, and smokers older than 35.

Absolute contraindications include liver disease (progesterone is metabolized through the liver, and liver function tests should be performed if there is any doubt regarding the woman's hepatic status), current or past thromboembolic disorders, pregnancy, and breast cancer.

Their major disadvantage is irregular bleeding, which ranges from very annoying daily spotting to complete amenorrhea, which may or may not be a perceived advantage for the woman.

Although each of these methods utilizes the same mechanism of action, the delivery systems are completely different, leading to distinct advantages and disadvantages. Contraception via the oral route can be started and stopped easily, providing the option of "trial" use. Its major disadvantage is patient noncompliance.

Injectable medroxyprogesterone acetate (Depo-Provera), 150 mg must be given intramuscularly every 12 to 13 weeks. There is great variability in duration of absorption, leading to unpredictability regarding abatement of side effects, return of fertility (which can take up to 18 months), and resumption of menses. It should be used with caution in women with depression, since adverse effects may last up to 6 months and be refractory to treatment.

The Norplant System consists of levonorgestrel in six silicone capsules that are placed under the skin of the upper, inner arm. It offers highly effective contraception for 5 years. In contrast to Depo-Provera, blood levels of hormone drop rapidly after removal of the implants, allowing for rapid resolution of any adverse effects and almost immediate return to baseline fertility levels.[10] The initial cost to the patient is quite high, and a surgical procedure is required for placement. Surgical removal of the capsules may be difficult and cause scarring.

Special Considerations

A frequently encountered concern with Depo-Provera is the management of contraception when either a dose is to be given late or the method is to be discontinued. This is because the woman may reamin amenorrheic for many months following even a single shot. If pregnancy can be excluded (by a negative highly sensitive pregnancy test following 2 weeks of abstinence), a repeat shot may be given, or another method, such as combined oral contraceptives, initiated.

Patient Education

As with all contraceptive methods, education is essential for success and acceptance of the method. This is particularly true of Norplant, which requires a well-thought-out 5-year commitment to this method if it is to be cost effective for the patient or third-party payer.

Future Trends

Injectable depo-medroxyprogesterone acetate was introduced into the United States as a contraceptive method in late 1992. It has become quite popular, and the trend is likely to continue. Norplant use has become less popular due to adverse publicity regarding its complications. Its future in a market where contraceptive choices are limited is unknown.

Intrauterine Devices

Despite being highly effective and requiring no compliance on the part of the contracepting couple after its insertion, IUDs are currently used by only 2 percent of U.S. women who are at risk for pregnancy.[11] Primary care clinicians who do not insert IUDs should be familiar with their advantages and contraindications, and where to refer those women who desire this method of contraception.

Absolute contraindications to IUD placement include pregnancy, extreme bleeding and cramping with menses that would be worsened with the IUD, risk factors for pelvic inflammatory disease (PID), and sensitivity to its components, particularly copper. The most important relative contraindication to IUD use is nulliparity, since IUD-related infection may lead to future infertility.

The ideal candidate for an IUD is a monogamous woman who has probably completed her child-bearing but does not want surgical sterilization for reasons of cost, convenience, or irreversibility. Many of these women choose hormonal or barrier methods of contraception, but some have contraindications to hormonal methods and want the greater effectiveness and spontaneity afforded by the IUD compared with less-convenient barrier methods.

Nulliparous women may find that their contraceptive options are limited. Many clinicians offer IUDs to highly motivated nulliparous women after careful informed consent regarding the possibility of future infertility. IUD candidates must be at low risk for developing PID, namely, having only one partner and no history of sexually transmitted infections. Nulliparous women must also understand that they are at increased risk for other IUD-associated problems, such as increased menstrual pain and cramping, difficulty with insertion, and the possibility of a spontaneous expulsion.

Types of IUDs

Although new devices are being investigated, only two types of IUDs are available in the United States. The Copper-T (as its name suggests, a copper-containing T-shaped IUD) is approved for the duration of up to 8 years after insertion. In cannot be used in the presence of copper allergy and carries the same warnings and contraindications of any IUD.

Progestasert is also T-shaped and slowly releases impregnated progesterone over a 1-year period. It then must be replaced. Theoretically, the release of progesterone increases the efficacy of the IUD and decreases bleeding and cramping.

Future Trends

Despite a sudden plunge in popularity associated with high rates of infection associated with some types of IUDs in the 1970s, this method will continue to be useful in a variety of clinical settings. IUDs with the highest complication rates have been removed from the market, and many manufacturers have discontinued distribution in U.S. markets.

Surgical Sterilization

Mechanical interruption of the fallopian tubes in women and of the vasa deferentia in men causes permanent sterilization of the individual with very low failure rates. Primary care clinicians should counsel patients who have clearly come to the decision to have no more children of the availability of tubal ligation and vasectomy options, and be familiar with referral sources for these procedures.

Vasectomy is a popular, widely available contraceptive method, often done in the practitioner's office under local anesthesia. The procedure varies, with some clinicians using a "no-scalpel method," while others utilize the traditional approach of small incisions through the scrotum to ligate the vas deferens. Success of the procedure in permanently ending the man's fertility approaches 100 percent, whereas mortality and major morbidity are extremely rare. Common complications, which occur in approximately 1 percent of procedures, are infection and hematoma. Rigorous attention must be paid to postsurgery sperm analysis, as fertility remains for at least 1 month following the procedure. This is due to sperm remaining in the vas deferens after ligation. Some clinicians recommend two analyses for presence and motility of sperm, one done 4 weeks after the vasectomy, and the second one done at 6 to 8 weeks. Until infertility is established, couples should continue to use an alternative form of contraception.[12]

Of the two surgical procedures, tubal ligation is a more invasive procedure. It requires more extensive anesthesia and has a greater surgical risk and cost, compared with vasectomy. For these reasons, many couples who are making a joint decision regarding family size select a vasectomy. Tubal ligation may be done at the same time as a cesarean birth, but must be done as a separate surgical procedure following vaginal birth. Vasectomy is also the more reversible of the two procedures, although this varies, and no man should have the procedure done unless he is truly committed to permanent sterilization.

Special Considerations

Primary care clinicians may be in better positions than the surgeons performing these procedures to select out patients who are not ready for an irreversible contraceptive method. As with all methods, every option must be discussed with each individual or couple to assure the best contraceptive decision.

REFERENCES

1. Hatcher RA, Trussel J, Stewart F, et al: *Contraceptive Technology,* 16th rev ed. New York, Irvington, 1994, p 182.
2. Hatcher RA, Trussell J, Stewart F, et al: *Contracep Technol Update* 17(4):37–41, 1996.
3. Hatcher RA, Trussell J, Stewart F, et al: *Contracep Technol Update* 16(9):105–110, 1995.
4. *Physician's Desk Reference,* 52nd ed. 1998. Adapted from product labeling information. Medical Economics, Montvale, NJ.
5. Hatcher RA, Trussell J, Stewart F, et al: *Contraceptive Technology,* 16th rev ed. New York, Irvington, 1994, p 263.
6. *Medical Lett* 37(946):36.
7. Hatcher RA, Trussell J, Stewart F, et al: *Contraceptive Technology,* 16th rev ed. New York, Irvington, 1994, pp 415–432.
8. Jick A, Jick SS, Gurewich V, et al: Risk of idiopathic cardiovascular death and nonfatal venous thromboembolism in women using oral contraceptives with differing progestogen components. *Lancet* 346: 1589–1593, 1995.
9. Spitzer WO, Lewis MA, Heinemann LAJ, et al: Third generation oral contraceptives and risk of venous thromboembolic disorders: An international case-control study. *Br Med J* 312:88–90, 1996.
10. Hatcher RA, Trussel J, Stewart F, et al: *Contraceptive Technology,* 16th rev ed. New York, Irvington, 1994, pp 285–322.
11. Hatcher RA, Trussel J, Stewart F, et al: *Contraceptive Technology,* 16th rev ed. New York, Irvington, 1994, p 341.
12. Smith DR: *General Urology.* Los Altos, CA, Lange Medical, 1984.

Chapter 12–15
PREECLAMPSIA AND ECLAMPSIA
Glen E. Combs

DISCUSSION

The diagnosis of preeclampsia is made with the occurrence of hypertension, proteinuria, and edema in pregnancy. The incidence of hypertension in pregnancy is 14 to 20 percent in primigravidas and 6 to 7 percent in multiparas.[1] Twin pregnancies have a higher incidence of preeclampsia than primigravidas. Ninety percent of all cases of hypertension in pregnancy are related to preeclampsia. In addition to marked hypertension, patients usually present with proteinuria, excessive sudden weight gain, and edema after the 20th week of gestation. Though elevated blood pressure is an important presenting sign of preeclampsia, it should be emphasized that symptoms including persistent headache, visual disturbances, and continuous epigastric pain are also important diagnostic symptoms of preeclampsia. By the time the patient begins experiencing headache, visual disturbances, or epigastric pain, the condition is usually severe. Therefore monitoring blood pressure and checking for proteinuria and sudden weight gain should become routine for all prenatal office visits to detect early warning signs of preeclampsia.

The major distinguishing sign that differentiates preeclampsia from eclampsia is the onset of tonic-clonic convulsions. A patient who experiences a seizure is considered eclamptic and should be immediately hospitalized for continuous monitoring and care. Eclampsia is primarily a disease of young primigravida patients, though its incidence is also increased in women older than 35 years. Low socioeconomic status appears to play a significant role in this condition with low-income nonwhite primigravidas having the highest incidence of eclampsia.

PATHOGENESIS

The actual cause of preeclampsia is unknown. There are multiple theories that have been used to explain the pathogenesis of preeclampsia. One theory suggests that preeclampsia is the result of blood vessel spasm.[2] Vessel spasm ultimately results in systemic problems including hypertension, edema, and proteinuria. Multiorgan vasospastic disease results in decreased sensitivity to angiotensin II and increased thromboxane/prostacyclin ratio and usually begins early in the pregnancy, producing physical signs after the 20th week of gestation. A consequence of vasospasm is cerebral vasoconstriction, which ultimately leads to cerebral edema, hypoxia, and irritation of the cerebral cortex. Severe headache and blurred vision are symptoms of this progressive disease and considered precursors to convulsions and coma.

SIGNS AND SYMPTOMS

The triad of signs for preeclampsia consist of (1) hypertension, (2) sudden weight gain, and (3) proteinuria. Most patients are not aware of two of the major presenting signs, namely, hypertension and proteinuria.

Hypertension

Diastolic pressure is considered a more reliable prognostic indicator than systolic pressure for preeclampsia. Diastolic pressures over 90 mmHg or more should be considered abnormal and warrant further investigation.

Sudden Weight Gain

Weight assessment at each prenatal visit is essential. In most cases, a sudden increase in weight will precede a condition of preeclampsia. Patients who have more than a 2-lb weight gain in any given week or have a 6-lb increase in a month need to be further evaluated for preeclampsia.

Proteinuria

The presence of proteinuria is not unusual in pregnancy. Proteinuria that is 1+ by dipstick by itself is not significant. Two consecutive 1+ or greater protein results in a 6-h interval should be considered abnormal. Urine specimens should be obtained either by clean midstream catch or by catheterization due to the possibility of contamination from vaginal discharge or blood, both of which could give a false-positive result. Proteinuria usually follows the advent of hypertension and sudden weight gain.

Other symptoms that are associated with preeclampsia include headache, abdominal pain, and visual disturbances. Headache pain is usually frontal and is not relieved by ordinary analgesics. A severe headache is an ominous symptom that may precede a seizure. Abdominal pain is usually felt in the epigastric region and in some circumstances localizes in the right upper quadrant as the result of expansion of the liver capsule from edema and hemorrhage. Visual disturbances may include blurring, scotomas, and progressive partial to complete blindness. It is thought that visual disturbances are caused by retinal ischemia, arteriolar spasm, and intraorbital edema. In some rare cases retinal detachments have been observed.

OBJECTIVE FINDINGS

The significant findings of the patient with preeclampsia consist of edema, proteinuria, and hypertension. These signs usually occur following the 20th week of gestation, and any one or combination of signs may be present. Edema that results in pitting of the face, hands, sacral area, abdominal wall, or legs should be of concern. Specifically, edema that does not disappear after 12 h of bed rest should give reason for further evaluation and diagnostic studies to confirm preeclampsia. Bed rest increases the patient's urinary output and lessens the intravascular dehydration and hemoconcentration.

LABORATORY FINDINGS

In the early stages of preeclampsia, proteinuria may be minimal or not present. In most cases proteinuria develops following hypertension and sudden weight gain. Careful blood pressure measurement, 24-h urine for protein and creatine clearance, complete blood cell count (CBC) with platelets, and uric acid are part of the routine laboratory studies needed to monitor the hospitalized patient. Elevated levels of aspartate aminotransferase (AST), bilirubin, and lactate dehydrogenase (LDH) should be anticipated.

OTHER DIAGNOSTIC CONSIDERATIONS

In addition to continuous observation of the mother, ultrasonography should be used to assess fetal growth and size, cardiac activity, amniotic fluid volume, and general well being. In severe preeclampsia, deterioration of both the maternal and fetal condition should be anticipated. Frequent monitoring of the mother and fetus is of the utmost importance. Maternal evaluation should include a daily platelet count and measurement of liver enzymes. Signs of fetal distress should be further evaluated with a daily biophysical profile.[3]

TREATMENT

Patients with sustained preeclampsia should be hospitalized with strict bedrest throughout most of the day. Treatment should be focused on the prevention of convulsions, control of severe hypertension, the limitation of intravenous fluids and steps to effect delivery. Delivery of the infant and placenta is considered the only known treatment of preeclampsia and eclampsia. Magnesium sulfate administered intravenously with a loading dose of 4 to 6 g should be initiated followed by 2 g/h for seizure prophylaxis. Patients receiving magnesium sulfate should never be unattended. Blood pressure, urine output, and assessment of reflexes should be measured frequently. Hydralazine (Apresoline) has become one of the frequently used drugs to control severe hypertension (diastolic pressure >100 mmHg).

SUPPORTIVE MEASURES

Managing a patient with preeclampsia involves monitoring vital signs, urine output, and magnesium sulfate serum levels. Ocular fundi should be examined for signs of increased intracranial pressure, and patellar tendon reflexes should be evaluated for hyperreflexia frequently. Hyperreflexia is a sign of cerebral cortex irritability and cerebral edema. In addition, electronic fetal monitoring should be undertaken to evaluate fetal status.

Magnesium sulfate when administered intramuscularly can be painful, and 1 percent procaine added to the mixture may help to relieve some of the discomfort associated with the injection. Patients who have had a convulsion should be cared for in a bed with padded side rails, and a padded tongue blade should be immediately available to place in the mouth to prevent tongue biting during a convulsion. The foot of the bed should be elevated to prevent the drainage of secretion and possible aspiration.

PATIENT EDUCATION

The incidence of sustained hypertension following preeclampsia or eclampsia or in subsequent pregnancies is not high enough to advise against future pregnancies, though women who have had an episode of preeclampsia should be advised to seek early prenatal care on a frequent basis for all future pregnancies. There is some evidence that the prevention or reduction in incidence may be affected with the use of nutritional supplementation of calcium, magnesium, zinc, and fish oils.[4]

Patients should be instructed that excessive weight gain needs to be avoided and that diet should be well balanced and include approximately 80 to 100 g of protein per day.

COMPLICATIONS

Magnesium toxicity should be monitored in all patients receiving magnesium sulfate. Signs of maternal respiratory distress, semiconsciousness and loss of deep tendon reflexes are important indicators of magnesium toxicity. At therapeutic levels magnesium sulfate slows neuromuscular conduction and depresses central nervous sytem irritability. At toxic levels (<9.6 mg/dL) patients may present with slurred speech, somnolence, loss of patellar reflex, paralysis, and respiratory difficulty followed by respiratory arrest. At the first sign of magnesium toxicity, the infusion should be discontinued. If respiratory distress occurs, the patient should be given calcium gluconate intravenously slowly over a 3-min period. Mechanical ventilation may be necessary if the patient further develops respiratory arrest. As a precaution, there should always be ready access to an ampule of calcium gluconate [1 g (10 mL of 10% solution)] and a syringe at the bedside of patients receiving magnesium sulfate. Magnesium sulfate therapy must be monitored with hourly urine output. Urine output should be optimally maintained at 30 mL/h during the periodic infusion of magnesium sulfate. In the event that urine output decreases below 100 mL in 4 h, the dose of magnesium sulfate should be reduced accordingly.

NOTES AND PEARLS

The most important management steps in treating severe preeclampsia include strict bed rest, prevention of convulsions, reduction of maternal high blood pressure, and the quick facilitation of a safe delivery. Once the patient is stabilized, cesarean section or induction should be initiated. Delaying the delivery only puts the mother and fetus at serious risk. In the event that a preterm infant (< 36 weeks) is anticipated, the mother should be transferred to a medical facility that has a neonatal intensive care unit to provide adequate support to the newborn.

Eclampsia should be considered a preventable complication of pregnancy.[5] Appropriate prenatal care should identify the patient at risk, and proper treatment should be initiated to prevent eclampsia. It should be acknowledged that eclampsia is the result of failing to diagnosis preeclampsia in a timely way or the result of inadequate treatment. Eclamptic patients should be closely monitored following delivery for blurred vision, severe headache, and scotomas. These symptoms may precede a convulsion, and it is advisable to continue magnesium sulfate therapy for at least 48 h postpartum.

REFERENCES

1. Gabbe SG, Niebyl JR, Simpson JL: *Obstetrics: Normal and Problem Pregnancies,* 2d ed. New York, Churchill Livingstone, 1995, p 995.
2. Gant NF, Cunningham FG: *Basic Gynecology and Obstetrics.* East Norwalk, CT, Appleton & Lange, 1993, p 427.
3. Gabbe SG, Niebyl JR, Simpson JL: *Obstetrics—Normal and Problem Pregnancies,* 2d ed. New York, Churchill Livingstone, 1995, pp 1015–1016.
4. Sibai BM, DeCherney AH, Pernoll ML: *Obstetric and Gynecologic Diagnosis and Treatment,* 8th ed. East Norwalk, CT, Appleton & Lange, 1992, p 386.
5. Gabbe SG, Niebyl JR, Simpson JL: *Obstetrics: Normal and Problem Pregnancies,* 2d ed. New York, Churchill Livingstone, 1995, pp 1033–1034.

Chapter 12–16
HYPEREMESIS GRAVIDARUM
Glen E. Combs

DISCUSSION

Hyperemesis gravidarum is a condition that consists of protracted vomiting following the first trimester of pregnancy. It is associated with electrolyte imbalance, weight loss, dehydration and, in some severe cases, hepatic and renal damage. This condition can persist throughout the pregnancy and is considered a challenging management dilemma requiring hospitalization for parenteral fluid and nutrient replacement. Early detection and routine prenatal care can prevent serious complications of this condition.

Some nausea and vomiting during the first trimester of pregnancy is common and is experienced in approximately 70 percent of all pregnancies.[1] Frequent bouts of nausea and vomiting causing dehydration, ketonuria, significant weight loss, and hypokalemia are generally referred to as hyperemesis gravidarum, which

is considered quite rare. Patients with true hyperemesis gravidarum usually require hospitalization to correct fluid and electrolyte imbalance. Negative protein balance and ketonemia can adversely affect fetal growth and development.

PATHOGENESIS

The cause of pregnancy-related nausea and vomiting is thought to be related to the rapidly rising human chronic gonadotrophin levels associated with the pregnancy. In addition, the emotional feelings coupled with the stress related to the repetitive bouts of nausea and vomiting can exacerbate the condition. The specific cause is somewhat unclear, although relaxation of the smooth muscle of the stomach probably plays a significant role. Steroid hormones associated with the pregnancy are also thought to contribute to this condition.

SIGNS AND SYMPTOMS

The major signs and symptoms of hyperemesis gravidarum consist of persistant vomiting, dizziness, presyncope, and signs of dehydration. Depending on the severity of the case, ketouria, and elevated creatinine and blood urea nitrogen (BUN) are also possible.

OBJECTIVE FINDINGS

In addition to the usual signs of pregnancy, patients with hyperemesis gravidarum exhibit signs of postural hypotension and weight loss. In severe cases of persistent vomiting, signs of dehydration are evident, namely, hypotension, dry mucous membranes, and collapsed neck veins.

Ominous findings may consist of hemorrhagic retinitis, liver damage, and CNS deterioration, which ultimately may lead to coma. Hemorrhagic retinitis caused by repetitive vomiting and retching is a serious sign that carries a 50 percent mortality rate.[2]

DIAGNOSTIC CONSIDERATIONS

The initial assessment of a pregnant patient with persistent nausea and vomiting should focus on the extent and severity of dehydration. With signs of dehydration, immediate steps should be taken to replenish fluids and nutrients and at the same time correct electrolyte imbalance. Diagnostic concern should be given to the possibility of multiple gestation or molar pregnancy. Certainly other underlying causes need to be excluded, including gastrointestinal problems, diabetes mellitus, peptic ulcer disease, hepatitis, and systemic infection.

Supportive measures that include hospitalization and fetal monitoring should be instituted with the goal of reversing fluid loss and correcting electrolyte imbalances.

LABORATORY TESTS

Pregnancy testing should be considered in patients of reproductive age who present with nausea and vomiting and a history of a missed menstrual period or menstrual irregularity. In severe dehydration, hemoconcentration and an elevated BUN or creatine are possible. Electrolyte imbalance including hypokalemia and metabolic alkalosis can accompany severe vomiting. The urine is usually concentrated with an elevated specific gravity and positive for ketonuria. In moderate to extreme cases, the initial baseline laboratory studies should include a pregnancy test, complete blood count, BUN, electrolyte panel, and urinalysis.

OTHER DIAGNOSTIC CONSIDERATIONS

Pregnancy alone is the usual cause of nausea and vomiting, though other conditions need to be considered while making the primary diagnosis of hyperemesis gravidarum. The differential diagnosis should include those conditions that are associated with nausea and vomiting, namely, cholecystitis, gastroenteritis, hepatitis, pancreatitis, peptic ulcer disease, and pyelonephritis. The customary diagnostic workup for these conditions may need to be modified in light of the pregnancy and potential harm to the fetus. It is important to consider multiple gestation or molar pregnancy as a cause of protracted vomiting, and diagnostic testing as well as ultrasonography may be indicated.

TREATMENT

Unfortunately, it is seldom that symptoms of nausea and vomiting can be completely abated with treatment, though symptoms can be diminished using various treatment modalities singularly or in combination. Conservative treatment for pregnancy-related nausea and vomiting consists of reassurance, psychological support, and avoidance of all foods that trigger nausea. Frequent small meals and in-between light dry snack foods have proved to be beneficial for some patients. It is important to instruct patients to eat small amounts of foods at frequent intervals. Patients should eat a little less than necessary to feel satisfied, and the feeling of fullness be avoided.

Most patients with hyperemesis gravidarum require hospitalization for treatment and care. Aggressive fluid replacement and the correction of electrolyte imbalance usually relieves or significantly diminishes the symptoms. Low-dose IV infusion of promethazine (Phenergan) has proved helpful, using 10 to 25 mg of promethazine per liter of fluid. The patient should be kept NPO and receive 5 to 6 L of fluid per 24-h period for 48 h following cessation of vomiting.[3] Potassium replacement should be given as needed and monitored closely. Renal function should be assessed for elevated BUN or creatine. All antinauseant drugs should be used sparingly, because of the potential adverse effects to the fetus. As a precaution, parental consent should be obtained and documented prior to administration of all medications that may have an adverse effect on the fetus.

SUPPORTIVE MEASURES

High-dose pyridoxine (vitamin B_6) therapy has proved helpful in reducing bouts of pregnancy-related nausea and vomiting. A dosage of 10 to 30 mg daily of pyridoxine is the usual daily amount prescribed. Maternal weight assessment is of importance in managing patients with hyperemesis gravidarum. In most cases the illness is self-limited with good prognosis if weight is maintained at more than 95 percent of the prepregnancy weight. Frequent feedings of low-fat meals and emotional support are important factors that should be stressed in the treatment regimen. Reducing pungent odors in the household may very well minimize the unpleasant symptoms of nausea. Some cooking odors can precipitate symptoms and should be avoided.

PATIENT EDUCATION

Nutritional guidance should be part of all preconception counseling appointments in anticipation of pregnancy-related nausea and vomiting. In the event of that "morning sickness" occurs, the patient should be encouraged to eat dry toast or soda crackers prior to getting out of bed and standing. Reassurance should be given that the unpleasant symptoms of nausea usually pass after the first trimester of pregnancy. Patients with persistent vomiting should be encouraged to seek medical attention and should use antinauseant medications only as a final measure.

DISPOSITION

Patients with persistent vomiting and ketonuria should be hospitalized for fluid replacement and correction of electrolyte imbal-

ance. Once the vomiting has been controlled and laboratory values have returned to normal, outpatient therapy may be initiated. Antiemetic suppositories may be of benefit and should be prescribed as needed.

COMPLICATIONS

Complications of hyperemesis gravidarum consist of severe electrolyte imbalance, dehydration, and CNS deterioration. Patients who experience a more than 5 percent weight loss are at risk for fetal intrauterine growth retardation and possible fetal anomalies.

NOTES AND PEARLS

Making the diagnosis of hyperemesis gravidarum is fairly straightforward, though other causes for vomiting during pregnancy should be explored. Consideration of infection, diabetes mellitus, and gastrointestinal problems should be part of any initial working differential. In addition, molar pregnancy and multiple gestation must be excluded as a underlying cause when completing the initial diagnostic workup.

Hyperemesis gravidarum is a serious condition that requires immediate attention to correct fluid loss and dehydration. Parenteral fluids need to be continued for at least 48 h once the patient has stopped vomiting to lessen the recurrence of symptoms. Maintenance support consists of frequent small low-fat meals plus light dry food snacks. The daily use of pyridoxine (vitamin B_6), 10 to 30 mg, may be of some benefit in minimizing the symptoms of nausea and vomiting. Maternal weight loss should be monitored and corrected to avoid potential fetal anomalies. Finally, it is important that emotional support and reassurance be provided to the expectant mother during the remaining time of her pregnancy.

REFERENCES

1. Gabbe SG, Niebyl JR, Simpson JL: *Obstetrics: Normal and Problem Pregnancies,* 2d ed. New York, Churchill Livingstone, 1994, p 127.
2. Dambro MR, Fields SA: *Griffith's 5 Minute Clinical Consult.* Baltimore, Williams & Wilkins, 1996, p 507.
3. Gabbe SG, Niebyl JR, Simpson JL: *Obstetrics: Normal and Problem Pregnancies,* 2d ed. New York, Churchill Livingstone, 1994, pp 127–128.

Chapter 12–17
MENOPAUSE
Laura Hess

DISCUSSION

During the next two decades, more than 40 million American women will pass through menopause, and by the year 2020, one of every three women will have to cope with this significant event in their lives. Menopause is defined as the complete cessation of menstruation caused by loss of ovarian function. The average age of women experiencing menopause is 51 years old, with smokers going through menopause 2 to 3 years earlier than nonsmokers. The ovaries actually begin to lose their function over a period of 10 years before a woman stops having regular menses, and this perimenopausal period is often referred to as the *climacteric*. During this time many women notice changes in their menstrual cycle, such as change in length of cycle or flow pattern. Menopause is not a clearly defined event, but a process that affects a woman physically, mentally, and emotionally.

PHYSIOLOGY

Menopause is associated with a decrease in density of primordial follicles. During the perimenopausal period, there is great fluctuation in ovarian steroids with production of estradiol in irregular bursts. The glandular secretion of estrogen diminishes steadily, even with regular menstrual cycles, for 5 years preceding menopause. As menopause progresses, the ovary requires higher amounts of follicle-stimulating hormone (FSH) to stimulate estrogen production and ovulation.[1] During this time oligoovulatory and anovulatory bleeding is common. Luteinizing hormone (LH) and FSH produced by the pituitary rise during the menopause.

SIGNS AND SYMPTOMS

Irregular menstrual bleeding is usually the first manifestation of menopause. After the cessation of menses, vasomotor instability becomes more prominent. Vasomotor symptoms are often a major disruption of a woman's life. The classic "hot flash" is a sudden transient sensation of heat and warmth that occurs most often on the chest, face, and head. It is accompanied by perspiration and can be followed by flushing. Hot flashes may last from 30 s to several minutes, and may occur repeatedly throughout the day and night.[1,10] Some women are more affected at night and complain of severe sweats and sleep disturbance. Nearly 75 percent of women experience hot flashes followed by the hot flush and/or night sweats. Women experiencing surgical menopause tend to have more hot flashes than those experiencing natural menopause. The prevalence of hot flashes or flushes is highest the first 2 years after menopause. However hot flashes can begin well before menopause and last for 10 years following cessation of menses.[1] Although it is unclear exactly what causes the hot flash, researchers have proved repeatedly that estrogen replacement can eliminate these troublesome symptoms.

Estrogen is also critical in maintaining vaginal and urethral tone. Woman who do not take estrogen often develop symptoms of atrophic vaginitis, such as dyspareunia (painful intercourse) and vaginal irritation. Urethral atrophy can lead to dysuria, nocturia, urinary frequency, and incontinence. Atrophy of the pelvic support from loss of estrogen predisposes to uterine prolapse, cystocele, rectocele, and stress incontinence. These genitourinary changes occur slowly over years following menopause.[2] Treating with estrogen early in menopause prevents or minimizes many of these conditions.

The loss of ovarian hormones is also the major risk factor of osteoporosis (see Chap. 5-2). Estrogen deficiency causes a increased rate of skeletal resorption that is greater than the rise in bone formation, leading to a weakening of cortical and trabecular bone. Bone loss is a subtle, long-term process with the most rapid loss occurring within the first 3 to 7 years following menopause. The weakened bone cannot tolerate normal stress and may fracture after even minor trauma. Osteoporotic fractures are most common in the spine (vertebral crush fractures), hip (femoral neck or intertrochanteric fractures—see Chap. 10-13), and wrist (Colles' fractures).[3] Currently, osteoporosis contributes to more than 1.5 million fractures in the United States each year. With the population aging, this number is expected to double by the year 2050. Other risk factors for osteoporosis include white or Asian race, body habitus, family history, smoking, alcohol use, physical inactivity or immobilization, medications (steroids, heparin, methotrexate), and certain disease states (hyperthyroidism and hyperparathyroidism). Preventing osteoporosis with estrogen replacement therapy may be especially important in women with these concomitant risk factors.

Because osteoporosis can be asymptomatic for decades, it is easy to overlook. Trabecular (spine) fractures begin at approximately age 60, followed by hip (cortical bone) fractures at about age 70. Osteoporosis and the resultant fractures are late physical manifestations of long-term estrogen deficiency following menopause. Early treatment with estrogen not only stops bone resorption but also produces a slight increase in bone density. The closer to menopause that estrogen is initiated, the greater the benefit.

Women frequently attribute their mood swings, irritability, and feelings of agitation to menopause. This area of menopause is challenging for the clinician and patient because the relationship between estrogen loss and certain mood states has not been proved. There is some evidence that estrogen in doses used to control menopausal symptoms can be therapeutic for women experiencing mild symptoms of depression and mood lability. However, hormone replacement therapy (HRT) has not been shown to be beneficial in women with mood disturbances indicating a major depression.[4]

PHYSICAL EXAMINATION

Most menopausal women have unremarkable physical findings. There may be some mild changes in the amount of vaginal secretions, indicating vaginal dryness and causing the woman to complain of dyspareunia. However, within 4 to 5 years after cessation of menses, a significant number of women show signs of atrophy in the vagina and urethra. In those women not using hormones who go on to develop osteoporosis, the physical examination may demonstrate loss of height with kyphotic changes in the spine.

DIAGNOSTIC CONSIDERATIONS

Generally, the clinical manifestations of menopause and associated age of the patient make it easy to determine that a woman is menopausal. However, other causes of amenorrhea include situational stress, excessive exercise, hypothyroidism, drugs (e.g., oral contraceptives), pituitary disorders such as hyperprolactinemia, or occasionally pregnancy. Polycystic ovary syndrome is an important cause of amenorrhea in younger women characterized by amenorrhea, irregular menstrual cycles, hirsutism, enlarged ovaries, and infertility (Chap. 12-9). Uterine causes of amenorrhea include endometrial scarring (Asherman's syndrome) as a consequence of septic abortion, overly vigorous curettage, radiation therapy, and cervical stenosis from scarring.[5]

LABORATORY AND RADIOLOGIC STUDIES

An increase of FSH production and decrease in estradiol are the only reliable biochemical markers of menopause. An FSH greater than 30 IU/L defines menopause biochemically. Additionally, the estradiol level is less than 50 ng/dl. In clinical practice, an elevated FSH level is the most important laboratory determinant of menopause. The FSH can be drawn at any point if the clinician needs documentation of menopause. However, complete cessation of menses for more than 6 months with the accompaniment of hot flashes, night sweats, and hot flushes is enough clinical evidence to determine that a woman is experiencing menopause. Checking a serum FSH may be most useful in women who have nonspecific symptoms that may be due to menopause, especially if they have undergone a hysterectomy without oophorectomy.

Bone densitometry of the spine and femoral neck may also be useful in some women to provide a quantitative measurement of bone mineralization. Bone density can be used to predict the risk of osteoporotic fractures of the spine and femoral neck. This test may be particularly helpful in women who are ambivalent about HRT.

CARDIOVASCULAR DISEASE AND MENOPAUSE

The potential for dramatically reducing deaths from coronary artery disease is now believed to be the major benefit in taking HRT (see Chap. 1-7). Statistically, coronary artery disease is the leading cause of death in women (36 percent of all deaths in women), far exceeding mortality rates for breast cancer (4 percent), osteoporosis (2.5 percent), or diseases of the ovaries and uterus (2 percent). The incidence of cardiovascular disease sharply rises in women following menopause, eventually matching that in men. The benefits of estrogen replacement therapy (ERT) on the cardiovascular system have been proved by a number of large-scale epidemiologic trials, including the Framingham Heart Study and the Nurses' Health Study. These studies demonstrated that women taking estrogens had a 50 percent reduction in cardiovascular disease, with a 35 to 45 percent reduced total mortality rate.[2] The more recent Postmenopausal Estrogen/Progestin Intervention (PEPI) trial found that estrogen, with or without a progestin, increased serum levels of high-density lipoprotein and lowered levels of low-density lipoprotein. Currently, it is thought that estrogen's positive effect on lipids accounts for 25 to 50 percent of its cardioprotection, with the remainder due to its direct effect on the blood vessel wall[2] (see Chap. 1-4). Estrogen reduces the adherence of WBCs to the vascular epithelium, has an antiproliferative effect on the smooth-muscle cells of the blood vessels, and enhances the normal contraction and relaxation of the blood vessel walls. Theoretically, all postmenopausal women could derive benefit from taking estrogens; however, those women with significant cardiac risk factors receive the greatest benefit.

RISKS AND CONTROVERSIES OF ESTROGEN THERAPY

Endometrial Hyperplasia and Cancer

Estrogen has a potent effect on the lining of the uterus. It has been shown that using unopposed estrogen, meaning estrogen without progesterone replacement, on a woman with an intact uterus increases the risk of endometrial cancer. This risk is proportional to the time that a woman is taking estrogen. After 10 to 15 years of unopposed estrogen use, a woman's risk of endometrial cancer is 10 times higher than that of a woman who is not on estrogen.[2] Adding progestin in a cyclic or continuous fashion to the hormone regimen eliminates the risk. Progestins oppose some of the action of estrogens and prevent endometrial hyperplasia. Progestins do, however, mitigate some of the benefits of estrogen by interfering with the elevation of HDL seen with estrogen alone. Because of this the American College of Obstetricians and Gynecologists (ACOG) recommend using the lowest effective dose of progestin. Medroxyprogesterone acetate (MPA) is the most commonly used progesterone in the United States, and the ACOG recommends using 5 mg/day of MPA for 12 to 14 days per month or 2.5 mg daily. Recent findings of the PEPI trial revealed that the use of micronized progesterone (MP) showed less adverse effects on the lipid profiles of women than other progestins. MP is not yet approved by the U.S. Food and Drug Administration (FDA), but is widely used in Europe. It is currently available only from specialty compounding pharmacies.[6]

Breast Cancer

The risk of breast cancer in women taking estrogens is one of the most controversial aspects of HRT (see Chap. 13-4). Some authors believe that estrogen is mitogenic and may accelerate the onset of breast cancer.[2] Others suggest that breast cancer is detected earlier in women taking hormones because regularly scheduled mammograms are done in this population. The controversy is exemplified by two studies published recently in reputable medical journals.[7,8] The first study reported an increase of breast cancer risk in the estrogen users versus nonusers. The increased risk was associated with length of use. The second study concluded that there was no increased risk of breast cancer in women who had been on HRT. Several meta-analyses have been done that show a slight overall increase in breast cancer.[10] This leaves clinicians with unanswered questions and emphasizes the importance of individualizing treatment by evaluating each woman's symptoms and risk factor profile before initiating therapy.[6] In counseling women, it is important to discuss risk factors in relationship to their likelihood of developing a disease. For example, a 50-year-old woman has a 10 percent lifetime probability of developing breast cancer with a 3 percent risk of dying of breast cancer. In contrast, this same 50-year-old woman has a 46 percent chance of developing heart disease with a 31 percent probability of death related to heart disease.[9] Since HRT can lower mortality rates from cardiovascular disease by 35 to 45 percent for a large number of women, the cardioprotective benefits of estrogen may outweigh the potential risks of developing breast cancer.

Other Risks

Estrogen replacement therapy appears to increase the risk of gallbladder disease in some women, requiring the need for cholecystectomy (see Chap. 6-10). The package insert warns of the risk of thromboembolic disorders; however, this association is based on studies of more potent synthetic estrogens used in oral contraceptives. The relative risk with estrogens used in HRT is quite low.

Some absolute and relative contraindications regarding the use of estrogens are found in Table 12-17-1.

TREATMENT

There is no one standard treatment regimen for hormone replacement therapy in menopausal women. Each regimen is tailored to fit the individual and focuses on providing the lowest dose of estrogen and progestin to fit the patient's age, risk of bone loss and cardiovascular disease, and symptom profile. Education is necessary to inform the woman of any expected bleeding pattern

Table 12-17-1. Contraindications to Use of Estrogens

Absolute contraindications
  Undiagnosed vaginal bleeding
  Suspected or known pregnancy
  Active thrombophlebitis or thrombosis
  Breast cancer
  Estrogen-dependent tumors
  Endometrial cancer
  Acute liver disease
Relative contraindications
  Chronic liver disease
  Gallbladder disease
  Hypertriglyceridemia
  History of migraines
  Endometriosis
  Uterine fibroids
  History of thrombosis or thrombophlebitis

Table 12-17-2. Estrogen Products Used for Hormone Replacement Therapy

Tablets, Creams, Capsules		
Brand Name	**Generic Name**	**Available Dosages**
Estinyl	Ethinyl Estradiol	0.02-mg tablet 0.05-mg tablet
Estrace	Estradiol	0.5-, 1-, 2-mg tablets 0.01% vaginal cream
Estratab	Esterified estrogens	0.3-, 0.625-, 1.25-, and 2.5-mg tablets
Estratest	Esterified estrogen + methyltestosterone	1.25- and 2.5-mg tablets
Estratest HS	Esterified estrogen + methyltestosterone	0.625- and 1.25-mg tablets
Ogen	Estropipate	0.625-, 1.25-, and 2.5-mg tablets; 1 5-mg/g cream
Ortho-est	Estropipate	0.625- and 1.25-mg tablets
Premarin	Conjugated equine estrogen (CEE)	0.3-, 0.625-, 0.9-, 1.25-, and 2.5-mg tablets; 0.625-mg/g cream
Premarin with methyltestosterone	CEE + methyltestosterone	0.625 mg CEE/5 mg testosterone; 1.25 mg CEE/10 mg testosterone
Premphase	CEE + medroxyprogesterone	0.625 mg CEE (14 tabs) + 0.625 mg CEE/2.5 mg progesterone (14 tabs)
Prempro	CEE + medroxyprogesterone	0.625 mg CEE/2.5 mg progesterone
Tace	Clorotrianisene	12 and 25 mg capsules
Patches		
Climara	Estradiol	0.05 mg/d, 0.1 mg/d, applied every week
Estraderm	Estradiol	0.05 mg/d, 0.1 mg/d applied twice a week
Vivelle	Estradiol	0.0375 mg/d, 0.05 mg/d, 0.075 mg/d, and 0.1 mg/d, applied twice a week
Fempatch	Estradiol	0.025 mg/d applied once or twice a week

as well as adverse side effects. Estrogen alone is prescribed for women who have had a hysterectomy. There is a wide array of oral estrogens and transdermal estrogens on the market now which are used for HRT (see Table 12-17-2).

The most common estrogen compounds used for HRT are the natural and equine estrogens such as micronized estradiol, estradiol valerate, estropipate, and the conjugated equine estrogens (CEE). All estrogen preparations are converted to estrone sulfate and rapidly metabolized by the liver. Within 1 week of therapy, there should be a steady state of estrone sulfate in the body and symptom relief should occur. The usual starting dose of CEE (Premarin), estropipate (Ogen), and esterified estrogens (Estratab) is 0.625 mg. Micronized estradiol (Estrace) has a starting dose of 1 mg.[6]

Larger starting doses are often required for women who have had a sudden menopause such as a surgical menopause. Other women who may need higher doses of estrogen are those who smoke more than 15 cigarettes per day, those who abuse alcohol, and those taking psychotropic drugs. The

estrogen patch is applied to the skin either once or twice weekly and provides controlled release of estradiol. The goal of all forms of therapy is to alleviate symptoms, prevent bone loss, and provide cardioprotection. Adverse effects of estrogens include breast tenderness, headaches, exacerbation of fibroids, and endometriosis. The patch can also cause skin irritation at the patch site.[6] For women who are unable to take estrogens, nonhormonal drug treatment which may sometimes alleviate hot flashes includes use of clonidine (Catapres) or ergotamine and phenobarbitol (Bellergal-S).

For women with an intact uterus, it is necessary to add a progestin to the hormone replacement regimen. MPA is the most widely used progestin for HRT in the United States, although there are a number of progestins available on the market. Progestins do interfere with the positive lipid benefits provided by estrogen, so it is important to use the lowest effective dose. Frequently the use of the progestin can cause some bothersome side effects for women such as bloating, weight gain, irritability, depression, and PMS-like symptoms. The cyclic use of progestins often causes a monthly withdrawal bleed, which is bothersome for some women and a major reason for lack of compliance. By giving a smaller dose of progestin daily, the monthly withdrawal bleeding pattern is avoided; however, there may be up to 6 months of erratic spotting with the regimen.[10]

Most women are on one of three regimens (see Table 12-17-3):

1. The first is the *cyclic regimen*, which consists of administering estrogen for the first 25 days of the month. A progestin is added on day 14 for a total of 10 to 12 days. Both drugs are stopped from day 26 until the end of the month. Then the estrogen is started again. On this regimen, a woman may expect to have a withdrawal bleed during the hormone-free interval. Withdrawal bleeding occurs in close to 80 percent of women taking HRT in this fashion. However over time the bleeding will taper off and often cease.

Table 12-17-3. Summary of Hormone Replacement Therapy Treatment Regimens

Regimen	Advantages	Disadvantages
Estrogen alone Estrogen daily	Simplest regimen	Only for women who have had hysterectomy, or who receive periodic surveillance endometrial biopsy to check for hyperplasia.
Cyclic Estrogen on days 1–25; progestin, 5–10 mg, for 10–12 days starting on day 14	The traditional method, which many women are still using	80% of women have withdrawal bleeding, but over time bleeding tapers off.
Continuous Estrogen every day; progestin, 5–10 mg, from day 1 to day 12	Simpler than traditional method Predictable withdrawal bleeding which may be helpful for women early in menopause	As with the cyclic regimen, withdrawal bleeding may continue indefinitely.
Continuous combined Estrogen daily; progestin 2.5 mg daily	Simple regimen After 6–9 months, no more bleeding for 70% of women	Initial bleeding is unpredictable. Women who have ongoing bleeding after 6–9 months may need alternative regimen.

2. The second is the *continuous regimen* in which estrogen is taken every day of the month with no break. Progestin is added from day 1 of the month through day 12 then stopped. A withdrawal bleed is expected shortly after the progestin is stopped. With both the cyclic and continuous regimens, a woman can usually predict when during the month she will have bleeding. The predictability of monthly bleeding is an attractive feature of these methods.

3. However, many women would like to eliminate bleeding postmenopausally. Therefore the third regimen, *continuous combined,* is often chosen and can eliminate bleeding in 60 to 70 percent of women. With the continuous combined regimen, both estrogen and a low-dose progestin are taken daily. Initially, spotting and irregular bleeding can occur, but after 6 months more than 50 percent of women have no bleeding at all. The continuous exposure of the uterus to progestin causes thinning and atrophic changes in the lining of the uterus. Despite the bothersome nature of the early spotting with this regimen, the benefit of not having regular menses makes it an attractive option to many postmenopausal women.

With all these regimens it is critical to educate women on what sort of bleeding pattern to expect. Any abnormality in bleeding patterns usually necessitates an endometrial biopsy to rule out endometrial hyperplasia or cancer. Therefore, education and timely follow-up is necessary to ensure compliance and monitor bleeding patterns.

NOTES AND PEARLS

It is important to document menopause before initiating HRT. Amenorrhea for 12 months and a FSH level of greater than 30 IU/L indicates a menopausal state. During perimenopause many women complain of symptomatic hot flashes despite having a normal FSH and estradiol level, as well as regular menses. These women are not candidates for HRT, but may do well on low-dose oral contraceptives, which both suppress and replace estrogen, and, it is hoped, alleviate some of their bothersome symptoms. Additionally, a complete history and physical examination should precede the initiation of HRT. Appropriate laboratory tests to order include a thyroid-stimulating hormone (TSH), complete blood cell count (CBC), lipid panel, and glucose. Clinicians should be aware that there is more evidence now demonstrating that ERT is associated with a lower risk of Alzheimer's disease (see Chap. 11-4, "Alzheimer's Disease.") There is also some evidence that estrogen helps to preserve the function of the hippocampus, the part of the brain that controls memory. Some controlled studies are needed to further verify these findings.

REFERENCES

1. Hammond CB: Menopause and hormone replacement therapy—an overview. *Obstet Gynecol* 87:2–13, 1996.
2. Gallagher J, Hulka B, Ravnikar V, Villablanca A: Why HRT makes sense. *Patient Care.* 30:166–192, 1996.
3. Lindsay R: The menopause and osteoporosis. *Obstet Gynecol* 87:16S–19S, 1996.
4. Shenvin BB: Hormones, mood and cognitive functioning in postmenopausal women. *Obstet Gynecol* 87:20S–25S, 1996.
5. Goroll AH, May LA, Mulley AG: Evaluation of secondary amenorrhea, in *Primary Care Medicine,* 3d ed. Philadelphia, Lippincott, 1995, chap. 112.
6. Scharbo-Dehaan M: Hormone replacement therapy. *Nurse Practit* Part 2 of 2 Supplement, Dec 1996, 1–15.
7. Colditz G, Hankinson S, Hunder D, et al: The use of estrogens and progestins and their risk of breast cancer in postmenopausal women. *New Engl J Med* 332(24):1589-1593, 1995.
8. Stanford J, Weiss N, Voight L, et al: Combined estrogen and progestin hormone replacement therapy in relation to risk of breast cancer in middle-aged women. *JAMA* 274(2):137–142, 1995.
9. Grady D, Rubin S, Pettiti D, et al: Hormone replacement therapy to prevent disease and prolong life in postmenopausal women. *Ann Intern Med* 117:1016–1037, 1992.
10. Hammond CB: Management of menopause. *Am Fam Phys* 55(5):1667–1673, 1997.

SECTION 13
Oncology

Chapter 13–1
ESOPHAGEAL CARCINOMAS
Anne P. Heinly

DISCUSSION

Compared with other carcinomas, esophageal carcinomas are relatively uncommon in the United States, but they are quite common in other parts of the world, especially China and Japan. An estimated 10,000 cases are reported yearly in the United States, primarily among men over 50 years old. Blacks and Asians seem to have a higher predisposition for this disease, although a specific genetic marker has not been found. Table 13-1-1 reviews the risk factors associated with squamous cell carcinoma, the most prevalent type of esophageal carcinoma. Adenocarcinoma, which is on the rise in this country, occurs almost exclusively secondary to Barrett's esophagitis, a severe complication of gastroesophageal reflux disease (GERD) (see Chap. 6-11). Ten years ago adenocarcinoma accounted for about 10 percent of esophageal carcinomas; today the incidence is closer to one-third, and the disease is being found earlier in white males.

PATHOGENESIS

Chronic irritation and inflammation provide the setting for squamous cell carcinoma of the esophagus. The resultant hyperplasia and the subsequent development of atypia are directly related to the tissue's attempt to protect itself from irritation. The most common site of squamous cell carcinoma is the midesophagus, followed by the distal esophagus. The thin layer of squamous epithelium and the absence of a serosa layer allow malignancies to invade the muscular layers readily and, from there, the rich lymphatics of the chest. Unfortunately, the degree of irritation from external sources such as alcohol and tobacco does not provide clues to the timing or extent of injury to the esophagus.

Adenocarcinoma is found primarily in the distal esophagus in association with an incompetent lower esophageal sphincter. The resultant chronic gastric reflux triggers the conversion of the squamous epithelium to a columnar cell–lined esophagus (similar to stomach lining) in an effort to protect itself from the increased acidity. There is no doubt that alcohol and tobacco abuse contribute to these changes in association with chronic GERD. Table 13-1-2 reviews less common esophageal tumors.

SYMPTOMS

Esophageal carcinomas present as mechanical obstructions, and thus progressive dysphagia is the first and most classic symptom. Initially the patient has difficulties with solid food, but over time (weeks to months) semisolids and then liquids become difficult. Early clues such as chest fullness or pressure, hiccups, cough, and hoarseness may be interpreted as benign by both the patient and the provider. Odynophagia (pain on swallowing) eventually occurs as a result of a narrowed, irritated lumen and metastasis to the surrounding nerve plexus. The pain generally is described as constant, deep, and penetrating.

Pulmonary symptoms may bring the patient to a practitioner before dysphagia occurs. Recurrent pneumonia and upper respiratory infections (URIs) are quite common because the tumor mechanically allows aspiration and fistula formations in the pulmonary tree. As the patient's immunologic status diminishes from weight loss, malnutrition, and electrolyte imbalance, the chances of severe pulmonary sequelae increase. Occult bleeding is common and can be readily demonstrated. Gross, profuse bleeding is uncommon but can occur if a major vessel is breached by the tumor.

As may be suspected from the symptoms, esophageal carcinomas generally are found well after they have metastasized. Dysphagia and weight loss are signs of large tumors producing symptoms through a mass effect. This severely affects the prognosis, and so it is imperative that the provider listen carefully and associate the possible risk factors so that the patient will have a fighting chance of recovery.

OBJECTIVE

Overt physical signs of esophageal carcinoma are rare. Only general evidence of disease will be present: anemia and weight loss. Careful examination may pick up a supraclavicular nodal enlargement (Virchow's nodes) or unilateral vocal cord paralysis. A thorough physical is mandated to help with the differential diagnosis.

DIAGNOSTIC CONSIDERATIONS

Any disease process that can cause dysphagia should be considered (Table 13-1-3). Extrinsic impression can occur as well and represents nongastrointestinal sources of dysphagia. The extrinsic type generally is not associated with significant weight loss or anemia.

LABORATORY TESTS

Hypercalcemia and its clinical manifestations are an all too common initial presentation. A patient with an elevated serum calcium will complain of a rapid onset of spreading weakness, nausea, sedation, and eventual stupor. A hypokalemic alkalosis may occur, and a hypochromic, microcytic anemia associated with chronic blood loss is commonly found. Specific laboratory tests do not exist to diagnose or define esophageal carcinomas. The

Table 13-1-1. Risk Factors for Squamous Cell Carcinoma of the Esophagus

Risk Factor	Effect
Smoking	Increases GERD, decreases mucosal blood flow, decreases prostaglandin synthesis, interferes with action of H_2 antagonists
Alcohol abuse	Alone, there is a questionable relationship; with tobacco, effects are increased
Chronic candidiasis	Persistent tissue irritation
Chemical ingestion (lye)	Corrosive injury, stricture formation
Achalasia	Relationship unsure; some studies quote 6% increase in cancer rates
Plummer-Vinson syndrome	Webs in upper esophagus associated with iron deficiency; over 90% are women
Exposure to radiation	Direct tissue damage, stricture formation

Table 13-1-2. Esophageal Tumors

Tumor	Description
Squamous cell carcinoma	Middle to distal esophagus; etiology unknown; risk factors include tobacco, alcohol, lye ingestion, candidiasis; poor prognosis
Adenocarcinoma	Distal esophagus; vast majority result from Barrett's esophagitis (GERD); poor prognosis
Small cell carcinoma	Rare, highly aggressive; survival usually less than a year
Malignant melanoma	Extremely rare; 6-month survival despite surgery
Leiomyosarcoma	Rare, noncancerous malignant tumor; survival after surgery 25%
Leiomyoma	Usually asymptomatic; those with symptoms can be ablated with laser therapy
Lipoma	Fatty, nonmalignant tumor; removed as a polyp if symptomatic

measurement of CA-19-9 in serum has not been a successful marker.

RADIOLOGIC (IMAGING) STUDIES

The gold standard for the initial workup is the barium swallow. The double-contrast study is preferred, and the potential findings include nodularity, sudden angularities in contour, stricture formation with lumen stenosis, ulcerations, and rigidity of movement. CT is valuable in looking for metastasis and establishing staging.

A careful esophagogastroduodenoscopy (EGD) should be performed to confirm the carcinoma by cytology. The tumor also can be visualized for size, location, spread, fistulas, bleeding, and ulcerations. Brush cytology is the recommended method because of its accuracy. Staining the mucosa with Lugol's iodine can define early lesions, and when it is used in conjunction with endoscopic ultrasound, local spread can be clearly defined.

Once cancer is diagnosed, staging is done to evaluate the extent of invasion and the development of a treatment regimen. Stage 0 is carcinoma in situ, affecting only a single layer of the esophagus. In stage I, the cancer is present in more than one layer but not in lymph nodes. In stage II, esophageal spread is extensive without metastases. Stage III includes the intrusion of the tumor into the chest lymphatics. In stage IV, there are metastases to other organs, such as liver and lung. Unfortunately, most esophageal carcinomas are found in stages III and IV.

TREATMENT

In China and Japan, where early screening is done, therapy is accomplished through the endoscope, using a variety of methods: laser ablation, bicap tumor probe, and sclerotherapy. If the tumor is in stage I or II, a cure is possible. However, in this country, where practitioners do not screen for esophageal carcinoma, the treatment is only palliative in the vast majority of cases.

Currently, the only curative procedure is esophagectomy. The most successful procedures involve the middle and distal esophagus. The surgery removes the cancerous section, and the remaining portion or a loop of intestine is anastomosed. This surgery has a grave prognosis, and despite the best efforts, 5-year survival is less than 10 percent.

Palliative therapies include laser ablation to relieve obstruction, stent placement, and chemotherapy to shrink tumor size (Table 13-1-4). Nutritional status must be maintained, and control of nausea, pain, and constipation is essential.

COMPLICATIONS

The most obvious complication of esophageal carcinoma is death. Long-term survival is poor. Complications after esophagectomy are many and include dumping syndrome, GERD, regurgitation, weight loss, muscle atrophy, malnutrition, and psychiatric illnesses.

PATIENT EDUCATION

The best hope in this country to affect the prevalence of this devastating disease is prevention. Alcohol and tobacco abuse should be stopped. Treatment of Plummer-Vinson syndrome, candidiasis, and GERD is essential. When a diagnosis of esophageal carcinoma is made, it is imperative to inform the patient about all available options and the prognosis. Several studies have shown that skilled clinicians often fall short in explaining a realistic prognosis to their patients.

Table 13-1-3. Differential Diagnosis of Dysphagia

Oropharyngeal	
Motor disorders	
Achalasia	Aperistalsis, esophageal dilation, chest pressure, inability to burp or vomit, weight loss
Scleroderma	Dysphagia with decreased peristalsis, other systemic manifestations
Myasthenia gravis	Dysphagia and cough; affects upper esophageal sphincter
CNS disease	Amyotrophic lateral sclerosis, parkinsonism, Huntington's chorea, polio, cerebrovascular accident: esophageal weakness, aperistalsis, drooling
Structural disorders	
Zenker's diverticulum	Outpouching through weakened muscular coat usually near the upper esophageal sphincter, regurgitation, halitosis, gurgling, and swelling at the neck
Chagas disease	Megaesophagus secondary to trypanosomiasis; seen in children, myxedema, congestive heart failure; restricted to the tropics
Esophageal body	
Motor disorders	Same as above
Infections (common in immunocompromised patients)	Candidiasis: severe odynophagia, drooling, oral thrush
	Herpes simplex: chest pain, odynophagia, bleeding, nausea/vomiting, leukocytosis
	Cytomegalovirus: serpiginous ulcers, odynophagia, chest pain, hematemesis
Obstructions	Carcinomas
	Reflux esophagitis: inflammation, strictures
	Prolonged nasogastric tube intubation: inflammation, strictures
	Ingestion of corrosives: inflammation, strictures
	"Pill" esophagitis: lodged medication causes inflammation and strictures
Lower esophageal sphincter	All the above and GERD
Extrinsic compression	Substernal thyroid goiter
	Aortic aneurysm (arch or descending)
	Double aortic arch
	Abnormal subclavian arteries
	Mediastinal masses or lymphadenopathy
	Arthritic bone spurs from cervical or thoracic spine

Table 13-1-4. Treatment Options for Esophageal Tumors

Photofrin	Chemotherapy, twofold therapy, ingestion of porfimer sodium that binds to plasma lipoproteins; in second step nonthermal red laser light is applied to the tumor; the light activates the lipoproteins and kills tumor cells; palliative only, with no extension of life expectancy
Neodymium:YAG laser	Thermal ablation provides palliation and some improvement in survival time
Cisplatin	The most commonly used chemotherapy alone and in combination; remission extremely rare with chemotherapy alone

PEARLS

When a patient comes in with a recurrent dry cough, hoarseness, or persistent URIs, think esophageal cancer after the pulmonary workup. The two systems often produce symptoms that mimic each other, and it takes an index of suspicion to catch esophageal carcinomas early. Keep in mind the risk factors for this consuming disease; the vast majority of cases may be prevented through healthy life-style changes.

BIBLIOGRAPHY

Photofron recommended as palliative for esophageal cancer, *Medical Science Bulletin* (Internet), Pharmaceutical Information Associates, November 1994.

Sleisenger MH, Fordtran JS: Esophageal cancer, in *Gastrointestinal Disease*, 5th ed. Philadelphia, Saunders, 1993, pp 115–118.

Chapter 13–2
PROSTATE CANCER
William A. Mosier

DISCUSSION

Adenocarcinoma of the prostate is the most common malignant neoplasm in men, accounting for 33 percent of all cancers diagnosed in men. The risk of acquiring cancer of the prostate (CaP) increases with age. CaP is the second most commonly occurring cancer in American men over age 65 years. Adjusted for age, 80 percent of all cases of CaP are diagnosed in men over age 65. It is the most frequently diagnosed carcinoma and accounts for about 15 percent of all deaths from cancer in the United States. One in every six men will eventually be diagnosed with CaP. Metastatic CaP is a leading cause of cancer-related deaths among men. The American Cancer Society (ACS) estimates that from 1980 to 1990 there was a 50 percent increase in the number of men diagnosed with this condition. This increase in the rate of diagnosis is due to the improved screening tools available and increased awareness of the importance of screening.

Only about 30 percent of prostatic cancers are potentially curable at the time of diagnosis. In fact, about 50 percent of all new cases include lymph node involvement or metastases by the time of diagnosis. This means that two-thirds of all cases of CaP are widespread and incurable by the time they are diagnosed. The resulting malignancy is usually responsive to hormonal manipulation, however. Therefore, the spread of disease can be controlled somewhat. Ten percent of tissues removed for the treatment of urinary obstruction resulting from prostatic hypertrophy are found to have malignant pathology. For an unknown reason, the incidence of CaP is highest among African-Americans in spite of the fact that it is rare in Africa. The incidence is lowest among Asians.

Although the etiology is unknown, CaP tends to run in families. Ninety-eight percent of all cases of CaP are adenocarcinomas that arise from the glandular acini and proximal ducts. Less common malignancies of the prostate include neuroendocrine tumors and sarcomas. Even less frequently occurring are transitional cell, squamous cell, and endometrioid carcinomas that originate from the distal ductal elements of the prostate.

PATHOGENESIS

The pathogenesis of CaP is not known. Initiating or promoting factors have not been determined.

SYMPTOMS

There are no symptoms per se of CaP. However, in the later stages a patient may experience urinary obstruction or bone pain from the spread of the cancer to the low back, pelvis, or thighs. Other symptoms of CaP may include impotence, hematuria, nocturia, a weak or interrupted stream, frequency, urgency, dysuria, and hesitancy. Of course the typical symptoms of cancer may also be present with more advanced CaP, such as nausea and vomiting, weight loss, fatigue, and persistent pain.

OBJECTIVE FINDINGS

Diagnosis is difficult for the detection of early CaP. Screening involves digital rectal examination (DRE) as part of a routine physical examination. Unfortunately, only about 10 percent of cases of CaP identified as nodules on rectal examination are sufficiently localized for cure. A cancerous prostate may present as a discrete hard nodule or diffuse induration of the prostate on DRE. The diagnostic evaluation of CaP is tied to a staging system that is outlined in "Other Diagnostics," below.

DIAGNOSTIC CONSIDERATIONS

In screening for CaP it is important to consider the possibility of metastases to other tissue, since over 60 percent of all cases of CaP have metastasized by the time they are diagnosed.

SPECIAL CONSIDERATIONS

More than 90 percent of cases of CaP remain latent and never metastasize. The prevalence of the pathology far exceeds its clinical incidence. It is detected in 30 percent of autopsies done on males who have died of unrelated causes. Currently there is no way to definitively determine which cancer will spread and which will not. Therefore, great care must be taken in weighing the potential merits of treatment against the risk of decreased quality of life potentially caused by the side effects of treatment.

LABORATORY TESTS

A laboratory assessment should include a complete blood count, serum acid phosphatase, alkaline phosphatase, lactic dehydrogenase, and renal and liver function tests. The prostate specific antigen (PSA) serum level also may be useful as an immunohistochemical marker when the primary site of a prostatic tumor is occult. A PSA level of 4 ng/mL or higher should be considered suspicious of cancer until proved otherwise. An increase in the PSA level generally is correlated with an advanced tumor stage.

Table 13-2-1. The American Urological Association System for Staging Prostate Cancer

Stage	Description
A1	A well-differentiated cancer present in no more than three resected chips
A2	A well-differentiated cancer present on more than three resected chips or a not-well-differentiated cancer
B	A well-differentiated nodule detectable on digital rectal examination
C	A local yet extensive tumor that penetrates past the prostate capsule into the seminal vesicles or bladder neck or through the lateral wall of the pelvis (these patients often present with symptoms of urinary obstruction)
D0	Indicates an elevated acid phosphatase level but no physical or radiographic evidence of metastases
D1	Cancer present on histology specimen, and lymph node samples positive below aortic bifurcation
D2	Lymph node involvement superior to aortic bifurcation, or bone, soft tissue, or visceral metastases present

SOURCE: Adapted from the American Urological Association system for staging PC.

An elevated PSA after radiotherapy for CaP can predict residual CaP or metastases. After hormonal therapy for metastatic disease has been initiated, PSA may return to normal limits. A persistent decrease in PSA may predict a favorable response to treatment.

Prostatic acid phosphatase is not useful as a screening test in early-stage CaP. However, it may be useful as a marker for treatment response, since it is found to be elevated in many patients with CaP when there is disease outside the prostate capsule.

RADIOLOGIC STUDIES

Computed tomography (CT) and magnetic resonance imaging (MRI) of the pelvis can be useful to detect metastases to pelvic organs and lymph nodes. Skeletal x-ray studies and a radionuclide bone scan are useful for assessing the degree and location of bone metastases. Either renal ultrasonography or intravenous pyelography should be included to assess for hydronephrosis. Despite the value of imaging techniques, they tend to underestimate the severity of tumors about 50 percent of the time.

OTHER DIAGNOSTICS

Transrectal ultrasonography (TRUS) is a useful screening device for early detection. However, it is not currently recommended for patients with a normal PSA level and a normal DRE.

A transurethral, transrectal, or transperineal ultrasound-guided needle biopsy of the prostate is indicated when there is a suspicion of cancer. It can detect CaP earlier than DRE can.

The level of severity of CaP generally is determined by DRE and the histology of prostate biopsy specimens in conjunction with whether lymph node samples are positive and metastases are identified. Staging is crucial in the investigation and appropriate treatment of CaP. The American Urological Association system for staging CaP is presented in Table 13-2-1.

TREATMENT

The treatment of CaP is dependent on the stage of cancer to which it has progressed:

- If the CaP is confined to stage A1, transurethral resection followed by watchful waiting is a typical therapy. (A serious limitation of watchful waiting is that there is a large margin of error with the currently available prognostic indicators.)
- If CaP is found to be at stage A2 or stage B, radical prostatec-

tomy or radical radiation therapy is considered. (When the cancer is confined to the prostate, radical prostatectomy can eradicate the tumor in 90 percent of patients.)

- If the cancer has progressed to stage C, radiation therapy alone is considered the first-line treatment. Once metastases have been confirmed, first-line therapy often is aimed at blocking the synthesis and action of androgens. Androgen deprivation can be achieved by orchidectomy or luteinizing hormone–releasing hormone analogues, often combined with androgen receptor antagonists (see "Medications," below).
- At stage D1, transurethral prostatectomy (TURP) or radiation is used if the patient is experiencing urinary obstruction. If the patient is asymptomatic at stage D1, watchful waiting or endocrine manipulation is tried. At stage D2, symptomatic patients are first treated with hormonal therapy. If the disease appears refractory to hormonal manipulation, chemotherapy is considered. Palliative radiation therapy may be used for symptomatic areas.
- If a patient at stage D2 is asymptomatic, watchful waiting is considered. A stage D patient with bilateral hydronephrosis or impending spinal cord compression should be considered for orchiectomy. However, in many patients with pain from bone metastases, androgen deprivation produced by medication therapy is equivalent to the androgen deprivation produced by bilateral orchiectomy. The option of adding antiandrogen drugs together with castration, which is called combination androgen blockade (CAB), may lengthen survival and improve the patient's quality of life.

MEDICATIONS

Hormonal therapy (HT) is often considered a first-line treatment for CaP. Some questions that have been raised about HT are as follows:

1. Can HT for CaP prolong patient survival?
2. Can HT improve a patient's quality of life?
3. Is complete androgen blockade superior to androgen reduction therapy?
4. Is preoperative HT more beneficial than postoperative HT?

Although these are unresolved questions, HT is considered a major therapeutic modality.

Typically, therapy for stage D1 or D2 disease consists of androgen deprivation. Because CaP is influenced by androgen hormones, androgen deprivation may improve the symptoms and even cause disease regression. The role of therapy is to reach castration levels of testosterone and dihydrotestosterone. Among the drugs currently used are the following:

- Diethylstilbesterol (DES), an exogenous estrogen
- LHRH analogues, such as Zoladex (a goserelin acetate implant), that inhibit the release of pituitary gonadotropins
- Antiandrogen blocking agents such as bicalutamide and flutamide (of the two, bicalutamide offers the convenience of once-a-day dosing and is better tolerated)
- Goserelin, a gonadotropin-releasing hormone (GnRH) analogue, which is better tolerated than DES.
- Cyproterone acetate (CPA), which has been demonstrated to be an alternative to orchiectomy in advanced cases of metastatic CaP

Second-line agents used in cases of advanced CaP include liarozole, ketoconazole, and aminoglutethimide. A once-a-month injection of the agent Lupron Depot (leuprolide acetate), another GnRH analogue, is also used as a safe and effective alternative to surgical castration.

SUPPORTIVE MEASURES

An increased intake of red meat and dietary fat may be correlated with a higher risk for CaP. Some studies suggest that a diet rich in soy products and vegetables may contain phytoestrogens that can exert a chemopreventive effect on the prostate gland. Decreased levels of vitamin D secondary to insufficient sun exposure and very high levels of vitamin D–binding proteins may also precipitate CaP.

PATIENT EDUCATION

All male patients should be instructed about the importance of a yearly DRE after age 40. Men 50 and older should be reminded to have a PSA test along with the annual DRE. Patients also should be reminded that a high-fat diet and a sedentary life-style are linked to an increased risk of CaP. Choosing the optimal therapy for each patient requires appropriate counseling of patients about the relative risks and benefits of each treatment option. Patients should definitely be counseled about the risks of impotence as a side effect of treatment.

DISPOSITION

Once CaP has been diagnosed, it is imperative to maintain close follow-up. The optimal treatment would provide a complete cure. However, since most cases of CaP have already metastasized by the time of diagnosis, much of the treatment may be palliative. Treatment decisions must be based on the probability of enhancing each patient's quality of life over a potential 10- to 15-year survival period.

COMPLICATIONS AND RED FLAGS

It should be noted that both radical radiotherapy and surgery tend to cause permanent impotence and often cause sphincter problems as well. If flutamide is used for total androgen suppression (TAS), liver function tests are required at regular intervals to guard against liver toxicity.

OTHER NOTES AND PEARLS

There are many opinions about how best to treat CaP. However, it is imperative to remember that one is treating people, not just a disease. Therefore, the patient must be drawn into all decision-making about his treatment and consideration must be given as to whether the treatment will truly benefit the individual patient.

Urinary excretion of pyridinoline and deoxypyridinoline appears to be a useful marker for evaluating the activity of bone metastases and their response to hormonal treatment in CaP. Current research is exploring the use of herpes simplex virus thymidine kinase gene transduction followed by ganciclovir (HSV-tk plus GCV) as cytotoxic gene therapy to treat locally advanced or metastatic CaP. Studies are under way in Japan to assess the efficacy of intraarterial chemotherapy for the treatment of advanced CaP, utilizing an implantable injection pump. Prostatic inhibin peptide (PIP) is being researched as a possible additional treatment option. Some studies suggest that vasectomy may be associated with an increased risk of CaP. Studies at the National Cancer Institute are investigating the oral intake of modified citrus pectin as a potential inhibitor of CaP metastases. Other studies suggest a possible relationship between the high consumption of green tea and the low incidence of prostate cancer among Asian men. Advances in gene therapy may represent the best chance for an eventual cure for CaP.

BIBLIOGRAPHY

American Urological Association: Prostate cancer clinical guidelines: Summary report on the management of clinically localized prostate cancer. *J Urol* 154:2144, 1995.

Armas OA: Clinical and pathobiological effects of neoadjuvant total androgen ablation therapy on clinically localized prostatic adenocarcinoma. *Am J Surg Pathol* 18(10):979–991, 1994.

Austin O, Ricer RE: Prostate cancer screening: An appraisal of the PSA test. *Fam Pract Recert* 18:81–91, 1996.

Baffa R, Moreno JG, Monne M, et al: A comparative analysis of prostate-specific antigen gene sequence in benign and malignant prostate tissue. *Urology* 47(6):795–800, 1996.

Bauer JJ, McLeod DG, Moul JW: Prostate cancer: Diagnosis, treatment, and experience at one tertiary-care military medical center, 1989 and 1994. *Mil Med* 161:646–653, 1996.

Boring CC: Cancer statistics 1994. *Ca Cancer J Clin* 44:7–26, 1994.

Denis L: Commentary on maximal androgen blockade in prostate cancer: A theory to put into practice? *Prostate* 27(5):233–240, 1995.

Dillioglugil O, Miles BJ, Scardino PT, et al: Current controversies in the management of localized prostate cancer. *Eur Urol* 28(2):85–101, 1995.

Garnick MB, Fair WR: Prostate cancer: Emerging concepts: part II. *Ann Intern Med* 125(3):205–212, 1996.

Gee WF, Holtgrewe HL, Albertsen PC, et al: Practice trends in the diagnosis and management of prostate cancer in the United States. *J Urol* 154(1):207–208, 1995.

Ikeda I, Miura T, Kondo I, et al: Pyridimium cross-links as urinary markers of bone metastases in patients with prostate cancer. *Br J Urol* 77(1):102–106, 1996.

Kolvenbag GJ, Blackledge GR: Worldwide activity and safety of bicalutamide: A summary review. *Urology* 47(suppl 1A):70–84, 1996.

Krongrad A, Lai H, Lamm SH, et al: Mortality in prostate cancer. *J Urol* 156(3):1084–1091, 1996.

Labrie F, Cusan L, Gomez JL: Combination of screening and preoperative endocrine therapy: The potential for an important decrease in prostate cancer mortality. *J Clin Endocrinol Metab* 80(7):2002–2013, 1995.

Rubenstein M: Induction of apoptosis by diethylstilbestrol in hormone-insensitive prostate cancer cells. *J Natl Cancer Inst* 388(13):908–917, 1996.

Williams TR, Love N: Treatment of localized prostate cancer: Choosing the best alternative. *Postgrad Med* 100(3):105–107, 111–112, 118–120, 1996.

Chapter 13–3
ORAL CANCER
Kathleen J. Dobbs

DISCUSSION

Oral cancers account for approximately 5 percent of all cancers. Although this appears to be a small proportion, oral cancers have a great impact on social interaction, individual identification, and well-being. Disfigurement of the face and alterations in speech and eating affect the ways in which patients interact with the world. All health care providers must be cognizant of the presentations of oral cancers to achieve an optimal outcome. Early recognition and treatment are essential.

Table 13-3-1. Structures of the Oral Cavity

Anatomic Structure	Location	Pearls
Lips	External structures at the entrance of the cavity	Most common site of oral cancer, particularly lower lip
Buccal mucosa	Lining of cheeks laterally from maxillary to mandibulary gingival borders	Carcinoma rare; common site for leukoplakia
Upper and lower alveolar ridges	Mounds in maxilla and mandible in which teeth are implanted	Carcinomas more common in mandibular versus maxillary, particularly in molar and premolar regions; most arise in edentulous areas[5]
Retromolar trigone	Area behind molars adjacent to tonsillar pillars and oropharynx	Bony involvement extension to adjacent structures common; difficult to visualize unless mouth opened wide
Oral tongue	Anterior two-thirds of tongue, commonly called mobile tongue	Second most common site of oral cancer
Hard palate	"Roof" of mouth	Cancers rare in this area; most are punched-out ulcerations
Floor of mouth	All tissue below oral tongue to lower alveolar ridges	Considered a "silent area," as it is rarely examined; at this site, cancers typically develop at junction of tongue in sublingual space

The oral cavity is made up of many structures (Table 13-3-1). Each area requires careful examination and consideration. The prognosis and treatment of each area within the oral cavity have been the topics of research for years. For the purposes of this chapter, they will be discussed collectively unless a specific oral cancer is highlighted.

The salivary glands, though not considered structures of the oral cavity, open into the oral cavity and can be the site of oral cancer, although quite rarely. The ductal openings of the three largest salivary glands (parotid, submaxillary, and sublingual) should be examined closely. With a rich blood and lymphatic supply, metastatic spread of all oral cancers can occur to adjacent structures, including the lymph nodes. The vast majority of oral cancers are squamous cell carinomas. The remaining 5 to 10 percent include a variety of cell types, such as melanoma, lymphoma, adenocystic carcinoma, adenocarcinoma, and sarcoma.

PATHOGENESIS

The cause of oral cancers remains obscure. However, there are risk factors that show a definite causal relationship. Other risk factors only suggest an increase in the incidence of developing oral cancers. The combination of large quantities of alcohol and smoking accounts for approximately three-fourths of all oral cancers in the United States.[1] This additive effect has a greater impact on the disease than does either of the risk factors alone. Cancer of the lip may occur in pipe smokers. The popularity of oral tobacco has been followed by an increase in oral cancers, especially in the buccal mucosa and the floor of the mouth. There is a clear relationship between the common practice of betel nut

chewing and the development of oral cancers in areas that are in contact with the quid or chewed mixture. Betel nuts, which are grown in India and southeast Asia, have a stimulant effect. Additional risk factors may include poor dental hygiene, loose or ill-fitting dentures, tertiary syphilis, the use of mouthwashes with a high alcohol content, a genetic predisposition, and previous radiation. Sunlight exposure and lip cancer are noted to have a higher incidence in men. The lower incidence in women may be secondary to lip protection from lipstick and other protective coverings. In past decades, radiation was used as therapy for many benign problems, such as tonsillitis, an enlarged thymus in newborns, chronic sialoadenitis, and acne. There is a correlation between treatment with radiation for benign conditions and cancer in adjacent areas in these individuals.

SIGNS AND SYMPTOMS

The typical oral cancer patient is male and between 50 and 60 years old. Despite this propensity, one should be prepared to look for the disease in both younger and older age groups and in both sexes, as it is not a rare occurrence. Among all cancers, the incidence in the oral cavity is approximately 5 percent in men and 2 percent in women.

Primary care clinicians and dentists are essential in recognizing oral cancers in the early stages. Early detection and treatment significantly improve the prognosis and decrease morbidity. Clinical acumen and vigilance may be necessary to appreciate many of the signs and symptoms. Occult oral cancers occur. The signs and symptoms may be vague or nonspecific in the oral cavity, with cervical lymphadenopathy as the presenting sign. Typically, oral cancers are symptomatic, with patients seeking medical attention for any of the symptoms listed below. An intraoral mass or a distortion in the usual architecture is common. Ulceration with or without bleeding, pain, halitosis, odynophagia (painful swallowing), dysphagia (difficulty swallowing), trismus, decreased tongue mobility, loosening of teeth, and poorly fitting dentures are possible presenting symptoms. Because of the extensive lymphatic system servicing the oral cavity, any neck mass present for 1 to 2 months should alert the practitioner to look for a cancer. An occult oral cancer may be present and merits a complete evaluation, particularly if the social history indicates tobacco and alcohol use. The presence of lesions in the oral cavity is also a red flag.

Leukoplakia and erythroplakia are strong indicators of premalignancy or carcinoma in situ. Leukoplakia appears as white patches in the oral cavity that cannot be removed with scraping. This lesion is thought to be precancerous and should be recognized and evaluated histologically. Erythroplakia is a velvet-like red patch that also cannot be removed by simple scraping. It has greater implications for the development of oral cancer than does leukoplakia. It is histologically considered a carcinoma in situ. Physical examination of the entire oral cavity and the cervical, supraclavicular, and infraclavicular nodes is essential.

Inspection and palpation are used to assess oral cancers. A good white light source allows the examiner to visualize all aspects of the lips and oral cavity, including under the tongue and along the gingival–buccal mucosal border back to the retromolar trigone. Patients with dentures or removable orthodontic equipment should have them removed to uncover any lesions or evidence of irritation, especially over the alveolar ridges. With a gloved hand the practitioner must palpate all the surfaces of the oral cavity, focusing on changes in consistency or texture. Attention should be given to signs of patient discomfort during palpation.

Attention to the opening of the major salivary glands into the oral cavity is mandatory. This can be a site for the development of cancer or an indicator of diseased salivary glands. Examination

Table 13-3-2. Diagnostic Considerations for Oral Lesions

Aphthous ulcers (canker sores)
Herpes simplex infection (cold sore, fever blister)
Herpes simplex gingivitis (seen in children)
Benign pemphigus
Erosive lichen planus
Plummer-Vinson syndrome (atrophic oral changes)
Oral candida infection
Fibroma
Papilloma (benign neoplasm, cause unknown)

of the tongue requires several maneuvers. The anterior surface is examined with bright light. Over 85 percent of lingual cancers arise in the lateral margins of the tongue.[2] Induration and ulceration are suggestive of cancer. Grasping the tongue with dry gauze while palpating the tissue with the other gloved hand is very effective for a complete examination. Viewing all the surfaces of the tongue is crucial. Neck examination completes the physical examination for oral cancer. The oral cavity has two lymphatic systems draining the area. Neck masses on the ipsilateral side occur most often. Lesions in the midline of the oral cavity drain into both sides, resulting in potentially bilateral lymphadenopathy.

DIAGNOSTIC CONSIDERATIONS

The differential diagnostic considerations in oral cancer vary with the signs and symptoms, the location of the mass or lesion, and concurrent medical problems. Ulcerations of a common aphthous ulcer or canker sore can mimic cancers of the tongue, gingiva, and buccal mucosa. Oral cancers can be mistaken for the painful and erosive lesions of herpes simplex infection, erosive lichen planus, and benign pemphigus. Oral candidiasis must be differentiated from leukoplakia.

Plummer-Vinson syndrome (iron-deficiency anemia) causes the oral mucosa to have an ash-gray color, and atrophic changes of the tongue have been implicated in the etiology of tongue cancer. Kaposi's sarcoma also may be identified with violaceous macules on the mucosa. Mass lesions such as fibroma and papilloma must be differentiated from malignant oral lesions (Table 13-3-2).

LABORATORY STUDIES

History and physical examination and in many cases an index of suspicion are the primary diagnostic requirements. Complete blood count (CBC) with differential, platelet count, prothrombin time, partial prothromboplastin time, chemistry profile, and ECG provide both baseline information and potential clues for a further diagnostic workup. Biopsy is the next essential step. Histologic examination and identification are imperative. Means of acquiring tissue include fine needle aspiration biopsy, excisional biopsy, and rarely incisional biopsy of the oral lesion. Cervical or supraclavicular node biopsy is not routinely done to establish a diagnosis.

RADIOLOGIC STUDIES

Magnetic resonance imaging (MRI) is useful in assessing soft tissue and bone detail. Computed tomography (CT) often is used to define anatomic relationships. Although both imaging studies are useful, CT may be used more often because of its lower cost and higher availability. Both of these diagnostic studies are very valuable in staging oral cancers. Ultrasonography has limited use; its primary benefits are distinguishing solid from cystic tumors and evaluating neck and thyroid tumors. When CT is unavailable, chest x-ray may be used to look for metastasis or a secondary primary. If oro- or nasopharyngeal lesions are suspected, referral to an otolaryngolist for direct examination of the nasopharynx, oropharynx, and larynx is necessary.

TREATMENT

Once the diagnosis and staging have been established, consideration must be given to treatment. Quality of life issues must affect treatment decisions. If a cure is the goal, total eradication of tumor with the best functional and cosmetic outcome is the strategy. If palliation is the best option, the priority shifts to limiting the expansion of the mass and providing optimal comfort. Surgery for the removal of the tumor and the affected lymph nodes, radiation therapy, chemotherapy, and a combination of these modalities are the current methods of treating oral cancer. Referral to a medical oncologist for the treatment of oral cancer is important. Often a multidisciplinary team includes the medical oncologist; ear, nose, and throat surgeon; dentist; and psychosocial support professionals working together to achieve the best possible outcome.

Early cancers of the lip, the floor of the mouth, and the retromolar trigone are highly curable. Cancers of the buccal mucosa, tongue, alveolar ridge, and hard palate can be cured if detected and treated early.[3] Eighty-one percent of oral cavity cancer patients survive 1 year after diagnosis. For all stages (I through IV) combined, the 5-year relative survival is 52 percent. The 10-year rate is 41 percent.[4] Recurrence of the development of a second primary after successful treatment of the first cancer can occur. The patient must be monitored periodically for any further cancers.

REFERENCES

1. Day GL: Cancer rates and risks: Oral cavity and pharynx, in *Risks for Major Cancers.* Cancer Statistics Branch Division of Cancer Prevention and Control, National Cancer Institute, 1996.
2. US Public Health Service: Cancer detection in adults by physical examination. *Am Fam Physician* 51(4): 1995.
3. National Cancer Institute: *CancerNet, Lip and Oral Cancer.* January 1997. http://www.nci.gov/oral
4. American Cancer Society: *Oral Cavity and Pharynx Cancer Statistics.* January 1997. http://www.cancer.org/oral.html
5. Lee KJ: *Essential Otolaryngology Head and Neck Surgery,* 6th ed. Norwalk, CT: Appleton & Lange, 1996.

BIBLIOGRAPHY

Alford BR: *Head and Neck Tumors Core Curriculum Syllabus.* January 1997. http://www.bcm.tmc.edu/oto/studs/hnt.html
Schuller DE, Schleuning II, Alexander J, et al: *Otolaryngology—Head and Neck Surgery,* 8th ed. St. Louis, Mosby, 1994.

Chapter 13–4
BREAST CANCER
Patricia Kelly

DISCUSSION

The term *breast cancer* refers to a group of neoplasms that usually but not always first present in the female breast. These neoplasms may be ductal (78 percent), lobular (9 percent), associated with other special histologies (12 percent), or inflammatory (1 percent). Breast cancer is a very heterogenous disease that grows at very different rates in different patients and is often a systemic disease at the time of presentation.[1] Tumor doubling time can vary from 25 to 500 days. Breast cancer is a subtle disease with great variability in its presentation and prognosis.

Prevalence

Breast cancer is the most common lethal malignancy in females. The annual incidence of this cancer increases with age. Statistics regarding its incidence can be manipulated to portray breast cancer as an epidemic disease in women of all ages. Slogans such as "One out of eight women will get breast cancer in her lifetime" reinforce this theme. Some epidemiologists prefer to identify the probability of developing breast cancer in specified age intervals, however. For example, there is a 2.53 percent chance that a white female will develop breast cancer between ages 35 and 55. The cumulative lifetime probability of developing breast cancer is 12 percent, and that of dying from breast cancer is 3.5 percent.[2]

Etiology and Risk Factors

New evidence is constantly presented regarding the etiology of and risk factors for breast cancer. Without doubt, there is a genetic component. First-degree relatives of breast cancer patients have a twofold to threefold risk of developing the disease compared with women without affected first-degree relatives. Additionally, the identification of three specific genes (BCRA1, BCRA2, and p53) linked with a marked risk of breast cancer explain the very high incidence of the disease in some family clusters. Relatively few breast cancer patients have these genetic mutations, however.

Women with a history of benign breast disease generally do not have a greater risk of breast cancer. However, there is one type of benign abnormality, hyperplasia with atypia, that is associated with a higher risk of subsequent malignancy. This is a diagnosis that can be made only by biopsy; it is not the same as "fibrocystic breast disease."

High-fat diets have been implicated, but to date there is no evidence that changing to a low-fat diet later in life lowers the absolute risk. Endogenous hormones are implicated in certain groups. Nulliparous women and women who bear the first child after age 31 have a threefold to fourfold increased risk of breast cancer compared with women who have the first child before age 18. However, since most women fall into an intermediate category, the usefulness of this finding is uncertain. Early menarche and late menopause (inferring longer hormone exposure) increase the risk somewhat; however, the parameters have not been defined, and the average age at both of these events has changed rapidly during the twentieth century, making epidemiologic correlation difficult.

Oral contraceptives generally are not thought to increase the risk of breast cancer and may confer some protection. Estrogen replacement therapy may confer a theoretical risk, since exogenous estrogen can enhance tumor growth; also, since tumors are not diagnosed when the first cancerous cells form, estrogen replacement may increase the doubling times of certain neoplasms. A causative effect, however, has not been documented.

It is known that surgical castration (removal of the ovaries) before age 37 without subsequent hormone replacement decreases the risk of breast cancer. This, however, can hardly be used as a preventive measure because of the marked increase in cardiovascular disease and osteoporosis that would result.

It appears that increased alcohol intake is associated with increased risk. The intake years that may be most important, however, are in early adulthood. There is no evidence to suggest that discontinuing alcohol intake after age 45 will reduce the risk, and alcohol is somewhat protective against cardiovascular disease at low doses. However, even a history of low alcohol intake in large cohorts of women has been weakly associated with an increased risk of breast cancer. The overall health benefits of low alcohol intake (one drink per day or less) in women are therefore controversial.

Diabetes mellitus also increases the risk, as does age greater than 40 and a previous history of cancer of the ovary, uterus, or colon. Smoking is a weak risk factor. Demographically, Asian women seem to have the lowest risk in the U.S. population.

If one reviews these risk factors in a congregate or additive fashion, erroneous conclusions can result. There is no group of females, even with multiple risk factors, whose cumulative incidence of breast cancer is higher than 30 to 40 percent, excluding BRCA1 and BRCA2 carriers and women with a mutation in the p53 gene. One could examine the risks of a 50-year-old nulliparous white woman who has a mother and sister with breast cancer, drinks alcohol, has a high-fat diet, and has experienced early menarche, late menopause, and estrogen replacement therapy. This woman would statistically have a cumulative lifetime incidence of breast cancer less than 40 percent and a risk of death from breast cancer less than 20 percent. In comparison, this woman has a cardiovascular mortality risk higher than 33 percent.

SIGNS AND SYMPTOMS

The following signs and symptoms are significant:

1. Breast lumps are found in the majority of these patients. They tend to be dominant, firm to hard, immobile, irregular, and adherent to skin and/or underlying tissue.
2. Serosanguinous, unilateral nipple discharge should greatly increase the clinical suspicion of a neoplasm.
3. Eczematous skin changes, especially unilateral, can be a sign of breast cancer and warrant further investigation.
4. Any irregularity or "dimpling," induration, or unilateral size change should be explored.
5. Axillary adenopathy that is not otherwise explained is strongly suspicious of breast cancer until another etiology is histologically identified.

Breast pain is seldom a presenting symptom. However, bone pain from previously unsuspected metastatic breast cancer can be the first symptom of disease.

DIFFERENTIAL DIAGNOSIS

"Fibrocystic disease," fibroadenomas, cysts, mastitis, and fibrous tumors often must be surgically evaluated before malignancy can be excluded.

DIAGNOSTIC EVALUATION OF SUSPICIOUS FINDINGS

Mammography is approximately 85 percent sensitive in diagnosing breast cancer. It is less sensitive, however, in women under age 40 with dense breast tissue. The specificity of mammography is markedly lower leading to a great number of invasive procedures. The specificity increases in direct proportion to age. A palpable mass that is negative on mammography should always be biopsied.

Surgical Evaluation

The accuracy of fine needle aspiration of solid masses is directly related to the degree of operator and cytopathology experience with this technique. If tissue unequivocally characteristic of a benign entity (such as a fibroadenoma) is found, the sensitivity is higher than 95 percent. However, if insufficient or nondiagnostic tissue is obtained, an excisional biopsy is mandatory. Many surgeons strongly urge excisional biopsy of all solid masses. Cystic structures may be aspirated. If the cyst remains palpable or bloody fluid is obtained, an excisional biopsy must be performed.

The Positive Biopsy

Staging is necessary to determine the appropriate treatment. The most important element of staging—lymph node status—can be obtained concurrently with mastectomy or local excision (lumpectomy). Further staging studies for all these patients include a complete blood count (CBC), liver function tests, serum calcium, alkaline phosphatase, a chest x-ray, and a mammogram, all obtained preoperatively. Further staging is deferred until the lymph node status is available. If lymph nodes are positive or if the tumor is over 2 cm in size, CT of the liver, a bone scan, and possibly a bone marrow biopsy are indicated. This further evaluation should be conducted after consultation with a medical oncologist.

Staging of Breast Cancer

The American Joint Committee for Cancer Staging and End-Results Reporting developed a staging system based on the standard TNM [T (tumor size), N (node status), and M (metastatic disease)] criteria.

True breast cancer is grouped into clinical stages I through IV. Less advanced cancer (smaller tumor size and lack of spread to lymph nodes) generally is staged into the first two groups. More advanced cancer, as indicated by increasing tumor size, invasion of lymph nodes, and/or distant metastatic lesions, is grouped into clinical stages III and IV. There is some overlap; women who have small tumors but one or two positive, small nonfixed lymph nodes may be classified as stage II. Women with tumors greater than 2 cm, even without positive lymph nodes, are considered stage III, and women with primary tumors larger then 5 cm in size and without evidence of nodal involvement may have stage IV disease and a poorer prognosis.

As a very general rule, women with stage I or stage II cancers have a relative survival rate >66 percent after 6 years; women with stage III or stage IV cancers have a relative survival rate <49 percent over the same time period.

Since many oncologists use slightly different staging systems, it is usually most helpful to describe the tumor by size, the number and location of involved nodes, and any metastatic lesions. It is more difficult to predict survival rates with the "intermediate" stages (II and III), and the percentages given above, especially those for stage IIb and IIIa cancers, should be viewed with extreme caution.

There are any number of other variables (hormone receptor positivity, DNA ploidy, S stage activity, histologic grade, etc.) that affect survival but have not been included in a universal staging system. Every case should be evaluated individually by a medical oncologist experienced in breast cancer treatment. Newer prognostic factors, such as estimating the percentage of cells in the S phase of replication, will play a larger role in defining the prognosis in the future.

Breast cancer does not play by the same "rules" as other cancers, and 5 or 10 years of survival is not considered a definitive cure.

TREATMENT
Local Treatment

Counterintuitively, local treatment involving mastectomy for tumor removal and adjuvant local radiation does not dramatically affect survival time or the occurrence of metastases. Breast cancer is frequently a systemic disease at the time of presentation. What-

ever their cause of death, 75 to 85 percent of patients with a history of breast cancer have evidence of tumor at the time of autopsy.[3] The standard at this time for surgical treatment is modified radical mastectomy or removal of the tumor with clear margins, node dissection, and postsurgical adjuvant radiation. These treatments are designed to provide local disease control and offer identical outcomes in terms of survival benefit.

Systemic Treatment

Women generally are divided into premenopausal and postmenopausal groups for treatment options. Premenopausal women with negative nodes generally are treated with adjuvant chemotherapy if their tumors are larger than 1 cm. Women with positive nodes also are treated with adjuvant chemotherapy. There has been a recent trend of treating premenopausal women with 5 years of tamoxifen after adjunctive chemotherapy, especially if their tumors are hormone-receptor-positive. Postmenopausal women with positive lymph nodes, who are hormone-receptor-positive, generally are treated with oral tamoxifen 20 mg daily for 2 to 5 years. Depending on age, degree of node positivity, and size of tumor, many clinicians also recommend adjuvant chemotherapy for these patients. Postmenopausal women with hormone-receptor-negative tumors should receive adjuvant chemotherapy. For premenopausal women with more than 10 positive lymph nodes, dose-intensive chemotherapy with autologous bone marrow transplantation should be considered. Metastatic disease, if it is life-threatening or symptomatic, should be treated with chemotherapy and with tamoxifen if it is hormone-receptor-positive. For asymptomatic metastatic disease that is hormone-receptor-positive, tamoxifen alone may be considered. Radiation can provide palliative control for bone, brain, and chest wall metastases.

The standard adjuvant chemotherapy includes cyclophosphamide, methotrexate, and 5-fluorouracil. There is some evidence that regimens containing doxorubicin (Adriamycin) may offer a slight advantage; however, doxorubicin can cause cardiomyopathy, which is its dose-limiting factor. A new cardioprotective drug that can be administered concomitantly with doxorubicin should prove useful in allowing longer and more intense regimens containing this agent.

Salvage Chemotherapy for Recurrent Disease

Chemotherapy, if it did not previously contain doxorubicin, should now include this agent in combination with other standard agents. A newer agent, taxol, has been studied extensively and is very valuable in salvage chemotherapy. A related drug, docetaxel, has been approved by the U.S. Food and Drug Administration for patients who have failed during or relapsed after Adriamycin-based therapies. Relatively lengthy remissions can occur with salvage chemotherapy, but a cure is not the goal of this treatment.

SPECIAL CONSIDERATIONS

With an increase in the incidence of mammography, improvements in technique, and increased radiologist expertise, noninvasive tumors (carcinoma in situ) can now be detected.

Ductal carcinoma in situ is clearly malignant and can be multicentric in more than 50 percent of patients. Mastectomy or lumpectomy with radiation therapy usually is indicated. However, some clinicians advocate lumpectomy alone for small, well-differentiated lesions that can be removed with generous margins.

Lobular carcinoma in situ is premalignant, affects primarily premenopausal females, and is commonly bilateral. The risk of developing invasive cancer is high, and these patients may benefit from bilateral mastectomy. Other options include extremely close follow-up; however, given the 15 percent false-negative rate for mammography, there are risks with this approach that should be understood clearly by the patient and the clinician.

SUPPORTIVE MEASURES

It is very important to convey to breast cancer patients a sense of optimism for the immediate future. Even stage IV disease can be controlled for up to 3 years. The earlier the cancer, the better the prognosis. Breast cancer can have a slow and indolent natural history even without treatment. Cures are possible and even likely in stage I and stage II disease; very long remissions with many cures can be expected in early stage III disease. During disease-free and treatment-free periods, the quality of life is excellent. All symptoms suffered during chemotherapy, except for hair loss, can be substantially lessened or prevented by talented clinicians. The newer antiemetic drugs and more sophistication with anti-emetic drug combinations have virtually eliminated acute nausea and vomiting. Pain from metastatic disease can be controlled with sophisticated analgesic regimens and palliative radiation. Quality time is achievable even with advanced metastatic disease.

PATIENT EDUCATION AND PREVENTION

Optimism concerning the treatability of breast cancer is necessary to achieve an acceptable rate of screening. Rates of screening will increase when various health agencies and authorities agree on appropriate screening mammography schedules. There are few or no data to support a baseline mammogram before age 40. Screening women between ages 40 and 50 can save lives but is costly. This is due to

1. The relatively low prevalence in this age group
2. The large number of false-positive mammograms in women between 40 and 50
3. The huge financial and emotional cost of positive screening mammograms and subsequent biopsies that reveal benign disease

Women age 50 and over clearly benefit from regular screening mammography. Their disease is easier to visualize, and if it is diagnosed at an early stage, their prognosis is better than that of premenopausal patients.

Breast self-exams and provider breast exams are inexpensive; self-examination has been shown to be efficacious. Surprisingly, routine provider breast examination has a very low positive yield. Better training and increased time spent on breast examination by clinicians have been shown to improve the yield.

DISPOSITION

Follow-up should be individualized. In general, these patients should be seen at least every 6 months for a physical examination and a thorough review of systems.

Mammograms should be done annually. From a survival standpoint, no routine laboratory test or imaging scan has been shown to be valuable in a patient without symptoms or abnormalities on physical examination, and frequent repeated studies tend to induce anxiety in patients, who fearfully await the results of routine x-rays, CBCs, and chemistry panels.

Other routine health care maintenance should be stressed. Patients should be screened for colon and ovarian cancer regularly; however, optimal schedules have not been demonstrated. Annual pelvic examinations and colonoscopy or flexible sigmoidoscopy every 3 to 5 years would be a reasonable approach, since breast cancer patients have an increased incidence of these neoplasms.

REFERENCES

1. Haskell CM, Casciato DA: Breast cancer, in Casciato DA, Lowitz BB: *Manual of Clinical Oncology.* Boston, Little, Brown, 1995, p 186.
2. Henderson IC: Breast cancer, in Isselbacher KJ, Braunwald E, Wilson JD, et al (eds): *Harrison's Principles of Internal Medicine,* 13th ed. New York, McGraw-Hill, 1994 p 1840.
3. Casciato DA, Lowitz BB: *Manual of Clinical Oncology.* Boston, Little, Brown, 1995, p 186.

BIBLIOGRAPHY

Clement KD, Conner PD: Breast cancer, in Taylor RB: *Manual of Family Practice.* Boston, Little, Brown, 1997 pp 461–463.

Harris JR, Lippman ME, Veronesi U, et al: Medical progress—breast cancer. *New Engl J Med* 5:325–327, 1992.

Harris JR, Merrow M, Bonadonna G: Cancer of the breast, in DeVita VT Jr, Hellman S, Rosenberg SA, et al (eds): *Cancer: Principals and Practice of Oncology,* 4th ed. Philadelphia, Lippincott, 1993.

Kennedy MJ: Systemic adjuvant therapy for breast cancer. *Curr Opin Oncol* 6(6):570–577, 1994.

Muss HB: The role of chemotherapy and adjuvant therapy in the management of breast cancer in older women. *Cancer* 74(suppl 7):2165–2171, 1994.

Olivotto IA, Bajdik CD, Plenferleith IH, et al: Adjuvant systemic therapy and survival after breast cancer. *New Engl J Med* 330(12):805–810, 1994.

Report of the Council on Scientific Affairs: Management of patients with node-negative breast cancer. *Arch Intern Med* 153(1):58–67, 1993.

Rosen PP, Groshen S, Kinne DW, et al: Factors influencing prognosis in node-negative breast carcinoma—analysis of 767 $T_1N_0M_0$ patients with long term follow-up. *J Clin Oncol* 11:2090, 1993.

Roy JA, Swaka CA, Prichard KI: Hormone replacement therapy in women with breast cancer: Do the risks outweigh the benefits? *J Clin Oncol* 14:997–1006, 1996.

Smith TJ, Hillner BE: The efficacy and cost-effectiveness of adjuvant therapy of early breast cancer in premenopausal women. *J Clin Oncol* 11:771, 1993.

Chapter 13–5
COLORECTAL CANCER
Patricia Kelly

DISCUSSION

Colorectal cancer is the second most lethal cancer in the U.S. population. However, its rate has been declining. Demographically, it is most common in the northeastern United States. The risk increases with age. There is a 5 percent lifetime prevalence rate in this country.

Heredity is an important risk factor; as many as 25 percent of cases may be related to genetic causes. There are several variants of familial polyposis syndromes, all of which are linked with an increased incidence of colorectal cancer. Some of these syndromes have a familial rate of colorectal cancer higher than 50 percent; prophylactic colectomy without colostomy is a consideration for some of these persons.

The geographic incidence had led to the study of diet in relation to colorectal cancer risk. It is clear that high-fat, low-fiber diets contribute to the incidence of colorectal cancer. Smoking also increases the risk to two to three times baseline.

Ulcerative colitis markedly increases the risk of colorectal cancer and requires annual screening colonoscopy (see "Screening and Prevention," below). Crohn's disease is associated with an increased incidence of this malignancy; afflicted persons have a 1.5-fold to twofold higher risk. Other risk factors include a personal or family history of other cancers, especially reproductive cancers in women. Exposure to asbestos may increase the risk slightly.

About 98 percent of true colorectal cancers are adenocarcinomas by histology. The distribution of malignant lesions throughout the colon is as follows: 66 percent left colon and 33 percent right colon; 20 percent of colorectal cancers occur in the rectum. Some patients have disease at more than one site.

SIGNS AND SYMPTOMS

The signs and symptoms are related to the size and location of the neoplasm. Tumors of the left side of the colon may present with changes in bowel habits, flank pain, bleeding, constipation, decreased stool diameter, and obstruction. Right-sided colon cancer results in varying degrees of abdominal discomfort, weight loss, and stools positive for occult blood.

Findings on physical examination may be absent, depending on tumor location and size. Tumor that has already metastasized to the liver may be palpable; infrequently, asymptomatic large colon masses may be palpated through the abdominal wall. Rectal cancer frequently can be detected on digital rectal examination. Stool for occult blood, depending on the technique, may be positive (see "Screening and Prevention," below). Visible bleeding is rarely noted. Weight loss is common in patients with advanced disease.

DIAGNOSTIC CONSIDERATIONS

In symptomatic patients, the causes of abdominal pain must be systematically evaluated. Right-sided pain may prompt consideration of gallbladder disease (see Chap. 6-10). Acute left lower quadrant pain is also seen in diverticulitis, which also can produce bleeding (see Chap. 6-8). Generally, diagnostic studies reveal intracolonic abnormalities that will prompt studies for a definitive diagnosis.

DIAGNOSTIC STUDIES

Laboratory studies should include a complete blood count (CBC) primarily to detect the severity of anemia and a chemistry panel that includes liver function tests to assist in ruling out metastatic disease.

A complete physical examination, including a digital rectal examination with testing of stool for occult blood, should be performed. A carcinoembryonic antigen (CEA) test should be ordered preoperatively if suspicion of colorectal cancer is strong. It may be included in the initial evaluation or deferred until disease is confirmed by colonoscopy and biopsy.

IMAGING AND ENDOSCOPIC STUDIES

The workup should then progress to a colonoscopy and biopsy for histologic confirmation. If a polyp is discovered and removed, the area should be marked and measured precisely so that further surgery for definitive resection with wide margins may be performed. A CEA is mandatory before the removal of the suspect lesion.

CEA is the best known marker to follow disease recurrence or progression, and so a baseline level must be established. However, some colorectal cancers do not produce CEA; therefore, a normal CEA should not preclude further evaluation if other findings are suspicious.

Table 13-5-1. Staging of Colorectal Cancer

Stage	Description
A1	Limited to mucosa; negative nodes
B1	Extension into muscularis propria; negative nodes
B2	Extension through entire bowel wall; negative nodes
B3	Extension into adjacent organs; negative nodes
C1	Positive nodes; lesion limited to muscularis propria
C2	Positive nodes; lesion extends through entire bowel wall
C3	Positive nodes with tumor invasion of adjacent organs (locally invasive)
D	Distant metastatic disease

If a neoplasm is discovered, it is staged preoperatively and postoperatively. The postoperative staging is of course more definitive. Preliminary (preoperative) treatment planning and final (postoperative) treatment planning are dependent on the stage of the disease.

STAGING OF COLORECTAL CANCER

The most widely used staging system is the modified Duke's-Astler-Coller method (Table 13-5-1).

Prognosis

A stage A cancer, perhaps represented by a completely excised polyp with tumor limited to the polyp itself, has a 90 to 100 percent 5-year survival rate. Node-negative cancers have 5-year survival rates that range from 55 to 85 percent. Node-positive disease is ominous even without distant metastatic lesions; without local invasion, the 5-year survival rate is between 25 and 50 percent. Locally invasive disease has a 5-year survival rate of 0 to 20 percent, and distant metastatic disease has a median survival rate of 6 to 12 months.[1]

TREATMENT

Unless distant metastatic disease exists, surgery is the initial management of choice. Partial colectomy with wide margins and adjacent lymph node removal is the standard procedure.

Permanent colostomy may or may not be needed but is performed frequently on a temporary basis to permit stool passage postoperatively. Upper and high middle rectal tumors are excised with an anterior resection of the rectum. Abdominal perineal resection generally is used for lower rectal lesions. Obstruction of the left side of the colon requires at least a temporary colostomy with deferred closure. Obstructive tumors of the right side of the colon frequently can be managed by wide resection with immediate anastomosis, without the need for even a temporary colostomy. High rectal lesions can be treated with the same approach. Perforation secondary to mass obviously requires excision and at least a temporary colostomy.

Adjuvant Chemotherapy and Radiation

Colon cancer with nodal spread is treated with adjuvant 5-fluorouracil and levamisole with various dosing schemes for up to 1 year. Three large, prospective randomized trials have demonstrated that 5-fluorouracil adjuvant therapy improves the 5-year survival rate approximately 10 to 15 percent. Clinical trials to find the optimal drugs, doses, and length of treatment are ongoing.

Rectal cancer is almost always treated postsurgically with adjuvant radiation therapy and concomitant 5-fluorouracil. After the completion of combination radiation therapy and chemotherapy, adjuvant therapy with 5-fluorouracil and levamisole is indicated for disease that has spread locally or to adjacent nodes. This aggressive treatment is necessary because of the technical difficulty of achieving adequate clear surgical margins after resection of a rectal cancer.

Recurrent and metastatic colorectal cancers generally are treated with 5-fluorouracil and folinic acid (Leucovorin). Long-term remission and survival rates are low, generally with a median survival less than 1 year. A new chemotherapeutic agent, irinotecan hydrochloride, a topoisomerase 1 inhibitor, recently was approved for patients with metastatic colorectal cancer who recur or progress after 5-fluorouracil therapy. A 15 percent response rate (complete or partial remission) was noted during premarketing trials, and survival data are being accumulated. This agent has a relatively severe side effect profile; quality of life must be considered in patients at this stage of illness.

DISPOSITION

In patients with resected colon cancer, CEA levels should be measured every 3 months for 24 months and every 6 months thereafter. Chest x-rays are recommended annually. Repeat colonoscopy should be performed 6 weeks postoperatively if the patient's condition permits and then annually. Most recurrences occur within 3 years.

Screening and Prevention

A low dose of aspirin daily may aid in the prevention of colorectal cancer. Low-fat, high-fiber diets are useful. Knowledge of a family history of colorectal cancer or female reproductive cancer is useful in the design of an individualized screening schedule.

Digital rectal examinations should be performed every 1 to 2 years in adults over 40. Stool testing for occult blood is 40 percent specific and <50 percent sensitive with one test result; a huge expense is generated by further workup. Efforts to increase the effectiveness of this test are ongoing, and large trials will determine whether annual screening is advisable and which groups will benefit most. Currently, annual tests for occult blood are recommended by the American Cancer Society for persons older than 50 years of age.

Flexible sigmoidoscopy or colonscopy every 3 to 5 years is recommended for individuals older than 50 without other known risk factors. Individuals with verified family histories or familial polyposal syndromes require more frequent examinations starting at a younger age. Some authorities recommend starting screening colonoscopy 10 years before the age of first occurrence in a relative if prophylactic surgery is not done for the more aggressive familial syndromes.

REFERENCES

1. Tabarrah EJ: Gastrointestinal tract cancers, in Casciato DA, Lowitz BB (eds): *Manual of Clinical Oncology.* Boston, Little, Brown, 1995, pp 145–182.

BIBLIOGRAPHY

DeCosse JJ, Tsioulias GJ, Jacobson JS, et al: Colorectal cancer—detection, treatment, and rehabilitation. *Cancer* 44:27, 1994.

Laurence G, Orientale E Jr: Colorectal cancer, in Taylor RB: *Manual of Family Practice.* Boston, Little, Brown, 1997, pp 385–388.

Moertel CG: Chemotherapy for colorectal cancer. *New Engl J Med* 330:1136, 1994.

Moertel CG, Fleming TR, MacDonald JS: Fluorouracil plus levamisole as effective adjuvant therapy after resection of stage III colon carcinoma—a final report, *Ann Intern Med* 122:321, 1995.

Rahman MI, Chagoury ME: Selections from current literature—screening for colorectal cancer. *J Fam Pract* 11(3):333–339, 1994.

Chapter 13–6
LUNG CANCER
Patricia Kelly

DISCUSSION

Lung cancer is the leading cause of cancer deaths in the United States. Most of these patients die within 1 year of the diagnosis. The peak incidence occurs between ages 55 and 65, although cases occur in smokers as young as 30. This is a disease that is almost completely preventable: Tobacco is the direct cause of approximately 90 percent of lung cancers.

There probably is an enhanced carcinogenic effect of tobacco combined with the pollutants present in modern society. However, tobacco is carcinogenic in and of itself.

Four major histologic types of cancer constitute 95 percent of primary lung tumors:

1. Squamous cell carcinomas
2. Small cell carcinomas
3. Adenocarcinomas
4. Large cell carcinomas

For purposes of treatment and prognosis, lung cancer is thought of as small cell or non-small cell. Small cell lung cancer generally goes into remission with appropriate chemotherapy, although recurrence within 2 years is the almost absolute rule. If non-small cell lung cancer is diagnosed very early, it potentially can be cured with complete resection. However, at the time of diagnosis, only one of five patients has local, resectable disease. Only 30 to 40 percent of patients with resected local disease, however, survive for 5 years.

SIGNS AND SYMPTOMS

About 10 percent of these patients are asymptomatic and are detected on screening radiography. Others present because of cough, hemoptysis, shortness of breath, weight loss, wheezing, or obstructive pneumonia. Later-stage patients may have lung abscess, tracheal obstruction, esophageal compression, hoarseness, or Horner's syndrome (enophthalmos, ptosis, miosis, and ipsilateral loss of sweat). Patients can develop superior vena cava syndrome with associated swelling of the head and jugular venous distention. Pancoast's syndrome (superior sulcus tumor) involves the eighth cervical and the first and second thoracic nerves, causing shoulder pain and rib destruction. Rapidly progressive bronchoalveolar carcinoma can obstruct the bronchi, causing hypoxemia and death. Metastatic cancer, of course, can produce multiple symptom complexes.

There may be abnormal wheezing, dullness, rales, and rhonchi on lung examination. Of course, these symptoms coincide with the findings of frequently concomitant chronic obstructive pulmonary disease and obstructive pneumonia secondary to a neoplasm. Generally, the patient experiences some weight loss and may have clubbing of the extremities.

DIAGNOSTIC CONSIDERATIONS

Patients with lung cancer may present with paraneoplastic syndromes characterized by anorexia, cachexia, weight loss, decreased immunity, hypercalcemia, hypophosphatemia, hyponatremia, and hypokalemia. Fatigue also may be present and can represent myasthenic Eaton-Lambert syndrome, which is found primarily in patients with small cell lung cancer. Hypercoagulable states also may ensue with all cancers. The syndrome of inappropriate excretion of antidiuretic hormone (SIADH) can be commonly found in patients with small cell lung cancer.

LABORATORY STUDIES

No laboratory test is especially indicative of lung cancer. Laboratory studies should be reserved for staging.

RADIOLOGIC STUDIES

Chest radiography and, if it is nondiagnostic, CT are necessary. Chest CT is especially valuable in localizing a tumor for the most important diagnostic test: the confirming biopsy for definitive cytology. CT of the thorax, down to the level of the liver and adrenals, also assists in staging and in excluding metastatic disease.

BIOPSY

Tissue must be obtained. Histology and the extent of spread determine treatment. Tissue can be obtained from fine-needle aspiration CT-guided biopsy of peripheral lesions, samples from bronchoscopy, nodal biopsy during mediastinoscopy, and video-assisted thoracoscopy. A positive sputum cytology, although diagnostic, is rarely obtainable, and false-negatives are the rule.

STAGING OF LUNG CANCER

Non-small cell lung cancers are staged according to the extent and position of nodal spread, the size and degree of invasion of the tumor itself, and any metastatic lesions that are present. Obviously, smaller tumors with absent or limited nodal spread or local invasion may be resectable. Tumors with nodal spread on both sides of the chest and tumor locally invasive to adjacent organs are usually, although not always, not resectable. Tumors with distant metastatic lesions are not resected. If a patient is believed to have a resectable cancer, after consultation with the thoracic surgeon, he or she will require pulmonary function tests and ventilation-perfusion scans to determine if he or she will have sufficient residual functional lung tissue postoperatively.

Frequently, the question of resectability is resolved only by open surgery. Recently, attempts have been made to "downstage" tumors by giving preoperative chemotherapy and radiation therapy. This is called *neoadjuvant treatment* and can be useful in certain well-motivated patients.

TREATMENT OF NONRESECTABLE LESIONS

Medical oncologists believe that chemotherapy for non-small cell lung cancer is essentially palliative in nature and may provide slightly longer survival than do other modalities of palliative care. This difference is small, and the increased survival is measured in weeks. There is controversy concerning offering patients chemotherapy for inoperative lung cancer, although a new agent (Navelbine) recently was approved by the U.S. Food and Drug Administration for use with traditional agents, primarily cisplatin and carboplatin, in patients with this disease.

Radiation therapy can be used for palliation of hemoptysis, superior vena cava syndrome, or other syndromes that would be amenable to local control. Radiation therapy with curative intent can be offered to patients with earlier stages of lung cancer who decline surgery or are not surgical candidates. The percentage of actual cure with this modality, however, is quite small. Longer courses of radiation therapy than are used for palliation can cause side effects, including radiation pneumonitis and decreased pulmonary function.

TREATMENT OF SMALL CELL LUNG CANCER

Small cell lung cancer is considered limited if the neoplasm is clinically confined to the hemithorax and the associated draining regional nodes at the original presentation. Other patients are considered to have "extensive" disease. Small cell lung cancer is very sensitive to both chemotherapy and radiation and is treated with those modalities sequentially or in combination. The drugs most frequently used for initial treatment are cisplatin-based derivatives and etoposide in combination.

Prophylactic whole-brain irradiation is controversial but sometimes is used to prevent the common occurrence of brain metastases. However, there is no survival advantage with this approach. If a patient fails to achieve a complete remission after six cycles of chemotherapy with or without radiation, the chemotherapy is changed to a salvage regimen and radiation therapy is added if it was not utilized previously. Most patients can achieve a complete response, and almost all have a partial response with a survival advantage. However, the disease usually recurs or relapses after 12 to 18 months. At that time, the patient can be treated with chemotherapeutic agents that were not previously used on that particular tumor. It is sometimes possible to induce another complete or partial remission. Entries into clinical trials should be encouraged at this stage, since the optimal salvage regimen has not been established.

Metastatic disease from small cell lung cancer is very amenable to radiation therapy, which should be used on bone and brain lesions.

Pain Management

Pain management is always a concern with any type of lung cancer. Adequate analgesia should be provided to patients who are receiving palliative care and patients who are receiving chemotherapy or radiation therapy but are experiencing pain. Respiratory depression can occur with adequate doses of opioid analgesia; however, this should not prompt the clinician to give a suboptimal dose. The "air hunger" of terminal, end-stage lung cancer is also effectively treated with larger doses of morphine, which reduce anxiety and the subjective feeling of shortness of breath. Patients and their families should receive appropriate education and support from their primary clinicians even after hospice referral. Optimal palliative treatment of end-stage cancer is in and of itself an extremely worthy goal that should be learned and practiced by all clinicians who deal with oncologic patients.

Prevention

Patients (or humans in general) should not be exposed to tobacco products. Children and adolescents must be educated at every opportunity about the dangers of tobacco. Most addicted smokers start smoking before age 18. Therefore, the illegal consumption of nicotine products should be dealt with as firmly as is the illegal consumption of alcohol and illicit drugs. Smoking in all public places should be forbidden. No one should smoke near children or even pets.

Every visit or communication with a smoking patient should include motivation and the offer of a plan for tobacco cessation. Self-help groups, nicotine replacement, and strong clinician support are associated with successful cessation attempts. The average former smoker attempted to stop twice before making the successful attempt. One should never give up on smoking patients.

Screening

There is no evidence that screening chest radiography of high-risk patients improves the detection of treatable lesions or improves survival. There is no current preventive medicine recommendation for routine chest radiography in the absence of symptoms. However, screening can and does encompass the assessment of all patients for firsthand or secondhand exposure to tobacco and appropriate subsequent education and medical support for smokers and persons exposed to secondhand smoke. Persons who have high-risk environmental exposures (e.g., asbestos) should be cautioned and informed that tobacco is especially risky for them.

BIBLIOGRAPHY

Adelstein DJ: Palliative chemotherapy for non-small cell lung cancer. *Semin Oncol* 22(suppl 3):35–39, 1995.

Elias AD: Future directions in lung cancer research and therapeutics. *Hematol Oncol Clin North Am* 11(3):519–527, 1997.

Ganz PA, Figlin RA, Haskell CM: Supportive care versus supportive care and combination chemotherapy in metastatic non-small cell lung cancer: Does chemotherapy make a difference? *Cancer* 63(7):1271–1278, 1989.

Green MR, Barkley JE: Intensity of neoadjuvant therapy in resectable non-small cell lung cancer. *Lung Cancer* 17(suppl 1):S111–S119, 1997.

Kessel KF, Hannigan JE Jr: Lung cancer, in Taylor RB: *Manual of Family Practice.* Boston, Little, Brown, 1997, pp 337–340.

Mulshine JL, Glatstein E, Ruckdeschel JC: Treatment of non-small cell lung cancer. *J Clin Oncol* 4(11):1704–1715, 1986.

Soda H, Tomita H, Kohno S: Limitation of annual screening chest radiography for the diagnosis of lung cancer—a retrospective study. *Cancer* 72(8):2341–2346, 1993.

Chapter 13–7
OVARIAN CANCER
Amelia Naccarto-Coleman

DISCUSSION

Ovarian cancer is the number one cause of gynecologic cancer deaths and the fifth leading cause of all cancer-related deaths among women in the United States. An estimated 26,000 new cases were diagnosed in the United States in 1995, and more than 14,000 women died as a result of this disease. Even though the incidence rate is low, overall survival rates, which have been unchanged for over 30 years, remain at 30 to 35 percent and drop to 4 percent in women with advanced disease. Widespread screening has been ineffective in detecting this malignancy in its early stages, when it is confined to the ovary. Unfortunately, more than two-thirds of women with documented ovarian cancer have advanced disease (stages III and IV) at the time of diagnosis. Mortality rates are stage-dependent and increase dramatically with age. Worldwide, ovarian cancer accounts for approximately 4 percent of all cancers in women. With the exception of Japan, this disease is more commonly found in highly industrialized and affluent countries, particularly North America and western Europe. The incidence of ovarian cancer peaks at two distinct ages: premenarchal and postmenopausal. It is prevalent in approximately 30 to 50 in 100,000 cases, with the lifetime incidence being 1 in 70 women.

Etiology and Risk Factors

The natural history and etiology of this disease remain unclear. The main theory proposes that incessant ovulation causes repetitive trauma to the ovarian surface, which may lead to the genesis of ovarian neoplasia by disrupting the germinal epithelium, thus inhibiting repair. The risk factors included in this hypothesis are advancing age, nulliparity, a history of infertility or delayed childbearing, early menarche, and late menopause. This theory is supported by evidence that shows that long-term suppression of ovulation actually decreases the lifetime risk by as much as 50 percent.

Oral contraceptive use, breast feeding, and multiparity have all demonstrated significant protection against the occurrence of ovarian cancer. Women with a family history of ovarian cancer have a significant lifetime risk of developing this disease. Proportionate to the number of first-degree relatives diagnosed with ovarian cancer, the highest risk appears to be in women who have two or more first-degree relatives in two successive generations. This subgroup of familial ovarian cancer is postulated to be an autosomal dominant inherited trait.

The three hereditary syndromes are

1. *Site-specific:* families with an increased risk for ovarian cancer only
2. *Breast and ovarian:* families with an increased risk of both
3. *Lynch type II syndrome* (also known as family cancer syndrome): clustering of endometrial, breast, ovarian, and early-onset colorectal cancers within families

Although age and family history are the two most important risk factors, other considerations currently being investigated include high dietary fat consumption, chemical exposure to talc or asbestos introduced into the peritoneal cavity by perineal dusting, white women, and, most recently, genetic linkages.

PATHOGENESES

Several different types of ovarian malignancies fall under the disease category ovarian carcinoma. Each of them has different characteristics, treatments, and survival rates and can be classified according to its histologic type. The four major categories are

1. Epithelial neoplasms
2. Germ cell tumors
3. Stromal/sex cord tumors
4. Metastatic disease from a distant primary site

Epithelial neoplasms are derived from the peritoneal covering of the ovary and account for more than 60 percent of all ovarian neoplasms. They are identified by the following subtypes: serous, mucinous, endometrioid, clear cell, transitional cell, and undifferentiated. More than 90 percent of these tumors are malignant. A subset of ovarian epithelial neoplasms are called borderline cystadenocarcinomas or tumors of low malignant potential. These benign tumors are histologically similar to their malignant counterparts and are clinically important because of the possibility of future transformation.

Germ cell tumors are seen predominantly in younger age groups and rarely after age 30. They account for less than 5 percent of all ovarian neoplasms. Their rapid growth and hemorrhagic nature are associated with acute abdominal symptoms, and they can easily be confused with appendicitis or pregnancy-associated complications. The prognosis is excellent, with a 5-year survival rate exceeding 85 percent.

Stromal cell tumors are characterized by the production of male, female, and adrenal steroid hormones. They account for less than 5 percent of all ovarian malignancies and can occur in all age groups. The secretion of large amounts of estrogen is associated with precocious puberty in younger girls and endometrial hyperplasia or vaginal bleeding in postmenopausal females. The prognosis is good, with 10- and 20-year survivals of 90 percent and 75 percent, respectively, after resection.

Metastatic carcinoma can present as bilateral adnexal masses and mimic primary ovarian cancer. This categorization can account for approximately 15 to 20 percent of all ovarian malignan-

Table 13-7-1. Characteristics of a Pelvic Mass

	Benign	Malignant
Physical examination	Mobile	Fixed
	Unilateral	Bilateral
	Cystic	Solid or firm
	Smooth	Nodular
Ultrasound	Simple cyst <10 cm	Solid cyst >10 cm
	Septations <3 mm	Multiple septations
	Unilateral	Bilateral
	Calcification	None seen
	Gravity-dependent contents	Ascites

cies and should be a major diagnostic consideration in all ovarian tumors. The most common primary sites are the breast, stomach, colon, and endometrium. The prognosis is dismal, with 5-year survival rates between 5 and 10 percent.

SIGNS AND SYMPTOMS

Since most of the symptoms are nonspecific and diverse, the key to diagnosis is a high index of suspicion and familiarity with the epidemiologic risk factors. The symptomatology in the early stages includes vague abdominal discomfort, painless swelling or bloating of the lower abdomen, dyspepsia, increasing flatulence, early satiety, mild gastrointestinal and bowel disturbances, and nonspecific pelvic discomfort. In the advanced stages, the symptoms generally become more specific and are related to the pain and pressure associated with an enlarging mass. The predominant finding in making a diagnosis is the detection of an adnexal mass on bimanual and rectovaginal examination.

OBJECTIVE FINDINGS

A pelvic mass usually is palpated on bimanual examination in patients with the advanced stages of the disease. Because of the deep, anatomic location of the ovary, early-stage tumors usually are not detected. Certain characteristics of the mass may offer additional clues to the etiology.

The diagnostic evaluation is influenced by the patient's age and menopausal status and the characteristics of the mass on pelvic examination and ultrasonography (Table 13-7-1).

Abdominal swelling or distention resulting from an ovarian enlargement or accumulation of ascitic fluid appears very late in the course of the disease. Other findings may include the effects of functional tumors that produce steroid hormones, causing postmenopausal bleeding or virilization.

LABORATORY STUDIES

If an ovarian malignancy is suspected, a general preoperative assessment should be performed, including a complete blood count (CBC), differential, and platelet count and a chemistry panel with hepatic and renal function tests and serum CA-125 levels. Elevated CA-125 levels are present in 80 percent of advanced epithelial ovarian cancers and are useful in monitoring treatment. They are not helpful in screening women for the detection of early-stage disease.

RADIOLOGIC AND IMAGING STUDIES

Sonographic imaging is extremely useful in the evaluation of a pelvic mass. Transabdominal ultrasound and transvaginal sonography (TVS) are used to estimate ovarian size, complexity, and morphology and the likelihood of malignancy. Color Doppler imaging (CDI) may offer additional prognostic information in the future but is still under investigation. Extensive imaging stud-

ies such as computer tomography (CT) and magnetic resonance imaging (MRI) are reserved for select cases and rarely provide additional clinical information. TVS has been shown to be the most efficient, accurate, and cost-effective modality in diagnosing ovarian disease.

When a malignancy is suspected, additional preoperative studies are considered to evaluate metastatic disease and the patient's general medical condition. These studies include a chest x-ray to exclude pleural effusion, ultrasound assessment of the abdomen and liver, intravenous pyelography, and a barium enema if colorectal disease is suspected. Because of the genetic association in familial cancer syndromes, a screening mammogram should be obtained.

OTHER DIAGNOSTICS

Ultimately, the evaluation of a pelvic mass under optimal conditions requires an exploratory laparotomy and a histologic review to diagnose ovarian cancer definitively. This is the only way to determine whether the tumor is benign or malignant, primary or metastatic. Diagnostic paracentesis is rarely indicated because of the high percentage of false-negative results in the presence of widespread disease and the possibility of introducing tumor cells into the peritoneal cavity through needle insertion.

SURGICAL STAGING FOR OVARIAN CANCER

Ovarian cancer can spread in three ways: direct extension, exfoliation of malignant cells, and lymphatic spread. Once the diagnosis of ovarian cancer has been established, determination of the extent of the disease or of the stage is made according to the Federation of Gynecology and Obstetrics (FIGO) system. Comprehensive surgical staging is carried out by meticulous examination of all peritoneal and retroperitoneal surfaces at risk of tumor spread.

DIAGNOSTIC CONSIDERATIONS

Epithelial ovarian cancer needs to be distinguished from functional ovarian cysts and benign adnexal masses. This differentiation can be achieved by evaluating the characteristics of the mass, the age of the patient, and the radiographic presentation. Benign adnexal masses as seen on ultrasonography are generally simple, mobile cysts that are unilateral, are under 10 cm in size, contain septations less than 3 mm in thickness, and often show signs of calcifications, especially teeth. Malignant masses are often solid, fixed nodular tumors that are bilateral, contain multiple septations larger than 3 mm in size, and present with ascites. Other gynecologic syndromes that simulate this disease are pelvic inflammatory disease, endometriosis, and pedunculated uterine leiomyomas. Nongynecologic causes include inflammatory or neoplastic colonic carcinomas, irritable bowel disease, and hepatic failure with ascites.

TREATMENT

Ovarian cancer generally is managed in five distinct phases:

- Initial laparotomy for cytoreduction and staging
- Postoperative adjuvant therapy with chemotherapy and radiation
- Reevaluation after treatment
- Salvage therapy for persistent or recurrent disease
- Palliative care

The primary treatment of early-stage disease consists of surgery, chemotherapy, and radiotherapy.

Surgery

Surgical intervention is usually aggressive and is best performed by a qualified gynecologic oncologic surgeon. However, if the woman is still in her reproductive years and wants to have more children, there is now the option of preserving some of her reproductive functions after surgical staging has been performed. The goals of treatment are optimal debulking of the tumor and accurate surgical staging and diagnosis.

For epithelial ovarian cancers, surgical procedures include total abdominal hysterectomy/bilateral salpingo-oophorectomy (TAH/BSO), omentectomy/debulking, and staging biopsies, including nodal sampling if indicated. For ovarian germ cell cancers, the procedures include salpingo-oophorectomy on the affected side only in young patients and careful staging and lymph node dissection. For sex cord stromal cancers, the procedures include adnexectomy of affected side with surgical staging in young patients and TAH/BSO and surgical staging in postreproductive women. For low malignant potential (LMP) tumors, the procedure is TAH/BSO with optimal staging and debulking in postreproductive women.

Chemotherapy

In advanced epithelial ovarian malignancies, systemic chemotherapy is the mainstay of treatment after surgery. It is most effective in patients who have had optimal cytoreduction and patients who present with minimal disease after resection. The treatment of choice is a platinum-based combination therapy given every 3 weeks for six to eight cycles. Either cisplatin or carboplatin is effective combined with cyclophosphamide (Cytoxan). Another drug used in this regimen is paclitaxel (Taxol). Clinical response rates range between 60 and 70 percent, with 5-year survivals of 10 to 20 percent. Because of the potential toxicities of these drugs, contraindications include patients with a history of impaired renal function, hearing loss, or neuropathy. Cisplatin has been associated with ototoxicity, renal toxicity, and peripheral neuropathy and usually is administered on an inpatient basis. Carboplatin can be given on an outpatient basis and has minimal renal toxicity and neurotoxicity. All these regimens cause some degree of bone marrow suppression but do not warrant the routine use of hematopoietic growth factors or bone marrow transplantation. Intraperitoneal chemotherapy in the treatment of ovarian cancers remains to be defined. Alternative drugs include various agents of the alkylating group, 5-fluorouracil, and doxorubicin.

Radiotherapy

Postoperative radiation therapy for advanced epithelial ovarian cancer has demonstrated long-term, relapse-free intervals in patients with stage II or stage III disease. However, whole abdominal irradiation is controversial and requires further study.

Follow-up Care

Management is still unclear in patients who are clinically disease-free and have had primary debulking surgery and chemotherapy. Generally, a second-look surgery is performed after the completion of chemotherapy to assess a patient's response to treatment. If there is evidence of residual disease, investigational therapy is attempted. Asymptomatic patients are currently monitored every 3 to 4 months with a complete history, a physical, a rectovaginal pelvic examination, and CA-125 levels. Monitoring of CA-125 levels is used to detect early recurrence of disease in women who had elevated levels before surgery. A sevenfold fall in the CA-125 level indicates a good response to treatment. However, a normal CA-125 level does not necessarily exclude the presence of disease, and a rising level is predictive of a relapse. After 2 years, longer follow-up intervals can be considered.

In patients who have relapsed after primary therapy, salvage therapy is not curative. In fact, even though the response rate to treatment is very high, there is no evidence that it prolongs survival. When the primary treatment consists of platinum chemotherapy, the response to a secondary platinum regimen is based on the interval to relapse. Patients who relapse within 6 months generally have a poor response to platinum-containing regimens. The drug of choice for relapsed therapy is paclitaxel. Relapses that occur the second time have almost no possibility for a cure. These patients receive no benefit in survival from the various chemotherapeutic agents and have a response rate of only 15 percent.

Palliative Therapy

Since the majority of these women are diagnosed with advanced-stage disease, it is important to keep the patient's quality of life in mind at all times. Supportive measures to control pain, establish good nutritional habits, maintain proper hydration, and relieve additional suffering are critical. Emphasis should be placed on comfort, symptom control, and pain management. Small bowel obstruction is commonly seen with progression of the disease. Gastrointestinal problems can be treated with frequent, small feedings and medication to improve gastric motility. Relief from malignant effusions is achieved by performing paracentesis to draw off as much ascitic fluid as possible. Another problem encountered is pleural effusion, which can be alleviated temporarily by thoracocentesis.

Terminally ill patients also develop psychiatric problems that can severely alter their quality of life. These psychiatric symptoms usually result from uncontrolled pain or the medical complications of the illness or treatment and disappear. Supportive psychotherapy and pharmacotherapy should be prescribed for patients who exhibit depression or anxiety. The shorter-acting benzodiazepines, such as lorazepam, alprazolam, and oxazepam, are the preferred choices in the treatment of anxiety. For depression, the use of tricyclics or fluoxetine (Prozac) or sertraline (Zoloft) is extremely beneficial. Pain is best controlled with opioid analgesics. Issues pertaining to death and dying are another area a health care provider needs to understand in the overall management of patients with advanced disease. Decisions about resuscitation, hospice care, and family matters need to be addressed despite being difficult to initiate. Empathetic listening is helpful in minimizing the fear of abandonment and death that most patients entertain during the course of the illness. When appropriate, enlisting support from the clergy can be beneficial to the patient, family, and medical staff. All these supportive measures ultimately allow the patient to regain a feeling of control over the remaining portion of her life.

BIBLIOGRAPHY

Altchek A, Deligdisch L: *Diagnosis and Management of Ovarian Disorders.* New York, Igaku-Shoin, 1996.

Baker TR, Fiver MS: Etiology, biology, and epidemiology of ovarian cancer. *Semin Surg Oncol* 10(4):242–248, 1994.

Beekmann C, Ling F, Barzansky B: *Obstetrics and Gynecology,* 2d ed. Baltimore, Williams & Wilkins, 1995, pp 459–463.

Berek JS, Hacker NF: *Practical Gynecology.* Baltimore, Williams & Wilkins, 1989.

Blackledge GRP, Jordan JA, Shingleton HM: *Textbook of Gynecologic Oncology.* London, Saunders, 1991.

Cohen CJ, Jennings TS: Screening for ovarian cancer—the role of noninvasive imaging techniques. *Am J Obstet Gynecol* 170(4):1088–1094, 1994.

DeCherney AH, Pernoll ML (eds.): *Current Obstetric and Gynecologic Diagnosis and Treatment,* 8th ed. Norwalk, CT, Appleton & Lange, 1994.

Hacker NF, Moore JG: *Essentials of Obstetrics and Gynecology,* 2d ed. Philadelphia, Saunders, 1992, pp 602–612.

Herbst AL: The epidemiology of ovarian carcinoma and the current status of tumor markers to detect disease. *Am J Obstet Gynecol* 170(4):1099–1105, 1105–1107, 1994.

John EM, Whittemore AS, Harris R, Itnyre J: Characteristics relating to ovarian cancer risk: Collaborative analysis of seven U.S. case-control studies: Epithelial ovarian cancer in black women: Collaborative Ovarian Cancer Group. *J Natl Cancer Inst* 85(2):142–147, 1993.

Osmers RGW, Osmers M, von Maydel B, et al: Preoperative evaluation of ovarian tumors in the premenopause by transvaginosonography. *Am J Obstet Gynecol* 2:428–434, 1996.

Ovarian cancer: Screening, treatment, and follow-up: NIH Consensus Conference. *JAMA* 273:491–497, 1995.

Ovarian cancer: Screening, treatment, and follow-up: NIH Consensus Statement Online 1994 April 5–7, 1994. [cited 96/18/10] 12(3):1–30.

Whittemore AS: Characteristics relating to ovarian cancer risk: Implications for prevention and detection. *Gynecol Oncol* 5:S15–9, 1994.

Chapter 13–8
PANCREATIC CANCER
Patricia Kelly

DISCUSSION

Ductal adenocarcinomas account for almost 90 percent of pancreatic neoplasms. Approximately 60 percent occur in the head of the pancreas, 9 to 10 percent in the body and 7 to 8 percent in the tail; approximately 20 percent are overlapping or occur in an unknown subsite. Uncommonly, anaplastic cancers may occur, and rare cases of adenosquamous pancreatic cancers have been reported.

It is well established that there is a 9 in 100,000 incidence of disease in the overall U.S. population. African-Americans have an increased risk at 15 per 100,000. Males and females are equally affected. The cause is not known. However, several risk factors have been found:

- Cigarette smoking increases the relative risk to 1.5.
- Diets high in fat and/or meat raise the incidence to an unspecified level.
- Partial gastrectomy increases the risk twofold to fivefold (relative risk 2 to 5).
- It seems likely that diabetes enhances the growth of pancreatic cancer.
- Toxic substances, especially occupational exposure to 2-naphthylamine, benzidine, gasoline derivatives, and DDT and its derivative compounds, can increase the relative risk to between 4 and 7.

Coffee has been investigated extensively, but it has not been demonstrated that any possible human level of coffee intake increases the risk of this cancer.

SIGNS AND SYMPTOMS
Signs

The signs include

- Cachexia
- Low serum albumin
- Palpable abdominal mass
- Jaundice
- Recurrent idiopathic deep venous thrombosis
- Normal examination (50 percent)

Common Symptoms

The common symptoms include

- Abdominal pain
- Anorexia
- Weight loss
- Early satiety
- Easy fatigability
- Weakness
- Nausea
- Vomiting
- Constipation
- Depression (up to 40 percent)

Physical Examination

Palpable abdominal masses and/or jaundice should lead the clinician to evaluate the pancreas for a neoplasm.

DIAGNOSTIC STUDIES

Abdominal ultrasound can detect pancreatic cancers in 60 to 90 percent of cases. CT is less operator-dependent and can demonstrate the degree of invasion and lymph node involvement. Twenty percent of pancreatic cancers cannot be found on CT; these are potentially resectable lesions less than 2 cm in size. MRI may offer an advantage when other studies are suspicious but nondiagnostic.

After these noninvasive studies are completed, endoscopic retrograde cholangiography (ERCP) is utilized to visualize tumors of the pancreaticobiliary junction and obtain biopsies of accessible tumors. For other tumors, percutaneous fine-needle aspiration (CT-guided) is safe. Positive results are diagnostic; negative results with suspicious masses or other studies may require rebiopsy. Tumor markers are not generally useful.

Staging of Pancreatic Cancers

Staging is most important because only resectable tumors have the possibility of being cured. The TNM system is utilized, with T denoting tumor size:

T1: tumor that is localized to the pancreas
T1a: tumor that is less than 2 cm in diameter
T2: tumor that indicates extension into the duodenum, bile duct, or stomach
T3: tumor that is unresectable

T2 tumors may be resectable with major surgery [pancreaticoduodenal resection with or without preservation of the pylorus (Whipple's procedure with modification)]. Preoperative evaluation with CT, angiography, and laparoscopy is necessary to spare patients with unresectable disease (T3) unnecessary major surgery with significant morbidity and mortality rates.

TREATMENT AND PROGNOSIS

Less than 20 percent of these patients have true resectable disease. Surgery also is utilized for palliation in the relief of jaundice or duodenal obstruction. Even patients with resectable disease who undergo surgery have a 5-year survival rate less than 25 percent. This rate is improved for a very small subset of patients without any evidence of lymph node involvement; their 5-year survival rate may approach 50 percent.

The average survival of patients with nonresectable disease is no more than 6 months. The majority of studies demonstrate that the median survival of patients who receive chemotherapy is no better than that of patients who receive the best supportive care. A new chemotherapeutic agent, gemcitabine, has received approval from the U.S. Food and Drug Administration for use in patients with unresectable pancreatic cancer either as a first-line treatment or for persons who have failed therapy with 5-fluorouracil. Gemcitabine is a nucleoside analogue with antitumor activity. This agent may slightly increase median survival time. Radiation therapy combined with chemotherapy for locally advanced but unresectable disease increases the median survival time to approximately 10 months; the side effects are significant, and quality of life must be considered.

Supportive Measures

Supportive measures include aggressive pain management with narcotics and consideration of percutaneous chemical neurolysis of the celiac ganglion. The patient must be instructed to insist on appropriate doses of analgesics to control pain, since some clinicians may be reluctant to prescribe the large amounts required for patients with advanced disease.

Prevention

Smoking cessation for all patients is a general rule of preventive medicine and may help decrease the incidence of pancreatic cancer. Special attention should be paid to occupational exposures to the certain solvents (see "Discussion").

DISPOSITION

Patients who have had successfully resected disease generally are imaged with abdominal CT every 6 months for at least 5 years. The cost-effectiveness of this approach, however, is questionable since there is no truly effective salvage therapy.

BIBLIOGRAPHY

Prandoni P, Lensing AW, Buller HR, et al: Deep vein thrombosis and the incidence of subsequent symptomatic cancer. *New Engl J Med* 327:1128, 1992.

Sarcina R: Cisplatin (CDDP) + 5-fluorouracil (5-FU) in the treatment of advanced pancreatic adenocarcinoma (meeting abstract). *Ann Oncol* 3(suppl 5):25, 1992.

Tabbarah HJ: Gastrointestinal tract cancers, in Casciato DA, Lowitz BB (eds): *Manual of Clinical Oncology.* Boston, Little, Brown, 1995, pp 145–182.

Tempero M: Dose escalation of gemcitabine in previously untreated patients with pancreatic adenocarcinoma (meeting abstract). *Proc Ann Meet Am Soc Clin Oncol* 13:A660, 1994.

Chapter 13–9
TESTICULAR CANCER
Patricia Kelly

DISCUSSION

Testicular cancer is the most common malignancy in males between 20 and 40 years of age. White people are six times more likely to develop testicular cancer than are African-Americans. Risk factors include cryptorchidism (10-fold to 40-fold increase) and testicular feminization syndromes. Ninety-five percent of testicular cancers originate from germ cells. Approximately 40 to 50 percent of germ cell tumors are seminomas and usually occur in a slightly older age range (30 to 50 years). Another 50 percent are embryonal carcinomas and teratomas, which are more frequently found in men between ages 20 and 30. In elderly males, lymphomas predominate.

SIGNS AND SYMPTOMS

These patients are frequently asymptomatic and are diagnosed when a small testicular mass is noted during a routine sports or preemployment examination. As testicular self-examination becomes more popular, early detection should increase. The testicular mass may be painless. In one-third to one-half of these patients, a mild discomfort or "heaviness" is noted.

Unfortunately, common entities such as acute epididymitis may mask the palpation of a distinct tumor in up to 25 percent of patients with an underlying mass. Other presenting signs and symptoms include gynecomastia and infertility in a small percentage of males. Back pain is most commonly encountered when metastasis has already occurred, especially to the retroperitoneal nodes. Rare patients may have rapid tumor growth with associated necrosis and bleeding that results in flank pain. Patients with nodal metastasis may have palpable contiguous or distant lymph nodes.

Physical Examination

It is important to palpate the testicle with both hands, using moderate pressure and a "rolling" motion. Any palpable abnormalities, including induration and irregularity, should prompt a further workup.

DIAGNOSTIC CONSIDERATIONS

Hydroceles are not frequently malignant, but approximately 10 percent of men with testicular cancer have an associated hydrocele. If aspiration of hydrocele fluid yields blood, exploratory surgery is indicated. Transillumination of a suspected hydrocele may aid in the diagnosis but cannot definitively rule out a malignancy. Ultrasound is helpful in this situation. Varicoceles are swollen veins in the spermatic cord; they have a characteristic feel on palpation that has been compared to "a bag of worms." When the scrotum is elevated, venous distention is decreased.

Epididymitis should not exclude suspicion of testicular cancer (see Chap. 18-4). Both can cause pain and testicular swelling. Dysuria and pyuria are more common with epididymitis than they are with testicular cancer. Episodes of recurrent epididymitis with a return to interval normal testicular examination usually exclude neoplastic disease. However, if the clinical abnormalities do not resolve completely with adequate antibiotic and supportive therapy, exploratory surgery is indicated to rule out malignancy. Translucent spermatoceles and inguinal hernias generally can be differentiated from testicular cancer on physical examination. Entities such as infectious orchitis, hematoma secondary to injury, and acute testicular swelling, however, generally require surgery to definitively rule out neoplastic disease.

LABORATORY STUDIES

Approximately 50 percent of testicular tumors in patients between 20 and 40 years of age are nonseminomatous germ tumors. Ninety percent of these men will have either positive β-human chorionic gonadotropin (β-hCG) or alpha fetoprotein. β-hCG should never be found in a normal male and strongly implicates testicular cancer. Alpha fetoprotein occasionally can be found with malignant or non-malignant liver disease, especially hepato-

Table 13-9-1. Stages and Histologic Diagnosis of Testicular
Cancer

Stage	Histology
Stage A	Tumor limited to testes and cord
Stage B	Tumor of testes and retroperitoneal nodes
Stage B1	≤ 5 nodes positive for tumor
Stage B2	> 5 nodes positive for tumor
Stage B3	Nodes >10 cm (bulky disease)
Stage C	Distant metastatic disease found on imaging study or node biopsy above diaphragm

cellular carcinoma, but most strongly suggests testicular cancer in a younger age group.

Other laboratory studies are not routinely diagnostically useful, although some clinicians measure placental alkaline phosphatase as a marker for a seminoma.

RADIOLOGIC STUDIES

Although frequently performed, testicular ultrasound is rarely more specific than is physical examination. At this time there is no role for MRI or CT imaging of the testes.

EXPLORATORY SURGERY AND HISTOLOGIC DIAGNOSIS

Transinguinal unilateral orchiectomy is the diagnostic procedure of choice for a suspicious lesion. Routine preoperative laboratory and imaging studies, especially chest x-ray and liver function tests, may suggest metastatic disease. It must be emphasized that any type of needle or partial excisional biopsy is unacceptable and contraindicated. If the lesion is malignant, other diagnostic modalities are used to stage the neoplastic process. Treatment is based on tumor type and the extent of disease spread.

Chest CT and abdominal CT are used to image metastatic pulmonary and retroperitoneal disease. Any palpable upper body lymph node should be biopsied.

TREATMENT

The prognosis and treatment are dependent on the disease stage and histology of the tumor (Table 13-9-1). This table should be used as a rough guideline, since staging systems for seminomas and nonseminomatous tumors can vary.

Staging Process and Treatment

Seminomas

After a positive histologic diagnosis of seminoma is made, stage A patients and stage B1–B2 patients should obtain bipedal lymphangiography to determine radiation ports. Seminomas are extremely radiosensitive, and patients without evidence of nodal involvement receive 2500 cGy to the retroperitoneal area. Stage B2 patients receive a 1000-cGy boost to positive nodes. Chemotherapy is indicated for stage B3 or stage C disease.

Nonseminomatous Tumors

Stage A patients require retroperitoneal lymph node dissection alone after the initial orchiectomy. Subsequently, alpha fetoprotein and β-hCG must be remeasured. If these markers remain positive, residual disease is assumed and the patient is treated with chemotherapy.

Stage B1 patients with micrometastatic disease in one to six nodes <6 cm as found on retroperitoneal lymph node dissection may be observed monthly with alpha fetoprotein and β-hCG. If they are elevated, these patients require chemotherapy. Many

clinicians opt to treat all B patients with combination chemotherapy regardless of marker levels. Patients with stage B2–B3 disease must be treated with adjuvant chemotherapy. All stage C patients also must be treated with chemotherapy.

Chemotherapy for Nonseminoma Testicular Cancer

Combination chemotherapy with bleomycin, etoposide, and cisplatin is administered every 3 weeks for three or four cycles. The patient is then reevaluated; approximately 70 percent of these patients have a complete remission that may be long-lasting for stage B patients. Those with obvious residual disease on imaging studies are considered for debulking surgery and two additional cycles of chemotherapy. Patients with persistently elevated markers should receive two additional cycles of chemotherapy even in the absence of visible disease.

If the tumor persists, salvage chemotherapy with cisplatin, vinblastine, and ifosfamide can be considered. High-dose intensive multiagent chemotherapy followed by autologous bone marrow transplantation may be useful in selected cases. Recurrent disease also may be treated with these protocols.

DISPOSITION

Seminomas

Chest x-ray and liver function tests are given twice yearly for 2 years and then annually. Most, although not all, recurrences occur before year 3 of follow-up.

Nonseminomas

Lymph node physical examination and markers for all patients who do not receive chemotherapy should be performed monthly for 1 year and then bimonthly for 2 years. A bimonthly chest x-ray should be done.

In patients who are receiving chemotherapy, markers and chest imaging studies should be performed at every clinical decision point regarding the cessation or continuation of chemotherapy, or the patient should be changed to a salvage protocol. When the tumor markers become negative, one should follow as if the patient had initially been a stage A patient and repeat the markers monthly for 1 year and bimonthly for 2 years, with bimonthly chest x-rays.

PROGNOSIS

Both seminomas and nonseminomas have an excellent prognosis, with a true cure rate greater than 90 percent when the patient has limited (stages A and B1) disease. Cure rates are lower with more advanced disease, but significant remissions can occur. If the disease does not recur within 5 years, the chances for a true cure are high.

Prevention

Death from testicular cancer is almost totally preventable. Integrating testicular self-examination with interval clinician examination at every routine physical would ensure the early diagnosis of local disease, with an attendant 97 to 98 percent cure rate.

Patient Education

The diagnosis of testicular cancer in a young male can be psychologically devastating. Thorough discussions concerning the usual efficacy of treatment and an expedited staging evaluation are excellent ways to enhance a patient's coping skills. Men must be reassured that reproductive function and testosterone production continue in the remaining testicle and that an implant can be inserted at the time of surgery. The specific details of chemotherapy and radiation therapy can, however, interfere with reproduction function in the long term, although not with sexual performance once the course of treatment is complete.

BIBLIOGRAPHY

Einhorn LH: Treatment of testicular cancer—a new and improved model. *J Clin Oncol* 8:1777, 1990.

Einhorn LH, Lowitz BB: Testicular cancer, in Casciato DA, Lowitz BB (eds): *Manual of Clinical Oncology.* Boston, Little, Brown, 1995, pp 228–236.

Vogt HB, McHale MS: Testicular cancer: Role of primary care physicians in screening and education. *Postgrad Med* 92(1):93–96, 99–101, 1992.

Chapter 13–10
THYROID CANCER
Patricia Kelly

DISCUSSION

Seventy percent of the thyroid cancers found in adults are papillary cancers. Among these cases, regional lymph nodes are involved in approximately half the patients. These are indolent cancers with late, less frequent distant metastases compared with other head and neck neoplasms. Approximately 20 percent of the malignancies are follicular; these cancers peak in early middle age. With follicular thyroid cancer, metastasis is usually distant rather than to adjacent lymph nodes. Approximately 10 percent of thyroid cancers have unusual histologies and generally aggressive courses.

Risk factors include environmental radiation exposure and, most specifically, neck radiation given for benign conditions. The incidence of papillary thyroid cancer is especially increased in these circumstances. Heredity and congenital risk factors are thought to be rare and do not play a large role, with the exception of medullary thyroid cancer, which can be part of a dominantly inherited syndrome. Iodine deficiency is a risk factor for follicular carcinoma. Females are at increased risk; for every 1 male with thyroid cancer, 2.6 females are afflicted.

SIGNS AND SYMPTOMS

These patients may notice hoarseness or an enlarging neck mass. Rarely, neck pain occurs. Generally, these patients are asymptomatic. On physical examination, masses larger than 1 cm usually can be palpated. These patients may have a diffuse enlarged multinodular thyroid, although it is more common to find a single mass. A thorough physical examination of the thyroid gland, asking the patient to swallow during thyroid palpation, is imperative. Adjacent neck structures and lymph nodes also require thorough examination.

DIAGNOSTIC CONSIDERATIONS

Thyroglossal duct cyst remnants may resemble a thyroid nodule, and cervical lymph nodes can be mistaken for an enlarged thyroid or mass.

LABORATORY STUDIES

Chest x-ray, liver function tests, and serum alkaline phosphatase should be obtained to rule out metastatic disease in the lungs, liver, and bones. If alkaline phosphatase is elevated, liver and bone scans and directed plain films of abnormalities on bone scan are indicated. Routine thyroid function tests are usually normal in thyroid cancer patients.

RADIOLOGIC AND IMAGING STUDIES

Thyroid scans reveal nonfunctional "cold" nodules in 9 of 10 of these patients; only 10 percent of the nodules are malignant. Thyroid ultrasound does not enhance the sensitivity or specificity of the diagnosis.

Thyroid scans should be obtained, however, to exclude functional lesions, although some clinicians omit this step and perform a fine-needle aspiration biopsy. These biopsies have a false-negative rate of 5 to 10 percent. Since most thyroid cancers are indolent, routine thyroidectomies to reduce this false-negative rate are not recommended.

TREATMENT
Surgical

Total or modified total thyroidectomy is the procedure of choice. Neck dissection is not routinely indicated. Thyroxine is then given to suppress thyroid-stimulating hormone (TSH) to subnormal levels and is monitored with routine thyroid function tests, much as it would be in patients with hypothyroidism (see Chap. 5-3).

Patients can receive ablative therapy with iodine 131 postoperatively to destroy any residual thyroid tissue. The true value of the treatment is not known. It seems to be most rational in patients with large, multiple, or locally invasive tumors. Since it has been standard practice for some time, there are no controlled trials to validate this belief.

Although most thyroid cancer is indolent, if it does relapse, it is not very amenable to radiation or chemotherapy. These modalities are used primarily for palliation.

SPECIAL CONSIDERATIONS

Hyperparathyroidism can complicate the clinical picture after thyroidectomy unless radioactive ablative therapy is used. Blood calcium levels should be checked 1 week after thyroidectomy, especially if iodine 131 is not utilized or if the signs or symptoms of hypocalcemia appear. These patients may require chronic calcium and sometimes vitamin D supplementation and regular monitoring of blood calcium levels and signs or symptoms of hypocalcemia (see Chap. 5-10).

DISPOSITION
Prognosis

Less than 15 percent of patients with thyroid cancer succumb to it. Even distant metastatic disease can remain relatively dormant for many years. The raw data suggest a 95 percent 10-year survival for patients under age 40 and a 75 percent 10-year survival for patients over age 40. Persons with papillary thyroid cancer rarely die from the disease. Follicular thyroid cancer has an impressive 75 percent 10-year survival rate. Most fatalities arise from the histologically unusual or rare thyroid cancer variants, including anaplastic giant cell and spindle cell cancers, medullary thyroid cancers, and Hürthle cell cancer.

Patients should be scanned initially postsurgically; repeat scans should be obtained every 6 months, along with a chest radiogram, for 1 year. Patients then can be followed annually with these imaging studies. Thyroid function studies should be performed every 3 months or, as clinically indicated, for the first year. After that period, thyroid function studies should be performed as clinically indicated. Thyroid scans must be done in a "hypothyroid" state, and so replacement therapy must be withdrawn 6 weeks before follow-up scans.

Prevention

Known preventive measures include limiting radiation exposure to safe levels and designing garments to shield the thyroid area of persons who could receive repetitive radiologic exposure.

Physical examinations of the thyroid should be performed carefully on all persons, especially those with a history of radiation exposure or iodine deprivation.

BIBLIOGRAPHY

Carlson HE, Lowitz BB, Casciato DA, et al: Endocrine neoplasms, in Casciato DA, Lowitz BB (eds): *Manual of Clinical Oncology.* Boston, Little, Brown, 1995, pp 268–287.

Mazzaferri EL: Management of a solitary thyroid nodule. *New Engl J Med* 328:553, 1993.

Sakiyama R: Thyroid disorders, in Taylor RB: *Manual of Family Practice.* Boston, Little, Brown, 1997, pp 616–621.

Chapter 13–11
HODGKIN'S DISEASE
Patricia Kelly

DISCUSSION

Hodgkin's disease is a cancer that generally originates in the lymphatic system. It accounts for about 1 percent of newly diagnosed cancers and is most common in young adults (20 to 30 years of age) and adults above the age of 50. It occurs occasionally in children. Males and females are at essentially equal risk, although some cell types show a male or female preference.

The cause of Hodgkin's disease has not been discovered. Clinically, the disease can present slowly or in a limited area or can progress rapidly and systemically. Current therapy has an approximate 70 percent cure rate across the board; the stage of disease markedly influences the prognosis.

Risk factors have not been well delineated. In the United States, the disease found in younger adults seems to be more common with increased affluence and smaller family size. Some researchers have hypothesized that an infectious agent may be responsible; several multiple-sibling episodes have been reported. However, there is no definitive evidence for this hypothesis, and Hodgkin's disease remains a disorder of unknown origin.

SIGNS AND SYMPTOMS

Hodgkin's disease almost always originates in a lymph node. The axial lymphatic system is almost always affected; involvement of peripheral nodes outside the cervical chain is less common. Hodgkin's disease demonstrates contiguous progression throughout the lymphatic tissue. Mediastinal lymph node enlargement is frequently the first sign, encountered on routine chest x-ray. Hilar node involvement often follows. Cervical and supraclavicular adenopathy is common. Retroperitoneal lymphadenopathy is seen late in the course of the disease if it has started above the diaphragm; however, it may be an early sign of disease that originates in the inguinal area. An extranodal site is frequently the spleen. Other extranodal sites are rare at the time of disease presentation but can include the liver and bone marrow.

Constitutional symptoms are present in some cases of Hodgkin's disease (the so-called B symptoms) and are important for diagnosis and staging. These symptoms include persistent fever over 38.5°C (101.3°F), night sweats, and a 10 percent weight loss over 6 months. The presence of B symptoms confers a worse prognosis.

DIFFERENTIAL DIAGNOSIS

Lymphadenopathy in a young adult should prompt a thorough evaluation. Metastatic cancer to regional lymph nodes should always be ruled out in persons with a single area of nodal involvement. Localized adenopathy of course also can indicate a bacterial infection. HIV, especially in the early stages of seroconversion, can mimic Hodgkin's disease and should be considered in all persons with generalized lymphadenopathy and constitutional symptoms. Serologic tests should be used to rule out viral infection (HIV, Epstein-Barr), which can be confused with the presentation of Hodgkin's disease.

DIAGNOSTIC STUDIES

Physical examination should include palpation of all nodal areas, palpation of the liver and spleen, and a general overview of the patient. Initial diagnostic studies may include a complete blood count (CBC), which can point toward viral or bacterial etiologies; specific serologic studies for virus; a chemistry panel to define hepatic abnormalities that may be present with certain viruses, especially Epstein-Barr and cytomegalovirus; and chest radiography to demonstrate the presence or absence of mediastinal and hilar adenopathy. Skin testing for tuberculosis, which can cause identical constitutional symptoms and sometimes mediastinal adenopathy, is helpful. Mediastinal adenopathy in the absence of peripheral adenopathy strongly argues for a neoplastic origin. If the initial tests are inconclusive for another etiology, the definitive diagnosis, is made by means of lymphatic biopsy. Generally, lymph nodes larger than 1 cm that are present for longer than 3 weeks warrant biopsy.

Characteristically, the presence of Reed-Sternberg cells provides conclusive evidence of Hodgkin's disease. These are giant multinucleated cells; however, they may make up less than 1 percent of the malignant "bulk." There are four common histologic subclassifications of Hodgkin's disease, although a particular histology usually does not alter the prognosis or treatment substantially.

After a positive biopsy, initial evaluation should include CT of the thorax, including the pelvis; bilateral bone marrow biopsies; and possibly a lymphangiogram. If there is any suggestion of hepatic or splenic involvement on imaging studies, a laparotomy usually is performed if it will change the proposed treatment. Although it has not been extensively studied, MRI may be useful in avoiding staging laparotomies.

Stages of Hodgkin's Disease

Following are the stages of Hodgkin's disease:

Stage I: Hodgkin's disease confined to a single lymph node group
Stage II: involves more than one lymph node group but confined to above or below the diaphragm
Stage III: involves nodes on both sides of the diaphragm or involvement of the spleen
Stage IV: indicates hepatic or marrow malignancy

An A designation is used for persons with no constitutional symptoms. A B designation denotes constitutional symptoms.

TREATMENT AND PROGNOSIS

Surgery is utilized for diagnostic and staging purposes not for treatment. Radiation therapy is used for most patients with limited (generally stage IA and stage IIA disease). Radiation fields are dependent on the location of disease.

Chemotherapy generally is utilized for persons with constitutional symptoms and persons with stage III disease or above. Chemotherapy is also effective for stage I and stage IIA disease but is rarely used because of the increased risk and poor tolerance. However, clinical trials are ongoing in an attempt to improve long-term survival. Survival rates for persons with Hodgkin's disease, regardless of extent, who do not have constitutional symptoms are above 80 percent at 10 years. Patients with stage IIIB and stage IVB disease have a 60 to 80 percent survival rate. Seventy-five percent of persons who receive radiation alone for stage I or stage IIA disease remain disease-free, and relapses can be managed effectively over 50 percent of the time with chemotherapy. Persons who have bulky disease, generally stage III and stage IV, especially in the mediastinum, may benefit from combined radiation and chemotherapy.

Persons with extensive or aggressive Hodgkin's disease that relapses months after chemotherapy may benefit from high-dose cytotoxic therapy followed by autologous or allogeneic bone marrow or peripheral stem cell transplantation. Fortunately, these patients constitute a minority of all Hodgkin's disease patients.

Prevention and Screening

Since the etiology is not known, there are no specific preventive measures. There is no cost-effective screening test, with perhaps the exception of a thorough lymph node palpation during a routine physical examination. Screening chest radiograms for mediastinal adenopathy are not recommended because of low disease prevalence.

DISPOSITION

Patients are at greatest risk for relapse in the first 3 years. Persons who have received radiation therapy or chemotherapy should be followed carefully. Many oncologists recommend follow-up every 2 months for the first 2 years, then every 3 months for 2 additional years, and then every 6 to 12 months. Examinations should include a standard CBC with sedimentation rate and chemistry panel and a chest radiogram. If mantle radiation was received, routine thyroid function tests are indicated.

COMPLICATIONS AND RED FLAGS

In a primary care setting, it is more common for practitioners to see persons with a history of Hodgkin's disease than to see patients presenting for the initial diagnosis or for oncologic management. Therefore, all providers should be familiar with the sequelae of chemotherapy and radiation treatment.

Elevated thyroid-stimulating hormone (TSH) can occur in almost 50 percent of persons with a history of mantle radiation. Persons who have received gonadal radiation can present with infertility, although the testes usually are shielded. Men who receive certain types of chemotherapy [mechlorethamine, Oncovin (vincristine), procarbazine, and prednisone (MOPP)] will almost always be infertile; sperm banking before therapy should be encouraged. Women, however, can be rendered infertile, especially if they are older than 25. Radiation pneumonitis generally is seen in the acute oncologic setting and should not be a concern in primary care. However, cardiac damage, including cardiomyopathy significant enough to require transplantation, can occur after the concomitant use of doxorubicin (Adriamycin) and mantle radiation or high-dose doxorubicin alone. Aseptic necrosis of the femoral heads after the high-dose steroid therapy used in

some chemotherapy regimens is not uncommon. Patients treated with certain chemotherapy regimens can develop secondary malignancies a decade after treatment. Acute myelogenous leukemia, epithelial cancers, sarcoma, breast cancer, and other solid tumors have an increased incidence. Some of this can be related to the radiation exposure; the etiology of other cancer incidence increases is unclear.

BIBLIOGRAPHY

Bhatia S, Robison LL, Oberlin O, et al: Breast cancer and other second neoplasms after childhood Hodgkin's disease. *N Engl J Med* 334(12):745, 1996.
Canellos GP, Anderson JR, Properk KJ, et al: Chemotherapy of advanced Hodgkin's disease with MOPP, ABVD, or MOPP alternating with ABVD. *New Engl J Med* 327(21):1478, 1992.
Devita VT Jr, Hubbard SM: Hodgkin's disease. *New Engl J Med* 328(8):560, 1993.
Urba WJ, Longo DL: Hodgkin's disease. *New Engl J Med* 326:678, 1992.

Chapter 13–12
MULTIPLE MYELOMA
Patricia Kelly

DISCUSSION

Multiple myeloma is a type of plasma cell dyscrasia that is characterized by monoclonal production of IgG, IgA, IgD, IgE, or free monoclonal light chain (Bence Jones) protein. It is the most common plasma cell dyscrasia.

Multiple myeloma occurs in 0.00005 percent of the population and is therefore not a common disease in any age group. It is almost unheard of in persons under age 20; the risk increases with age. The highest risk is seen in those age 60 and older; men and women are equally afflicted. African-Americans have a higher incidence of this disease in the United States and have an earlier age of onset on average. Radiation exposure and chemical exposure (pesticides, petroleum products, and asbestos) add to the risk.

SIGNS AND SYMPTOMS

The early symptoms are quite nonspecific and include fatigue, weakness, decreased appetite, and sometimes weight loss. Further into the disease course, patients may present with bony pain, anemia, renal function abnormalities, neurologic symptoms, and repeated bacterial infections.

The physical findings can include skeletal pain on palpation, bruising with petechiae and purpura, epistaxis, numbness, pallor, wasting, and frank neurologic deficits.

Patients with the form of multiple myeloma characterized only by the production of Bence Jones proteins are prone to acute renal failure. Many multiple myeloma patients demonstrate mild to moderate renal insufficiency.

Multiple myeloma patients are functionally immunodeficient and frequently succumb to encapsulated organisms such as *Streptococcus pneumoniae* because they cannot synthesize normal specific antibody after antigen exposure. On hematologic examination, the complete blood count (CBC) frequently shows a normochromic, normocytic anemia and an elevated sedimentation rate. Leukopenia and thrombocytopenia are seen less commonly. If large numbers of plasma cells are seen in the peripheral blood, very aggressive disease or plasma cell leukemia must be suspected.

LABORATORY AND RADIOLOGIC STUDIES

Routine chemistry and a CBC are indicated. A protein immunoglobulin electrophoresis is also recommended. Approximately 50 percent of those patients show an IgG spike; 25 percent demonstrate an IgA spike, and almost 25 percent demonstrate Bence Jones proteinuria only.

Skeletal lesions are perhaps the most common finding on radiologic examination, which often is prompted by complaints of bony pain. These are osteolytic lesions produced by focal accumulations of plasma cells. The margins of these lesions are sharply defined and sometimes described by radiologists as "punched out." They may be present anywhere but are more common in the skull, ribs, spine, and pelvis.

Diffuse and generalized osteoporosis also may occur even in the absence of characteristic lytic lesions. This frequently leads to pathologic fractures, including compression fractures of the spine that cause neurologic deficits. Hypercalcemia is a common metabolic complication and can be seen on routine chemistry examinations. Increased levels of serum protein are also suspicious for this malignancy.

DIFFERENTIAL DIAGNOSIS

The characteristic symptoms of multiple myeloma are vague. Laboratory findings on routine chemistry and hematologic tests tend to be equally vague. If the diagnosis is suspected, electrophoresis can guide a clinician to the appropriate diagnosis rapidly. If characteristic lytic lesions or extreme osteoporosis is visualized radiographically, protein electrophoresis should be utilized to exclude multiple myeloma as an etiology before other, more invasive or expensive procedures or imaging techniques are used.

TREATMENT

Supportive care of the abnormalities characteristic of multiple myeloma is a cornerstone of treatment. Anemia can be corrected, bony pain can be treated palliatively, and hypercalcemia should be corrected with fluids and/or medication if necessary.

Transfusions of platelets may be appropriate. If renal failure is a prominent component, dialysis should be discussed with the patient as an option.

Immunodeficiencies can be corrected with intravenous gamma globulin; however, this is of limited usefulness. Febrile patients, especially neutropenic febrile patients, should be treated promptly and empirically with a wide-spectrum intravenous antibiotic combination.

Oral administration of melphalan and prednisone is the most common initial chemotherapy. It should be used intermittently and guided by symptomatic improvement. The response to chemotherapeutic agents includes relief of symptoms and improvement in hematologic parameters. For patients unresponsive to initial therapy, various intravenous chemotherapeutic agents have proved helpful but can induce multiple toxicities. In extreme cases, younger patients may benefit from bone marrow transplantation.

DISPOSITION

Prognosis

Without treatment, median patient survival is approximately 1 year. Careful, intermittent use of chemotherapy and other symptomatic measures can increase life expectancy significantly to almost 5 years. The natural tempo of each individual's disease greatly influences the prognosis and follow-up. Persons who present with advanced disease (poor performance status, hematocrit less than 30 percent, severe hypoalbuminemia and leukopenia, or marked renal insufficiency) have a very poor prognosis, with an expected survival of approximately 6 months; treatment may not alter this course substantially. In contrast, some individuals may have a disease course that appears to wax and wane and appear asymptomatic for longer periods. However, progression is the rule, and even if indolent disease is observed, treatment is indicated.

These persons most likely will be followed by an oncologist. If the primary care practitioner is seen during periods of indolent disease, routine hematologic and serum chemistry testing is appropriate. If disease progression is suspected, repeated immunoglobulin electrophoresis can provide a rough guide to disease progression and help direct oncologic therapy.

Screening and Prevention

Other than an "index of suspicion" on routine clinical encounters, there is no cost-effective screening test for multiple myeloma. Patients over age 50 who present with diffuse multisystem signs and symptoms and have characteristic hematologic and chemistry findings should undergo serum protein electrophoresis to rule out multiple myeloma. Prevention involves avoiding the environmental hazards, such as pesticides, petroleum products, and radiation, that are implicated in this and many other malignancies.

BIBLIOGRAPHY

Alexanian R, Dimopoulos MA: Management of multiple myeloma. *Semin Hematol* 32:20, 1995.
Seiden MV, Anderson KC: Multiple myeloma. *Curr Opin Oncol* 6:41, 1994.

Chapter 14–1
GLAUCOMA
Wesley T. Ota
Francis J. Sousa

DISCUSSION

Glaucoma is a disease of the optic nerve caused by intraocular pressure. It is one of the leading causes of blindness in the elderly population. There are two categories of glaucoma: open-angle and angle-closure. The first (90 to 95 percent of cases) tends to be chronic with slowly progressive visual field loss. This does not become apparent to the patient until late in the course of the disease. Angle-closure glaucoma (5 to 10 percent of cases) tends to have acute episodes that are symptomatic.

The exact pathophysiology of glaucoma is not well understood, but it is known to be more common in people older than 40 years, of African-American heritage, or with a family history of the disease.

Most people think that the intraocular pressure must be elevated (greater than 21 mmHg) for glaucoma to be present, though this is not always true.

SIGNS AND SYMPTOMS

Open-Angle Glaucoma

This is an asymptomatic disease until very late in the process. It is characterized by irreversible pericentral and peripheral visual field loss that, when advanced, patients notice as marked peripheral visual field loss. On examination, the eye may appear essentially normal with normal visual acuity, but the optic cup is enlarged, the intraocular pressure is elevated (greater than 21 mmHg), and visual field testing reveals characteristic visual field loss. Unfortunately, early visual field loss is difficult to detect on routine physical examination. This leaves the primary care provider with screening for elevated pressure and enlarged optic cups as the methods of diagnosis.

Patients older than 40 years old, especially if they are African-American or have a positive family history, should be screened yearly and referred to an eye doctor if the diagnosis is suspected.

Angle-Closure Glaucoma

This disease presents with ocular pain, decreased vision, halos around lights, and sometimes nausea and abdominal pain. The intraocular pressure is usually markedly elevated (greater than 40 mmHg), the conjunctiva is injected, the cornea is cloudy, and the pupil is in the middilated position and minimally reactive. Visual acuity is reduced.

Glaucoma is usually a disease of the elderly, becoming clinically significant after the age of 40. It is most often a bilateral condition that leads to slowly progressive visual loss. In glaucoma, the visual loss is not characterized by visual blurring, but by loss of the peripheral visual field. The disease is usually asymmetric, and the patients become symptomatic only late in the course of the disease.

OBJECTIVE FINDINGS

The objective findings in glaucoma are an enlarged optic cup, visual field defects, and usually an increased intraocular pressure. Unfortunately, sensitive visual field testing is difficult to perform routinely, making the importance of the optic cup evaluation and measurement of intraocular pressure crucial.

DIAGNOSTIC CONSIDERATIONS

The differential diagnosis of glaucoma is that of other diseases causing peripheral visual field loss, including retinitis pigmentosa, tumors, and stroke. The prevalence of this disease is so great that it should be the primary consideration when field loss is being considered.

SPECIAL CONSIDERATIONS

Glaucoma is more common in the elderly, African-Americans, and those with a family history.

TREATMENT

The treatment of glaucoma consists of medications, laser therapy, and surgery.

Open-Angle Glaucoma

The goal of therapy is to lower the intraocular pressure to the point that visual field loss is arrested. Medications, laser treatment, and surgery are used, generally, in this order.

Medications

The agent of first choice depends upon the patient. The following medications are used:

- Beta-blockers (timolol, betaxolol, levobunolol) (0.25/0.5%, usually have yellow-top bottles) work to decrease production of the aqueous leading to lower intraocular pressures (IOPs). Contraindications are asthma, chronic obstructive pulmonary disease (COPD), or any breathing problems; slow heart rate or heart block; and depression.
- Dipivefrin (0.1%, purple-top bottle) decreases production and increases outflow of aqueous. Contraindications include the fact that Dipivefrin may cause chronic follicular conjunctivitis.
- Dorzolamide (2%, orange-top bottle) is a topical carbonic anhydrase inhibitor that decreases production of aqueous. Contraindications include a sulfa medication allergy.
- Pilocarpine (1, 2, 4%, green-top bottle) increases outflow of aqueous to lower IOP. Contraindications are that it may cause fluctuations in vision, stinging, or brow ache.
- Apraclonidine (0.5%, white-top bottle) may work on trabecular meshwork to increase outflow.
- Latanaprost (0.005%, white-top bottle) is thought to work on the uveal-scleral outflow system.

Laser (Laser Trabeculoplasty)

In many patients treatment of the anterior chamber trabecular meshwork with approximately 50 laser burns increases outflow and lowers IOP. This is usually done over 180° of the anterior chamber angle. After 6 weeks, if the pressure is not significantly reduced, the other 180° of the anterior chamber angle may be treated.

Note: (1) The treatment is not a miracle. It may control pressures in patients that were not controlled on medications alone. (2) Generally, medications must be continued, although it may reduce the number of medications that a patient needs to take. (3) It may have just a transient effect, or no effect at all.

Surgery (Trabeculectomy)

If medications or medications in combination with laser do not control the pressure and if visual field loss is progressive, surgery may be required. By far the most common procedure performed is trabeculectomy, in which a new channel or hole for fluid to leave the eye is made, allowing flow of fluid from the anterior chamber to the subconjunctival space.

Also, in some cases tubes with control valves are implanted into the episcleral space. The tube allows flow of fluid from the anterior chamber of the eye to the subconjunctival space, just as the trabeculectomy does.

Angle-Closure Glaucoma

The treatment in this condition is to lower the IOP to a level near normal and then to create an alternative pathway for the aqueous to get to the trabecular meshwork from the posterior chamber without passing through the pupil. After IOP reduction has been achieved, the argon laser, or more recently the yttrium-aluminum-garnet (YAG) laser can be used to make an opening in the iris that allows this flow. The focusing of the laser allows the hole to be made in the iris without harming the cornea or lens.

SPECIAL CONSIDERATIONS

If acute uveitis is suspected, the patient should be asked about systemic diseases, especially arthritis, bowel disease, and skin disease. Although many different systemic diseases can be associated with uveitis, there are some that are more common: rheumatoid arthritis, ankylosing spondylitis, Reiter's syndrome, ulcerative colitis, and psoriasis. Sarcoidosis, syphilis, herpetic disease, and other systemic inflammatory problems may also be causes of uveitis.

LABORATORY TESTS

On the first episode of uveitis extensive laboratory testing is usually not indicated. If the history leads the practitioner to suspect a certain disorder, for example, ankylosing spondylitis, then testing may be performed to confirm or disprove this suspicion by obtaining sacroiliac joint x-rays and an HLA-B27 typing.

TREATMENT

The treatment of uveitis should always be under the supervision of an eye doctor. Usually a topical cycloplegic agent (e.g., homatropine, 5% drops tid, scopolamine, 0.25% drops bid) and topical prednisolone, 1% drops every 1 to 4 h, are prescribed. Patients are followed regularly by the eye doctor and tapered off the medications as the disease resolves.

Chapter 14–2
UVEITIS

Wesley T. Ota
Francis J. Sousa

DISCUSSION

Uveitis is inflammation of the uveal tract, the main vascular coat of the eye (the iris, the ciliary body, or the choroid). The disease is usually divided into anterior uveitis (iritis or iridocyclitis) and posterior uveitis (choroiditis). The etiology is often unknown, although trauma, infection, and autoimmune reactions can be related. It can be acute or chronic, and it can be recurrent. The most common form of uveitis is acute, anterior uveitis.

SIGNS AND SYMPTOMS

The classic triad of acute uveitis is redness, pain, and photophobia. The conjunctiva is injected, and often the distribution of the redness is most prominent around the cornea at the limbus. This is often referred to as ciliary flush. The pain is intraocular boring pain that can be throbbing at times. The photophobia is true intraocular pain when the eye is exposed to light (as opposed to glare, when the eye is overwhelmed by glare).

On slit-lamp examination the anterior chamber (AC) has inflammatory cells (clumps of white blood cells) and flare (protein) that has leaked in the AC. On the posterior cornea there may be deposits of white blood cells called keratic precipitates, or KPs. The pupil may be small. Vision may be decreased.

Chapter 14–3
AGE-RELATED MACULAR DEGENERATION

Wesley T. Ota
Francis J. Sousa

DISCUSSION

Age-related macular degeneration (AMD) is one of the leading causes of new blindness in older adults. It is a disorder that involves central vision (visual acuity) and is bilateral, although often asymmetric. The pathophysiology of the condition is not well understood, but it is thought to be a disorder of metabolism of the retina and choroid.

SIGNS AND SYMPTOMS

The symptom associated with AMD is central visual loss. Usually, this begins with mild to moderate decrease in visual acuity (20/40 to 20/60), but may progress to marked, severe central visual loss (20/200 to less than 20/400). Fortunately, peripheral vision is spared so that the patient can navigate with mild to moderate difficulty.

There are two stages of the disease process:

1. *Dry AMD* This is characterized by scattered yellow deposits in the macular area (called drusen) and associated areas of pigment atrophy (white areas) and pigment clumping (dark areas).

2. *Wet AMD* This is characterized by the above findings as well as by new blood vessels growing under the retina (subretinal neovascularization) which leak and bleed causing exudate and hemorrhage as well as causing a dark membrane under the retina.

DIAGNOSTIC CONSIDERATIONS

The differential diagnosis of age-related macular degeneration is that of central visual loss including refractive error, cataract, diabetes, and optic nerve disease. Also, the conditions that can cause macular deposits and/or macular hemorrhage must be considered, such as branch retinal vein occlusion, hypertension, diabetes, bleeding disorders, and arteriosclerosis.

SPECIAL CONSIDERATIONS

AMD should strongly be considered in elderly people with progressive central visual loss.

TREATMENT

The treatment of AMD is based on early diagnosis and patient education. It is crucial that patients play an active role in the daily monitoring of their vision so that they can detect treatable changes.

Most patients do not progress from the dry form to the wet form, but the disability can be devastating to those who do. Daily checking of central visual acuity is important using the Amsler grid. This allows the patient to detect early changes in central vision such as distortion or micropsia (images becoming smaller) that may be the first signs of a subretinal neovascular membrane (SRNVM). If this is detected, a fluorescein angiogram can be performed to diagnose whether the membrane is present and its exact location. If the membrane does not invade the foveal region, it can sometimes be treated with laser photocoagulation.

Unfortunately, by the time the diagnosis is made, the disease is often untreatable and will follow its natural course.

Recently, the use of medical therapy including vitamins, zinc, and antioxidants has been proposed as a possible medical therapy to prevent the progression of AMD to the wet stage in which central vision is lost completely due to SRNVM. These are still being studied, and definitive evidence of their effectiveness has not been shown.

Chapter 14–4
CATARACT
Wesley T. Ota
Francis J. Sousa

DISCUSSION

Cataract is defined as any opacity of the lens of the eye. This means that a cataract is a milkiness of the lens inside the eye, and not a growth over the surface of the eye, as many patients may believe. It is one of the leading causes of visual loss in adults. Vision can usually be restored with cataract surgery and intraocular lens implantation.

SIGNS AND SYMPTOMS

Cataract is usually a disease of aging, becoming clinically significant usually after the age of 50. It is most often a bilateral condition that leads to slowly progressive visual loss including blurring, distortion, and loss of color perception. Although the disease is bilateral, cataracts are almost always asymmetric so that the patient will complain of one eye being the particularly bad eye.

OBJECTIVE FINDINGS

Cataracts are detected on physical examination with the slit lamp and/or flashlight, but are most commonly and easily found objectively as shadows or black spots in the red reflex with an ophthalmoscope.

DIAGNOSTIC CONSIDERATIONS

The differential diagnosis of cataract includes any cause of progressive visual loss. The most common of these diseases are refractive errors, age-related macular degeneration (AMD), diabetic retinopathy with macular edema, and optic nerve disease.

Refractive errors can be detected on physical examination using a Snellen chart and a pinhole. If the vision improves significantly with the use of a pinhole occluder, then the cause of visual loss is probably due to an uncorrected spectacle error.

Even though the history of slowly progressive asymmetric visual loss may be very similar in AMD, it can be differentiated from a cataract by the appearance of the macular region of the retina. In AMD the maculae have scattered yellow spots (called *drusen*) and other pigment irregularities, including pigment dropout and pigment clumping. In severe forms of AMD, the macula may also be found to have exudate and hemorrhage. This form is usually accompanied by severe visual loss.

In diabetic retinopathy, visual loss can also be bilateral and asymmetric. Diabetic visual loss is differentiated by the presence of macular edema. Unfortunately, macular edema is extremely difficult to detect with the direct ophthalmoscope. Therefore, the history of diabetes control, fluctuations in vision, and the presence of the dot and blot hemorrhages, as well as hard exudates, are important for diagnosis.

Optic nerve disease is usually acute, but progressive lesions can present similarly to cataract. To differentiate optic nerve disease, the appearance of the optic nerve head (temporal pallor), the results of pupillary testing (positive afferent pupillary defect), and color vision are used.

SPECIAL CONSIDERATIONS

Although cataract can occur at any age, it occurs most commonly in the geriatric population. Therefore, when evaluating the significance of cataract and the benefits of treatment, it is particularly important to take a detailed history of the patient's visual needs and abilities, as well as disabilities. Systemic diseases must be taken into consideration, and the physical ability of the patient to tolerate surgery must be determined.

TREATMENT

The most common treatment of cataract is surgical removal of the lens with implantation of an intraocular lens. The procedure is performed electively as an outpatient procedure and has one of the highest success rates of any surgery. An increasingly common technique for performing cataract surgery is phacoemulsification. In this procedure, high-frequency sound waves are used to break up and remove the cataract.

Lasers are not used to perform cataract surgery, although many patients will ask about this. Sometimes, after cataract surgery, vision may slowly decrease due to opacification of the posterior capsule. When this occurs, the yttrium-aluminum-garnet (YAG) laser can be used to create an opening in the opacity. This procedure takes just a few minutes to perform as an outpatient procedure and can significantly improve vision.

After cataract surgery, patients are usually placed on a topical antibiotic for 1 to 2 weeks and a topical steroid for 1 to 2 months.

COMPLICATIONS

Although uncommon, infection, bleeding, inflammation, or retinal detachment may occur after the cataract operation, leading to visual loss. In general, anytime a patient complains of pain, redness, or blurred vision after a cataract operation, the surgeon who performed the procedure should be contacted immediately for evaluation and diagnosis.

Chapter 14–5
BLEPHARITIS

Wesley T. Ota
Francis J. Sousa

DISCUSSION

Blepharitis is a chronic inflammation of the eyelid margins. There are two categories of blepharitis: seborrheic and staphylococcal. Usually, a combination of both types occurs in most patients.

PATHOGENESIS

Blepharitis is an inflammatory reaction of the eyelids that can be caused by seborrhea, infections, and often a mix of the two. Infections are most commonly caused by the *Staphylococcus* organism, specifically *Staphylococcus aureus* or *Staphylococcus epidermidis,* but can be caused by other bacterial, viral, or fungal origins. Seborrheic blepharitis is associated with dermatologic conditions of the scalp and face. This occurs more commonly in elderly persons. More recent studies consider the inflammatory process to be a delayed or type IV hypersensitivity reaction to the exotoxins of the microorganism. This is a sterile autoimmune response.

The disease starts with telangiectasia and thickening of the eyelids. The chronicity of the disease creates a smoldering low-grade irritation and erythema of the eyelids. Crusting of lipid debris and eczema along the base of the lashes, madarosis (loss of lashes), trichiasis (misdirected lashes), and ulceration develop in the more severe stages of inflammation. Finally, conjunctivitis and keratitis can develop because of their apposition against the lids. A history of dandruff, atopy, and clogged eyelid glands (chalazia) is common with this disease.

SIGNS AND SYMPTOMS

The most common symptoms of blepharitis are burning and itching sensations of the eyelids and the eyes. Dry eye symptoms are also experienced with lid margin inflammation. There is no effect on vision. Affected patients usually report irritation and crusting worse on awakening in the morning, but it persists throughout the day. Redness of the eyelid margins and the eye is a common sign of this chronic disease.

OBJECTIVE FINDINGS

Examination of the eyelids reveals accumulation of debris such as scales and crusting on the base of the eyelashes. The eyelashes may be misdirected (trichiasis) or missing (madarosis) as the disease becomes chronic. There is often a thickened and hyperemic lid margin because of inflammation. This can sometimes develop into superficial ulcerations. Eczematous skin around the eyes and on the forehead and ears is commonly found with seborrheic blepharitis. The bulbar conjunctiva may be injected as the inflammation spreads to the globe.

DIAGNOSTIC CONSIDERATIONS

Active infection of the eyelid margins can occur from various etiologies, most commonly *Staphylococcus, Streptococcus,* gram-negative microorganisms, mites, herpes simplex, and herpes zoster.

PHARMACOLOGIC TREATMENT

There are no medications that cure blepharitis. Because it is a chronically occurring disease, only supportive measures are beneficial in keeping the inflammation under control.

SUPPORTIVE MEASURES

The treatment of blepharitis primarily involves eyelid hygiene, since eyedrops alone do not resolve the symptoms. The goal is to remove or minimize the offending organism or antigenic cause, thereby reducing the chronic disease process.

Eyelid hygiene should be performed first by placing a warm compress over the eyelid margins for a few minutes to soften and loosen the debris. Next, a cotton-tipped applicator should be dipped into a mixture of half baby shampoo and half water. The upper and lower eyelid margins and eyelash base should be scrubbed with the applicator, followed by a rinsing with regular tap water. This should be performed twice a day, and symptoms will diminish in approximately 2 weeks. Because this is usually a chronic problem, lid scrubs should be performed on a regular basis even after the symptoms have resolved. There are commercial lid scrub mixtures that can be purchased that serve the same purpose (Eye-Scrub, Ocusoft). Artificial tears can be used in addition to lid hygiene to reduce dry eye symptoms. Cold compresses can be used to decrease inflammation and promote vasoconstriction. Hypertonic saline solution soaks against the eyelid can reduce edema.

Treatment of seborrheic blepharitis should also include dermatologic management of the face and scalp.

PATIENT EDUCATION

Patients should be advised that this is a chronic disease and symptoms will recur unless lid hygiene is done on a regular basis. It is important that the lid scrubs are done properly, emphasizing scrubbing at the base of the lashes, as most failures occur when the skin of the eyelid is scrubbed and not the margins. Symptoms will be relieved after approximately 2 to 3 weeks of regular lid hygiene.

DISPOSITION

A follow-up should be done in 1 month to determine if symptoms and signs have regressed. A review of proper steps in lid hygiene should be emphasized.

COMPLICATIONS AND RED FLAGS

Severe chronic blepharitis can potentially cause corneal ulcerations that can impair vision. Any patient who complains of ocular surface pain should seek consultation with an eye doctor. Steroids should not be considered as part of the treatment plan by primary care health providers. There can be severely detrimental outcomes if steroids are used inappropriately.

Chapter 14–6
ORBITAL CELLULITIS
Wesley T. Ota
Francis J. Sousa

DISCUSSION

Orbital cellulitis is an acute infection of the orbital tissue of the eye. It is a very ominous infection that requires prompt treatment and hospital admission. It can cause permanent vision loss, intracranial infection, and potentially death if not treated appropriately.

PATHOGENESIS

Orbital cellulitis is an infection that occurs through vascular extensions to the orbit, vascular channels connecting to the adjacent sinuses, or postocular surgery. The most common cause of orbital cellulitis is paranasal sinusitis. The sinuses form the walls of the orbit except for the lateral aspect. The frontal sinus is found above, the ethmoid and sphenoid sinuses medially, and the maxillary sinus on the floor of the orbit. They are potential entrance ports of mucosal infections. A sheet of fascia called the orbital septum is the anterior-most aspect of the orbital cavity. It is a protective tissue that lines the walls of the orbit and extends to the tarsus of the eyelid. The orbital septum inhibits infections entering the orbit from the eyelids and the surrounding sinuses. Trauma can cause a break in the skin and create an opening through the orbital septum to cause an orbital cellulitis. Because the venous system of the orbit does not have valves, there are open communications with vessels of the nasal cavity, the face, and the sinuses potentially leading to infections.

SIGNS AND SYMPTOMS

The common symptoms of orbital cellulitis are acute pain and warmth around the eyes, decreased vision, and double vision. There may be signs of a purulent discharge because of the infection, diffuse lid swelling, conjunctival hyperemia, and often a febrile illness.

OBJECTIVE FINDINGS

Initially, eyelids are tender, warm, and erythematous. The patient commonly possesses a febrile illness because of the infection and usually presents to the office with a unilateral swollen and closed eyelid. Purulent discharge is often present. The eyelid must be raised to determine visual acuity. Vision can be reduced in orbital cellulitis as the disease progresses, but is not affected in a similar appearing inflammation called preseptal cellulitis. As orbital cellulitis progresses, the eye becomes more proptotic, ocular motility becomes limited causing double vision, and pain intensifies because of inflammatory reactions.

DIAGNOSTIC CONSIDERATIONS

The organisms most commonly involved with orbital cellulitis are *Staphylococcus* (*aureus, pyogenes*), *Streptococcus pneumoniae,* and *Haemophilus influenzae* (most common in children, exclusively in children under 5 years).

The *etiology* of the orbital cellulitis can result from paranasal sinusitis (most common cause), orbital trauma (causing injury to and penetration through the orbital septum), dental infections (through the maxillary sinus), eye surgery complications (retinal reattachment, strabismus), and bacteremia.

Differential diagnoses include preseptal cellulitis (infection limited anterior to the orbital septum with normal ocular motility and vision, absence of proptosis), orbital pseudotumor (purulent discharge absent), and chalazion (localized nodular swelling of the eyelid).

SPECIAL CONSIDERATIONS

The most frequent cause of orbital cellulitis in children is ethmoiditis. The ethmoid air cells are widely open at a young age, predisposing that sinus to nasal infections. A child presenting with fever, a swollen lid, eye pain, and proptosis is highly suspected of orbital cellulitis secondary to an extension of a nasal mucosal infection.

LABORATORY AND RADIOLOGIC STUDIES

Cultures and smears are taken to determine the causative organism and to tailor antibiotic treatment. A neurologic consult is obtained if meningitis is suspected.

A CT scan of the orbit should be performed to detect sinusitis, foreign bodies, and orbital abscesses.

PHARMACOLOGIC MANAGEMENT

The treatment of orbital cellulitis involves the early identification of the microorganism and aggressive administration of antibiotics. The patient should be admitted to the hospital for IV administration of broad-spectrum antibiotics until improvement. Paranasal sinus decongestion can be reduced with local sprays such as phenylephrine hydrochloride (Neo-Synephrine) or oxymetazoline hydrocholoride (Afrin), oral decongestants, and antihistamines.

SUPPORTIVE MEASURES

In cases of corneal exposure due to proptosis, antibiotic ointment (erythromycin, bacitracin) or lubricating ointment (Refresh PM, HypoTears) can be used to prevent exposure keratopathy. A cool compress can be used to decrease the inflammation if the patient is uncomfortable.

PATIENT EDUCATION

The patient should be instructed to complete the antibiotic therapy as prescribed to reduce the risk of recurrence and infection of a more virulent strain.

DISPOSITION

Progress is monitored by body temperature, visual acuity, ocular motility, and degree of proptosis. As definite improvement is seen in the orbital cellulitis, an oral antibiotic regimen can replace the intravenous treatment. The patient is examined every 2 to 4 days until resolution of the infection.

COMPLICATIONS AND RED FLAGS

In some cases, an orbital cellulitis infection progresses even after aggressive intravenous antibiotic therapy. This can occur with intraorbital abscesses and, less commonly, meningitis and cavernous sinus thrombosis. A CT scan of the orbit should be repeated to look for an abscess.

Immediate surgical drainage of an abscess should be performed under general anesthesia followed by additional intravenous therapy.

Chapter 14–7
CORNEAL ABRASION AND FOREIGN BODY

Wesley T. Ota
Francis J. Sousa

DISCUSSION

Corneal abrasions are superficial irregularities of the cornea caused by a foreign object. The object itself may still be present in the eye, or it may have merely scraped the cornea as in the case of a fingernail or a mascara brush. Pain, photophobia, and redness are the usual symptoms and signs related to the corneal insult.

PATHOGENESIS

The corneal epithelium, the most superficial layer of the cornea, is prone to abrasions by sharp objects or objects with significant force applied to the cornea. The insult causes a disruption of the smooth epithelial surface. Because there is an abundance of pain fibers in the cornea originating from the trigeminal nerve (cranial nerve V), intense pain, redness, and tearing occur with even minor abrasions. The epithelial insult stimulates an inflammatory process of the eye. Because the cornea is essentially avascular, no significant changes are observed. However, the conjunctiva and periorbital area become hyperemic and edematous. Pain thresholds are reduced. All these factors are associated with the release of inflammatory chemical mediators such as prostaglandins, histamine, and bradykinins. The metabolism of the cornea is so high that many superficial corneal abrasions will heal within 1 day as cells multiply and slide over to cover the defect. Deeper or larger abrasions may take 4 to 5 days, depending on the severity.

SIGNS AND SYMPTOMS

The hallmark symptom of a foreign body or corneal abrasion is acute pain because of the abundant number of pain receptors in the cornea. As the cornea becomes traumatized, these pain receptors are enhanced, which leads to heightened pain. The patient may experience less pain if the eyelid is lifted above the cornea. This can occur because of two reasons: there is minimal contact of the eyelid with the disrupted cornea, causing less insult to this area, or the foreign object under the upper lid will not cause additional insult to the cornea as it is raised. Photophobia (pain induced by light), hyperemia, and increased tearing are commonly associated with corneal abrasions and foreign bodies.

OBJECTIVE FINDINGS

Visual acuity can be decreased if the central cornea is affected. The patient commonly presents to the clinic with the eye closed because of pain and sensitivity to light. Profuse tearing is usually associated with corneal abrasions. The bulbar conjunctiva is diffusely hyperemic on external examination. If the patient is unable to open the eye because of pain, a topical ophthalmic anesthetic drop can be used to reduce discomfort so that the eye can be examined. This is recommended as a final resort, since a patient with residual foreign bodies in the eye may be asymptomatic until the anesthetic effect is diminished. This usually occurs after the patient leaves the clinic and has returned home. In cases of disrupted corneal epithelium, the crisp reflection of a penlight will be irregular on external examination.

Upon application of a fluorescein strip, the disrupted corneal epithelium will stain green under a cobalt blue or black light. The appearance of the stain may be linear, usually vertically oriented, in foreign body tracks from an object under the upper lid. A pooling of fluorescein will occur around an object embedded in the cornea. Generalized staining will occur in a corneal abrasion with its pattern being dependent on the object that caused the abrasion. For example, a blunt object will cause a wide epithelial stain, whereas a fingernail will cause a narrow and linear stain. The lids should be everted and evaluated if the history and findings support evidence of a foreign body in the eye. The magnification of a biomicroscope (slit lamp) is used for the best evaluation of the cornea. Burton lamps with fluorescein strips, ocular lens loupes, and gross observation are other methods of corneal evaluation.

DIAGNOSTIC CONSIDERATIONS

The differential of an acute painful red eye includes iritis (injection localized at the limbus, miotic pupil, and decreased vision) and angle-closure glaucoma (diffuse red eye, a middilated pupil, corneal edema, and high intraocular pressures).

PHARMACOLOGIC MANAGEMENT

The goal of management of a corneal abrasion is to promote reepithelialization. The corneal epithelium is the protective layer of the eye. During the interim, the cornea must be protected from bacterial infection entering the disrupted epithelium, and the patient kept comfortable. If there is pain involved with the abrasion, pressure patching the eye for 24 h will increase comfort as well as increase the rate of healing. The patch should be applied with adequate pressure rather than loosely so that the eyeball cannot move and further disrupt the cornea. The use of a pressure patch is optional and used for comfort only.

A topical antibiotic ointment (bacitracin, erythromycin, tobramycin) is used prophylactically under the eye patch to prevent secondary infections. A secondary iritis can develop from spasm of the ciliary body muscle which is a reflex from eye pain. A topical drop of a cycloplegic agent (scopolamine 0.25%, homatropine 5%, cyclopentolate 10%) is instilled prior to patching to paralyze the muscle and reduce the risk of iritis. This also decreases intraocular pain caused by ciliary muscle spasm. A side effect of this drop is a dilated pupil and should cause no alarm in follow-up of the patient.

If there is a foreign body present in the eye, a sharp object such as a 22-gauge needle or a pin can be used to flick the object off and away from the cornea. A sharp, rather than blunt, object is used to reduce further epithelial disruption from iatrogenic causes when attempting to remove the foreign body. There are battery-operated instruments, such as an Alger brush, which have a high spinning tip that can dislodge the foreign body from the eye. If the object is away from the cornea, a blunt object such as a cotton-tipped applicator can be used to remove the foreign body.

SUPPORTIVE MEASURES

Oral analgesics such as aspirin, acetaminophen (Tylenol), and ibuprofen (Advil, Motrin) can be considered for the pain. More potent analgesics such as tramadol hydrochloride (Ultram) or acetaminophen with codeine (Tylenol 3) can be used for more severe symptoms.

PATIENT EDUCATION

The patient should be instructed to wear the eye patch continuously overnight until the follow-up appointment without removal. The patient should be instructed not to drive or operate dangerous machinery with any eye patching, because of loss of depth perception. Should pain increase after leaving the office, the patient should contact the office or an eye doctor for evaluation. Any corneal abrasion that does not appear to be improving on follow-up should be seen by an eye doctor as well. Patients with foreign bodies should be instructed to use protective eyewear when engaging in causative activities.

DISPOSITION

A mandatory follow-up evaluation should be performed the next day. The patch should be removed in the office. Visual acuity should be measured. Acuity may be slightly decreased because of residual epithelial disruption or the applied antibiotic ointment. The pain should be significantly less than the previous day. Inspection of the cornea should be performed in the same manner as the initial evaluation. Continue patching with a cycloplegic drop and an antibiotic ointment if significant epithelial disruption still persists or if the patient is still slightly symptomatic. If significantly resolved, use a broad-spectrum antibiotic drop (Polytrim, Tobramycin) qid for 3 to 4 days.

COMPLICATIONS AND RED FLAGS

If pain has not decreased, or if there is no improvement of the epithelium, a consultation with an eye doctor is recommended. Additional foreign bodies, secondary infections, or iritis can be the cause of nonresolving symptoms and signs. Corticosteroids should not be used in corneal abrasions because they can allow easier access of bacteria and viruses through the cornea and into the eye.

Chapter 14–8
DIABETIC RETINOPATHY

Wesley T. Ota
Francis J. Sousa

DISCUSSION

Diabetic retinopathy is the retinal manifestation of the systemic disease diabetes mellitus. (See Chap. 5-1, "Diabetes Mellitus.")

It is the leading cause of blindness among working-age adults in the United States. The risk of retinopathy increases with the duration of the disease and the patient's age. Type I diabetics commonly have more complications associated with diabetic retinopathy in their lifetime. The Diabetic Control and Complication Trial (DCCT) found the progression of diabetic retinopathy in type I diabetics was significantly reduced if the blood glucose levels were in strict control. Glucose levels less than 200 mg/dL significantly decreased the frequency of microvascular complications.

PATHOGENESIS

Diabetic retinopathy is essentially a disease of microvascular occlusion. As vessel walls tend to weaken, some develop microaneurysms while others close off, causing the surrounding tissue to die. The early stage of the disease is called *nonproliferative diabetic retinopathy.* The initial changes may be invisible, but continued deterioration results in visible blood or blood components in the retina such as hemorrhages, hard exudates (lipid accumulation), and edema (serum). Further in the disease process, hypoxia will result in cotton-wool spots (focal infarction).

The disease can progress and lead to a stage called *proliferative diabetic retinopathy.* Hypoxic tissue releases an angiogenesis factor, triggering the growth of new vessels to supply oxygen. This is known as neovascularization. These new vessels are fragile and can break, resulting in a vitreous hemorrhage. In conjunction with the neovascularization, there are fibrocytes that proliferate and contain contractile proteins which shrink the fibrovascular stalk growing into the vitreous. They cause traction of the retina that can lead to a retinal detachment or a vitreous hemorrhage.

SIGNS AND SYMPTOMS

There are usually no symptoms in patients with nonproliferative or proliferative diabetic retinopathy. Visual acuity may be decreased if significant leakage of blood vessels occurs in the macula. Many patients notice daily changes in their vision as their blood sugar fluctuates. This causes changes in the thickness of crystalline lens of the eye resulting in non-vision-threatening refractive error shifts. In cases of acute retinal detachments in severe diabetic retinopathy, patients may experience loss of vision, flashing lights, or an increasing number of new floaters in the eye. Vitreous hemorrhages can also cause the same symptoms.

OBJECTIVE FINDINGS

Visual acuity may or may not be affected in diabetic retinopathy. On fundus examination, hemorrhages (red), exudates (yellow), and cotton-wool spots (white) can be scattered throughout the fundus. Decreased visual acuity and an absence of a red reflex may occur with a retinal detachment or vitreous hemorrhage. A thorough evaluation can be done only through a dilated pupil.

DIAGNOSTIC CONSIDERATIONS

In addition to diabetic retinopathy, hemorrhages in the retina can be caused by a variety of other vascular diseases, most commonly central retinal vein occlusions (CRVO), branch retinal vein occlusions (BRVO), hypertensive retinopathy, and blood hyperviscosity syndrome.

TREATMENT

Diabetic changes may occur in the peripheral retina, which cannot be seen solely through a direct ophthalmoscope. Diabetic retinopathy is best monitored and managed by an eye care practitioner. They have the topical ophthalmic agents available to dilate the eye as well as additional instruments to view the entire fundus. Patients should be asked when their last dilated fundus examination was performed. If they are unsure, ask if they received dark glasses upon leaving the office. Confusion exists if patients are asked if drops were placed in the eye because eyedrops that are commonly used to measure intraocular pressures do not dilate the eyes.

The following are the recommended guidelines for retinal evaluations in diabetics.

Examination frequency involves one of two types of dilated retinal evaluation:

1. Five years after diagnosis, at puberty if diagnosis is prior to that, and at least annually thereafter
2. Upon diagnosis and at least annually thereafter

With surgical treatment, laser instruments are used to cauterize leaking blood vessels or to reduce the oxygen demand of the retina. In cases of retinal detachments or vitreous hemorrhages, surgical vitrectomy and retinal attachment are performed in an attempt to restore as much visual function as possible.

PATIENT EDUCATION

Regulating blood sugar to acceptable levels is crucial in reducing risk of complication of diabetic retinopathy as well as other organ problems. The importance of routinely scheduled dilated retinal examinations by eye care practitioners, at least annually, should be emphasized to the patient. Symptoms that require immediate referrals are listed under "Complications and Red Flags," below, and should be explained to the patient.

DISPOSITION

Proper education should be reviewed, emphasizing a dilated fundus examination at least annually and more frequently if recommended by the eye care provider.

COMPLICATIONS AND RED FLAGS

Diabetic retinopathy is the leading cause of blindness among the working age population in the United States. There are certain symptoms that require immediate referral to an eye doctor. These are symptoms of retinal detachment or vitreous hemorrhage.

The following conditions warrant immediate eye care practitioner referral:

1. New onset of floaters
2. Sudden decreased vision (centrally or peripherally)
3. Flashes of light

In cases where loss of functional vision has developed, consultation with a low-vision specialist is recommended. They are eye care practitioners who can prescribe magnifiers, telescopes, and other optical and nonoptical aids to assist the patient who has visual impairment related to diabetes or other visually impairing eye diseases.

Diabetes is a disease of multiorgan complications. A team approach and communication between all involved health care providers are crucial in minimizing complications created by this potentially debilitating disease.

Chapter 14–9
ENTROPION AND ECTROPION

Wesley T. Ota
Francis J. Sousa

DISCUSSION

Entropion and ectropion are abnormal appositions of the eyelid margins. Entropion occurs when the eyelid margin is turned *inward,* toward the eyeball. Ectropion is the opposite situation, where the eyelid margin is turned *outward,* away from the eyeball.

PATHOGENESIS

Entropion most commonly occurs due to an involutional change (age). A complex change of the fascia takes place, leading to stretching and disinsertion. Cicatricial causes create a shrinkage and foreshortening of the conjunctiva, resulting in a pulling of the lid margin inward.

In ectropion, the most common cause is involutional. This results from a lengthening of the lower medial and lateral aspect of the eyelid margin. In cicatricial ectropion, there is a shortening of the laminar portion of the skin on the eyelid. Trauma, such as burns or scars, can cause the shrinkage of this tissue. Palsy of the facial nerve can paralyze the lower lid muscles and give them a laxity, causing ectropion.

SIGNS AND SYMPTOMS

Entropion and ectropion can both cause irritation of the eye. There can be excessive tearing and sensitivity to light, as well as foreign-body sensation of the eye. In some occasions, the patient may be asymptomatic. The eye is commonly red because of dryness or irritation.

OBJECTIVE FINDINGS

The diagnosis can be made on the external examination of the eye. In entropion, the entire lid margin, most commonly the lower, is rolled inward toward the eye. A portion or entire row of eyelashes can be hidden since the margin is turned inward. Eyelashes can commonly be seen against the eyeball itself since they are rolled inward. Redness and tearing can occur from irritation of the eyelashes against the cornea producing a foreign body insult. Tear dysfunctions can also occur because of the interruption of the tear layer by the eyelashes and lid margin against the eye.

In ectropion, the lower lid margin droops outward, away from the globe. The pink palpebral conjunctiva is often visible because there is poor apposition of the eyelid to the globe. This does not occur in the upper eyelid since gravitational forces allow the lid to rest on the eyeball. There is often a false sign of excessive tearing because the tear drainage channel of the lower nasal puncta is not in proper position. Rather than flowing out through the puncta, the tears flow over the lid margin. However, excess tearing and irritation of the eye can occur, since the inferior globe and inner eyelid are exposed to air and cause dryness. This can produce a reflex hypersecretion of tears to offset the dry eye. The cornea can show irregularities on evaluation with fluorescein stain because of exposure to air. As the irregularity progresses, keratinization of the conjunctiva can develop secondary to the chronic severe exposure and dryness.

Visual acuity should not be affected in pure entropion and ectropion conditions. Keratopathy may develop as a secondary complication and should be assessed with a fluorescein strip and a cobalt blue light.

DIAGNOSTIC CONSIDERATIONS

Entropion, or the inwardly turned eyelid, can occur from the following causes: aging, spastic (caused by acute lid swelling and resolves after swelling decreases), congenital, and cicatricial (caused by trauma, chemical injuries, inflammatory processes such as trachoma; the conjunctiva develops submucosal scarring and vascularization resulting in conjunctival shrinkage and loss of mucus-producing cells.)

Ectropion, or the outwardly turned eyelid, can be precipitated by the following causes: aging, facial nerve palsy (cranial nerve VII), congenital, cicatricial.

The differential diagnosis of entropion includes trichiasis. The same type of symptoms can occur, but the cause is the misdirection of eyelashes toward the globe with a regular lid margin. Trichiasis commonly occurs with chronic inflammation of the eyelids known as blepharitis. (See Chap. 14-5, "Blepharitis.")

PHARMACOLOGIC MANAGEMENT

Artificial tears should be used in both situations to keep the eye lubricated. Because of the frequent applications, a preservative-free artificial tear product should be considered. Carboxymethyl-cellulose 1% (Celluvisc) is often used because of its preservative-free and viscous characteristics. An ocular ointment should be applied at bedtime for lubrication as well. This can be used in place of artificial tear supplements during the day but will impair vision because of its oily properties.

In cases of keratopathy, antibiotic ointments (bacitracin, erythromycin) should be applied qid to protect the cornea from secondary infections. Aminoglycoside ointments such as tobramycin (Tobrex) are not recommended because of their toxicity to the cornea during long-term use.

SUPPORTIVE MEASURES

In both situations, taping the eyelid into normal position can minimize secondary ocular symptoms and complications. In entropion, the lid margin should be everted so that the eyelashes are directed away from the globe prior to taping the eyelid. In ectropion, the lid margin should be positioned against the globe before taping. Epilation of the eyelashes in entropion cases significantly decreases the foreign-body sensation and corneal complications. Cool soaks can be used in both situations to decrease swelling and inflammation.

SURGICAL INTERVENTION

Surgical repair of the lid is required if the condition persists and the patient is symptomatic. A consultation with an oculoplastic surgeon is recommended if this procedure is considered. Spontaneous resolution should be considered prior to surgical intervention in cases such as facial nerve palsy and spastic entropion.

PATIENT EDUCATION

Patient education is important in explaining the cause of irritation as well as the management needed to prevent severe ocular complications. The importance of constant lubrication of the eye should be emphasized to protect the cornea from scarring, which can lead to vision loss.

DISPOSITION

Follow-up should be done as needed in mild cases of entropion or ectropion. If the patient is symptomatic, evaluation should be done in 1 to 2 weeks or sooner if the problem worsens. Patients should be instructed to return if an acute red or painful eye develops. A referral to an oculoplastic surgeon should be considered if the problem cannot be managed by supportive measures.

Chapter 14–10
HERPES SIMPLEX KERATITIS
Wesley T. Ota
Francis J. Sousa

DISCUSSION

The herpesviruses, HSV-1 and HSV-2, are DNA viruses whose natural reservoir is human. The transmission of the virus occurs through direct contact. It is the most ubiquitous communicable infectious virus in humans. Herpes simplex is the leading cause of infectious corneal blindness in the United States.

PATHOGENESIS

Approximately 70 to 90 percent of the population show evidence of previous HSV infection by age 15 and 97 percent by age 60. Primary illness is clinically manifested in only approximately 1 to 6 percent of cases. The virus then becomes latent and remains in the trigeminal ganglion. Infection of the eye is uncommon in primary herpes simplex. Almost all herpes simplex keratitis infections present in the recurrent stage and are predominantly of HSV-1 type. As the virus replicates on the corneal epithelium, further breakdown of the epithelium occurs. If the infection progresses, deeper corneal tissues become inflamed and can eventually cause an iridocyclitis which is an inflammation of the iris and ciliary body.

SIGNS AND SYMPTOMS

The symptoms of herpes simplex keratitis can include tearing, irritation, photophobia, and decreased visual acuity. These symptoms can occur on their own or in conjunction with the others. Hyperemia of the conjunctiva is a common sign of herpes simplex keratitis.

OBJECTIVE FINDINGS

The objective findings of herpes simplex keratitis can vary with each presentation. In primary infections, acute follicular conjunctivitis and preauricular adenopathy are present. There are usually vesicular eruptions of the periocular skin. This should be differentiated from the vesicular eruption of the entire first branch of the trigeminal nerve, which occurs with herpes zoster ophthalmicus. There is usually diffuse bulbar conjunctival injection of the affected eye, and corneal sensation is commonly reduced. In recurrent infections, many of these findings may not be present. Often the disease is confined to the cornea. The corneal findings on fluorescein evaluation classically reveal dendritic lesions with minute terminal bulbs at the ends of the branches, but in some cases, the disease may present as minute, diffuse, punctate lesions or as a large geographic lesion.

Table 14-10-1. Topical Antivirals for Herpes Simplex Keratitis

Medication	Dosage	Comments
Trifluridine 1% (Viroptic)	1 gt. q2h max 9×/d until reepithelialized; cont. additional 1 gt. qid × 7d	Treatment of choice because of lowest toxicity of topical antivirals
Vidarabine 3% (Vira-A)	Apply 1/2″ strip to affected eye q3h 5×/d	Will impair vision because of ointment form; can be used h.s. in addition to trifluridine
Idoxuridine 0.1% sol or 0.5% ung (Herplex, Stoxil)	Sol: 1 gt. q1h during the day and q2h at night; ung: apply 1/2″ strip to affected eye q4h 5×/d	Generally not used unless other antivirals are not effective or create allergic reactions

NOTE: sol = solution; ung = ointment; gt. = drop; h.s. = at bedtime.

DIAGNOSTIC CONSIDERATIONS

There are various factors which can induce activation of the herpesvirus, most commonly sunlight, fever, immunodeficiency, heat, local trauma, and emotional stress.

SPECIAL CONSIDERATIONS

Any person who has a red or irritated eye should be questioned about a previous herpes keratitis, recent trauma, or any predisposition to cold sores. Any dendritic corneal lesion or decreased corneal sensitivity should be considered herpes simplex keratitis until proved otherwise. Pseudodendritic lesions and decreased corneal sensation can occur in herpes zoster ophthalmicus. Pseudodendrites can occur in contact lens wear secondary to contact lens solution preservatives which create toxicity of the cornea. Although most cases of primary herpes are subclinical, herpes simplex keratitis should be considered in any acute red eye in children or teenagers.

PHARMACOLOGIC MANAGEMENT

Various antiviral agents are presently being used to treat herpes simplex keratitis. The treatment of choice is trifluridine ophthalmic drops 1% (Viroptic) used nine times a day for 10 to 14 days until lesions resolve (see Tables 14-10-1 and 14-10-2). The eyedrop is then tapered according to corneal findings. Trifluridine, in comparison to the other topically applied antivirals, is found to be least toxic to the corneal epithelium. Because the use of drops can be difficult in uncooperative children, a topical ointment, vidarabine 3% (Vira-A), can be applied five times a day for 10 to 14 days until lesions resolve. Idoxuridine (Herplex) is not commonly used because of its high corneal toxicity, but

can be applied in case of allergic reactions to the previously discussed medications. The topical ophthalmic form of cidofovir is currently being investigated for the treatment of herpes simplex, varicella zoster, and adenovirus.

The use of oral acyclovir (Zovirax), 400 mg PO five times a day; valacyclovir (Valtrex), 500 mg PO tid; or famciclovir (Famvir), 500 mg PO bid for 7 days can be taken in cases where topical agents cannot be applied, or if bilateral eye infections exist. Acyclovir classification of drugs is contraindicated in pregnant women and persons with renal disease.

SUPPORTIVE MEASURES

Cool compresses can relieve some of the inflammation if the patient is symptomatic.

PATIENT EDUCATION

Patients should be informed about the recurrent nature of the disease and the importance of seeking eye care when significant irritation, redness, or photophobia develop. When seeking eye care for an inflamed eye, the patient should inform the office while making the appointment that there is a history of herpes infection of the eye. Patients should be educated on the possible causes of recurrence such as stress, trauma, and sun exposure.

COMPLICATIONS AND RED FLAGS

The treatment of ocular herpes infection can be challenging. This, and any corneal infections, should be managed by an eye doctor who has the proper equipment and time to closely follow the patient. An iritis can occur in association with herpes simplex keratitis which manifests with symptoms of decreased vision and photophobia. *The use of topical steroids is contraindicated in herpes simplex keratitis infections* because it predisposes the cornea to further breakdown and increased infection. Steroids have been found to inhibit formation of substances needed for the integrity of corneal structure and enhance collagenolytic enzymes causing thinning and possible perforation of the cornea. Any use of oral, inhaled, or topical corticosteroids should be discontinued by the patient during epithelial infection if safe to do so. Corneal stromal or uveitic involvement, which is a secondary complication of the eye, may require treatment with topical corticosteroids prescribed by an eye doctor.

Table 14-10-2. Oral Antivirals for Herpes Simplex Keratitis

Medication	Dosage	Comments
Acyclovir (Zovirax)	400 mg PO 5×/d × 7d	Generically available in reduced price, making it cost-effective
Valacyclovir (Valtrex)	500 mg PO tid × 7d	Pro-drug of acyclovir but no major benefits except less frequency of dosage
Famciclovir (Famvir)	500 mg PO bid × 7d	Less frequency of dosage compared with acyclovir but no other major advantage. Treatment of choice in herpes zoster because it diminishes the extent of postherpetic neuralgia

Chapter 14–11
LEUKOCORIA

Wesley T. Ota
Francis J. Sousa

DISCUSSION

Leukocoria means "white pupil." When the normally black pupil is seen as white, or the red-reflex as darkened on the ophthalmoscopic examination, the diagnoses of retinoblastoma, congenital cataract, persistent hyperplastic primary vitreous, and retinopathy of prematurity should be considered.

Retinoblastoma

Retinoblastoma is the most common intraocular malignant tumor in children. It occurs in about 1 in 20,000 live births causing about 1 percent of childhood deaths from cancer. It may present at birth, but usually presents between 8 months and 3 years of age. The genetics of retinoblastoma is very complex. It may occur either as a dominantly inherited disorder or sporadically. About 30 percent of all cases have a genetic basis. Bilateral cases are thought to be genetic, even if the family history is negative. The disease is hereditary with an autosomal dominant pattern. The disease can be unilateral or bilateral and asymmetric.

OBJECTIVE FINDINGS

Retinoblastoma occurs in small children, making the evaluation of visual acuity difficult. The most common presenting findings are leukocoria and/or strabismus. Ophthalmoscopy reveals often calcified, multifocal retinal tumors in one or both eyes. The eyes are of normal size.

DIAGNOSTIC TESTS

Ocular ultrasound revealing intratumoral calcification is helpful in confirming the diagnosis of retinoblastoma.

SPECIAL CONSIDERATIONS

The early pediatric age group is almost exclusively afflicted. When the disease is bilateral, it is devastating and genetic counseling should be considered.

TREATMENT

Referral to a specialist in eye tumors is strongly recommended. Once the diagnosis of retinoblastoma is confirmed, treatment depends on if it is unilateral or bilateral. In the unilateral cases, the involved eye is enucleated, and careful examination of the other eye is performed regularly to ensure that subclinical involvement does not manifest itself. In bilateral cases, the more seriously involved eye is enucleated and the less involved eye is treated with radiation therapy. Because of the incidence of secondary tumors, especially osteosarcoma, careful follow-up must be part of the long-term management of these patients.

Congenital Cataract

Congenital cataract is opacity of the lens that is present at birth. It can be unilateral or bilateral, and the etiology is variable, from birth trauma to intrauterine infection. Because vision develops in the first years of life, the visual prognosis in patients with congenital cataracts is very poor.

OBJECTIVE FINDINGS

Visual acuity is generally difficult to evaluate because of the age of these patients. The pupil examination is usually normal, and there is no afferent pupillary defect. On ophthalmoscopy there is a defect in the red reflex, which may present as various degrees of darkness or shadow in the normally orange pupil.

DIAGNOSTIC TESTS

Generally, no special testing is required, but the ophthalmologist may wish to perform an ultrasound examination to evaluate the eye behind the cataract.

SPECIAL CONSIDERATION

Because of the age of these patients and their developing vision, it is particularly important to refer them to an eye doctor immediately, since permanent visual loss may develop from amblyopia.

TREATMENT

The treatment of congenital cataracts depends on the severity or density of the opacities in the lenses and the threat to the development of amblyopia. Bilateral congenital cataracts are treated, when indicated, with cataract surgery. Unilateral cataracts have a particularly poor prognosis, but some studies do show clinical improvement with early surgery.

Persistent Hyperplastic Primary Vitreous

The vitreous of the normal eye is formed in the prenatal period and is actually the secondary vitreous. The primary vitreous consists of the blood vessels and lymphatics that supply the anterior segment of the eye, including the lens during fetal development. This primary vitreous usually atrophies as the secondary vitreous forms, but in patients with persistent hyperplastic primary vitreous (PHPV) this does not occur properly and the primary vitreous remains. Subsequently the lens is often opaque and the secondary vitreous is not clear.

OBJECTIVE FINDINGS

Vision is usually irreversibly lost in these eyes. The condition is usually unilateral, and the involved eye is smaller (the horizontal corneal diameter can be measured relatively easily.) The red reflex is compromised with varying degrees of darkness, depending on the prominence of the PHPV.

TREATMENT

Unfortunately, surgical removal of the opaque vitreous material does not bring the vision back to any significant degree. These eyes are abnormal in other ways, often showing foveal hypoplasia or lack of development of central visions. Therefore, surgical intervention is usually not indicated or beneficial.

Retinopathy of Prematurity

Retinopathy of prematurity (ROP) is the condition that was historically known as retrolental fibroplasia (RLF). It is a condition of premature babies who have almost always been on high percentages of inspired oxygen (FIO_2) due to abnormal pulmonary development. In premature babies the retinal blood vessels have not completely formed (especially on the temporal side of the retina). For some reason, when these developing blood vessels are exposed to high FIO_2, they cease growth and new blood vessels form from the retina out into the vitreous. When this occurs and becomes more severe, the new blood vessels (neovascularization) pull the retina off and a total retinal detachment with blindness may result. The condition may be unilateral, or bilateral and asymmetric.

OBJECTIVE FINDINGS

These are premature infants. On routine examination of the eyes, the only observation that may be present is a persistent pupillary membrane (persistent tunica vasculosa lentis). This is the group of blood vessels that surround the lens embryologically and which atrophy with development.

SPECIAL CONSIDERATIONS

All premature infants, especially those on high FIO₂ for pulmonary dysfunction, should be evaluated by an eye doctor regularly.

TREATMENT

Fortunately, now that the etiology of ROP is better understood, pediatricians monitor arterial blood gases regularly and attempt to keep FIO₂ as low as possible while still keeping the infant's respiratory system oxygenating the blood sufficiently. This has greatly decreased the incidence of ROP. Even after the early condition is diagnosed, many cases spontaneously regress and vascularize normally.

For those cases that continue to progress, many different therapies have been attempted. Cryotherapy, scleral buckling, and laser treatment are all modalities that have shown some success, but preventing or reversing the condition is the best alternative in the management of these patients.

Chapter 14–12
STRABISMUS

Wesley T. Ota
Francis J. Sousa

DISCUSSION

Strabismus is the condition of the eyes when the lines-of-vision (visual axes) of the two eyes are not aligned simultaneously on the object of regard. By far the most common etiology of strabismus is hereditary or unknown, but it can also occur as a result of trauma, stroke, thyroid disease, tumor, and many other systemic problems. It is most common in young children and requires evaluation by an eye doctor because it can lead to permanent vision loss called *amblyopia*. Visual acuity continues to develop until the age of 8 to 10 years. Until this time a strabismus can cause amblyopia, or "lazy eye," to occur.

SIGNS AND SYMPTOMS

The most common presentations of strabismus are *esotropia* (cross-eyed) and *exotropia* (wall-eyed).

Esotropia can be present at birth or shortly thereafter. This is called congenital esotropia. It may present later, between ages 6 months and 7 years (usually about 2 to 3 years old) and often

has an accommodative component. In either case, one eye may not develop good visual acuity and develop amblyopia, or lazy eye.

Exotropia may be present at birth or it may be a progressive problem with age. Often, one of the eyes has a tendency to wander out, and this becomes apparent only when a patient is tired, ill, or compromised in some way. This occasional wandering out is called *intermittent exotropia.* As time goes by, in many of these patients, the eye wanders more frequently and longer in duration. Eventually, it may lead to the eye being "out" all the time. This is called *constant exotropia.*

SCREENING ON PHYSICAL EXAMINATION

When performing a physical examination on a child, it is critical to screen for strabismus. This can be done using a variety of methods, but perhaps the two most practical are the Hirschberg light reflex test and the cover-uncover test.:

- The *light reflex test* is performed by shining the penlight simultaneously at both corneas. The light should reflect off each of the two corneas in the same relative location (usually a little to the nasal side of the center of the pupil). If this is the case the eyes are probably aligned properly.
- The better and preferred method for examining for strabismus is the *cover-uncover test.* This is performed in a well-lit room with the patient fixing his or her gaze at a target, using both eyes. (*Hint:* In young children, it is often handy to carry various finger puppets or other interesting objects so as to assure fixation.) With both eyes attempting to fixate on the object, one eye is covered using an occluder of any kind; often a hand is the least threatening. The eye that is not being covered is observed. If the eye moves, it was not pointed at the object to begin with. If it moves temporally to see the object of regard, the patient is esotropic. If it moves nasally to see the object of regard, the patient is exotropic. Make sure to test each eye.

Regardless of the method used, if there is any doubt as to whether strabismus is present, the patient should be referred to an eye doctor for further evaluation.

TREATMENT

Strabismus should always by treated by an eye doctor. The treatment of strabismus is twofold. The first goal is to preserve or restore the vision in each eye. This is done by evaluating visual acuity and then, if amblyopia is present, patching the good eye. Patching forces the patient to use the amblyopic eye, promoting visual development. Patching must be watched carefully so that there is no regression of vision in the better eye. Also once the vision is restored, it is important not to lose it again from the strabismus.

After any amblyopia has been corrected, the treatment aim becomes cosmetic. When and if the patient or the parents think that it is socially and psychologically important, surgery can be performed to straighten the eyes. This surgery rarely allows the eyes to work together perfectly, but it can do much to make the patient's eye alignment appear normal and it may result in the patient regaining some degree of fusion.

Strabismus can be caused later in life by trauma, stroke, or tumor among other causes. In patients with the onset of strabismus causing diplopia, the treatment goal is to reduce the double vision. A late onset of strabismus often causes diplopia. The main etiologies are trauma, stroke, and those listed previously. The treatment goal in these cases is to reduce the double vision. This may be facilitated with surgical procedures, but often prisms in spectacles or an eye patch is preferable.

Chapter 14–13
SUBCONJUNCTIVAL HEMORRHAGE
Wesley T. Ota
Francis J. Sousa

DISCUSSION

Subconjuctival hemorrhages are areas of blood located under the conjunctiva. Although it is an alarming visual observation, this is a benign, non-vision-threatening presentation that gradually resolves in 10 to 14 days. Subconjunctival hemorrhages can occur at any age but more commonly in the elderly population as vascular wall integrity diminishes.

PATHOGENESIS

Subconjunctival hemorrhages develop from an insult to the conjunctival blood vessels of the eye. As a break develops in a conjunctival vessel, blood flows freely through the loose space between the clear conjunctival tissue and the white sclera beneath. Because the conjunctival tissue is strongly attached only to the limbus, where the sclera meets the cornea, an initially focal area of hemorrhage most often spreads and expands prior to its resolution, giving the false suspicion of progression. A traumatic subconjunctival hemorrhage can often obstruct the view of the entire sclera. As the hemorrhage resolves, the color of the blood becomes reddish brown, the borders become more feathery, and the hemorrhage becomes less dense. Depending on the extent of the hemorrhage, the entire process resolves in approximately 1 to 2 weeks.

SIGNS AND SYMPTOMS

Other than a mild irritation in some cases, a subconjunctival hemorrhage is generally asymptomatic. There may be eye pain if there was a traumatic cause. A striking red hemorrhage of the bulbar conjunctiva is the only sign alerting the patient to this presentation. Its appearance can be frightening to a patient.

OBJECTIVE FINDINGS

There is no decrease in visual acuity associated with a subconjunctival hemorrhage. On external evaluation of the eye, an area of blood would be observed under the conjunctiva obstructing the view of the sclera. There can be some elevation of the conjunctiva, especially visible at the limbus, as blood fills the loose space below and displaces the conjunctiva forward. There should not be any blood in the anterior chamber, the area behind the cornea of the eye. This would occur in a hyphema, which is an entirely different and visually compromising presentation.

DIAGNOSTIC CONSIDERATIONS

The etiology of the insult for a subconjunctival hemorrhage can be idiopathic, or it can result from trauma, valsalva maneuvers (lifting, sneezing, defecating), bleeding disorders (systemic or secondary to medications), or hypertension.

A list of differential diagnoses includes hyphema (blood behind the cornea), scleritis (injection and redness of the conjunctiva with no free blood), and conjunctival Kaposi's sarcoma (red area usually elevated in a patient with AIDS).

LABORATORY TESTS AND WORKUP

Blood pressure should be taken on suspicion of hypertension. A thorough history should be taken regarding trauma, Valsalva maneuvers, and medications. Patients who are on anticoagulants should be questioned on proper medication levels and follow-up by their medical provider. Laboratory tests for bleeding disorders should be considered for patients with recurrent presentations.

PHARMACOLOGIC MANAGEMENT

There are no pharmacologic treatments for subconjunctival hemorrhage.

SUPPORTIVE MEASURES

Artificial tears can be prescribed for patients who have mild ocular irritation. A patient who is on daily aspirin should consider its discontinuation for a few days, if safe, to increase resolution time. Vasoconstrictors have no beneficial effect on subconjunctival hemorrhages.

PATIENT EDUCATION

Patient reassurance is essential. If the patient is having anticoagulation therapy, questioning about proper monitoring of medication levels is recommended.

DISPOSITION

No follow-up is necessary for a benign subconjunctival hemorrhage. The patient should be reassured of gradual resolution over the next 10 to 14 days. If the presentation does not improve by that time, the patient should be reevaluated.

Chapter 14–14
SUDDEN VISUAL LOSS IN ONE EYE
Wesley T. Ota
Francis J. Sousa

DISCUSSION

When any visual loss occurs suddenly and for no apparent reason, the etiology is almost always a vascular compromise. The four major vascular diseases that cause sudden visual loss are as follows:

1. Central retinal artery occlusion (CRAO)
2. Central retinal vein occlusion (CRVO)
3. Anterior ischemic optic neuropathy (AION)
4. Vitreous hemorrhage (associated with diabetes mellitus)

Although the history is very similar in these four conditions, the physical or objective findings make them relatively easy to diagnose and differentiate.

Central Retinal Artery Occlusion

Central retinal artery occlusion is an obstruction of the blood flow into the retina of the eye. This causes infarction of the retina and marked visual loss.

OBJECTIVE FINDINGS

Visual acuity is usually lowered to 20/200 or worse. Although the external eye may appear relatively normal, the pupil of the involved eye exhibits an afferent pupillary defect, or a positive swinging flashlight test. The visual fields are markedly constricted. The most dramatic findings will be on ophthalmoscopy, which reveals a pale retina around the optic nerve and macular area, except in the immediate fovea which remains bright red (called a cherry-red spot); narrowed or irregularly constricted retinal arterioles; an optic nerve that may have somewhat indistinct margins; and perhaps intravascular refractile plaques(s) at the bifurcation of the retinal arterioles (Hollenhorst plaques). This appearance of a pale, poorly vascularized retina with a central red spot is quite distinctive.

The carotid arteries should be palpated to evaluate their pulse and auscultated to evaluate for bruits which may be associated with carotid obstruction from arteriosclerotic plaques. The status of the heart, such as previous myocardial infarctions or valvular heart disease, should also be evaluated as a source of emboli.

SPECIAL CONSIDERATIONS

Often this disease occurs as the result of an embolus from the carotid artery or the heart. It is particularly common in patients with arteriosclerotic vascular disease that is associated with hypertension, diabetes, hypercholesterolemia, and smoking.

TREATMENT

Unfortunately, if these patients do not reach medical care within the first few minutes to hours after the onset of their visual loss, the final visual outcomes are usually very poor.

When the diagnosis is made, probably the most beneficial treatments that carry the lowest risks are having the patient rebreathe into a brown paper bag, which increases the percentage of inspired CO_2 in an attempt to dilate the retinal arterioles, and placing intermittent firm pressure on the eyelids for 10 to 20 s with quick release, which increases intraocular pressure and suddenly decreases it in an attempt to loosen the obstruction.

An immediate consultation with an eye doctor for further evaluation and possible treatment is mandatory. Various treatment modalities that are used by specialists include having the patient breathe a 5% CO_2/95% O_2 mixture, performing anterior chamber paracentesis, which involves inserting a needle through the cornea to decompress the globe, and/or giving retrobulbar injections of a vasodilating substance.

Perhaps the most important treatment is to ensure that the underlying diseases are properly addressed by the primary care provider.

Central Retinal Vein Occlusion

Central Retinal Vein Occlusion is obstruction of the blood flow out of the retina. This causes increased pressure in the venules of the eye, hemorrhage, and varying degrees of hypoxia and ischemia—usually severe.

OBJECTIVE FINDINGS

Visual acuity is usually lowered to 20/200 or worse. Although the external eye may appear relatively normal, the pupil of the involved eye will exhibit an afferent pupillary defect or positive swinging flashlight test. The visual fields are markedly constricted.

As with CRAO, the most dramatic clinical objective findings are seen on ophthalmoscopy, revealing diffuse hemorrhages throughout the retina involving many different layers of the retina. This is called a "blood and thunder" fundus because of the extent and dramatic appearance of the hemorrhages. The appearance is unique and the diagnosis follows.

SPECIAL CONSIDERATIONS

As with CRAO, these patients often have an extensive history of peripheral vascular disease and diseases that accelerate vascular disease.

TREATMENT

Unfortunately very little can be done to intervene when a CRVO has occurred. Many different therapies have been attempted over the years, including anticoagulation to break up any clot that might be present, but these have proved to be of little or no benefit.

It is important to refer these patients to an eye doctor for thorough evaluation and follow-up. Unfortunately, because of the profound ischemia which is longstanding, new blood vessel formation (neovascularization) may occur within the first few months. This usually occurs on the iris (rubeosis iridis) and may lead to a very severe form of glaucoma (neovascular glaucoma) which can destroy the little remaining vision and be very painful. Therefore, careful follow-up by the eye doctor is indicated. Usually it is treated medically and with laser therapy to the retina to destroy the ischemic retinal tissue, called pan-retinal photocoagulation (PRP).

Anterior Ischemic Optic Neuropathy

Anterior ischemic optic neuropathy is the obstruction of blood flow through the small arterioles feeding the anterior portion of the optic nerve.

OBJECTIVE FINDINGS

Visual acuity usually is lowered to 20/50 or worse, but this may vary and be less severe. Although the external eye appears relatively normal, the pupil of the involved eye will exhibit an afferent pupillary defect or positive swinging flashlight test. The visual fields show a dense central scotoma.

The most dramatic findings are seen on ophthalmoscopy. The optic nerve is swollen, showing elevation, blurred disk margins, very small or no cup, and obscured vessels on and near the nerve owing to the fluid, and eventually, pallor. This appearance of a pale, swollen nerve with visual loss makes the diagnosis of AION.

SPECIAL CONSIDERATIONS

AION is most often associated with arteriosclerotic disease. An extensive vascular history should be taken and any underlying conditions treated. A special situation that occurs most often in the geriatric age group is AION associated with temporal arteritis. This is important because the diagnosis is easy to miss and must be considered. These patients are usually older than 65 years old (prevalence accelerates into the 70s, 80s, and 90s) with the clinical syndrome of temporal arteritis or polymyalgia rheumatica. Remember to ask about weight loss, temporal tender headache, jaw claudication, general malaise, fever, night sweats, and proximal muscle myalgias. If the diagnosis is at all suspected clinically, obtaining an erythrocyte sedimentation rate (ESR) which will be elevated and referring the patient for evaluation by a rheumatologist immediately is indicated. This disease can cause blindness in the other eye as well as severe systemic problems.

TREATMENT

The treatment of the arteriosclerotic disease is one of controlling the underlying diseases. Extensive research has been done to evaluate the role of steroid use in this disease, and the studies are equivocal.

The arteritic form must be treated aggressively with systemic steroids to control the temporal arteritis, which is a systemic disease. The vision will probably not improve in the affected eye, but the other eye must be spared, as well as the remainder of the body.

Treatment is usually under the management of the rheumatologist and consists of high-dose steroids (prednisone 80 mg/day), which is tapered as the patient's symptoms improve and the ESR comes down into a more normal range. The rheumatologist may request a temporal artery biopsy to confirm the diagnosis.

Vitreous Hemorrhage

Vitreous hemorrhage is a usually sudden leakage of blood into the vitreous cavity causing obscuration of the clear vitreous and decreased vison. Although there are many conditions that can cause blood vessels to break and bleed into the vitreous, the most common is diabetes mellitus (see Chap. 14-8, "Diabetic Retinopathy," and Chap. 5-1, Diabetes Mellitus.")

Objective Findings

The visual acuity is decreased to varying degrees, but may be profound. The external eye is relatively normal in appearance. The pupils are normal. The visual fields are constricted.

The most dramatic physical findings once again are in ophthalmoscopy, which reveals an abnormal red reflex and inability to see the retina clearly or at all. "The patient sees nothing and the clinician sees nothing" would often be an appropriate phrase for this condition.

SPECIAL CONSIDERATIONS

Although diabetes is the most common etiology, consider other causes of neovascularization such as sickle cell disease and previous vascular occlusions of the eye. Also, a retinal tear may break a blood vessel causing hemorrhage.

TREATMENT

The initial treatment is to have the patient sit up and stay as relaxed as possible so that the blood can layer in the eye with gravity and the source of the bleeding can be identified.

Referral to an eye doctor is mandatory in this condition so that treatment is not delayed. Often a retinal specialist is the best person to manage the problem and treat the underlying condition. In the case of systemic diseases, of course they must be optimally managed.

Chapter 14–15
CHALAZION AND HORDEOLUM (STYE)
Suzanne Warnimont

DISCUSSION

A chalazion is a granulomatous inflammation of a meibomian gland of the eye. It is a common non-vision-threatening condition of the eye that can distort vision if the lesion is large enough to press on the cornea.

A hordeolum (stye) is a staphylococcal abscess of the meibomian gland (internal hordeolum) or of the glands of Zeis or Moll around the lashes (external hordeolum).

SIGNS AND SYMPTOMS

With chalazion, there is a visible, hard, sometimes tender swelling near the lid margin. The surrounding conjunctiva may be red and elevated.

With hordeolum, there is a red, swollen, tender area on the upper or lower lid margin. An internal hordeolum may point to the internal or external lid; an external hordeolum points externally.

DIAGNOSTIC CONSIDERATIONS

Preseptal cellulitis is associated with an abrasion or site infection and fever. Sebaceous cell carcinoma should be suspected with recurrent chalazion. It causes thickening of both upper and lower lid margins and loss of eye lashes. Biopsy establishes the diagnosis. Pyogenic granuloma may develop after trauma or surgery. Basal cell carcinoma appears as dimpled or ulcerated and pearly. A firm appearance increases the likelihood of malignancy (see Chap. 2-7).

SPECIAL CONSIDERATIONS

History should include inquiries regarding a past chalazion excision. Everting the lid may allow better visualization of the nodule caused by a chalazion.

LABORATORY AND RADIOLOGIC STUDIES

There are no appropriate laboratory and radiologic studies for chalazion and hordeolum.

Chalazion

TREATMENT

Use warm compresses for 20 min qid with light massage. If chalazion does not disappear within 3 to 4 weeks of conservative treatment, it may be removed by incision and curettage by an ophthalmologist.

Topical antibiotics (erythromycin ophthalmic ointment bid) may be administered directly behind the lid because penetration through the skin is poor. Steroids may be injected into the lesion, especially if the lesion is near the lacrimal apparatus. Use triamcinolone, 40 mg/mL, 0.2 to 1.0 mL (depending on the size of the lesion), injected into and around the lesion.

PATIENT EDUCATION

If the lesion does not resolve in 3 to 4 weeks with conservative treatment, the patient may choose to have the lesion incised or injected (see above).

COMPLICATIONS OR RED FLAGS

Steroid injection can cause skin depigmentation or localized atrophy at the injection site and should be done only by those skilled with this intralesional procedure.

Hordeolum

TREATMENT

Use warm compresses for 20 min qid. In the acute stage, antibiotic ointment is instilled into the conjunctival sac with excess rubbed onto the eyelids every 3 h.

A variety of ophthalmic antibiotic ointments are acceptable, including sodium sulfacetamide (Sulamyd), neomycin sulfate (Neosporin), gentamicin sulfate (Garamycin), and erythromycin.

PATIENT EDUCATION

A nonresponsive lesion may require incision and curettage by an ophthalmologist.

COMPLICATIONS OR RED FLAGS

Hordeolum may lead to diffuse superficial lid infection or preseptal cellulitis.

BIBLIOGRAPHY

Cullom, RD, Chang B: *The Wills Eye Manual,* 2d ed. Philadelphia, Lippincott, 1994, pp 133–134.

Goldberg S: *Ophthalmology Made Ridiculously Simple.* Miami, FL, MedMaster, 1994, pp 9, 22.

Goroll AH, May LA, Mulley AG: *Primary Care Medicine,* 3d ed. Philadelphia, Lippincott, 1995, pp 958–959.

Tierney LM Jr, McPhee SJ, Papadakis MA (eds): *Current Medical Diagnosis and Treatment,* 35th ed. Stamford, CT, Appleton & Lange, 1996, p 160.

Chapter 14–16
CONJUNCTIVITIS

Wesley T. Ota
Francis J. Sousa

DISCUSSION

Acute conjunctivitis is a self-limiting inflammation of the conjunctiva, which is the mucous membrane lining of the eye. It is the most common eye disease in the western hemisphere and is determined by the causative agent. The duration of acute conjunctivitis is less than a month.

PATHOGENESIS

One function of the conjunctiva is to protect the eye from foreign objects and infectious organisms. Because it contains a rich vascular supply and many inflammatory cells such as lymphocytes and plasma cells, the conjunctiva often becomes a common site of irritation. Acute conjunctivitis can develop from three main causes: bacterial infections, viral infections, and allergies. This chapter focuses the discussion of viral infections on the adenoviral strains although the herpesvirus is another form of infection. The herpes simplex virus is discussed in a separate chapter (See Chap. 2–16.)

Conjunctivitis begins with a causative agent that invades the eye. This stimulates the inflammatory cells to migrate to the conjunctival epithelial surface from the stroma. The cells combine with mucus and fibrin and create the exudate that is secreted from the eye. The inflammatory cells involved differ, depending on the type of conjunctivitis. Bacterial conjunctivitis has a preponderance of polymorphonuclear cells. Adenoviral infections contain monocytes and lymphohcytes, and the majority of cells found in allergic reactions are eosinophils. All these conjunctivitides are self-limiting because of the high number of lymphocytes to fight the infection, the flushing and diluting action of the tears, and the antigen entrapping capability by the production of exudate.

SIGNS AND SYMPTOMS

The symptoms of conjunctivitis can vary depending on the etiology. Having variable amounts of diffuse conjunctival redness (hyperemia) is the most obvious sign of conjunctivitis. All types can have symptoms of foreign-body sensation, periocular edema, and tearing. The discharge secreted can vary depending on the type of conjunctivitis, as is explained in the following section. In allergic conjunctivitis, the hallmark symptom is itchiness. Many times the symptoms of allergic conjunctivitis significantly outweigh the objective findings.

OBJECTIVE FINDINGS

Objective findings are the most important factors in diagnosing the type of conjunctivitis. A purely conjunctival inflammation with no corneal involvement should have no effect on visual acuity. Photophobia can occur when there is corneal involvement.

A *bacterial conjunctivitis* will present with a purulent or mucopurulent discharge. The discharge is very often greenish white in color with a sticky consistency. The lashes are matted with

Table 14-16-1. Categories of Acute Conjunctivitis

Category	Discharge	Itching	Preauricular Adenopathy	Cytology
Viral	Serous, occasionally mucous strands	Minimal	Common	Monocytes, lymphocytes
Bacterial	Purulent, mucopurulent	Minimal	Uncommon	Bacterial, PMNs
Allergic	Mucoid, stringy	Severe	Absent	Eosinophils

NOTE: PMN = polymorphonuclear neutrophil leukocytes.

this substance as well. There is usually some chemosis of the conjunctiva. Preauricular adenopathy is uncommon in bacterial conjunctivitis. The injection of the conjunctiva is a beefy red color and increases in intensity from the limbus toward the palpebral conjunctiva. The presentation of a bacterial conjunctivitis is initally monocular. The other eye typically becomes involved in approximately 48 h. The infection is self-limiting and commonly resolves in 4 to 7 days with topical antibiotic drops, but can resolve without treatment within 10 to 15 days. Acute bacterial conjunctivitis is caused by various microorganisms, most commonly *Staphylococcus aureus*, *Streptococcus pneumoniae*, and *Haemophilus* spp.

Viral conjunctivitis is generally more common than bacterial conjunctivitis. A viral conjunctivitis has a serous, clear discharge but often elicts increased tearing. Many viral cases develop occasional mucous strands caused by irritation to the eye. The bulbar conjunctiva is diffusely pink in color versus dark red in bacterial infections. There are follicles, which are lymphocyte germinal centers, present in the inferior palpebral conjunctiva. Preauricular adenopathy is usually present. The history commonly includes a runny nose, upper respiratory infection or contact with a person who had these symptoms. The onset is commonly unilateral with a duration of 10 to 21 days, depending on the adenovirus strain. The conjunctivitis typically worsens for the first 5 to 7 days prior to improving. There is often inoculation of the other eye in approximately 5 to 7 days because of the highly contagious nature of viral infections.

Allergic conjunctivitis presents with a stringy white discharge that has an elastic characteristic. Patients commonly report excessive tearing and itchiness in allergic conjunctivitis as well. There is usually chemosis of the bulbar conjunctiva and often chemosis of the periocular area. Papillae, which are focal areas of serous fluid caused by the inflammatory process, are found in the superior palpebral conjunctiva. The onset of allergic conjunctivitis usually occurs bilaterally as opposed to unilaterally in viral and bacterial infections (see Table 14-16-1).

DIAGNOSTIC CONSIDERATIONS

The cause of acute conjunctivitis can stem from various etiologies, most commonly bacterial, viral, seasonal allergies, chemicals, hay fever, atopy, and medicamentosa.

SPECIAL CONSIDERATIONS

Any inflammation which involves the cornea should warrant consultation with an eye doctor. This can be determined if there is discharge on the cornea or any irregularity in corneal clarity. The involvement of the cornea would produce a decrease in visual acuity as well. A hyperacute purulent discharge occurs with gonococcal or pseudomonal conjunctivitis. These are serious infections with a severely purulent discharge and should be sent for an eye consult as well. Gonococcal and pseudomonal conjunctivitis can cause corneal perforations and require oral medications and close monitoring. They may require hospitalization. Any person who has a prior history of herpes simplex infection of the eye requires evaluation by an eye doctor (see Chap. 14-10). Any person who has a herpes zoster presentation that affects the first branch of the trigeminal nerve should consult an eye doctor for ocular involvement.

LABORATORY TESTS

Cultures of the conjunctiva are typically not performed in clinical settings unless there is no improvement in the viral infection or acute bacterial infection with antibiotic treatment. Chronic, hyperacute, and neonatal conjunctivitides deserve cultures.

TREATMENT

Pharmacologic Management

The main indication for the treatment of conjunctivitis is to protect the cornea from infection that can lead to visual compromise. Bacterial conjunctivitis should be treated with a broad-spectrum

Table 14-16-2. Antibiotics Used for Bacterial Infections

Antibiotic	Dosage	Comments
Polymyxin B sulfate-trimethoprim (Polytrim)	1 gt. q3h × 7 d	Broad spectrum with minimal allergic reactions. Treatment of choice.
Tobramycin sulfate ((Tobramycin or Tobrex) Tobrex avail. in ung	Sol: 1 gt. q4h × 7 d ung: apply 1/2-in. strip to affected eye qid × 7 d	Broad spectrum with corneal toxicity on chronic use.
Ciprofloxacin (Ciloxan)	1 gt. q2h × 2 d, 1 gt. q4h × 5 d thereafter	Recommended for severe conjunctivitis if other antibiotics are not effective and for the treatment of corneal ulcers. Temporary white crystalline precipitates can develop with use of the medication.
Erythromycin (AK-Mycin, Ilotycin)	Apply 1/2-in. strip to affected eye qid × 7 d	Rare allergic or toxic reactions. Excellent as a prophylactic coverage. Used if allergic reactions to other antibiotics.
Bacitracin (Bacitracin, AK-Tracin)	Apply 1/2-in. strip to affected eye qid × 7 d	As with erythromycin, used if allergic reactions occur with other antibiotics. Excellent as a prophylactic coverage.

NOTE: ung = ointment; gt. = drop.

Table 14-16-3. Treatment of Allergic Conjunctivitis

Medication	Dosage	Comments
Levocabastine hydrochloride 1% (Livostin), topical antihistamine	1 gt. qid as needed up to 2 wk	Very effective fast-acting treatment of allergic symptoms. Do not use while wearing soft contact lenses.
Naphazoline hydrochloride/pheniramine maleate (Opcon-A, AK-Con A, Naphcon A), decongestant-antihistamine combination	1 gt. qid as needed	Not intended for chronic regular use since rebound hyperemia may develop. Side effect of pupillary dilation. Contraindicated in patients at risk for or with narrow angle glaucoma.
Naphazoline hydrochloride/antazoline phosphate (Vasocon-A), decongestant-antihistamine combination	1 gt. qid as needed	Not intended for chronic regular use since rebound hyperemia may develop. Side effect of pupillary dilation. Contraindicated in patients at risk for or with narrow angle glaucoma.
Cetirizine hydrochloride (Zyrtec), oral antihistamine	10 mg (1 tab) PO qd	Very fast acting antihistamine. Has recently been released in the U.S. Minimizes drowsiness. No known adverse reactions used in conjunction with macrolide and imidazole derivatives.
Terfenidine (Seldane), oral antihistamine	60 mg (1 tab) PO q8–12h for adults (see insert for children's dosage.)	Minimizes drowsiness. Can have adverse cardiac effects with macrolide and imidazole derivatives.
Chlorpheniramine maleate (Chlortrimeton), OTC oral antihistamine	4 mg (1 tab) PO q8–12h	Causes drowsiness.
Diphenhydramine hydrochloride (Benadryl), OTC oral antihistamine	25–50 mg PO tid-qid for adults. 12.5–25 mg PO tid-qid for children over 20 lbs	Causes drowsiness.

antibiotic qid for 7 to 10 days. A combination topical drop consisting of trimethoprim and polymyxin B (Polytrim) is an excellent antibiotic. Aminoglycosides, such as tobramycin (Tobrex), can also be used but are known to be more toxic to the cornea on extended use.

Sulfacetamide drops are not regularly used in eye care since there is a high resistance to this antibiotic as well as a large population allergic to sulfa medications. The drops tend to burn, and patients, especially children, tend to resist subsequent doses.

Ointments can be applied to the eye for bacterial infections, but impair vision when applied. Because of its prolonged contact time compared with drops, ointments can be considered in difficult cases such as an uncooperative child or an elderly individual who requires assistance in treatment. Ointments can be fairly effective on a bid dose. Tobramycin (Tobrex), erythromycin, bacitracin, or polymyxin B are ophthalmic ointments available for use in the eye.

There are no medical treatments for adenoviral conjunctivitis at the present time. Research is currently being performed on a topical form of cidofovir to treat adenovirus infections. Artificial teardrops can be used to relieve some of the discomfort as well as dilute the antigen. OTC antihistamine-decongestant combination used qid can minimize redness and decrease irritation as well.

Acute allergic conjunctivitis can best be treated with levocabastine (Livostin) which is a powerful H_1 receptor blocker used qid × 7 days to minimize itchiness. OTC antihistamine-decongestants (Naphcon-A, Opcon-A, Vasocon-A) can be used qid for mild allergic symptoms. This should not be used on a chronic basis because rebound hyperemic effects often occur. OTC oral antihistamines such as chlorpheniramine maleate (Chlor-Trimeton) or diphenhydramine hydrochloride (Benadryl) can be used as directed. Prescription oral antihistamines (Zyrtec, Seldane) can be considered and have minimal side effects of drowsiness that can occur with the OTC antihistamines (see Tables 14-16-2 and 14-16-3).

Supportive Measures

The use of cool compresses can relieve discomfort created by irritation from any of the conjunctivitides. This will decrease the inflammatory process of swelling and pain sensitivity that commonly occurs. If inflammatory symptoms are absent, the use of warm compresses can increase vascular circulation to the affected area in viral and bacterial infections. This will stimulate the body's own immune response to accelerate the recovery time of the infection.

PATIENT EDUCATION

The contagious aspect of bacterial and viral conjunctivitis should be a vital part of patient education. Prior to the antibiotic treatment of a bacterial infection, or during any viral infection, the infection can be transmitted to the other eye as well as other people. Generally, viral infections are more highly contagious than bacterial infections. Patients with bacterial conjunctivitis should be cautioned against social interactions until 24 h after antibiotic treatment. Patients with viral conjunctivitis should be very careful throughout the term of conjunctivitis because no treatment is available to eradicate the virus. These patients should be informed not to share towels, pillows, or cosmetic eye products with other people. The use of contact lenses should be discontinued until the conjunctivitis resolves. Allergic conjunctivitis is not a contagious type of inflammation. Most allergic conjunctivitides are caused by seasonal or hay fever stimuli. If this is not the case, the antigen should be identified and avoided in the future.

Chapter 15–1
PEDIATRIC NUTRITION
Kimberly Brown Paterson

DISCUSSION

Growth may be defined as an increase in size. Physiologic growth depends on a variety of nutrients in the food a child eats. The goal of nutrition is appropriate growth and development along with the avoidance of deficiency states. Requirements vary with stages of development as well as the genetic and metabolic differences that exist among individuals. Nutrient needs also depend on body composition. For example, in term neonates the brain accounts for 10 percent of body weight and 44 percent of total energy needs under basal conditions. This indicates that the brain accounts for a generally high percentage of basal energy requirements.[1]

Nutritional requirements change with the composition of new weight gain. Fat accounts for 40 percent of weight gain between birth and age 4 months but only 3 percent between 24 and 36 months, making constant reassessment of infant and pediatric nutritional intakes important. The stages reviewed in this chapter include infant feeding (e.g., breast versus bottle feeding) and toddler or childhood nutrition to age 12:

- *Infant feeding:* birth to 1 year
- *Premature infant:* gestation less than 270 days or weight less than 2500 g (5.5 lb)
- *Small for gestational age (SGA):* full term but have experienced intrauterine growth failure and have low birth weights along with general growth retardation

Premature infants require special care in regard to feeding. Extra attention must be paid to the type of milk and the method of feeding. The body composition of premature infants differs from that of term infants in that "preemies" have

1. More water and less protein and minerals per kilogram of body weight
2. Little subcutaneous fat
3. Poorly calcified bones
4. An underdeveloped neuromuscular system, making sucking difficult
5. Inadequate iron stores
6. Limited digestive and absorption abilities[1]

The merits of breast feeding versus bottle (formula) feeding have been debated; fortunately, premature babies do well on both. Breast milk may be more desirable with its higher protein and mineral content and more easily digested fat. It provides immunoactive immunologic factors, including secretory IgA, lysozyme, lactoferrin, and macrophages, to provide protection against upper respiratory and gastrointestinal infections as well as allergic disorders. However, many new formulas have been developed and provide excellent nutritional value for premature infants (Table 15-1-1).

There are some contraindications to breast feeding. Maternal tuberculosis and galactosemia in an infant are absolute contraindications. Concern about HIV transmission by nursing mothers is certainly warranted. It has been suggested that HIV-positive mothers in developing countries use alternative methods of feeding even though recent evidence suggests that breast feeding may not be a route of transmission.[1]

Additional contraindications to breast feeding include maternal septicemia, nephritis, eclampsia, profuse hemorrhage, chronic poor nutrition, substance abuse, and severe psychological disturbances.

More information regarding the composition of formulas and special formulas for all infants can be found in standard reference texts.[1]

PEDIATRIC NUTRITION AGE 1 TO 2

The 1-year-old birthday is a milestone in itself. Major development has occurred since the infant has come home from the hospital. One-year-olds use sippy cups and have become accustomed to a schedule of three meals a day with snacks in between. Independence is being suggested, with toddlers beginning to select foods and feed themselves. Some doubt may arise about whether a balanced diet is being taken. However, children have the ability to select a balanced diet over the course of several days.

A point to emphasize to parents regarding feeding at this time is that the need for kilocalories during this stage decreases. At 1 year of age children need about 1000 kcal, which increases to 1300 to 1500 kcal by age 3. It is important to offer a variety of foods in smaller amounts to provide key nutrients. Two to three cups of milk provide protein and iron in this stage. Single foods and finger foods such as raw fruits and vegetables cut into finger-sized pieces can be a great source of nutrition for children who have a decreasing appetite (Table 15-1-2).

CHILDHOOD NUTRITION TO AGE 12

Nutritional habits are formed early in life; therefore, dietary intervention can be effective when started early in childhood.

Dietary Guidelines for Children Age 2 Years and Older

The following recommendations are appropriate for these children:

1. The diet should be nutritionally complete and include a variety of foods.
2. Carbohydrates (CHO) should provide 60 percent or more of the daily caloric intake, with 50 percent or more in the form of complex carbohydrates.
3. A high-fiber diet is encouraged.
4. A low salt intake is advised.
5. Total fat should constitute less than 30 percent of caloric intake, with saturated fats and polyunsaturated fats providing less than 10 percent each. Monounsaturated fats should provide 10 percent or more of the caloric intake from fat.
6. Cholesterol intake should be less than 100 mg/1000 kcal/d to a maximum of 300 mg/d.[1]

Table 15-1-1. Number and Quantity of Feedings per 24 Hours

Age	Average Quantity Taken in Individual Feedings, oz	Average Number of Feedings in 24 h
Birth–2 weeks	2–3	6–10
3 weeks–1 month	4–5	6–10
2–3 months	5–6	5–6
3–4 months	6–7	4–5
4–7 months	7–8	4–5
8–12 months	7–8	3

USEFUL PEDIATRIC NUTRITION CALCULATIONS

Energy Requirements

After age 4 energy requirements expressed on a body weight basis fall to 40 kcal/kg/d by the end of adolescence. Energy requirements are calculated with a base of 1000 kcal. At age 1 year, it is necessary to add 100 kcal/year. For example, for a child up to age 6 years, a base of 1000 kcal plus 600 kcal (100 kcal/year) equals a 1600-kcal energy requirement for a child age 6.

The basal energy requirement for premature infants is 120 kcal/kg/d.[2]

PARENT INFORMATION GUIDELINES

The following outline is helpful in discussions with parents about feeding and nutrition:

- Discuss feeding behaviors in infancy and early childhood bottle feeding.
- Do not place the infant in the crib with his or her bottle.
- Discourage the use of a bottle of milk or juice as a pacifier.
- Explain that the nursing bottle carries possible risk of otitis media.
- Begin to think about offering a cup for water or juice when appropriate.

The following age milestones should be discussed:[1,2]

2 to 4 weeks	Breast or formula feeding, vitamin D in breast-fed infants, and fluoride supplements.
2 to 4 months	Introduce solid food at 4 to 6 months. Consider an iron supplement in premature infants.
6 months	Solid foods: iron-fortified cereal as well as fruits and vegetables should be added to the diet at this time. Meals may be given two to three times a day. It is acceptable for commercially prepared infant cereals to be the chief source of dietary iron.
12 months	Encourage table foods.
18 months	Wean from the use of bottles.
3 years	Stress a balanced diet. Avoid low-nutrition foods.

Table 15-1-2. Food Choices for Toddlers

Vegetables and Fruits	Breakfast	Lunch	Dessert
Apples	Cereal	Pizza	Ice cream
Corn	French toast	Spaghetti	Cookies
Carrots	Pancakes	Macaroni and cheese	Brownies
Oranges	Eggs	Hamburger	Gelatin
Bananas	Doughnuts	Chicken tenders	Pudding
Watermelon		Peanut butter and jelly	

5 years	Establish a pleasant atmosphere at mealtimes. Encourage good eating habits. Limit empty carbohydrate snacks.
6 years	Maintain appropriate weight.

REFERENCES

1. Wilson JD et al (eds): *Harrison's Principles of Internal Medicine*, 12th ed. Companion Handbook. New York, McGraw-Hill, 1991, pp. 740–747.
2. Hathaway WE et al (eds): *Current Pediatric Diagnosis and Treatment*, 11th ed. Norwalk, CT, Appleton & Lange, 1993, pp 236–261.

Chapter 15–2
COLIC
Richard Dehn

DISCUSSION

Colic is an infant syndrome of excessive crying in the absence of a physical disorder. It is characterized by lengthy incidents of severely increased crying accompanied by a characteristic "pained" look on the infant's face, abduction of the knees to the abdomen accompanied by abdominal distention, and increased flatus. The crying typically begins in the late afternoon, and efforts to comfort the child are usually ineffective. Infant colic is rarely present before the third week of life and in most cases begins to improve by the fourth month, although occasionally it can last through the first year.

The diagnosis can be challenging, since the crying of normal infants increases from birth until about 6 weeks of age and then gradually decreases until it reaches a steady state at about age 4 months. A normal infant averages about 3 h per day of crying at 6 weeks of age. Parents unaware that this is typical infant behavior may feel that the child is abnormal or that something is wrong.

The general rule for making the diagnosis of infant colic is the rule of threes:

- A healthy child who cries for a minimum of three h per day
- At least 3 days per week
- For at least 3 weeks

A prospective study of 1221 families showed a colic incidence of 13 percent using this criterion. The mean amount of total crying was 241 min per day for the colicky group compared with 112 min per day for the noncolicky group, with a mean age of 5 weeks. The survey also had parents quantify the quality of crying by indicating how many minutes of "colicky" crying (inconsolable crying) the infant exhibited each day. The colicky group was reported to exhibit a mean of 122 min per day of colicky crying compared with a mean of 19 min per day in the noncolicky group.

The crying of a colicky infant is often so distressing to parents that it is hard for them to believe that the child does not have a serious medical malady. In this regard it is imperative that the clinician rule out any pathology that might explain the behavior, thus making colic a diagnosis of exclusion. A careful physical examination and close monitoring of growth parameters are useful tools to help exclude other causes of crying.

The effects of a colicky child on its family can be significant. The inconsolable nature of the crying can cause the parents to question their ability to nurture the child, especially when a colicky child is the firstborn. Siblings can find the chaos generated by a colicky child destabilizing at a time when the addition of a new child has already generated family stress. Friends, neighbors, and relatives who normally interact with the parents and siblings find the environment too chaotic for visiting, thus isolating the family. Sleep disturbances created by the inconsolable crying contribute to psychological depression, reducing the family's functional ability to cope with the colicky infant's care demands.

PATHOGENESIS

The cause of infant colic is unknown, though many theories exist. Because these children appear to be suffering from gastrointestinal symptoms (thus the name *colic*), the most popular theory proposes that the crying is due to immaturity of the gastrointestinal (GI) system. As the GI system matures, the painful symptoms resolve, explaining the eventual normalizing of the crying. A few studies have shown that colicky infants have measurable differences in specific organ functions (a recent study showed differences in gallbladder function); however, it is not known whether these differences are the cause of the colic or are secondary to it.

Sensitivity to substances in the diet is also a popular theory. Commonly implicated foods include cow's milk–based formulas, eggs, wheat, and nuts. In bottle-fed infants, this hypothesis can be tested by eliminating cow's milk–based formulas from the diet. In breast–fed infants, the mother must eliminate those foods from her diet. While some infants improve after the dietary changes, the vast majority are unchanged, leading to the conclusion that food sensitivities may be an etiologic factor in only a small percentage of colicky infants.

Another theory is that psychological traits of the parents and their manifestation during pregnancy have a bearing on an infant's coping mechanisms. Several retrospective studies have shown poorer psychological rating scores in the parents of colicky infants than in those of normal infants. However, those studies are not able to show whether the poor scores are a determinant of colicky behavior or a result of it.

Yet another theory is that a colicky infant's neurologic system is immature compared to that of a normal infant and that this affects a colicky infant's ability to make the transition from an awake state to a crying state to a sleep state. A related theory is that colic is caused by lack of establishment of a melatonin nocturnal secretion rhythm that would be maintained by the infant's pineal gland. The hypothesis is that some infants need 12 months to establish a circadian rhythm, having had only 9 months in utero to do so, and thus have 3 months of colic symptoms.

Sensory integration theory hypothesizes that abnormalities in vestibular function decrease an infant's ability to integrate sensory stimulation into appropriate motor responses. Several sensory integration theory researchers have found a positive correlation between a history of infant colic and later sensory integration disturbances such as sensory defensiveness. Treatment of sensory integration disorders involves vestibular stimulation, and this may explain why some colicky infants improve when in motion.

LABORATORY TESTING

Since infant colic is a diagnosis of exclusion, no available laboratory test is useful in making the diagnosis.

TREATMENT

The first step in the treatment of colic is confirmation of the diagnosis and education of the parents about the expected characteristics and time-limited nature of the syndrome. Parents often are relieved to learn that a child does not have a "serious" illness. It is important that the provider evaluate the psychological and social support structure of the family, as family resources are the most important factor in managing colic. The practitioner should carefully monitor the status of the support systems over the course of the syndrome and suggest interventions when necessary. Occasionally the family stresses generated by a colicky infant result in child abuse.

Suggestions for increasing the social and psychological support of affected families include getting friends and relatives to give the parents occasional relief from the overwhelming responsibilities of caring for a colicky infant. Finding good-quality child care to allow the parents a few hours away from the inconsolable crying is quite valuable. Extra support is also needed for the other siblings, who have temporary feelings of neglect.

Dietary changes can be suggested, keeping in mind that improvement is not a common result. Bottle-fed infants can be switched to soy formula, and the mothers of breast-fed infants can avoid dairy products, wheat, and nuts. Frequent small feedings occasionally improve the abdominal distention; however, it is also important to advise the parents to make sure all the air is expelled from the stomach after feedings. Medications are not useful for controlling colic symptoms. Simethicone has not proved to be any more effective than placebo, and aluminum-containing antacids have been implicated in two cases of rickets.

Occasionally exposure to motion improves colicky symptoms. Some infants improve when placed in an infant swing or taken for a car ride. Carrying a child in a front-style infant carrier while walking is sometimes helpful.

Generally, the overall approach to treatment involves supportive measures directed toward the whole family unit while monitoring for evidence of child abuse. The guiding philosophy should be one of helping the family survive this difficult self-limited syndrome and preventing long-term residual effects on the individuals in the family.

BIBLIOGRAPHY

Goldson E: *Current Pediatric Diagnosis and Treatment,* 12th ed. Appleton, WI, Appleton & Lange, 1995.

Hill DJ: A low allergen diet is a significant intervention in infantile colic: Results of a community-based study. *J Allergy Clin Immunol* 96(61):886–892, 1995.

Lehtonen L: Infantile colic. *Arch Pediatr Adolesc Med* 149(5):533–536, 1995.

Metcalf TJ: Simethicone in the treatment of infant colic: A randomized, placebo-controlled, multicenter trial. *Pediatrics* 94(1):29–34, 1994.

Pivnick EK: Rickets secondary to phosphate depletion: A sequela of antacid use in infancy. *Clin Pediatr* 34(2):73–78, 1995.

Rautava P: Psychosocial predisposing factors for infantile colic. *Br Med J* 307(6904):600–604, 1993.

Weissbluth L: Infant colic: The effect of serotonin and melatonin circadian rhythms on the intestinal smooth muscle. *Med Hypotheses* 39(2):164–167, 1992.

Chapter 15–3
NEONATAL CYANOSIS
David P. Asprey

DISCUSSION

Cyanosis is a visually observable bluish discoloration of the skin or mucous membranes. It can be either peripheral or central.

This distinction is an important one for a clinician to make and is determined by the oxygen level of the arterial blood. If the oxygen level in the arterial blood is low, it is defined as central cyanosis; if it is normal, it is defined as peripheral cyanosis. While peripheral cyanosis may be a normal physical examination finding, central cyanosis is always considered abnormal.

It is important that a clinician be able to distinguish peripheral from central cyanosis. Inspection of the mucous membranes is the most reliable way to determine the presence of central cyanosis on the physical examination. Cyanosis that is observable on inspection of the mucous membranes is indicative of central cyanosis. Mild degrees of cyanosis are very difficult to detect. To maximize the examiner's ability to detect the presence of mild cyanosis, the patient should be examined in natural rather than artificial lighting. Utilization of a cutaneous pulse oximeter to measure the patient's oxygen saturation is beneficial when this is available. In patients with normal hemoglobin who have observable central cyanosis, the arterial saturation is typically less than 85 percent.

SYMPTOMS

Cyanosis is a common presenting symptom in neonates and requires a very thorough investigation for its etiology. Peripheral cyanosis (acrocyanosis) is a common finding in the first 48 to 72 h of life. It usually results from slower blood flow through the distal aspect of an extremity, resulting in a large arteriovenous oxygen difference. In most instances, peripheral cyanosis is not indicative of pathology in a neonate.

Central cyanosis occurs when the absolute concentration of unoxygenated or reduced hemoglobin in the arterial blood exceeds 3 g/dL. It is important to recall that adult and fetal hemoglobin differ in regard to their binding capacities for oxygen. The hemoglobin-oxygen dissociation curve is diagrammed and well described in most standard human physiology texts. In fetal hemoglobin, the curve is shifted to the left so that at the same oxygen partial pressure the oxygen saturation is higher in fetal blood than in a child's or adult's blood. Consequently, a neonate develops cyanosis at a lower oxygen partial pressure than older children do.

When the total hemoglobin concentration is low (i.e., anemia), a higher percentage of unsaturated hemoglobin is needed to develop visible cyanosis. In a normal neonate, the typical hemoglobin concentration is 17 g/dL. In this instance, when the oxygen saturation is approximately 82 percent, more than 3 g/dL of unoxygenated hemoglobin is present and cyanosis results (the oxygen partial pressure necessary to produce cyanosis in this case is approximately 38 to 39 mmHg). Premature infants may have hemoglobin concentrations as low as 12 g/dL or less. In this instance, the level of unoxygenated hemoglobin has to be 25 percent (or saturation levels as low as 75 percent with an oxygen partial pressure as low as 30 mmHg) to result in a level of reduced or unoxygenated hemoglobin greater than the 3 g/dL needed to produce cyanosis.[1]

Once the presence of central cyanosis has been established, the potential causes must be considered and the specific etiology must be identified. Generally the pathophysiologic mechanisms of cyanosis can be considered to consist of the following five categories: alveolar hypoventilation, right-to-left shunting of blood, ventilation-perfusion inequality, impaired oxygen diffusion, and decreased affinity of hemoglobin for oxygen. In some patients multiple factors may be present simultaneously, resulting in multiple pathophysiologic mechanisms that contribute to the presence of the cyanosis.

Alveolar hypoventilation occurs with conditions that decrease the alveolar ventilation, resulting in an accumulation of carbon dioxide in the alveoli. Consequently, the alveolar oxygen tension is decreased and there is incomplete oxygenation of arterial blood.

Right-to-left shunting results when a portion of the venous blood is mixed into the arterial system without circulating through the lungs to undergo oxygenation. The admixture of venous blood into the arterial system results in desaturation of the arterial blood supply. This can occur as a result of intracardiac lesions or extracardiac (vascular) lesions and through intrapulmonary mechanisms.

Ventilation-perfusion inequality can occur when there is a mismatch between the ventilation and the perfusion in each area of the lung. Decreased ventilation with normal or increased perfusion results in incomplete oxygenation of the blood. The admixture of this incompletely oxygenated blood with oxygenated blood results in a partially desaturated arterial blood supply.

Impairment of diffusion of gases from the alveoli to the pulmonary capillary blood can result in clinical cyanosis. Any condition that results in an accentuated cardiac output may contribute to this problem. The excess volume of blood may result in accelerated blood flow through the pulmonary capillary beds and thus prohibit the full exchange of gases at this level.

Abnormalities of the hemoglobin structure may interfere with its ability to bind with oxygen, resulting in incomplete oxygen saturation. An example of this is methemoglobinemia, which can occur with exposure to oxidants, such as nitrates (in untreated water supplies), that are converted to nitrites. The nitrites bind with the hemoglobin, displacing the oxygen molecules.

The most likely causes of central cyanosis in a neonate are respiratory or cardiac in origin. However, there are numerous potential etiologies for cyanosis, and in many instances the degree of cyanosis may result from a combination of causes. Table 15-3-1 provides a list of common clinical conditions that may result in central cyanosis in a neonate.

MEDICAL HISTORY

A careful medical history should be obtained for the infant and the mother. The infant's gestational and birth history may provide important diagnostic clues to potential causes of cyanosis. A description of the presentation of the symptoms also may provide important information. The timing and occurrence of the cyanosis, precipitating events, and the duration of the cyanosis may give the clinician critical clues to the etiology.

PHYSICAL EXAMINATION FINDINGS

A thorough physical examination should be completed with the patient in a quiet, warm environment, utilizing natural lighting when possible. The examination should first be conducted with the patient on room air when possible. The clinician should first attempt to distinguish peripheral from central cyanosis. Careful inspection of the skin for plethora may provide evidence of polycythemia. One should observe capillary refilling of the extremities for indications of decreased peripheral blood flow.

Decreased muscle tone and activity and the response to noxious stimuli may suggest CNS disease, sepsis, or severe shock. The presence of a murmur, a single second heart sound, and diminished pulses may be indicative of congenital heart disease. However, it should be noted that significant heart disease may be present in the absence of these findings. A careful evaluation of the respiratory system is often the most productive aspect of the physical examination. One should note the tracheal position for evidence of pneumothorax or space-occupying lesions. It is necessary to determine the respiratory rate and pattern and the degree of respiratory effort and observe for evidence of retractions and other signs of respiratory distress (nasal flaring, grunting, etc.).

Table 15-3-1. Common Clinical Conditions Associated with Neonatal Cyanosis

Alveolar hypoventilation
  Parenchymal disease
    Atelectasis, respiratory distress syndrome: diffuse
    Aspiration syndrome: blood or meconium
    Infection: pneumonia
    Pulmonary hypoplasia
  Space-occupying lesions
    Pneumothorax
    Lobar emphysema
    Diaphragmatic hernia
    Pleural effusion
    Diaphragmatic elevation: ascites, etc.
  Obstructive lesions
    Choanal atresia
    Vocal cord paralysis
    Vascular rings
    Tracheal or bronchial stenosis
  Excessive lung fluid
  Pulmonary hemorrhage
  Diaphragmatic paralysis: phrenic nerve palsy
  Cardiovascular
    Congestive heart failure
    Persistent pulmonary hypertension: persistent fetal circulation
  Central nervous system
    Infection
    Hemorrhage
    Arteriovenous malformations
    Seizure disorders
    Apnea
  Polycythemia
  Methemoglobinemia
  Metabolic
    Hypoglycemia
    Hypocalcemia
Right-to-left shunting
  Congenital heart disease (with admixture-type defects)
  Parenchymal disease
    Respiratory distress syndrome
    Aspiration syndrome: blood, meconium, etc.
    Infection: pneumonia
  Pulmonary hypertension
Ventilation-perfusion inequality
  Parenchymal disease
    Atelectasis: diffuse respiratory distress syndrome or localized (bronchial mucus plugs)
    Aspiration syndrome: blood, meconium
    Infection: pneumonia
  Polycythemia
Impaired diffusion
  Aspiration syndrome: blood, meconium
  Pulmonary hemorrhage
Decreased affinity of hemoglobin for oxygen
  Methemoglobinemia

SOURCE: Modified from Kitterman.[2]

DIAGNOSTIC CONSIDERATIONS

In many instances the etiology of cyanosis may be readily apparent. An arterial blood gas should be obtained to assess the severity of the patient's clinical condition, establish the etiology, and guide the treatment of the cyanosis. However, differentiating cardiac from respiratory causes of cyanosis may be challenging. A particularly useful tool in differentiating respiratory from cardiac causes is an oxygen challenge test. This test is conducted by measuring the arterial partial oxygen pressure on room air. The patient is then administered 90 to 100% oxygen for approximately 15 min, and the partial oxygen pressure is repeated. In patients with congenital heart disease and right-to-left shunting, only minimal increases (10 to 15 mmHg) in the partial oxygen pressure will be achieved. However, if the partial oxygen pressure improves considerably (50 percent or more) while 100% oxygen is inspired, a pulmonary etiology is likely. A low partial oxygen pressure with a low or normal partial carbon dioxide pressure is indicative of the right-to-left shunting of blood that can occur with congenital heart disease, pulmonary hypertension, and other forms of pulmonary disease.

LABORATORY STUDIES

The following laboratory studies may be useful in assessing patients with cyanosis: a complete blood count to assess hemoglobin and hematocrit levels, cutaneous oxygen saturation monitoring, arterial blood gases to assess the partial oxygen pressure and carbon dioxide levels, electrolyte levels including calcium, and the glucose level.

RADIOLOGIC STUDIES

A chest x-ray may be useful in providing diagnostic clues to the etiology of central cyanosis in a neonate. Many findings associated with respiratory disease and in some instances congenital heart disease are associated with abnormal findings on chest x-ray. One should observe the x-ray for evidence of pneumonia, infiltrates, space-occupying lesions, air leaks, respiratory distress syndrome, increased pulmonary blood flow, and cardiomegaly.

OTHER DIAGNOSTIC STUDIES

An ECG may be useful in establishing the diagnosis of dysrhythmias and some types of congenital heart disease. Echocardiography is an extremely useful and sensitive tool to assess patients with suspected congenital heart disease. A careful study by a skilled pediatric echocardiographer can identify congenital heart disease, persistent fetal circulation, pulmonary hypertension, and the presence of right-to-left shunting through intracardiac and some extracardiac lesions.

TREATMENT

Central cyanosis in a neonate should be treated as a medical emergency. If the specific etiology of the cyanosis is not readily apparent, supportive treatment should be initiated until the etiology can be established and treated appropriately. This treatment includes ensuring the patency of airways, administering oxygen, ensuring an appropriate core body temperature, and correcting abnormal electrolyte, calcium, and hemoglobin levels. In cases of severe cyanosis, intubation and mechanical ventilation may be necessary. In addition, if the oxygen challenge test results in a neonate suggest a cardiac etiology of the cyanosis, consideration should be given to treating the patient with prostaglandin E_1 to maintain the patency of the ductus arteriosus.

Once a specific etiology has been identified, the treatment should be directed at correcting the underlying clinical condition causing the cyanosis. A full discussion of the treatment options for each of the clinical conditions that can cause cyanosis is outside the scope of this chapter. A more detailed discussion of treatment may be found by looking up the specific clinical condition in the index.

PEARLS

When the initial assessment of the patient fails to provide a likely etiology of the cyanosis, one should consider methemoglobinemia. This condition results when infants ingest well water containing high levels of nitrates. The nitrate ion is converted to nitrite in the intestine. After this ion is formed, it is absorbed and reacts with hemoglobin to form methemoglobin. Methemoglobin competes with normal hemoglobin for nonreduced oxygen, thus creating cyanosis. A careful history often reveals that a child has been ingesting water from an untreated well with an excessive nitrate level.

REFERENCES

1. Rudolph AM, Kamei RK: *Rudolph's Fundamentals of Pediatrics.* Norwalk, Conn. Appleton & Lange, 1994, p. 102.
2. Kitterman JA: Cyanosis in the newborn infant. *Pediat Rev* 4(1):19, 1982.

Chapter 15–4
REYE'S SYNDROME
Thomas J. Schymanski

DISCUSSION

Reye's syndrome is an acute and potentially fatal encephalopathy of unknown etiology that is emerging as one of the more common causes of death in childhood. Little is known about the pathogenesis of this syndrome, but it is believed that the major site of injury is the mitochondrion. The reasons for this mitochondrial dysfunction are unknown. It is thought to be precipitated by salicylates during episodes of chickenpox or influenza–upper respiratory infection (URI). The circumstances in which salicylates serve as a cofactor (or comitochondrial toxin) in a susceptible host during a viral infection remain to be determined. This most often occurs in children 4 to 12 years old, with a peak incidence at about 6 years of age.

Reye's syndrome is a multisystem disease that affects the liver, brain, heart, kidneys, pancreas, and muscle tissue. Pathologic findings in the brain include cerebral edema with or without herniation; anoxic neuronal changes are most severe in the cerebral cortex. The liver appears swollen and yellow or reddish yellow. Light microscopy reveals a fine vacuolization of the parenchymal cells resulting from intracellular lipid. Glycogen is absent, and there is no evidence of inflammation. Electron microscopy reveals mitochondrial abnormalities consisting of ameboid and spherical structural deformation, loss of dense bodies and cristae, and swelling of the mitochondrial matrix.

The kidneys are pale with a slight yellowish tinge and a widening of the cortices. Light microscopy reveals fatty degeneration of Henle's loops and proximal convoluted tubules. The glomeruli, vessels, and interstitium appear to be normal. Examination of the heart reveals epicardial petechiae in many cases. Light microscopy reveals Oil Red O–positive material in the ventricles and especially in the atria. Electron microscopy reveals mitochondrial swelling and fragmentation of the cristae.

Most cases occur in the late fall and winter. Widespread outbreaks have occurred in association with regional influenza epidemics. Varicella virus, the enteroviruses, Epstein-Barr virus, and the myxoviruses have been associated with sporadic cases.

The question remains whether Reye's syndrome is a new disease or whether affected children previously were classified as having "postviral encephalopathy." It is very likely that mild cases are missed and that these patients recover without any significant medical event. In any case, Reye's syndrome may be the most common potentially lethal virus-associated encephalopathy in the United States.

Table 15-4-1. Clinical Staging of Reye's Syndrome

Grade	Symptoms at Time of Admission
I	Usually quiet, lethargic, and sleepy; vomiting; lab evidence of liver dysfunction
II	Deep lethargy, confusion, delirium, combative, hyperventilation, hyperreflexic
III	Obtunded, light coma, with or without seizures, decorticate rigidity, intact pupillary light reaction
IV	Seizures, deepening coma, decerebrate rigidity, loss of oculocephalic reflexes, fixed pupils
V	Coma, loss of deep tendon reflexes, respiratory arrest, fixed dilated pupils, flaccidity and decerebrate (intermittent) posturing, isoelectric EEG

SIGNS AND SYMPTOMS

The severity of the disease varies greatly but is characterized by a biphasic illness: Initially a viral infection, usually a URI (occasionally exanthematous), is followed on about day 6 by the onset of nausea and vomiting and a sudden change in mental status.

When associated with varicella, the encephalopathy usually develops on the fourth to fifth day of the rash. The changes in mental status may vary from mild amnesia and noticeable lethargy to intermittent episodes of disorientation and agitation that often progress rapidly to deepening stages of coma manifested by progressive unresponsiveness, decorticate and decerebrate posturing, seizures, flaccidity, fixed dilated pupils, and respiratory arrest. Focal neurologic findings are usually not present.

The clinical features are best reflected in the system of clinical staging (Table 15-4-1); grades I through III represent mild to moderate illness, while grades IV and V indicate severe illness. The majority of affected children have mild illness without progression.

OBJECTIVE FINDINGS

Characteristically, an antecedent viral illness is followed by vomiting and progressive lethargy (noted from the history). Physical examination reveals tachypnea, fever, and lethargy, and stupor and coma are typical findings. Signs of elevated intracranial pressure (ICP) and seizures also may be noted.

DIAGNOSTIC CONSIDERATIONS

The differential diagnosis includes other causes of coma and hepatic dysfunction, such as sepsis or hyperthermia (especially in infants), salicylism, drug ingestion, head trauma, bacterial and viral infections of the central nervous system, and hepatitis.

LABORATORY TESTS AND RADIOLOGIC STUDIES

Elevated serum heptatocellular enzyme assays (serum glutamic-oxaloacetic transaminase, serum glutamate pyruvate transaminase, lactic dehydrogenase) and elevated serum ammonia (arterial) are the laboratory hallmarks; one also may see metabolic acidosis and respiratory alkalosis as well as hypoglycemia and prolongation of the prothrombin time (PT) and partial thromboplastin time (PTT). A liver biopsy generally is performed when the diagnosis is in question but is not essential for the clinical diagnosis. The data gained are crucial in the precise definition of the syndrome. Biopsy should be carried out in atypical or severe cases to rule out other disorders, such as metabolic or toxic liver disease, especially in patients under 1 year of age. CT may be necessary to rule out an intracranial mass.

TREATMENT

Since the cause of the syndrome is uncertain and widespread metabolic derangements are present, there is no universally accepted therapy. Early diagnosis and prompt institution of intensive supportive care are the mainstays of treatment. Meticulous and constant attention to neurologic, electrolyte, metabolic, cardiovascular, respiratory, and fluid status is essential to cope with rapid changes. Treatment includes intravenous fluid and electrolyte solutions containing glucose, usually 5 to 10% but occasionally up to 50%; the judicious use of nonabsorbable antibiotics (such as neomycin 100 mg/kg/d orally every 6 h); and vitamin K 5 mg/d intravenously or intramuscularly. Increased ICP must be controlled with agents such as mannitol 0.5 to 1 g/kg given intravenously over 45 min and dexamethasone 0.5 mg/kg/d intravenously; close monitoring of ICP may help guide this therapy. Common procedures include monitoring blood gases, blood pH, and blood pressure by means of arterial catheters; inserting an endotracheal tube; and controlling ventilation.

SUPPORTIVE MEASURES

The medical professionals who are usually involved in the care of a patient with Reye's syndrome include pediatricians, neurologists, gastroenterologists, and physical and respiratory therapists. The ability to serially monitor arterial blood gases, central venous pressure, and electroencephalography (EEG) and 24-h intensive care nursing and physician coverage are imperative. Throughout the course of the illness, the primary care provider is an indispensable member of the team, interpreting procedures and progress for the family. After recovery, long-term follow-up by the primary care team is of great importance and involves coordinating care as required for the management of neurologic and psychological sequelae and recognizing and treating patient and family stresses that have resulted from the illness.

Patient Education

One should avoid the administration of salicylates in children with a viral illness. Printed patient information can be obtained from the National Reye's Syndrome Foundation, (800) 233-7393.

Disposition

The overall majority of these patients have mild illness without progression of the condition. The prognosis is related to the degree of cerebral edema and the ammonia level on admission.

Possible neurologic complications include problems with attention, concentration, speech, language, and fine and gross motor skills. These complications necessitate the involvement of medical providers, psychologists, and physical, occupational, and speech therapists.

COMPLICATIONS

Potential complications are as follows:

- Aspiration pneumonia
- Respiratory failure
- Cardiac dysrhythmia or arrest
- Diabetes insipidus
- Cerebral edema
- Inappropriate vasopressin excretion

OTHER NOTES AND PEARLS

Reye's syndrome does not always follow a typical clinical pattern. Vomiting may not occur.

BIBLIOGRAPHY

Nelson R, Behrman RE, Kliegman RM, Arvin, AM: *Nelson's Textbook of Pediatrics,* 15th ed. Philadelphia, Saunders, 1996, pp 1144–1155.
Rakel E: *Conn's Current Therapy 1995.* Philadelphia, Saunders, 1994, pp 845–848.
Rakel RE: *Textbook of Family Practice,* 5th ed. Philadelphia, Saunders, 1995, pp 388, 462, 644, 1031, 1057.

Chapter 15–5
TEETHING
Richard Dehn

DISCUSSION

Teething is the common term for problems associated with the development and eruption of teeth in children. Teething problems are common in the first 18 months of life, with folklore attributing to teething numerous symptoms, including fever, diarrhea, mouth lesions, rashes, and drooling. In the nineteenth century, teething was thought to be the leading cause of infant death.

In a paper presented at an 1896 meeting of the American Medical Association, Dr. S. W. Foster stated:

The [teething] child becomes wakeful, restless, and fretful, refuses nourishment; the alimentary canal becomes more active, diarrhea follows, and if relief is not given, relaxation of the vital forces follows, and we have nausea, vomiting, convulsions, paralysis, and not infrequently, death.

The formation of teeth begins in the second gestational month. Primary mandibular and maxillary incisors can appear as early as age 3 months but usually erupt at around 6 months. The lower central incisors often appear first at 5 to 7 months of age, followed by the upper central incisors at 6 to 8 months. These usually are followed by the upper lateral incisors at 9 to 11 months and the lower central incisors at 10 to 12 months. Generally the first molars appear next at 12 to 16 months, then the cuspids at 16 to 20 months, and finally the second molars at 20 to 30 months. The eruption of all the primary teeth usually is completed by age 3. The eruption of permanent teeth commonly begins at about 6 years of age. Medical practice in underdeveloped areas that do not record birth dates sometimes utilizes a method of estimating a child's age by counting the teeth: The age in months equals the number of teeth plus 6 months for children under age 3.

Occasionally children are born with teeth or have the eruption of teeth in the first month of life, and these children often have a family history of early tooth eruption. Some controversy has emerged about whether these teeth should be extracted, since they may lead to tongue lacerations, feeding difficulties, and abrasions to the mother's nipples during breast feeding. Delayed eruption is sometimes present in patients with Down syndrome, hypothyroidism, hypopituitarism, achondroplastic dwarfism, and other syndromes that involve the delayed development of organ systems.

Typically the pending eruption of a tooth in an infant produces discomfort and tenderness, which lead to irritability and a compulsion by the infant to chew on relatively hard objects. The chewing activity can stimulate increased salivation, which may account for the drooling characteristically described by parents.

Diarrhea often has been associated with teething, but no studies have confirmed a relationship. The development of oral lesions also has been associated with teething, but it is thought that these may be herpetic gingivostomatitis lesions. Fever commonly has been associated with teething; however, studies are unclear about whether there is a relationship. It has been observed that an infant's temperatures are slightly elevated [37 to 38°C (98.6–100.4°F)] the day before the eruption of the first tooth, but no studies have shown that teething is associated with greater temperature elevations. The association of fever might be a manifestation of the development of a coincidental viral gingivitis, which might then produce lesions, fever, irritability, drooling, and diarrhea, all of which are folkloric symptoms of teething.

PATHOGENESIS

It is thought that the physical pressure of erupting teeth may create physical pressure on nearby structures. This could produce temporary discomfort and a local sensation of irritability that induces a need to manipulate or stimulate the affected area. Increased chewing resulting from this need can increase salivation, which over time can produce an atopic rash below the lower lip and at the corners of the mouth.

DIAGNOSTIC CONSIDERATIONS

Symptoms attributed to teething by folklore should be considered to be possibly secondary to other causes. Infectious diseases that are common in this age group should be ruled out, along with pathology secondary to trauma. Teething is essentially a diagnosis of exclusion.

LABORATORY TESTS

Since teething is a diagnosis of exclusion, no laboratory testing is useful in making the diagnosis. The diagnosis usually is made in light of the history and physical examination findings, sometimes with additional support from the negative results of laboratory tests used to rule out other disorders.

TREATMENT

The most common treatment for teething is the application of a topical anesthetic (teething gel) to the affected areas. Several compounds are available without prescription that contain ethylaminobenzoate (Benzocaine) in a gel formulation that can be applied with cotton, a cotton swab, or a fingertip. For infants and children 4 months to 2 years of age, compounds containing 7.5 to 10% Benzocaine can be applied up to four times a day. Products containing 7.5% Benzocaine include Anbesol Baby, Num-Zit Gel, Orabase Baby, and Orajel Baby. Products containing 10% Benzocaine include Numzident, Orajel, Orajel Nighttime Formula Baby, and Rid-A-Pain. Benzocaine teething jel should be used with caution in infants and young children, since absorption may result in methemoglobinemia. Benzocaine products can produce allergic sensitivity to other local anesthetics, and overuse can suppress the gag reflex and inhibit the swallowing mechanism, with potentially serious results.

Analgesics such as acetaminophen and ibuprofen are considered safer and are thought to be more effective than teething gels for the treatment of teething discomfort. Teething toys are useful mainly for distraction and should be evaluated primarily with safety in mind.

The general approach to the treatment of teething problems first consists of the exclusion of other causes of the symptoms. The expected course of normal tooth eruption should be explained to the parent, and the use of systemic analgesics should be encour-

aged. The parent should be cautioned about the use of teething gels and encouraged to monitor teething toys and devices for safety. Like many minor childhood problems, teething difficulties eventually go away regardless of what treatment, if any, is provided.

BIBLIOGRAPHY

Abrams RB, Mueller WA (eds): *Current Pediatric Diagnosis and Treatment,* 12th ed. Appleton, WI, Appleton & Lange, 1995.
Castiglia P: Teething. *J Pediatr Health Care* 6(3):153–154, 1992.
Coreil J: Recognition and management of teething diarrhea among Florida pediatricians. *Clin Pediatr* 34(11):591–598, 1995.
Jaber L: Fever associated with teething. *Arch Dis Child* 67(2):233–234, 1992.
King DL: Herpetic gingivostomatitis and teething difficulty in infants. *Pediatr Dentistry* 14(2):82–85, 1992.
King DL: Teething revisited. *Pediatr Dentistry* 16(3):179–182, 1994.
Kowitz AA: Paediatric dentistry: Fauchard and before. *Int Dent J* 43(3):239–244, 1993.

Chapter 15–6
GROWTH AND DEVELOPMENT IN INFANCY AND EARLY CHILDHOOD
Jill Reichman

DISCUSSION

To provide comprehensive health care for infants and children, a clinician needs to monitor their growth and development. Although significant variation in the rate of growth and development may occur among children, an accepted range of normal has been established by statistically comparing children of the same age and sex. Growth charts are developed by using these data to create percentiles. Plotting growth data for an infant or child allows a clinician to compare that infant or child with the statistical norm and assign a percentile. Conscientious surveillance can identify infants and children who are outside this normal range as well as those who have sudden changes in their growth patterns. Once identified, these children can be closely monitored and referred as needed for further evaluation.

The most basic evaluation of growth and development involves the measurement of height and weight along with head circumference in children age less than 3. Using and maintaining data on growth charts help a clinician visually map growth and quickly identify abnormalities and changes in growth curves. Growth charts are available for recording the length and weight of infants and toddlers age 0 to 36 months and for recording the height and weight of toddlers and older children age 2 to 18 years (Figs. 15-6-1 and 15-6-2). A separate chart can be completed to record head circumference in infants and children under age 3 (Fig. 15-6-3). All these charts are available with appropriate percentiles for both boys and girls.

Several other parameters should be evaluated during the routine examination, including neonatal reflexes, gross motor skills,

BOYS: BIRTH TO 36 MONTHS
PHYSICAL GROWTH
NCHS PERCENTILES*

NAME _____ RECORD # _____

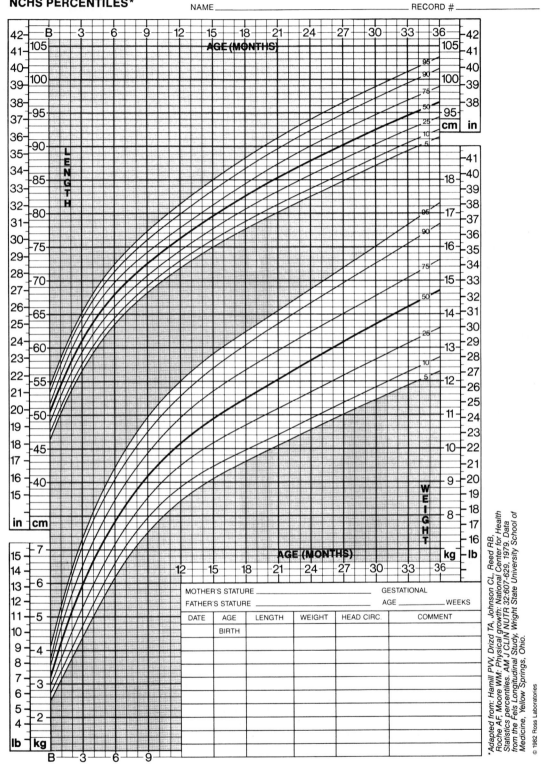

FIGURE 15-6-1. Growth chart for recording length and weight for boys 0 to 36 months.

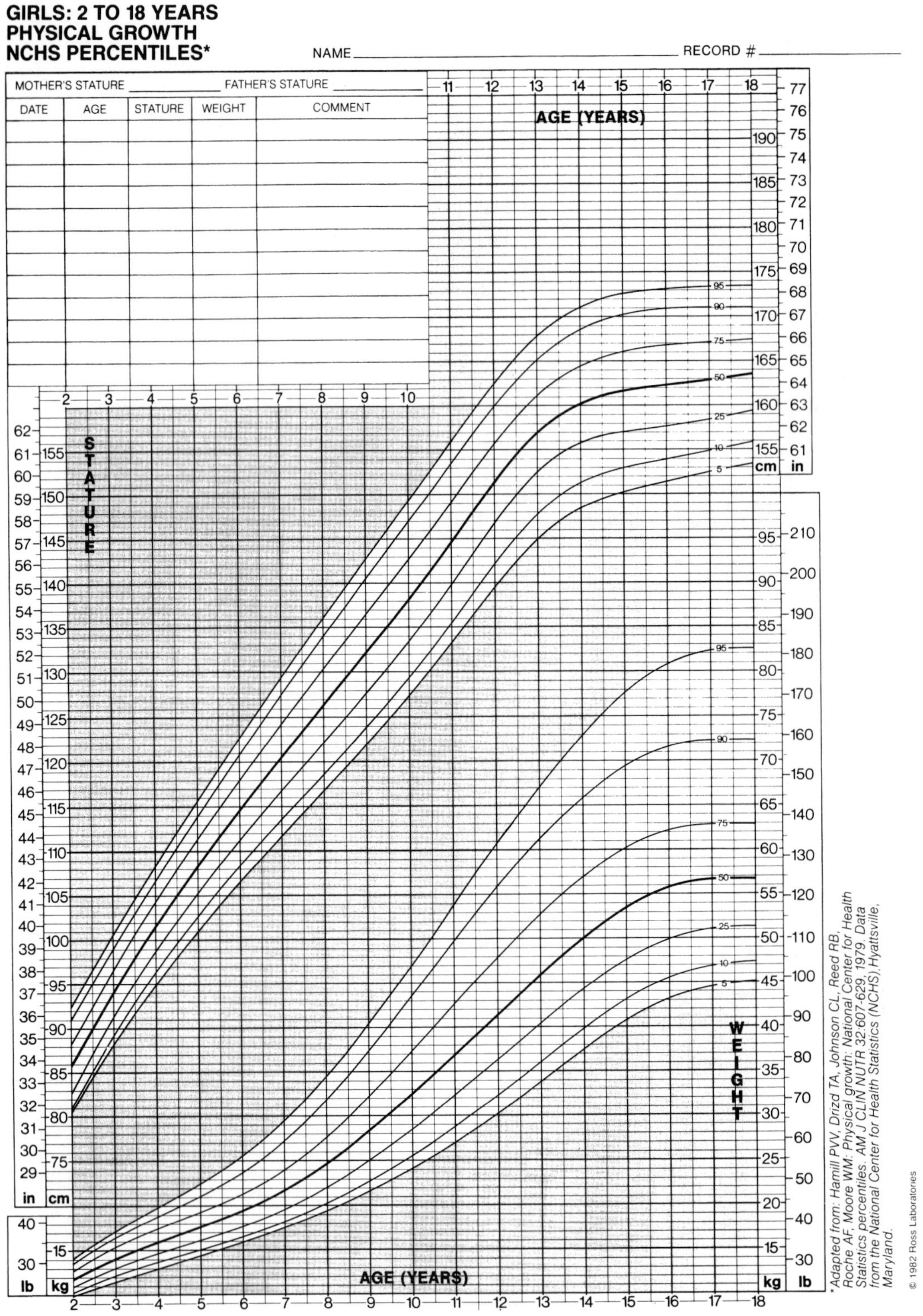

FIGURE 15-6-2. Growth chart for recording height and weight for girls 2 to 18 years.

**BOYS: BIRTH TO 36 MONTHS
PHYSICAL GROWTH
NCHS PERCENTILES***

NAME _____   RECORD # _____

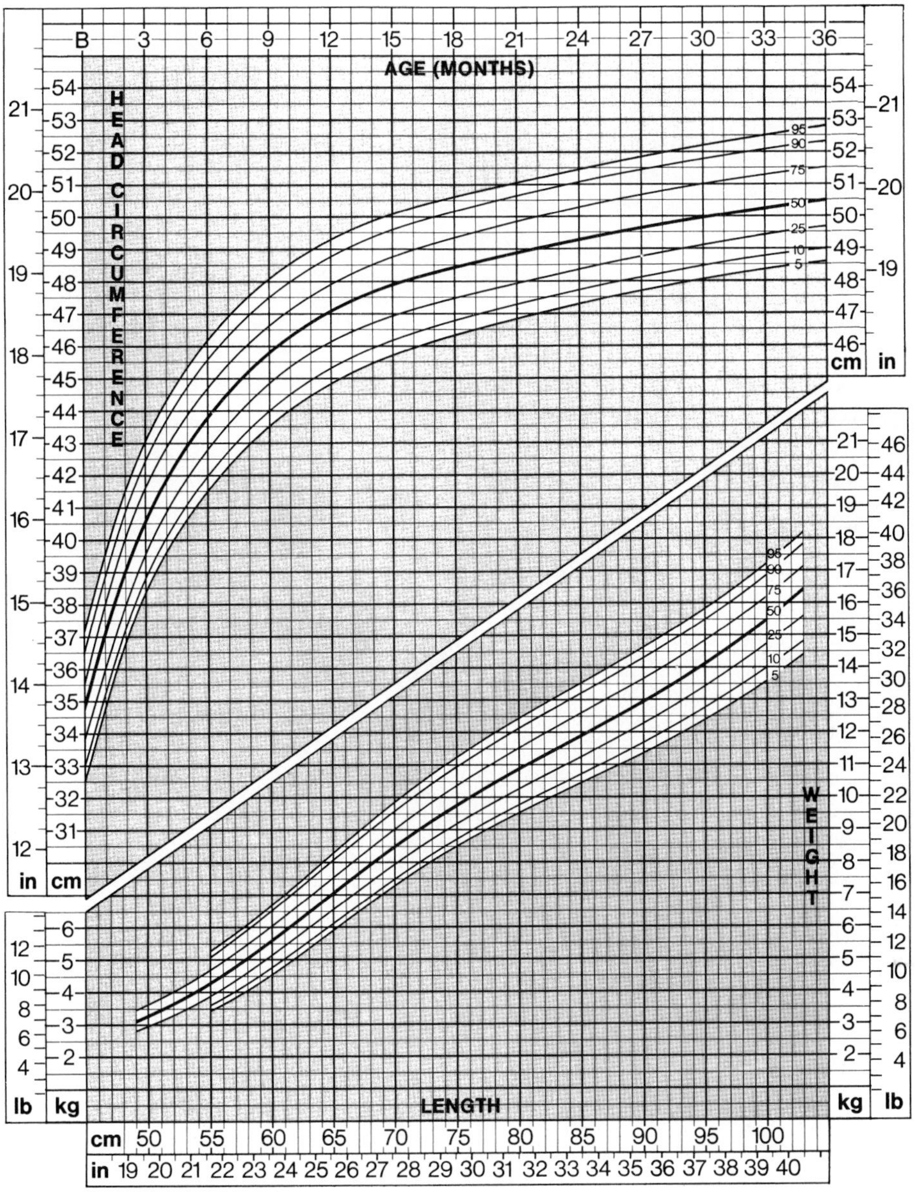

*Adapted from: Hamill PVV, Drizd TA, Johnson CL, Reed RB,
Roche AF, Moore WM: Physical growth: National Center for Health
Statistics percentiles. AM J CLIN NUTR 32:607-629, 1979. Data
from the Fels Longitudinal Study, Wright State University School of
Medicine, Yellow Springs, Ohio.

© 1982 Ross Laboratories

DATE	AGE	LENGTH	WEIGHT	HEAD CIRC.	COMMENT

SIMILAC® WITH IRON
Infant Formula

ISOMIL®
Soy Protein Formula with Iron

Reprinted with permission
of Ross Laboratories

FIGURE 15-6-3. Growth chart for recording head circumference, length, and weight for boys 0 to 36 months.

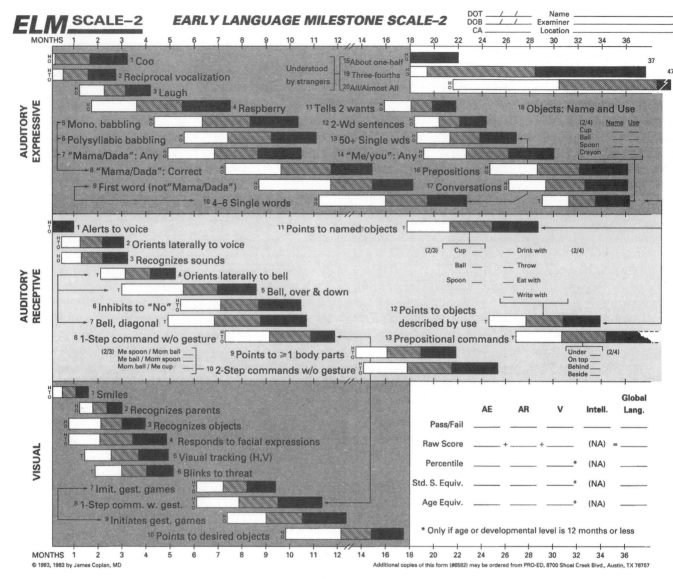

FIGURE 15-6-4. Early Language Milestone (ELM) Scale–2.

fine motor-adaptive skills, social skills, and language skills. Monitoring developmental milestones in infants and children allows a clinician to screen for children who need further evaluation.

DEVELOPMENTAL MILESTONES

Neonatal Reflexes

Early milestones of development include the appearance and disappearance of neonatal, or primitive reflexes. Infants are born with most of the primitive reflexes, which slowly disappear between 5 weeks and 6 months of age. These reflexes are involuntary motor responses elicited by environmental stimuli. Table 15-6-1 describes some of the reflexes that can be evaluated during a routine examination. The absence or persistence of these reflexes suggests a dysfunction of the central nervous system and requires referral.

Gross Motor Development

Milestones in gross motor development can be observed in a newborn and continue to occur throughout childhood. In the first

2 years of life, gross motor development is dramatic, transforming an infant with little head control into a toddler who runs and jumps. From ages 2 through 6, gross motor development seems less dramatic to the observer, but this is a time when the coordination of gross motor skills is achieved. It is also a time when injuries tend to occur as children venture forth and experiment with new motor skills and abilities. The clinician should be aware of the range of normal abilities and should inform parents about injury prevention. Table 15-6-2 describes the major gross motor milestones as they occur chronologically.

Fine Motor-Adaptive Skills

Fine motor skills involve the use of smaller muscles in the hands and fingers and correspond to the development of adaptive skills that require hand-eye coordination. These skills are present in infants but are most notable after age 4, when children begin to manipulate small objects easily and perform complicated tasks such as putting together a puzzle. By age 6 most children can tie their shoes and write their names. Toddlers spend much of their

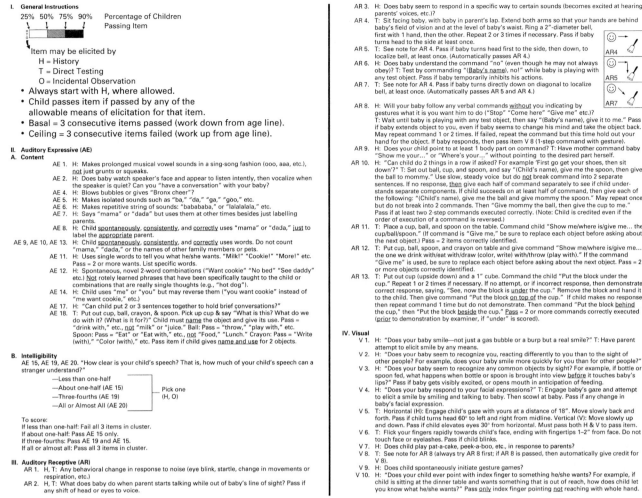

FIGURE 15-6-4 (*continued*). Early Language Milestone (ELM) Scale–2.

time practicing fine motor skills by using paper and pencils or crayons. Parents should be reminded about the need for supervision of these activities to prevent injuries in young children. Table 15-6-3 describes the major fine motor-adaptive skills in infants and children.

Language Development

Like motor skills, speech and language develop with recognizable milestones that can be evaluated by a clinician. In most cases, problems are identified by the parents and brought to a clinician for evaluation. Understanding the range of normal helps a clinician appropriately reassure the parents that the child's development is within the range of normal or, alternatively, initiate a workup and referral for a child with suspected delayed language development. Because delayed language development may be due to hearing impairment, the evaluation of hearing is a critical part of the workup. Careful assessment of language ability may be aided by the use of a screening test such as the Early Language Milestone (ELM) Scale. This allows the screening of language development in children under 36 months of age. The ELM allows a clinician to evaluate expressive, receptive, and visual language through parental reporting and direct observation of the child (Fig. 15-6-4).

The development of language requires three basic abilities: expression, reception, and articulation. Expressive skills can be appreciated very early in life as the vocalizations of infants. Re-

ceptive skills involve the ability to hear and react to sound. Later, more sophisticated language skills allow a child to convey meaning and understand language. This can be seen as early as 9 to 12 months of age, when most infants begin to use language meaningfully by saying "mama" or "dada." These single-word expressions eventually become multiword expressions, whole sentences, and ultimately groups of sentences strung together to express complex ideas. Table 15-6-4 reviews the developmental milestones in language skills as they occur chronologically.

The referral of young children with a suspected delay in language development is aided by the use of tools such as the ELM. There are, however, specific guidelines for referral that should be followed, including the following:

1. Lack of response to sound at any age
2. Lack of babbling by 9 months
3. Inability to understand and/or respond to simple requests by age 2
4. Speech predominantly unintelligible by age 3
5. Stuttering, poor voice quality, and/or poor ability to articulate after age 5

The Development of Social Skills

Social skills are abilities that allow children to care for themselves and interact with others. As children grow older, some of these skills are molded by cultural or societal norms. These skills start

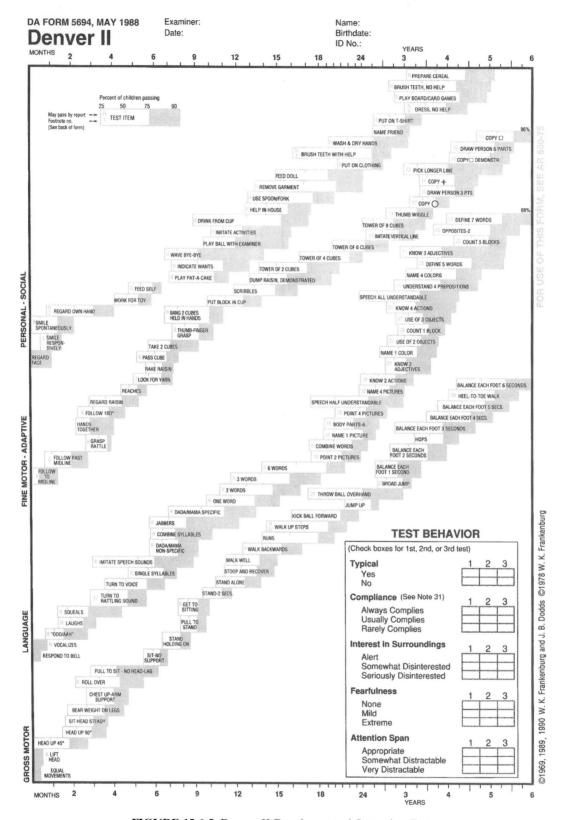

FIGURE 15-6-5. Denver II Developmental Screening Test.

DIRECTIONS FOR ADMINISTRATION

1. Try to get child to smile by smiling, talking or waving. Do not touch him/her.
2. Child must stare at hand several seconds.
3. Parent may help guide toothbrush and put toothpaste on brush.
4. Child does not have to be able to tie shoes or button/zip in the back.
5. Move yarn slowly in an arc from one side to the other, about 8" above child's face.
6. Pass if child grasps rattle when it is touched to the backs or tips of fingers.
7. Pass if child tries to see where yarn went. Yarn should be dropped quickly from sight from tester's hand without arm movement.
8. Child must transfer cube from hand to hand without help of body, mouth, or table.
9. Pass if child picks up raisin with any part of thumb and finger.
10. Line can vary only 30 degrees or less from tester's line.
11. Make a fist with thumb pointing upward and wiggle only the thumb. Pass if child imitates and does not move any fingers other than the thumb.

  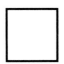

12. Pass any enclosed form. Fail continuous round motions.
13. Which line is longer? (Not bigger.) Turn paper upside down and repeat. (pass 3 of 3 or 5 of 6)
14. Pass any lines crossing near midpoint.
15. Have child copy first. If failed, demonstrate.

When giving items 12, 14, and 15, do not name the forms. Do not demonstrate 12 and 14.

16. When scoring, each pair (2 arms, 2 legs, etc.) counts as one part.
17. Place one cube in cup and shake gently near child's ear, but out of sight. Repeat for other ear.
18. Point to picture and have child name it. (No credit is given for sounds only.)
    If less than 4 pictures are named correctly, have child point to picture as each is named by tester.

 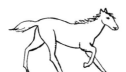   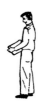

19. Using doll, tell child: Show me the nose, eyes, ears, mouth, hands, feet, tummy, hair. Pass 6 of 8.
20. Using pictures, ask child: Which one flies?... says meow?... talks?... barks?... gallops? Pass 2 of 5, 4 of 5.
21. Ask child: What do you do when you are cold?... tired?... hungry? Pass 2 of 3, 3 of 3.
22. Ask child: What do you do with a cup? What is a chair used for? What is a pencil used for? Action words must be included in answers.
23. Pass if child correctly places <u>and</u> says how many blocks are on paper. (1, 5).
24. Tell child: Put block **on** table; **under** table; **in front of** me, **behind** me. Pass 4 of 4. (Do not help child by pointing, moving head or eyes.)
25. Ask child: What is a ball?... lake?... desk?... house?... banana?... curtain?... fence?... ceiling? Pass if defined in terms of use, shape, what it is made of, or general category (such as banana is fruit, not just yellow). Pass 5 of 8, 7 of 8.
26. Ask child: If a horse is big, a mouse is __? If fire is hot, ice is __? If the sun shines during the day, the moon shines during the __? Pass 2 of 3.
27. Child may use wall or rail only, not person. May not crawl.
28. Child must throw ball overhand 3 feet to within arm's reach of tester.
29. Child must perform standing broad jump over width of test sheet (8 1/2 inches).
30. Tell child to walk forward, ⟨⟩ heel within 1 inch of toe. Tester may demonstrate. Child must walk 4 consecutive steps.
31. In the second year, half of normal children are non-compliant.

OBSERVATIONS:

Catalog #2115

FIGURE 15-6-5 (*continued*). Denver II Developmental Screening Test.

Table 15-6-1. Selected Neonatal Reflexes

Reflex	Description
Moro (startle)	Occurs when the neck and limbs contract in response to allowing infant's head to fall backward suddenly or when the infant is startled by a sudden noise or jerk. Generally disappears by age 4 months
Rooting	Elicited in response to touching cheek or corner of mouth and results in turning of head and opening of mouth. Facilitates breast feeding and usually disappears by age 3 to 4 months
Sucking	Elicited by placing an object in infant's mouth; results in sucking movements of lips. Along with rooting reflex, helps facilitate feeding
Palmer grasp	Occurs when object or finger is placed in infant's hand, causing infant to grasp object or finger tightly. Usually disappears by age 2 to 3 months
Tonic Neck	Seen in supine infant when head is turned to one side, causing infant to extend extremities on same side and flex extremities on opposite side. Although often present at birth, may not appear until 2 months and usually disappears by 4 months
Placing	Elicited when dorsal aspect of foot is allowed to touch edge of a table, causing infant to flex at hip and knee and place foot onto tabletop. Disappearance is variable but may occur by 1.5 to 2 months
Stepping	Elicited when infant is held upright and leaning forward; this causes movements of the legs that look like walking. Usually disappears by 1.5 to 2 months

SOURCE: Adapted from Berkowitz.[2]

at just a few weeks of age as a simple preference for the human face. Later, children shift from playing side by side (parallel play) to engaging in interactive play that requires communication with and consideration of others. Children learn to toilet train, bathe, and dress themselves with the encouragement and modeling of their caretakers.

The psychologist Erik Erikson developed a theory of child development that emphasizes the psychosocial focus of each developmental stage throughout childhood. His theory suggests that at each stage of development a child must successfully navigate a critical period. This accomplishment leads to a healthy sense of self and the development of positive social skills. Table 15-6-5 gives a brief overview of social development in childhood and includes Erikson's stages of psychosocial development.

SCREENING TESTS

There are numerous screening instruments that allow a clinician to look at most or all of the developmental parameters through the use of a single tool. The Denver Developmental Screening Test (DDST), originally published in 1967, has been used worldwide, and it was revised and restandardized in 1989 to make it more accurate. The new Denver II allows a clinician to monitor development in the following areas: gross motor, language, fine motor-adaptive, and personal-social (Fig. 15-6-5). It also includes a test behavior rating scale that offers an opportunity to evaluate variables such as attention span, fearfulness, and compliance.

The authors "emphasize that the Denver II is a screening test, the results of which should be integrated with everything else that one knows about the child, the family, the community, the educational experiences, and the culture in which the child has grown up."[1] The Denver II is not a diagnostic or predictive tool. It is designed to identify children who are not performing as expected for age so that they can be referred for further evaluation.

The Denver II is most effectively administered by a trained clinician. Denver Developmental Materials, Inc., of Denver, Colorado, offers training materials that include a technical manual

Table 15-6-2. Gross Motor Milestones

Age	Ability
Newborn	Moves head from side to side
1 month	Raises chin, lifts head when prone, makes lateral head movements
2 months	Raises chest with arms when prone
3 months	Holds head steady when upright, sits on lap with support
4 months	No head lag when pulled to sitting, rolls from front to back
5 months	Sits alone momentarily, rolls from back to front
6–7 months	Sits alone steadily
7–9 months	Creeps or crawls, pulls to standing
9–11 months	Cruises, walks when led with support
12–15 months	Stands alone, walks a few steps independently
18 months	Walks backward, walks up stairs with support, starts running
2 years	Runs, jumps down from a low object
3 years	Begins throwing and catching with assistance, walks up stairs using alternating steps, rides a tricycle, begins hopping
4 years	Begins skipping, walks down stairs using alternating steps, refines running and hopping
5 years	Running speed increases; further refines jumping, hopping, and skipping
6 years and older	Skillful hopping and skipping, mature throwing pattern, catches with hands only

Table 15-6-3. Fine Motor-Adaptive Skills

Age	Skill
1 month	Hands closed most of the time; can follow object to midline
2 months	Can follow object past midline and vertically
3 months	Hands more often open than closed; can follow object 180°
4 months	Regards hands; reaches for bright object; hands come together; brings objects to mouth
5 months	Grasp now voluntary; combs for objects with hands
6 months	Transfers objects from one hand to other
7 months	Can grasp with three-finger pincer motion
9–12 months	Grasp now two-finger pincer; bangs objects together in midline; releases objects voluntarily; plays pat-a-cake
15 months	Makes tower of three cubes; can draw line with crayon
18 months	Makes tower of four cubes; can scribble
2 years	Makes tower of seven cubes; copies vertical and horizontal lines
3 years	Makes tower of 10 cubes; copies a circle
4 years	Can build bridge from model; copies cross and square; draws person with two to four parts besides head
5 years	Copies triangle; draws person with three parts
6 years	Draws person with six parts; writes name

Table 15-6-4. Milestones in the Development of Language Skills

Age	Expressive Skills	Receptive Skills
0–2 months	Cries, begins gurgling sounds (cooing, vowel-like sounds)	Is aware of sound; turns toward sound; prefers human voice
3–4 months	May start to laugh or chuckle; cooing sustained	Seems to be listening; looks at speaker; reacts differently to different types of speech, e.g., angry versus happy
5–6 months	Cooing includes sounds of consonants, and babbling begins	Responds to own name; begins to understand other familiar words
9–12 months	Sounds start to be repeated, and "words" appear, e.g., *mama, dada*	Responds to *no* or other simple verbal commands by stopping activity or using other gestures to communicate
14–16 months	Vocabulary 10–50 words; speaks using jargon (actual words mixed with nonsense words)	Can point to familiar named objects or body parts
18–24 months	Vocabulary 50–75 words; speaks in two-word phrases, e.g., *my doll, thank you*	Responds to two-step command, e.g., "Come to Mommy and bring the book"; understands complex sentences and simple questions
2–3 years	Fast-growing vocabulary up to 1000 words; speaks in short (three-word) sentences; speech most often intelligible	Can follow a story in a picture book; understands prepositional commands
3–4 years	Vocabulary up to 1500 words; speech intelligible; speaks in four-word sentences	Responds to three-step commands
4–5 years	Language well established; conversation mature; large vocabulary; defines simple words; uses five-word sentences	Responds to four-step commands
5–6 years	Has adult speech pattern; articulation continues to improve	Responds to five-step commands; can follow story told without picture book; begins to understand more subtle nuances of language, e.g., that same word may have two meanings

Table 15-6-5. An Overview of Social Development in Childhood

Age	Social Skills	Erikson's Developmental Stage
1 month	Preference for human face; begins to smile	Stage 1: Trust versus mistrust (0–1.5 years)
2 months	Responds to voice; coos	Focus of this stage is trust and social support. Infant learns to trust or mistrust that his or her needs will be met by caregiver. This is determined by consistency of care infant receives from caregiver. Erikson's theory supports idea that this early developmental period sets groundwork for future socialization. Trust is necessary to achieve healthy social interactions. Successful resolution of this stage sets stage for healthy interactions later in life.
6 months	Laughs; interacts with caregiver	
9 months	Prefers mother to others; may show stranger anxiety	
12 months	Plays games; peek-a-boo, pat-a-cake; waves bye-bye on command; may cooperate with dressing; drinks from cup	
18 months	Starts to feed self with spoon; communicates some needs with gestures and words; hugs and kisses	
2 years	Cooperates with dressing; communicates verbally with caregivers; helps in bathing self	Stage 2: Autonomy versus shame and doubt (1.5–3 years)
3 years	Parallel plays; begins to help with dressing—may button and unbutton; washes and dries hands; may be toilet trained	Focus of this stage is establishment of independence and sense of self. During this phase, much of a child's time is spent practicing self-control. Sense of autonomy and well-being is achieved as child successfully completes this stage. If child feels unsuccessful, he or she is likely to experience feelings of shame. Healthy limits provided by caregiver help the child through this stage.
4 years	Plays interactively with others; models behavior of others	Stage 3: Initiative versus guilt (3–6 years)
5 years	Dresses self; often plays by role modeling; asks questions and when comfortable interacts with others, often enthusiastically	Focus of this stage is learning to care for oneself. During this stage children are eager to learn and begin to understand social rules and appropriate behavior. Successful resolution of this stage helps child be enthusiastic and industrious. Difficulty in this stage can lead to feelings of guilt. As in previous developmental periods, healthy limits set by caregiver help child be successful.

and training videotapes. Appropriate training in the administration of the Denver II helps assure the reliability of the test outcome.

Screening is the process by which a clinician can identify children who need further evaluation. Using standardized screening tools, such as growth charts and developmental testing instruments, a properly trained clinician can perform this task with the greatest reliability. In this way, physician assistants can fill a critical role in the early identification and referral of children with suspected developmental delays.

REFERENCES

1. Frankenburg WK, Dodds J, Archer P, et al: The Denver II: A major revision and restandardization of the Denver Developmental Screening Test. *Pediatrics* 89:91–97, 1992.
2. Berkowitz CD: *Pediatrics: A Primary Care Approach.* Philadelphia, Saunders, 1996, pp. 49–58.

BIBLIOGRAPHY

Bates B: *A Guide to Physical Examination and History Taking,* 6th ed. Philadelphia, Lippincott, 1995, pp 555–633.
Behrman R: *Nelson Textbook of Pediatrics,* 14th ed. Philadelphia, Saunders, 1992, pp 413–443.
Gormly A, Brodzinsky D: *Lifespan Human Development,* 4th ed. Fort Worth, TX, Holt, Rinehart and Winston, 1989, pp 10–258.
Hay W, Groothuis J, Hayward A, et al: *Current Pediatric Diagnosis and Treatment,* 12th ed. Norwalk, CT, Appleton & Lange, 1995, pp 65–82.
Rudolph A, Kamei R: *Rudolph's Fundamentals of Pediatrics.* Norwalk, CT, Appleton & Lange, 1994, pp 1–25.
Tanner JM: *Fetus into Man.* Cambridge, MA, Harvard University Press, 1978.

Vaughan V, Litt I: *Child and Adolescent Development: Clinical Implications.* Philadelphia, Saunders, 1990, pp 145–227.
Walker D, Gugenheim S, Downs M, et al: Early Language MilestoneScale and language screening of young children. *Pediatrics* 83:284–288, 1989.

Chapter 15–7
DISRUPTIVE AND NEGATIVISTIC BEHAVIOR PROBLEMS IN CHILDREN AND ADOLESCENTS

Kelly E. Naylor

DISCUSSION

Conduct disorders carry significant social and monetary costs. These disorders are the most common reason for juvenile referrals in clinical settings, with prevalence estimates ranging from 30 to 50 percent of clinical populations. Since minor conduct problems disappear with age, it generally is accepted that limited youthful delinquent or resistant behavior is normative and developmentally appropriate. Nevertheless, clinicians must be prepared to examine the severity, frequency, longevity, onset pattern, and consequent level of life disruption of delinquent behaviors to help identify youths at higher risk for persistent antisocial behavior. This is particularly important, since many of these youths will not be adequately treated before becoming personally involved with the juvenile justice system, an event that suggests decreased success of treatment. Furthermore, early intervention seems prudent in light of calls for increasingly punitive treatment of juvenile offenders.

In the presence of antisocial acts committed by minors that are severe enough to be the focus of clinical attention, three major diagnoses should be considered. The selection of a diagnosis will of course shape the treatment plan selected. These diagnoses are

1. Child or adolescent antisocial behavior
2. Oppositional defiant disorder
3. Conduct disorder

The second and third conditions result from a mental disorder. Extreme caution should be used in the diagnosis of disorders associated with children's oppositional and delinquent behaviors. Some authors suggest that these diagnoses are significantly overused and too easily assigned.[1] This observation has serious implications for youth. A label such as *conduct disorder* probably will follow a young person throughout his or her academic career and may influence that person's school performance and attendance. Youths with serious conduct disorders have the potential to be a danger to themselves and/or others and must be identified in order to receive whatever remediation, however limited, may be available. In addition, the early identification of such youths is likely to increase their ability to benefit from treatment.

Antisocial Behavior

The descriptor *antisocial behavior* may be used when a child or teenager needs to receive treatment because of antisocial acts that do not reach the severity levels of more advanced disordered behavior. These behaviors are isolated and singular incidents and do not reflect a pattern of antisocial behaviors. In addition, they are not precipitated by an underlying mental disorder, although they cause significant familial and/or personal disruption. It is important to note that these types of "acting-out" behaviors may indicate a seemingly unrelated problem or stressor in the family or school setting, and a thorough social history is requisite. Thus, the presence of an adjustment disorder with disturbance of conduct should be ruled out on the basis of the recent occurrence of a stressor to which the child has not adjusted. Impulse control disorders, mood disorders, and attention disorders may produce conduct problems and often co-occur with disorders of conduct (see Chap. 16-4). Thus, treatment may include alleviating environmental stressors or addressing comorbid psychological problems. The clinician should assess whether the act or acts were committed alone or in a group, and what type or types of delinquent acts were attempted or completed. As a general rule, acts committed alone and acts that include confrontation with or harm to other people should be considered more serious and should alert the clinician to the need for continued monitoring of the patient's behavior.

Oppositional Defiant Disorder

Oppositional defiant disorder is often a precursor of conduct disorder, but there is not a perfect predictive relationship. This disorder is usually present by age 8 years and rarely has an onset after early adolescence. Prevalence estimates range from 2 to 16 percent. These children are resistant, hostile, and defiant in the home but can display such behavior in other settings. They argue with adults, refuse to comply with rules, and behave in angry, spiteful, vindictive, annoying, and/or overly sensitive ways. These children often lose their temper and blame others for their problems. To be considered clinically significant, these behaviors must persist for at least 6 months, cause a clear functional impairment, and occur more often than would be expected for the child's age (e.g., children under 3 years of age are frequently, and developmentally appropriately, defiant). Conduct disorder should be ruled out, which includes repeated violations of rules or the rights of others. Mood disorders, psychotic disorders, developmental disabilities, and impulse control problems and attention disorders can mimic or co-occur with oppositional defiant disorder. Furthermore, as with other conduct symptoms, this behavior can result from environmental stressors that may best be detected through a full social history and assessment of a child's current life circumstances and coping resources. Family functioning also must be assessed. Often clinical intervention with the family is necessary, and if the youth is still attending school, behavioral school intervention is warranted.

Conduct Disorder

Etiology

The development of conduct disorder has been linked to a number of factors, including familial dysfunction,[2] poverty,[3] impulsivity,[4] antisocial attitudes,[5] intellectual limitations,[6] victimization and early childhood trauma,[7] and inadequate prenatal and perinatal care.[8]

Genetic factors have been implicated in the development of conduct disorder. Although these results are suggestive, they are often difficult to interpret since genetic causality overlaps with environmental factors. Neurologic issues appear to contribute to impulse control problems, such as associated attention deficit hyperactivity disorder (ADHD) symptoms. Neurotransmitters have not been conclusively shown to contribute to this disorder; however, youths with conduct disorder tend to have lower overall levels of physiologic arousal,[9] and serotonin levels have been linked to aggression and violent behaviors.[10,11]

Prevalence and Onset

Conduct disorder may occur as early as age 6, but is more likely to be recognized in later childhood and early adolescence. Onset is rare after age 16 years. Prevalence estimates suggest that males under 18 years old are more likely to receive the diagnosis than are females (6 to 16 percent versus 2 to 9 percent). In addition, the prevalence of conduct disorder has increased over time, and it occurs more frequently in urban populations.[12] An early onset of delinquent behaviors may predict more severe acts over longer periods of time.[13] Childhood onset (before 10 years of age) or adolescent onset should be diagnostically specified.

Comorbidity

Physician assistants should note that children and adolescents with conduct problems are at increased risk for a broad spectrum of health problems and are far more likely to engage in health-deleterious behaviors than are typical youths.

Research indicates that conduct-disordered youngsters are

- More likely to engage in unprotected sexual activities that could result in early pregnancy and/or sexually transmitted diseases, including HIV infection
- More likely to use and abuse illicit and legal substances
- More susceptible to injury and to being seen in an emergency room
- More likely to fail in school
- More likely to be socially alienated and/or incarcerated
- At higher risk for a variety of mental health problems

SIGNS AND SYMPTOMS

These children view the world as a hostile place. As a result, they may misperceive others' actions as aggressive despite good intentions and react in "justifiably" aggressive ways. The diagnostic criteria stated in the *Diagnostic and Statistical Manual*[12] (DSM-IV) for conduct disorder include a repeated and lasting pattern of behaviors that are violations of the norms and rules of conduct expected for the child's age or violate the rights of others. To be considered conduct-disordered, a youth must demonstrate three problematic behaviors in the prior 12 months, with at least one behavior occurring in the past 6 months. According to the DSM-IV, the presence of the following behaviors is included in those that should be used to build a case for the treatment of conduct disorder:

1. Aggressive behaviors such as threatening or intimidating people, initiating physical fights, using a weapon with a high level of lethality or injury-causing potential (e.g., gun, knife, broken bottle), physically harming animals and/or people, stealing in the presence of the victim (e.g., face-to-face extortion, mugging, armed robbery), and forcing someone into unwanted sexual activity
2. Destruction of property, including setting intentional fires and perpetrating other types of deliberate damage to property
3. Deceitfulness or theft such as breaking into someone else's car, house, business, or building; stealing an item of value without confronting the victim (e.g., shoplifting); and lying to obtain things or avoid responsibilities (e.g., "conning" others)
4. Serious rule violations, including frequently staying out at night despite parental prohibitions beginning before age 13, running away from home overnight more than once or for long periods, and being truant from school beginning before age 13

In addition to the exhibition of these types of behaviors, the symptom severity must be of sufficient magnitude to cause serious impairment in the individual's functioning. Often among these youths there is a major discord in the family related to a child's attitudes and behaviors, and school failure, suspension, or expulsion occurs. A substantial proportion of individuals who are diagnosed with conduct disorder are later diagnosed with antisocial personality disorder in adulthood, a disorder that shares with conduct disorder a number of factors, such as lack of empathy or concern for the rights of others, lying, substance abuse, and legal transgressions. In addition, these youths are at risk for adult substance abuse problems.

Male and female patients with conduct problems may or may not present differently. In general, females tend to show internalizing delinquent behaviors, such as substance abuse, early sexual promiscuity, and/or pregnancy. However, more recently females have been showing an increased frequency of committing externalizing acts similar to those of males (e.g., physical fights and interpersonal violence, stealing, weapons use). It is rare to find a youth displaying conduct problems who does not use or abuse mood-altering substances.

What is notable about the types of behaviors considered diagnostic of conduct disorder is the vast range of severity. Clearly, a child who in the last year has verbally intimidated other children, shoplifted a pack of chewing gum, and lied several times to avoid chores has a level of disorder severity different from that of a child who has stolen a neighbor's automobile, set the school gymnasium on fire, and forced a female acquaintance to perform oral sex on him. A clinician must be aware of the broad range of behavior that may support a diagnosis of this disorder and judiciously choose when another diagnosis or no diagnosis is warranted. The general view is that one should use a diagnostic label only when it is fully justified. In the case of conduct disorder, quasi-normative delinquent behaviors that are likely to abate with age must be separated from a repetitive pattern of predatory and/or antisocial behavior in the assignment of a diagnosis. This is a difficult task, and a competent mental health professional can be a useful ally in the diagnostic process. Furthermore, it is helpful to differentiate the disorder as mild, moderate, or severe.

Solitary and Group Activities

A further differentiating factor in understanding conduct disorder may be whether the individual acts delinquently in the presence of others or alone; however, research to date is inconclusive. Clinical views of the solitary versus the group type of violator tend to paint the group type of perpetrator as more likely to be a victim of social facilitation or mob rule who may be swept along with whatever delinquent acts his or her peers are engaged in at the time. Thus, this individual is not a premeditator, and the rewards for the behavior are largely social, consisting of peer recognition and status. Solitary or unsocialized perpetrators, by contrast, are considered more pathologic and as drawing the reward from the commission of the illegal act or the domination or humiliation of another person. However, certain group acts are of such a heinous nature that they suggest the highly pathologic composition of packs of antisocial youth (e.g., "gang" rapes). Both solitary and group-type perpetrators may act impulsively, show little remorse, and lack empathy.

Gangs

Some clinicians believe that all gang members are delinquent or conduct-disordered, but this is not the case. Some youths are nominal members of gangs only, for instance, as a result of their recruitment by a relative who is a member or to be able to use recreational facilities in their neighborhoods that they would otherwise be banned from accessing as nonmembers. Some youths identify with gangs for personal protection. Others find that gangs serve as a surrogate family and/or workplace that provides relatively clear role expectations and support for gang-normative behavior. Problems arise for youths who are engaged in gang-related criminal activity, since the norms of the gang collide with the norms of society. Thus, while gang membership, style of dress, and tattoos may be red flags for potential antisocial behavior and conduct disorder, a thorough psychosocial history using a number of information sources should be used to affirm or disaffirm the practitioner's suppositions.

OBJECTIVE FINDINGS

A full psychosocial history is needed to adequately establish whether a youth is at risk for or can be diagnosed with conduct-related disorders. Psychological testing by a psychologist may be warranted to determine the intelligence level and functional level. It is essential to obtain a history from a parent or caregiver, who may be less likely to "sugar coat" the facts; however, youngsters often hide criminal activity from their parents, and therefore the youth may be the best informant in certain areas of inquiry. These youths are less likely to display attitudinal correlates of opposition or argumentativeness with strangers (such as during a first meeting with a clinician) than with family members, and observation of the patient in other settings and with authority figures is essential to diagnosis and treatment planning. Furthermore, some of these youths have had considerable practice at distorting the truth and are quite successful at hiding their antisocial attitudes and behaviors when it is in their best interest to do so. Often red flags occur in the individual's story, such as school problems, early and/or frequent sexual activity, early and/or frequent substance abuse, and a clear failure to empathize with others whom they have victimized and/or acknowledge the needs of anyone other than themselves. It is helpful to question the origins of any visible scars or other physical evidence of injuries, which may reveal a history of fighting or abuse. In the examining room, these youths may be disrespectful to the practitioner or may refuse to speak. In addition, the practitioner may feel hostile toward or fearful of them.

Formal measurement of delinquent behavior or prediction of conduct disorders is difficult. The Youth Self-Report Scale[14] and the Child Behavior Checklist teacher- and parent-reported versions may help identify youths who more frequently engage in aggressive and delinquent behaviors, but these scores are not considered clinical cutoff scores.

Documented criminal acts and self-reported and other-reported delinquent acts are often the best clinical indicators of potential conduct problems and are the most accessible to physician assistants. It should be noted that poor early school achievement and prior neglect and/or abuse are seen as being related to later conduct problems.

TREATMENT

Research findings are mixed on the effectiveness of various treatments for disruptive disorders. All treatments must be tailored to the individual child and family. The best treatments probably are multimodal and comprehensive, including the family, children, school, community, and peers.[15] Behavioral, family-based interventions hold promise and need additional evaluation.[16,17] These programs teach parents how to reward positive, prosocial behaviors and remove rewards for problem behavior in a manner that does not provide the child with any power (e.g., the ability to upset parents). Residential treatment often is used for more severe disorders, with varying results. The most effective programs include token economy systems that teach youths how to obtain rewards through their behavior and how to delay gratification and also teach social skills with peers and adults to reduce social rejection.

The Role of the Physician Assistant

It is essential to recall that these patients are children who probably have experienced significant trauma, lack a stable home life, or have been exposed to parental criminal behavior. However, these youths also have the potential to perpetrate serious offenses. A clinician can provide these youngsters with much-needed aid. It is important to provide good mental health referrals when indicated (e.g., enough offenses have occurred to warrant concern and impair the youth's ability to function). If the child is already in a group home or another out-of-home court-ordered placement, he or she probably is receiving mental health services in the residential setting. The practitioner's intervention should vary with the severity of the disorder. Clearly, youngsters who are incarcerated are a different population than youths who infrequently commit less serious offenses. Incarcerated youths are most likely serious violent offenders, repeat offenders of less serious crimes, or both violent and repeat offenders. It is important to be mindful that arrest and/or incarceration typically occur in a youth's life after numerous undetected crimes have occurred, although this is not always the case.

A physician assistant's therapeutic role with such children should include

- Serving as a stable adult figure who shows genuine concern for their welfare
- Serving as an adult figure who keeps his or her agreements and can be trusted
- Serving as an adult who is not easily duped but is willing to believe and trust the youngster within limits
- Modeling and requiring respectful interpersonal behavior
- Indicating to youths that one can and will help them as long as they comply with clinic rules (no smoking on the premises, no stealing supplies, etc.)
- Indicating that they have worth and bolstering their self-esteem
- Empathizing with their difficult experiences
- Empowering them to take control of their futures and change them

It may be useful to discuss with adolescents the career paths they have chosen. If they are engaged in serious offenses, they often spontaneously acknowledge that the path they are now on is likely to lead them to be an exceptional criminal and resident of a penitentiary in adulthood. Most of the time this image does not fit with some of their more positive aspirations. At this point, the practitioner can begin to discuss how to train for a new career if they would like to (e.g., get the GED, look into community college, explore job training programs). The practitioner also must debunk the myth of having a record "wiped clean" at 18 years of age. This is a hope that many of these youths hold dear. Although the opportunity to "stay clean" as an adult and have no record to follow them should be acknowledged, the practitioner must emphasize that the changes that can allow staying clean to happen must occur now. In other words, some youths believe that once their records are expunged, so is their risk of committing crimes. This belief should be challenged, and success should be linked to slow, painstaking behavioral changes. One should support and reward prosocial behaviors and, if possible, allow the child to experience success in his or her contact with the practitioner. These simple steps can be accomplished through verbal praise of appropriate behavior in the waiting and examination rooms and the setting of easily attainable goals that the youth can reach and receive attention for completing. However, each should be an act that the practitioner can easily document when it occurs (e.g., being on time for an appointment). These goals can be set to be progressively more difficult as a relationship develops. A fine line must be observed in developing such goals. The youths must be included in the development of the goals or they are sure to resist and fail. Also, the clinician should avoid being too authoritarian with these youths, as this can reduce their responsiveness. However, one should keep in mind that most children who are out of control are desperately seeking structure and guidance. Their acting-out behaviors often require the structure and guidance of the state juvenile justice and/or social services systems. Thus, once a relationship is established, the use of some authority is appropriate.

Simultaneously, the practitioner should assure the youth that he or she is giving the youth no less than his or her best job despite the discomfort. This is often a rare experience for them with adults.

Children who have had scholastic difficulty must be reintegrated into a targeted, often limited, school setting as quickly as possible—a setting in which they can experience success.

Alternative, safe circumstances must be designed for children in abusive homes and homes in which the parents are partially functional (e.g., poorly managed mental illness in a parent or active addictions). Social services agencies should be notified if there is abuse or neglect.

Pharmacologic Management

The use of medication may be indicated if a youth exhibits certain features, such as hyperactivity, mood fluctuations, and psychotic symptoms. Drug therapy should never be used as an independent treatment without additional interventions.

As was previously noted, youths with conduct problems also often display ADHD symptoms or syndromes. Under these circumstances, the use of stimulant medication can reduce not only inattention but also aggression, oppositional behaviors, and impulsivity. Some research suggests the usefulness of lithium (1 to 6 mg/d) and haloperidol (500 to 2000 mg/d).[18] For youngsters with depressive episodes, antidepressant medications may be indicated.[19] Beta blockers may be indicated for patients with rage reactions or neurologic problems.[20] Carbamazepine may be useful in adolescents with impulsive aggression with emotional irritability or lability, abnormal EEG, or suggested epileptic symptoms.[21]

There is some risk of misuse or abuse involved in prescribing drugs to youngsters with conduct problems, not only among the youths themselves but often among a patient's peers and family members. Thus, although it has been suggested that certain psychoactive medications may improve conduct problems, caution should be exercised in prescribing pharmacologic agents, and close monitoring by a psychiatrist is recommended, particularly when noncompliance is a problem.

NOTES AND PEARLS

The identification and treatment of conduct problems in youth must be directed by normative developmental expectations of behavior. Clinicians must guard against the random assignment of such diagnostic labels yet be responsive to troubled youths who need help in reducing delinquent behaviors. The role of the primary care provider should focus on extensive history taking that allows early suspicion, confirmation, and treatment of these disorders. All treatments for conduct problems should involve the individual youth, the educational system, the family, the medical system, and, if indicated, the legal and social services system. Pharmacotherapy may be indicated in certain cases.

REFERENCES

1. Lewis DO: Conduct disorder, in Lewis M (ed): *Child and Adolescent Psychiatry: A Comprehensive Textbook.* Baltimore, Williams & Wilkins, 1991.
2. Farrington DP: The family backgrounds of aggressive youths, in Hersov LA, Berger M, Shaffer D (eds): *Aggression and Antisocial Behavior in Childhood and Adolescence.* Oxford, UK, Pergamon Press, 1978.
3. Fergusson DM, Horwood LJ, Lynskey M: The childhoods of multiple problem adolescents: A 15 year longitudinal study. *J Child Psychol Psychiatry* 35(6):1123–1140, 1994.
4. Pfefferbaum B, Wood PB: Self-report study of impulsive and delinquent behavior in college students. *J Adolesc Health* 15(4):295–302, 1994.
5. Hoge RD, Andrews DA, Leschied AW: Tests of three hypotheses regarding the predictors of delinquency. *J Abnorm Child Psychol* 22(5):547–549, 1994.
6. Rantakallio P, Myhrman A, Koiranen M: Juvenile offenders, with special reference to sex differences. *Soc Psychiatry Psychiatr Epidemiol* 30(3):113–120, 1995.
7. Schwartz IM, Rendon JA, Hsieh CM: Is child maltreatment a leading cause of delinquency? *Child Welfare* 73(5):639–655, 1994.
8. Penzerro RM, Lein L: Burning their bridges: Disordered attachment and foster care discharge. *Child Welfare* 74(2):351–366, 1995.
9. Raine F, Venables P, Williams M: Relationships between central and autonomic measures of arousal at age 15 and criminality at age 24 years. *Arch Gen Psychiatry* 47:1003–1007, 1990.
10. Mann JJ: Psychobiological predictors of suicide. *J Clin Psychiatry* 48(12):39–43, 1987.
11. Virkkunnen M, DeJong J, Bartko J, et al: Relationship of psychobiological variables to recidivism in violent offenders and impulsive fire setters: A follow-up study. *Arch Gen Psychiatry* 46:600–603, 1989.
12. *Diagnostic and Statistical Manual of Mental Disorders*, 4th ed. Washington, DC, American Psychiatric Association, 1994.
13. Tolan PH, Thomas P: The implications of age of onset for delinquency risk: II. Longitudinal data. *J Abnorm Child Psychol* 21(2):157–181, 1995.
14. Achenbach TM: *The Manual for the Youth Self-Report and 1991 Profile.* Burlington, University of Vermont, Department of Psychiatry, 1991.
15. Henggeler SW, Borduin CM: *Family Therapy and Beyond: A Multisystemic Approach to Treatment of the Behavior Problems of Children and Adolescents.* Pacific Grove, CA, Brooks/Cole, 1990.
16. Patterson GR: *Families: Applications of Social Learning to Family Life.* Champaign, IL, Research Press, 1975.
17. Forehand RL, McMahon RJ: *Helping the Non-Compliant Child: A Clinician's Guide to Parent Training.* New York, Guilford Press, 1981.
18. Campbell SB, Small AM, Green WH, et al: Behavioral efficacy of haloperidol and lithium carbonate: A comparison in hospitalized aggressive children with conduct disorder. *Arch Gen Psychiatry* 41:650–656, 1984.
19. Puig-Antich J: Major depression and conduct disorder in prepuberty. *J Am Acad Child Adolesc Psychiatry* 42:511–517, 1982.
20. Williams DT, Mehl R, Yudofsky S, et al: The effects of propranolol on uncontrolled rage outbursts in children and adolescents with organic brain dysfunction. *J Am Acad Child Adolesc Psychiatry* 21:129–135, 1982.
21. Evans RW, Clay TH, Gualtieri CT: Carbamazepine in pediatric psychiatry. *J Am Acad Child Adolesc Psychiatry* 26:2–8, 1987.

Chapter 15–8
PEDIATRIC INNOCENT (FUNCTIONAL) HEART MURMURS
David P. Asprey

DISCUSSION

The terms *innocent murmur* and *functional murmur* refer to the audible sound that results from the flow of blood through a structurally normal heart and vascular system. Primary care clinicians are repeatedly confronted with the diagnostic dilemma of distinguishing innocent heart murmurs from pathologic ones. Pathologic murmurs result from turbulent blood flow caused by an underlying cardiac defect. As many as 90 percent of all children have an audible heart murmur at some point in time.[1] However, the incidence of congenital heart disease has been estimated to be less than 1 percent of all live births. Consequently, the vast majority of children with murmurs have murmurs that are innocent or functional. This chapter focuses on distinguishing innocent heart murmurs from pathologic murmurs. An understanding of the various types of common innocent (normal) murmurs is essential to avoid the mistaken diagnosis of organic heart disease. A discussion of the murmurs associated with common congenital heart defects appears in Chap. 1-1 and 1-2.

The clinician's responsibility is to distinguish an innocent murmur from a pathologic murmur that is indicative of a cardiovascular defect. The most common pediatric innocent heart murmurs are discussed in this chapter, including

1. Vibratory, or Still's, murmur
2. Pulmonary flow murmur
3. Peripheral pulmonary artery stenosis murmur
4. Supraclavicular arterial bruit murmur
5. Venous hum

The unintentional mislabeling of an innocent heart murmur as pathologic may have adverse effects on the psychosocial well-being of a child and family by inducing unnecessary concern about the child. In addition, unnecessarily prescribed subacute bacterial endocarditis (SBE) prophylaxis can result in adverse side effects. Finally, this may make obtaining certain types of employment difficult or impossible and securing reasonably priced life and health insurance very difficult.

Failure to diagnose a child with congenital heart disease when the child has a heart defect can be even more problematic. Often children with congenital heart disease are instructed to observe SBE prophylaxis to reduce the risk of acquiring a serious infection of the endocardium. In addition, some children require medical or surgical treatment of a cardiac defect to prevent irreversible damage (i.e., pulmonary hypertension) from occurring.

Primary care clinicians can effectively distinguish murmurs with a pathologic origin from the innocent variety. The ability to make this distinction with a high degree of accuracy is dependent on the clinician's ability to appropriately utilize the history, physical examination, and laboratory data in a systematic fashion.

SIGNS AND SYMPTOMS

The first and often the most important step in distinguishing between innocent and pathologic murmurs is to take a thorough and careful history. Symptoms that may be indicative of congenital heart disease include cyanosis, decreased exercise tolerance, fatigue, shortness of breath or tachypnea, chest pain, syncope, palpitations, diaphoresis, and failure to thrive. In addition, collecting a careful prenatal and postnatal history may provide additional clues to the likely presence of congenital heart disease. A family history is useful in establishing any increased risk the patient may have for congenital heart disease.

OBJECTIVE FINDINGS

The physical examination is a very powerful tool in distinguishing innocent heart murmurs from pathologic murmurs. Many syndromes are associated with a high incidence of congenital heart disease. Consequently, the general assessment begins with an inspection of the patient, which may reveal dysmorphic features and/or the presence of a syndrome. Common syndromes associ-

ated with cardiac defects and abnormalities include trisomy 21 (Down syndrome), trisomy 18, and trisomy 13 and Turner's, Noonan's, VATER, Williams, DiGeorge, and Marfan syndromes. The assessment of the general appearance also may reveal tachypnea or respiratory distress, cyanosis, pallor, and diaphoresis, each of which may be a sign of underlying congenital heart disease.

Palpation should include the precordium and the peripheral pulses. A palpable lift or heave may be indicative of pressure of volume-overload cardiac defects such as aortic stenosis, aortic insufficiency, and defects resulting in a large left-to-right shunting of blood (atrial septal defects, ventricular septal defects, and patent ductus arteriosus). Palpation also should be carried out to assess the presence of a thrill. A thrill is the palpable vibratory sensation that results from turbulent blood flow in the cardiovascular system. Typically, the presence of a thrill suggests obstructive defects (such as pulmonic stenosis and aortic stenosis) or a shunt defect between two chambers with a large pressure difference (such as a ventricular septal defect). Peripheral pulses should be assessed carefully for amplitude, intensity, and symmetry. Diminished left arm or leg pulses compared to the right arm suggest coarctation of the aorta. Bounding pulses suggest the presence of a large patent ductus arteriosus or severe aortic insufficiency.

Finally, because many patients do not have any signs or symptoms of their disease except the presence of a murmur, auscultation of the patient's heart becomes critical to accurately distinguish between many innocent murmurs and pathologic murmurs. Each of the five commonly occurring pediatric innocent murmurs is discussed in "Diagnostic Considerations," below.

Even in the absence of pertinent findings from the medical history, identifiable syndromes, or dysmorphic features, certain auscultatory findings should be considered abnormal until proved otherwise. These findings include diastolic murmurs, any systolic murmur associated with a thrill, pansystolic murmurs, continuous murmurs that cannot be suppressed (see below), systolic clicks, opening snaps, fixed splitting of the second heart sound, an accentuated P_2 component, and S_4 gallops. If any of these findings are present, the child should be referred to a pediatric cardiology clinician for further evaluation.

DIAGNOSTIC CONSIDERATIONS

It is important to adopt and utilize a systematic approach to performing the auscultatory examination to help ensure that no important information is inadvertently left out. Auscultation of the heart should be performed with the patient sitting, sitting and leaning forward, supine, and in the left lateral decubitus position. In each position the examiner should listen to several heartbeats through a few respiratory cycles at the aortic, pulmonic, tricuspid, and mitral areas at a minimum. In each position the examiner should utilize the diaphragm and bell capabilities of the stethoscope to increase the likelihood of hearing all important sounds of high and low pitch. At each site the clinician should specifically listen to and assess the first heart sound, the second heart sound, extra sounds in systole (clicks, etc.), extra sounds in diastole (S_3, S_4, opening snaps, etc.), murmurs in systole, and murmurs in diastole.

If a murmur is detected, the clinician should note the following characteristics: timing, location of maximal intensity, radiation, intensity (grade), pitch, and quality. If a murmur of extra heart sound is present, special maneuvers, such as listening to the change in the timing or quality of the murmur while the patient squats, stands, or performs a Valsalva maneuver, may help distinguish various murmurs.

Innocent heart murmurs have a distinct set of features that a clinician can become very skilled at identifying. Studies have shown that pediatric cardiologists can differentiate innocent from pathologic murmurs by clinical examination alone with high degrees of sensitivity and specificity.[2] Each of the five innocent heart murmurs identified in this chapter has characteristic findings that most clinicians will be able to develop confidence in diagnosing after getting adequate experience in examining children with murmurs.

The vibratory, or Still's, murmur is a low-pitched vibratory (i.e., has a musical quality) midsystolic murmur that is heard maximally at the lower left sternal border. This murmur is most prevalent in children between 3 and 6 years of age. Typically it is grade II to grade III/VI in intensity. It decreases in intensity with the Valsalva maneuver and when the patient is in a sitting or standing position. The intensity will increase with any high-output state, such as fever, anxiety, anemia, and exercise. The primary differential diagnosis of this murmur is a small ventricular septal defect or subvalvular left ventricular outflow tract stenosis such as a subaortic membrane or idiopathic hypertrophic subaortic stenosis.

The pulmonary flow murmur is an early to midsystolic ejection murmur that is middle- to high-pitched and is heard maximally at the upper left sternal border. It is usually grade I to grades II to VI in intensity and is louder during inspiration and when the patient is in a supine position. Typically this murmur is present in older children between the ages of 8 and 14 years. It increases in intensity during times of increased cardiac output. This murmur usually has very little radiation. The primary differential diagnosis is pulmonic stenosis (generally associated with a pulmonic click in valvular pulmonic stenosis) or atrial septal defect, which is associated with a fixed, split second heart sound.

The peripheral pulmonary artery stenosis murmur is most common in the newborn period, especially in premature infants and infants with low birthweight. This is a short midsystolic murmur that is generally of middle pitch and intensity, seldom louder than grade II/VI. This murmur is usually transient and resolves spontaneously by approximately 6 months of age. The murmur often is heard loudest over the lung fields rather than the heart and radiates throughout the lung fields. There should be no ejection click present. The primary differential for this murmur is supravalvular stenosis, which is very rare in isolation. If the murmur does not diminish in intensity or resolve by 6 months of age, another cause should be sought.

The supraclavicular arterial bruit murmur is a harsh, relatively low-pitched (best heard with the bell) systolic murmur that usually is heard maximally just above the clavicles and typically is louder on the right side. This murmur is usually grade II to grades III to VI in intensity and can be made softer by hyperextending the shoulders during auscultation. It is generally present in older children but is reported in children of all ages. The primary differential diagosis for this murmur is supravalvular aortic stenosis. The examiner should be certain to check for the presence of a suprasternal notch thrill. The presence of this type of thrill suggests a pathologic cause of the murmur.

The venous hum murmur is a common, continuous murmur that is present at either the upper right or the upper left sternal border and is usually grade II to grade III/VI in intensity when the child is in a sitting position. It results from the turbulence created by venous return from the head and neck through the jugular vein. This murmur can be decreased in intensity or even obliterated by having the child rotate the head to a position of maximal rotation in either direction, by digital compression of the jugular venous system just above the clavicles, or by placing the patient in a supine position. This murmur is common among children between 3 and 8 years of age. The primary differential diagnosis is a patent ductus arteriosus. The murmur associated with patent ductus arteriosus is continuous and is heard maximally at the upper left sternal border. However, this murmur is not reduced in intensity or eliminated by the maneuvers described above.

LABORATORY STUDIES

In most children with murmurs laboratory data are of little benefit. However, electrocardiography may provide additional information about the heart and the likelihood of a heart defect. However, some studies have indicated that ECGs do not help clinicians distinguish between innocent and pathologic murmurs.[3]

RADIOLOGIC STUDIES

There is considerable debate regarding the usefulness of chest x-rays in distinguishing innocent heart murmurs from pathologic murmurs. Many pediatric cardiology clinicians perform chest x-rays only on children less than 2 years of age when they are referred for an initial evaluation of a murmur.

OTHER DIAGNOSTIC STUDIES

Echocardiograms are utilized only in situations in which pathology is suspected or when the diagnostic evaluation does not provide a clear differentiation of a patient's condition.

TREATMENT

Patients diagnosed with innocent heart murmurs have a normal heart. Therefore, no treatment is necessary.

Patient Education

Educating the patient and family about the meaning of an innocent heart murmur is extremely important. It is a natural reaction for patients to assume that if a child has a murmur, there is something wrong with the child's heart. It is important that the clinician assure the patient and family that this is a normal finding. The patient can be advised that many times the murmur resolves on its own as the child gets older but that if it does not, it is of no consequence because the heart is normal. If the patient was started on SBE prophylaxis, care should be taken to inform the patient that it is not indicated in persons with innocent heart murmurs. It may be useful to explain to the child and family that anything that results in increased cardiac output (anxiety, fever, etc.) will make the murmur louder and that clinicians unfamiliar with the child's examination may interpret the intensity of the murmur as a sign of heart disease.

Disposition

No follow-up is necessary for patients diagnosed with an innocent heart murmur.

NOTES AND PEARLS

Often it is very challenging to obtain an adequate period of quiet time to perform a complete cardiac examination that includes the auscultation of potentially subtle sounds in small children. If you are unable to perform an adequate cardiac examination because of the activity level of a child, schedule another appointment for the child or ask the parents to drop in at the clinic at a time when the child is sleeping. The absence of evidence does not always equate with the evidence of absence. In other words, unless you have been able to listen carefully and convince yourself that the sounds in question are not present, it is not wise to assume that they do not exist.

REFERENCES

1. Harris JP: Evaluation of heart murmurs. *Pediatr Rev* 15(12):490, 1994.
2. McCrindle BW, Shaffer KM, Kan JS: Cardinal clinical signs in the differentiation of heart murmurs in children. *Arch Pediatr Adolesc Med* 150(2):171–173, 1996.

3. Birkebaek NH, Hansen LK, Oxhoj H: Diagnostic value of chest radiography and electrocardiography in the evaluation of asyptomatic children with a cardiac murmur. *Acta Paediatr Scand* 84(12):1379–1381, 1995.

Chapter 15–9
PEDIATRIC ARRHYTHMIAS
David P. Asprey

DISCUSSION

Abnormal cardiac rhythms are a fairly common problem among children. Potential etiologies of arrhythmia are congenital, toxin-induced, medication- or drug-induced, and the sequelae of the surgical repair of congenital heart disease. In evaluating children with an arrhythmia, the distinguishing features are the presence of significant symptoms and the presence of structural heart disease. The vast majority of children who have an arrhythmia but no underlying heart disease or significant symptoms do not require treatment. Conversely, children with an arrhythmia who have a structurally abnormal heart or significant symptoms should receive immediate evaluation and treatment. Typically, serious symptoms (light-headedness, near syncope, syncope) result from diminished cardiac output that may be secondary to tachycardia, profound bradycardia, or cardiac standstill.

In this chapter the discussion of the various pediatric arrhythmias is conducted by category. The use of broad groupings of arrhythmias for the purpose of discussion results in the following categories: sinus rhythm variations, atrial-originating arrhythmias, ventricular-originating arrhythmias, and atrioventricular conduction disturbances.

Sinus Rhythm Variations

Several physiologic variations of sinus rhythm exist and occur commonly in the pediatric population. Sinus arrhythmia is a physiologic phasic variation in the timing of the electric impulse that is discharged from the sinoatrial (SA) node. The result is a rhythm that appears to change rate from beat to beat. Because the discharged electric impulse travels through the normal conduction mechanism, it results in normal sinus rhythm. The observable variation correlates with the respiratory cycle. While this finding may occur with respiratory distress or increased intracranial pressure, most often it is associated with a normal heart. This variation of sinus rhythm does not require treatment.

Sinus bradycardia occurs when the underlying rhythm of the heart is sinus but the heart rate is lower than the normal range for the patient's age. Normal resting heart rates are age-dependent; as a rule, the normal newborn range is 110 to 150 beats per minute (bpm), at 2 to 3 years it is 85 to 125 bpm, at 4 to 6 years it is 75–115 bpm, and over 6 years of age it is 60 to 100 bpm. Sinus bradycardia may be caused by athletic conditioning, vagal stimulation, increased intracranial pressure, hypothyroidism, hypoxia, and hyperkalemia and as a side effect of drugs such as digitalis and beta-adrenergic blockers. If marked bradycardia is present, adequate cardiac output may not be maintained, resulting in the development of symptoms. Typically, in otherwise healthy children, sinus bradycardia is without significance and does not require treatment.

Sinus tachycardia occurs when the underyling rhythm of the heart is sinus but the rate exceeds the upper limits of the established normal range for the child's age. The causes of sinus tachycardia include anemia, hypovolemia, anxiety, fever, congestive heart failure, and catecholamines. The treatment of sinus tachycardia involves treating the underlying cause.

Atrial-Originating Arrhythmias

Several abnormal heart beats or rhythms originate from the atrium. Wandering atrial pacemaker is the phenomenon that occurs when the origination point of the electric impulse within the atrium varies from one beat to the next. This is manifested in the ECG by a changing P-wave axis and morphology. This is a normal finding and is not indicative of cardiac disease; consequently, no treatment is indicated.

Premature atrial contractions (PACs) occur when the SA node or another region of the atrium generates an organized atrial contraction that occurs earlier than anticipated in the cardiac cycle. Often the electric impulse is generated from an area of the atrium other than the SA node; thus, the morphology and axis of the P wave are abnormal. In most instances, the QRS complex is normal in duration and morphology as the conduction of the electric impulse through the ventricles occurs through the normal mechanism. A distinguishing feature of a PAC compared with other premature beats is that there is an incomplete compensatory pause. PACs may be a normal finding in newborns and children. In addition, they may occur as a result of trauma to the atrium (cardiac surgery, catheter stimulation, etc.) or in response to drug toxicity or inflammation. Isolated PACs are not hemodynamically significant and usually are undetectable by the patient. No treatment is required unless they are determined to result from a correctable underlying etiology.

Supraventricular tachycardia (SVT) is the most common tachyrhythmia in children. It is characterized by a regular and very rapid heart rate that may range from 180 to nearly 300 bpm. Both the onset and the cessation of SVT tend to be abrupt. Consequently, a careful history to elicit the onset and cessation is useful in establishing this diagnosis. Episodes of SVT may last as little as a few seconds and as long as several hours. Some children are unaware of the rapid heart rate, and others describe their hearts as racing or fluttering. This arrhythmia generally does not result in significant symptoms associated with decreased cardiac output. The ECG reveals a normal (narrow) complex QRS with regular R-to-R intervals.

While the specific etiology of an SVT is often undetermined, the most common mechanism is reentry within the atrioventricular (AV) node. SVT occurs when a premature atrial beat is conducted through the AV node via a bypass tract. As the impulse proceeds through the ventricle and back to the AV node, it is transmitted back up to the atrium in a retrograde manner through the AV node bypass tract. This impulse is then transmitted through the atrium and back to the AV node, and an accelerated rhythm occurs.

The specific cause of SVT is not identifiable in more than 50 percent of the cases that occur in children. Wolff-Parkinson-White syndrome may be present in as many as 20 percent of all children with SVT; however, this diagnosis can be established only from an ECG taken when a child is not experiencing tachycardia. SVT is associated with Ebstein's anomaly of the tricuspid valve and corrected transposition of the great arteries. SVT may be precipitated by caffeine ingestion and the sympathomimetic amines commonly utilized in decongestants. If SVT is sustained for long periods, it may result in congestive heart failure secondary to diminished cardiac output.

The treatment of SVT that is not associated with significant symptoms is conservative initially. This treatment includes vagal stimulation. In infants, a bag of ice water applied to the face may abort an episode of SVT. Children may be taught how to perform self-administered vagal stimulation maneuvers, such as carotid massage, the Valsalva maneuver, and drinking ice water. If these conservative treatments are unsuccessful, pharmacologic treatment should be initiated. Adenosine is most effective in the acute setting, when the mechanism of SVT is presumed to be a result of an AV reentry bypass tract. It is administered rapidly as an intravenous bolus followed with a saline flush. The starting dose is 50 μg/kg and is increased in increments of 50 μg/kg every 1 to 2 min up to a maximum of 250 μg/kg.[1] Once the SVT is interrupted, digitalization may be necessary to prevent its reoccurrence. Other treatments include primary digitalization, propranolol, and verapamil. In addition, transesophageal pacing wires may be utilized to achieve overdriving of the rhythm and subsequent conversion to sinus rhythm. Finally, in acute symptomatic cases, cardioversion may be indicated.

Atrial flutter is characterized by a very fast atrial rate that is described as a "sawtooth" pattern on the ECG. The atrial rate may approach 300 bpm, with ventricular response rates varying from 2:1 to 5:1. Most patients who are old enough to verbalize their symptoms describe palpations and occasionally light-headedness.

The causes of atrial flutter include myocarditis, digitalis toxicity, congenital heart disease that results in atrial dilation, and atrial trauma from surgery or another intracardiac intervention. Digitalization acts to decrease the ventricular response rate. Cardioversion may be necessary to convert some cases of atrial flutter. Anticoagulation therapy is indicated before the cardioversion to prevent systemic embolization.

Atrial fibrillation also is characterized by a very rapid atrial rate between 300 and 500 bpm. Unlike atrial flutter, there is no distinct "sawtooth" pattern representing the atrial activity on the ECG. However, as with atrial flutter, an irregular ventricular rate is typically present. The causes of atrial fibrillation are the same as those associated with atrial flutter; the treatment of atrial fibrillation thus is the same as that of atrial flutter. It should be noted that even when cardioversion is initially successful, it often converts back to atrial fibrillation.

Ventricular-Originating Arrhythmias

Premature ventricular contractions (PVCs) occur when an ectopic focus in the ventricles generates an impulse that results in the contraction of the ventricles at a point earlier than expected in the cardiac cycle. With a PVC the electric impulse is generated in and transmitted through the myocardium of the ventricle and is not transmitted through the normal conduction system. The transmission of the impulse is slower, and thus the morphology of the QRS complex is widened. It is important to realize that some patients may have a wide QRS from a bundle branch block or another conduction abnormality, making it difficult to identify conduction abnormalities. A distinguishing feature of PVCs compared with PACs with aberrancy (which appear as a widened QRS) is that a patient with a bundle branch block experiencing a PVC usually has a full compensatory pause, while those with PACs have an incomplete compensatory pause.

PVCs may be classified into different categories on the basis of the uniformity of the QRS complexes and their relationship to other PVCs. If each of the QRS complexes appears the same throughout the tracing, they are described as uniform or unifocal, implying that the electric impulse generating the PVC consistently arises from the same area within the ventricular myocardium. Conversely, if each of the QRS complexes is different in appearance, they are described as multiform or multifocal PVCs. This pattern implies that the electric impulses generating the PVCs arise from different areas within the ventricular myocardium each time.

PVCs may vary in their timing and relationship to other PVCs. A single PVC on a tracing without other PVCs on the strip being reviewed is described as an isolated PVC. If the PVC alternates with a normal QRS complex so that every other beat is a PVC, this is described as bigeminy. If every third complex is a PVC, this pattern is known as trigeminy. When two PVCs occur in succession, this is a couplet. If three PVCs occur in succession, this is referred to as a triplet.

PVCs may be a normal finding in newborns and children. In addition, they may occur as a result of trauma to the ventricle (cardiac surgery, catheter stimulation, etc.), myocarditis, cardiomyopathy, myocardial ischemia, drug toxicity, and inflammation. Isolated PVCs are not hemodynamically significant and are usually undetectable by the patient. Occasional PVCs are believed to be benign in children, particularly if they are suppressed by exercise and are uniform or unifocal.

In children without underlying congenital heart disease, occasional uniform PVCs do not warrant extensive investigation. Children and infants with frequent PVCs, bigeminy, or trigeminy should be evaluated with ECG, echocardiography, and exercise stress testing. If each of these tests is normal, no further evaluation is indicated. If these tests are abnormal or unavailable, referral to a pediatric cardiologist should be considered. Children and infants with ventricular couplets, triplets, or multiform PVCs should undergo an evaluation that includes ECG, echocardiography, exercise stress testing, and 24-h Holter monitoring. No treatment is required for PVCs unless they are associated with significant symptoms or result from a treatable underlying etiology. When indicated, pharmacologic treatment options include lidocaine as an intravenous bolus and beta blockers, among others. Agents that are known to prolong the QT interval should be avoided.

Ventricular tachycardia (VT) is quite rare in the pediatric age group. It is described as three or more PVCs in succession with a rate greater than 120 bpm (normally 120 to 200 bpm). The QRS complexes in VT are wide and have a characteristic morphology analogous to that of the QRS complexes associated with PVCs. The presence of sustained VT constitutes a medical emergency. Sustained VT is usually an unstable condition that has the potential to progress to ventricular fibrillation. Torsade de pointes is a characteristic type of VT that on ECG appears as VT with rapidly changing QRS morphology and amplitude.

The presence of VT is always abnormal. It usually is associated with abnormalities of the ventricular myocardium such as myocarditis, cardiomyopathy and myocardial tumors or in conjunction with severe forms of congenital heart disease. Torsade de pointes may be associated with a long QT syndrome and drugs that prolong the QT interval. Symptoms associated with VT usually occur as a result of decreased cardiac output.

Treatment of VT in the acute symptomatic setting (patient unconscious or profoundly symptomatic) should include synchronized cardioversion using approximately 1 J/kg. In a conscious patient, a lidocaine bolus given intravenously at a rate of 1 mg/kg over the course of 1 to 2 min followed by an intravenous drip often is effective. Bretylium tosylate given at 5 mg/kg intravenously over the course of 10 min also may be effective. In all cases of confirmed VT the clinician should strive to identify the underlying cause and treat any correctable causes.[2]

Ventricular fibrillation (VF) is very rare in children and infants and occurs when the electrical activity of the heart fails to generate a synchronized contraction of the ventricles. Consequently, the cardiac output is dramatically decreased and is typically incompatible with life. The ECG shows only fine variations in the amplitude of the baseline waveform and often may appear as artifactual electrical activity. When specific waveform activity correlating with the ventricular contractions is identifiable, it is typically very rapid and of varying morphology.

VF is an emergency and if untreated is fatal as a result of inadequate cardiac output. It may occur as a result of myocardial ischemia, electrolyte imbalance, myocarditis, digitalis, quinidine, catecholamine and other drug toxicities, and some postoperative states. Because this rhythm is fatal, immediate treatment with cardiopulmonary resuscitation (CPR) and electrical defibrillation (2 J/kg) is required. When the development of VF is witnessed, a precordial thump may be administered immediately as the first-line attempt to reestablish sinus rhythm. However, if an initial attempt is unsuccessful, CPR should be started immediately until cardioversion can be performed.

Atrioventricular Conduction Disturbances

An AV block can occur at different regions in the normal conduction system, resulting in varying degrees of heart block. Heart block is divided into three broad categories: first degree, second degree, and third degree. First-degree heart block occurs when there is a delay in the conduction of the impulse generated in the SA node (or another region of the atrium) and its transmission to the ventricles, resulting in ventricular contraction. This manifests itself on ECG as a prolongation of the PR interval beyond the uppper limits of normal for age. Normal PR intervals are age- and heart rate–dependent, and normal ranges should be determined by consulting published standardized tables.

The causes of first-degree heart block include idiopathy in healthy children and infants, certain forms of congenital heart disease, acute rheumatic fever, cardiomyopathies, cardiac surgery or trauma, and digitalis toxicity. No hemodynamic compromise is associated with first-degree heart block, and no treatment is necessary.

Second-degree heart block occurs when only some of the atrial electric impulses result in a ventricular contraction. Thus, ECG demonstrates some P waves that are not followed by a QRS complex. Three different forms of second-degree heart block have been well described. Mobitz type I, also known as the Wenckebach phenomenon, manifests itself on the ECG tracing by a PR interval that becomes increasingly prolonged until the P wave fails to produce a QRS (dropped beat) and is eventually followed by the succeeding P wave. This form of second-degree heart block suggests AV node disease. Patients with this condition should undergo 24-h Holter monitoring. Treatment includes correction of the underyling conditions.

Mobitz type II second-degree heart block is characterized on ECG by consistent PR intervals but has occasional P waves that do not result in QRS complexes; thus, a beat is dropped and the P wave is followed by the subsequent P wave. Conduction through the AV node is normal, or the impulse is blocked completely. This block is believed to occur at the level of the bundle of His. In addition, this form of second-degree heart block may progress to third-degree, or complete, heart block. Patients with this condition should undergo periodic 24-h Holter monitoring to determine whether periods of bradycardia or third-degree heart block are occurring.

A final type of second-degree heart block is described by its ratio of P waves to QRS complexes. This form manifests itself by a series of P waves followed by a QRS complex. Thus, it may be described as a second-degree heart block with a 2:1 or 3:1 AV block. This form of second-degree heart block usually occurs at the level of the bundle of His. These patients should be followed with periodic 24-h Holter monitoring. Treatment involves correction of the underlying problems.

The causes of all three types of second-degree heart block are similar and include idiopathy in healthy children, cardiac ischemia, myocarditis, cardiomyopathy, cardiac surgery, and digitalis and other drug toxicities.

Finally, third-degree, or complete, heart block occurs when the atrial activity and ventricular activity function completely independently of each other. Because the atrial activity is not influencing the ventricular response, the ventricular response rate may become quite slow. Third-degree heart block may be congenital or acquired. Congenital causes include some forms of congenital heart disease and infants who are born to mothers with systemic lupus erythematosus. The most common etiologies of acquired third-degree heart block include cardiac surgery and myocardial ischemia. Children with third-degree heart block should undergo periodic 24-h Holter monitoring to assess their heart rate during sleep. Treatment may require permanent pacemakers in symptomatic patients and patients with congestive heart failure.

REFERENCES

1. Park MK: *The Pediatric Cardiology Handbook*, 2d ed. St. Louis, Mosby Years Book, 1997, pp 203–204.
2. Behrman RE, Kliegman R, Arvin AM, Nelson WE: *Nelson's Textbook of Pediatrics*, 15th ed. Philadelphia, Saunders, 1996, p 1341.

Chapter 16–1
EATING DISORDERS: ANOREXIA AND BULIMIA

Meredith Davison

DISCUSSION

Both anorexia nervosa and bulimia are eating disorders affecting primarily young women in societies that place a high value on slimness as a characteristic of beauty. *Anorexia nervosa* is characterized by fear of obesity, distorted body image, obsession with thinness, and eventually secondary physiologic abnormalities. *Bulimia* occurs when individuals consume large quantities of food in a short period of time, and then self-induce vomiting or abuse laxatives to compensate. Since these eating disorders are often seen in the same individual, some believe the two are different manifestations of the same underlying entity. About 40 to 50 percent of anorexics have a history of binge eating. However, each disorder is described separately in the *Diagnostic and Statistical Manual of Mental Disorders*, fourth edition (DSM-IV), and bulimia is further divided into purging and nonpurging types.

ETIOLOGY

The exact cause of anorexia nervosa and bulimia is unknown. Current understanding suggests that multiple psychological, biologic, and cultural factors are involved in an interactive fashion. Individuals may have a physiologic or genetic predisposition and early childhood experiences which interact with current societal influences. Both of these eating disorders tend to cluster in families with other psychopathologic conditions, particularly emotional disorders and alcohol abuse.

EPIDEMIOLOGY

The worldwide incidence of anorexia nervosa is estimated to be 1 per 100,000, but in Western countries the incidence in white adolescent females may be as high as 1 per 200. Evidence suggests that anorexia nervosa has increased during the last 20 years. Anorexia nervosa occurs predominantely in females with a sex distribution of approximately 10 : 1. Age of onset is usually between 10 and 25 years.

Risk factors for anorexia nervosa include female, slightly overweight, white, adolescent, feelings of low self-esteem, achievement-oriented middle-to-upper-income family, a culture that equates female beauty with thinness, and an intense interest in diet and physical fitness. Although females account for 90 to 95 percent of anorexia nervosa cases, there is evidence of an increased incidence in males.

The onset of bulimia is similar to that of anorexia nervosa, usually during late adolescence or early adulthood. Prevalence of bulimia is estimated to be between 1 and 3 percent of adolescent women in Western industrialized societies. Risk factors for bulimia are similar to those of anorexia nervosa. In addition, some studies suggest a possible genetic predisposition for the development of bulimia, since a higher concordance rate has been found in monozygotic twins. Bulimia also tends to cluster in families with other psychopathologic conditions, particularly affective disorders and alcohol abuse. Other physiologic changes that develop in the course of the eating disorder may exacerbate the condition. Recent studies suggest some bulimic patients may have impaired satiety responses. Pain thresholds may also be altered. These changes suggest some underlying abnormalities in biologic processes may predispose some individuals to the development and maintenance of this disorder.

SIGNS AND SYMPTOMS

The most common presenting signs and symptoms of anorexia nervosa are weight loss, amenorrhea, hyperactivity, social isolation, depression, and preoccupation with food. Symptoms secondary to weight loss include hair loss, yellow skin, fatigue, and gastrointestinal complaints (nausea, vomiting, constipation, bloating, epigastric pain).

Most patients with bulimia exhibit relatively normal body weight, and the marked physical changes associated with starvation found in anorexia nervosa are not present. The most obvious sign of bulimia is episodic binge eating. The patient also senses a lack of control over eating during the binge episode. Characteristics of binge eating include eating the food very quickly, eating without chewing, eating large amounts of high caloric food, frequently experiencing guilt and remorse after the binge, and hiding the episodes.

OBJECTIVE FINDINGS

Most objective findings in anorexia nervosa result from weight loss and are similar to the findings in starvation. They include decreased weight, decreased temperature, hypotension, bradycardia, edema, dry skin, yellowish discoloration of the skin, nail changes, lanugo hair, systolic murmurs, and short stature.

Patients with bulimia ordinarily present with weakness and fatigue, swelling of hands and feet, headaches, abdominal fullness, and nausea. Other signs include skin changes, primarily on the hand secondary to self-induced vomiting, enlargement of the salivary glands, and dental erosions. Dental erosions occur in the lingual, palatal, and posterior occlusal surfaces of the teeth. Recurrent vomiting causes decalcification of the dental surfaces exposed to the vomitus. Dental fillings or amalgams often project above the surface of the teeth. Females with both anorexia nervosa and bulimia frequently present with either primary or secondary amenorrhea, depending on their age.

Psychosocial features of patients with eating disorders frequently include low self-esteem, depression, perfectionistic attitude, overachieving, and social withdrawal. These patients also display a disturbed body image where the body size is overestimated, as well as a misperception of physical sensations. They often deny fatigue following excessive exercising and have a distorted awareness of hunger.

Families of patients with eating disorders generally present with obvious economic, social, and academic success. Beneath the family facade, there may be issues of overprotectiveness, rigidity, emotional coldness, and lack of communication. Although no typical family pattern predisposing to the development of eating disorders has been discovered, the eating disorder itself often disrupts the family.

Table 16-1-1. DSM-IV Characteristics of Anorexia Nervosa

Diagnostic Criteria

1. Refusal to maintain body weight at or above a minimally normal weight for age and height (e.g., weight loss leading to maintenance of body weight less than 85 percent of that expected; or failure to make expected weight gain during period of growth, leading to body weight 85 percent of that expected)
2. Intense fear of gaining weight or becoming fat, even though underweight
3. Disturbance in the way in which one's body weight, size, or shape is experienced, undue influence of body weight or shape on self-evaluation, or denial of the seriousness of the current low body weight
4. In postmenarcheal females, amenorrhea, i.e., the absence of at least three consecutive menstrual cycles (A woman is considered to have amenorrhea if her periods occur only following hormone, e.g., estrogen, administration.)

Types

Restricting type: During the current episode of anorexia nervosa, the person has not regularly engaged in binge eating or purging behavior (i.e., self-induced vomiting or the misuse of laxatives, diuretics, or enemas).

Binge-eating/purging type: During the current episode of anorexia nervosa, the person has regularly engaged in binge eating or purging behavior (i.e., self-induced vomiting or the misuse of laxatives, diuretics, or enemas).

SOURCE: American Psychiatric Association: *Diagnostic and Statistical Manual of Mental Disorders,* 4th ed. Washington, DC, American Psychiatric Association, 1994, pp 544–545. Used with permission.

DIAGNOSTIC CONSIDERATIONS

The diagnosis of eating disorders is based on the criteria of the *Diagnostic and Statistical Manual of Mental Disorders,* listed in Tables 16-1-1 and 16-1-2. Differential diagnoses include other behavioral disorders associated with weight loss, such as severe depression, psychological reactions to food, and psychotic disorders. Physical disorders to be rule out are inflammatory bowel disease, diabetes mellitus, malabsorptive states, hypo- and hyperthyroidism, brain tumors (especially of the fourth ventricle), collagen vascular disease, and Addison's disease.

SPECIAL CONSIDERATIONS

Males

Although less common, anorexia nervosa does occur in males, and the signs and symptoms resemble those in females. Some have suggested that male adolescents with anorexia nervosa may present with more severe medical abnormalities because of a delay in establishing the diagnosis. An increase in bulimia has been reported recently in males, especially those who try to maintain specific weights for sports events (e.g., wrestling).

Young Children

A recent review of anorexia nervosa in children under 13 years of age found that younger children had a higher severity of illness, a delay in diagnosis, and a higher incidence of family psychiatric history. Since bulimia tends to have a slightly later onset than anorexia nervosa, it is seldom observed in young children.

LABORATORY TESTS

The evaluation of anorexic patients should include: complete blood count and platelet count, erythrocyte sedimentation rate

(ESR), blood urea nitrogen (BUN) and creatinine, urinalysis, serum electrolytes, liver function tests, serum calcium and phosphate, serum albumin, carotene, T_4, and a chest x-ray. Other tests that may be of interest are stools for occult blood and fat, upper GI tract series, barium enema, and a computed tomography or magnetic resonance imaging of the head. Fluid and electrolyte abnormalities are frequently revealed by laboratory tests (see Chaps. 4-2 and 4-3). Metabolic alkalosis, hypochloremia, and occasionally hypokalemia are most commonly seen.

NUTRITIONAL ASSESSMENT

The nutritional assessment of anorexia nervosa should involve weight, height, triceps circumference, skinfolds, midarm circumference, and a calculation of percentage body fat.

TREATMENT

Medical Management of Anorexia Nervosa

Treatment of eating disorders first focuses on normalization of the nutritional status, particularly in patients with severe symptoms of malnutrition. Hospitalization should be considered in patients who have the following:

1. Severe medical complications
2. Severe depression, particularly with the risk of suicide
3. Mental instability, including failure to comply with outpatient treatment
4. Severe bingeing and/or purging behavior

Oral feeding to increase weight should be tried first. Some patients, however, require nasogastric feeding or intravenous hyperalimentation. Following diagnosis and stabilization in the hospital, long-term therapy should focus on both individual and family psychotherapy.

Table 16-1-2. DSM-IV Characteristics of Bulimia Nervosa

Diagnostic Criteria

1. Recurrent episodes of binge eating. An episode of binge eating is characterized by both of the following:
   A. Eating, in a discrete period of time (e.g., within any 2-h period), an amount of food that is definitely larger than most people would eat during a similar period of time and under similar circumstances.
   B. A sense of lack of control over eating during the episode (e.g., a feeling that one cannot stop eating or control what or how much one is eating).
2. Recurrent inappropriate compensatory behavior to prevent weight gain, such as self-induced vomiting; misuse of laxatives, diuretics, enemas, or other medications; fasting; or excessive exercise.
3. The binge eating and inappropriate compensatory behaviors both occur, on average, at least twice a week for 3 months.
4. Self-evaluation is unduly influenced by body shape and weight.
5. The disturbance does not occur exclusively during episodes of anorexia nervosa.

Types

Purging type: During the current episode of bulimia nervosa, the person has regularly engaged in self-induced vomiting or the misuse of laxatives, diuretics, or enemas.

Nonpurging type: During the current episode of bulimia nervosa, the person has used other inappropriate compensatory behaviors such as fasting or excessive exercise, but has not regularly engaged in self-induced vomiting or the misuse of laxatives, diuretics, or enemas.

SOURCE: American Psychiatric Association: *Diagnostic and Statistical Manual of Mental Disorders,* 4th ed. Washington, DC, American Psychiatric Association, 1994, pp 549–550. Used with permission.

Pharmacotherapeutics

Antidepressant drugs are helpful in eating disorders, particularly in patients with bulimia. The results of numerous placebo-controlled double-blind antidepressant trials have demonstrated that these drugs have a potent and significant suppressant effect on binge eating and purging behavior. Studies suggest that individuals who are not depressed at baseline may respond equally well to antidepressant treatments. Fluoxetine hydrochloride (Prozac), a serotonin reuptake inhibitor, is the drug of choice. Although antidepressants can be quite useful, research indicates that relapse is high with discontinuation of the drugs. The combined use of psychotherapy with antidepressants may be the best treatment for bulimia.

Antidepressants have also been found to be effective in treating the depression often associated with anorexia nervosa. Antidepressant medications can be of help in medically stable anorectics.

PSYCHOTHERAPY

The treatment of eating disorders is at best difficult. Treatment begins with an open acknowledgment to the patient and family that, although the striving for thinness and control is obviously very important, it has serious dangers, including physical illness, psychologic morbidity, and even death.

The most effective psychotherapy approach is cognitive behavioral therapy techniques delivered in either group or individual formats. The core cognitive distortion in eating disorders is the patient's belief that the only way to feel good about his or her own competence is to be in rigid control of body weight. There are a number of elements common in successful treatment programs:

1. There is a strong emphasis on nutritional counseling.
2. Behavioral techniques are used to control binge eating and challenge irrational beliefs.
3. Alternative ways of dealing with disruptive emotions, such as anger and depression, are taught.
4. Family treatment accompanies individual psychiatric care. The focus is on decreasing parental overprotectiveness, fortifying intergenerational boundaries, and minimizing the child's role as a peacemaker in the family.

PROGNOSIS

The course and outcome for eating disorders are highly variable. Recent studies of prognosis were completed by Gilbert et al. (1994) and Steinhausen and Seidel (1993). The results of their investigations suggest mortality rates for anorexia nervosa between 0 and 22 percent. They found that the percent of former eating disorder patients who were eating normally at follow-up ranged from 15 to 82 percent. Depressive symptoms were still common. Factors related to a good prognosis for anorexia nervosa are young age of onset, high educational achievement, supportive family, improvement in body image after weight gain, and good initial ego strength. A poor prognosis is associated with late age of onset, premorbid obesity, self-induced vomiting or purging, laxative abuse, long duration of disorder, low social class, disturbed parental relationship, marked depression, and obsessional behavior.

Generally, bulimia appears to have a better outcome than anorexia nervosa. A review of seven studies by Herzog et al. (1988) found an absence of mortality and normal body weight in most patients but a high incidence of depression and 29 to 87 percent still having binge eating episodes. Self-induced vomiting and laxative abuse were still present in some bulimics.

OTHER NOTES OR PEARLS

The most important ingredient in the diagnosis of eating disorders is a high degree of suspicion. These patients usually present with a lack of insight into the severity of their weight loss, sometimes still maintaining that they are overweight. The patient may wear loose, baggy clothes to hide the extent of emaciation. As many as 50 percent of anorexic patients have an associated major depressive syndrome.

BIBLIOGRAPHY

Bassoe H: Anorexia/bulimia nervosa: Treatment and the outcome of the disease. *Acta Psychiatricia Scand* 82:7, 1990

Gillberg IC, Rastam M, Gillberg C: Anorexia nervosa outcome: Six-year controlled longitudinal study of 51 cases including a population cohort. *J Am Acad Child Adoles Psychiatry* 33:729, 1994.

Herzog DB, Keller MB, Lavori PW: Outcome in anorexia nervosa and bulimia nervosa: A review of the literature. *J Nerv Ment Dis* 176:131, 1988.

MacKenzie R, Neinstein LS: Anorexia nervosa and bulimia, in Neinstein LS (ed): *Adolescent Health Care: A Practical Guide*, 3d ed. Baltimore, Williams & Wilkins, 1996, pp 564–593.

Olivardia R, Pope HG Jr, Mangweth B, et al: Eating disorders in college men. *Am J Psychiatry* 152:1279, 1995.

Steinhausen HC, Seidel R: Outcome in adolescent eating disorders. *Int J Eat Disord* 14:487, 1993.

Yates A: Biological considerations in the etiology of eating disorders. *Pediatr Ann* 21:739, 1992.

Chapter 16–2
SLEEP DISORDERS (INSOMNIA)
William A. Mosier

DISCUSSION

Sleep is a complex physiologic function. The variations in depth and length are markedly pronounced. The range of sleep period, in healthy adults, is 4 to 10 h. Insomnia can be defined as an involuntary sleeplessness severe enough to interfere with daytime alertness and energy level. Insomnia should be thought of as a symptom of some other underlying problem and not a disease in itself. There is an increased rate of mortality in individuals who sleep fewer than 4 h or more than 10 h per night. Throughout the life span, total sleep time, in a 24-h period, declines. It is highest during infancy and declines with age. The average newborn sleeps 18 h a day. The average total sleep time in an elderly individual is 6.5 h. Of all the factors that can modify normal sleep architecture, age is the strongest influence; however, contrary to common perception, the need for sleep does not significantly decrease with age. However, because of changes in individual circadian rhythms, a decrease in sleep regulation may occur with advancing age. Individuals deprived of sleep for as little as 60 h tend to experience increased fatigue and irritability and decreased concentration. With longer periods of sleep deprivation, illusions and even hallucinations can impair consciousness. One of three Americans reports difficulty sleeping. About 40 million Americans (9 percent) suffer from chronic sleep disorders. Insomnia is the most commonly reported symptom of premenstrual syndrome (PMS). Forty percent of women experiencing menopause suffer from insomnia for 2 to 5 years after the onset of menopause.

Table 16-2-1. Common Sleep Problems

Chronic insomnia
Narcolepsy
Sleep apnea
Sleepwalking
Changes with advanced age
Body clock disorder (e.g., jet lag)
Disturbances caused by shift work changes
Restless leg syndrome
Periodic leg movement disorder

Insomnia is generally classified into two categories: primary (no apparent cause) and secondary (a cause can be identified). Sometimes, insomnia is classified as transient (lasting only a few nights), short-term (lasting up to 3 weeks), or long-term (lasting more than 3 weeks).

The three most commonly occurring insomnia patterns are the following:

1. Sleep onset insomnia (taking more than 30 min to fall asleep).
2. Sleep maintenance insomnia (frequent wakening during the night).
3. Early morning awakening (having a pattern of awakening about 2 h prior to normal waking time).

Other sleep disturbances are sleep apnea, narcolepsy, body clock disorder, changes due to aging, periodic limb movement disorder, problems caused by shift work, restless leg syndrome, and sleepwalking (see Table 16-2-1).

Approximately, 50 percent of patients presenting with the complaint of insomnia have previously been diagnosed with a psychiatric disorder. Only about 15 percent of individuals diagnosed with psychiatric disorders have no sleep complaints. The most common psychiatric disorders associated with sleep complaints are depression and anxiety disorder. Alcohol and other drug abuse disorders (including tobacco use) reflect a positive relationship to increased rates of insomnia. Approximately 90 percent of patients hospitalized for depression demonstrate electroencephalogram (EEG) verified sleep disturbance. In fact, 90 percent of all patients diagnosed with major depression complain of insomnia. Less than 10 percent complain of hypersomnulance. Approximately, 25 percent of patients complaining of chronic insomnia are diagnosed with an anxiety disorder.

Psychophysiologic or chronic primary insomnia (also referred to as conditioned or learned insomnia) usually involves both sleep-onset and maintenance of sleep difficulties. Conditioned insomnia usually results from a somatized anxiety-tension state and poor sleep hygiene.

PATHOGENESIS

The sleep-wake cycle is controlled by the circadian system. This internal biologic clock is thought to be located in the suprachiasmatic nucleus (SCN) of the hypothalamus. Two of the neurotransmitters that promote sleep associated with slow-wave sleep activity are serotonin and gamma-aminobutyric acid (GABA). The human body moves through five stages during a normal sleep period. The typical sleep period consists of 4 to 6 sleep cycles. Each cycle lasts about 90 min in the nonelderly adult. A cycle consists of two different types of sleep:

1. Nonrapid eye movement (NREM) sleep
2. Rapid eye movement (REM) sleep

NREM sleep is divided into four different stages:

1. *Stage I* is a brief transition from wakefulness to sleep. It is characterized by slow, rolling eye movements identifiable on electrooculogram (EOG), low-voltage, mixed frequency electroencephalogram (EEG) activity, and moderately high amplitude discharges recorded on electromyogram (EMG). Stage I sleep tends to increase in the elderly.
2. *Stage II* generally constitutes the onset of true sleep. It is characterized by a moderately low-voltage EEG, interspersed with brief, high-voltage discharges (referred to as K complexes), as well as vertex waves, interspersed with low- to moderate-amplitude discharges (referred to as sleep spindles).
3. *Stage III* is considered deep sleep. It is characterized by high-amplitude background activity of delta and theta waves, as well as K complexes and sleep spindles.
4. *Stage IV* is also referred to as a deep sleep phase. It is characterized by high-voltage delta waves.

Eye movements are infrequent or totally absent during stages III and IV. Low-voltage muscle potentials occur during stages II, III, and IV. The secretion of growth hormone (GH) is elevated during NREM sleep. The immune system is also more active during this slow-wave sleep. Stage III and stage IV tend to decrease in the elderly.

Stage V (REM) sleep is the stage at which dreams that can be remembered occur. Heart rate, blood pressure, and respirations are similar to waking state during REM sleep. It is characterized by an abrupt change in EEG pattern; it appears as a low-voltage, fast-frequency activity resembling the pattern observed during wakefulness or stage I sleep. It may resemble a sawtooth wave pattern of moderately high amplitude or a triangular-shaped waveform. REM sleep demonstrates an absence of deep tendon reflexes. During REM sleep there is also a markedly suppressed or totally absent EMG activity. Positron emission tomography (PET) studies indicate that the brain's use of glucose during REM sleep is within the same range as that recorded during wakefulness. REM sleep constitutes about 25 percent of a person's total sleep time.

Patients manifesting generalized anxiety disorder (GAD) typically demonstrate the following:

- Prolonged sleep onset latency (time from laying down to sleep to actual onset of sleep)
- Increased stage I and stage II sleep
- Decreased slow-wave sleep
- Lower REM sleep percentage

The sleep architecture associated with major depression includes the following:

- Shortened REM sleep latency (time from sleep onset to the onset of REM sleep)
- Increased REM sleep density (frequency of eye movements)
- Reduced total sleep time
- Reduced sleep efficiency
- Increased awakenings
- Decreased slow wave sleep
- Increased duration of first REM sleep period

The only apparent gender difference associated with insomnia is a decreased slow-wave sleep pattern identified in men diagnosed with major depression.

SYMPTOMS

Insomnia associated with mood disorders is common. The presenting complaints may be problems of sleep onset, middle of

Table 16-2-2. Medications Known to Produce Insomnia

OTC Agents	Prescription Agents	
Alcohol	Antiparkinson agents	NSAIDs
Caffeine	Amantadine HCl	Flurbiprofen
Cough, cold, allergy	Diphenhydramine HCl	Indomethacin
preparations	Pergolide mesylate	Ketoprofen
Actifed	Cardiovascular agents	Naproxen
Alka-Seltzer Plus	Acebutolol	Psychotropics
Benadryl	Atenolol	Alprazolam
Benylin Cough	Betaxolol	Clozapine
Belix	Captopril	Isocarboxazid
Comtrex	Diltiazem HCl	Muscle relaxants
Contac	Guanfacine HCl	Cyclobenzaprine
Coricidin	Metoprolol	H_2 blockers
Dimetapp	Nifedipine	Ranitidine
Drixoral	Pindolol	Asthma preparations
Robitussin Night	Propranolol HCl	Aminophylline
Relief	Conjugated estrogens	Theophylline
Sudafed		
Triaminic		

the night awakenings, and/or early morning awakenings. [It is useful to remember that all three of these presenting disturbances may commonly occur in patients meeting the *Diagnostic and Statistical Manual of Mental Disorders,* fourth edition (DSM-IV) criteria for major depression.] Because of the sleep maintenance difficulties involved with insomnia, many patients also complain of daytime fatigue and lethargy.

OBJECTIVE FINDINGS

Asking the patient detailed questions about the quality and quantity of sleep can greatly assist in getting an accurate picture of the origin of the insomnia. The following questions are useful to ask:

1. How long does it take you to fall asleep once you have gone to bed?
2. Do you remain asleep all night?
3. Do you awaken feeling well rested in the morning?

DIAGNOSTIC CONSIDERATIONS

A patient with a presenting complaint of insomnia should be screened for the other core symptoms of major depressive disorder. When differentiating between depression and anxiety, it is helpful to remember that the anxious patient may have more difficulty falling asleep, whereas the depressed patient may fall asleep more readily but experience early morning awakenings. If the depression and anxiety screening prove negative, then thyroid disorders should be ruled out. If untreated, hyperthyroidism may cause irritability, tension, and insomnia. The chemical replacement therapy for hypothyroidism can also produce symptoms of insomnia. Cystitis in women and benign prostatic hypertrophy (BPH) in men can cause nighttime awakening and disrupt restful sleep, resulting in fatigue the following day. Other organic causes of insomnia can be angina, arthritis, asthma, back pain, chronic sinusitis, diabetes, dementia, epilepsy, heart disease, and ulcers. Some medications can produce a side effect of insomnia, including some antidepressants, tranquilizers, diuretics, and even some high-potency vitamin supplements (see Table 16-2-2).

SPECIAL CONSIDERATIONS

Age-related changes in sleep physiology correspond to patient complaints of disrupted sleep. Sleep disorders are particularly prevalent among the elderly. Approximately half of all individuals over the age of 65 suffer from insomnia. Although they constitute only 25 percent of the U.S. total population, persons over 50 years of age account for 50 percent of all prescribed sleep medications. Insomnia in the elderly is usually secondary to some other underlying condition or event. Taking a complete medical, psychiatric, and medication history is necessary to evaluate insomnia in any patient, but especially in an elderly patient. Although transient insomnia can be resolved when the stressors are removed or modified, chronic insomnia requires a comprehensive evaluation and treatment plan to address the underlying causes.

DIAGNOSTIC TESTS

Diagnosis is usually based on symptoms that can be identified from taking a thorough history. However, it is sometimes helpful to have the patient undergo sleep studies in a sleep laboratory, to aid in the search for an underlying cause of the insomnia. In psychophysiologic insomnia, sleep EEG studies typically demonstrate delayed sleep onset or frequent nocturnal awakenings but otherwise no specific changes in sleep architecture or REM sleep abnormalities. However, in insomnia associated with depression, early morning awakenings (at least 2 hours before the usual time for awakening) as well as the typical REM sleep findings associated with depression are useful for identifying depression-based insomnia. (See "Pathogenesis," above, for EEG findings associated with depression.)

TREATMENT

The goal of treatment should be uninterrupted sleep and improved daytime function. Short-term use of the sedative-hypnotic drugs may be useful. However, long-term use can be habit forming, lead to decreased efficacy, and result in rebound insomnia. By matching specific drugs to specific sleep problems, treatment for insomnia can be tailored to each patient's needs. Insomnia is best managed by treating the underlying disorder. It must be emphasized that alteration of sleep is a hallmark symptom of affective disorders such as depression. Therefore, treatment with antidepressants and careful monitoring is warranted as first-line treatment for insomnia if depression is suspected. When no underlying condition can be uncovered, treatment should begin with behavior modification strategies followed by conservative use of medication only when necessary.

Regardless of their effect on depression, antidepressants can differ greatly in their effects on sleep. Research substantiates that both sedating and nonsedating antidepressants can decrease insomnia as a result of decreasing a patient's overall symptoms of depression. Antidepressants that produce an immediate prolongation of REM sleep latency, a reduction of total REM sleep time, and a reduction of total REM density appear to provide a better clinical response to the treatment of insomnia. Antidepressants that tend to stimulate REM sleep at the onset of sleep episodes and stimulate shorter REM sleep episode duration are associated with an increased risk of insomnia relapse. If a mood disorder or anxiety disorder is the underlying cause of the sleep disturbance, medications most often utilized are tricyclic antidepressants, buspirone, selective serotonin reuptake inhibitors (SSRIs), or sedative hypnotics.

Sedative-hypnotic agents should generally be limited to 7 to 10 days of use. Reevaluation of the patient is recommended if treatment continues for more than 3 weeks.

The benzodiazepines can be useful in the treatment of insomnia because they seem to bind to the omega receptors which are part of the GABA receptor complex. The benzodiazepines along with the first of a new class of nonbenzodiazepine sleep agents commonly prescribed for insomnia are listed in Table 16-2-3 along with their half-life, common dosages, and typical onset of action.

Table 16-2-3. Common Sleep Agents Used to Treat Insomnia

Drug	Half-life	Dosage	Onset of Action
Benzodiazepines			
Quazepam (Doral)	2–4 d	7.5–15 mg	Intermediate
Flurazepam (Dalmane)	2–3 d	15 mg	Intermediate
Estazolam (ProSom)	14 h	1 mg	Fast
Temazepam (Restoril)	10–20 h	15 mg	Intermediate
Lorazepam (Ativan)	12–18 h	0.5–1 mg	Intermediate
Oxazepam (Serax)	5–10 h	10–15 mg	Intermediate
Triazolam (Halcion)	2–4 h	0.25 mg	Fast
Nonbenzodiazepine			
Zolpidem tartrate (Ambien)	2.5 h	5–10 mg	Fast

The benzodiazepines are only a temporary solution to the problem of insomnia. They should be prescribed only for the shortest possible time. It should also be remembered that because they cause depression to the central nervous system, eventually they may worsen the insomnia. Contrary to common perception, the benzodiazepines with the longer half-life may actually be safer, as evidenced by a decrease in observed rebound. Quazepam (Doral) has not been documented as demonstrating rebound phenomena. However, extreme care must be taken to monitor for the effects that long half-life may have, such as impairment of daytime function if dosed too high. Of note is the nonbenzodiazepine hypnotic agent zolpidem tartrate (Ambien). It is the first of a new class of imidazopyridine agents that is chemically distinct from benzodiazepine. Zolpidem tartrate is indicated for the short-term treatment of insomnia. An improvement over the benzodiazepine hypnotics, zolpidem tartrate tends to preserve the deep sleep of stage III and IV NREM sleep.

SUPPORTIVE MEASURES

Relaxation therapy such as muscle relaxation techniques, biofeedback, breathing exercises, and meditation have been found to be useful for enhancing sleep induction ability. Stimulus-control therapy is also a valuable adjunct treatment to improve sleep hygiene. Patients should be taught techniques to refine their bedtime habits. A patient who is unable to fall asleep should get out of bed and go do another activity until tired. The patient should be instructed about the importance of discontinuing the drinking of coffee and other caffeinated beverages. The use of tobacco and alcohol should also be discouraged. Patients should be reminded that these substances actually interfere with normal sleep patterns and can cause a person to awaken during the night. Sugary snacks and heavy, late-evening meals can stimulate metabolism, making it difficult to fall asleep and/or sleep restfully. Moderate daily exercise reduces anxiety and therefore may improve a patient's sleep pattern as well.

PATIENT EDUCATION

Patients should be instructed to avoid the habit of watching television or reading a book in bed, if they have difficulty falling asleep. Taking the time to teach healthy bedtime habits can help patients understand the relationship between sleep hygiene and the inability to fall asleep. Patients should also be instructed about how the abuse of sleeping pills can actually cause insomnia to worsen.

DISPOSITION

When prescribing a hypnotic for the treatment of insomnia, use the lowest possible dose, dispense a limited number of doses, monitor for side effects, monitor for cognitive or behavioral changes, monitor for effectiveness, and plan for a follow-up office visit in 2 to 3 weeks.

COMPLICATIONS AND RED FLAGS

Short-term memory problems and rebound insomnia can be side effects of the benzodiazepines. It is important to remember that the helpful effects of the benzodiazepines may diminish over time. The risk of addiction is a major concern if the dose must be increased to control the insomnia. Mixing the benzodiazepines with alcohol can result in death. Although triazolam (Halcion) is currently available in the United States, it is associated with rebound insomnia and amnesia. It has been removed from the market in the United Kingdom based on the recommendations of the Committee on Safety of Medicines in the United Kingdom. Therefore, it should probably not be considered as a first-line choice.

OTHER NOTES OR PEARLS

Sleep complaints should not be automatically treated with hypnotic agents. Careful evaluation of each patient's insomnia must be performed to uncover and treat any underlying condition, such as a mood disorder. In general, hypnotics should be prescribed for the short term only. In cases of chronic insomnia they should be combined with other therapeutic approaches. Because REM latency appears to be reduced in individuals suffering from depression, the following question is postulated: Is insomnia a consequence of depression or an indicator of vulnerability to depression or a predictor of depression in individuals at risk for manifesting depression? Not every patient with insomnia has major depressive disorder. However, if a patient complains of insomnia, it is most prudent to inquire about other core symptoms of depression before prescribing a sedative hypnotic. The old adage: "The anxious patient can't fall asleep; the depressed patient can't stay asleep" is probably an oversimplification. However, any sleep disturbance is a possible marker for underlying anxiety or depression.

BIBLIOGRAPHY

American Psychiatric Association: *Diagnostic and Statistical Manual of Mental Disorders,* 4th ed. Washington, DC, American Psychiatric Association, 1994.

American Sleep Disorders Association: *The International Classification of Sleep Disorders Diagnostic and Coding Manual.* Rochester, MN, 1990.

Bachman DL: Sleep disorders with aging: Evaluation and treatment. *Geriatrics* 47(9):53–61, 1992.

Becker PM, Jamieson AO: Common sleep disorders in the elderly: Diagnosis and treatment. *Geriatrics* 47(3):41–52, 1992.

Brunton SA: When your patient can't sleep. *Fam Prac Recert* 14:149–170, 1992.

Feinsilver SH, Hertz G: Sleep in the elderly patient. *Clin Chest Med* 14:405–411, 1993.

Hales RE, Rakel RE, Rothschild S: Depression: Practical tips for detection and treatment. *Patient Care* 28(18):60–80, 1994.

Monane M: Insomnia in the elderly. *J Clin Psychiatry* 53(6, suppl):23–28, 1992.

Monjan AA: Sleep disorders of older people: Report of a consensus conference. *Hosp Comm Psych* 41(7):743–744, 1990.

Simon GE, VonKorff M: Recognition, management, and outcomes of depression in primary care. *Arch Fam Med* 4:99–105, 1995.

Ware JC, Morewitz J: Diagnosis and treatment of insomnia and depression. *J Clin Psychiatry* 52(6, suppl):55–61, 1991.

Wooten V: Sleep disorders in psychiatric illness, in Chokroverty S (ed): *Sleep Disorders Medicine.* Stoneham, MA, Butterworth-Heinemann, 1993, pp 337–347.

Chapter 16–3
ANXIETY AND PANIC DISORDERS
Don St. John

DISCUSSION

Anxiety disorders are the most prevalent psychiatric disorders, affecting 12 percent of the population at any given time. Patients with anxiety-related complaints represent 20 to 30 percent of patients in a primary care setting. The majority of patients with anxiety disorders are seen in a medical setting, especially in primary care. These patients usually present with somatic complaints and, for this reason, the diagnosis is often missed.

Table 16-3-1 lists the anxiety disorders described in the *Diagnostic and Statistical Manual of Mental Disorders,* fourth edition (DSM-IV). There are a number of factors involved in the etiology of anxiety disorders, ranging from psychosocial (e.g., adverse early environment) to behavioral (e.g., learned response) to biologic and genetic (e.g., abnormalities of the locus ceruleus).

SYMPTOMS

The symptoms of anxiety vary according to the specific disorder, but there is much overlap of symptoms as well as comorbidity. General symptoms of anxiety include a sense of apprehension, worry, tension, uneasiness, emotional lability, and hypervigilance. Somatic symptoms include palpitations, chest pain, nausea, dizziness, motor tension (tremor, twitches, muscle aching), insomnia, and autonomic hyperactivity (diaphoresis, tachycardia, diarrhea). The possibility of an anxiety disorder should be considered and communicated to the patient early in the evaluation of such symptoms.

Anxiety may also contribute to the morbidity of medical conditions such as chronic obstructive pulmonary disease, coronary artery disease, gastrointestinal ulcers, ulcerative colitis, asthma, hypertension, urticaria, and seizure disorders. Some anxiety disorders mimic physical conditions (e.g., panic disorder), and physical disorders (e.g., hyperthyroidism)and certain substances (e.g., caffeine) often give rise to anxiety symptoms. Table 16-3-2 gives a differential to consider when evaluating anxious patients.

TREATMENT CONSIDERATIONS

Although many anxiety disorders are acute reactions to circumstances, others are chronic disturbances with fluctuating course. Long-term treatment may be required for patients who fail to achieve full resolution of symptoms with brief interventions. Psychopharmacologic management varies according to the specific

Table 16-3-1. Anxiety Disorders

> Panic disorder with or without agoraphobia
> Agoraphobia without panic disorder
> Generalized anxiety disorder
> Social phobia
> Specific phobia
> Obsessive-compulsive disorder
> Adjustment disorder with anxiety
> Acute stress disorder
> Posttraumatic stress disorder
> Substance-induced anxiety disorder
> Anxiety disorder due to a general medical condition

SOURCE: From American Psychiatric Association.

Table 16-3-2. Differential Diagnosis of Anxiety Disorders

Cardiac
  Ischemic heart disease
  Mitral valve prolapse
  Dysrhythmias
  Pericarditis
Endocrine and metabolic
  Hyperthyroidism
  Hypoglycemia
  Pheochromocytoma
Gynecologic
  Menopause
  Premenstrual syndrome
Neurologic
  Transischemic attacks
  Cerebrovascular accident
  Psychomotor epilepsy
  Postconcussion syndrome
  Delirium
Nutritional
  Deficiencies of thiamine, pyridoxine, folate, iron
Respiratory
  Asthma
  Chronic obstructive pulmonary disease
Pharmacologic
  Caffeine
  Alcohol use or withdrawal
  Sympathomimetics
  Yohimbine
  Amphetamines
  Cocaine
  Benzodiazepine withdrawal
  Corticosteroids
  Illicit drugs, especially marijuana, phencyclidine, and organic solvents

disorder being addressed. Attention must be paid to development of coping skills and improvement of social support systems and interpersonal relationships. Depression is frequently comorbid with all anxiety disorders, especially in the presence of chronic and severe symptoms and other comorbidity, such as low assertiveness, high generalized anxiety, and severe agoraphobia.

SPECIAL POPULATIONS
Children

Symptoms of anxiety in children include physiologic hyperarousal, hypervigilance, and temperamental fearfulness, often demonstrated by behavioral restraint. Pediatric patients who develop an anxiety disorder may be irritable as infants, shy and fearful as toddlers, and cautious, quiet, and introverted during school years. Separation anxiety and school refusal (phobia) are associated with the development of adult anxiety disorders. Children with anxiety are more likely to develop anxiety and other psychiatric disorders in adult life.

Behavioral inhibition is a strong predictor of the later development of anxiety. Parental anxiety may be a marker for at-risk children. Children appear to respond to psychopharmacologic management like adults, though studies of specific agents are few. Other therapy methods used in children include contingency management, in vivo exposure, and cognitive restructuring. Involvement of parents is important in treating children with anxiety disorders.

Elderly

Anxiety disorders are common in the elderly, often in association with physical illness. Psychopharmacologic treatment must begin with low doses, gradually increasing to therapeutic response, as tolerated by the individual patient.

Benzodiazepines should be avoided in patients with dementia because of the risks of confusion, incoordination with falls, paradoxical reactions, and behavioral disinhibition. Many drugs have altered metabolism and are likely to accumulate in elderly patients. Buspirone, trazodone, selective serotonin reuptake inhibitors, and beta blockers have been effective in this special group of patients.

Generalized Anxiety Disorder

PREVALENCE AND ETIOLOGIC FACTORS

Personal suceptibility and life stressors appear to play an important role in the etiology of generalized anxiety disorder (GAD). GAD tends to occur in persons with high levels of trait anxiety, that is, temperamental tendencies to react to stressful circumstances with anxiety symptoms. GAD is usually seen by primary care practitioners, not by psychiatrists. Lifetime prevalence is 8.5 percent; 1-year prevalence is 3 percent. Women are twice as likely to develop GAD as men.

SIGNS AND SYMPTOMS

GAD symptoms often begin gradually and early in life. Despite an early onset, often in childhood, the average age of presentation for treatment may be years later. GAD tends to run a chronic or recurrent course.

Symptoms include chronic worrying out of proportion to the situation (the principal feature of GAD), difficulty concentrating, dizziness, insomnia (especially difficulty falling asleep), unrestful sleep, emotional tension, easy distractibility, irritability, and restlessness. Physical symptoms include dry mouth, palpitations, flushing, frequent urination, headache, and fatigue.

Signs may include diaphoresis, tachycardia, and diffuse muscular tension. Discrete episodes or attacks of anxiety are absent.

The worry of GAD is diffuse, unfocused, and ongoing. Patients tend to believe they have little control over situations, especially aversive situations. Patients also tend to selectively attend to threatening or potentially threatening information in both their internal and external environments.

DIAGNOSTIC CONSIDERATIONS

Differential diagnosis includes many physical conditions. A representative list can be found in Table 16-3-2. Patients with hyperthyroidism may have a fine tremor and heat intolerance (see Chap. 5-4). Hypoglycemia tends to be episodic, predictably occurs several hours after meals, and is reversed by glucose ingestion. A history of head trauma with amnesia surrounding the event may suggest postconcussion syndrome. Patients with delirium exhibit an altered level of consciousness and cognitive dysfunction.

Many psychiatric disorders have prominent anxiety symptoms. A diagnosis of GAD is not made in the presence of another, diagnosed primary anxiety disorder. In other anxiety disorders, the focus of anxiety is on the principal feature of the disorder. Panic attacks are discrete episodes of intense anxiety. There is a specific focus of anxiety in specific phobic disorders. Anxiety occurs in social contexts with social phobia. A hypochondriacal patient fears disease and exaggerates the danger of physical signs and symptoms.

One-third of patients with GAD have other axis I disorders, most commonly depressive disorders and substance abuse. There

may be considerable symptom overlap between depression and GAD. Schizophrenic patients may display disorganized thinking and constricted affect and may be distrustful if paranoid. Twenty-five percent of patients have comorbid panic disorder and/or major depressive disorder. Ninety percent of elderly patients with GAD may have comorbid depression. GAD symptoms are often prodromal to panic disorder. Substance abuse is common in patients with GAD and may begin as a form of self-treatment. Axis II disorders are also commonly present.

TREATMENT

Pharmacologic Management

Patients with GAD may require long-term pharmacotherapy, since symptoms tend to recur with medication discontinuation. Benzodiazepines (BZDs) are the treatment of choice for acute and time-limited therapy, though there are many patients who may require chronic use. BZDs are especially effective in patients who have panic attacks. Tolerance to the adverse effects (especially drowsiness, dizziness, and slowed responses) often develops after 6 to 8 weeks of treatment. However, impairment of short-term memory and learning sometimes persists. Because of this, BZD use may interfere with psychological therapy. BZD use is also associated with a higher dropout rate from concurrent psychological therapy. Abuse tends to occur in those patients who abuse other drugs, especially alcoholics. Escalation of dosage, initiated by the patient should alert the practitioner to potential for abuse. As the patient responds, the benzodiazepine dose may be slowly tapered and discontinued. The half-life of longer-acting agents may be prolonged in elderly patients. Table 16-3-3 lists commonly used BZDs with dosage ranges. Table 16-3-4 lists significant potential drug interactions.

All of the currently available antidepressants, appear to be effective for the treatment of GAD, especially for more severe or chronic symptoms, or when dependence is a concern. Tricyclics have been studied the most. Serotonergic drugs, especially fluoxetine, may initially increase anxiety symptoms. Beginning with low doses and gradually increasing to dosages used to treat depression may be helpful in developing tolerance to side effects. Among the selective serotonin reuptake inhibitors (SSRIs), fluvoxamine appears to be the most sedating, followed by paroxetine, sertraline, and fluoxetine, which tends to be more activating. Bupropion is likely to worsen anxiety symptoms, especially at the onset of therapy, but can be an effective treatment.

Buspirone has been shown to be as effective as tricyclics in the treatment of GAD, and, at higher dosages, may also be effective in treating comorbid depression. Buspirone is well tolerated by most patients and has few significant drug interactions. Patients who have been previously treated with benzodiazepines tend not to respond as well to buspirone. As with antidepressants, it often takes 2 to 6 weeks before effectiveness is realized, and onset of action may be gradual. Buspirone cannot be used on an as-needed basis, does not treat benzodiazepine withdrawal symptoms, and cannot be directly substituted for benzodiazepines. Buspirone may be used to augment the action of antidepressants, though concurrent use of serotonergic agents may lead to a serotonin syndrome if instituted too rapidly. Side effects are uncommon and usually remit with continued use. Dizziness may occur 30 to 60 min after a dose and usually does not last longer than 20 min. Headache may occur and responds to OTC analgesics. Other possible side effects include drowsiness, nausea, insomnia, and nervousness (especially when first instituted). As with all serotonergic agents, buspirone should not be given with monoamine oxidase inhibitors (MAOIs) because of the possibility of serotonin syndrome.

Table 16-3-3. Benzodiazepines

Drug	Half-Life, h	Dose Equivalent, mg	Onset	Dosage Range, mg/d
Low-potency				
Diazepam	20–50	5	Fast	2–40
Chlordiazepoxide	5–30	25	Slow	10–40
Clorazepate	36–200	3.75	Intermediate	7.5–60
Prazepam	48–78	10	Slow	20–60
Oxazepam	5–10	30	Slow	40–120
High-potency				
Alprazolam	12–15	0.25	Fast	0.75–8
Clonazepam	18–50	0.5	Slow	1–8
Lorazepam	10–20	1	Fast	1–10

Beta blockers have been used to treat the peripheral autonomic symptoms of anxiety, especially tachycardia and tremor. Antihistamines may be used short-term for the elderly, with appropriate caution regarding sedation and potential anticholinergic effects. Antipsychotics should be avoided because of potentially serious adverse reactions, such as tardive dyskinesia, and the dysphoria often associated with their use. Caffeine and alcohol should be avoided, as well as illicit drugs, during treatment of GAD.

Supportive Measures

The patient should be informed of the fluctuating and chronic nature of GAD and the tendency for symptoms to wax and wane in response to stressors. Patients may find anxiety support groups helpful. Some patients respond to specific bibliotherapy recommendations.

Many patients find supportive counseling effective in treating their anxiety symptoms. Patients may be aided in identifying stressors and developing more effective means of coping with the stresses of their lives. Nondirective forms of therapy are often not as effective as more directive forms such as cognitive-behavioral therapy (CBT). Insight-oriented therapy may be helpful for some patients in exploring the meaning and function of anxiety in their lives.

Specific interventions include relaxation training, meditation, imagery, social skills training, problem-solving training, and biofeedback. Relaxation is used to reduce arousal and should be practiced daily. Patients should be encouraged to enter situations where avoidance has taken place, using their relaxation skills to manage situation-specific anxiety.

In cognitive therapy, patients are taught to identify, evaluate, and modify chronically worrisome and danger-related thoughts

Table 16-3-4. Potential Benzodiazepine Drug Interactions

All may potentiate CNS depression when used with any other CNS depressant.
 Diazepam
  Theophylline and rifampin may decrease effects.
  Cimetidine, valproate, and fluoxetine may increase effects.
 Chlordiazepoxide
  Effects of levodopa increased.
  May increase serum levels of phenytoin.
  May alter levels of anticoagulants.
 Prazepam
  Cimetidine and MAOIs may potentiate.
 Alprazolam
  Effects of digoxin may be potentiated.
  May increase levels of imipramine and desipramine.
  Potentiated by other drugs metabolized by CYP450 enzyme system 3A4.

and behaviors and develop more rational responses. Anxious thoughts are replaced by more positive, realistic, and functional thoughts.

Panic Disorder
PREVALENCE AND ETIOLOGIC FACTORS

Panic disorder (PD) is believed to be a genetically influenced disease in which biologic factors play an important role. Biologic factors may include abnormalities involving the nucleus ceruleus, dorsal raphe nucleus, hippocampus, and the cerebral noradrenalin system, and overactivity of the cerebral serotonergic system. Findings of 20 percent of patients with a first-degree relative with panic, and monozygotic/dizygotic concordance of 5:1, point to a genetic component. Psychological etiologic factors may include anxious attachment caused by aberrant family patterns, repression of unconscious conflicts, and childhood trauma.

Childhood anxiety may predispose to the development of panic disorder. Half of patients have a history of a childhood anxiety disorder, especially separation anxiety and school phobia. Patients appear to have a preexisting tendency to fear and misinterpret physical and emotional sensations. Exposure to frightening situations, scary stories, the sudden loss of a loved one, poor parental relationships, and threats of harm during childhood may also predispose to the development of panic disorder.

Women are two to three times as likely to develop panic disorder as men, with a lifetime prevalance rate of 2 to 3 percent for women and 0.5 to 1.5 percent for men.

Panic disorder usually begins in the late teens and early twenties, with 20 to 40 percent of patients having their first attack before age 20. PD rarely begins before age 12 or after age 40. Median age of onset is 25 for men, 28 for women. Initial attacks commonly follow an adverse life event. Occasionally attacks occur in thyroid disorders, the immediate postpartum period, or with use of marijuana, cocaine, or amphetamines. Late-onset panic disorder is unusual and presents with fewer panic symptoms, less avoidance, and less somatization.

Caffeine may cause attacks in some patients. Shame may prevent patients from seeking evaluation and treatment in Western cultures, that value self-reliance and view fear as weakness.

SIGNS AND SYMPTOMS

Though panic disorder and agoraphobia may be independent syndromes, they are treated as related and similar syndromes in this section. The key characteristic of panic disorder is recurrent panic attacks with subsequent fear of recurrence.

Symptoms include palpitations, tachycardia, diaphoresis, tremor, shortness of breath or choking sensation, hyperventilation, chest pain, nausea and abdominal pain, dry mouth, dizziness, weakness, presyncope, paresthesias, chills or hot flashes, and derealization or depersonalization. Many of these symptoms can be attributed to adrenergic excess. During attacks, patients irrationally fear losing control, going crazy, or dying. Panic attacks have a sudden onset, peak within minutes, and last 5 to 30 min. Attacks occur without warning or in agoraphobic situations. Panic attacks often awaken patients from sleep, resulting in anticipatory bedtime anxiety and insomnia.

The initial panic attack is usually well remembered and alarming. Patients may display increased general anxiety and apprehensive preoccupation with everyday difficulties prior to the initial attack. Each attack magnifies fear of future attacks. Patients begin to worry about the implications or consequences of a panic attack, especially public humiliation, and anxiety rises in anticipation of future attacks. Significant behavioral changes (primarily avoidance) may occur in response to repeated attacks. Left untreated, PD progresses from limited-symptom attacks to full panic attacks, hypochondriasis, limited phobic avoidance, extensive phobic avoidance, then development of secondary depression. The disorder may evolve rapidly, over days to weeks, or slowly, over months to years.

Agoraphobia is fear of being in a place or situation where escape may be difficult, or a fear of separation from one's source of security. This fear leads to phobic avoidance of places and situations where attacks have occurred in the past or where the patient fears an attack may occur. Agoraphobic patients commonly avoid crowded places, travel, and being alone. Some eventually become house-bound.

Patients with panic disorder often have self-perceptions of poor physical and/or emotional health, and may complain of marital and financial concerns not apparent to others. They often view themselves as overanxious, emotionally overly dependent on others, unassertive, and lacking self-confidence. They may express shame and humiliation regarding their dependence, especially if house-bound. Their sense of security may be fragile and closely bound to their family environment. Patients are often fearful of the medical profession and medications, with heightened sensitivity to adverse medication effects. Patients often have good work records and maintain their marriages, though sexual adjustment tends to be poor and there is a higher rate of divorce and separation among patients with panic disorder.

DIAGNOSTIC CONSIDERATIONS

Panic attacks occur in other disorders, such as depression (where 20 percent have panic attacks without panic disorder), other anxiety disorders, and certain personality disorders, especially borderline personality disorder. They are not usually accompanied by anticipatory anxiety between attacks.

The most common complications of panic disorder are depression and substance abuse, especially alcohol dependence. Seventy percent of patients may develop a secondary depression. These patients tend to respond better to antidepressants than benzodiazepines. About 15 to 30 percent of patients abuse drugs, especially alcohol and benzodiazepines. Patients with panic disorder are also at increased risk for committing suicide and for sudden death due to coronary artery disease. There may be an increased risk of peptic ulcer disease and hypertension among patients diagnosed with panic disorder. Dependent personality traits are common among patients with panic disorder, as is social phobia.

Panic disorder is not a diagnosis of exclusion. When symptoms are of recent onset, other treatable disorders should be ruled out before making the diagnosis of panic disorder. Evaluation should include a complete history and physical examination and may include a complete blood count, general blood chemistry screen, electrolytes, thyroid function studies, serum cortisol, electrocardiogram, and pulmonary function studies. The differential diagnosis can be found in Table 16-3-5.

Table 16-3-5. Differential Diagnosis for Panic Disorder

Cardiopulmonary
  Pulmonary embolus
  Dysrhythmia
    Supraventricular tachycardia (sudden increase then decrease in heart rate, with other symptoms secondary to tachycardia)
  Silent myocardial infarction (especially in diabetics)
  Mitral valve prolapse
  Angina
  Hypoxia
  Asthma
Neurologic
  Temporal lobe epilepsy/partial complex seizure disorder (sudden paroxysmal episodes of fear with derealization, depersonalization, nausea, and behavioral automatisms)
  Meniere's disease
  Transischemic attack or cerebrovascular accident
  Atypical migraine
  Small tumor of the temporal lobe (rare)
Endocrine
  Pheochromocytoma (rare, with marked episodic elevation of blood pressure and vasomotor lability)
  Hypoglycemia (probably overdiagnosed)
  Hyperthyroidism, especially thyrotoxicosis
  Carcinoid syndrome
  Diabetes mellitus
  Addison's or Cushing's disease
Psychiatric
  Posttraumatic stress disorder
  Separation anxiety
  Social phobia
  Generalized anxiety disorder
  Nightmare
  Sleep terror disorder
  Personality disorder, especially borderline, dependent, avoidant
  Adjustment disorder with anxious mood
Other
  Severe pain
  Severe anemia
  Labyrinthitis
  Chronic fatigue syndrome
Drug-induced
  Caffeine
  Aminophylline or theophylline
  Sympathomimetic agents
  Monosodium glutamate
  Psychostimulants and hallucinogens
  Thyroid supplementation
  Antipsychotics
  Hydroxyzine
  Levodopa
  Nicotine
Drug withdrawal
  Alcohol, antihypertensives, barbiturates, nicotine, benzodiazepines, tricyclic antidepressants

TREATMENT

The goal of treatment is the cessation of panic attacks. A 70 percent reduction in symptoms constitutes a good response to treatment. Patients often respond best to a combination of medications and psychological therapy. Patients should be informed about the diagnosis and prognosis, especially the propensity for fluctuation in the course of the disorder. Many patients respond well to self-help materials. The National Institute of Mental Health has educational materials and may be reached at 1-800-64-PANIC. Drug therapy may facilitate cognitive-behavioral therapies; however, BZDs may reduce motivation for exposure and other psychological therapies. Because panic disorder is chronic, patients often require long-term treatment.

Pharmacologic Management

Patients with panic disorder are often sensitive to medication effects. They may also fear that medication will lead to loss of control. Drugs should be started at low doses and very gradually increased to therapeutic doses as tolerated. Elderly patients may require half the usual starting dose than younger patients. Patients should be warned against sudden discontinuation of drugs. No medication should be discontinued until the patient has been panic-free at least 6 months. The most common reason for treatment failure is use of inadequate dosages for inadequate lengths of time.

Antidepressants are effective in treating panic disorder. Patients should be warned that symptoms may temporarily increase the first 1 to 2 weeks of therapy, and with each dose increase. Patients should remain on medication for at least 6 to 12 months, then may be very slowly tapered (over a 1- to 5-month period) to the least effective dose that prevents relapse. More detailed information on antidepressants can be found in Chap. 16-5.

All the tricyclics are equally effective in treating panic disorder. Nortriptyline tends to have the fewest anticholinergic side effects. Protriptyline may be activating to some patients. Tricyclics may be given in divided doses or once daily, usually at bedtime. Three to four weeks at a therapeutic dose may be needed to attain an antipanic effect. Remission may be maintained at a dosage lower than that initially needed to attain cessation of panic symptoms.

Serotonergic agents are useful in treating panic disorder. Patients with panic disorder may be more sensitive to activating side effects, especially with fluoxetine, though many patients find this drug effective.

Monoamine oxidase inhibitors affect both the noradrenergic and serotonergic systems and are effective in treating panic disorder, but many patients are reluctant to take them because of the restrictive diet potential side effects. Bupropion, which may be activating, may worsen panic symptoms.

Benzodiazepines are often started to provide rapid (often within a week) relief of symptoms. Table 16-3-3 lists BZDs used in the United States, their potency, dosage range, etc. Table 16-3-4 lists some important drug interactions. Therapeutic efficacy is equal to that of antidepressants when adequate doses are used, and all of the BZDs appear to be equally effective. Shorter half-life agents may be associated with interdose rebound or breakthrough panic attacks during sleep.

Once the patient has been panic-free at least 3 months, the BZD may be slowly tapered and discontinued. Patients should be warned of a possible temporary increase in anxiety with each dosage reduction. Often the last reductions are the most difficult. Although BZDs are most often used short-term, some patients require more long-term use. Driving ability may be impaired the first 1 to 2 weeks of therapy, but tolerance to sedative effects often develops rapidly. BZD use should be monitored closely or avoided in the elderly because of memory impairment and increased risk of falling. Physical dependence may occur in as little as 1 to 2 weeks, especially with higher doses, and patients should be warned of serious withdrawal symptoms with sudden discontinuation. As a rule, patients with panic disorder do not develop psychological dependence, and often take less than an effective dose because of fear of addiction. Buspirone is not effective for treatment of panic disorder, though it may be helpful in treating other comorbid or underlying anxiety disorders, and may augment the effectiveness of antidepressants.

Psychological Therapies

Up to 15 percent of patients are panic-free following cognitive-behavioral therapy. The risk of relapse is lower following CBT than medication treatment alone. Techniques used include somatic management (breathing and other relaxation training), distraction, exposure (to both internal and external cues), cognitive restructuring (confronting catastrophic thinking and overestimation of danger), and relapse prevention (preparation for potential panic-evoking situations). Patients respond best once symptoms have been partially controlled by medications. Some patients find supportive and interpersonal therapy helpful. These therapies can be expensive, they are not always covered by insurance, and qualified professionals may not be easily accessible. Individual and group therapy appear to be equally effective.

PROGNOSIS

As a rule, the earlier treatment is instituted in the disease process, the better the outcome. A substantial minority of patients achieve remission by the end of the first year of treatment, but relapse is frequent following medication discontinuation, and many patients require long-term maintenance treatment. Poor response is associated with psychiatric comorbidity, especially personality disorders, avoidance behaviors, anxiety sensitivity, and a history of childhood anxiety.

Obsessive-Compulsive Disorder
DISCUSSION

The exact etiology of obsessive-compulsive disorder (OCD) is unknown, but appears to involve abnormal serotonin neurotransmission and basal ganglia dysfunction. OCD appears to be a genetic disorder with 70 percent concordance of monozygotic and 50 percent concordance of dizygotic twins. There is a 25 percent chance that a first-degree relative will also have OCD.

About 2 to 3 percent of the U.S. population develops OCD. Males and females are at equal risk, though males tend to develop the disorder earlier than women. Avoidant and dependent personality disorders are common among OCD patients but tend to improve with treatment of OCD symptoms. Failure to marry and an inability to sustain interpersonal relationships is common.

SIGNS AND SYMPTOMS

Obsessions are persistent, disturbing thoughts or impulses that the patient experiences as intrusive or inappropriate and finds illogical, but irresistible. Obsessions go beyond excessive worries about real-life problems and are recognized by patients as products of their own mind. Patients consider their obsessions absurd and actively attempt to resist them. Patients often attempt to ignore or suppress obsessional thoughts or neutralize them with other thoughts. There is often some form of pathologic doubting behind obsessions.

Compulsions are repetitive, purposeful, intentional behaviors or mental acts that a patient feels driven to perform in response to obsessions, and according to rules that must be rigidly applied. They are aimed at preventing or reducing the distress of obsessions or preventing some dreaded event or situation.

Obsessions and compulsions must cause marked distress, markedly interfere with the patient's functioning, and be significantly time-consuming to be pathologic. Most patients recognize that they are excessive and/or unreasonable. Attempts to resist the obsessions and compulsions may produce extreme anxiety. Common types of obsessions and compulsions are listed in Table 16-3-6.

Two-thirds of patients with OCD have the onset of significant symptoms before age 15, with onset typically during adolescence or early adulthood. Five percent of patients with OCD have a

Table 16-3-6. Types of Obsessions and Compulsions

Washer	The patient fears contamination and has cleaning compulsions.
Checker	The patient demonstrates repetitive checking (such as door locks, the stove or oven, or other appliances) secondary to pathologic doubting.
Doubter and sinner	The patient fears something terrible may happen if everything is not perfect. Some patients may become paralyzed into inaction.
Counter and arranger	The patient compulsively arranges things into very specific patterns or obsessively counts (such as being able to cross a threshold only after taking a specific number of steps or not being able to speak until the number of words spoken by another party are counted). Patients often display magical thinking and superstition.
Hoarder	The patient believes something terrible may happen if something is discarded and may save unusual items, such as wrappers or used gum.

comorbid tic disorder, and 50 percent of patients with Tourette's syndrome have comorbid OCD, especially males. OCD is generally a chronic disorder in which symptoms tend to develop quickly (in fewer than 30 days) and then may fluctuate, worsening with stressors.

Patients should be informed that OCD is a lifelong illness, with symptoms waxing and waning throughout their lifetime. Because of embarrassment or fear of "being crazy," many patients do not volunteer OCD symptoms, but present with anxiety or depressive symptoms, which are common in OCD. All patients with anxious or depressive symptoms should be specifically asked about obsessions or compulsions so treatment may be directed toward the primary problem.

DIAGNOSTIC CONSIDERATIONS

The differential diagnosis includes "normal" routines or rituals (e.g., perfectionistic behaviors, habits of dressing or grooming a certain way), which are not distressing or time-consuming; excessive and/or impulsive gambling, eating, or sexual behaviors; major depressive disorder; organic mental disorders (e.g., brain tumor, head injury); Tourette's syndrome; schizophrenia; and obsessive-compulsive personality disorder. All but the last two may be comorbid with OCD. Schizophrenic delusions are not recognized by the patient as excessive or unreasonable and are usually not considered by the patient as illogical.

Eighty percent of patients with OCD develop a secondary depression. These patients tend to present with the depressive symptoms. Thirteen percent of patients with OCD have a comorbid eating disorder, and 15 percent have comorbid trichotillomania, which is often resistant to pharmacologic management.

TREATMENT

Pharmacologic Management

Effective psychopharmacologic agents increase serotonin activity. Currently available drugs are the selective serotonin reuptake inhibitors (i.e., fluoxetine, fluvoxamine, paroxetine, sertraline), venlafaxine, and clomipramine, all of which appear to be equally effective in the treatment of OCD. Patients may respond best to dosages that are higher than generally used to treat depression, titrated rather rapidly. An adequate trial, 4 months in the upper

dosage range, should be undertaken before considering changing to a different agent. Since a given patient may respond to one SSRI over another, a different agent should be tried if there is no response to the first.

Clomipramine reaches steady-state plasma levels in 1 to 3 weeks. Blood levels are accurate and may be used to ensure adequate dosage and compliance if the patient has not responded, or to rule out toxicity if the patient has excessive side effects. Tobacco, alcohol, and antipsychotics may raise the level of clomipramine's major metabolite. Common side effects include dry mouth, dry skin, and constipation. Orthostatic hypotension, sexual dysfunction (loss of libido, anorgasmia, and/or erectile dysfunction), tremor, ataxia, rigidity, dizziness, sedation, and headache may also occur. Clomipramine may be given once daily or in divided doses.

Fifty to 70 percent improvement in symptoms is a good pharmacologic response. Response is measured by the patient spending less time with symptoms, finding it easier to ignore symptoms, and experiencing less distress. Those who respond usually do so within 4 months of initiation of treatment. Any improvement occurring after the initial 4 months tends to be slight and very gradual. Seventy percent of patients show some response to pharmacologic treatment, but most will have residual symptoms.

Patients should be informed that medications may need to be taken lifelong, since symptoms tend to rapidly recur with discontinuation. Most patients require the initial treatment dose for long-term use.

Augmentation may be considered for patients who respond poorly or not at all to single agents. Patients with comorbid tic disorders and schizotypal personality disorder may respond to augmentation with a neuroleptic. Other augmentation strategies include lithium, pindolol, trazodone or nefazodone, risperidone, olanzapine and fenfluramine. Women tend to respond best if estrogen levels are stabilized. Cingulotomy has been used successfully in some patients with severe, treatment-resistant OCD.

Psychological Therapies

Patients respond best when a combination of cognitive-behavioral therapy and medications are used. Techniques include graded exposure, response prevention, and thought-stopping. These interventions should be administered by clinicians experienced in the psychotherapy of OCD. Support groups provide education and destigmatize patients.

Phobic Disorders
ETIOLOGY AND PREVALENCE

Current ideas regarding the etiology of phobic symptoms include the use of repression and displacement as defense mechanisms, learned behavior, and classic conditioning. Agoraphobia and specific phobias are two to three times prevalent in women than men. Social phobia appears to affect the sexes equally. Social phobias tend to begin during adolescence.

SIGNS AND SYMPTOMS

A *phobia* is an irrational dread of and compelling desire to avoid a specific object, situation, or activity. The fear is excessive and disproportionate to any actual danger, always anticipated, and, never spontaneous. Apart from contact with the feared stimulus, the patient is usually free of symptoms. Patients rarely present for treatment of phobic symptoms. Anticipatory anxiety quickly develops, followed by avoidant behaviors, often taken to extremes. Phobic symptoms become a phobic disorder when they cause undue distress and impair a patient's function.

Common specific phobias include fear of animals, storms, heights, flying, closed places, etc. Phobias usually have their onset in childhood or early adolescence and cease within 5 years in 50 percent of patients. Specific phobias tend to remit spontaneously with age. If they persist into adulthood, they may become chronic, but are rarely disabling. Certain phobias may interfere with medical care, such as fear of needles or blood, or claustrophobia, which may interfere with CT scans, MRI, and other specialized medical procedures.

Social phobia is the excessive fear of embarrassment in social situations and of being scrutinized and judged by others. Social phobia is more than a fear of public speaking and may generalize to many or all social encounters. The mean age of onset is 15 to 19. Social phobia has a lifetime prevalence of 13 percent, making it the third most common mental disorder. Patients may fear and avoid eating and writing in public, or use of public toilets. In such situations, patients fear being unable to perform and embarrassing themselves. Substance abuse, mood disorders, and suicidal ideation and attempts may occur. Sixteen percent of relatives of social phobics are also diagnosed with social phobia. Unfortunately, without early therapy, social phobia runs a chronic and unremitting course throughout the patient's lifetime.

DIAGNOSTIC CONSIDERATIONS

Patients with schizophrenia often have negative symptoms similar to social phobia prior to the onset of positive symptoms. Patients with paranoid delusions fail to see the irrationality of their fears. Patients with clear obsessive-compulsive disorder and phobic symptoms are given only the OCD diagnosis. Patients who avoid social situations as a result of posttraumatic stress disorder have a specific and identical past stressor. Depression may be comorbid or secondary to phobic disorders. The fears some depressed patients demonstrate may initially appear to be phobias, but clear as the depression clears. Phobias are common in patients with borderline, paranoid, and avoidant personality disorders. Patients with avoidant personality disorder display a general discomfort in social situations and require continual reassurance. They do not identify fears of scrutiny and judgment as the cause of their social avoidance.

TREATMENT: PHARMACOLOGIC MANAGEMENT

Beta blockers have been used to treat "stage fright" when given in single doses an hour before performance. Benzodiazepines may also be used as needed for anticipated stressful social situations, though their use may interfere with psychotherapy, especially exposure techniques. Monoamine oxidase inhibitors work well for social phobias, as do many other antidepressants. Patients with social phobia are prone to developing dependence on alcohol or sedative drugs, especially if psychotherapy is not concurrently used. Buspirone has not demonstrated efficacy in treating phobic disorders. Medications are not effective in treating specific phobias.

The most effective treatment of specific phobias is psychotherapy. Exposure is essential to successful therapy, and includes such techniques as flooding, graduated exposure, and systematic desensitization. Relaxation training is usually the first step in treatment. Patients with social phobia often benefit from assertiveness training, social skills training, and cognitive therapy for their dysfunctional thoughts. Cognitive therapy is most effective when the fear of negative evaluation is targeted. Utilizing a combination of techniques tends to be more effective than using one technique alone.

Posttraumatic Stress Disorder
ETIOLOGY

By definition, posttraumatic stress disorder (PTSD) follows a severe and extraordinary stressor. The stressor need not be a single event (i.e., a natural disaster such as a tornado or earthquake), but may be repetitive and/or ongoing severe traumas such as military combat or past childhood sexual abuse.

The most common cause of PTSD for men is military experience. Increased risk of developing PTSD is associated with young age, less military training, prior emotional or physical abuse, and the presence of psychiatric symptoms prior to the stressor. For women the most common causes of PTSD are rape and sexual and physical abuse. Increased risk of developing PTSD symptoms is associated with the use of physical force, display of a weapon, and physical injury.

SIGNS AND SYMPTOMS

PTSD symptoms may begin hours, months, or even years following the stressor. The stressful event is one in which the patient experiences, witnesses, or is confronted with actual or threatened death or serious injury, producing intense fear, helplessness, and/or horror. The event is usually beyond the ordinary traumas of human experience. Dissociative symptoms often appear after the event and include a subjective sense of numbing and detachment, a reduction in the awareness of one's surroundings, derealization, depersonalization, and dissociative amnesia surrounding the event. The event is then persistently reexperienced in recurrent images, thoughts, dreams, affect, or a sense of repeatedly reliving the experience. Stimulation of any of the senses may cause this reexperiencing, such as sound (e.g., a helicopter used in battle), smell (e.g., the cologne of one's attacker), touch (e.g., cold metal reminiscent of a gun used), or sight (e.g., dark clouds present just prior to a tornado).

As a result, the patient may begin to avoid all stimuli that may arouse recollection of the trauma. The patient eventually develops persistent symptoms of anxiety, hypervigilance, and increased arousal. These symptoms must cause the patient significant distress or impairment of function to be pathologic.

PTSD tends to occur in *two stages*:

1. In the *avoidance phase,* the patient may experience psychic numbing, minimization of the effect of the experience, affective detachment, poor interests, and a constricted affect.
2. During the *reexperiencing phase,* the patient may demonstrate hypervigilance, intrusive memories, poor sleep, poor concentration, rumination, and affective instability.

Occupational or interpersonal impairment is common in patients suffering with PTSD. Substance abuse, mood disorders, panic attacks, or phobic disorders may also develop in response to PTSD symptoms.

Acute PTSD lasts less than 3 months. Chronic PTSD lasts longer than 3 months. Delayed-onset PTSD does not emerge until at least 6 months after the trauma, and may even emerge years later, such as with childhood sexual abuse. This last type carries the worst prognosis.

The intensity of the physiologic response to the original trauma appears to be the most significant predictor of poor outcome and chronic course. Ongoing life stressors may slow recovery. A protracted course may also be associated with dissociative symptoms, emotional constriction, and drug abuse.

DIAGNOSTIC CONSIDERATIONS

Acute stress disorder is diagnosed when PTSD symptoms occur within 4 weeks of the event, but last only 2 days to 4 weeks. The type of event and symptoms are otherwise the same as with PTSD. Schizophrenic patients may experience hallucinations or delusions, but without a past identified stressor. Dissociative disorders occur more often as a result of childhood abuse and may represent a special type of PTSD. Dissociation may also be a symptom associated with borderline personality disorder. Up to 85 percent of patients with bipolar disorder have a history of childhood sexual abuse. An adjustment disorder may occur in response to more ordinary trauma (death of a loved one, loss of a significant relationship, etc.), in which the patient demonstrates a brief but strong affective response. Other considerations include temporal lobe epilepsy, malingering, other anxiety disorders (especially panic disorder), major depressive disorder, and compensation neurosis. Substance abuse commonly develops in response to PTSD symptoms and may worsen symptoms during acute intoxication or a "bad trip."

TREATMENT

Pharmacologic Management

Any of the antidepressants may be used for symptom control, but some clinicians have found the monoamine oxidase inhibitor phenelzine especially useful. Carbamazepine or valproic acid may be used for behavioral control, especially irritability and aggression. Beta blockers, trazodone (especially in divided doses), and buspirone may also be used for anger management. Trazodone (25 to 100 mg) may be useful for treating insomnia. Benzodiazepines should be used with caution, since they may cause disinhibition or lead to dependence.

Supportive Measures

Immediate debriefing following a severely traumatizing event may be helpful in preventing the development of PTSD. Such debriefing should include repetitive disclosure of the event in detail, exploration of troubling reactions, identification of coping strategies, exploration of feelings about leaving the disaster site, and a specific and workable plan of transition and referral.

Support groups may be helpful to reinforce normal reactions; address common fears, concerns, and traumatic memories; increase the capacity to tolerate disturbing emotions; and share coping strategies. Cognitive behavioral techniques, such as exposure and cognitive restructuring, may be helpful. Psychodynamic therapy has been helpful for some patients.

BIBLIOGRAPHY

American Psychiatric Association: *Diagnostic and Statistical Manual of Mental Disorders,* 4th ed. Washington, DC, American Psychiatric Association, 1994.

Andreasen NC, Black DW: *Introductory Textbook of Psychiatry.* Washington DC, American Psychiatric Press, 1995.

Baughan DM: Barriers to diagnosing anxiety disorders in family practice. *Am Fam Pract* 52(2):447–450, 1995.

Coryell N, Winokur G: *The Clinical Management of Anxiety Disorders,* New York, Oxford, 1991.

Davis M et al: *The Relaxation and Stress Reduction Workbook.* Oakland, CA, New Harbinger, 1995.

Katon N: *Panic Disorder in the Medical Setting.* National Institute of Mental Health, DHHS Pub No (ADM) 89-1629. Washington, DC, U.S. Government Printing Office, 1989.

McGlynn TJ, Metcalf HL: *Diagnosis and Treatment of Anxiety Disorders: A Physicians' Handbook,* 2d ed. Washington, DC, American Psychiatric Press, 1991.

Noyes R, Holt CS: Anxiety disorders, in G Winokur (ed):*The Medical Basis of Psychiatry.* 2d ed. Philadelphia, Saunders, 1994, pp 139–160.

Pollack MH, Otto MW (eds): Anxiety disorders: Longitudinal course and treatment. *Psychiatric Clin North Am* 18:4, 1995.

Weinstein RS: Panic disorder. *Am Fam Pract* 52(7):2055–2063, 1995.

Chapter 16–4
ATTENTION DEFICIT DISORDER
Anita D. Glicken

DISCUSSION

Attention deficit disorder (ADD), which has a subtype that includes hyperactivity (ADHD), is the most commonly diagnosed childhood mental disorder. Recent estimates suggest that between 3 and 9 percent of children have the disorder, accounting for one-third to one-half of all pediatric mental health referrals. In population-based studies, boys are three times more likely than girls to have the disorder; however, the ratio is 6 : 1 in clinical studies. The majority of children with ADHD demonstrate hyperactive and impulsive motor behavior. Much less frequently (one in seven children with ADHD), inattention may be the predominant symptom without increased motor behavior. Symptoms, often first identified in the preschool years, are exhibited in a variety of settings and are consistent over time.

ETIOLOGY

During the past 10 to 15 years, multiple causes have been suggested for ADHD, which was originally labeled *minimal brain dysfunction (MBD).* There is some evidence that these children do demonstrate a greater incidence of neurologic "soft signs." For example, they may experience increased difficulty with fine and gross motor coordination or balance. This has led researchers to explore prenatal and postnatal risk factors in these children such as maternal age, smoking history, alcohol consumption, and length of labor, all of which may also increase the occurrence of soft neurologic damage. At this time, however, no consistent association of this historical data with ADHD has been demonstrated.

During the 1970s, the popular media supported the notion that food additives or sugar might play an important role in the etiology of ADHD. Many studies have addressed this possibility, and those remain controversial.

Additional avenues of exploration examine how acquired problems, such as otitis media, may be related to ADHD. (See Chap. 3-2, "Otitis Media.") Other research studies continue to explore localized areas in the central nervous system or the role of neurotransmitter mechanisms. The latter research is due, in part, to the fact that a number of these children have a positive response to stimulant medication.

Although no definitive answer has emerged on the etiology of ADHD, recent studies suggest it may be an inherited disorder.

SIGNS AND SYMPTOMS

The core clinical features of ADHD include impulsivity, distractibility, inability to sustain attention and/or concentration, and developmentally inappropriate activity levels.

Table 16-4-1. Summary of DSM-IV Criteria for Attention-Deficit and Hyperactivity Disorders

- The patient has six (or more) identified symptoms of either inattention, hyperactivity-impulsivity, or both that have been present for 6 months, is maladaptive, and is inconsistent with developmental level.
- Inattention includes symptoms such as poor attention to detail, frequent forgetfulness, distractibility, difficulty organizing tasks and responsibilities, and difficulty in maintaining attention or sustained mental effort in play, school, or work situations.
- Hyperactivity-impulsivity includes symptoms such as frequent motor restlessness, excessive talking, difficulty remaining seated when necessary, interrupting others, and difficulty taking turns.
- Some symptoms must be present before the age of 7.
- Impairment from symptoms must be present in two or more settings (e.g., school and home).
- There must be evidence of clinically significant impairment in social, academic, or occupational functioning.

SOURCE: American Psychiatric Association: *Diagnostic and Statistical Manual of Mental Disorders*, 4th ed. Washington, DC, American Psychiatric Association, 1994.

The Diagnostic and Statistical Manual of Mental Disorders, fourth edition (DSM-IV), criteria for ADHD are summarized in Table 16-4-1.

OBJECTIVE FINDINGS

There are no consistent, specific neurologic or physical findings that establish a diagnosis of ADHD, although it should be noted that some children do demonstrate neurologic soft signs. Recent authors have stated that a positive response to methylphenidate is indicative of a diagnosis.

DIAGNOSTIC CONSIDERATIONS

The DSM-IV criteria are helpful in establishing the PA's differential; however, diagnosis is often confounded by several factors. This includes the commonality between these psychiatric criteria and descriptions of normal childhood behaviors. ADHD also has a comorbidity rate with a number of other childhood disorders, including oppositional defiant disorder, conduct disorder, mood disorders, anxiety disorders, and learning problems. These comorbid conditions, and associated problems with academic and social functioning, add to the complexity of diagnosis and treatment for ADHD.

SPECIAL CONSIDERATIONS

The majority of the literature on ADHD focuses on the school-age child. However, it is often the developmental issues of preschoolers and adolescents that make diagnosis and treatment difficult in these age groups. Caution should be exercised in diagnosing a child under the age of 5 with ADHD due to normal overactivity and inattention in 3- and 4-year-olds. Because of these normal developmental issues, 12 months' duration of symptoms should be observed for this age group, rather than the six recommended in the DSM-IV.

Adolescents with ADHD are often underdiagnosed. They typically demonstrate impaired concentration and attention and difficulty structuring time and activities. These behaviors may also be misinterpreted as normal developmental behavior. Additional confusion also exists related to those adolescents previously diagnosed with ADHD as a child. Although there is considerable research that demonstrates that ADHD may decrease in only one-third of children during adolscence, many health care providers and educators still believe that ADHD disappears with puberty. ADHD in adults has only recently become an area of interest and is also often misdiagnosed. Comorbid disorders among adults may include antisocial personality and substance abuse.

LABORATORY TESTS AND OTHER DIAGNOSTIC CONSIDERATIONS

No laboratory or radiologic studies can be used at this time to identify ADHD. Several behavioral rating scales, which have proved effective in gathering a thorough clinical history and observational data from families and schools, are widely available. The Conner's Parent Rating Scale requires approximately 10 min to complete and consists of 48 items. Another commonly used scale is the Child Behavior Checklist (CBCL). The CBCL is broader than Connor's scale and assesses nine domains of childhood psychopathology. In addition to identifying ADHD, the CBCL also uncovers childhood depression and somatization. Separate self-report measures are also available for adolescents and teachers. The Child Attention Problems instrument assesses classroom behavioral changes in children on stimulant medication. This scale, as well as the Iowa Conner's Teacher Rating scale, may aide in the recognition of ADHD in adolescents.

TREATMENT

Treatment for ADHD is multifaceted and includes medication, counseling, cognitive therapy, behavior management, school-based interventions, family therapy, and social skills training in various combinations. Psychostimulants, however, remain the most common treatment for ADHD. Approximately 70 percent of ADHD children treated with stimulants show significant improvement in hyperactivity, inattention, and impulsivity. Methylphenidate hydrochloride (Ritalin) and dextroamphetamine (Dexedrine) are the most commonly prescribed drugs. Dextroamphetamine increases dopamine and norepinephrine neurotransmission and inhibits monoamine oxidase activity, whereas methylphenidate releases stored dopamine, decreases dopamine reuptake, and inhibits monoamine oxidase activity. The two drugs, equally effective in therapeutic doses, demonstrate a behavioral effect within 30 to 60 min, usually lasting 3 to 6 h. Most patients require a second dose at noon. The sustained release forms have a greater delay in the onset of action, and their effect does not last as long as a second dose of standard medication, but they eliminate the problems associated with the administration of the drug during the school day. The recommended starting dose for methylphenidate is 5 mg and for *d*-amphetamine it is 2.5 mg. For young children, one-half of this amount is recommended, and the *d*-amphetamine elixir may simplify use. The effective daily dose of the stimulant medication varies. The recommended average daily dose of methylphenidate ranges from 10 to 40 mg.

The third available stimulant is magnesium pemoline (Cylert). It is occasionally prescribed for patients who do not respond to methylphenidate. Like the slow-release drugs mentioned above, it has a longer half-life and is generally only given in the morning. Pemoline is absorbed and metabolized at varying rates. As a result, behavioral changes may not be seen for up to 2 weeks and often exhibit a small acute effect and a substantial delayed effect. The initial daily dose is 18.75 mg, with increasing weekly increments of 18.75 mg up to a total of 75.0 mg daily. Older children and adolescents may require a slightly higher dose. Patients receiving pemoline should be monitored for possible liver toxicity. It should be noted that all medications have side effects, of which most are dose-related. Possible adverse effects include insomnia, anorexia, irritability, nausea and vomiting, mood alterations, and an increase in heart rate or blood pressure.

Alternative medications should be considered for children and adolescents when the adverse effects of stimulant treatment are not tolerable. Tricyclic antidepressants are the most frequent alternative. Imipramine (Tofranil or Janimine), desipramine

(Norpramin or Pertofrane), and amitriptyline (Elavil) are believed to potentiate adrenergic synapses by blocking uptake of dopamine at nerve endings and increasing local dopamine levels. Their most common side effect is drowsiness, which can be mitigated by giving the medication at bedtime. Although the clinical onset of the effects of tricyclics can be slower, possible advantages are a longer duration of action, feasibility of a single dose, absence of symptom rebound or insomnia, and less risk of abuse or dependence. Onset of the drug action is gradual, and it may be several weeks before significant changes are seen. The initial dose for all three drugs is 25 to 50 mg a day up to 5 mg/kg/day. Doses in excess of 3.5 mg/kg have been associated with mild diastolic hypertension, tachycardia, and electrocardiograph conduction anomalies. Plasma levels must be monitored to avoid toxicity.

Several other medications have also been found useful in managing the impulsivity, hyperactivity, or distractibility of ADHD. These include carbamazepine, bupropion, nomifensine, fluoxetine, and clonidine. Clonidine (Catapres), an antihypertensive drug in adults, based on teachers' and parents' ratings, was found to be as effective as methylphenidate in decreasing motor activity, improving frustration tolerance, and enhancing cooperation and compliance.

Clonidine may be a suitable option for children with ADHD who have a poor response to stimulants, tic disorders, extreme overactivity, oppositional or conduct disorder, or hyperarousal. A combination of clonidine and methylphenidate is often considered for those children who do not respond to either drug alone and seems to be particularly effective for children who are easily distracted and hyperaroused.

In summary, there is strong evidence that stimulant medication has short-term benefit in normalizing many of the clinical symptoms of ADHD. Pharmacologic treatments appear less reliable in producing any long-term benefits. Also, stimulants appear to have unreliable therapeutic effects on many of the secondary problems of children with ADHD such as academic or emotional difficulties. These considerations have led several authors to suggest that sound clinical practice in the treatment of ADHD should include multimodal treatment strategies that combine multiple forms of intervention. Interventions include an individualized approach for the ADHD child and family that incorporates judicious use of stimulant medication along with psychosocial interventions. Psychosocial interventions might include social skills and cognitive training, parent training and home-based programming, classroom-based behavior modification techniques, as well as individual and family counseling. The National Institute of Mental Health (NIMH) has recently launched a 5-year multisite, multimodal treatment study of children with ADHD, its associated comorbid conditions, and its social-emotional and academic impairments. The findings of this important project should shed some light on any synergistic or additive effects of stimulant and psychosocial treatments.

PATIENT EDUCATION

Parents of children with ADHD need to recognize that their child's inattentiveness and distractibility are not willful behaviors and are generally beyond the child's control. This recognition may help the parent depersonalize the child's behaviors and assist them in supporting treatment endeavors. Families of all individuals with ADHD need education about the disorder and a clear explanation of treatment options. Individuals and families should also be informed of their legal rights with respect to the Americans with Disabilities Act (ADA, PL 101-336) and the Individuals with Disabilities Education Act (IDEA, PL 101-476). Although IDEA does not at this time possess a separate classification for ADD, many states have chosen to include children with that diagnosis for special education and related services. These laws

promote the rights of persons with disabilities. For example, ADA's definition of disability, which includes attention deficit disorder, may assist an individual in obtaining reasonable accommodations in an employment setting.

DISPOSITION

Proactive and thoughtful management allows most patients with ADHD to be treated successfully by their primary care provider. Children being treated with medication for ADHD, should be closely followed with periodic data gathered from teachers and parents. Observational data should be utilized for adjusting dosages. All patients should be carefully monitored for the previously noted side effects. Patients should have their height and weight checked regularly, and heart rate and blood pressure should be monitored during treatment, particularly after an increase in dosage.

COMPLICATIONS, RED FLAGS, AND INDICATIONS FOR REFERRAL

With many patients the clinical indications for a diagnosis of ADHD are ambiguous. Parents and teachers supply much of the data in the form of verbal reports, which may be distorted by their own needs. Further confusion may result when a diagnosed child does not respond to medication. A PA may also suspect a comorbid disorder or learning disability. Referral to a mental health professional for differential diagnosis, including psychoeducational assessment, may help detect learning disabilities or a comorbid condition.

The PA should be aware that methylphenidate and dextroamphetamine are controlled substances and potential drugs of abuse. They also have an illicit street value if sold. Requests for dosage adjustments, early refills, and replacement of lost or stolen medication should alert the prescriber to the possibility of medication abuse. Other family members may be using these drugs for their stimulant effects.

OTHER NOTES OR PEARLS

A multidimensional, systematic approach to the differential diagnosis of ADHD is critical prior to the implementation of any treatment regimen. Since normal children demonstrate improved attention with methylphenidate, a drug response should not be the sole criteria for diagnosis. The use of drugs alone, without other kinds of therapy, often is inadequate to resolve educational difficulties or social skills deficits. Important questions remain unanswered with respect to which subgroups of individuals with ADHD will receive differential benefit from particular treatments. Optimal results will be achieved by those physician assistants who thoughtfully integrate current knowledge, skills, and experience with available treatment methodologies and resources in a consistent and compassionate manner. Future research should prove critical in improving the efficacy and efficiency with which this disorder is treated.

BIBLIOGRAPHY

American Psychiatric Association: *Diagnostic and Statistical Manual of Mental Disorders,* 4th ed. Washington, DC, American Psychiatric Association, 1994.

Barkley RA, Fischer M, Edelbrock C, Smallish L: The adolescent outcome of hyperactive children diagnosed by research criteria, III: Mother-child interactions, family conflicts and maternal psychopathology. *J Child Psychol Psychiatry* 32:233–255, 1991.

Richters JE, Arnold LE, Jensen PS, et al: NIMH collaborative multi-site multimodal treatment study of children with ADHD: I. Background and rationale. *J Am Acad Child Adoles Psychiatry* 34(8):987–1000, 1995.

Searight HR, Nahlik JE, Campbell DC: Attention-deficit/hyperactivity disorder: Assessment, diagnosis, and management. *J Fam Pract* 40(3):270–279, 1995.

Simeon JG, Wiggins DM: Pharmacotherapy of attention-deficit hyperactivity disorder. *Can J Psychiatry* 38(6):443–448, 1993.

Vinson DC: Therapy for attention-deficit hyperactivity disorder. *Arch Fam Med* 3(5):445–451, 1994.

Chapter 16–5
DEPRESSION

Don St. John

DISCUSSION

Depression is the third most common mental disorder seen in the general population and the most common disorder seen by psychiatrists. Unfortunately, many patients with depression in the United States are incorrectly diagnosed, untreated, or inadequately treated. Depression is the most salient risk factor for suicide. Adequately treating depression results in a lower suicide rate. About 25 percent of high users of primary care services meet the criteria for a major depressive disorder, with two-thirds having a lifetime history of a major depressive episode.

ETIOLOGY

Depression appears to be a final common pathway syndrome with several potential etiologic factors. Affective disorders run in families. Twin and adoption studies demonstrate a genetic component. Biologic factors include a deficit of norepinephrine at central nerve terminals (the catecholamine hypothesis), abnormal serotonin function, dysregulation of the acetylcholine system, increased cholinergic sensitivity, and abnormalities of the hypothalamic-pituitary-adrenal axis.

Cognitive factors include significant tangible loss, especially early in life, expectation of loss, self-esteem–lowering events, reversal in object valuation, depression in close family members, severe punishment by parents, overprotection by parents, strict parental rules, extremely critical parenting, and isolation from others. The cognitive triad of depression is a negative view of self, world, and future.

Behavioral factors include learned helplessness and modeling by depressed family members. Psychodynamic factors include anger turned inward and early severe loss. Adverse life events may precipitate a depressive episode, especially separation from important persons. In depressive spectrum disorder, females with milder forms of depression have higher numbers of female relatives with mild depression and male relatives with alcoholism and antisocial personality disorder.

RISK FACTORS

Depression has been associated with a number of medical problems, especially stroke, multiple sclerosis, epilepsy, and dementia.

Table 16-5-1. Physical Illnesses Associated with Depression

Metabolic	Cancer
Dehydration	Pancreatic
Azotemia, uremia	Occult carcinomas
Acid-base disturbance	Infections
Hypoxia	AIDS
Hypo- and hypernatremia	Postviral syndromes
Hypo- and hyperglycemia	Lyme disease
Hypo- and hypercalcemia	Syphilis
Endocrine	Influenza
Hypo- and hyperthyroidism	Hepatitis
Addison's disease	Pneumonia
Cushing's disease	Urinary tract infections
Hypo- and hyperparathyroidism	Endocarditis
Diabetes mellitus	Tuberculosis
Neurologic	Brucellosis
Sleep apnea	Cardiovascular
Parkinson's disease	Congestive heart failure
Brain tumors	Myocardial infarction
Dementia	Pulmonary
Meningitis	Chronic obstructive pulmonary
Neurosyphilis	disease
Normal pressure hydrocephalus	Malignancy
Subarachnoid hemorrhage	Gastrointestinal
Cerebrovascular accident and	Malignancy
transient ischemic attack	Irritable bowel syndrome
Seizure disorder	Chronic abdominal pain
Multiple Sclerosis	Other
Genitourinary	Heavy metal toxicity
Urinary incontinence	Deficiencies of B_{12}, thiamine,
Musculoskeletal	folic acid
Arthritis	
Osteoporosis	
Polymyalgia rheumatica	
Paget's disease	
Fibromyalgia	
Collagen vascular	
Systemic lupus erythematosus	
Hematologic	
Anemia	
Leukemia	

(See Table 16-5-1.) There is a strong relationship between economic stress and depressive disorders. Depression is twice as common in urban areas as in rural areas. Higher risk is associated with loss of either parent in the first 5 years of life, poor or absent support network, and a history of sexual, physical, or emotional abuse, especially early in life. Also at risk for developing depression are young women with children and minimal support, and women widowed when young or middle-aged.

EPIDEMIOLOGY

Approximately 15 percent of Americans develop depression at some time in their life, with 5 percent of the population meeting criteria for major depressive disorder at any given time. The incidence of depression appears to be increasing for each decade since World War II, with a progressively earlier age of onset. The lifetime prevalence of dysthymia may be from 3 to 13 percent, making it the third or fourth most common psychiatric disorder in the United States.

Depression is twice as common in women as men, though the course of illness appears to be similar for men and women. Bipolar disorders are much less common than unipolar disorders.

SIGNS AND SYMPTOMS

The basic abnormality in depression is an abnormal alteration in mood. Depressed mood must be present most of the day, every

Table 16-5-2. Primary Depressive Symptoms That Make Up
SIG: E-CAPS

Sleep
Interests
Guilt
Energy
Concentration
Affect or appetite
Psychomotor agitation or retardation
Suicidal ideation

day for at least 2 weeks to make a diagnosis of major depressive disorder. The primary depressive symptoms may he remembered by the mnemonic SIG: E-CAPS ("prescribe energy capsules"), as shown in Table 16-5-2.

Symptoms may be conceptualized as encompassing a pervasive disturbance of mood (sadness, crying, anxiety, brooding, irritability, paranoia), dysphoria or anhedonia, and disturbances in perception of self, world, and future (resulting in social withdrawal, decreased libido, feelings of worthlessness, excessive fears, self-reproach, delusions, hallucinations, passivity, and excessive criticism of self and others). Negative thinking is common regarding the past (guilt), present (low self-esteem), and future (hopelessness).

Vegetative symptoms include insomnia (initial, middle, and/or terminal) or hypersomnia, psychomotor agitation (more common among elderly patients, such as purposeless pacing, wringing hands) or retardation (more common among younger patients, characterized by speech latency or catatonia), fatigue and anergia, changes in appetite and weight, difficulty concentrating, and constipation. In many patients, unique diurnal variations of symptomatology occur, especially with symptoms worse in the morning, and improve throughout the day. Anxiety is commonly present in depressive disorders. Suicidal ideation is more likely to be passive (wishing one were dead) than active (planning and/or carrying out a suicide attempt). Frequent thoughts of death are common.

An abnormal suppression of cortisol secretion following dexamethasone administration may be present. About half of patients show a blunted response of thyroid-stimulating hormone to thyrotropin-releasing hormone administration. EEG abnormalities include decreased delta sleep, decreased REM latency, and increased REM density. Interviews and pen and paper tests to screen for depression include the Beck/Depression Inventory, the Hamilton Depression Rating Scale, and Structured Clinical Interview for the *Diagnostic and Statistical Manual (SCID).*

TYPES OF DEPRESSION

Melancholia used to be called endogenous depression. Vegetative symptoms are more prominent and include anhedonia for all activities, diurnal variation of symptoms with symptoms worse in the morning, terminal insomnia (early morning awakening), psychomotor retardation or agitation, anorexia and weight loss, and excessive guilt. Melancholia tends to respond better to somatic therapies and may be more prominent in older patients.

The presence of delusions and/or hallucinations distinguishes *psychotic depression.* In some studies, up to half of depressed patients develop psychotic symptoms. Delusions or hallucinations are usually mood-congruent (content consistent with depressive themes), but may be mood-incongruent (inconsistent with typical depressive themes). Relapse and recurrence tend to be more common, and neuroleptics are usually required for treatment.

Motor immobility or excessive motor activity (purposeless), extreme negativism or mutism, peculiarities of voluntary move-

ment (such as posturing), stereotyped movements, echolalia, or echopraxia are catatonic features sometimes present. Depression with catatonic features tends to respond better to electroconvulsive therapy (ECT).

Atypical features include increased appetite and weight gain, hypersomnia, leaden paralysis, and interpersonal rejection sensitivity leading to significant social or occupational impairment. This type of depression is more difficult to treat and tends to respond poorly to tricyclic antidepressants and ECT, responding better to serotonergic agents and best to monoamine oxidase inhibitors (MAOIs).

Postpartum depression occurs within 4 weeks postpartum, and is more likely to lead to a bipolar disorder. Postpartum depression is associated with *seasonal depression,* where there exists a temporal relationship between symptoms and the time of year. Seasonal depression may respond to phototherapy.

Depression is *masked* when the patient does not complain of a depressed mood, but has enough other criteria for a diagnosis to be made. *Bipolar depression* occurs in the context of a bipolar disorder. (See "Diagnostic Considerations," below.) Patients with bipolar depression tend to be depressed longer, relapse more frequently, display more depressive symptoms, have more severe symptoms, be more likely to be delusional or hallucinate, be more likely to commit suicide, and be more incapacitated by the depression. Depression is *chronic* when full criteria for major depressive disorder are present continuously for at least 2 years.

Depression may be conceptualized as *endogenous* (no precipitant) or *reactive* (identified precipitant), *primary* (spontaneous) or *secondary* (occurring after the onset of another illness or drug), *unipolar* (no history of mania or hypomania) or *bipolar* (history of mania or hypomania), and *psychotic* (psychotic symptoms present) or *neurotic* (psychotic symptoms absent).

COURSE OF DEPRESSION

The onset of depression usually occur after puberty, with a median age of onset of 37. Age of onset tends to be earlier with a positive family history of affective disorders or alcoholism. Untreated episodes last 3 to 9 months, with 85 percent remitting within a year. Up to 80 percent of patients fully recover from a depressed episode. Predictors of a favorable prognosis include few stressful life events and positive social support, especially intimate friendships.

Episode length tends to remain constant for an individual patient. Longer episodes are associated with delay in treatment, older age, lower socioeconomic status, and prior history of a long episode. Ten to fifteen percent of patients with unipolar depression will eventually have a manic or hypomanic episode, converting their diagnosis to a bipolar disorder. Women tend to have more episodes than men.

Half of patients never have another episode. For the other half, depression recurs or becomes chronic, with the chance of recurrence increasing dramatically with each subsequent episode. Twelve percent of patients with major depressive disorder fail to recover within 5 years, 7 percent within 10 years. *Recurrence* is defined as a new depressive episode following a period of at least 2 months without depressive symptoms. Each recurrence results in decreasing length between episodes and increasing treatment resistance. The risk of recurrence is greatest the first 4 to 6 months following recovery and decreases with time. Increased risk of recurrence is associated with dysthymia, substance abuse, comorbid anxiety, comorbid personality disorder, older age of onset, and greater number of previous episodes. Predictors of *relapse* (meeting full criteria for a major depressive episode following a partial response to treatment of a major depressive episode) include greater number of prior episodes, secondary depression, and increased length of prior episodes.

A patient is *refractory* to treatment when symptoms persist despite an accurate diagnosis, patient compliance, and treatment at an adequate dosage for an adequate time period (at least 6 to 8 weeks for most drugs). Serum levels of antidepressants should be obtained when available to document an adequate trial.

COMPLICATIONS AND RED FLAGS

The most serious complication of depression is suicide, which occurs in 15 percent of depressed patients. Risk of suicide is especially high after discharge from inpatient treatment (see Chap. 16–7).

Of the top 10 major medical disorders, depression and cardiac disease have the most negative impact on social, occupational, family, and physical function. Patients with depression are four times more likely to die from physical illness. Depressed patients are at greater risk for developing substance abuse problems.

Patients show impaired judgment and may make poor decisions when depressed. Occupational and academic failure are common. Complications extend beyond the depressed patient, with 40 percent of children of depressed patients developing long-lasting major impairments.

DIAGNOSTIC CONSIDERATIONS

Other Affective Disorders

In *dysthymic disorder,* the patient has a depressed mood most of the day for more days than not, for at least 2 years. Dysthymic patients have fewer vegetative signs (i.e., changes in appetite and sleep) and more fatigue, social-motivational, and cognitive symptoms than patients with major depressive disorder (MDD). The onset is insidious and usually during adolescence. Many patients say they have always been depressed. Dysthymia is more relenting, but less consuming than MDD. The most discriminating factor is its persistence. Patients frequently describe feeling chronically unhappy and miserable, with irritability, anger, and self-pity commonly present.

It is rare for a dysthymic patient not to have a comorbid psychiatric or medical problem. The course tends to wax and wane, typically dependent on environmental stressors. Only 50 percent of patients fully recover. Seventy percent of patients will eventually develop an episode of MDD, which decreases their chance of recovery to only one-third. *Double depression* refers to an episode of MDD concurrent with ongoing dysthymia. Double depression leads to high rates of relapse and treatment resistance. Patients may require at least 2 years of treatment, but most will require lifelong antidepressant pharmacotherapy.

Seasonal affective disorder refers to a regular temporal relationship of symptom onset, with full remissions during each year over a 3-year period.

Depressed mood is an expected and common symptom in uncomplicated bereavement; however, MDD occurs in 10 percent of grieving patients and is characterized by depressed mood lasting more than 3 months, worsening of symptoms over time, and biologic symptoms. Grief-related depression that results in significant impairment of function should be treated as MDD. Treatment of grief-related depression does not interfere with the grieving process.

Bipolar variants include *bipolar I disorder* (diagnosed when the patient has had at least one manic episode), *bipolar II disorder* (when the patient has had at least one hypomanic episode), *cyclothymia* (dysthymia with hypomanic episodes), and *mixed episodes* (the presence of depressive and manic symptoms at the same time). Patients with bipolar variants tend to have more atypical features. Family history of bipolar disorder is often present. Bipolar patients tend to be more sensitive to changes in sleep-wake cycle, diet, exercise, work, and time zone travel.

Other Psychiatric Disorders

Depression may develop as a secondary illness during many other psychiatric disorders, especially substance abuse, panic and other anxiety disorders, and cluster B personality disorders. The presence of depression tends to worsen the primary psychiatric disorder, and the primary disorder tends to worsen the secondary depression, making treatment challenging. Patients with *somatization disorders* somatize whether they have a depressed mood or not, whereas depressed patients somatize only when depressed.

When a patient has been abusing a substance, a diagnosis of depression is deferred until the patient has been drug-free for at least 4 to 6 weeks. Depression is more likely primary when depressive symptoms were present prior to substance use, depression persists during abstinence, depressive symptoms are chronic, there is a positive family history for affective disorders, and there is a profound suicidal ideation. The presence of substance abuse significantly increases treatment resistance, but ongoing substance use is not necessarily a contraindication to antidepressant therapy.

Depression has been triggered by attempts to stop smoking. Caffeine withdrawal can look like depression with symptoms including somnolence, lethargy, and headache.

Depression may be misdiagnosed as *dementia* in elderly patients (pseudodementia). Depressive symptoms tend to be more acute, present with a past history of depression, include self-reproach, are worse in the morning, and involve both recent and remote memory problems. Depressed patients have normal psychometric testing, selectively remember negative events, and show concern for their memory loss (demonstrate insight into their disorder). Dementia has a more insidious onset, with no self-reproach, and is worse at night, with recent memory loss greater than remote memory problems. (See Chap. 11–5.)

Negative symptoms of *schizophrenia* may be misdiagnosed as depression. Patients with schizophrenia do not experience depressed mood as painful, tending to have more apathy and emptiness than dysphoria. Delusions and hallucinations occurring in the context of an affective disorder tend to be briefer and less bizarre than in schizophrenia.

DEPRESSION SECONDARY TO OTHER MEDICAL PROBLEMS

Table 16-5-1 lists medical problems associated with depression. Depressive symptoms associated with medical problems tend to be more resistant to treatment. Characteristics of a secondary depression include absence of family history of affective disorder, greater cognitive impairment, more severe initial episode, and poorer response to treatment. Table 16-5-3 lists other medications associated with depression.

Patients with comorbid anxiety disorders tend to respond better to antidepressants than anxiolytics. Avoidant, dependent, and borderline personality disorders are commonly comorbid with depressive disorders.

Depressed patients tend to attribute negative events to internal causality and believe consequences are irreversible or permanent, with pervasive or global impact. Patients with comorbid personality disorders may be less well equipped to handle life stressors and tend to be at higher risk for experiencing them. The diagnosis of a personality disorder should be suspended until the depression has cleared.

Table 16-5-3. Medications Associated with Depression

Antihypertensives
  Reserpine (15%)
  Methyldopa
  Propanolol (8%)
  Clonidine
  Hydralazine
  Guanethidine
Psychotropics
  Sedatives
    Barbiturates
    Benzodiazepines
    Meprobamate
  Antipsychotics
  Hypnotics
Antiparkinsonian
  Levodopa
Analgesics
  Narcotics
  Indomethacin
Cardiovascular
  Digitalis
  Diuretics
Antimicrobials
  Antiarrhythmic agents
  Sulfonamides
  Isoniazid
Steroids
  Corticosteroids (20%)
  Estrogens (90% have pyridoxine deficiency and respond to
    replacement)
Others
  Cimetidine
  Cancer chemotherapeutic agents
  Alcohol
  Oral hypoglycemic agents
  Stimulant medication withdrawal
  Smoking (nicotine) cessation
  Caffeine withdrawal

Many depressed patients have a comorbid medical diagnosis. Depression is especially common in chronic obstructive pulmonary disease (COPD), myocardial infarction, chronic fatigue syndrome, and HIV infection. About 25 to 50 percent of patients develop MDD after a stroke, and in some patients, depression appears to be causally related to the brain injury. One-third of patients with Parkinson's disease develop depression (see Chapter 11–7). Elevated thyroid-stimulating hormone (TSH) is more common in depressed patients, and some treatment-resistant depressed patients have subclinical hypothyroidism (see Chap. 5–3).

SPECIAL POPULATIONS

Adolescents tend to have more acting out behaviors when depressed, and have fewer introspective abilities. It is important to obtain clinical information and support from significant others (parents, teachers, adult leaders, friends) when dealing with adolescents.

Elderly patients have the highest rates of suicide, especially single, elderly, white males. They also have higher rates of masked depression and become more impaired faster than younger patients. Depression risk increases with concomitant medical illnesses, and the elderly have higher rates of primary medical problems. Elderly patients have more losses and fewer individual and social resources. Older patients are as treatable as younger patients, though they have increased sensitivity to medication side effects and may require more time to respond to antidepressants. The cognitive impairment with pseudodementia does respond to appropriate antidepressant therapy.

TREATMENT

Depression is a treatable disorder, and treatment can be lifesaving. The stance to take with depressed patients is warm, real, and accepting. Depressed patients have a negative cognitive bias and will easily recognize frustration and hopelessness in the provider.

Psychopharmacotherapy and psychotherapy are both effective treatments for depression with a combination of medication and psychotherapy working better than either treatment alone. Suicide risk must be frequently assessed. Understanding cultural differences in the expression and experience of mood and depression assists in assessing response. Patients should be informed that response to treatment tends to be saw-toothed, not linear.

It is important to establish hope early in the treatment of depressed patients. Patients should be followed frequently for reassurance and support until they demonstrate a good response to treatment. Practitioners should take a collaborative approach with patients, encouraging them to take whatever responsibilities they can handle. The depression should be validated at the same time as the patient is encouraged that efforts are being made toward achieving remission of symptoms.

Significant others should be involved in monitoring and providing support. Increasing contact with others may help to stimulate a socially withdrawing patient. Structure and security should be provided in the environment, and the patient should be discouraged from making major life decisions while actively depressed. Contributing psychological stressors should be determined and addressed.

Pharmacologic Management

About 60 to 75 percent of patients achieve complete remission with pharmacologic therapy alone. Less than 30 percent fail to respond to antidepressants. Good response is associated with vegetative symptoms, hypersomnia, melancholia, acute onset, absence of family dysfunction, history of prior response to antidepressants, and family history of mood disorders. Medications are often chosen by matching side effects to individual patient symptoms. Patients tend to respond to medications previously found helpful or to medications found to be effective in family members or friends.

Response may not be seen for weeks after achieving therapeutic doses. Patients with psychotic depression may require higher doses of antidepressants. Potential side effects should be discussed with patients when therapy is instituted. Antidepressants (especially the tricyclic antidepressants) used to treat bipolar depression may lead to induction of mania or increased cycling. Augmenting agents should be used for 2 to 3 months, then tapered.

There is a 50 percent chance of relapse if antidepressants are discontinued before 6 months, so therapy should be continued for at least 6 to 12 months. When discontinuation is considered, it should occur gradually. Longer prophylaxis should be considered with history of recurrence, greater severity, later age of onset, and longer depressive episodes. Maintenance doses are often the same as those needed to achieve remission.

Tricyclic Antidepressants

There are no differences in efficacy among the tricyclic antidepressants (TCAs), with 60 to 70 percent of moderately to severely depressed patients demonstrating response. Predictors of good response to TCAs include insidious symptom onset, upper socioeconomic class membership, presence of biologic symptoms (anorexia, weight loss, middle and late insomnia, psychomotor disturbance), and orthostatic hypotension in response to treatment. Predictors of poor response include the presence of neurotic,

Table 16-5-4. Comparison of Antidepressants

Drug	Usual Dose, mg/d	Dose Range, mg/d	Half-life, h	Antichol-inergic	Drowsiness	Insomnia	Hypo-tension	CYP450 System	Weight Gain	Cardiac
Amitriptyline	150–300	75–300	9–46	++++	++++	0	++++	3A4 2D6	++++	+++
Nortriptyline	75–150	40–150	18–56	+	+	0	++	3A4 2D6	+	++
Protriptyline	15–40	15–60	54–198	++	+	+	++	3A4 2D6	0	++
Imipramine	150–300	75–300	6–28	+++	+++	+	++++	3A4 2D6	+++	+++
Desipramine	150–300	75–300	12–28	+	+	+	++	3A4 2D6	+	++
Clomipramine	150–300	100–300	15–62	+++	++	+	++	3A4 2D6	++	++
Trimipramine	150–200	75–300	16–40	+	++++	0	++	3A4 2D6	+++	++
Doxepin	150–300	75–400	8–25	+++	++++	0	++	3A4 2D6	+++	++
Trazodone	200–400	50–600	6–13	0	++++	+	++	3A4	−	+
Nefazodone	200–600	200–600	3–18	0	++	+	+	3A4	0	+
Amoxapine	75–300	75–600	9–14	++	++	++	++		+	+++
Maprotiline	75–225	75–225	27–50	++	++++	0	0		++	+
Fluoxetine	5–20	10–80	48–96	0	0	++	0	2C9 2D6 3A4	−	0
Sertraline	50–100	25–200	26	0	+	++	0	2C9 2D6 3A4	+/−	0
Paroxetine	20–30	10–60	20	0	+	++	0	2D6	+	0
Fluvoxamine	50–150	50–300	20	0	++	++	0	1A2 2C9 2D6 3A4	−	0
Bupropion	150–300	150–450	10–21	0	−	++	0		−	+
Venlafaxine	75–225	150–375	4–10	+	++	+	+	2D6	0	+
Phenelzine	60–90	30–90	2	+	+	++	++		++	0
Tranylcypromine	30–60	30–60	2	+	+	++	++		++	0
Mirtazepine	15–45	15–60	20–40	+	+++	+	++++	2D6 1A2 3A4 2C9	++	++
St. John's Wort	200	300–1000	25	0	+/−	0	0		−	0
Hypericin	1.0	0.4–2.7	25	0	+/−	0	0		−	0

hypochondriacal, and hysterical traits; history of multiple prior episodes; presence of delusions; and atypical symptoms (hypersomnia, hyperphagia, profound anergy, mood reactivity, rejection sensitivity, and nocturnal worsening of mood).

Dosage may be increased by 25 to 50 mg every 3 to 5 days as tolerated by the patient, until therapeutic dosage is attained. The dose-response curve for TCAs tends to be linear. After 1 week on a fixed dose, plasma levels (obtained 12 to 14 h after last dose) should be assessed for patients not responding to usual therapeutic doses. Ingestion of food has no effect on bioavailability. Obese patients may require higher doses, since TCAs are highly lipophilic, with less than 1 percent of drug present in the vascular compartment. TCAs are excreted in breast milk.

Table 16-5-4 provides a comparison of antidepressants by dosage and side effects. Anticholinergic side effects include dry mouth, constipation, urinary retention, and blurred vision. TCAs may impair pulmonary toilet in patients with chronic respiratory disorders. Cardiovascular side effects include orthostatic hypotension, tachycardia, prolonged ventricular conduction, prolonged PR interval, and an antiarrhythmic effect. Heart failure can slow TCA clearance. Diabetic patients may be more sensitive to hypotensive side effects because of autonomic insufficiency. Other side effects include drowsiness, insomnia, sexual dysfunction, and weight gain. TCAs should be gradually discontinued because withdrawal symptoms occur in 70 percent with abrupt discontinuation. Withdrawal symptoms include nausea, headache, giddiness, coryza, chills, weakness, musculoskeletal pain, and increased dreaming and nightmares.

TCAs are demethylated by the CYP450 3A4 system, and hydroxylated by CYP450 2D6. Table 16-6-5 lists important drugs metabolized by the P450 system. Increased plasma levels are increased with aging, smoking, liver disease (especially alcoholic), oral contraceptives, methylphenidate, chloramphenicol, haloperidol, phenothiazines, cimetidine, disulfiram, and selective serotonin reuptake inhibitors (especially fluoxetine). Decreased plasma concentrations occur with smoking, acute alcohol ingestion, and use of barbiturates, carbamazepine, chloral hydrate, phenytoin, and trihexyphenidyl.

Heterocyclics

Trazodone is available in generic form, and therefore may be less expensive than many other antidepressants. It is compatible with most other antidepressants, though the serotonin syndrome is a potential complication when used with other serotonergic agents. It may not be as effective in treating depression as other agents, but it is frequently used to treat insomnia because of its short half-life and sedative side effect. Other side effects include orthostatic hypotension, headache, nausea, dry mouth, and constipation. A unique and potentially serious side effect is priapism in 1 in 6000 men. It also does not cause sexual dysfunction.

Table 16-5-5. Potential Cytochrome P450 Interactions

1A2
    Haloperidol
    Phenytoin
    Theophylline
    Caffeine
2C9
    Phenytoin
    Diazepam
    Tolbutamide
2D6
    Tricyclic antidepressants
    Haloperidol
    Perphenazine
    Thioridazine
    Clozapine
    Risperidone
    Beta blockers
    Type IC antiarrhythmics
3A4
    Tricyclic antidepressants
    Carbamazepine
    Alprazolam
    Triazolam
    Terfenadine
    Astemazole

Nefazodone is chemically similar to trazodone, but has additional neurotransmitter activity (antagonism of $5HT_2$ receptors), which may make it more effective as an antidepressant. Food may delay absorption, and it may seriously interact with MAOIs because of its serotonergic activities. Adverse side effects include headache, drowsiness, dizziness, hypotension, dry mouth, nausea, constipation, diarrhea, increased appetite, pharyngitis, and blurred vision.

Selective Serotonin Reuptake Inhibitors

Selective serotonin reuptake inhibitors (SSRIs) are the drugs of first choice for treating depression, because they are well tolerated, as effective as TCAs, and relatively safe in overdose. Despite their high cost, they may be more cost-efficient than TCAs because they are so well tolerated and demonstrate nonlinear pharmacokinetics, making dosing relatively uncomplicated. Unlike TCAs, increasing doses does not necessarily lead to enhanced therapeutic effect. There appear to be more similarities than differences among the four current choices. SSRIs may be less effective than TCAs in treating melancholia, but appear to be more effective in treating dysthymic disorders and atypical symptoms, especially irritability, anger, and fatigue.

Potential side effects include headache, nervousness, insomnia, drowsiness, fatigue, anorexia, weight loss, tremor, nausea, diarrhea, constipation, dry mouth, a modest decrease in heart rate, sweating, inhibited libido, anorgasmia, and impotence. All but the last three side effects tend to be transient, often improving as the antidepressant effects become noticeable. Sexual side effects may be dose-related, but are transient in a minority of patients. Treatment approaches for SSRI-induced sexual dysfunction include using a shorter-acting agent and taking drug holidays (not effective for fluoxetine because of its very long half-life), or adding bupropion, buspirone, cyproheptadine, yohimbine, or amantadine. Fluoxetine has the greatest potential for activation, and fluvoxamine has greatest potential for drowsiness, with sertraline and paroxetine demonstrating equal potential for drowsiness and activation. Patients with AIDS appear to be sensitive to developing akathisia, especially with fluoxetine. SSRIs may stimulate respiratory drive in patients with chronic pulmonary disease.

SSRIs need to be completely washed out before switching to a monoamine oxidase inhibitor because of the potential for a hypertensive reaction, especially with fluoxetine, which can take as long as 6 to 7 weeks to clear. SSRIs may increase prothrombin time with concurrent warfarin therapy. They may also inhibit the metabolism of TCAs and carbamazepine.

Monoamine Oxidase Inhibitors

The monoamine oxidase inhibitors are generally avoided by non-psychiatrists because of the dietary and pharmacologic restrictions required to prevent hypertensive crises; however, they are highly effective, well-tolerated antidepressants.

MAOIs are the antidepressants of choice for atypical depression. Predictors of a good response to MAOIs include atypical features (symptoms worse in the evening, initial insomnia, increased appetite and weight gain, hypersomnia), presence of dysthymia, preexisting anxiety (especially with agoraphobia), and bipolar variants. Abrupt discontinuation may lead to vivid and frightening dreams, so gradual withdrawal is usually recommended.

Side effects include hypotension, primarily the first two months of treatment, hepatic damage, peripheral neuropathy, ataxia, hyperacusis, hyperirritability, muscle tension, myoclonic jerks, sexual dysfunction, and acute hypertensive crisis associated with foods and medications found in Table 16-5-6. Symptoms of a hypertensive crisis include a soaring blood pressure, severe head-

Table 16-5-6. Foods and Drugs to Be Avoided When Using MAOIs

Foods

Cheeses
  English Stilton, blue, 3-year-old white, extra-old, old cheddar, Danish blue, mozzarella, Swiss gruyere, Canadian muenster, Canadian old colored, feta, Italian grated parmesan, Italian gorgonzola, brie (Yogurt, cottage cheese, cream cheese, American cheese are okay.)
Fish
  Pickled herring, fish roe, caviar, schmaltz herring in oil, smoked or pickeled fish, shrimp paste
Meat
  Salami, beef or chicken liver, bologna, aged sausage, smoked meat, corned beef, pepperoni, summer sausage
Fruit
  Banana peel or stewed bananas, canned or overripe figs, raisins, avocados
Yeast extracts
  Marmite concentrated yeast extract, brewer's yeast, packet soups (Yeast in baked goods is okay.)
Alcoholic drinks
  Beer, sherry wine, chianti wine
Other
  Products containing fermented bean curd (soya beans), soya paste, soy sauce, fava or broad beans, large amounts of caffeine or chocolate

Drugs

Sympathomimetics
  Amphetamines, dopamine, ephedrine, epinephrine, isoproterenol, metaraminol, methylphenidate, norepinephrine, phenylephrine, phenylpropanolamine
Dopamine precursors
  L-dopa
Narcotic analgesics
  Synthetic narcotics (e.g., meperidine), dextromethorphan (Morphine, oxycodone, codeine, and NSAIDs cause no infraction.)
Serotonergic antidepressants
  Fluoxetine, sertraline, paroxetine, fluvoxamine, trazodone, nefazodone, venlafaxine, buspirone
Tricyclic antidepressants
  Imipramine, clomipramine, trimipramine, desipramine, amitriptyline, nortriptyline, protriptyline, doxepin, etc.
Other
  Barbiturates, reserpine, succinylcholine

ache, chest pain, fever, and vomiting. It may be treated with sublingual nifedipine. Seizures may occur with concomitant pyridoxine deficiency, so many practitioners recommend vitamin supplementation. Hypoglycemia may occur when given with insulin and oral hypoglycemic agents. Use with succinylcholine may lead to prolonged muscle relaxation.

Other Antidepressants

Bupropion is a unique agent that which structurally resembles the amphetamines and tends to be more activating than other antidepressants. Maximum daily dose is 450 mg because of the potential for seizure induction, and it must be given in divided doses, with the doses 6 h apart. Bupropion does not appear to induce rapid cycling in bipolar disorders. It induces its own metabolism as well as the metabolism of other hepatically metabolized agents, such as carbamazepine. It is also effective in treating attention deficient disorder in adults, and binging and purging, though use in bulimia has been associated with increased seizure risk, probably related to nutritional deficiencies (see Chap. 16–1).

Adverse effects include dry mouth (14 percent), nausea and vomiting, insomnia, rash, orthostatic hypotension, hypertension, excitement and agitation, seizures (in 0.4 percent, especially in patients with a history of seizure disorder), and weight loss (30 percent). Because it may enhance dopaminergic transmission, it could worsen psychotic symptoms and has been associated with psychotic side effects. Adding bupropion to an SSRI may increase the risk of seizure and delirium. Patients with AIDS may also be at greater risk for seizure. Other potential drug interactions may occur with warfarin, phenytoin, carbamazepine, phenobarbital, and cimetidine. Bupropion may stimulate respiratory drive in patients with chronic pulmonary disease.

Venlafaxine is unique in that it increases both synaptic norepinephrine and serotonin by inhibiting reuptake. It may be a better antidepressant for patients showing only partial response to SSRIs, though its effectiveness may diminish within 3 months of use. One-third of treatment-resistant patients respond to venlafaxine, but half of these eventually relapse. As with TCAs, abrupt discontinuation may lead to withdrawal symptoms, and use with MAOIs may be associated with a hypertensive crisis. Potential side effects include dizziness, insomnia, nervousness, headache, somnolence, dry mouth, nausea, constipation, anorexia, and anorgasmia.

Mirtazapine is a strong blocker of alpha/adrenoceptors, resulting in increased noradrenalin and serotonin activity. Its anxiolytic effect at 15 mg/day equals that of diazepam at 10 mg/day. Mirtazapine demonstrates linear pharmacokinetics.

Potential side effects include dry mouth, drowsiness (especially at 15 mg/day), increased appetite and weight gain, benign elevation of liver function tests, and increased cholesterol and triglycerides. Most side effects are mild and transient. *St. John's wort* is an herb commonly used in Europe to treat mild to moderate depression. The mechanism of action is unknown. It appears to inhibit noradrenalin, serotonin reuptake, increase dopamine and noctural melatonin, and inhibit prolactin. Hypericin (one clinical found in St. John's wort) is an MAOI, but not at doses currently used.

St. John's wort is very well tolerated, with no reported significant drug interactions or toxicity. Valerian root may potentiate an antidepressant effect.

Other Medications

Used alone, *lithium* has an antidepressant effect, but its main use in affective disorders is as a mood stabilizer, and as an augmenting agent. (See Chap. 16–6.) About 70 percent of bipolar patients and 50 percent of unipolar patients respond to lithium. Predictors of good response include bipolar symptoms, family history of bipolar disorder, mood lability, history of postpartum depression, hypersomnia, hyperphagia, and early age of onset. About 74 percent of partially responding patients on a TCA demonstrate a 50 percent or better improvement in symptoms within 48 h of adding lithium. Half of partially responding patients on an SSRI demonstrate symptomatic improvement. Use with bupropion increases seizure risk.

Buspirone is a serotonergic anti-anxiety agent (see Chap. 16–3). It has antidepressant properties when given in higher doses and may be used to augment the effect of antidepressants, especially in the presence of concurrent anxiety symptoms. More than half of patients who partially respond to fluoxetine improve with the addition of buspirone.

Stimulants are not effective first-line agents for the treatment of depression, but are used in augmenting antidepressants. They are especially useful in elderly and medically ill patients, and for symptoms of amotivation and lethargy, often working within 1 to 2 days.

Triiodothyronine (T_3) is as effective as an augmenting agent and more effective than thyroxine. T_3 may be used in augmentation for both unipolar and bipolar disorders, in either phase.

Onset of TCA antidepressant action is accelerated when T_3 is started simultaneously with the TCA.

Other augmentation strategies include adding an antidepressant with a different mechanism of action, pindolol, carbamazepine, meclobemide, selegeline, lamotrigine, inositol, dexamethasone, bromocriptine, and antiglucocorticoids. There are numerous other agents currently under investigation for treating depression. Consultation with a provider familiar with these new agents is indicated prior to their use.

Other Somatic Treatments

Electroconvulsive therapy is the gold standard in the treatment of depression, with 80 percent of patients responding. Current indications include severe depression, treatment resistance, psychotic depression, high suicide risk, the presence of cardiovascular disease precluding use of antidepressants, and pregnancy. ECT causes short-term memory loss and confusion. There is no evidence of permanent brain damage or permanent memory loss. Patients are at high risk for relapse if maintenance antidepressant pharmacotherapy is not instituted.

Phototherapy, especially when used in the morning, is effective for both treatment and prevention of seasonal depression, and is only effective when used during the winter months. Patients respond within 1 to 2 weeks, and efficacy tends to remain stable over time. The only adverse effect is a slight risk for precipitation of mania. Continued use of phototherapy during high-risk periods decreases the risk of recurrence.

Psychotherapy

Psychotherapy is as effective as medication in the treatment of mild to moderate depression, though individual response varies widely. Formal therapy may be time-consuming, expensive, and not widely available, especially in rural areas.

Intense exploration into personal problems during an acute depressive episode is contraindicated, as it may heighten negativity and hopelessness. Patients with melancholic and psychotic depressions and patients with poor insight may not respond as well to psychotherapeutic techniques. Therapeutic factors associated with effectiveness include an active and directive therapist, focus on current problems, emphasis on changing current behavior, self-monitoring of change and progress, use of homework, and a predetermined number of sessions.

Cognitive-Behavioral Therapy

Cognitive-behavioral therapy (CBT) has been the most studied in the treatment of depression. It also decreases the likelihood of relapse. Cognitive interventions include identifying dysfunctional automatic thoughts, challenging cognitive distortions, cognitive restructuring, and problem solving. Common cognitive distortions present in depressed patients include all-or-nothing thinking, overgeneralization, selective abstraction, emotional reasoning, personalization, disqualifying the positive, jumping to conclusions, magnification or minimization, labeling, and arbitrary inferences (i.e., mind reading, fortune telling).

Behavioral interventions include activity scheduling, development of mastery and pleasurable activities, graded task assignments, and assertiveness training. Formal CBT should be performed by caregivers specifically trained in these techniques.

Other Psychotherapies

In interpersonal therapy (IPT), patients are assisted in developing functional strategies to deal with specific problem areas such as grief, interpersonal disputes, role transitions, and interpersonal deficits. Attention is placed on relationships, using the therapeutic relationship as an example.

Family therapy enhances support and compliance. Marital therapy may be helpful for support and in mild depression associated with marital strife. Dysthymia tends to respond best to social skills training, problem solving, and a focus on the present. Group therapy appears to be as effective as individual therapy, and is more cost-effective.

BIBLIOGRAPHY

Andreason NC, Black DW: *The Introductory Textbook of Psychiatry.* Washington, DC, American Psychiatric Press, 1995.

Beck AT, Rush AJ, Shan BF, Emery G: *Cognitive Therapy of Depression.* New York, Guilford, 1979.

Hornig-Rohan M, Amsterdam JD (eds): Treatment-resistant depression. *Psychiatr Clin North Am* 19:2, 1996.

Keller MB (ed): Mood disorders. *Psychiatr Clin North Am* 19:1, 1996.

Macimen JS, Ward NG: *Essential Psychopathology and Its Treatment.* New York, Norton, 1995.

Paykel ES: *Handbook of Affective Disorders.* New York, Guilford, 1992.

Sansone RA, Sansone LA: Dysthymic disorder: The chronic depression. *Am Fam Phys* 53(8):2588–2594, 1996.

Winokur G, Clayton PJ (eds): *The Medical Basis of Psychiatry.* Philadelphia, Saunders, 1994.

Chapter 16–6
MANIC DISORDERS
Don St. John

DISCUSSION

Mania is the defining symptom of bipolar affective disorders (BPADs), which have a 1 percent lifetime prevalence, and equal distribution in men and women. Age of onset is usually late adolescence to the middle of the fourth decade. An affective disorder can be found in a first-degree relative in more than 50 percent of patients with BPAD.

Diagnostic and Statistical Manual of Mental Disorders, fourth edition (DSM-IV), criteria for a manic episode are:

1. A distinct period of abnormally and persistently elevated mood, lasting at least 1 week
2. Three or more of the following symptoms: inflated self-esteem, decreased need for sleep, more talkativeness than usual, flight of ideas, distractibility, increase in goal-directed activity, excessive involvement in pleasurable activities
3. Sufficient severity to cause marked impairment in functioning

Mania tends to occur in three stages. *Hypomania* is characterized by mild euphoria or irritability, expansive speech, and reduced sleep. *Classic mania* is characterized by grandiosity, euphoria, excessive energy, impulsivity, and insomnia. *Psychotic mania* includes hallucinations, delusions, confusion, agitation, and/or catatonia.

SIGNS AND SYMPTOMS

Increased goal-directed behavior and thoughts are distinguishing symptoms of mania. Decreased attention occurs to both internal and external cues, and the patient may be easily distractible, rapidly going from one activity to another. There is often an increase in energy with psychomotor hyperactivity. Psychomotor agitation may also be present. Weight loss may occur in response to both increased physical activity and inattention to nutritional needs.

Disinhibition may be exhibited by increased sexual thoughts and appetite, overfamiliarity and demanding demeanor towards caregivers, overspending, fast driving, and aggression.

Mood changes are often abrupt, over hours or a few days. Mood is always and persistently elated, angry, and/or irritable. Though usually not recognized as abnormal by the patient, both during the manic phase and in retrospect.

Grandiose ideas and delusions are common. Predominant themes may be religious, sexual, financial, political, and/or persecutory. Often one or two themes predominate. Eutonia (a subjective sense of well-being), inflated self-esteem, or grandiosity is frequently present. Thought and perception appear to the patient unusually sharp or brilliant.

A significant decrease in need for sleep is often present, and the patient may find brief periods of sleep refreshing.

Speech may be pressured, loud, rapid, and/or difficult to interrupt. The manic patient may switch topics abruptly and even talk when alone.

Twenty to fifty percent of acutely manic patients have psychotic symptoms. Delusions are usually of grandeur, but may be paranoid. Delusions tend not to be as fixed and persistent as in schizophrenia. Hallucinations, usually auditory, tend to reflect prevailing delusions.

The manic patient often demonstrates poor insight, even after recovery from a manic episode. Mania may last a few days to months, with an average duration (untreated) of 3 to 6 months. In bipolar patients, mania often follows a period of depression.

Atypical mania is characterized by dysphoria, rapid-cycling, mixed symptoms, organic etiology and lithium nonresponsiveness.

DIAGNOSTIC CONSIDERATIONS

Schizophrenia

In BPAD, personality and general functioning are normal between episodes. There is more disturbance of mood, more overactivity and physical agitation, and more elation with mania. Mania tends to have a more abrupt onset. The triad of manic mood, rapid or pressured speech, and hyperactivity is a robust finding in mania. There is less formal thought disorder in mania, and delusions and hallucinations tend to reflect the mood disturbance. Affective and schizophrenic family histories tend to be distinct, with schizophrenic patients rarely reporting either mania or bipolar illness in the family history.

Other Disorders

Truly manic patients tend to have a more abrupt onset and offset of manic behavior, with more stable premorbid states than patients with personality disorders. Symptoms of attention deficit disorder tend to be more chronic, with less clear onset and offset of symptoms, no expansive mood, and lack of psychotic symptoms. Other conditions to rule out include delirium, hypoglycemia, seizure disorders, and anticholinergic psychosis.

Mania can be precipitated by drug withdrawal (especially rapid discontinuation of lithium) stressful life events (especially if associated with sleep deprivation), antidepressant therapy (though this is controversial), seasonal changes (mania is more likely during the spring months), sleep deprivation, hormonal changes (especially the postpartum period), and light exposure.

Comorbidity

Higher rates of obsessive-compulsive disorder occur in bipolar patients. Comorbid impulse control disorder may predate the onset of BPAD. Patients with BPAD have the highest rates (50%) of comorbid drug and alcohol abuse.

Mania Due to Secondary Causes

Mania is more likely to be secondary or organic if the first episode occurs after age 40 or before puberty, or if there is no family history of affective disorders. The mood tends to be more irritable, patients are less likely to be psychotic, and there is better therapeutic response to antiseizure medications.

Drugs most likely to cause mania include all stimulants and sympathomimetics, steroids, anticholinergic agents, baclofen, and L-dopa. Medical conditions associated with manic states include organic mood disorders; head injuries, especially involving right subcortical or cortical structures, the hypothalamus, thalamus, and caudate; multiple sclerosis; hyponatremia; both hyperthyroidism and hypothyroidism; both Addison's and Cushing's diseases; AIDS; and several other neurologic conditions and infections.

Thyroid function studies, complete blood count, blood glucose, drug and alcohol screen, head scan (CT or MRI, depending on neurologic findings and suspicions), EEG, and a thorough physical examination, with special attention given to the neurologic examination should be considered to rule out secondary causes of a manic episode.

TREATMENT

Pharmacologic Management

Mood Stabilizers

Lithium is most effective for the treatment of classic mania, demonstrating improvement in 70 percent of manic patients, with average doses of 1200 to 2400 mg/day. Twelve-hour blood levels should be targeted at 0.9 to 1.4 mg/dL during acute manic episodes. Steady state is achieved in 4 to 5 days. Once the patient is stable, the dose may be given once daily. Lithium clearance is increased during acute mania, so levels may rise as the patient responds to treatment.

Signs of lithium toxicity include tremor, nausea and vomiting, diarrhea, and confusion. There is a 4 to 12 percent risk of congenital malformation when given during pregnancy. The elderly may respond to a lower dose. Predictors of poor response to lithium include atypical presentation, history of more than three lifetime manic episodes, and prior poor response to lithium. Three weeks at a therapeutic serum level constitutes an adequate therapeutic trial.

Valproic acid [or divalproex sodium (Depakote)] is more effective for atypical mania and overall as effective as lithium. Valproate may be started at 750 mg/day in divided doses and increased 250 to 500 mg/day until a therapeutic level of 50 to 120 μg/mL is achieved. Once the patient is stable, valproate may be administered once daily. Valproate may also be initiated at 20 mg/kg/day. Steady state occurs in 2 days. Benign liver function test (LFT) elevation occurs in 5 to 15 percent and does not predict hepatic failure, which is a rare complication.

Carbamazepine is given at 400 to 1000 mg/day to a therapeutic 12-h serum level of 6 to 12 μg/mL, with steady state achieved in 3 to 4 days. Carbamazepine is also more effective in atypical mania and overall as effective as lithium. About 10 to 20 percent of patients display a fall in WBC, which is not predictive of aplastic anemia or agranulocytosis, a rare side effect. Benign LFT increases occur in 5 to 15 percent. Carbamazepine induces its own metabolism, so blood levels must be checked frequently and the dosage adjusted accordingly during the first several months of use. Carbamazepine also induces the metabolism of several other drugs, especially antipsychotics.

Antipsychotics

High- and low-potency antipsychotics and atypical antipsychotics (Risperidone, Olanzapine, and Clozapine) are equally effective as the three thymoleptics discussed above in treating the symptoms of flight of ideas, delusions, psychomotor agitation, and combativeness of manic states. Patients may require high doses. Patients with affective disorders may be at a higher risk for developing tardive dyskinesia. Therefore, discontinuation should be considered following symptom resolution and adequate tymoleptic therapy. Some patients may require continued use of neuroleptics. Depot neuroleptics have been used successfully in patients who have mainly manic episodes (rather than depressions) and have been difficult to manage.

Benzodiazepines

Benzodiazepines are useful in decreasing psychomotor agitation, aggression, and logorrhea. They tend to normalize sleep, which is therapeutic during a manic episode. Tapering of these drugs should be considered as behavior normalizes, though continued use is associated with a lower relapse rate in some patients. Typical doses would be clonazepam, 1 mg every 4 to 6 h, or lorazepam, 2 to 4 mg orally or intramuscularly every 2 h.

Other Drugs

Other drugs reported to be effective in treating manc symptoms in small studies and case reports include verapamil, clonidine, fenfluramine, thyroid supplementation, and the antiseizure medications gabapentin and lamotrigine.

Electroconvulsive Therapy

Electroconvulsive therapy (ECT) is highly effective in treating mania and may be considered when mood stabilizers are relatively contraindicated, such as during pregnancy, in the elderly, in patients with epilepsy, or in patients with severe cardiovascular disease. Remission or significant clinical improvement occurs in 80 percent of patients, including 50 to 60 percent of nonresponders to standard mood stabilizers. Lithium should be discontinued prior to ECT treatments, as concomitant use may be associated with a higher risk of organic brain syndrome. Maintenance ECT has been effective in controlling otherwise intractable bipolar illness.

Other Treatments

Psychosocial management is not possible during an acute manic state because of the patient's poor insight. Patients should be protected from the consequences of their actions. Avoid confining manic patients in a small space. Restrict telephone use to avoid huge bills. Maintain the environment with as little stimulation as possible. Set limits in an unambivalent and firm manner.

Antidepressants should be discontinued unless past history suggests otherwise. Sleep should be induced quickly to prevent escalation of manic symptoms. Clinicians should be aware of the potential for aggressive and assaultive behavior, especially when the patient exhibits suspiciousness and agitation or excitement.

Hospitalization should be considered when the patient is unable to cooperate with treatment, is at risk for suicidal or homicidal behavior, lacks a good social support system, is pregnant, or when protection from the consequences of poor judgment is necessary. The patient may be discharged when there has been a significant reduction in symptoms and a commitment to continued mood-stabilizer therapy.

Mood stabilizers must be continued on an outpatient basis for at least 4 to 6 months, usually at the dose required for control of acute symptoms. Indefinite continuation of mood-stabilizer therapy should be considered after three or more manic episodes.

COMPLICATIONS AND RED FLAGS

Potential complications of a manic episode are primarily social and include marital discord and divorce, business difficulties, financial extravagance, sexual indiscretions and sexually transmitted diseases, drug or alcohol abuse, suicide, homicide, and death from physical exhaustion or participation in dangerous activities.

BIBLIOGRAPHY

American Psychiatric Association: *Diagnostic and Statistical Manual of Mental Disorders*, 4th ed. Washington, DC, American Psychiatric Association, 1994.

Andreason NC, Black DW: *Introductory Textbook of Psychiatry*. Washington, DC, American Psychiatric Press, 1995.

Clayton P: Bipolar illness, in *The Medical Basis of Psychiatry,* Winokur G, Clayton P (eds): Philadelphia, Saunders, 1994, pp 47–68.

Gerner RH: Treatment of acute mania. *Psychiatr Clin North Am* 16(3):443–460, 1993.

Wender SF: An update on the diagnosis and treatment of mania in bipolar disorder. *Am Fam Phys* 51(5):1126–1136, 1995.

Chapter 16–7
SUICIDE

Don St. John

DISCUSSION

Suicide is a growing problem worldwide. At least 20 percent of the population has seriously considered or attempted suicide. Approximately 1 percent of the population will complete a suicide. There are 30,000 suicides per year in the United States, making it the second leading cause of death in the 15- to 24-year-old age group, and the ninth leading cause of death overall in the United States. The suicide rate for adolescents tripled between 1952 and 1992.

Suicide rates tend to diminish during war, rise during times of economic stress, increase with media coverage of suicide, and peak during the spring.

Suicidality may be thought of on a continuum, from consideration to ideation, planning, attempting, and completion. Survivors (those with a significant relationship with the victim) may be considered the final phase of this continuum. Baechler has defined suicide as occurring "when people are using their own deaths instrumentally to try to solve their problems of living."[1]

Completed suicide is an act that results in the death of the victim. Attempted suicide (parasuicide) does not result in death.

A variety of classifications of suicidal patients have been put forth. One scheme classifies victims into four categories: hopeless, psychotic, histrionic or impulsive, and rational.

Hopeless patients have such psychic pain that they can see no alternative solution to the situation. In this category are patients who are depressed, chronically ill (especially with poorly treated pain) and those with toxic pride, who are unable to cope with feelings of depression secondary to perceived failure, such as the straight-A medical student who obtains a first "C" and is then unable to face family and friends.

Psychotic patients may commit suicide in response to a command hallucination or delusion.

Histrionic or impulsive patients may commit suicide to punish themselves, obtain revenge or attention, provide stimulation and excitement, or symbolically kill or punish another.

Some see suicide as a "rational" solution to a terminal or progressive illness.

The *attempted suicide* (parasuicide) rate is 10 times that of completed suicide. Attempts may be a "cry for help" or used as a cathartic (to provide relief from a stressful situation), are more likely in women who tend to be impulsive, and are often associated with substance use. The most common method attempted is drug ingestion (or overdose) (see Chap. 4-8). A personality disorder (usually cluster B) is present in 40 percent of attempters. The motivation behind an attempt is often interpersonal and meant to affect other individuals, make a statement, or create some change in a relationship.

Completers are more likely to be older and male, take precautions not to be discovered, have a plan, have high suicidal preoccupation and intent, use a more lethal method, leave a note, be socially isolated, and be self-directed in motivation. Attempters are more likely to be young and female, take more precautions to be discovered, be impulsive, have low suicidal preoccupation and intent, use a less lethal method, and often have an interpersonal motivation for the attempt.

RISK ASSESSMENT

It is not possible to predict with any clinically useful degree of accuracy the risk of a patient committing suicide, despite the availability of several assessment tools and the large body of data concerning suicide risk factors. However, it is possible to assess an individual's risk factors to be addressed during the treatment phase.

Sex

Males tend to use more lethal methods, though females (especially those over age 65) are using increasingly lethal methods, such as firearms. Males complete suicide four times more often than females.

Age

The highest risk age categories are those under 19 and over 45, but especially men over 65, which is the age group with the highest suicide rate. This older, at-risk group may be more sensitive to normal losses associated with aging, and often have lifelong evidence of poor adaptive skills. Ninety percent of older males will complete a suicide with their first attempt. Adolescent suicide is often associated with family conflict, exposure to violence (especially a suicide in the family), and a depressed father.

History of Suicide Attempts

Past history of suicide attempt(s) is one of the most robust predictors of suicide. Thirty to forty percent of suicide victims have a past history of at least one attempt. The risk of completing a suicide is 1 percent within 1 year of an attempt. Ten to fifteen percent of attempters will eventually complete a suicide.

Family History of Suicide

Up to 11 percent of suicide victims have a first-degree relative who committed suicide. Exposure to suicide in the family is associated with increased risk, perhaps by modeling suicide as an acceptable problem-solving method. Exposure of adolescents to the suicide of a family member is associated with a stronger attraction to death.

Presence of a Psychiatric Disorder

More than 90 percent of completers have a major psychiatric illness, usually depression. Fifteen percent of patients with depression will eventually commit suicide, which is five to seven times the risk of the general population. The most at-risk period may be just as the patient begins to respond to treatment. Only 17 percent of these depressed patients are being adequately treated at the time of their depression. Adequately treating depression is the single most effective intervention in the prevention of suicide.

Forty percent of schizophrenic patients attempt suicide, 30 percent of whom succeed with their first try; 10 percent of all schizophrenics eventually complete a suicide. The suicidal schizophrenic tends to be young, male, white, single, and socially isolated, with a chronic and relapsing illness and high expressed emotion in the family. The suicide is often committed during the first 10 years of the illness, often during a relatively nonpsychotic phase.

The majority of suicidal patients with a personality disorder also have a current axis I depressive illness and/or substance abuse at the time of the suicide. Suicide is rare in cluster A disorders and does not differ from the general population in cluster C disorders. At-risk patients with cluster B disorders tend to have borderline or antisocial personality disorders and often have a history of prior attempts and substance abuse.

Substance Abuse

Eighteen percent of all alcoholics eventually commit suicide, usually late in the disease process. Alcoholics who have been excluded from their marriages and families are at particularly high risk for completing suicide. Victims tend to use substances to disinhibit themselves prior to the act. Forty percent of suicide victims have alcohol in their blood at the time of death.

Hopelessness

A sense of hopelessness is the most robust psychological factor present in suicidal patients. Cognitive disorders associated with hopelessness include dysfunctional assumptions, dichotomous thinking, cognitive rigidity, poor problem-solving abilities, a negative self-concept and traumatizing self-denigration, a sense of isolation, poor concept of the future, and the use of aggression in problem solving.

Psychosocial Stressors

Stressors frequently found at the time of a suicide include a disruptive close interpersonal relationship, social isolation (e.g., a recent geographic move, separation, divorce, or widowhood), recent bereavement (especially of a spouse), unemployment or retirement, residence in a violent area, low socioeconomic status, and the presence of medical problems (especially chronic, severe, and/or debilitating).

Suicidal Ideation

Chronic suicidal ideation is highly associated with suicide risk. Up to 15 percent of victims give some clue just prior to the act, usually a verbal warning. One in six leave a note. The majority of suicide victims have visited a health care practitioner within a month of committing suicide.

The more lethal and detailed the plan, the greater the risk of completion. Access to and familiarity with the chosen method also increases the risk of a completed suicide. The mere presence of a firearm in the home increases risk significantly.

A rather abrupt appearance of an attitude of peace and calm displayed by a chronically suicidal patient may be a warning sign that the patient has finally accepted suicide as the method to deal with life's problems. The patient may display an attitude of finality with visits, using such phrases as "Thanks for trying" and "Goodbye" instead of the usual "See you next week."

TREATMENT AND INTERVENTION

The primary goal of suicide intervention is to protect the patient from self-harm. Risk factors are assessed, the act is physically prevented by appropriate means, ethical and moral barriers to committing suicide are strenghtened, and underlying distress is treated. Supports are improved or developed, vulnerabilities are reduced, and the patient is given hope that the current suicidal crisis will pass. An enhanced sense of self-control and personal effectiveness is developed as the patient is assisted in choosing to live. Past failures and losses are not addressed during the crisis intervention phase.

Characteristics of the Intervenor

Effective treatment begins with the establishment of a trusting collaborative therapeutic relationship. Take an active and problem-solving stance. Patients should be approached with confidence, empathy, support, and a nonjudgmental attitude. Promote an open and honest discussion about patients' suicidal thoughts, letting them known the clinician takes their suicidal feelings seriously.

Suicidal crises should be prepared for in advance, as with all potential emergency situations. Referral sources should be developed and available before a crisis occurs. Clinicians should understand their limits of training and experience, as well as their comfort level with suicidal patients. Countertransference is dealt with by clinicians asking themselves such questions as, How am I reacting? To what am I reacting? What are my feelings telling me about this patient?

Open and Thorough Discussion

All depressed patients should be screened for suicidal ideation. Most patients are relieved to be able to discuss their suicidal thoughts and feelings, since many are actually frightened by them. Exposing and discussing this ambivalence are important in establishing alternative solutions. Sample questions to use are listed in Table 16-7-1.

Confidentiality

Patients should be informed of the limits regarding confidentiality. General rules of medical confidentiality may be broken when the patient's life is in danger. The patient should be informed when others are notified and the patient's clinical condition is discussed with other health care providers, family, and/or friends. They should be reassured that this is for their safety. Permission

Table 16-7-1. Interviewing the Suicidal Patient

Opening questions
  Does it ever seem like life is not worth living anymore?
  Have you been thinking about hurting yourself or taking your life?
  Many patients who are depressed think about suicide. Have you had thoughts like these?
Follow-up questions
  Have you ever attempted or seriously considered suicide before?
  If you were to commit suicide, how would you do it?
  What is the problem you are trying to solve by committing suicide?
  Why commit suicide now?
  Why not commit suicide now?
  Will you work with me?
  Will you be safe?
  Who else needs to know you are thinking about suicide?
Other questions to consider
  What reasons does the patient have for contemplating suicide?
  Is there a specific psychiatric illness present?
  What substances is the patient using?
  What is the degree of depression and hopelessness?
  Does the patient feel the predicament is intolerable and requires an immediate solution?
  What is the degree of suicidal intent?
  What situational or social factors contribute to the suicidal thinking?
  What adaptive coping capabilities does the patient have?
  What resources and supports are available for this patient?
  What is the patient's attitude toward death and suicide?
  Does the patient have reason(s) to live . . . to not commit suicide?

Table 16-7-2. When to Admit a Suicidal Patient

Need to shelter patient from self-harm
Need to develop supports sufficient to justify outpatient treatment
Need to examine the patient in an undrugged state
Need to observe the patient to adequately determine the risk of suicide
Need to remove the patient from a stressful situation
Need to stabilize the patient's emotional state
Need to reassess outpatient treatment

for such sharing of information may be sought, but is not required during a suicidal situation.

The PA may need to be quite directive. Help patients organize their thinking and behavior. If the suicidal threats are being used in a manipulative manner, the suicidal talk may be confronted and challenged.

Support Systems

Organize a supportive environment. This may be done on an outpatient basis if safety can be assured. The ultimate safe and supportive environment may be the inpatient psychiatry ward, though safety can never be completely guaranteed. Involve family and supportive friends. Give precise instructions to the patient's social network regarding care and supervision. Have someone stay with the patient until the suicidal crisis has passed. Do not allow the patient to be alone.

Identify the patient's personal strengths and emphasize them to the patient. Protective factors include religious faith and religious prohibitions to committing suicide, loved objects, a perceived future, and empathy toward potential survivors.

If the patient is to be treated as an outpatient, provide a 24-h emergency telephone number. A written contract may not provide legal protection, but can be used as a negotiation tool. The contract should stipulate that the patient will call the 24-h number (which is written on the contract) if there is any worsening of the suicidal crisis. The contract should be in force for a specified and brief time period, renewable at the end of the period. The patient should call in daily to review safety procedures. Family and friends should be involved in both the negotiation and fulfillment of the contract.

Cognitive-Behavioral Therapy

The goal of crisis intervention is to decrease the suicidal potential by the end of the session. Most suicidal patients hold some ambivalence toward committing suicide, and this should be capitalized

on. The motive for the patient's suicide should be challenged and hopefully destroyed.

Accept the person and the pain, but not suicide as a method of dealing with the situation. Make the patient aware of ignored factors in the seemingly hopeless situation, remaining aware that a depressed affect biases the memory to selectively recall in a negative and hopeless manner.

Cognitive distortions should be gently but firmly challenged. Common distortions include futility and hopelessness regarding the situation, a sense of inadequacy and failure as a human being, and an intense feeling of guilt for real or imagined wrong.

Identify negative thinking and reframe in a more positive and realistic manner. Keep alert to such distortions as overgeneralizations, exaggerations, and selective abstractions. Help patients to reality-test their appraisal of the situation and reinterpret their experiences more realistically.

Inpatient Treatment

Most patients with suicidal thoughts can be treated on an outpatient basis. Indications for inpatient treatment can be found in Table 16-7-2. Hospitalization (especially if involuntary) should be conceptualized as a show of concern, not a threat or punishment. Patients do commit suicide even when hospitalized. The most common methods are jumping out of a window on nonpsychiatric units, and hanging within locked psychiatric units.

It is important to know the policies of each institution and the laws of the state regarding involuntary commitment before clinicians find themselves in such a situation. If commitment is necessary, it should be carried out as rapidly as possible. The risk of suicide and need for suicidal precautions must be clearly communicated to every professional treating the patient, and the reasons for suicidal precautions and/or involuntary commitment must be clearly and thoroughly documented in the chart.

Other Considerations

Consultation is strongly recommended when dealing with a suicidal patient. Underlying conditions, especially depression, should be adequately treated. Firearms should be removed from the patient's environment. Any other preferred method identified by the patient should be contained. Patients taking an overdose tend to take whatever (and all) medications they can find, so all medications (including over-the-counter) should be kept and dispensed by a responsible adult. Finally, contagion should be contained by avoiding publicity.

Failure to protect the patient from self-harm may lead to the demise of the patient as well as a lawsuit. Most states provide immunity from legal action if involuntary commitment proceedings and breaching of ordinary confidences are performed in good faith. Use the same usual and reasonable degree of care given to all patients and document, document, document. To a jury, if it is not documented, *it was not done.*

REFERENCE

1. Baechler J: *Suicides.* New York, Basic Books, 1979,

BIBLIOGRAPHY

Bongar B (ed): *Suicide—Guidelines for Assessment, Management, and Treatment.* New York, Oxford, 1992.

Dattilio FM, Freeman A (eds): *Cognitive-Behavioral Strategies in Crisis Intervention,* New York, Guilford, 1994.

Freeman A, Reinecke MA: *Cognitive Therapy of Suicidal Behavior.* New York, Springer, 1993.

Hoffman DP, Dubarsky SL: Depression and suicide assessment, in Kercher EE, Moore GP (eds): *Emergency Medical Clinics of North America,* Philadelphia, Saunders, 1991.

Maris RW, Berman AL, Maltsberger JT, Yufit RI (eds): *Assessment and Prediction of Suicide,* New York, Guilford, 1992.

Murphy GE: Suicide and attempted suicide, in Winokur G, Clayton P (eds): *The Medical Basis for Psychiatry,* Philadelphia, Saunders, 1994.

St. John D: The suicidal patient—identifying, evaluating, and intervening. *J Am Acad Phys Assist* 9(6):58–76, 1996

Tanney B, Tierney R, Lang W: *The Suicide Intervention Handbook,* Calgary, Canada, Living Works Education, 1994.

Respiratory

Chapter 17–1
ASTHMA
David A. Luce

DISCUSSION

Asthma is a respiratory disease whose hallmark is intermittent, reversible obstruction of the airways. The resulting airflow obstruction usually results in cough, wheezing, dyspnea, and chest tightness. Although the disease has several precipitating characteristics, increased recognition of the role of airway inflammation is revolutionizing asthma management.

Since 1979, asthma prevalence in the United States and the rest of the world has been increasing. Approximately 10 million people, or 3 to 5 percent of the U.S. population, have asthma. In spite of vastly improved pharmacologic treatment, there is a disturbing trend of rising numbers of outpatient visits, hospitalizations, and asthma-related deaths. Although this trend is partially due to better reporting and more accurate diagnoses, the cause remains unknown.

Patients at increased risk of dying from asthma include (1) elderly persons, (2) African-Americans, (3) those with previous life-threatening, acute asthma episodes or asthma-related hospitalization within the past year, (4) those with poor general medical care or lack of access to medical care, and (5) those with psychological or psychosocial problems. A primary care clinician must look for those patients to prevent unnecessary asthma-related deaths.

Asthma is one of three diseases under the umbrella classification of chronic obstructive pulmonary disease (COPD). However, COPD more commonly refers to the other two diseases: emphysema and chronic bronchitis. Although there is significant overlap among the three diseases, asthma differs substantially from the other two. Mild to moderate asthma symptoms are usually episodic and reversible. Cigarette smoking is not a primary etiologic factor, and the pathogenesis occurs in the airways themselves. Emphysema and chronic bronchitis symptoms are much more chronic and demonstrate little reversibility. Cigarette smoking is almost always causative for emphysema and chronic bronchitis, and the underlying pathologic changes occur in the lung parenchyma.

Asthma's basic pathophysiologic changes occur in the airways. Those changes fall into three categories:

1. *Airway inflammation:* more evident in severe asthma but plays a role in all cases
2. *Airway obstruction:* extensive narrowing and marked restriction of airflow that reverses spontaneously or with treatment
3. *Airway hyperresponsiveness:* exaggerated response to a multitude of stimuli, such as allergens, environmental irritants, viral infections, cold air, and exercise

The pathophysiologic process of airway hypersensitivity, inflammation, and obstruction is uniform in all types of asthma. There are several different ways to classify the disease. For exam-

ple, asthma often is classified as acute or chronic and as mild, moderate, or severe. It also is classified as intrinsic or extrinsic. Extrinsic asthma results from inhaled allergens that trigger IgE-mediated airway reactions; intrinsic asthma results from other, nonallergic stimuli.

There are several different subsets of asthma syndromes:

- *Exercise-induced asthma (EIA):* bronchospasm beginning 5 to 10 min after one begins aerobic activity.
- *Sampter's triad, or triad asthma:* a combination of asthma, aspirin sensitivity, and nasal polyps.
- *Drug-induced asthma:* asthma precipitated by many common inhaled and oral agents, such as aspirin, other nonsteroidal anti-inflammatory drugs (NSAIDs), beta blockers, histamine, methacholine, acetylcysteine, aerosolized pentamidine, and any other nebulized medication.
- *Occupational asthma:* asthma caused by exposure to specific offending agents in the workplace. Causes such as laboratory animals and over 200 other sensitizing agents are commonly present in workplace environments.
- *Baker's asthma:* a form of occupational asthma caused by flour in small bakeries.
- *Cardiac asthma:* wheezing of congestive heart failure (CHF) probably caused by vasodilation in the small airways.
- *Status asthmaticus:* severe, acute asthma exacerbtion that is unresponsive to aggressive emergency treatment.

SIGNS AND SYMPTOMS

The most common symptoms are episodic wheezing, cough, chest tightness, and dyspnea. The symptoms are often more prevalent at night and most severe in the early morning hours as a result of circadian changes in bronchomotor tone and airway reactivity. As an attack becomes more severe and prolonged, fatigue and sweating become evident.

OBJECTIVE FINDINGS

Diffuse wheezing on auscultation is the most common physical finding in patients with bronchospasm. Tachypnea and tachycardia may be evident. Prolonged expiration is present on auscultation. More severe episodes result in the use of accessory muscles in breathing, intercostal retractions, hyperresonance, and distant breath sounds. Ominous findings during a severe attack include increasing fatigue, diaphoresis, pulsus paradoxus (>25 mmHg), diminishing wheezing, inaudible breath sounds, and cyanosis.

DIAGNOSTIC CONSIDERATIONS

It is important to differentiate asthma from several other diseases and clinical entities in which wheezing occurs. The differential diagnosis of asthma includes COPD (emphysema, chronic bronchitis, α_1-antitrypsin deficiency, cystic fibrosis), left ventricular failure, pulmonary embolism, anatomic upper airway obstruction such as abscess, tumor or epiglottitis, large airway obstruction as in bronchogenic carcinoma or foreign body aspiration, functional upper airway obstruction, drug side effects, parasitic infections such as *Strongyloides* spp., and bronchopulmonary aspergillosis.

Table 17-1-1. Asthma Medications

Drug	Dose	Comments
Bronchodilators		
Beta$_2$-adrenergic agonists		
Albuterol (Proventil, Ventolin)	MDI: 1–4 puffs q 4–6 h	The most widely-used of the beta$_2$ agonists
	Nebulized solution (0.5%): 0.5 mL with 2.5 mL normal saline q 4–6 h	Patients can use home nebulizers; young children can use masks
	Unit dose solution (0.083%): one dose (3 mL) q 4–6 h	For use in home nebulizers
	Powder (Ventolin Rotocaps): inhale one capsule q 4–6 h	For use with a plastic Rotohaler; device is breath-actuated
	Tablets and syrup: 2–4 mg orally q 6–8 h	Proventil Repetabs 4 mg q 12 h; Volmax 4 or 8 mg q 12 h
Bitolterol (Tornalate)	MDI: 2–3 puffs q 6–8 h	Slightly longer duration of action than albuterol
	Nebulized solution: 1.25 mL q 6–8 h	
Metaproterenol (Alupent, Metaprel)	MDI: 1–4 puffs q 3–4 h	Shorter duration of action but more rapid onset of action
	Nebulized solution: 0.3 mL with 2.5 mL normal saline q 3–4 h	For use in home nebulizers
	Unit dose solution: one 2.5-mL dose q 4–6 h	For use in home nebulizers
	Tablets and syrup: 10–20 mg orally q 6–8 h	CNS symptoms such as nervousness and tremor common with oral preparations
Pirbuterol (Maxair, Maxair Autohaler)	MDI: 2 puffs q 4–6 h	Most cardioselective of the beta$_2$ agonists; Autohaler is breath-actuated
Salmeterol (Serevent)	MDI: 2 puffs q 12 h	Longest-acting beta$_2$ agonist for maintenance; has longer onset of action and should not be used for acute therapy
Terbutaline (Brethaire) (Brethine, Bricanyl)	MDI: 2–3 puffs q 4–6 h	
	Tablets: 2.5–5 mg orally 3 times a day	Nervousness and tremor common in oral preparations
	Subcutaneous injection: 0.25 mg SC; may repeat once in 30 min	Less cardioselective than other beta$_2$ agonists; slower onset of action and fewer side effects than SC epinephrine
Other sympathomimetics		
Epinephrine	Subcutaneous injection: 0.3–0.5 mL 1:1000 solution SC; may repeat once in 30 min	No more effective than inhaled beta$_2$ agonists; α and β stimulation cause tremor, nervousness, palpitations, and vomiting
Anticholinergics		
Ipratropium bromide (Atrovent)	MDI: 2–4 puffs q 6 h	Particularly useful in COPD; helps dry secretions; very few side effects
	Unit dose solution: one 2.5 mL dose q 6–8 h (may be mixed with albuterol nebulized solution)	
Theophyllines		
Theophylline, oral (several brands, short-acting and long-acting)	Sustained-release tablets and capsules; short-acting tablets and capsules: 200–600 mg orally q 8–12 h	Used for maintenance therapy; serum theophylline levels must be maintained at 5–15 μg/mL; available in 24-h preparations
Aminophylline	Intravenous injection: loading dose of 6 mg/kg over 10 min in patients who haven't received theophylline in past 24 h	Not recommended for initial, acute emergency care; may be useful in acute care of hospitalized patients when inhaled beta$_2$ agonists haven't been effective
Anti-inflammatory agents		
Corticosteroids		
Beclomethasone dipropionate (Beclovent, Vanceril, and Vanceril Double Strength)	MDI: 2–4 puffs q 6–12 h	Rinsing mouth after use and spacer devices help prevent oral candidiasis
Flunisolide (Aerobid)	MDI: 2–4 puffs q 12 h	Rinsing mouth after use and spacer devices help prevent oral candidiasis
Fluticasone propionate (Flovent 44 μg, 110 μg, 220 μg)	MDI: 88–880 μg twice daily	Available in 3 dosage strengths; rinsing mouth after use and spacer devices help prevent oral candidiasis
Hydrocortisone sodium succinate	Intravenous injection: 4 mg/kg q 6 h	Treats late-phase asthmatic response and usually doesn't act immediately
Methylprednisolone sodium succinate	Intravenous injection: 0.5–1 mg/kg q 6 h	Treats late-phase asthmatic response and usually doesn't act immediately
Prednisolone liquid (Prelone, 15 mg/5 mL, Pediapred 5 mg/5 mL)	Oral liquid: 40–60 mg q 24 h for acute exacerbations	
Prednisone	Tablets: 40–60 mg q 24 h for acute exacerbations	Should be used for very short courses of 7–10 days; long-term use only when absolutely necessary and at lowest dose possible daily or every other day.
Triamcinolone acetonide (Azmacort)	MDI: 2–6 puffs q 6–12 h	Rinsing mouth after use and spacer devices help prevent oral candidiasis

Table 17-1-1. Asthma Medications (*continued*)

Drug	Dose	Comments
Anti-inflammatory agents (*continued*)		
Leukotriene inhibitors		
Zafirlukast (Accolate)	Tablets: 20 mg twice daily	Indicated for prophylaxis and chronic treatment of asthma in adults and children 12 or older; use with caution in patients on oral warfarin anticoagulant therapy as prothrombin times increase
Zileuton (Zyflo Filmtabs)	Tablets: 600 mg 4 times daily	Indicated for prophylaxis and chronic treatment of asthma in adults and children 12 or older; contraindicated in patients with active liver disease or elevated liver enzymes
Mast cell stabilizers		
Cromolyn sodium (Intal)	MDI: 2–4 puffs 4 times daily	Not effective in acute episodes, but may be used 15–20 min before exertion to prevent EIA
	Nebulized solution: 20 mg 4 times daily	For use in home nebulizers
Sodium nedocromil (Tilade)	MDI: 2 puffs 4 times daily	

SPECIAL CONSIDERATIONS

The diagnosis and management of asthma in infants and young children are often much more difficult since pulmonary function tests are not feasible. A nebulizer or a spacer with a face mask is necessary to deliver inhaled medications to young children. Coexisting respiratory or cardiac conditions often complicate the diagnosis and management of asthma in elderly patients. Many medications for other illnesses exacerbate asthma symptoms in older patients. Asthma medications are likely to produce particularly troublesome side effects in the elderly. Pregnant patients should understand that most asthma medications are relatively safe and that poorly controlled asthma greatly increases the risk of perinatal mortality, prematurity, and low birth weight. Asthma patients have a greater risk of complications during and after major surgical procedures. They should have a thorough preoperative clinical assessment, including pulmonary function testing. If FEV_1 values are below 80 percent of a patient's prior personal best results, the patient should receive a short course of oral corticosteroids before the procedure. If patients have taken systemic corticosteroids within the last 6 months, they should receive intravenous or oral corticosteroids the night before, the day of, and the day after surgery.

LABORATORY TESTS

During acute episodes of bronchospasm the total white blood cell count often is elevated. Eosinophilia is almost always present in patients with asthma unless they are taking or have recently taken systemic corticosteroids. Microscopic examination of the sputum may show eosinophils, mucus casts of the small airways (Curschmann's spirals), or Charcot-Leyden crystals from eosinophilic cellular matter. Early in an asthmatic episode the arterial blood gases reveal respiratory alkalosis and hypoxemia. Normalizing P_{CO_2} and developing respiratory acidosis are ominous signs that may indicate impending respiratory failure and the necessity for mechanical ventilation.

RADIOLOGIC STUDIES

To rule out other possible causes of bronchospasm, it is essential to order a routine baseline chest film for every patient with asthma. It is also critical to identify treatable complicating conditions such as pneumonia and pneumothorax. However, it is not necessary to get a chest x-ray routinely every time a patient has an uncomplicated acute episode of wheezing, as it usually shows only hyperinflation.

OTHER DIAGNOSTICS

Routine pulmonary function testing in asthma patients is rapidly becoming as important as routine capillary blood glucose monitoring in diabetics. Because the severity of bronchospasm often does not correlate with the intensity of symptoms or the degree of wheezing on auscultation, pulmonary function tests yield objective, "hard" data that lead to much more effective diagnosis and management. The forced vital capacity (FVC) and the forced expiratory volume after 1 s (FEV_1) are excellent indicators of airflow obstruction and reversibility. A decreased midexpiratory flow rate (MMEF or FEF_{25-75}) is very specific for narrowed small airways and points toward an asthmatic process rather than an obstructive, large airway, or parenchymal process. The peak expiratory flow rate (PEFR) is also a reliable indicator of airway function and is easy to measure at home. A patient with suspected asthma and consistently normal pulmonary function tests should undergo methacholine or histamine bronchial provocation testing to confirm the diagnosis. Skin testing or radioallergosorbent testing (RAST) in a patient with extrinsic allergic asthma often can identify the offending allergens.

TREATMENT
Medications

Each patient's therapy should be unique and specific. The lowest dose of medication that prevents symptoms that interfere with a normal, active life-style and maintains optimum measures of pulmonary function is the goal. The best classification of chronic asthma management is a stepwise approach in which first-line through fourth-line agents are added as the severity increases.

Step 1: Intermittent asthma (symptoms < 1 time/week, nocturnal symptoms < 2 times/month, PEFR > 80 percent of personal best with < 20 percent variability. An as-needed beta$_2$ agonist metered-dose inhaler (MDI) works very well as the first-line reliever agent.

Step 2: Mild persistent asthma (symptoms > 1 time/week, nocturnal symptoms > 2 times/month, PEFR > 80 percent of personal best with < 20 to 30 percent variability. A daily anti-inflammatory MDI is a good second-line agent after the beta$_2$ agonist. Either of the mast cell stabilizers (milder, few side effects) cromolyn sodium and nedocromil, an inhaled corticosteroid (more potent, more side effects, starting dose of 200 to 800 μg/d), or an oral leukotriene inhibitor is an appropriate maintenance controller medication.

Step 3: Moderate persistent asthma (symptoms daily, nocturnal symptoms > 1 time/week, PEFR 60 to 80 percent of personal best with 20 to 30 percent variability. The corticosteroid MDI dose should be increased to 800 to 2000 μg/day. Sustained-release theophylline, an oral long-acting beta$_2$ agonist, an inhaled long-acting beta$_2$ agonist, an anticholinergic MDI, or an oral leukotriene inhibitor is the appropriate third-line agent. Patients on theophylline should have serum concentrations between 5 and 15 μg/mL.

Step 4: Severe persistent asthma (symptoms variable and continuous, nocturnal symptoms frequent, PEFR < 60 percent of personal best with > 30 percent variability. The corticosteroid MDI dose should be increased to > 800 to 2000 μg/day. A sustained-release theophylline, an oral long-acting beta$_2$ agonist, an inhaled long-acting beta$_2$ agonist, an anticholinergic MDI, oral leukotriene inhibitor supplements as needed, or a short-acting beta$_2$ agonist is the appropriate third-line agent. Long-term oral corticosteroids daily or every other day in the lowest possible daily doses are a fourth-line agent.

Exercise-Induced Asthma

An MDI 15 to 20 min before exercise is effective in patients with EIA, a relatively mild form of asthma. A beta$_2$ agonist, cromolyn sodium, and nedocromil work well. When a single agent alone fails to prevent wheezing on exertion, a beta$_2$ agonist and cromolyn sodium or nedocromil is a potent combination.

Acute Asthma Exacerbations

An inhaled, short-acting beta$_2$ agonist given by MDI or nebulizer is the first-line agent in the office or emergency department for acute episodes. More severe episodes require higher doses. A patient should start oral or parenteral corticosteroids as quickly as possible since these medications require several hours to take effect (they treat the late-phase response). Subcutaneous epinephrine and intravenous aminophylline offer no advantage over inhaled beta$_2$ agonists and add little to initial outpatient management unless anaphylaxis is present. More severe episodes require oxygen. Monitoring should be close and regular (hourly PEFR or FEV$_1$, pulse oximetry, arterial blood gases, and a chest x-ray if underlying pulmonary pathology is suspected). Admission to the intensive care unit may be necessary if an episode does not resolve or there are signs of increasing respiratory effort or fatigue.

Adult medication regimens (childhood doses are lower) are given in Table 17-1-1.

Supportive Measures

Preventive measures such as decreasing exposure to allergens and irritants in the outdoor, indoor, and workplace environments are crucial. Eliminating exposure of infants and young children to passive smoking may decrease asthma morbidity rates. Helping patients avoid starting or helping them quit active smoking is vital, improved maternal care, smoking cessation, and improved nutrition help prevent prematurity and small size at birth (a risk factor for developing asthma during childhood or adolescence). Preventive measures to decrease the frequency of viral respiratory infections that lead to recurrent bronchitis or bronchiolitis may make the development of asthma less likely in young children.

Patient Education

Education in asthma self-management empowers a patient to achieve the optimum level of wellness. Because improving compliance and guiding self-management are essential to improved outcomes, many local and national organizations and support groups promote asthma education. Patients with mild to moderate asthma should have active lives at school, home, and work, including sports and recreation. High-quality training in proper inhaler technique, using slow inhalation of MDIs over 4 to 12 s (depending on lung volume), is critical to the medication's adequate deposition in the small airways. Learning to keep a daily record of PEFRs with a home peak flowmeter can greatly increase asthma control. Any drop in the PEFR is an early warning of decreasing pulmonary function. A patient can add or increase prescribed medications according to a prearranged plan, using an asthma management zone system. Knowing whether a patient is in the "green, yellow, or red zone" enables a clinician to monitor and adjust the care plan. This prevents prolonged exacerbations that cause missed days from school and work or hospitalization.

Disposition

Regular follow-up visits facilitate the monitoring of progress and the assessment of home PEFR results and symptom records in order to adjust the care plan. In an allergic patient who has documented positive results on skin testing or RAST, immunotherapy may lead to a marked improvement.

COMPLICATIONS AND RED FLAGS

Asthma that does not respond to aggressive medical management should stimulate a search for the underlying causes and possible specialty evaluation. During acute exacerbations, increasing symptoms and signs of respiratory fatigue indicate the need for hospitalization for continuous monitoring.

OTHER NOTES AND PEARLS

Asthma severity cannot be assessed by signs and symptoms alone; objective measurements of lung function are essential. Thorough, ongoing education and training in proper MDI technique, spacer device use, and home peak flow monitoring empower patients to self-manage their asthma and literally change their lives. The aggressive use of short courses of oral corticosteroids prevents prolonged exacerbations, missed school and work, hospitalizations, and asthma deaths. Because of the uncertainty of high-dose, inhaled corticosteroids' long-term effects on growth, children with mild to moderate persistent asthma merit an initial trial of inhaled cromolyn sodium or nedocromil as an anti-inflammatory agent.

BIBLIOGRAPHY

Fishman MC, Hoffman AR, Klausner RD, Thaler MS: *Medicine*, 4th ed. Philadelphia, Lippincott-Raven, 1996.

Global Initiative for Asthma: Global Strategy for Asthma Management and Prevention, NHLBI/WHO Workshop Report (Based on a March 1993 Meeting). Bethesda, MD, National Institutes of Health and National Heart, Lung, and Blood Institute Publication Number 95-3659, January 1995.

Guidelines for the Diagnosis and Management of Asthma. National Asthma Education Program, Expert Panel Report. Bethesda, MD, U.S. Department of Health and Human Services, Public Health Service, National Institutes of Health Publication Number 91-3042, August 1991.

McPhee SJ, Vishwanath RL, Ganong WF, Lange JD: *Pathophysiology of Disease: An Introduction to Clinical Medicine*. Stamford, CT, Appleton & Lange, 1995.

Stobo JD, Hellmann DB, Ladenson PW, et al: *Principles and Practice of Medicine*, 23d ed. Stamford, CT, Appleton & Lange, 1996.

Tierney LM Jr, McPhee SJ, Papadakis MA: *Current Medical Diagnosis and Treatment*, 36th ed. Stamford, CT, Appleton & Lange, 1997.

Chapter 17–2
ACUTE BRONCHITIS IN PREVIOUSLY HEALTHY INDIVIDUALS

Maureen MacLeod O'Hara

DEFINITION

Acute bronchitis in a previously healthy individual is defined as an inflammation of the large airways of the tracheobronchial tree caused by an infectious agent. The large airways of the lower respiratory tract are defined as the part of the trachea below the vocal cords to the intermediate bronchi. Infection of the smaller airways is termed *bronchiolitis* and is considered a disease of infants. The anatomic dividing line between the upper and lower respiratory tracts is the vocal cords, which are above the cricoid cartilage (Fig. 17-2-1).

ETIOLOGY AND EPIDEMIOLOGY

Acute bronchitis is the ninth most common ambulatory illness in the United States and is most prevalent during the winter and early spring. This coincides with the peak incidence of viral respiratory illness, the most common cause of acute bronchitis. The most common viruses responsible for this infection include adenovirus, influenza virus A and B, coronavirus, rhinovirus, respiratory syncytial virus, and parainfluenzavirus. Bacterial

pathogens are less commonly the primary cause of acute bronchitis and are considered a secondary cause of infection. Among the causative agents are *Haemophilus influenzae, Mycoplasma pneumoniae, Moraxella catarrhalis, Chlamydia pneumoniae, Chlamydia psittaci, Streptococcus pneumoniae, Staphylococcus aureus,* and pneumococci. *Bordatella pertussis* and *Corynebacterium diphtheriae* are considerations in nonimmunized children. The lower respiratory tract is usually sterile in healthy individuals, and the mechanism of infection is considered to be aspiration of organisms from the nasopharanx. Inhalation is not a usual route of entry for organisms into the lower respiratory tract, except for *Legionella pneumophilia* and *Mycobacterium tuberculosis.* Reflux from the stomach and subsequent aspiration may be a source of enteric pathogens. Acute bronchitis usually follows an upper respiratory illness (URI), which can strike anybody over age 1.

ASSESSMENT

Clinical Findings

History

The chief complaint is a cough preceded by the signs and symptoms of a URI, such as nasal congestion with discharge, sore throat, malaise, muscle aches, headache, slight fevers, chills, and sneezing for a few days to 2 weeks. Signs and symptoms of URI in children also include hyperemic pharynx and tonsils and injected tympanic membranes. Patients complain of a productive or nonproductive cough and possible hemoptysis secondary to the cough. Purulent sputum is suggestive of bacterial infection. Persistent fevers lasting more than 3 to 5 days may indicate pneumonia. Dyspnea is a rare complaint. Generally speaking, bacterial illness

Figure 17-2-1. The anatomic dividing line between the upper and lower respiratory tracts is the vocal cords, which are above the cricoid cartilage.

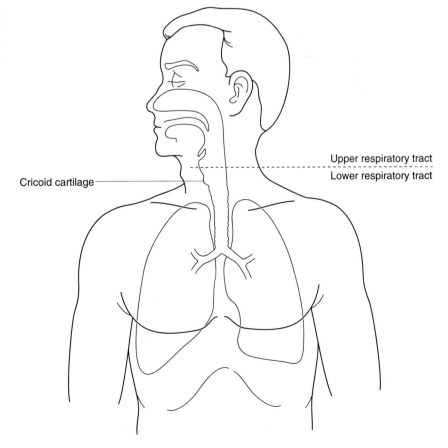

Upper respiratory tract
Lower respiratory tract
Cricoid cartilage

is characterized by fevers of 38.9°C (102°F) or more and chills, whereas viral illness tends to be milder.

Physical Examination

In addition to the findings of URI, the lung examination may demonstrate scattered rhonchi or possibly crackles and wheezes.

LABORATORY FINDINGS

Chest x-ray (CXR) is usually normal and is obtained to rule out pneumonia. A complete blood count (CBC) is not obtained routinely but may show increased white cells, especially if the patient has a URI or pneumonia. Sputum Grain stain may demonstrate many polymorphonuclear cells and can be misleading because of the presence of normal flora. Culture and sensitivity are reserved for hospitalized patients and usually are not obtained for outpatients.

DIFFERENTIAL DIAGNOSIS

The differential diagnosis includes bronchiectasis, pneumonia, asthma, chronic bronchitis, tuberculosis, cystic fibrosis, aspiration, a retained foreign body, inhalation of noxious agents, and lung cancer. Recurrent episodes of bronchitis in children may indicate asthma and should be evaluated.

TREATMENT

Treatment generally includes supportive measures, rest, cough suppressants for sleep (e.g., benzonatate, dextromethorophan, codeine), oral hydration (3 to 4 L per day to thin mucous secretions), and antipyretic measures. Expectorants (e.g., guiafenesin) may or may not be helpful. Because of the inflammation of the airways, inhaled bronchodilators may be helpful for dyspnea or persistent dry cough. If patients are suffering from a URI, decongestants may be helpful. Patients can expect to be symptomatic for 1 to 2 weeks, although as was mentioned above, a dry cough may persist for 3 to 6 weeks.

If a bacterial etiology is suspected, antibiotics are indicated for 5 to 10 days. For both adults and children, amoxicillin, cephalosporins, and erythromycin are good choices. Patients who are at risk, such as those with asthma, chronic bronchitis, diabetes, congestive heart failure, and immunosuppression, should be considered for antibiotic therapy.

PATIENT EDUCATION

Patients who smoke are at risk for recurrence of acute bronchitis and possible chronic bronchitis. This may provide another opportunity to encourage smoking cessation. Since influenza A and influenza B are implicated as a cause of bronchitis, consideration should be given to annual flu vaccination in the fall.

BIBLIOGRAPHY

Berkow R (ed): *The Merck Manual of Diagnosis and Therapy,* 16th ed. Rahway, NJ, Merck Research Laboratories, 1992.

Cho-Chou K, Jackson LA, Campbell LA, et al: *Chlamydia pneumoniae* (TWAR). *Clin Microbiol Rev* 8(4):451–461, 1995.

George RB, Light RW, Matthay MA, Matthay RA (eds): *Chest Medicine: Essentials of Pulmonary and Critical Care Medicine,* 3d ed. Baltimore, Williams & Wilkins, 1995.

Griffith HW, Dambro MR, Griffith J: *The 5 Minute Clinical Consult.* Philadelphia, Lea & Febiger, 1994.

Henry D, Ruoff GE, Jackson R, et al: Effectiveness of short-course therapy (5 days) with cefuroxime axetil in treatment of secondary bacterial infections of acute bronchitis. *Antimicrob Agents Chemother* 39(11):2528–2534, 1995.

Hueston WJ: Albuterol delivered by metered-dose inhaler to treat acute bronchitis. *J Fam Pract* 39(5):437–440, 1994.

Labus JB: *The Physician Assistant Medical Handbook.* Philadelphia, Saunders, 1995.

Loughlin GM, Eigen H (eds): *Respiratory Disease in Children: Diagnosis and Management.* Baltimore, Williams & Wilkins, 1994.

Mainous AG, Zoorob RJ, Hueston WJ: Current management of acute bronchitis in ambulatory care: The use of antibiotics and bronchodilators. *Arch Fam Med* 5:79–83, 1996.

Myint S, Taylor-Robinson D (eds): *Viral and Other Infections of the Human Respiratory Tract.* London, Chapman & Hall, 1996.

Murray JF, Nadel JA: *Textbook of Respiratory Medicine,* 2d ed, vol 1. Philadelphia, Saunders, 1994.

Nolan TE: Upper respiratory and pulmonary problems. *Clin Obstet Gynecol* 38(1):147–155, 1995.

Thom DH, Grayston JT, Campbell LA, et al: *Eur J Clin Microbiol Infect Dis* 13(10):785–792, 1994.

Vogel F: A guide to the treatment of lower respiratory tract infections. *Drugs* 50(1):62–72, 1995.

Chapter 17–3
BRONCHIECTASIS
Catherine J. Heymann

DISCUSSION

The word *bronchiectasis* is derived from the Greek *bronchos* ("windpipe") and *ektaus* ("extension" or "stretching"). It is an abnormal, irreversible structural deformity of the medium-size and large bronchi that results in decreased mucus clearance, ciliary dysfunction, and dilated bronchi. Increased, pooled, and often purulent secretions produce the primary symptom: a chronic productive cough. Pooled secretions become a breeding ground for the growth of pathogens, culminating in recurrent pulmonary infections that are difficult to resolve and often involve unusual or resistant organisms.

Bronchiectasis may be acquired, congenital, or primary. Acquired bronchiectasis is either focal or diffuse in distribution and usually is acquired in childhood through recurrent pulmonary infections before the bronchial tree is fully developed. The current use of antibiotics for respiratory infections and immunizations for pertussis, measles, and influenza has significantly reduced the incidence of acquired bronchiectasis in the United States. Bronchiectasis acquired in adulthood is unusual and results from a severe necrotizing pulmonary infection such as tuberculosis. Primary congenital bronchiectasis is rare and results from genetically induced developmental abnormalities of the bronchial tree. However, several genetic disorders are associated with the development of primary bronchiectasis, including cystic fibrosis (50 percent of all cases),[1] primary ciliary dyskinesia (PCD), alterations in the immune system, yellow nail syndrome, congenital tracheobronchial anomalies, α_1-antitrypsin deficiency (AAD), and reactive airway disease (RAD).

PATHOGENESIS

Bronchiectasis begins with bronchial tube and/or interstitial tissue inflammation that is initiated by an infection at the epithelial surface. Once it has been initiated, the process is perpetuated by interaction between inflammatory, immune, and resident cells of the airway, resulting in airway damage, hyperactivity, tissue reorganization, and/or obstruction of the bronchi and the adjacent tissue. The walls of the bronchi become dilated and show inflammatory damage, chronic inflammation, increased mucus production, loss of cilia function, and decreased mucus clearance. Adjacent or distal to the bronchi, there may be alveolar, interstitial tissue, cartilage, muscle, or elastic tissue damage. Normal components of lung tissue are replaced by fibrous material, causing traction on the bronchial walls, further dilation of the bronchi, and loss of lung volume. As the disease progresses, increased vascularity of the bronchial walls may result in an anastomosis between pulmonary veins and arteries. Ultimately, right-to-left shunts may occur, causing hypoxia, cor pulmonale, and pulmonary hypertension.

Acquired Bronchiectasis

Bronchiectasis usually results from repeated infective episodes that cause direct bronchial destruction or mechanical obstruction before the bronchial tree has fully matured. Modern antibiotics, immunizations, and diagnostic techniques have reduced the incidence of acquired bronchiectasis in childhood. RAD, severe infection, obstruction (foreign body, tumor, lymph node enlargement), inhaled irritants (cigarette smoke, immunologically active substances such as silica, talc, Bakelite, and asbestos), and aspiration of gastric contents are rare causative agents of bronchiectasis in adults.

Primary Bronchiectasis

Primary bronchiectasis is often comorbid with congenitally acquired diseases. Damage to the immature bronchi usually results from altered host defense mechanisms that are unique to the specific genetic abnormality.

Cystic fibrosis (CF) is an autosomal recessive genetic disorder that manifests itself in childhood or infrequently in adolecence or early adulthood. The lungs of a newborn with CF are normal but soon deteriorate as a result of diffuse destruction of the small bronchi from abundant, very viscous secretions (see Chap. 7-1).

Primary ciliary dyskinesia (PCD) is an autosomal recessive disorder with incomplete penetrance that produces an abnormal ultrastructure of the cilia and poor mucociliary transport in all bodily systems. PCD produces a diffuse bronchiectasis from recurrent upper and lower respiratory infections. PCD may be present in up to 11 percent of children who present with chronic respiratory diseases. Young's syndrome and Kartagener's syndrome are subgroups of PCD, with the primary site of cilia dysfunction in the sinuses or genital tract and less frequently affecting the bronchial tree.

Immunodeficiency states may result in an abnormal response to a pathogen or allergen, causing bronchial damage through an accelerated infectious inflammatory response and decreased clearance of bronchial secretions. Immunodeficiencies include panhypergammaglobulinemia, common variable immune deficiency, and selective IgA, IgM, and/or IgG deficiencies.

AAD is a genetic disorder that classically presents as emphysema, cirrhosis, and/or pancreatitis in adolescence or early adulthood. Damage to tissues is caused by an imbalance between protease and protease inhibitors, causing a reduction in tissue elasticity.

Yellow nail syndrome (YNS) is thought to be a congenital hypoplasia of the lymphatic system characterized by primary lymphedema, exudative pleural effusion, and thick, curved yellow-green nails. Up to 40 percent of YNS patients develop bronchiectasis.[1,2]

Congenital tracheobronchial anomalies include tracheobronchomegaly and a complete or partial absence of bronchial cartilage beyond the segmental bronchi (Williams-Campbell syndrome).

The pathology of any underlying abnormality that results in the chronic pulmonary changes associated with bronchiectasis must be considered in selecting treatment options.

Microbiology

The pathogens associated with the development or exacerbation of bronchiectasis are numerous and may be related to comorbid diseases.

Necrotizing pneumonia from Klebsiella spp., staphylococci, influenza virus, fungi, anaerobes, atypical mycobacteria, or mycoplasma may be responsible for bronchiectasis. Severe pneumonia may complicate measles, pertussis, or adenovirus infections, causing significant pulmonary damage and bronchiectasis, especially in children. In third world countries, tuberculosis is the most common infection that initiates the pulmonary damage that causes bronchiectasis (see Chap. 9-31).

Allergic bronchopulmonary aspergillosis (ABPA) is an allergic reaction to a fungus in the bronchial lumen and a rare cause of acquired bronchiectasis.

Aspergillus fumigatus is the most common pathogen isolated. Histoplasmosis (see Chap. 9-32), coccidioidomycosis (valley fever) (see Chap. 9-7), cryptococcosis (see Chap. 9-8), blastomycosis, paracoccidioidomycosis (South America), and mucormycosis are less common and are found in specific geographic regions or immunologically compromised patients. In early CF, *Staphylococcus aureus* is a common pathogen. Later in the disease, *Pseudomonas aeruginosa* and *Pseudomonas cepacia* are more frequently isolated.

SYMPTOMS

A persistent cough, often with purulent mucus production, is the most frequently reported symptom. Occcasionally a dry chronic cough that is intermittently productive is the presenting complaint. Hemoptysis occurs infrequently but may be substantial (>200 to 600 mL/24 h). A few patients remain asymptomatic. With progression of the disease, disabling dyspnea, fatigue, weight loss, anemia (or polycythemia), cyanosis, clubbing of the nails, and hemoptysis may occur.

A fever with increased or a new onset of hemoptysis and/or purulent sputum indicates an infectious exacerbation of the underlying process or an adjacent pneumonia.

OBJECTIVE FINDINGS

Chest auscultation is quite variable. Abnormal inspiratory and/or expiratory rales and low-pitched expiratory rhonchi are common over the affected area. Fine inspiratory crackles may denote infection, interstitial disease, early pneumonia, or chronic heart failure. Coarse inspiratory crackles are indicative of late pulmonary disease and/or pneumonia. Diminished breath sounds and dullness to percussion may be noted over areas of severe inflammation, pooled secretions, or mucus plugging. Egophony (A to E sounds) and decreased tactile fremitus can be appreciated in areas of consolidation. Diaphragmatic movement and chest contour may be unchanged. Later signs of bronchiectasis include clubbing and cyanosis, but these signs usually do not appear until large areas

Table 17-3-1. Differential Diagnosis of Chronic Cough

Angiotensin-converting enzyme inhibitor: adverse reaction
Chronic sinusitis and/or rhinitis
Congestive heart failure
Cystic fibrosis
Esophageal disease
   Esophageal reflux
   Achalasia
   Zenker's diverticulum
Inhaled irritants (e.g., smoker's cough)
Mechanical irritants (e.g., postnasal drip)
Pericardial inflammation
Post-bronchitis syndrome
Postnasal drip:
   Psychogenic throat clearing
   Chest cough
Psychogenic cough
Pulmonary abscess
Pulmonary emboli
Pulmonary sequestration
Reactive airway disease
Respiratory infections
Tracheobronchial neoplasms
Tracheobronchial obstruction

of the bronchi and lung parenchyma are involved. Signs and symptoms of cor pulmonale or right ventricular failure are seen with massive lung involvement, pulmonary fibrosis, and arteriovenous shunting.

DIAGNOSTIC CONSIDERATIONS

A chronic cough defined by persistent or recurrent coughing can last for weeks or months. Establishing the cause of a chronic cough is essential in guiding therapy. Is the cough the result of an acute illness, a complication of another disease, bronchiectasis, or all three? The differential diagnosis for a persistent cough is large (Table 17-3-1).[1-5]

SPECIAL CONSIDERATIONS

Damage to the bronchi and the adjacent interstitial tissue may be initiated in childhood by viral or bacterial pneumonia, adenoviruses, foreign body obstruction, asthma, and influenza. With more children in day-care settings, exposure to potential pathogens has increased. Immunizations and appropriate antibiotic therapy for community-acquired infections constitute good preventive medicine.

LABORATORY STUDIES

Multiple causes of bronchiectasis and the necessity of treatment for any contributing disease provide a plethora of laboratory tests to utilize. Testing for an infective process includes a complete blood count (CBC) with differential to detect a "left shift" and a Gram stain of sputum with culture and sensitivity to identify an offending pathogen. Normochromic, normocytic anemia of chronic disease and polycythemia of chronic hypoxia also may be noted on a CBC.

Tests for genetic disorders that may induce bronchiectasis are more expensive and complicated. CF is diagnosed through a sweat chloride test (quantitative pilocarpine iontophoresis), with a result of >60 meq in a child or >80 meq in an adult considered abnormal. Primary ciliary dyskinesia can be diagnosed by abnormal cilia ultrastructure with electron-microscopic studies. Congenital immunologic deficiencies can be diagnosed by testing IgA, IgM, IgE, and IgG subclasses.

ABPA is recognized by "golden plugs" with hyphae in sputum, peripheral eosinophilia, rapid to intermediate skin reactivity to *Aspergillus* antigen, precipitating antibodies to *Aspergillus* antigen, and/or a markedly elevated IgE level. One should consider ABPA if a patient presents with pulmonary infiltrates and/or central bronchiectasis and a clinical history of asthma. AAD is diagnosed by α_1-trypsin phenotype and quantitation. Since this is a genetic disorder, all family members should be tested.

RADIOLOGIC STUDIES

High-resolution thin-section (1.5 mm) computed tomography (CT) has been reported to have high sensitivity (96 percent) and specificity (93 percent) in the diagnosis of bronchiectasis.[2] CT has replaced bronchography in most circumstances as the "gold standard" for diagnosis. The appearance of thick-walled circular cavities with or without fluid ("honeycombing") or thin parallel lines ("tram tracks") is diagnostic. Chest radiography can be normal in the early stages of disease, but the later stages may show changes similar to those seen on CT. The distribution of affected lung tissue may be an indicator of the contributing diagnosis in bronchiectasis (Table 17-3-2).[1,2]

In Kartagener's syndrome, a subclass of PCD, radiography also reveals dextrocardia and situs inversus.

Classically, three variations of bronchiectasis may be seen on x-ray or CT. Varicose bronchiectasis demonstrates an irregular, beaded pattern of dilated bronchi resembling varicose veins. Cystic or saccular bronchiectasis displays large sacs without recognizable structures distally. Cylindrical bronchiectasis shows dilated bronchi with blunt end-points where mucus obstructs the airway. Determination of the specific type of bronchiectasis has limited clinical significance and no impact on treatment modalities.

OTHER DIAGNOSTICS

Pulmonary function testing (PFT) may demonstrate obstructive or combined restrictive-obstructive disease that may improve with bronchodilators. If obstruction is suspected, fiberoptic bronchoscopy may visualize a foreign body, a tumor, or another localized tracheal or endobronchial abnormality. In severe disease or an acute exacerbation, oximetry helps define the degree of O_2 saturation and hypoxia. Arterial blood gases and assessment of P_{CO_2} define lung ventilatory function and CO_2 retention.

Table 17-3-2. Diagnostic Clues by Distribution of Bronchiectasis

Upper lobes
   Allergic bronchopulmonary aspergillosis
   Tuberculosis
   Histoplasmosis
   Histocytosis X
   Cystic fibrosis
Middle lobes
   Tuberculosis
   Cancer
   Middle lobe syndrome
Lower lobes
   Primary ciliary dyskinesia
   Swyer-James syndrome
   Cancer
   Sequestration
   Cystic fibrosis
   Diffuse bronchiolitis
   Infections
   Immune deficiencies

Table 17-3-3. Selection of Antibiotics for the Initial Treatment of Bronchiectasis

Amoxicillin 500 mg tid
Ampicillin 250–500 mg qid
Tetracycline 250–500 mg qid
Trimethoprim (160 mg)-sulfamethoxazole (800 mg) 1 tablet q 12 h
Amoxicillin-clavulanate 500 mg tid

TREATMENT

The major goals of treatment for bronchiectasis include

1. Detecting and treating any underlying cause
2. Improving clearance of tracheobronchial secretions
3. Controlling or preventing recurrent infections
4. Reversing airflow obstruction
5. Controlling or preventing complications

Treatment modalities encompass medications, chest physical therapy, patient education, and infrequently surgical resection or transplantation.

Pharmacologic management includes the use of antibiotics for acute infections, prophylactic antibiotics to prevent recurrent infections, and medications to manage restrictive-obstructive airway disease. Pathogens are usually mixed gram-negative and gram-positive, necessitating the use of a broad-spectrum antibiotic. Appropriate empiric antibiotic therapies are listed in Table 17-3-3.[1,2,6]

Further treatment should be guided by the isolation and identification of an organism or organisms by sputum smear, culture, and sensitivity. If no specific pathogen can be identified, alternating cycles of two or three antibiotics may be employed for 2 to 4 weeks. Since the most common pathogen for CF patients with recurrent infections is *P. aeruginosa* or *P. cepacia,* the initial therapy may consist of a quinolone (dose must be individualized) combined with an aminoglycoside (dose must be individualized) until another pathogen is isolated.

If restrictive and/or obstructive airway disease is present, additional pharmacologic treatments may include a combination of a beta agonist, theophylline, ipratropium bromide, and oral or inhaled corticosteroids. The use of these therapies is covered in Chap. 17-1.

Bronchopulmonary aspergillosis requires glucocorticoids to reduce bronchial inflammation. Prednisone (0.5 mg/kg/d) is preferably given in a single morning dose to reduce the incidence of adrenal suppression. Several weeks of therapy may be needed before one can taper to alternate-day dosing and discontinue the steroids. The addition of bronchodilators is useful, especially in acute episodes. No antibiotics are needed unless a secondary infection is suspected.

AAD can be treated effectively with gene therapy and should be referred to a qualified specialist. Gene therapy is now in clinical trials for CF patients.

Supportive measures include chest physical therapy and expectorants to facilitate the clearance of tracheobronchial secretions. Traditional chest physical therapy (PT) includes postural drainage, clapping, and vibration. CF patients may require chest PT one or more times per day chronically. Bronchiectasis patients without CF may need chest PT only on an intermittent basis.

Patient education should include cautions against smoking, secondhand smoke, exposure to known inhalant irritants and asthmatic triggers, and the use of antitussives or sedatives (depress pulmonary function). Advice regarding a healthy diet, exercise, and stress reduction is an important component of patient education.

Disposition includes follow-up on a routine basis for basic medical care, monitoring for any deterioration in pulmonary status, and reevaluation of the treatment plan. At the first signs and/or symptoms of an upper respiratory infection, intensive antibiotic therapy should be instituted. A follow-up visit should be scheduled within 7 to 10 days to assure resolution of the infection. Routine influenza immunizations and one-time Pneumovax are appropriate for patients with compromised pulmonary status.

COMPLICATIONS AND RED FLAGS

Intensive management of upper respiratory infections and bronchiectasis may prevent or slow the progression of the disease and reduce the severity of complications such as protracted dyspnea, cyanosis, respiratory acidosis, obstruction, recurrent pneumonia, chronic infections, cor pulmonale, pulmonary hypertension, and pulmonary fibrosis. Infection in bronchiectasis patients rarely results in septicemia or a localization of an abscess at a remote site (e.g., brain).

Hemoptysis may be massive and life-threatening. Surgical resection of areas of bleeding pulmonary tissue may be required. Surgery or heart-lung transplantation may be considered if a patient has disabling hypoxia and/or significant localized disease.

NOTES AND PEARLS

Low-grade bronchiectasis probably is underdiagnosed. A chronic cough or bronchial infection that does not clear with standard therapy is a red flag for further evaluation. The threshold for suspicion of bronchiectasis should be lowered in patients with risk factors for pulmonary disease or congenital or acquired diseases associated with bronchiectasis. As with any chronic disease capable of disabling a patient without optimal control, an evaluation and a consultation with a specialist (pulmonologist) are desirable.

REFERENCES

1. Fauci AS, Braunwald E, Isselbacher KJ, et al (eds): *Harrison's Principles of Internal Medicine,* 14th ed. New York, McGraw-Hill, 1998.
2. Marwah OS, Sharma OF: Bronchiectasis. *Postgrad Med* 97:149–159, 1995.
3. Adler SN, Lam M, Gasbarra DB, Conners AF: *A Pocket Manual of Differential Diagnosis,* 3d ed. Boston, Little, Brown, 1994.
4. Greenberger NJ, Agee KR, King TM, Newson M: *The Medical Book of Lists,* 3d ed. St Louis, Mosby Year Book, 1990.
5. *Drug Facts and Comparison,* 50th ed. New York, Wolter Kluwer, 1996.
6. Stauffer JL: Lung, in *Current Medical Diagnosis and Treatment,* 34th ed. Stamford, CT, Appleton & Lange, 1995, pp 203–225.

BIBLIOGRAPHY

Barker AF: Bronchiectasis. *Semin Thorac Cardiovasc Surg* 7(2):112–118, 1995.
Berge E, Os I, Skjorten F, Svalander C: Alpha I-antitrypsin deficiency—not only pulmonary and hepatic involvement. *Tidsskr Nor Laegeforen* 115(7):8232–8236, 1995.
Berkow R (ed): *The Merck Manual of Diagnosis and Therapy,* 16th ed. Rahway NJ, Merck, 1992.
Curiel DT, Pilewski JM: Gene therapy approaches for inherited and acquired lung disease. *Am J Respir Cell Mol Biol* 14(1):1–18, 1996.
Knoell DI, Wewers MD: Clinical implications of gene therapy for alpha I-antitrypsin deficiency. *Chest* 107(2):535–545, 1995.
Lee PH, Carr DH, Rubens MB, et al: Accuracy of CT in predicting the cause of bronchiectasis. *Clin Radiol* 50(12):839–841, 1995.
Patrick H, Patrick F: *Comm Med Prob Ambulatory Care* 79:361–372, 1995.
Rabassa AA, Schwartz MR, Ertan A: Alpha I-antitrypsin deficiency and chronic pancreatitis. *Dig Dis Sci* 40(9):1997–2001, 1995.
Ray D, Saha K, Date A, Jairaj PS: Raised serum IgE levels in chronic inflammatory lung diseases. *Ceylon Med J* 40(1):14–18, 1995.

Reiff DB, Wells AU, Carr DH, et al: CT findings in bronchiectasis: Limited value in distinguishing between idiopathic and specific types. *AJR Am J Roentgenol* 165(2):261–267, 1995.

Shelhamer JH: Airway Inflammation. *Ann Intern Med* 123:288–304, 1995.

Tasaka S, Kanazawa M, Mori M, et al: Long-term course of bronchiectasis and bronchiolitis obliterans as late complication of smoke inhalation. *Respiration* 62(1):40–42, 1995.

Chapter 17–4
LARYNGOTRACHEOBRONCHITIS (CROUP)

John P. Donnelly

DISCUSSION

Viral laryngotracheobronchitis (LTB), or croup, is one of the most common childhood illnesses of the upper respiratory tract. LTB primarily affects children age 6 months to 6 years, with the peak incidence occurring at age 2.[1,2] LTB has a seasonal affinity, with peaks in the fall and winter. Parainfluenza viruses appear to be the main isolate in LTB. Other viruses, such as influenza virus, rhinovirus, and respiratory syncytial virus, also can be causative agents, though to a lesser degree. LTB causes airway obstruction through inflammation and edema of the subglottic region of the larynx. Most cases of LTB are mild; however, 1.5 to 15 percent of cases[3] require hospitalization for management of the airway. Because LTB is very common, practitioners sometimes forget that some infants require intubation as part of their management.

PATHOGENESIS

Transmission of LTB occurs by direct contact[1,4] with an incubation period of 2 to 5 days. Children often have an antecedent history of an upper respiratory infection for several days before the office visit. LTB is characterized by the typical barking cough, low-grade fever, and inspiratory stridor. The male to female ratio is about even at 1.5 : 1.[3] The main pathologic feature of LTB is the mucosal edema that causes the characteristic barking cough, which can progress to severe respiratory distress. As a result of the small size of an infant's larynx, slight edema, as is seen in LTB, can create marked changes in the lumen available for airflow. Stridor and retractions become severe with small increases in the relative edema of the subglottic regions. It has been suggested that a 1-mm increase in edema of the subglottic region of an infant's airway can result in a 50 percent reduction of the diameter of the trachea.[4] LTB may affect the small airways as well. This may result in respiratory distress from both narrowing of the upper airway at the level of the cricoid and parenchymal lung and small airway inflammation.

SIGNS AND SYMPTOMS

LTB usually presents with an antecedent history of an upper respiratory illness for 1 to 3 days. Symptoms include nasal discharge and congestion followed by the typical barking cough and hoarseness. A low-grade fever may be present, typically higher than 37.8°C (100°F).

Stridor, when present, tends to be high-pitched and is more severe in inspiration. Retractions may be present when stridor is severe. Stridor at rest with retractions is an indication for hospitalization.[2] The respiratory rate is commonly increased to 35 to 40 breaths per minute but is usually less than 50. This helps distinguish LTB from bronchiolitis. Symptoms in LTB can fluctuate in severity from morning to evening or from hour to hour.

OBJECTIVE FINDINGS

The typical patient with LTB exhibits a barking cough with or without inspiratory (and less commonly expiratory) stridor and hoarseness. These patients also may exhibit wheezing and a prolonged expiratory phase secondary to lower airway involvement. Retractions may be present when airway obstruction progresses secondary to subglottic edema. Examination of the chest may reveal typical coarse breath sounds or wheezing when small airways are involved. Hypoxia may be present in more severe cases and is best evaluated by pulse oximetry. Anteroposterior and lateral x-rays of the neck usually reveal the subglottic narrowing with the typical "pencil tip or steeple sign."

DIFFERENTIAL DIAGNOSIS

During the evaluation of a child with LTB one must be sure to distinguish between LTB and epiglottitis (see Chap. 4-5). Epiglottitis is one of the most dangerous and rapidly progressive pediatric airway infections. Patients with epiglottitis are acutely ill and may have a muffled voice, dysphagia, and drooling. X-rays of the neck are usually sufficient to differentiate between these two illnesses. Epiglottitis involves the supraglottic structures, and the pencil or steeple sign on x-ray is absent (although there is some controversy regarding the reliability of x-rays in the acute setting). The epiglottis is normal in LTB but is markedly erythematous and edematous in epiglottitis. Direct evaluation of the throat in suspected cases of epiglottitis should be carried out by specialists in a hospital setting because of the incidence of acute airway obstruction and the need for intubation. LTB is accompanied by the typical barking cough, which is absent in epiglottitis. Epiglottitis is most commonly caused by *Haemophilus* spp. and is less frequently seen now that vaccines (HibTITER, PedvaxHIB, ProHIBiT) have become widespread. Other possible agents in epiglottitis include pneumococcal, staphylococcal, and streptococcal bacteria.

Bacterial tracheitis (also called membranous laryngotracheobronchitis and membranous croup) is caused by *Staphylococcus aureus, Haemophilus influenzae* type B, or group A beta-hemolytic streptococci. Bacterial tracheitis is rare and may be more difficult to rule out. The child generally appears more toxic but has cough and stridor similar to those seen in viral LTB. Pharyngitis and progressive stridor follow a gradual onset and usually necessitate hospitalization to manage the airway. Hospitalization and endotracheal intubation are required in 80 to 85 percent of all cases of bacterial tracheitis. In suspected bacterial tracheitis, endoscopy in a controlled setting should be considered to manage the airway and remove the tenacious secretions that accompany this illness.

Spasmodic croup presents with symptoms similar to those of LTB, but the patient is generally without fever or a barking cough. The cause of spasmodic croup is unclear, but the croup may be due to allergic mediation or a virus. Differentiation from

LTB on a clinical basis is difficult. Spasmotic LTB resolves in 3 to 6 h, and no specific treatment is needed. Children with repeated bouts of LTB often are diagnosed with spasmodic croup.

SPECIAL CONSIDERATIONS

LTB may progress to severe stridor and respiratory distress. Hospitalization may be required to manage the airway. Endotracheal intubation (ETT) may be necessary for a short time until the subglottic edema subsides. Infants who are HIV-positive may have more severe LTB and a greater degree of subglottic narrowing. These patients should be admitted to the hospital for careful airway management. In children with hypoxia, parenchymal involvement must be assumed whether it is observed on chest x-ray or not.

LABORATORY TESTS

There are no specific laboratory assays to diagnose LTB. The disease is usually viral in nature, and the white blood cell count is usually normal. Pulse oximetry or arterial blood gases may be helpful in patients with severe stridor and retractions to rule out hypoxia.

RADIOLOGIC STUDIES

X-rays of the neck are helpful in distinguishing between LTB and epiglottitis or bacterial tracheitis. LTB presents with the typical pencil sign of subglottic narrowing. Bacterial tracheitis (membranous LTB) presents with irregular subglottic densities caused by the tenacious secretions. If epiglottitis is suspected, the evaluation should be confirmed by direct examination of the supraglottic larynx in a hospital setting.

TREATMENT

Humidification is widely used as a first-line treatment of LTB. Children often appear to improve after sitting in a steamy bathroom or breathing cool nighttime air. However, there are no proven benefits to this therapy. Bourchier[5] failed to show a therapeutic benefit in the first 12 h using humidification only. The child may derive indirect benefit from the calming effect of being held by a caring parent, thus reducing crying and the increased stridor it produces. Supplemental oxygen is important for hypoxemic patients with a $Pa_{O_2} < 60$ mmHg.

Epinephrine has become the cornerstone of treatment for exacerbations of LTB. Racemic epinephrine delivered by a nebulizer has both alpha- and beta-adrenergic activity. The alpha-adrenergic activity constricts the subglottic mucosal and submucosal capillaries; the beta-adrenergic activity acts on smooth muscle in the lower respiratory tract.[4] Recommended doses are 0.25 mL of a 1 : 1000 solution of epinephrine for children younger than age 6 months. Older children may receive 0.5 mL. Nebulized epinephrine lasts approximately 2 h and may be associated with a rebound effect. Studies have suggested that it does not improve arterial oxygen levels.

The necessity of hospitalizing children after nebulized epinephrine because of the rebound effect is somewhat controversial. Cressman and Myer[4] stated that any child who receives a treatment should be admitted for observation because a relapse or rebound effect may occur. Bank and Krug[1] stated that studies have shown that the rebound phenomenon does not exist. Rather than a worsening of pretreatment symptoms by a rebound effect, some authors[6,7] have demonstrated that children who have received nebulized racemic epinephrine tend to return to their pretreatment levels of distress when the medication wears off in 2 to 3 h. Therefore, the current data support outpatient treatment of mild to moderate croup with nebulized epinephrine. Hospitalization solely because of epinephrine use may not be necessary.

Nebulized epinephrine also has been shown to decrease the need for an artificial airway.[8,9] The side effects of epinephrine are rare, but great caution should be used in patients with left ventricular outflow obstruction such as idiopathic subaortic stenosis and tetralogy of Fallot. Children who receive racemic epinephrine also should be treated with steroids to prevent the need for further treatments.

Steroid use in the treatment of LTB is widespread but remains controversial. Most experts agree that the trials and studies thus far have been inadequate. Compared with controls, children who received steroids were less likely to require intubation and had a somewhat more rapid resolution of the stridor.[1] The consensus appears to favor the utilization of dexamethasone 0.6 to 1.0 mg/kg intramuscularly, intravenously, or orally. The oral route is preferable as it is less likely to produce crying and agitation. No adverse effects have been reported with the use of steroids in the management of croup. Children who receive nebulized epinephrine should receive steroids regardless of their disposition.[1]

Children are candidates for outpatient therapy for LTB when they

1. Do not appear toxic
2. Are well hydrated and able to handle fluids and secretions
3. Have minimal or no stridor or retractions at rest or for at least 2 to 3 h after the first nebulized epinephrine treatment
4. Have reliable parents who can transport them to a hospital if the condition worsens[1,3]

Parents should be informed that the condition may worsen and require hospitalization or further outpatient therapy.

The need for airway support in LTB is rare, but when medical therapy fails to resolve respiratory distress, intubation must be considered. Patients who exhibit changes in mental status caused by hypoxia or hypercarbia and those who require treatments with epinephrine more frequently than every 1 to 2 h are candidates for intubation. In intubating an LTB patient, it is necessary to use a tube with a diameter 0.5 mm smaller than what would be used for a normal child in an effort to reduce the risk of subglottic stenosis.[4] When intubation is required, the nasotracheal route is preferable.

A convenient algorithm by Bank and Krug[1] for the treatment of LTB divides the symptoms into mild and moderate to severe.

REFERENCES

1. Bank DE, Krug SE: New approaches to upper respiratory airway disease. *Emerg Med Clin North Am* 13(2):473–487, 1995.
2. Wright AL, Taussig LM, Ray CG, et al: The Tucson Children's Respiratory Study II: Lower respiratory tract illness in the first year of life. *Am J Epidemiol* 129(6):1232–1246, 1989.
3. Skolnik N: Croup. *J Fam Pract* 37(2):165–170, 1993.
4. Cressman WR, Myer CM III: Diagnosis and management of croup and epiglottitis. *Pediatr Clin North Am* 41(2):265–276, 1994.
5. Bourchier D, Dawson KP, Fergusson DM: Humidification in viral croup: A controlled trial. *Aust Paediatr J* 20:289–291, 1984.
6. Kelley P, Simon J: Racemic epinephrine use in croup and disposition. *Am J Emerg Med* 10:181–183, 1992.
7. Wussow K, Krug SE, Yamashita T: Duration of clinical response to racemic epinephrine in children with croup. *Pediatr Emerg Care* 8:306, 1992.
8. Adair JC, Ring WH, Jordan WS, et al: Ten year experience with IPPB in the treatment of acute laryngotracheobronchitis. *Anesth Analg* 50:649–655, 1971.
9. Taussig LM, Castro O, Beaudry PH, et al: Treatment of laryngotracheobronchitis (croup): Use of intermittent positive pressure breathing and racemic epinephrine. *Am J Dis Child* 129:790–793, 1975.

Chapter 17–5
PNEUMOTHORAX

Barry A. Cassidy

DISCUSSION

The pathophysiology and consequences of pneumothorax are better understood after review of the mechanisms of respiration. For the lung to exchange gases properly, it must be capable of expanding. Lung inflation is maintained by a negative pressure differential between the pleural space and the alveoli. Downward contraction of the diaphragm creates a bellows-like effect that

1. Increases the area of the lung
2. Passively moves air into the lung
3. Generates a negative pressure differential between the lung and the outside atmosphere[1]

The visceral pleura and parietal pleura separate alveolar tissues from the chest wall. During embryologic development, the pleura envelops the lungs, separating them from the heart and mediastinum, and then folds back on itself, covering the chest wall cavity and creating the pleural space. Pleural fluid in the intact pleural space allows the visceral pleura and parietal pleura to move on each other without friction.[2]

Any mechanism (external or internal) that interrupts the integrity of the pleural space, allowing air to enter, disrupts the negative pressure differential between the lungs and the outside atmosphere and results in a pneumothorax (air in the thorax). Pneumothorax is a common entity and is characterized as primary (spontaneous and not related to an underlying lung disorder) or secondary (related to an underlying lung disorder).

A high degree of suspicion for pneumothorax can be based on the patient's situation:

1. Penetrating trauma to the chest can cause a pneumothorax.
2. Patients, particularly smokers, with chronic obstructive pulmonary disease (COPD) develop spontaneous ruptures of blebs, resulting in secondary pneumothorax.
3. Iatrogenic pneumothorax occurs secondary to the attempted insertion of central venous lines, after lung biopsies, after chest surgery, etc.
4. Patients receiving positive-pressure ventilation from a ventilatory treatment such as intermittent positive-pressure breathing (IPPB) or intubated and on a positive-pressure ventilator are prone to develop pneumothorax.

Less likely etiologies of pneumothorax include menstruation (catamenial), blunt trauma from diving injuries or being near large explosions, pressurization changes during descent in an airplane, and deceleration injuries from automobile accidents. Spontaneous secondary pneumothorax is reported to occur in anywhere from 2.5 to 18 per 100,000 persons and is more commonly found in males than in females. The burden falls on the clinician to determine how the air got into the pleural space and what, if anything, should be done about it.

Understanding the mechanism of injury helps prevent a clinician from making the life-threatening mistake of missing a tension pneumothorax or performing a needless and dangerous invasive procedure. In most cases, the clinician relies on the chest x-ray to diagnose pneumothorax and determine a therapeutic plan. However, a chest x-ray can be a major cause of misdiagnosis. The following scenarios have all happened to this author:

- In an emergency department, a chest x-ray clearly showed a large tension pneumothorax. A chest tube was placed by a first-year resident. The physical findings, however, did not fit the noncommunicative patient's presentation (the x-ray technician put the wrong name on the x-ray; the patient in the room across the hall had the tension pneumothorax).
- A patient with chronic bullous emphysema had an overpenetrated x-ray that appeared to show a significant pneumothorax. The house staff was poised to place a chest tube, but the attending physician asked that CT be performed since the patient was stable (the CT revealed that the area in question was a large bulla, not a pneumothorax).
- An intubated unconscious patient on a ventilator developed respiratory distress. The supine portable chest x-ray revealed what appeared to be a collapsed lung with the edges of the pleura visible and no visible lung markings peripheral to the pleura. The placement of a chest tube did not improve the patient's condition, and air was not seen in the air leak chamber when the tube was inserted (in reality, what appeared to be pleura was actually a fold in the bedsheet; the patient improved with vigorous suctioning of the endotracheal tube).

It is imperative to make sure the patient's presentation fits the x-ray. The patient's history often reveals the disease process. For instance:

1. Trauma to the chest can lead to the suspicion that the integrity of the parietal pleura has been compromised.
2. A history of emphysema with acute respiratory distress may lead to the assumption that the integrity of the visceral pleura has been compromised as a result of a ruptured bleb.
3. A history of bullous emphysema with chronic dyspnea alerts the practitioner to watch for large bullae that may masquerade as a pneumothorax.
4. A large area of radiolucency of the left lung field with no evidence of atelectatic lung near the inferior mediastinum may represent severe gastric distention into the thorax with displacement of the lung into the apex of the thoracic cavity.

OBJECTIVE FINDINGS

Although the physical examination of a patient with a pneumothorax follows a logical pathway, it is not pathognomonic. In the presence of pneumothorax, one might predict such things as asymmetric chest expansion, tympany on percussion, absent breath sounds, and significant dyspnea if the pneumothorax is substantial in size. However, many of these findings can be present with other conditions, such as large bullae, atelectasis, a pulmonary embolus, lobar consolidation, effusion, and a hiatal hernia.

The chest x-ray serves as the most valuable tool in making the diagnosis of pneumothorax. If the patient is stable, an end-expiration view will show the smaller pneumothorax better than will an end-inspiration view. Lateral decubitus views help find an anterior air collection often missed on the anteroposterior (AP) and posteroanterior (PA) chest x-ray views and differentiates pneumothorax from skin folds in obese patients. Experienced clinicians, however, do not underestimate the importance of historic and physical findings.

DIAGNOSTIC CONSIDERATIONS

On inspection, the patient's general status reveals much about the seriousness of the disease process. Severe dyspnea, tachypnea, tachycardia, jugular venous distention, extreme agitation, asymmetric chest expansion, tracheal deviation, poor oxygen saturation, signs of cyanosis, and hemodynamic instability in patients who are at high risk for pneumothorax (sustained recent chest trauma, post-central line insertion, on a ventilator or with chronic pulmonary disease, etc.) are symptoms highly indicative of tension pneumothorax.

A tension pneumothorax occurs when air is allowed to enter the pleural space but cannot egress (creating a one-way-valve situation). In this setting, pressure continues to increase, causing collapse of the ipsilateral lung, depression of the diaphragm, shifting of the mediastinum, obstruction of the inflow of blood (vena cava) into the right atrium, decreased cardiac output, cardiac arrhythmias, and ultimately electromechanical disassociation. Thus, a tension pneumothorax is a medical emergency and requires immediate treatment. The placement of a chest tube to water-seal suction is the treatment of choice; however, if the materials are not immediately available, placement of a large-bore (12- to 14-gauge) Intracath needle into the chest wall (generally the second intercostal space in the midclavicular line) will temporarily release the pressure of a tension pneumothorax until the pleural space can be controlled with a chest tube. A plastic Intracath needle should be used so that the sharp needle bore can be removed before it punctures the expanding lung after insertion.[3]

SPECIAL CONSIDERATIONS

The insertion of a needle is not an innocuous procedure, and the clinical index of suspicion of tension pneumothorax should be high before the procedure is done. If a pneumothorax is not present (particularly in a patient with emphysematous disease), the insertion of a needle into the chest wall can puncture the lung, probably create an air leak resulting in a pneumothorax, and potentially infect the pleural space, possibly leading to the development of an empyema.

Patients on ventilators who have a sudden desaturation of blood and develop dysrhythmias recalcitrant to DC cardioversion should be suspect for possible pneumothorax (the dead air space will not conduct the electric current).

RADIOLOGIC STUDIES

Pneumothorax on chest x-ray is often reported in terms of a percentage of thoracic space filled by lung. A 10 percent pneumothorax implies that 90 percent of the lung remains inflated while the remaining 10 percent of the thoracic cavity is filled with air. This method of measurement is somewhat arbitrary and has led some researchers to suggest that a pneumothorax should be reported in terms of actual measurement of the area of air seen on the AP or PA and lateral (LAT) chest films (e.g., 2 cm by 10 cm). This method seems preferable, particularly if a physician assistant is describing x-ray findings on the phone.

TREATMENT

Roentgenographic findings of pneumothorax can be coincidental. Patients admitted to the hospital may be found to have small pneumothoraces; others are found on routine chest x-rays for workups of coughs or illnesses. The difficulty for the clinician is to decide what, if any, therapy to offer the patient. The cause, size, and changes of the pneumothorax determine in large part what treatment will be given.

A patient who develops a pneumothorax after an attempted invasive procedure (e.g., placement of a central venous line) probably will get a chest tube. Certainly this type of patient must be watched closely. The cause of such a pneumothorax is the needle puncturing the lung. The hole in the lung allows air to leak into the pleural space, and if this is allowed to continue, the increased pressure will collapse the lung. The pleural space cannot seal a break in the integrity of the pleura if the visceral and the

parietal pleura are not in contact. Therefore, air leaks that occur from the lung parenchyma itself usually require the placement of a chest tube. Once the negative pressure is reestablished in the pleural space by means of water-sealed suction, the pleura can heal itself.

One should note the type of air leak present in the air leak chamber after the insertion of a chest tube. An air leak (bubbles in some systems and fluttering valves in others) should be present upon expiration. (The air leak chamber consists of several small columns of water in most pleural drainage systems and should not be confused with the single water seal chamber that indicates centimeters of water pressure and slowly bubbles.) If a continuous air leak is present (on both inspiration and expiration), one should first look for a major system leak in the tubing. If no system leak is found, a thoracic surgeon should be called immediately, as there is a massive hole in the lung or a bronchial leak. This can be extremely critical, particularly if the patient has undergone recent thoracic surgery.

Sometimes small leaks can occur that manage to seal themselves. In this situation, the size of the pneumothorax remains the same and the patient can be observed without the placement of a chest tube as long as no significant increase in the pneumothorax occurs. When the source of the air leak is stopped, the remaining air in the pleural space is reabsorbed in a matter of a days to weeks.

A spontaneous pneumothorax should be watched closely. If the area of air seen on the chest x-ray is small and the leak continues, a chest tube should be placed. Ironically, a larger pneumothorax (provided that there is no tension pneumothorax) adds to the safety of the chest tube placement, as the air collapses the lung and protects the examiner from hitting the lung with the instruments. A trocar (a heavy metal skewer with an angled point) is inserted into some chest tubes and used to push through the pleura. Many physicians feel that trocar chest tubes are dangerous, particularly in the hands of an inexperienced user. A much safer means of insertion involves cutting down with a scalpel to the chest wall in a controlled manner, taking a Kelly clamp or scalpel, puncturing or cutting the pleura, introducing a finger to widen the incision, and then inserting the chest tube; this method protects any nearby organs and those stuck to the chest wall. A great deal of damage can be done if one is not familiar with chest tube insertion.

Patients on ventilators who develop pneumothorax probably will need the placement of a chest tube. The positive pressure probably will cause a continuous air leak, and placement of the chest tube will be essential. Generally, chest tubes placed while a patient is on a ventilator are left in until the ventilator is removed or the amount of positive pressure can be decreased significantly. Chest tubes that have been in place for an extended period may become clogged with fibrous material and become nonfunctional. There is no advantage to leaving a nonfunctioning chest tube in place.

A stable outpatient who complains of shortness of breath or an episode of sharp pleuritic chest pain and is found to have a pneumothorax can pose a treatment dilemma. Not all patients require chest tubes. Patients with recurrent pneumothorax should be referred to a thoracic surgeon. Treatment of recurrent pneumothorax can be accomplished by the instillation of a chemical irritant. These agents work by causing a chemical irritation of both the visceral and the parietal pleura. This inflammatory reaction induces the formation of adhesions that hold the pleural spaces together and cause eventual obliteration of the pleural space. Unfortunately, chemical pleurodesis, although very easy to perform, particularly with a chest tube in place, causes severe pain to the patient. There are a variety of "cocktails" to do chemical pleurodesis, such as doxycycline, talc, cisplatin, and tetracycline. Most contain a local anesthetic such as lidocaine. Regardless of the type of local anesthetic used, this remains a very painful procedure. Ironically, the more the procedure hurts, the more likely it is that the lung will remain adherent. Ample premedication should be given, and the patient should be warned that the procedure will be painful.

In most cases, chest tubes are left in until 12 to 24 h after the air leak stops. Some patients may have persistent air leaks, and their chest tubes are left in place for 3 weeks. At the end of the 3-week time frame, most lungs become adherent to the chest wall.

Some clinicians remove the chest tube after chemical or mechanical pleurodesis and insert a new chest tube if the lung collapses. Compliant patients may be sent home with continuous air leaks after the placement of a Heimlich tube (a "flutter" valve attached to the chest tube that lets air exit the pleural space and not reenter it) and followed on an outpatient basis until the air leak stops.

Mechanical pleurodesis is another alternative and can be accomplished via thoracoscopic surgery or through the traditional thoracotomy incision. The pleura is rubbed briskly with Brillo-type pads or with instruments that irritate it. This requires a general anesthetic but is much more comfortable for the patient. Once pleurodesis has been performed (either chemical or mechanical), the lung should become adherent to the chest wall. This adds risk and difficulty to any future lung surgery. The patient should be told to inform future physicians that pleurodesis has been performed.

REFERENCES

1. Witten ML: General overview of the pulmonary system. http://www.physiol.arizona.edu, 1996.
2. Lewis CE, Colt HG: Pleural effusion from diagnostic thoracentesis to thoracoscopy. *Phys Assist* 20(5):68–83, 1996.
3. Pluth JR: Personal communication, July 12, 1996.

Chapter 17–6
PNEUMOCYSTIS CARINII PNEUMONIA
Claire Babcock O'Connell

DISCUSSION

Controversy over the classification of *Pneumocystis* still exists; most microbiologists classify the organism as a fungus, but many clinicians believe it is a protozoon. Regardless, *Pneumocystis carinii* pneumonia (PCP) remains the most important respiratory condition and the most common AIDS-defining illness in HIV disease. The first cluster of opportunistic respiratory disease in gay men in San Francisco and New York in the early 1980s proved to be PCP. The incidence and mortality of PCP have declined since the development of advanced diagnostic and therapeutic methods; however, it remains the most common threat to patients with HIV. When untreated, PCP is uniformly fatal in HIV-positive patients.

Pneumocystis carinii is a ubiquitous microbe, and infection in humans is common. Serologic studies show that virtually all children have been exposed to the organism within the first few years of life. Inhalation of the cyst form is the most common route of transmission. Disease in immunocompetent persons is rare. It is not known whether the infection lies dormant or if a new infection causes disease in an immunosuppressed host. Outbreaks in late winter or after epidemics of other respiratory illnesses and clusters of infection in groupings of immunosuppressed hosts suggest that the organism is spread from human to human.

The organism exists in the lungs in two forms—the trophozoite and the cyst—that can be viewed with special staining. Propagation is slow and causes the accumulation of foamy alveolar exudates. Cell membrane permeability is altered, leading to impaired gas exchange and a reduction in diffusing capacity and lung compliance. Pneumocystic therapy also is associated with a release of tumor necrosis factor α and interleukins from the alveoli, which causes a further inflammatory reaction. Alveolar hypertrophy, interstitial edema, and fibrosis occur, which further compromise respiratory function.

More than 90 percent of PCP infections occur with CD4+ T-cell counts below $100/\mu L^3$. PCP also is encountered in patients with higher T-cell counts if the count has been rapidly declining or in the presence of opportunistic infections such as thrush.

SYMPTOMS

PCP typically presents with a chronic, nonproductive cough and dyspnea. The onset is insidious, and fever is common. Fatigue and weight loss are not unusual. The symptoms are usually very subtle, but the presentation can be quite variable. Symptom duration does not correlate with severity or prognosis.

OBJECTIVE FINDINGS

The lung examination in patients with PCP is generally normal. Some patients (<40 percent) may have rales, usually late in the course of the illness. Cyanosis, tachypnea, retractions, and wheezing are less common and may indicate severe disease.

Arterial blood gases reveal hypoxemia and respiratory alkalosis. Pulmonary function testing confirms hypoxemia in almost all patients. The level of hypoxemia often is used as an indicator of disease severity. Pao_2 is <80 mmHg in over 80 percent of cases. Other abnormalities include an increased alveolar-arterial oxygen gradient and a reduced carbon monoxide diffusing capacity.

Bronchoalveolar lavage is very sensitive and has become the cornerstone of diagnosis. Sampling from involved sites carries a very high yield of organisms. Transbronchial biopsy and sputum induction also may aid in the diagnosis of PCP.

DIAGNOSTIC CONSIDERATIONS

The differential diagnosis of PCP includes many other respiratory pathogens and conditions. Many other diseases may be evident concurrently. Table 17-6-1 provides a list of conditions commonly seen in HIV-positive patients that should be included in the differential.

LABORATORY TESTS

CD4+ T-cell counts below $100/\mu L^3$ are typical with PCP infection. Elevated lactic dehydrogenase (LDH), although nonspecific, can be used to aid in the differentiation of PCP from other respiratory illnesses in HIV-positive patients. Very high levels of LDH are correlated with an increased risk of death. Therapy for PCP can be monitored through decreasing LDH values.

RADIOLOGIC STUDIES

The typical chest x-ray in a PCP patient demonstrates a bilateral interstitial infiltrate, although the radiographic appearance of

Table 17-6-1. PCP Differential Diagnoses to Consider in HIV-Positive Patients

Mycobacterium tuberculosis
Haemophilus pneumoniae
Cryptococcus neoformans
Invasive cytomegalovirus pneumonitis
Kaposi's sarcoma
Streptococcus pneumoniae
Staphylococcus aureus
Mycobacterium avium
Legionella pneumophila
Coccidioidomycosis
Nocardiosis
Mycoplasma pneumoniae
Blastomycosis
Histoplasmosis
Aspergillosis
Lymphoid interstitial pneumonitis
Other mycobacterial species
Carcinoma
Chlamydia spp.
Toxoplasmosis
Strongyloides spp.

PCP can be highly variable. The changes usually are seen initially in the perihilar area and spread to the lower and then the upper lobes. The apices typically are spared unless the patient has received aerosolized pentamidine treatment. The infiltrate is typically diffuse, although specific areas of infection may be seen. Nodules, cavitary lesions, and pleural effusion may occur; if found, they should prompt a definitive diagnosis to prevent a misdiagnosis.

Gallium scans may show increased uptake in areas of infection, especially in patients who are suspected to be infected but present with normal chest x-rays. However, scans are not specific to PCP, and the rate of false-positives is high. Computed tomography also reveals diffuse alveolar infiltrates and bronchial wall thickening.

DIAGNOSIS

Identification of the organism is necessary for a definitive diagnosis. The cyst form is easily identified from induced sputum or bronchoalveolar lavage specimens using special stains (Giemsa, cresyl echt violet, methenamine silver). Diff-Quik and Papanicolaou stains help identify trophozoites. Immunofluorescence and polymerase chain reactions are also helpful for identifying both the cyst form and the trophozoite. Induced sputum specimens that are negative do not rule out the diagnosis in patients suspected to have PCP. Repeat sputum or bronchoscopy is recommended. There is no useful technique for culturing the organism.

TREATMENT

Pharmacologic Management

PCP is treated with pentamidine or trimethoprim-sulfamethoxazole [TMP-SMX (Bactrim, Septra)]. Both drugs are effective against the organism. Mild to moderate disease is commonly treated with 15 mg/kg/d TMP and 75 mg/kg/d SMX in three to four divided doses given orally for 21 days. If the patient is unable to tolerate oral drugs, the same dose is given intravenously, or intravenous pentamidine can be given in a single dose of 4 mg/kg.

Clinical improvement of PCP in HIV-positive patients is usually slow, and radiographic evidence of improvement is delayed. Often patients show a worsening of clinical status in the early part of treatment as a result of the increasing inflammatory reaction in the lungs. If no improvement is seen at the end of 1 week of treatment, alternative therapies should be considered, including trimethoprim plus dapsone, clindamycin plus primaquine, atovaquone, and trimetrexate. Aerosolized pentamidine once was used commonly as an alternative to TMP-SMX but is not often recommended because of its propensity to cause refractory apical illness.

The side effects of TMP-SMX include a delayed rash that is usually mild and can be treated with an antihistamine. The most serious side effect is neutropenia. The development of neutropenia is dose dependent; therefore, it is recommended that the lowest possible dose be given. Other side effects include fever and abnormal liver enzymes. Pentamidine can cause a rash, neutropenia, renal toxicity (especially if given with aminoglycosides or amphotericin B), hypotension, hypoglycemia, nausea and vomiting, arrhythmias, and pancreatitis. Dapsone may cause nausea and vomiting, rash, fever, hemolysis, and methemoglobinemia. Clindamycin is associated with diarrhea, rash, fever, neutropenia, and methemoglobinemia. Atovaquone may cause rash, elevated liver enzymes, and nausea and vomiting or diarrhea.

Adjunctive corticosteroids (prednisone 40 mg orally bid followed by systematic weaning) are recommended for moderate to severe disease. Mortality is reduced significantly if steroid therapy is instituted within 72 h of the initiation of the anti-PCP regimen. Studies have shown that steroid therapy results in improved survival, a reduction in respiratory failure [adult respiratory distress syndrome (ARDS)], and less pulmonary damage as a result of the anti-inflammatory action of steroids. If steroid therapy is administered to a patient who has been misdiagnosed with PCP and in fact has a fungal infection, the patient may initially show improvement but the condition will ultimately worsen. Steroids also may exacerbate tuberculosis, Kaposi's sarcoma, and other bacterial pneumonias.

Supportive Measures

Adequate oxygenation and hydration are very important, especially in patients with severe PCP, to ensure a good response to treatment. Many patients will benefit from continuous positive airway pressure in an intensive care unit setting. Maintenance of electrolyte balance and good nutritional intake also are beneficial.

Patient Education and Disposition

Patients should be instructed to seek medical care and treatment for any change in respiratory status. Prophylaxis is recommended for any HIV-positive patient with a history of prior PCP, unexplained fever, esophageal thrush, or a CD4+ T-cell count below $200/\mu L^3$. Prophylaxis most commonly consists of TMP-SMX in a single dose (160 mg TMP and 800 mg SMX). Recent studies have shown that a dose given three times per week may be equally effective. The alternative prophylactic regimen is dapsone 100 mg orally qid. Dapsone 50 mg orally qid with pyrimethamine 50 mg orally once weekly may be more effective than dapsone alone.

COMPLICATIONS

Pneumothorax and cavitation were commonly encountered in patients treated with aerosolized pentamidine but may be seen in HIV-positive patients with the first bout of PCP. Extrapulmonary *Pneumocystis* may be seen in up to 3 percent of these patients. Common sites of infection include the external ear, mastoid, choroid, skin, small intestine, peritoneum, liver, spleen, thyroid, lymph nodes, and blood. Disseminated infection has been documented with organisms also found in the pancreas, stomach, adrenals, heart, kidneys, and central nervous system. Lesions outside the lung are frequently calcified, the symptoms are nonspecific, the diagnosis is difficult, and the prognosis is poor. Death results from multiple organ failure.

BIBLIOGRAPHY

Bennet JC, Plum F (eds): *Cecil Textbook of Medicine,* 20th ed. Philadelphia, Saunders, 1996.
Dobkin F: Opportunistic infections and AIDS. *Infect Med* 12(Suppl A):58–70, 1995.
Fauci AS, Braunwald E, Isselbacher KJ, et al (eds): *Harrison's Principles of Internal Medicine,* 14th ed. New York, McGraw-Hill, 1998.
Muma RD, Lyons BA, Borucki MJ, Pollard RB: *HIV Manual for Health Care Professionals.* Norwalk, CT, Appleton & Lange, 1994.

Chapter 17–7
PNEUMONIA

JoAnn Deasy

DISCUSSION

Pneumonia is an infection of the lower respiratory tract that is characterized by inflammation and consolidation of lung tissue. The alveoli fill up with exudate, resulting in the exclusion of air and solidification of part of the lung. Pneumonia may be caused by a wide spectrum of infectious disease agents. Those agents gain entry to the lower respiratory tract most often through the inhalation of aerosolized material or the aspiration of upper airway normal flow. Less frequently, infectious disease agents may be seeded in the lungs through the blood (hematogenous spread). Only a hundred-thousandth of an inch separates the air environment in the lungs from the bloodstream.

PATHOPHYSIOLOGY

The surface area of the lungs is approximately 150 m^2, almost the size of a tennis court. Each day over 10,000 L of air passes in and out of the respiratory tract. This air contains particles from the environment. Normally, the lungs are quite resistant to infection. Pneumonia occurs when the offending microbe overwhelms the host's defenses. When a person is challenged with an infectious disease agent, the outcome depends on microbial virulence, the quantity of infectious inoculum, and host susceptibility.

The alterations in host defense that may predispose a person to pneumonia occur at different levels. Protective defense mechanisms include nasal clearance, which removes organisms through sneezing and blowing anteriorly and posteriorly; also, the nasopharynx traps particles, which are then swallowed. The larynx expels many particles via the cough reflex. The beating mucociliary action of the tracheobronchial tree moves particles toward the oropharynx, where they are then swallowed or expectorated. Bacteria or other particles making their way to the alveoli are phagocytized by alveolar macrophages. Respiratory secretions contain antimicrobial substances. General immune defenses such as antibodies, leukocytes, and the local blood supply are also protective against pneumonia.

If the protective barriers are passed and microbes make their way to the lungs, some organisms produce a typical inflammatory response to the alveoli while others may produce tissue destruction and cavitation. Viruses generally produce inflammation between the alveoli as opposed to directly in the air spaces. Influenza viruses and viruses that cause the "common cold" impair host defenses by damaging respiratory epithelium and cilia, resulting in an increased frequency of pneumonia after these viral infections. Acute pneumonia that develops in nonhospitalized patients is referred to as community-acquired pneumonia (CAP). Pneumonia acquired in the hospital (nosocomial pneumonia) may be caused by bacteria that are more virulent, and the patient may have coexisting illnesses and impaired immune defenses.

Community-Acquired Pneumonia
SYMPTOMS

The symptoms that are suggestive of pneumonia are fever, chills, pleuritic chest pain, dyspnea, cough, and sputum production. Ten to thirty percent of patients with pneumonia complain of headache, nausea, vomiting, abdominal pain, diarrhea, myalgia, and arthralgia.[1] In the elderly (over 65 years of age) the classic symptoms of pneumonia are less commonly noted; instead, nonrespiratory symptoms such as confusion and other mental status changes may predominate. If a fever is present in the elderly, it is usually a low-grade fever. In children, upper respiratory symptoms usually precede fever and cough.

OBJECTIVE FINDINGS

Vital signs that are predictive of pneumonia include fever higher than 37.8°C (100°F), pulse rate over 100 beats per minute, and respirations more than 25 per minute. The presence of crackles on auscultation of the chest and locally decreased breath sounds are strongly associated with pneumonia. In the elderly, an increased respiratory rate may be the only objective finding.

DIAGNOSTIC CONSIDERATIONS

Bronchitis, especially in persons with chronic lung disease, may present similarly to pneumonia. Other infectious processes, such as *Mycobacterium tuberculosis* and fungal infections, may mimic CAP. A number of noninfectious processes may present a picture that is clinically similar to pneumonia, including congestive heart failure, pulmonary fibrosis, pulmonary emboli, pulmonary edema, and myocardial infarction.

LABORATORY AND RADIOLOGIC STUDIES

The chest x-ray is considered the gold standard for the diagnosis of pneumonia. The presence of a new or progressive infiltrate supports the diagnosis. Because an opacity on chest radiography may represent infection, blood, edema fluid, malignancy, or inflammation caused by noninfectious processes, the radiograph must be interpreted in conjunction with the medical history and the physical examination findings.

In addition to the chest x-ray, diagnostic tests that may be performed in the outpatient setting include a complete blood count (CBC), looking for leukocytosis and a shift to the left, and a sputum Gram's stain. The Gram's stain should be examined for the presence of neutrophils and the identification of the predominant bacteria. The presence of large numbers of squamous epithelial cells suggests that the specimen represents saliva rather than sputum. Pulse oximetry can be done as a measure of oxygenation. Oximetric Sao_2 levels below 91 percent indicate poor oxygen delivery in patients without long-standing pulmonary disease. In a patient who is hospitalized with pneumonia, blood cultures should be done. Although the yield is low, a positive culture usually indicates the etiology of the pneumonia and is a marker of more serious disease. The value of a sputum culture remains controversial, but it is usually performed when a patient is hospitalized. If a specific etiology of the pneumonia is suspected, other organism-directed tests can be done. More advanced tests should be reserved for patients who fail to improve on treatment.

MICROBIOLOGY

Streptococcus pneumoniae is the most common cause of CAP in all age groups. *Mycoplasma pneumoniae* may account for 20 to 30 percent of pneumonias in adults under 30 years of age but less than 3 percent in those over age 60. *Moraxella catarrhalis* and *Haemophilus influenzae* are increasingly seen as important pathogens. Enteric gram-negative bacilli may be a more common cause of CAP than was previously thought. The epidemiology of *Legionella pneumophila* and seems to vary with the geographic location. *Chlamydia pneumoniae* and viruses are also responsible for CAP.

TREATMENT

The ideal way to treat pneumonia would be to know the causative infectious disease agent and direct treatment against that agent. However, even among hospitalized patients in whom extensive studies are done, in as many as 50 percent of pneumonia patients no etiologic agent is identified. Therefore, treatment is usually empirical. Pneumonia was previously divided into atypical and typical pneumonia. Atypical preumonia referred to *Mycoplasma, Legionella,* and *Chlamydia* pneumonias. In reality, both the clinical and the radiologic findings are nonspecific and this division has little predictive value. This does not diminish the importance of a thorough history and physical examination in an attempt to ascertain the most likely etiology. However, it has been determined that if empirical treatment is to be initiated, it should be based on (1) the severity of illness, (2) the most common pathogens in published studies, and (3) the age of the patient and coexisting morbidities. Using these criteria, the American Thoracic Society (ATS) publishing recommendations for the treatment of CAP (Table 17-7-1).[2] These recommendations exclude patients at risk for HIV. The newer macrolides, clarithromycin and azithromycin, should be considered in patients intolerant of erythromycin and to treat *H. influenzae* in smokers.

The use of these guidelines for initial empirical therapy may result in the patient being treated with an antibiotic with a broader spectrum of coverage than is necessary. If diagnostic testing reveals the etiology of the pneumonia, the antibiotic can be changed. Generally, pneumonia is treated for 10 days. Patients with *M. pneumoniae* and *Legionella* spp. may require 14 days of therapy. In addition to antibiotics, outpatients should be encouraged to maintain a good fluid intake, monitor their temperature, and rest. The overuse of cough suppressants should be avoided.

In some cases, the clinical features may strongly suggest a

Table 17-7-1. ATS Guidelines for the Initial Treatment of Adults with CAP

Group	Organism	Treatment
Outpatient without comorbidity 60 years of age or younger	*S. pneumoniae* *M. pneumoniae* Respiratory viruses *C. pneumoniae* *H. influenzae* Miscellaneous: *Legionella* sp., *S. aureus, M. tuberculosis,* endemic fungi, aerobic gram-negative rods (GNR)	Erythromycin or tetracycline*
Outpatient with comorbidity and/or age 60 or older	*S. pneumoniae* Respiratory viruses *H. influenzae* Aerobic gram-negative bacilli *S. aureus* Miscellaneous: *Moraxella catarrhalis, Legionella* sp., *M. tuberculosis,* endemic fungi	Second-generation cephalosporin or trimethoprim-sulfamethoxazole or β-lactam/lactamase inhibitor and erythromycin or other macrolide if *Legionella* is suspected
Inpatient without intensive care	*S. pneumoniae* *H. influenzae* Polymicrobial (including anaerobic bacteria) Aerobic GNR *Legionella* sp. *S. aureus* *C. pneumoniae* Respiratory viruses Miscellaneous: *M. pneumoniae, M. catarrhalis, M. tuberculosis,* endemic fungi	Second-or third-generation cephalosporin or β-lactam/β-lactamase inhibitor and erythromycin or an other macrolide if *Legionella* is a concern
Inpatient with severe CAP (intensive care)	*S. pneumoniae* *Legionella* sp. Aerobic GNR *M. pneumoniae* Respiratory viruses Miscellaneous: *H. influenzae, M. tuberculosis,* endemic fungi	Macrolide† plus third-generation cephalosporin with anti-*Pseudomonas* activity or other anti-*Pseudomonas* agent (imipenem/cilastatin, ciprofloxacin

* Many isolates of *S. pneumoniae* are resistant to tetracycline, and it should be used only if the patient is allergic to or intolerant of macrolides.
† Rifampin may be added if *Legionella* sp. is documented.

Table 17-7-2. Selected Etiologic Agents of Pneumonia

Organism	Characteristics
Streptococcus pneumoniae (pneumococcus)	Onset of pneumonia often abrupt with sudden chill, fever, cough, and pleuritic chest pain. Rust-colored or yellow sputum. May follow upper respiratory infection (URI) Gram stain: gram-positive diplococci Chest x-ray (CXR): lobar consolidation Treatment: penicillin or erythromycin
Mycoplasma pneumoniae	Onset gradual with nonproductive cough. May be associated with sore throat and earache. More prevalent in younger age groups Gram stain: polymorphonuclear neutrophils (PMNs), no predominant bacteria CXR: patchy infiltrates Complement fixation test: rise in specific antibody Treatment: erythromycin (tetracycline)
Haemophilus influenzae	May follow URI. More common in older age group (>60 years) and those with chronic cardiopulmonary disease Gram stain: gram-negative coccobacilli CXR: lobar consolidation Treatment: second-generation (or third) cephalosporin
Moraxella catarrhalis	More common in elderly with preexisting lung disease and immunocompromised persons. Presents with cough, weakness, and dyspnea Gram stain: gram-negative diplococci or coccobacilli CXR: patchy infiltrate or lobar consolidation Most strains produce B-lactamase Treatment: second-generation cephalosporin or amoxicillin-clavulanic acid or trimethoprim-sulfamethoxazole
Klebsiella pneumoniae	More common in the elderly, alcoholics, diabetics, and nosocomial setting. Presents with fever, chills, purulent sputum, and pleuritic chest pain Gram stain: plump gram-negative rods CXR: lobar consolidation Treatment: cephalosporin plus aminoglycoside
Staphylococcus aureus	Uncommon. Occurs in debilitated persons, nosocomial setting, and after influenza infection. High fever, chills, cough, pleuritic chest pain. High mortality rate Gram stain: gram-positive cocci in clumps CXR: patchy infiltrates Treatment: vancomycin or cephalosporin
Chlamydia pneumoniae (TWAR agent)	Affects young adults. Clinical presentation similar to *Mycoplasma* spp. Gram stain: not helpful CXR: patchy or interstitial infiltrate Serologic studies available Treatment: tetracycline
Legionella pneumophila	Associated with environmental water sources. No person-to-person transmission. More common in elderly, smokers, and alcoholics. Dry cough; gastrointestinal and CNS symptoms may be present. Progresses to respiratory failure in 30 percent Gram stain: few polymorphonuclear neutrophils, no predominant bacteria CXR: patchy or lobar consolidation. Various studies available, including direct immunofluorescent stain of sputum, rise in antibody titer, urine antigen test
Aspiration pneumonia	Predisposing factors include neurologic damage, esophageal diseaes, alcohol or drug abuse. Etiology includes anaerobes and aerobes. Slow onset, less fever. Weight loss, malaise-, and fatigue common Gram stain: mixed flora CXR: dependent segments of lung most often involved Lung abscess may form Treatment must include anaerobic coverage
Pneumocystis carinii	Found in persons with AIDS and other immunosuppressive states. Sudden onset of fever, cough, dyspnea, and tachypnea typical. Gram stain: not helpful Diffuse interstitial and alveolar infiltrates Special stains of sputum or bronchoalveolar lavage fluid may identify cysts Treatment: trimethoprim-sulfamethoxazole or pentamidine

specific etiology (atypical versus typical). Table 17-7-2 presents what have been described as the characteristic clinical findings associated with various etiologic agents of CAP. Recent analyses of published data show that there is a considerable overlap of clinical symptoms among etiologic pathogens.

HOSPITALIZATION

The majority of patients with CAP are treated as outpatients. The decision to hospitalize is based on clinical judgment. Certain risk factors, physical findings, and laboratory findings are associated with a complicated course and may be indications for hospitalization. These factors include age over 65; coexisting illnesses, such as chronic obstructive pulmonary disease (COPD), diabetes mellitus; congestion heart failure (CHF), and alcholism; alteration in vital signs; leukopenia or marked leukocytosis; evidence of respiratory distress; septic appearance; and lack of a support system.

COMPLICATIONS AND RED FLAGS

Infectious complications include meningitis, arthritis, endocarditis, pericarditis, peritonitis, and empyema. Noninfectious complications include renal failure, heart failure, multisystem organ failure, and adult respiratory distress syndrome (ARDS).

DISPOSITION

Patients with pneumonia who are treated as outpatients should return to the clinic for a recheck or receive a phone call 2 to 3 days after starting antibiotic therapy. Patients who are not improving at 72 h or are actually deteriorating should be reevaluated. The antibiotic regimen may need to be changed, or the patient may be a candidate for hospitalization. In previously healthy persons, fever is generally gone in 2 to 4 days and leukocytosis resolves by day 4 or 5 of therapy. It is not unusual for abnormal physical findings to persist for 7 days. Cough and fatigue may persist for several weeks. Radiographic resolution of pneumonia lags behind clinical resolution. In younger (<50 years of age) and previously healthy patients, x-ray resolution of pneumonia occurs within 4 weeks.

Patients should be seen at the end of treatment to confirm the clinical cure. This is an appropriate time to administer pneumococcal vaccine. The chest x-ray should be repeated 4 weeks after the initiation of therapy to confirm resolution.

PREVENTION

Streptococcus pneumoniae vaccine is a capsular polysaccharide vaccine that contains the 23 most prevalent types. It is recommended for all persons over 65 years of age and all patients over 2 years of age who have chronic disorders of the pulmonary or cardiovascular system as well as some other chronic diseases, such as diabetes. Persons with compromised splenic function or splenectomy and those who are HIV-positive also should be vaccinated. Yearly influenza vaccine should also be administered to those at risk for pneumonia.

Hospital-Acquired (Nosocomial) Pneumonia

DISCUSSION

Hospital-acquired (nosocomial) pneumonia is defined as a pneumonia occurring more than 48 h after admission to the hospital. Colonization of the pharynx is promoted by instrumentation of the upper airway in a hospitalized patient as well as by the use of broad-spectrum antibiotics that change the flora and promote the emergence of resistant organisms. Inhalation of contaminated aerosols and hematogenous dissemination of microbes also may play a role in the development of nosocomial pneumonia. It is especially common in patients who require intensive care and mechanical ventilation. Host factors such as advanced age, comorbidities, and immunosuppression also promote nosocomial pneumonia.

The bacteria most often responsible for hospital-acquired pneumonia include gram-negative rods, *Streptococcus* spp., and *Staphylococcus* spp. *Pseudomonas aeruginosa* and *Acinetobacter* spp. are responsible for nosocomial pneumonia in the most debilitated patients. Nosocomial pneumonia may represent a polymicrobial infection.

SIGNS AND SYMPTOMS

Fever and purulent sputum are the clinical findings most often associated with nosocomial pneumonia.

LABORATORY AND RADIOLOGIC STUDIES

The minimum workup usually includes a complete blood count for leukocytosis, a chest radiograph for a new pulmonary infiltrate, two blood cultures for bacteremia, and a sputum Gram stain and culture. Thoracentesis for pleural fluid examination should be performed in patients with pleural effusion when nosocomial pneumonia is suspected.

TREATMENT

Treatment is empiric and should be started as soon as nosocomial pneumonia is suspected (after blood cultures) because of the high mortality rate associated with hospital-acquired pneumonia. There is no consensus about the best antibiotic regimen. A third-generation cephalosporin with antipseudomonal coverage combined with an aminoglycoside is often used.

REFERENCES

1. Marrie TJ: State of the art clinical article: Community-acquired pneumonia. *Clin Infect Dis* 18:501–515, 1994.
2. Niederman MS, Bass JB Jr, Campbell GD, et al: Guidelines for the initial management of adults with community acquired pneumonia: Diagnosis, assessment of severity, and initial antimicrobial therapy. American Thoracic Society, Medical Section of the American Lung Association. *Am Rev Respir Dis* 148:1418–1426, 1993.

Chapter 17–8
PULMONARY EMBOLUS
Barry A. Cassidy

DISCUSSION

In 1969 at the old Duke University Hospital, one could find pasted to the ceiling of an internal medicine ward a simple note that stated "Think PE." The note was a tribute to the evasive quality of the often deadly disorder known as pulmonary embolism (PE). Almost 30 years later the diagnosis of PE remains a practitioner's nightmare. By definition, an embolus constitutes a moving thrombus, and in the case of PE, the embolus occurs on the right side of the closed cardiovascular circulation circuit.

The circuit can be viewed as having two sides: the low-pressure right side and the high-pressure left side. Anatomically, the low-pressure right-sided venous system begins at the level of the postcapillary venule and terminates at the distal branches of the pulmonary arterial system. The left-sided system (in this description it would actually start at the postalveolar pulmonary venous system) can be conceptualized as starting in the high-pressure left ventricle and terminating at the precapillary arterioles.

Conceptualizing a closed right-sided and left-sided vascular system helps one view embolic events on the basis of their expected anatomic end-point symptomatology (right-sided events terminate in the central venous circulation, the right side of the heart, or the lung parenchyma, whereas left-sided events manifest in any organ system, including the heart, brain, abdominal viscera, mesentery, and extremities).

ETIOLOGY AND RISK FACTORS

Both sides of the closed cardiovascular system can develop thrombi that are susceptible to embolism. Multiple factors increase the risk of thrombus formation in the right-sided circulation:

- Hypercoagulable states, particularly carcinogenic states[1]

- Pregnancy and oral contraceptives[2,3]
- Recent surgical procedures with general anesthesia, particularly orthopedic, neurosurgical, and gynecologic surgery[2]
- Recent major trauma (head injuries, spinal cord injuries, complex pelvic fractures, and hip fractures; long bone fractures are also a common source of fat emboli)[4]
- Atrial fibrillation causing the formation of a clot in the right atrium[5]
- Right ventricular myocardial infarction[5]
- Immobilization, particularly casting of the lower extremities and also including long airplane rides[6]
- Nonthrombotic embolization occurring in the right-sided circulation from amniotic fluid emboli–post-therapeutic abortion, fat emboli, after long bone fracture, and iatrogenic air emboli secondary to invasive venous procedures[7]

Thrombosis formation is inversely proportional to flow; thus, the slower the flow state (pressure of flow), the higher the risk of thrombosis. Consequently, the low-pressure right-sided circulation is more susceptible to thrombosis formation than is the high-pressure left side. Any condition that causes venous status increases the likelihood of thrombus formation. Clinicians can heighten their awareness of the possibility of PE by thinking physiologically. For instance, inflammatory processes in the venous system resulting from trauma or infection affect flow through the veins and set the stage for thrombus development.

The most likely origin of PE is the deep venous system of the extremities and the veins in the pelvic area. One can be misled and feel secure that deep venous thrombosis is not present in the setting of a superficial phlebothrombosis or thrombophlebitis. However, it has been pointed out that the presence of superficial venous disease must be considered a risk factor for deep venous thrombosis and should be treated as such.[8] Although emboli arising from the superficial venous system are filtered out before they get into the deep system, one is obligated to make sure that the underlying process causing the superficial venous abnormality is not present in the deep venous system.

PREVALENCE

Galvin and Choi estimated that 500,000 patients suffer annually from PE and that 10 percent (50,000) of those patients die.[9] A multicenter study done at the Henry Ford Heart and Vascular Institute looked at the prevalence of acute PE among 51,645 patients hospitalized over a 21-month period. Four hundred four autopsies were performed in this group of patients, and PE was observed in 14.6 percent (59) of the autopsies. Among patients at autopsy who died from PE, the diagnosis was unsuspected in 70 percent.[10] Morpurgo and Schmid similarly found in 92 postmortem examinations revealing PE that 72 percent of cases were not diagnosed before death.[11]

Morgenthaler and Ryu from the Mayo Clinic did a retrospective study of 2427 autopsies performed over a 5-year period in an attempt to determine the clinical characteristics of hospitalized patients who died of confirmed PE at autopsy. Ninety-two patients (3.8 percent) were judged to have died of PE, among whom 11 patients (12 percent) had no risk factors for PE. Prophylaxis against thromboembolism was instituted in slightly less than half the 92 patients (46 percent); presumably, the others were undiagnosed or not suspected of having PE before death. Classic symptoms were often absent: Dyspnea was reported in 59 percent, chest pain in 17 percent, and hemoptysis in 3 percent. Pulmonary embolism was entertained as a diagnosis in 49 percent.[12] Giuntini and associates[1] suggested that venous thromboembolism is the third most common acute cardiovascular disease after cardiac ischemic syndromes and stroke.

SIGNS AND SYMPTOMS

The classic triad of hemoptysis, pleuritic chest pain, and dyspnea occurs in less than 20 percent of patients with PE.[9] One might incorrectly assume that those who develop hemoptysis, pleuritic chest pain, and dyspnea are more likely to die. In fact, the classic symptoms occur when the PE is located in the very periphery of the pulmonary arteries, where the mortality rate is the lowest. However, the classic symptoms should be considered a "heralding sign" for the major embolus that frequently follows.

The diagnosis of PE is based more on suspicion than on pure quantitative facts.[12a] Swan and associates at the University of Arizona Health Sciences Center did an interesting study that supports the infrequency of symptoms in PE. They studied the use of thrombectomy with deliberate pulmonary embolization of thrombus after initial thrombolysis for occluded hemodialysis catheters. Thirty-one patients with 43 acutely thrombosed prosthetic hemodialysis fistulas were treated with thrombolysis and/or thrombectomy. Perfusion lung scans were obtained in 22 patients. Forty-one of the 43 patients (95 percent) had no clinical signs or symptoms, yet 59 percent of the lung scans were consistent with PE.

Over the years, authorities have reasonably speculated that symptoms with PE are more likely if the embolus is more peripherally located. One confusing factor in PE is that it occurs as a comorbid partner of many serious illnesses. The diagnosis of PE does not lend itself to a laundry list of signs and symptoms. When a patient experiences hemodynamic difficulties, begins acting strangely, becomes dyspneic with or without chest pain, or in general experiences a major change in clinical status, one should think of PE. Once the question has been raised, one should establish a strategy for ruling out the possibility that PE exists.

DIAGNOSTIC CONSIDERATIONS

The best way to diagnose PE is to be able to see its presence. Consequently, the best test is autopsy or surgery, followed by pulmonary angiography. Since deep venous thrombosis (DVT) is the most common source of PE, venography is another invasive yet helpful diagnostic test. The risk of invasive procedures is real but is warranted when the suspicion of PE is high; they become less attractive when the suspicion is moderate to low. The goal has been to find a noninvasive or minimally invasive test to stratify the likelihood of PE as a diagnosis.

Looking at risk factors, diffusion of gases, and functional abnormalities is helpful when PE becomes a diagnostic consideration.

Risk Factors

Listing risk factors helps an examiner quantitate the suspicion of possible PE. For instance, a previous history of PE, recent trauma to an extremity, birth control pills, smoking history, a history of cancer, a recent operation, superficial thrombophlebitis, and invasive central venous lines in place, separately or combined, allow a graphic representation of one's suspicions.

Diffusion of Gases

Blood gas diffusion as measured by arterial blood gases (ABGs) provides helpful but not absolute data. Large (or multiple) PEs block O_2 diffusion, and one would expect a lowering of the Pa_{O_2}. Calculation of the expected Pa_{O_2} requires knowing the concentration of oxygen and the barometric pressure in the site where the test is being performed. Once the expected Pa_{O_2} is calculated, it can be compared to the measured Pa_{O_2} of the patient. (The patient's normal baseline ABG must be known to determine whether any change has occurred.) This yields the A–a (alveolar-arteriolar) gradient that is reported on most arterial gas reports.* An A–a gradient >15 to 20 suggests that gas diffusion is impaired. The ABG findings commonly found in PE patients are a low measured Pa_{O_2} < 60 mmHg and a low P_{CO_2} < 40 mmHg with resultant respiratory alkalosis. The lowering of the P_{CO_2} probably is related in part to the tachypnea that results from dyspnea or pain.

ABGs unfortunately are of indiscriminate predictive value in permitting the exclusion of PE. Stein and associates used data from the National Heart, Lung and Blood Institute's Prospective Investigation of Pulmonary Embolism Diagnosis (PIOPED) to study 768 patients (438 with and 330 without prior cardiopulmonary disease) and looked at the predictive value of diagnosing PE on the basis of the results of their ABGs. Their conclusions showed PE could not be excluded in more than 30 percent of patients with no prior cardiopulmonary disease and in no more than 14 percent of patients with prior cardiopulmonary disease.[13] There is a place, however, for the measurement of blood gases to determine the possibility of PE. Abnormal ABGs in concert with other tests can increase suspicion, leading to more definitive invasive tests.

The chest x-ray affords an indirect anatomic view of the status of the lung parenchyma. Once thought to be of little value in the diagnosis of PE except to exclude other cardiopulmonary disorders, the chest x-ray gives a great deal of information to a skilled radiographer. Chest x-ray findings (present in more than 80 percent of patients with known PE[7]) generally are not specific to PE but are found in other disorders as well. Chest x-ray findings that are fairly specific to PE (Westermark's sign, dilation of the pulmonary artery, and Hampton's hump, a triangular or rounded pleural-based infiltrate with its apex toward the hilum) are not likely to be appreciated by a nonradiologist. This points out that the evaluation of suspected PE should be multidisciplinary in nature. One pitfall germane to primary practitioners is that radiographic changes may take 12 to 24 h to manifest and therefore may not show on the initial chest x-ray.

The lung scan and ventilation-perfusion ($\dot{V}/\dot{Q}$) scan probably offer the most suggestive information among all noninvasive studies. Worsley and Alavi reviewed data from the PIOPED study regarding $\dot{V}/\dot{Q}$ scan interpretation. A helpful fact concluded from this study was that a normal $\dot{V}/\dot{Q}$ scan excludes the diagnosis of PE. Second, scans that are highly suggestive have definite clinical value and should be responded to accordingly. However, the intermediate group of $\dot{V}/\dot{Q}$ scans requires additional supporting data to warrant more invasive diagnostic procedures.[14]

Functional Abnormalities

A large portion of patients who develop PE do so from DVT of the lower extremities. Patients at high risk for PE and those with complaints of DVT should have noninvasive ultrasound evaluation of the lower extremities. Positive ultrasonography results in the lower extremities indicate immediate treatment to prevent or limit PE. When clinical suspicion for PE is high, pulmonary angiography should be considered.

The D-dimer test has received interest as a possible predictor of PE. When fibrin monomers bond to form a thrombus, factor XIII acts to bond their D domains. This bond is resistant to plasmin, and thus this degradation fragment is the D-dimer. Elevated levels of D-dimer indicates that fibrinogen has been acted on to form a fibrin monomer and that this was lysed by plasmin. D-dimer fragments can be easily measured in plasma. Unfortunately, there is not universal acceptance of the reliability of D-dimer as a prognostic test for PE.[15,16]

Venography is the gold standard of diagnosing DVT. Unfortunately, it is a very uncomfortable procedure and is reserved as a last option. Similarly, the true gold standard for diagnosing PE is pulmonary arteriography. The pulmonary angiogram is invasive, although not as painful to the patient as a venogram, and carries a number of risks: Anaphylaxes may delay the onset of treatment and increase pulmonary pressures, and the manipulation of the heart may cause ventricular fibrillation. The angiogram helps determine if an operation is an option (particularly in large "saddle emboli") and answer the question of whether the PE is significant. The angiogram is particularly helpful in the setting of moderate- to high-probability $\dot{V}/\dot{Q}$ scans when comorbid conditions can account for filling defects on the scan.

Other Diagnostic Considerations

The electrocardiogram (ECG) has been reported to have a number of findings attributable to PE. The usefulness of the ECG as a predictor of PE is dubious, since PE is so often associated with other cardiopulmonary disorders. The classic ECG findings in PE are S_1-Q_3-T_3 (an S wave in lead 1, a Q wave in lead 3, and a T-wave abnormality in lead 3), sinus tachycardia, nonspecific ST-T wave changes, right or left bundle branch block, atrial fibrillation, and premature atrial contractions or premature ventricular contractions.

TREATMENT

The treatment of PE falls into two categories: (1) attempting to prevent PE and (2) responding to PE. Patients who are at high risk and develop DVT should be treated immediately with anticoagulation, hospitalization, and bed rest. Patients who develop PE should be anticoagulated as well but may require much more supportive treatment and are best managed in an intensive care unit.

Types of Anticoagulation

The gold standard of therapy for PE is heparinization. Historically, unfractionated heparin has been used intravenously to achieve immediate anticoagulation. Generally patients are given a bolus of 5000 to 10,000 units of heparin and are maintained at 800 to 1000 units/h titrated on the basis of activated partial thromboplastin time (aPTT) values obtained every 4 to 6 h (aPTT values are kept to 1.5 to 2.5 times the normal baseline). Heparin's advantage over other anticoagulants lies in its relatively immediate onset of action. However, it has additional advantages in the setting of PE. Heparin has both anti-inflammatory and vasodilatory effects on arteries. The exact nature of these effects is not clearly understood, but recent studies suggest that heparin may mediate its anti-inflammatory effects by inhibiting the passage of leukocytes through the subendothelial basement membrane.[17] The effectiveness of heparin therapy is well known. Agnelli reported a 60 to 70 percent reduction in the incidence of fatal pulmonary embolism in heparin-treated patients.[18] Generally heparin is administered for 4 to 7 days, and an oral anticoagulant [warfarin (Coumadin)] is started concurrently once the heparin dose has been stabilized. Warfarin takes 36 h to begin exerting its anticoagulant effects; consequently, it is not an adequate choice for immediate treatment. Once the warfarin is stabilized, the heparin can be discontinued. Anticoagulation should continue for 3 to 6 months, depending on the individual case.

Unfortunately, there are times when heparin is contraindicated or patients prove resistant to its effects. Agnelli reviewed a cause of heparin resistance as follows:

Unfractionated heparin presents an aspecific "nonfunctional" binding to plasma proteins such as fibrinogen, factor VIII, vitronectin, and fibronectin. This aspecific binding limits the anticoagulant effect of unfractionated

---

* The formula for calculating the A–a gradient is $(F_{I_{O_2}})$ (barometric pressure − 47) − $[(1.2)$ measured $Pa_{CO_2}]$.

heparin and is responsible for the heparin resistance observed in some patients with pulmonary embolism as well as of the high intersubject variability of the heparin-induced anticoagulant effect.[18]

A problem related to heparin that is particularly germane in today's cost-conscious atmosphere is that patients must be hospitalized to be safely anticoagulated with heparin. Some promising studies indicate that subcutaneous (SQ) heparin may be as effective as intravenous heparin. Berkowitz at Duke University suggests that subcutaneous heparin is as efficacious as intravenous heparin.[19] Experimentation on new low-molecular-weight heparins is bringing the promise of developing a therapy for DVT at home. When a significant embolus has occurred or a significant DVT exits, one should be cautious about deviating from the known and acceptable standard to hospitalize patients and give intravenous heparinization for at least 3 days. Clinicians may be pushed to try alternative treatment plans for patients with suspected PE, but the condition requires constant professional surveillance, and to do otherwise would be unwise.

The aPTT reagents have been found to have a fair amount of variability. Gibaldi and Wittkowsky suggested that practitioners base their titration of heparin on serum concentrations of heparin of 0.2 to 0.4 U/mL.[20] Other forms of long-term anticoagulation were offered in the past. The combination of warfarin and aspirin has been advanced because of its dual action on the clotting mechanism. This combination is used particularly in neurologic disorders that feature both platelet emboli and thromboemboli. The combination has the advantage of preventing thrombus formation and platelet aggregation but has distinct disadvantages, including potential hemorrhage and compliance difficulties. Lotke and associates at the University of Pennsylvania did a prospective randomized study of 388 patients having total hip or knee replacement surgery. They found no difference between the aspirin and warfarin groups in regard to the incidence of changes in $\dot{V}/\dot{Q}$ scans or bleeding complications.[21]

Postoperative complications of PE have been addressed by preventing the stasis of blood in the lower extremities with the use of elastic support stockings or pneumatic compression stockings (PCS); others have used subcutaneous heparin administration every 12 h as a prophylaxis. Recent data from St. Luke's Hospital in Chesterfield, Maryland, support the concept that subcutaneous heparin and PCS used together are superior to these agents used individually.[22]

Patients at high risk for or with documented large DVT can be treated with the insertion of a filter in the inferior vena cava. Trauma patients at high risk for PE may be considered for the prophylactic insertion of vena caval filters.[23]

Patients admitted to the hospital for PE should be administered oxygen even if the Pa_{O_2} is >60 mmHg. Oxygen has a salutary effect on pulmonary hypertension, which is a consequence of PE. This is important to remember, as justification probably will be needed for insurance purposes. It is recommended that one make a statement to that effect in the chart to avoid unnecessary hassles.

Thrombolytic therapies such as urokinase and streptokinase have been utilized for years at major centers for PE documented by angiography.[5] They have had problems with significant bleeding and have not gained favor as a routine therapy for PE.

Future Therapies

Patients allergic to heparin, those who fail heparin prophylaxis, and those who have contraindications to anticoagulation present serious management problems. New investigations show promise in the drug Ancrod, which is a fibrinogen-depleting agent produced from snake venom.[24] New experimental drugs such as CGP-39393, which is a recombinant hirudin, show great promise as prophylactic agents for the prevention of postoperative thromboembolism.[25]

Improved protocols for the use of thrombolytics such as tissue plasminogen activator, alteplase, anistreplase, urokinase, and streptokinase may yield improved strategies for the management of PE. The use of these agents in other countries has been encouraging. Simpler forms of administration, control of posttherapeutic bleeding problems, and decreasing costs will make these agents beneficial and practical for use in the United States.[26]

Finally, there probably will be a small place for surgery as an option for treating patients with acute PE, particularly those who are hemodynamically unstable and cannot wait for other therapies and agents to act. Thoracic and cardiovascular surgery consultations[27] should be obtained as quickly as possible in this select group of patients.

REFERENCES

1. Giuntini C, Di Ricco G, Marini C, et al: Pulmonary embolism: Epidemiology. *Chest* 107(suppl 1):3S–9S, 1995.
2. Rosenow EC: Venous and pulmonary thromboembolism: An algorithmic approach to diagnosis and management. *Mayo Clin Proc* 70(1):45–49, 1995.
3. World Health Organization: Venous thromboembolic disease and combined oral contraceptives: Results of international multicentre case-control study. *Lancet* 346(8990):1575–1582, 1995.
4. Hofmann S, Huemer G, Kratochwill C, et al: Pathophysiology of fat embolisms in orthopedics and traumatology. *Orthopade* 24(2):84–93, 1995.
5. Spittell JA, Pluth JR: Pulmonary embolism, in Juergens JL, Spittell JA, Fairbairn JF (eds): *Peripheral Vascular Diseases*, 5th ed. Philadelphia, Saunders, 1980, p 757.
6. Levy Y, George J, Shoenfeld Y: The occurrence of thromboembolic events following airplane flights—"the economy class syndrome." *Isr J Med Sci* 31(10):621–623, 1995.
7. Baer GR: The approach to diagnosis of pulmonary embolism. *Phys Assist* 6:21–50, 1996.
8. Guex JJ: Thrombotic complications of varicose veins: A literature review of the role of superficial venous thrombosis. *Dermatol Surg* 22(4):378–382, 1996.
9. Galvin JR, Choi BS: *Electronic Differential Multimedia Laboratory.* Iowa City, University of Iowa College of Medicine, Department of Radiology, 1995.
10. Stein PD, Henry JW: Prevalence of acute pulmonary embolism among patients in a general hospital and at autopsy. *Chest* 108(4):978–981, 1995.
11. Morpurgo M, Schmid C: The spectrum of pulmonary embolism: Clinicopathologic correlations. *Chest* 107(suppl 1):18S–20S, 1995.
12. Morgenthaler TI, Ryu JH: Clinical characteristics of fatal pulmonary embolism in a referral hospital. *Mayo Clin Proc* 70(5):417–424, 1995.
12a. Swan TL, Smyth SH, Ruffenach SJ, et al: Pulmonary embolism following hemodialysis access thrombolysis/thrombectomy. *J Vasc Intervent Radiol* 6(5):683–686, 1995.
13. Stein PD, Goldhaber SZ, Henry JW, Miller AC: Arterial blood gas analysis in the assessment of suspected acute pulmonary embolism. *Chest* 109(1):78–81, 1996.
14. Worsley DF, Alavi A: Comprehensive analysis of the results of the PIOPED Study: Prospective investigations of pulmonary embolism diagnosis study. *J Nucl Med* 36(12):2380–2387, 1995.
15. Becker DM, Philbrick JT, Bachhuber TL, Humphries JE: D-dimer testing and acute venous thromboembolism: A shortcut to accurate diagnosis? *Arch Intern Med* 156(9):939–946, 1996.
16. Van Beek EJ, Schenk BE, Michel BC, et al: The role of plasma D-dimers concentration in the exclusion of pulmonary embolism. *Br J Haematol* 92(3):725–732, 1996.
17. Bartlett MR, Cowden WB, Paris CR: Differential effects of the anti-inflammatory compounds heparin, mannose-6-phosphate, and catanospermine on degradation of the vascular basement membrane by leukocytes, endothelial cells, and platelets. *J Leukoc Biol* 57(2):207–213, 1995.
18. Agnelli G: Anticoagulation in the prevention and treatment of pulmonary embolism. *Chest* 107(suppl 1):39S–44S, 1995.
19. Berkowitz SD: Treatment of established deep vein thrombosis: A review of the therapeutic armamentarium. *Orthopedics* 18(suppl):18–20, 1995.

20. Gibaldi M, Wittkowsky AK: Contemporary use of and future roles for heparin in antithrombotic therapy. *J Clin Pharmacol* 35(11):1031–1045, 1995.
21. Lotke PA, Palevsky H, Kennan AM, et al: Aspirin and warfarin for thromboembolic disease after total joint arthroplasty. *Clin Orthop* (324):251–258, 1996.
22. Ramos R, Salem BI, De Pawlikowski MP, et al: The efficacy of pneumatic compression stockings in the prevention of pulmonary embolism after cardiac surgery. *Chest* 109(1):82–85, 1996.
23. Rogers FB, Shackford SR, Ricci MA, et al: Routine prophylactic vena cava filter insertions in severely injured trauma patients decreases the incidence of pulmonary embolism. *J Am Coll Surg* 180(6):641–647, 1995.
24. Cole CW, Shea B, Bormanis J: Ancrod as prophylaxis or treatment for thromboembolism in patients with multiple trauma. *Can J Surg* 38(3):249–254, 1995.
25. Eriksson BI, Ekman S, Kalego P, et al: Prevention of deep-vein thrombosis after total hip replacement: Direct thrombin inhibition with recombinant hirudin, CGP39393. *Lancet* 347(9002):635–639, 1996.
26. Goldhaber SZ: Contemporary pulmonary embolism thrombolysis. *Chest* 107(suppl 1):45S–51S, 1995.
27. Marder VJ: Thrombolytic therapy: Overview of results in major vascular occlusions. *Thromb Haemost* 34(1):101–105, 1995.

Chapter 17–9
PLEURISY

Randy Trudeau

DISCUSSION

Pleurisy is a term used to describe inflammation or irritation of the pleura. The pleura is a thin two-layer membrane that lines the lungs and the chest cavity. The parietal pleura lines the inner surface of the chest wall, diaphragm, and mediastinum, while the visceral pleura covers the outer surface of the lungs and lines the fissures.

Etiology

Pleurisy is not a disease but a manifestation of a disease or diseases. Pleural inflammation may be caused by many different etiologic factors, including trauma, infection, irritation, and neoplastic processes. Pleural trauma is most notably caused by rib fractures. Infection is most commonly related to pneumonia, either viral or bacterial. Irritant substances include noxious agents that affect the pleura via the bloodstream or lymphatics or by crossing the conductive respiratory tissue. Examples include asbestos-related diseases, pleural effusions secondary to tuberculosis, drug ingestion, and collagen vascular disease. Neoplastic cells can invade the pleura in a similar fashion.

Pathophysiology

Typically, the pleura first becomes congested and edematous. This is followed by cellular infiltration and fibrous exudates that develop on the pleural surface. Exudates may be absorbed or organized into fibrous tissue, resulting in pleural adhesions. Pleural exudate follows as a result of an outpouring from damaged vessels of fluid rich in plasma proteins. Occasionally some diseases (e.g., coxsackievirus B causing pleurodynia) may run their course without significant exudation of the fluid from the inflamed pleura, thus leaving a dry and fibrous pleurisy.

SIGNS AND SYMPTOMS

The onset is usually sudden, but this may be variable, depending on the etiology. Pain, which is the dominant symptom, may vary from vague discomfort to an intense stabbing sensation. Aggravating factors include deep inspiration, coughing, laughter, and any activity that results in sudden movements of the thoracic cavity. The discomfort usually occurs over the area of pleural inflammation and can be accentuated by moving the affected side.

The pain associated with pleurisy results from inflammation of the parietal pleura, which is innervated by the intercostal nerves. The pain, however, can be referred to distant regions. Irritation of the posterior and peripheral portions of the diaphragmatic pleura, which is supplied by the lower sixth thoracic nerves, may cause pain referred to the lower chest or abdomen and may simulate an intraabdominal process. The central portion of the diaphragmatic pleura is innervated by the phrenic nerve; thus, pain may be referred to the neck or the ipsilateral shoulder. The visceral pleura is supplied by the visceral afferent nerves and is mostly anesthetic; therefore, it does not produce sharp and localized pain.

The physical examination of the pleura seeks evidence of pleural adhesions, increased pleural thickness, pleural inflammation, and the presence of air or excessive fluid in the pleural cavity. Respirations may be noted to be shallow and rapid. The patient may splint the affected side.

A pleural friction rub is pathognomonic in pleurisy, though it often may be absent and quite frequently is heard only 24 to 48 h after the onset of pain. This friction rub varies from intermittent sounds that may simulate crackles to fully developed harsh grating, leathery, or creaking sounds synonymous with respiration. Pleuritis, which is adjacent to the heart (pleural pericardial rub), varies with cardiac pattern as well as respiration, and the clinical picture varies with the underlying disease.

If fluid develops at the site of inflammation between the two membranes, the liquid is called a *pleural effusion.* As a pleural effusion develops, pleuritic pain usually subsides; however, increasing dyspnea may be noted. Accompanying the dyspnea, percussion dullness, decreased or absent breath sounds, absent tactile fremitus, and egophony at the upper border of the fluid are noticeable. If superficial tenderness to light palpation is present, it may be of musculoskeletal origin. Fever generally is not present unless the primary etiology is an infectious source.

LABORATORY STUDIES

The diagnosis of pleurisy is generally one of exclusion. Diagnostic studies focus more on the cause of the pleurisy.

A complete blood count (CBC) will help the evaluation for acute infectious problems. The erythrocyte sedimentation rate (ESR), although nonspecific, may help in determining inflammatory or metastatic causes. A blood urea nitrogen/creatinine study is elevated in uremic pleurisy.

RADIOLOGIC STUDIES

Chest x-rays are of limited value in diagnosing pleurisy. Pleural lesions generally cause no shadow; however, pleural effusions, though typically small, may confirm that acute inflammation of the pleura is present.

An x-ray is useful to rule out a potential pneumonia, evaluate trauma to the chest wall, and rule out neoplasms or associated pulmonary or chest wall lesions.

A ventilation-perfusion ($\dot{V}/\dot{Q}$) scan may be ordered if a pulmonary embolus is considered in the differential diagnosis.

DIAGNOSTIC CONSIDERATIONS

The following diagnoses and conditions can result in pleurisy:

- Chest wall trauma, e.g., rib fracture
- Neoplasm, e.g., primary lung cancer or metastases
- Vascular: pulmonary embolus
- Metabolic: uremia
- Infection (e.g., pneumonia)
- Abdominal disease
- Intercostal neuritis
- Herpetic neuritis
- Myocardial infarction
- Spontaneous pneumothorax
- Pericarditis
- Chest wall lesions
- Inflammatory (e.g., lupus/rheumatoid arthritis)

TREATMENT

Treatment of the underlying disease is essential. If no underlying cause is found, treatment is aimed at relieving the discomfort. Although this is controversial, chest pain may be relieved by wrapping the entire chest with two or three 6-in-wide nonadhesive elastic bandages. The bandages should be removed several times a day, and the patient should be encouraged to take deep breaths. This maneuver is an attempt to expand the patient's lungs fully and prevent atelectasis. Pain from coughing can be relieved by having the patient hold a pillow firmly against the chest wall when coughing.

Idiopathic pleuritic pain may be controlled with the use of acetaminophen, although nonsteroidal anti-inflammatory drugs (NSAID) may be preferable because of their anti-inflammatory effects. Codeine-containing analgesics (30 to 60 mg every 4 to 6 h) are useful in combating more severe pain. It is important to remember the cough suppressant properties of codeine when using this analgesic. A patient taking narcotics should be urged to breathe deeply and cough when pain relief from the drug is maximal.

Antibiotics and aqueous aerosol inhalations along with bronchodilators should be considered where there is associated bronchitis and to prevent a complicating pneumonia.

COMPLICATIONS

The following complications may be found:

- Scarring from adhesions at the site of inflammation
- Lung collapse or compression secondary to effusion or fibrosis
- Impaired breathing secondary to lung collapse or more subtle decreases in vital capacity
- Pneumonia, which may be a cause of pleurisy or a complication of the pain of pleurisy, producing insufficient coughing that suppresses the expulsion of bronchial secretions.

SPECIAL CONSIDERATIONS

The patient should notify the office if he or she develops increased fever or pain, prolonged or worsening dyspnea, cough that becomes dry and nonproductive, changes in nail beds, or bloody sputum.

BIBLIOGRAPHY

Berkow R, Fletcher AJ: *The Merck Manual,* 16th ed., Merck, 1992.
DeGowin RL: *DeGowin and DeGowin's Diagnostic Examination,* 6th ed. New York, McGraw-Hill, 1994.
Fauci AS, Braunwald E, Isselbacher KJ, et al (eds): *Harrison's Principles of Internal Medicine,* 14th ed. New York, McGraw-Hill, 1998.
Griffith AW: *Instructions for Patients,* 5th ed. Philadelphia, Saunders, 1995.
Labus JB: *The Physician Assistant Medical Handbook.* Philadelphia, Saunders, 1995.

Chapter 17–10
OCCUPATIONAL PNEUMOCONIOSIS
Pamela Moyers Scott

DISCUSSION

Occupational pneumoconiosis (OP) is a chronic lung disease caused by inhalation of dust particles through exposure at work. The name of the specific occupational pneumoconiosis is derived from its etiologic dust. The three most common forms are silicosis, coal worker's pneumoconiosis (CWP), and asbestosis, which are caused by exposure to silica (or quartz) dust, coal dust, and asbestos fibers, respectively.

Other occupational pneumoconioses and offending agents include berylliosis (beryllium dust), byssinosis (cotton dust), bagassosis (dust from the pressed stalks of sugarcane), baritosis (barium sulfate dust), siderosis (iron sulfate dust), stannosis (tin oxide dust), and farmer's lung (dust from moldy hay).

Although information on the actual incidence of individuals affected with occupational respiratory diseases is difficult to obtain, the U.S. Department of Labor has estimated that annually in the United States, 65,000 individuals develop an occupational respiratory disease and 25,000 die from it.[1]

Millions of Americans are exposed to potentially disease-producing dusts regularly through their employment. The individuals who will develop a disease process and the severity of the disease cannot be determined in advance. Several variables determine the toxicity of the inhaled dust. These variables include the physical, chemical, and mechanical properties of the dust particles, including their size, shape, penetrability, concentration, solubility, form, acidity, fibrogenicity, and antigenicity.[2] Additionally, the individual worker's immune status and ventilation rate and depth are important factors.[2]

SIGNS AND SYMPTOMS

Initially, all affected individuals with occupational pneumoconiosis are generally asymptomatic. As the disease progresses, a mild productive cough and exertional dyspnea occur. These symptoms may continue to worsen until the patient experiences dyspnea at rest. Signs and symptoms associated with complications from occupational pneumoconiosis may be the presenting complaint (e.g., pneumonia, cor pulmonale, congestive heart failure).

OBJECTIVE FINDINGS

Early in the course of the disease, the physical examination is generally unremarkable. Depending on the severity of the occupational pneumoconiosis and the presence of complicating disease processes, the patient may have any of the following: diminished breath sounds, rhonchi, wheezing, rales, fever, edema, jugular vein distention, clubbing, cyanosis, and varying degrees of dyspnea. There are no physical findings specific for occupational pneumoconiosis.

DIAGNOSTIC CONSIDERATIONS

The differential diagnosis includes any chronic respiratory condition, such as emphysema, chronic bronchitis, asthma, and lung cancer.

SPECIAL CONSIDERATIONS

Cigarette smoking appears to have an additive detrimental effect on the development and progression of the disease.

LABORATORY STUDIES

There are no specific laboratory tests to diagnose occupational pneumoconiosis. However, if patients are on a theophylline preparation, periodic serum levels are necessary. A complete blood count (CBC) may be useful in individuals suspected of having a coexisting infection or polycythemia.

RADIOGRAPHIC STUDIES

Early in the course of the disease, the chest x-ray (CXR) is often normal. In fact, recent studies indicate that pulmonary function abnormalities may be demonstrated in the absence of radiographic findings.[3] The first visible finding of occupational pneumoconiosis on CXR is the presence of small (<5 mm), round parenchymal opacities (Fig. 17-10-1). If the disease progresses, these nodules coalesce, forming larger, irregular lesions referred to as progressive massive fibrosis (PMF) (Fig. 17-10-2).

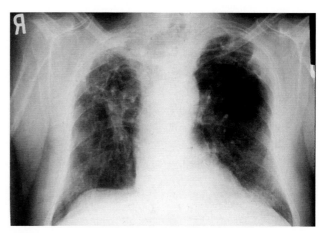

Figure 17-10-2. Complicated occupational pneumoconiosis evident by the appearance of progressive massive fibrosis and bullous formation.

An accurate occupational history is the only definite means to distinguish the various occupational pneumoconioses from one another, as the radiographic evidence is virtually identical. However, some features are more suspicious for specific disease processes. Asbestosis is more often associated with the following: pleural plaques (Fig. 17-10-3), an indistinct cardiac border (ground-glass appearance), and coalescence of parenchyma and obliteration of the acinar units (honeycombed lung). Hilar lymph node calcification may produce the characteristic eggshell pattern of silicosis.

OTHER DIAGNOSTICS

Pulmonary function testing (PFT) can reveal an obstructive, restrictive, or mixed pattern. An obstructive pattern is defined as a normal or decreased forced vital capacity (FVC) associated with a decreased forced expiratory volume (FEV). A restrictive pattern is characterized by a decreased FVC and a normal or increased FEV. A mixed pattern reveals a normal or decreased FVC and FEV, depending on the specific occupational disease that is present. Coal worker's pneumoconiosis is initially seen as an obstructive pattern whereas asbestosis and silicosis are initially restrictive.

Oxygen saturation as determined with a pulse oximeter is decreased in accordance with the severity of the pulmonary impairment.

Arterial blood gases (ABGs) also reveal hypoxemia that is consonant with the severity of the pulmonary impairment.

TREATMENT

Pharmacologic Management

First-line treatment of occupational pneumoconiosis generally consists of inhaled beta agonists, such as pirbuterol (Maxair), albuterol (Ventolin, Proventil), and metaproterenol (Alupent). These medications act by stimulating the beta receptors of the smooth muscles surrounding the airways, causing them to relax and hence causing bronchodilation to occur. Generally, these drugs are delivered by a metered-dose inhaler (MDI) at a dosage of two inhalations 4 times/day qid. Individuals with less severe disease may benefit from using MDIs on an as-needed basis only. However, if the patient requires them more than two or three times a week, he or she will probably benefit from using them regularly to prevent bronchospasms instead of treating them when they occur. Regardless, individuals who use beta-agonist

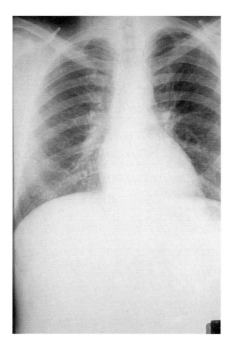

Figure 17-10-1. Simple occupational pneumoconiosis evident by the appearance of small, round parenchymal opacities.

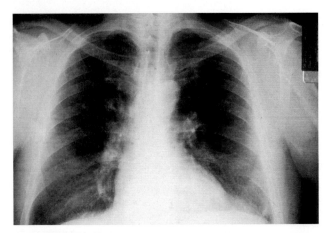

Figure 17-10-3. Probable asbestosis based on the presence of bilateral pleural thickening along with the parenchymal opacities.

MDIs must be cautioned never to exceed the recommended dose because of the potential for cardiac arrhythmias.

Salmeterol (Serevent) is the only currently approved long-acting beta agonist MDI available in the United States. The dose is two inhalations bid. Salmeterol has the same potential for fatal cardiac arrhythmias as the shorter-acting preparations and is not indicated for acute symptom relief.

Since many individuals have difficulty using MDIs properly, breath-activated devices are available to enhance patients' ability to receive an accurate dose of medication: pirbuterol (Maxair Autohaler), albuterol (Ventolin Rotacaps), and salmeterol (Servent Diskus). Many of the beta agonists are also available in a solution with normal saline for delivery by an ultrasonic nebulizer. Spacers also appear to be effective in enhancing the delivery of the desired MDI dose to the lungs.

An ipratropium bromide (Atrovent) MDI is also useful in treating OP. It induces bronchodilation through its anticholinergic effects on the muscarinic receptors of the bronchial smooth muscle. The usual dose is two inhalations qid.

Because ipratropium induces bronchodilation by a mechanism different from that of the beta agonists, the two can be used together. Ipratropium bromide also can be used independently to treat OP.

Theophylline probably induces bronchodilation by relaxing the smooth muscles surrounding the bronchial tree and pulmonary blood vessels. It is not used as much today as in the past because of its side effect profile, potential for toxicity, potential for drug interactions, and the need for serum monitoring.

Oral beta agonists are also available; however, they are used infrequently because the topical inhaled formulations tend to be much better tolerated. Examples of oral beta agonists include albuterol (Volmax, Ventolin) and terbutaline (Brethine).

Corticosteroids are occasionally beneficial in the treatment of OP by decreasing the amount of inflammation in the airways. Whenever possible, inhaled medications are preferred because they reduce significantly, if not eliminate entirely, the possibility of serious side effects. Inhaled corticosteroids include triamcinolone (Azmacort) and beclomethasone (Beclovent, Vanceril).

Home oxygen is necessary when the oxygen partial pressure (Po_2) is less than 55 percent and in individuals with severe complications such as pulmonary hypertension, right-sided heart failure, and cor pulmonale. Depending on the severity of the disease, the dosing schedule can be continuous (24 h/d), at night (8 to 10 h/d), or as needed. Care must be taken not to exceed 2 L/min via nasal cannula because the respiratory drive of OP patients could be based on O_2, not CO_2, and higher flow rates could result in respiratory depression and arrest.

SUPPORTIVE MEASURES

All individuals with OP should drink at least 8 to 10 8-oz glasses of water a day. This will keep them adequately hydrated as well as serve as a mucolytic.

Individuals with mild disease who continue to work should be moved to an area of reduced dust exposure and/or use protective equipment regularly. Additionally, they should have annual CXRs and pulmonary function tests (PFTs) to monitor the progression of disease.

Immunizations

All patients with occupational pneumoconiosis should receive the influenza vaccine annually. They should receive immunization against pneumococcus at least once and boosters at 5-year intervals if they are considered to be at high risk for fatal pneumococcal disease. Additionally, they should receive a tuberculosis skin test annually.

Patient Education

According to the American Lung Association, studies indicate that practically all dust-induced respiratory diseases can be prevented.[4] Primary prevention results from employers, employees, and health care providers working together to minimize the effects of occupational dusts. These efforts should include emphasizing the hazards of the job, encouraging the use of protective equipment, stressing the importance of annual CXRs and PFTs, and smoking cessation.

Disposition

Follow-up of a patient with OP depends on the severity of the disease and the associated complications. All these individuals should be seen at least annually for a history and physical update, CXR, PFT, tuberculosis skin test, influenza vaccine, and appropriate health maintenance and education.

COMPLICATIONS AND RED FLAGS

Complications from any occupational pneumoconiosis may include progressive massive fibrosis (PMF), cor pulmonale, right-sided heart failure, pulmonary hypertension, chronic bronchitis, pneumonia, tuberculosis, and death.

Specifically related to CWP is Caplan's syndrome, which is characterized by PMF and rheumatoid arthritis. Chronic lymphocytic alveolitis and lung cancer have been reported in individuals with silicosis. Asbestos exposure has been linked with many carcinomas, including lung, laryngeal, renal, and gastrointestinal cancers, as well as metheliomas.

REFERENCES

1. Anderson M: Introduction to occupational lung diseases, in American Lung Association: *Occupational Lung Diseases: An Introduction*. New York, ALA, 1986, pp 1–7.
2. Speizer F: Environmental lung disease, in Wilson JD, Braunwald E, Isselbacher KJ, et al (eds): *Harrison's Principles of Internal Medicine*, 12th ed. New York, McGraw-Hill, 1991, pp 1056–1060.
3. Attfield M, Hodous T: Pulmonary function of US coal miners related to dust exposure estimates. *Am Rev Respir Dis* 145:605–608, 1992.
4. American Lung Association: *Facts about Dust Diseases: Lung Hazards on the Job*. New York, ALA, 1988.

Chapter 17–11
CHRONIC OBSTRUCTIVE PULMONARY DISEASE: EMPHYSEMA AND CHRONIC BRONCHITIS
Maureen MacLeod O'Hara

EPIDEMIOLOGY

The term *chronic obstructive pulmonary disease* (COPD) refers to the obstructive airflow disorders of emphysema and chronic bronchitis. Up to 70,000 patients a year die from COPD, making it the fifth leading cause of death in the United States. It accounts for more than 17 million office visits and 2 million hospitalizations annually. The National Heart, Lung, and Blood Institute estimates that the annual cost of treatment for COPD is $18 billion. Approximately 2 million Americans have emphysema, and 14 million have chronic bronchitis. COPD is approximately three times more prevalent in white persons and approximately two times more prevalent in men. The incidence in women seems to be increasing as a result of higher numbers of women smokers in recent years.

Cigarette smoking is the primary risk factor 80 to 90 percent of the time for both emphysema and chronic bronchitis. These patients give a history of symptoms for 10 to 15 years and a history of smoking one or more packs per day for 25 years or more. It is not clear, however, why only 10 to 15 percent of smokers eventually develop COPD. In 1990, 28 percent of men and 22 percent of women over age 20 (i.e., 45 million people) smoked cigarettes in the United States. According to a 1995 study by the Centers for Disease Control and Prevention, 29 percent of boys and 26 percent of girls ages 12 to 21 smoke, and so the potential for developing respiratory diseases remains significant. Pipe and cigar smokers, along with those who have quit smoking, have a higher rate of COPD than do nonsmokers but a lower rate than those who still smoke.

The risk of developing COPD is approximately 10 to 30 times greater in smokers than in nonsmokers, indicating that there are risk factors for nonsmokers to develop COPD, including respiratory problems as children (viral infections and asthma), exposure to environmental or occupational dust, air pollution, and secondhand smoke. Among COPD cases, 0.5 to 2 percent are due to α_1-antitrypsin deficiency, suggesting a genetic predisposition. α_1-Antitrypsin deficiency should be suspected in persons who develop emphysema in their late thirties to early forties. If patients develop COPD from any of these factors and smoke cigarettes, the disease process may accelerate.

Survival rates for severe COPD are estimated at 50 percent after 5 years and 25 percent after 10 years. After the first episode of respiratory failure, 66 percent of these patients will die within 2 years.

PATHOPHYSIOLOGY

Emphysema is defined as "abnormal stretching and destructive changes in the alveoli" by the American Thoracic Society (ATS) and is a pathologic diagnosis made at autopsy. It is an assumed diagnosis in a living patient. Emphysema affects lung parenchyma distal to the terminal bronchioles and is characterized by destruction of alveolar walls and an abnormal, irregular enlargement of air spaces. This progressive destruction from the peripheral to the terminal airways accounts for the loss of alveolar capillary surface area and a disturbance in the capacity of the lungs to diffuse gases. Since there is a loss of both air space and blood vessels, emphysema demonstrates less of a ventilation-perfusion mismatch than does chronic bronchitis.

Elements in cigarette smoke are known to stimulate elastase enzymatic activity, causing degenerative changes in elastin and alveolar structures. These elements also interfere with antielastase activity and the repair process of elastin fibers. These substances also cause the release of cytotoxic oxygen radicals from white blood cells in lung tissue. The destruction of alveolar walls causes a loss of elasticity and an increase in lung compliance, resulting in obstruction of expiratory airflow. Because of this increased compliance, the work of ventilation is less intensive and may result in less CO_2 retention early in the disease process.

There are several patterns of tissue destruction in emphysema. In centrilobular or centriacinar emphysema, the most severe destruction appears in the central portion of the lobule or acinus with sparing of the alveolar ducts and alveoli (Figs. 17-11-1 and 17-11-2). Centrilobular emphysema is most often seen in the apex but spreads to the base of the lobe as the disease progresses. Mild destruction in the apices causes little or no lung dysfunction. Centrilobular is the most common type of tissue destruction and is seen most often in smokers.

Panlobular or panancinar emphysema affects the terminal bronchiole with its alveolar ducts and alveolar sacs, causing air trapping, and seems to be more prominent in portions of the lower lobes (Fig. 17-11-3). Centrilobular and panlobular emphysema may coexist in the same lung. Paraseptal emphysema involves destruction of the alveolar ducts and sacs as well as the interlobar walls. It is more common in the peripheral lobules (Fig. 17-11-4).

Bullous emphysema describes large cystic areas of destruction where air spaces have diameters greater than 1 cm, giving an appearance of Swiss cheese. By comparison, normal lung tissue appears to have a fine texture similar to that of bread. The air spaces or bullae gradually increase in size from the forces of the elastic recoil of other areas with greater elasticity, causing a loss of lung parenchyma volume.

Chronic bronchitis is a clinical diagnosis and is defined by the ATS as "excessive sputum production with chronic or recurring cough on most days for a minimum of 3 months of the year for at least 2 consecutive years." It includes smooth-muscle hypertrophy, inflammation, mucosal edema, narrowing of airways, goblet and squamous cell metaplasia, mucus plugging of small airways (less than 2 to 3 mm), and peribronchial fibrosis. As chronic bronchitis worsens over time, the airflow resistance (obstruction), which starts with the small airways, comes to involve larger peripheral airways as well.

The obstruction of small airways from any of the causes mentioned above results in CO_2 retention and hypoxemia from ventilation-perfusion mismatch. Hypoxemia and acidemia (from respiratory acidosis) cause constriction of pulmonary arteries and increased pulmonary arterial pressure, leading to pulmonary hypertension. *Cor pulmonale* is a term used to describe right ventricular enlargement caused by a disease of the lung. COPD is an underlying cause of pulmonary hypertension. Emphysema contributes to pulmonary hypertension by increasing vascular resistance from the loss of capillary beds. Chronic bronchitis contributes to pulmonary hypertension as a result of hypoxemia and acidemia. In advanced disease, cor pulmonale manifests more often in chronic bronchitis-dominant patients as polycythemia and evidence of fluid retention, such as dependent edema and jugular venous distention.

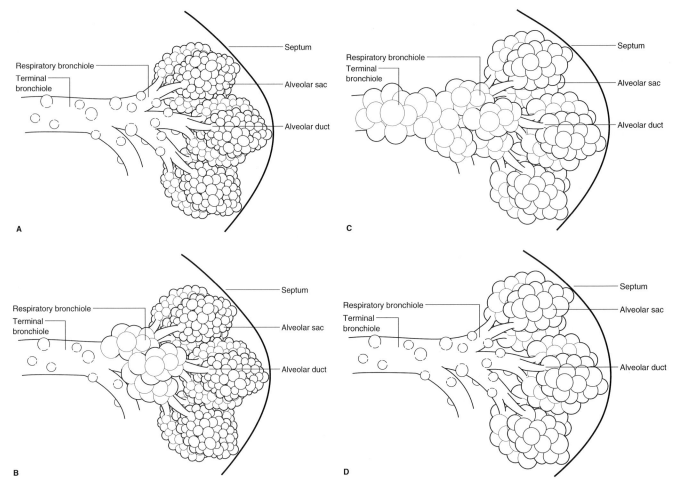

Figure 17-11-1. Tissue destruction in emphysema. *A.* Normal acinar (lobar) unit. *B.* Centriacinar (centrilobular) emphysema. *C.* Panacinar (panlobular) emphysema. *D.* Paraseptal emphysema. (*From Calverley and Pride, 1995; George et al, 1995; West, 1987.*)

ASSESSMENT

COPD is a diagnostic challenge for clinicians since approximately one-third of office visits are for respiratory complaints. Patients may have a predominance of emphysema or chronic bronchitis but usually have a mixture of both diseases. The diagnosis is based on the history, physical examination, and laboratory findings, since there is not a single pathognomonic hallmark for COPD.

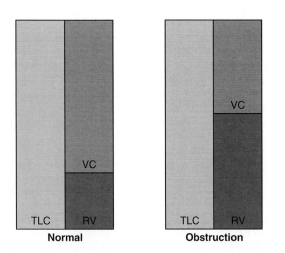

Figure 17-11-2. Lung volumes. (*From Fishman et al, 1985; O'Hara, 1995.*)

CLINICAL FINDINGS

History

Early detection of COPD is difficult because of its slow, progressive, insidious nature. Symptoms may be present for several years before patients seek treatment. Coughing and wheezing are early symptoms and may be easily overlooked or dismissed as a "smoker's cough," since dyspnea may not be present. Practitioners may not note the connection between a series of respiratory infections and the onset of COPD. Also, clinicians may not have the opportunity to see trends developing if patients do not maintain long-term therapeutic relationships as a result of changes in health insurance carriers or loss of coverage caused by downsizing of the economy. Patients may complain of cough, wheezing, or recurring respiratory infections, which may be attributed to disease entities other than COPD, but it is shortness of breath (dyspnea) or, more specifically, dyspnea on exertion, described as "breathlessness," that usually causes patients to seek medical attention. Patients may describe breathlessness while performing activities of daily living such as cleaning, making the bed, and dressing. Dyspnea is a late symptom and usually indicates 20 to 30 percent irreversible lung tissue destruction (Table 17-11-1).

Physical Examination

Depending on the severity of the progression of the disease process and the relative degrees of predominance of emphysema and chronic bronchitis, the physical findings vary. Physical examinations may be normal for many years, but the most prominent feature of the physical examination is prolonged expiration. A

Age	86 years	Room temp/pressure	23° C/760 mmHg				
Gender/race	F/black	Height	64 in./163 cm				
Weight	125 lb/57 kg	Spirometry and lung volumes at BTPS					
			Pre ℞			**Post ℞**	
		Predicted	**Best**	**%Predicted**	**Best**	**%Predicted**	**%Change**
	SPIROMETRY						
FVC	Liters	2.35	1.22	52*	1.32	56*	8
FEV$_1$	Liters	1.56	0.70	45*	0.70	45*	0
FEV$_1$/FVC	%	80	57		53		
FEF$_{25 \text{ to } 75\%}$	L/sec	1.08	0.32	30*	0.30	28*	−6
PEF	L/sec	5.08	2.36	46*	2.73	54*	−16
			Pre ℞				
		Predicted	**Average**	**%Predicted**			
	LUNG VOLUMES						
VC	Liters	2.35	1.22	52*			
TLC	Liters	4.69	4.76	102			
RV	Liters	2.08	3.54#	170*			
RV/TLC	%	44	74#				
FRC N$_2$	Liters	2.94	3.69	126			
	DIFFUSION						
DL$_{CO}$	mL/min/mmHg	15.3	6.5#	43*			

* = Outside normal range.

\# = Outside 95% confidence interval.

Calibration: Predicted: 3.30 Actual: Expired 3.37 Inspired 3.28

BTPS = Body temperature, ambient pressure and saturation with water vapor; PEF = Peak expiratory flow.

Figure 17-11-3. Example of a pulmonary function test.

simple measure of obstruction can be obtained by having the patient take a deep breath and forcefully exhale as fast as possible. Using a peak flowmeter (as a device for the patients to blow into) or listening to the trachea with a stethoscope, the practitioner times the length of the exhalation. Longer than 4 to 6 s is considered abnormal and indicates obstruction. The Snider match test is a screening test that is considered positive if the patient is unable to blow out a match held 15 cm from the mouth.

Type A, or emphysema-predominant, patients usually are able to maintain adequate oxygenation for a longer time during their disease. This slows the onset of the pulmonary hypertension and right-sided heart failure that are common in chronic bronchitis. These patients are labeled "pink puffers" because of their pursed-lip breathing, pink skin color, and thin body habitus. Type B, or chronic bronchitis-dominant, patients are often cyanotic from

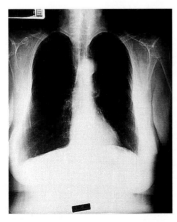

Figure 17-11-4. Example of a chest x-ray in a 65-year-old white female with COPD.

decreased oxygen saturation and being overweight, giving them the label "blue bloaters."

Pedal edema is common in type B patients because of pulmonary hypertension. COPD patients become dyspneic almost immediately upon lying down, whereas patients with congestive heart failure become orthopneic in a few hours. Pitting edema that does not clear with leg elevation should make one suspicious of right-sided heart failure. Digital clubbing is unusual in COPD patients and may indicate a neoplasm, infection, or interstitial lung disease (Table 17-11-2).

LABORATORY FINDINGS

Pulmonary Function Tests

Pulmonary function tests (PFTs) are used to characterize the pattern of the airway defect, quantify the airway obstruction, assess the reversibility of the airway obstruction, and monitor the progression of the disease. In normal lungs, vital capacity (VC), or the total amount of air a person can exhale after a maximal inspiration, exceeds the residual volume (RV), or the amount of air that remains in the lung after a full exhalation, by a ratio of 3:1. COPD causes difficult and incomplete emptying of the lungs, resulting in an increase in RV and a decrease in VC, so that the ratio approaches 1:1 (Fig. 17-11-2). Any reduction of vital capacity will impair the ventilatory capacity of the lungs. Spirometry employs a machine to measure lung volumes, flow rates, and diffusion capacity, providing information regarding lung function. The values given in this chapter are approximations of normal and abnormal, since lung function has been shown to vary with age, gender, race, height, and weight. Normal values are individualized for each patient on the basis of these variables and are reported as predicted normal values (PNVs). Variation from PNVs is considered abnormal for the patient.

The volume of air forcefully exhaled in 1 s is called the 1-s

Table 17-11-1. History Questions and Usual Responses

History Question	Emphysema	Chronic Bronchitis
Quantity and length of smoking Date of cessation	One or more packs per day for 25 years or more	
Cough	Minimal	Almost daily
Productive/nonproductive	Scant sputum	Thick, copious: 2 oz to 1 cup per day, worse in morning
Sputum color Noninfected		White, tan, gray
Infected		Yellow, green, brown, red
Frequency of respiratory infections	Occasional	Frequent
Dyspnea	Frequent	Intermittent
Wheezing	Minimal	Frequent
Hemoptyses	Rare	Occasional
Weight change	Loss	Gain
Duration of symptoms before office presentation	10 to 15 years	10 to 15 years
Age at presentation of complaints	50–55	35–40

SOURCE: Griffith, Dambro, and Griffith, 1994; Hahn, 1996; Johannsen, 1994; Kelley, 1994; Labus, 1995; Peterson, et al, 1995; Scientific American, 1995.

forced expiratory volume (FEV_1). In obstructive disease, the rate of exhalation slows down because of narrowing of the airways. FEV_1 may be prolonged as much as 15 to 20 s compared to a normal value of 3 s. The airway obstruction component of chronic bronchitis is considered reversible if the FEV_1 improves at least 15 percent or 200 mL after the administration of an aerosol bronchodilator. It is not unusual for nonsmokers to lose 20 to 25 mL of FEV_1 per year, while heavy smokers may lose 40 to 50 mL per year. Nonsmokers who have α_1-antitrypsin deficiency may lose 80 mL of FEV_1 per year, while smokers with α_1-antitrypsin deficiency may lose 150 mL per year. Forced vital capacity (FVC) is the total air forcefully exhaled. The normal value of the ratio of FEV_1 to FVC is 75 to 80 percent. A reduced FEV_1 with a reduced FEV_1/FVC ratio is considered the most indicative of obstructive disease. Forced expiratory flow ($FEF_{25-75\%}$) measures the flow of air in the middle of an exhalation. This is helpful information, since the obstructive process affects the small airways first and their collapse can be detected by the low flow volume. Total lung capacity (TLC) is the amount of air in the lungs after a full inspiration (RV + VC). In emphysema the TLC may actually increase as a result of hyperinflation from the increased lung compliance and loss of elastic recoil. An increased RV/TLC ratio may indicate air trapping. Functional residual capacity (FRC) is the amount of air remaining in the lung after a normal resting expiration. It is a measure of the balance between lung elastic recoil and chest wall recoil. FRC increases in emphysema as the elastic recoil of the lung decreases and gives an indication of the severity of hyperinflation. In chronic bronchitis, the mechanism for increased FRC is increased airway resistance from mucus plugging and inflammation. FRC also increases with

an increase in the respiratory rate. Hyperinflation increases the work of breathing as inspiratory capacity is reduced by an increase in RV. This is demonstrated by an increase in breathlessness. There are several methods to measure FRC with spirometry, but the most common techniques use helium or nitrogen gas. Inspiratory and expiratory lung volumes also may be recorded by flow-volume loops in a graphic presentation. These loops have characteristic shapes that depend on the type of respiratory disorder.

The spirometer can measure the inequality of ventilation by analyzing the nitrogen concentration expressed as the percentage of nitrogen per liter of expired air, called a single-breath nitrogen test (SBN_2). In normal subjects the inspired oxygen will attempt to equilibrate with the nitrogen from the dead spaces of the lung. In persons with obstructive disease, the dead spaces may be larger and unevenly distributed so that the inspired oxygen is not enough to dilute the nitrogen from the poorly ventilated areas of the lung, causing the nitrogen concentration to be increased. Helium is another gas that can be used to make these measurements.

In spirometry, reduced diffusing capacity of the lung for carbon monoxide (DL_{CO}) is a measure of ventilation. DL_{CO} is decreased more in emphysema than in chronic bronchitis because of the destruction of the pulmonary capillaries in the avleolar walls. In chronic bronchitis DL_{CO} is reduced by thickening of tissues in small airways (Table 17-11-3 and Fig. 17-11-3). If patients with COPD continue to smoke, their PFTs should be checked annually to measure the decline. For patients who are nonsmokers, the interval can be longer. When FEV_1 falls to less than 50 percent of the predicted normal value, an arterial blood gas should be obtained.

Table 17-11-2. Usual Physical Findings

	Type A: Emphysema-Predominant, "Pink Puffer"	Type B: Chronic Bronchitis–Predominant, "Blue Bloater"
General	Thin, cachectic, pursed-lip breathing, accessory muscle use, barrel chest	Obese, cyanotic
Vital signs	Tachypnea (> 18 respirations/min), occasional tachycardia (> 100 beats per min)	
Cardiovascular	Cor pulmonale rare	Cor pulmonale common
		Jugular venous distention, right-sided heart failure, right ventricular heave (pulmonary hypertension), S_3 murmur (tricuspid insufficiency)
Gastrointestinal		Hepatomegaly, ascites (right-sided heart failure)
Pulmonary	Dyspnea, prolonged expiration, minimal wheeze, hyperresonant to percussion, decreased breath sounds, reduced diaphragmatic excursion, low position of diaphragm	Minimal dyspnea, prolonged expiration, coarse rhonchi, wheeze, minimally decreased breath sounds
Extremities		Pedal edema

SOURCE: Braunwald et al, 1988; Griffith, Dambro, and Griffith, 1994; Hahn, 1996; Johannsen, 1994; Labus, 1995; *Scientific American*, 1995.

Table 17-11-3. Pulmonary Function Values

Measurement	Normal	Mild	Moderate	Severe
FEV_1	4 L/s	1.2 to 1.5 L/s (may be dyspneic)	1.0 L/s (may be sedentary) <1.0 L/s (may show signs of hypoxemia, hypercapnia, cor pulmonale)	≤ 500 mL/s (may be bed-bound)
		≥ 50% PNV	39–49% PNV	< 35% PNV
FEV_1/FVC	75–80%	60%		
FVC	5 L/s		Decreased	
$FEF_{25-75\%}$	3.5 L/s		Decreased	
TLC	6.58 to 9.25 L		Increased in emphysema	
RV/TLC	30–40%			
DL_{CO}			Decreased in emphysema > chronic bronchitis	
Single-breath nitrogen washout			Increased nitrogen concentration	

SOURCE: Fishman et al, 1985; Hahn, 1996; Johannsen, 1994; O'Hara, 1995a; West, 1987.

Peak Flow

The peak expiratory flow rate (PEFR) as measured by a handheld peak flowmeter is an estimate of ventilatory status for patients with asthma. The peak flowmeter has not proved helpful in COPD. Because of the prolonged exhalation, these patients cannot make a good expiratory effort. Also, because of the reduced FEV_1, the scale on a peak flowmeter is not sensitive enough to register very low volumes. FEV_1 as measured by spirometry is considered a more accurate measure of ventilatory status in COPD patients.

IMAGING
Chest X-Ray

X-ray abnormalities may be minimal and can be negative in up to one-third of these patients. Typical findings in emphysema-predominant patients are overinflation, flat diaphragm, low position of diaphragm at or below the seventh rib, and increased retrosternal air space (defined as an increase in radiolucency of 2.5 cm or more between the sternum and the most anterior margin of the ascending aorta) on the lateral view. Chronic bronchitis is difficult to see on x-ray and may be suggested by cardiac enlargement, lung field congestion, increased lung markings, and thickening of bronchial walls (parallel or tram lines). The chest x-ray is useful in ruling out other respiratory diseases (Fig. 17-11-4).

Computer Tomography

CT is exceptional for showing anatomic details and particularly useful in demonstrating lung parenchyma and interstitial disease. CT provides direct visualization of emphysematous areas without interference from overlapping structures so that a pathologic diagnosis of emphysema can be made in a living patient. This is helpful when early diagnosis is useful, such as in the diagnosis of α_1-antitrypsin deficiency, and to demonstrate extensive upper lobe emphysema when the patient does not have PFT abnormalities.

Arterial Blood Gas

Hypoxemia with or without carbon dioxide (CO_2) retention is common in COPD because of the uneven ventilation-perfusion of the lung. Emphysemia-predominant patients typically have mild to moderate hypoxemia with oxygen tension (Pa_{O_2}) levels of 65 to 70 mmHg and normal CO_2 tension levels (Pa_{CO_2}) of 35 to 40 mmHg. Chronic bronchitis-predominant patients typically have severe hypoxemia with Pa_{O_2} levels of 45 to 60 mmHg and hypercapnia with Pa_{CO_2} levels of 50 to 60 mmHg. Some patients

can compensate for the increased CO_2 retention. Their kidneys can slowly retain bicarbonate so that the pH will remain constant. Compensated respiratory acidosis can be seen in patients when FEV_1 drops below 1.0 L/s. The arterial blood gas (ABG) should be checked yearly once Pa_{O_2} falls to 55 mmHg or FEV_1 drops to 1.0 L/s (Table 17-11-4).

Pulse Oximetry

Pulse oximetry can be used to periodically check oxygen saturation (Sa_{O_2}). Oximetry is an indirect measure of Sa_{O_2} with an accuracy of 3 to 5 percent for Sa_{O_2} values greater than 70 percent at sea level. An Sa_{O_2} of 90 percent approximates a Pa_{O_2} of 60 mmHg. Sa_{O_2} should be 95 percent or more for adequate tissue oxygenation. Pulse oximetry should not be used to replace ABG but to monitor patients, keeping in mind that it gives no information on Pa_{CO_2}.

Electrocardiogram

The ECG is normal early in the course of the disease. Later in the course of the chronic bronchitis component there may be right axis deviation (QRS axis +90° and +180°), tall R waves in lead V_1 or V_2 (≥ 6 mm), and deep S waves in lead V_5 or V_6 (≥ 10 mm). During exacerbations tall P waves (≥ 2.5 mm) may be seen. There is not a good correlation, however, between these findings and pulmonary hypertension or cor pulmonale. Only one-third of COPD patients are found to have hypertrophy of the right ventricle at autopsy.

Complete Blood Count

The complete blood count is usually normal but may show polycythemia later in the course of chronic bronchitis-predominant dis-

Table 17-11-4. Values of Arterial Blood Gases and Hemoglobin and Hematocrit

Arterial measurements	Normal range on room air at sea level	
Pa_{O_2}	80–100 mmHg	
Pa_{CO_2}	35–45 mmHg	
pH	7.35 to 7.45	
Oxygen saturation (Sa_{O_2})	96 to 100%	
Venous measurements		
Hemoglobin	Men 16 g/dL ± 2	Women 14 g/dL ± 2
Hematocrit	47% ± 5	42% ± 5
Definitions		
Adequate hemoglobin saturation		Pa_{O_2} > 60 mmHg
Hypercapnia		Pa_{CO_2} > 45 mmHg
Hypoxemia		Pa_{O_2} < 60 mmHg

SOURCE: O'Hara, 1995a.

Table 17-11-5. Beta Agonist Medications

Medication	Route	Dose
Short-acting		
Albuterol sulfate	Oral	2–4 mg tid to qid
(Proventil, Ventolin)	0.5% solution	0.5 mL in 3 mL normal saline q 4 to 6 h
	MDI	2 puffs qid (90 μg/puff)
Metaproterenol sulfate	Oral	20 mg tid to qid
(Alupent, Metaprel)	5% solution	0.3 mL in 3 mL normal saline q 4 to 6 h
	MDI	2 puffs qid (650 μg/puff)
Terbutaline sulfate	Oral	5 mg tid
(Brethine, Bricanyl)	MDI	2 puffs qid (200 μg/puff)
Long-acting		
Salmeterol xinafoate	MDI	1 puff bid (42 μg/puff)
(Serevent)		

SOURCE: O'Hara, 1995b.

ease as a result of hypoxemia. The hemoglobin may drop below 16 percent from oxygen desaturation, and the hematocrit may be elevated to 50 to 60 percent in chronic bronchitis patients. The hematocrit value is usually three times the hemoglobin value.

DIFFERENTIAL DIAGNOSIS

Other bronchopulmonary diseases can coexist or be confused with COPD. The differential diagnosis includes upper airway obstruction (neck mass, upper airway narrowing), tuberculosis, lung cancer, cystic fibrosis, asthma, acute bronchitis, pneumothorax, bronchiectasis, chronic pulmonary embolism, and heart failure.

TREATMENT

Bronchodilators

Bronchodilators are the first-line treatment for COPD.

Beta Agonists

Inhaled beta-adrenergic agonists (BAAs) are used to reverse bronchospasm, addressing the chronic bronchitis component of COPD. Short-acting inhaled BAAs such as albuterol sulfate (Proventil, Ventolin) and metaproterenol sulfate (Alupent) have fewer side effects of skeletal muscle tremor, palpitations, nervousness, tachycardia, and hypertension because less is absorbed into the systemic circulation. They can be conveniently self-administered with a metered-dose inhaler (MDI). The onset of action occurs within minutes, and the duration is 3 to 6 h. The use of a spacing device allows the patient to inhale the aerosolized particles from a reservoir to improve delivery of the medication. Oral BAAs have more systemic side effects and are used by patients who cannot coordinate the use of a MDI. Nebulization is another delivery method for inhaled BAAs. Nebulizer treatment takes 5 to 15 min and is a more expensive delivery method than MDI mainly because of the greater amount of medication required in solution for aerosolization. The advantages of this delivery method are greater deposition of medication in the large and small airways and ease of use, especially by the elderly, for whom inspiratory effort and coordination of the puff from the inhaler may be a problem.

Salmeterol xinafoate (Serevent) is a long-acting selective inhaled beta$_2$ receptor agonist that was introduced into the United States in 1994 for chronic asthma. Patients with stable moderate to severe COPD have shown benefit from salmeterol. For breakthrough symptoms, rescue medication with short-acting inhaled BAAs up to eight puffs per day can be used in acute exacerbations. Patients must understand that salmeterol is used only for chronic treatment (Table 17-11-5).

Anticholinergic Agents

Inhaled anticholinergic agents cause bronchodilation by inhibiting the release of acetylcholine from the vagus nerve in respiratory smooth muscle. Anticholinergic agents have a slightly later onset of action than do BAAs (45 min) and a duration of 6 to 12 h. They are considered first-line therapy for emphysema. Ipratropium bromide (Atrovent) is available in MDI form, while atropine sulfate and glycopyrrolate (Robinul) are used for nebulization. The side effects are minimal but include dry mouth, flushing of the skin, blurred vision, tachycardia, and urinary retention. Atropine seems to dilate large airways more effectively than do BAAs primarily because of the greater number of cholinergic (muscarinic) receptors in the central airways compared with the peripheral airways. BAAs seem to have better dilatory effects on small airways because the density of the beta$_2$ receptors increases as the peripheral airways narrow. This may account for the synergistic effects of BAAs and anticholinergic agents. Studies show that stable COPD patients do better with routine doses of both drugs administered together two to four times a day. BAAs and anticholinergic solutions may be mixed together in the chamber of a handheld nebulizer for ease of delivery (Table 17-11-6).

Methylxanthenes

Theophylline is a weaker bronchodilator than are the BAAs, but there is evidence that it has some anti-inflammatory properties as well as the ability to improve respiratory muscle strength, increase diaphragmatic contractility, increase right and left ventricular contractility, and act as a pulmonary vasodilator to decrease pulmonary hypertension and increase cardiac output. Even at therapeutic levels (10 to 20 mg/L), theophylline has a significant potential for adverse effects and drug interactions and should be monitored for toxicity. One should check levels 2 to 5 days after a change in dose or when symptoms of toxicity are present, in particular nausea, vomiting, tachycardia, hypertension, and tremor. Theophylline is considered an adjunct with routine doses of BAAs and anticholinergic agents in the treatment of stable COPD patients and is particularly useful for nocturnal dyspnea (Table 17-11-7).

Corticosteroids

For patients with a greater predominance of the chronic bronchitis component, corticosteroids may be helpful in reducing inflammation in the airways. Corticosteroids are available in varying potencies and formulations based on a comparison with hydrocortisone.

Because of the variety of responses to corticosteroids, there are several approaches to their use. Oral prednisone is four times more potent than hydrocortisone in anti-inflammatory action and can be used for acute exacerbations or chronic treatment in conjunction with bronchodilators and theophylline. Patients can be given 40 to 60 mg of oral prednisone per day; if at the end of 2

Table 17-11-6. Anticholinergic Drug Dosing

Medication	Route	Dosing
Atropine sulfate	Nebulizer	1–3 mg in 3 mL normal saline q 6 to 8 h (can be mixed with BAA dose)
Glycopyrrolate (Robinul)	Nebulizer	0.2–1.0 mg in 3 mL normal saline q 6 to 10 h (can be mixed with BAA dose)
Ipratropium bromide (Atrovent)	MDI	2 puffs qid (18 μg/puff)

SOURCE: O'Hara, 1995b.

Table 17-11-7. Theophylline Side Effects, Interactions, and Dosing

Side effects
  Headache
  Anxiety
  Tremulousness
  Hypokalemia
  Hypercalcemia
  Nausea
  Vomiting
  Gastroesophageal sphincter relaxation
  Tachycardia
  Arrhythmias
  Levels > 40 mg/L
    Seizures
    Death
Drug interactions
  Erythromycin
  Cimetidine (Tagamet)
  Phenytoin (Dilantin)
  Quinolones (e.g., Cipro)
  Propranolol (Indural)
  High-dose allopurinol
  Rifampin
  Barbiturates
  Lithium
Dosing
  Sustained-release products
    Theo-Dur 200–300 mg qh or bid
    Slo-bid 200–300 mg qh or bid (check levels appropriately)

SOURCE: Johannsen, 1994; O'Hara, 1995b.

Table 17-11-9. Inhaled Corticosteroid Dosing

Metered-Dose Inhaler	Dose
Beclomethasone dipropionate (Beclovent, Vanceril; inhaler includes spacer)	4 puffs (42 μg/puff) bid to qid
Dexamethasone sodium phosphate (Decadron)	3 puffs (84 μg/puff) bid to qid
Flunisolide (Aerobid)	2 puffs (250 μg/puff) bid to qid
Triamcinolone acetonide (Azmacort; inhaler includes spacer)	4 puffs (100 μg/puff) bid to qid

SOURCE: O'Hara, 1995b.

to 3 weeks FEV_1 improves 20 to 30 percent compared to baseline, consideration should be given to long-term therapy. Patients can be tapered from the 40 to 60 mg per day to 20 mg over 1 to 2 weeks and then to less than 10 mg daily (5 to 7 mg per day or 15 to 20 mg on alternate days). Side effects of prednisone may develop if the daily dose is greater than 10 mg for longer than 3 weeks (Table 17-11-8). Studies show that the improvement in FEV_1 may last as long as 6 months, after which a decline is seen. The annual decline in FEV_1 with corticosteroids, however, is slower than that with bronchodilator treatment alone.

Inhaled corticosteroids (ICSs) can be used alone or in conjunction with oral prednisone. The advantage of ICSs is that they have the anti-inflammatory potency of oral corticosteroids with minimal systemic side effects. The maximum dose of an ICS is about 1.5 to 2.0 mg per day, which is equivalent to 10 mg of oral prednisone. The therapeutic effects of an ICS begin in 6 to 12 h, and maximum efficacy is achieved in 2 to 4 weeks. If patients respond well to ICS, it may be possible to lower the dose of oral corticosteroids or withdraw them altogether (Table 17-11-9).

For acute exacerbations, a short course of oral prednisone can be helpful for patients with or without long-term low-dose oral prednisone or ICS treatment. The onset of action takes a few hours, but the effects of one dose may last 16 to 36 h. A short course may prevent a relapse (Table 17-11-10).

Patients can be started on bronchodilators, theophylline, and corticosteroids individually or in combination, depending on which symptoms of emphysema or chronic bronchitis predominate. Medications can be maximized in a stepwise fashion. Patients may feel better on a regimen of a combination of medications, even though there may not be a significant improvement in FEV_1.

Other Anti-Inflammatory Agents

Cromylin sodium (Intal) and nedocromil sodium (Tilade) have been used in the treatment of asthma. Their use may be helpful in conjunction with respiratory tract allergies in association with COPD, but their use in COPD has not been proved to be effective.

Mucokinetics

Mucokinetic agents may be helpful for patients with chronic bronchitis predominance. They facilitate mucociliary clearance by increasing mucus production while decreasing the viscosity and tenaciousness of mucus. Oral iodides have antiallergic and anti-inflammatory properties. They serve as an expectorant by stimulating the vagal-gastropulmonary reflex and as a mucolytic by splitting mucoproteins. Guiafenesin is a common iodinated glycerol that is available in liquid or tablet form. It also can be found in combination with other ingredients for cough and

Table 17-11-8. Corticosteroid Side Effects

Short course (> 10 mg for less than 3 weeks)
  Increased appetite
  Acne
  Fluid retention
  Mood alterations
  Hyperglycemia in susceptible persons
Long-term effects (> 10 mg for longer than 3 weeks)
  Hypertension
  Diabetes mellitus in predisposed persons
  Osteoporosis
  Cushingoid obesity
  Poor wound healing
  Personality changes
  Glaucoma
  Cataracts
  Dyspepsia
  Suppression of the hypothalamic-pituitary-adrenal axis

SOURCE: O'Hara, 1995b.

Table 17-11-10. Oral Prednisone Burst

No previous oral prednisone use: 30 mg/d for 1 to 2 weeks
Previous oral prednisone use: 60 mg/d for 1 to 2 weeks
With or without previous oral prednisone use
  40–60 mg/d for 5 to 7 days
  40–80 mg/d for 5 to 7 days, then taper
Tapering suggestions
  40 mg 40×2 days, 30×2 days, 20×2 days, 15×2 days, 10×2 days, 5×2 days
  60 mg 60×1 day, 50×1 day, 40×1 day, 30×1 day, 20×1 day, 15×1 day, 10×2 days, 5×2 days

SOURCE: O'Hara, 1995b.

Table 17-11-11. Mucokinetic Drugs

Drug	Route	Dose
Guaifenesin	Tablets	200–400 mg q 4 h up to 2400 mg/24 h
Organidin NR	Elixir, 1.2%	1 teaspoon qid
Humibid LA	Tablets	600 mg, 1 or 2 bid up to 2400 mg/24 h

SOURCE: *Physicians' Desk Reference*, 1995.

rhinorrhea. BAAs and the methylxanthenes also have mucociliary clearance properties (Table 17-11-11).

Oxygen

Supplemental oxygen (O_2) therapy has been shown to improve survival and quality of life. Patients at rest with a Pa_{O_2} less than 55 mmHg with or without signs of cor pulmonale or an Sa_{O_2} less than 88 percent benefit from supplemental O_2. Low-flow O_2 by nasal cannula of 1 to 3 L raises Pa_{O_2} to 60 to 80 mmHg and Sa_{O_2} to approximately 90 percent. Patients are encouraged to use the O_2 15 to 24 h a day because survival is so significantly improved with continuous use. O_2 helps reduce hypoxemia, which in turn reduces pulmonary hypertension. The purpose of supplemental O_2 therapy is to enhance physiologic delivery of O_2 to the tissues. There are concerns that O_2 therapy will cause the Pa_{CO_2} to increase, blunting the chemoreceptors for respiratory drive. It is theorized that the increase in Pa_{CO_2} is due to the increased ventilation of the anatomic dead space. If the Pa_{CO_2} stabilizes and does not lead to increased respiratory acidosis, it is considered more dangerous to withdraw or withhold O_2 than to prevent the increasing Pa_{CO_2}. Only hypoxemia is treated; hypercapnia is not treated but is monitored for respiratory acidosis.

Patients who desaturate during exercise to less than 88 percent also benefit from supplemental O_2. It is documented that COPD patients desaturate when sleeping, especially during rapid eye movement (REM) sleep, and may experience periods of apnea. The supine position increases hypoxemia and decreases the respiratory drive. Sleep studies have shown diaphragmatic pauses and irregular breathing in association with REM sleep. Sa_{O_2} may drop 10 to 50 percent for more than 30 min during REM sleep (Table 17-11-12).

Diuretics, Digitalis, and Phlebotomy

Patients with COPD may exhibit pedal edema even without right-sided congestive heart failure. Diuretics may provide symptomatic relief. Digoxin is a weak inotropic stimulant for the right ventricle by itself and should be used in a patient who has both right and left ventricular failure. In the past phlebotomy was used

Table 17-11-12. Indications for Oxygen Therapy

Continuous therapy
  At rest on room air
    Pa_{O_2} 55 mgHg*
    Pa_{O_2} 55–59 mmHg with peripheral edema (cor pulmonale), polycythemia (hematocrit > 55%), congestive heart failure
    Sa_{O_2} < 88%*
    Hematocrit > 55%
Intermittent therapy
  Nocturnal hypoxemia
    Pa_{O_2} < 55 mmHg*
    Sa_{O_2} < 88%*
  Exercise-induced hypoxemia
    Pa_{O_2} < 55 mmHg*
    Sa_{O_2} < 88%*

* Will be reimbursed by Medicare.

SOURCE: Fei and Murata, 1994; *Scientific American*, 1995.

in patients whose hematocrit was above 55 to 60 percent. It was thought that the increase in blood viscosity contributed to right-sided heart strain. Now supplemental O_2 therapy is used.

Antibiotics

COPD patients are at risk for lower respiratory infections as a result of reduced mucociliary clearance. These patients probably are afflicted more often with viral illnesses that go on to become secondarily superimposed with bacterial infections. COPD patients should be considered for antibiotic treatment for 7 to 10 days when there is an increase in dyspnea, increased sputum production, and purulent sputum. The organisms most often recovered from the sputum of COPD patients are *Haemophilus influenzae* and *Streptococcus pneumoniae*. *Mycoplasma pneumoniae* and *Moraxella* (*Branhanella*) *catarrhalis* are also common. The literature does show an improvement in acute exacerbations in ambulatory patients with antibiotic treatment, but antibiotic prophylaxis consisting of 1 week of oral medication per month is controversial. If sputum cultures are not taken, consideration for empiric treatment should be given on the basis of the common organisms, and if there is no improvement in 2 days, one should consider a broader-spectrum agent to cover the less common organisms (Table 17-11-13).

Vaccinations

Patients with COPD are recommended to have influenza vaccinations annually to prevent lung damage from viral infections. Amantadine (Symmetrel syrup 50 mg/5 mL, 100 mg bid) may help decrease the severity of the symptoms of influenza A. Pneumovax 23 (Merck) is a pneumococcal vaccine that is effective against 23 types of pneumococcal strains responsible for 85 to 90 percent of pneumococcal infections. It is recommended that COPD patients be vaccinated at least once and that consideration be given to revaccination every 6 years.

Antiprotease Therapy

α_1-Antitrypsin deficiency is an inherited disorder that causes destruction of interstitial elastin fibers in alveolar walls by elastase. The deficiency can be detected by serum levels of α_1 antitrypsin < 11 μM. The ATS recommends recombinant antiprotease replacement therapy consisting of injections of purified α_1 antitrypsin weekly (60 mg/kg) or monthly (250 mg/kg) for selected candidates. This therapy is costly and controversial and is under clinical investigation.

SURGICAL TREATMENT

Lung Transplantation

The first successful single-lung transplantation was performed in 1983 for pulmonary fibrosis. Since that time single-lung transplant has been used for patients with end-stage emphysema. The majority of transplant patients are those with α_1-antitrypsin deficiency. Since they are younger than patients with smoking-induced COPD, in general they are better surgical candidates. Bilateral lung transplants have been performed on patients with chronic bronchitis. In spite of problems with the availability of donors, postoperative infections, organ rejection, and immunosuppression, survival rates have been reported to be as high as 93 percent, at 1 year, 74 percent at 3 years, and 50 percent at 5 years. Significant improvement in pulmonary function has made lung transplantation a viable therapeutic option for end-stage disease.

Reduction Pneumoplasty

Reduction pneumoplasty or bullectomy is another treatment option for bullous emphysema. The volume of one lung or both

Table 17-11-13. Examples of Antibiotic Coverage and Dosing for Outpatients

Drug	Brand Name	Dose	Covered Organisms or Particular Indication
Penicillins			
Penicillin*	Pen V	250 mg tid or 500 bid	*S. aureus, S. pneumoniae, S. pyogenes, S. viridans* group
	Bicillin C-R	2.4 million units IM, then use oral agent	Same as penicillin
	Wicillin	1.0 million units IM, then use oral agent	Same as penicillin
Ampicillin		250–500 mg qid	Same as penicillin, some gram-negatives, *H. influenzae* (not β-lactam-producing)
Amoxicillin		250–500 mg tid	Same as ampicillin
Amoxicillin/clavulanate potassium	Augmentin	250–500 mg tid	Same as penicillin, *H. influenzae* (β-lactam-producing), *M. catarrhalis*
Cephalosporins			
First generation			
Cefadroxil	Duricef	500 mg bid	*S. aureus, S. epidermidis, S. pneumoniae, S. pyogenes, M. catarrhalis*
Cephalexin	Keflex	250–500 mg qid	Gram-positives, some gram-negatives
Second generation			
Cefaclor	Ceclor	250–500 mg tid	*S. pneumoniae, S. pyogenes, H. influenzae, M. catarrhalis,* some gram-negatives
Cefuroxime	Ceftin	250–500 mg tid	Same as cefaclor
Third generation			
Cefixime	Suprax	400 mg qd	Gram-positives, *H. influenzae, M. catarrhalis,* gram-negatives (including *Pseudomonas aeruginosa*)
Ceftriaxone	Rocephin	1 to 2 g IM, then use oral agent	Gram-positives, *H. influenzae, M. catarrhalis,* gram-negatives (± *P. aeruginosa*)
Macrolides			
Erythromycin		250 mg qid or 500 mg bid	Beta-hemolytic streptococci, *S. aureus, S. pneumoniae, S. pyogenes, S. viridans,* ±*H. influenzae, Legionella pneumophilia, M. catarrhalis, Mycoplasma pneumoniae*
Clarithromycin	Biaxin	250–500 bid	Erythromycin-resistant organisms, β-lactam-producing *H. influenzae, M. catarrhalis*
Azithromycin	Zithromax	500 mg day 1; 250 mg days 2 through 5	Same as clarithromycin
Tetracyclines			
Tetracycline		500 mg bid to qid	Gram-positives, *H. influenzae, M. pneumoniae, M. catarrhalis*
Doxycycline	Vibramycin	100 mg bid	Same as tetracycline
Quinolones			
Ciprofloxacin	Cipro	500–750 mg bid	Gram-positives, resistant gram-negatives, methicillin-resistant *S. aureus, P. aeruginosa*
Ofloxacin	Floxin	400 mg bid	Same as ciprofloxacin
Sulfa			
Trimethoprim-sulfamethoxazole	Bactrim	Double-strength bid	Gram-positives, *Diplococcus pneumoniae, S. pneumoniae,* gram-negatives (except *P. aeruginosa*), *H. influenzae, L. pneumophilia, M. catarrhalis*

* All medications given orally unless indicated.

SOURCE: Dantzker, MacIntyre, and Bakow, 1995; Johannsen, 1994; Sanford, Gilbert, and Sande, 1995.

lungs is reduced by 20 to 30 percent in the hyperinflated areas. Respiratory mechanics are improved because the chest wall and diaphragm return to a more normal position. The FEV_1/FVC ratio is greatly improved, and the majority of patients do not need supplemental O_2. Even though mortality rates are as high as 15 percent, survival rates are greater than they are with lung transplantation because there are fewer postoperative complications.

Pulmonary Rehabilitation

Pulmonary rehabilitation is a multidisciplinary approach whose goal is to maximize functional capacity in activities of daily living and quality of life. It includes respiratory therapy, physical therapy, nutrition, psychology, and social work. The goals of pulmonary rehabilitation are to increase exercise tolerance, teach respiratory muscle training techniques, teach energy conservation techniques, provide psychosocial support, and give the patient information regarding the disease process, the use of medications, and smoking cessation. The best candidates for pulmonary reha-

bilitation are those who are motivated to improve their health status. All patients can benefit from pulmonary rehabilitation, but those with mild to moderate disease probably benefit the most.

ACUTE RESPIRATORY FAILURE

Acute respiratory failure is defined as a decrease in Pa_{O_2} 10 to 15 mmHg from the baseline ABG values or an increase in Pa_{CO_2} with pH ≤ 7.3 (acidemia). Hypoventilation at the level of the alveoli and pulmonary capillaries is the mechanism of failure in obstructive disease, causing an increase in the ventilation-perfusion mismatch. These patients may complain of headache, visual disturbance, memory loss, confusion, and palpitations. Reversal of hypoxemia corrects the acidemia. Respiratory failure calls for admission to an intensive care unit. The criteria for intubation and mechanical ventilation include altered mental status, labored breathing (tachypnea > 30 breaths per minute), hypoxemia not responsive to O_2 therapy, and rising hypercapnia.

Table 17-11-14. Instructions for Using Metered-Dose Inhalers

Without Spacer	Alternative Method without Spacer	With Spacer
1. Put inhaler together and shake canister		Put inhaler together with spacer and shake canister
2. Take cap off and close lips around mouthpiece. Be sure tongue is away from opening. Hold canister with index finger on top and thumb on bottom	Take cap off and hold mouthpiece approximately 1 in. (3 cm) from open mouth. Hold canister with index finger on top and thumb on bottom	Close lips around tubing of spacer mouthpiece. Be sure tongue is away from the opening. Hold canister with index finger on top and thumb on bottom
3. Exhale completely through the mouth		
4. Begin to inhale slowly and squeeze canister		
5. At end of inhalation, hold breath for 4 to 10 s if possible		
6. Wait 1 min before inhaling any more puffs		
7. Use bronchodilators before using inhaled corticosteroids		
8. Rinse out mouth after steroid use		

The mortality rate of any patient who undergoes mechanical ventilation for any reason is as high as 38 percent.

PATIENT EDUCATION

Smoking Cessation

Since there is no cure for COPD, quitting smoking is the number one intervention to help slow the deleterious effects and reduce the complications of COPD. Nicotine substitution in gum or patch form is available to help patients with smoking cessation.

Environmental Concerns

Patients with hypoxemia should avoid high altitudes, which may lower Pao_2 levels. Patients should live at altitudes lower than 3500 to 4000 ft and may need supplemental O_2 when traveling at high altitudes. Extremes of temperature and humidity may exacerbate airway hyperreactivity and bronchospasm. Patients should be advised to use air-conditioning in the summer and humidifiers in the winter. Particulate matter from air pollution or ozone (more than 0.12 parts per million) may irritate the airways. Patients should be advised to curtail outdoor activities on days of poor air quality. Efforts should be made to eliminate allergens from a patient's environment.

Advance Directives

All Medicare and Medicaid providers are required to inform all patients about their right to make choices regarding health care under provisions of the Self-Determination Act, which became effective on December 1, 1991. Discussion should be initiated regarding do not resuscitate orders and a living will or durable power of attorney for health care when patients are not critically ill. Patients can designate another person to make health care decisions if they are incapacitated and/or can document their wishes regarding resuscitation and life support measures.

Exercise

Exercise should be encouraged to maintain cardiovascular fitness and skeletal muscle tone. Walking is recommended. Exercise also raises self-esteem, increases the capacity to maintain the activities of daily living, reduces breathlessness, and increases the exercise capacity.

Nutrition

The work of breathing imposes high metabolic demands and requires high caloric expenditure. There can be an increase in resting energy expenditure of 10 to 20 percent without the matching caloric intake to counteract weight loss. The loss of more than 50 percent of ideal weight puts a patient at risk for nutritional deficiencies and decreased muscle strength of the diaphragm. A high-fat, high-protein (20 percent of total calories), low-carbohydrate diet is recommended because of the increased CO_2 from the by-products of the breakdown of carbohydrates. Adequate hydration of 2 L of water per day helps keep mucus secretions thin, even in those with right-sided heart failure.

Depression

Depression is seen in 42 percent of patients with COPD. It is described as an adjustment disorder with depressed mood because of identifiable stressors. These patients exhibit low self-esteem and lack confidence and spontaneity. The tricyclic antidepressant medications have been shown to produce improvement in patients with depression and COPD. The tricyclics have atropine-like properties that promote bronchodilation and decrease obstruction. Nortriptyline and desipramine have been commonly used.

Follow-up

One must make sure that patients understand the correct technique for the use of their inhalers (Table 17-11-14). Patients can

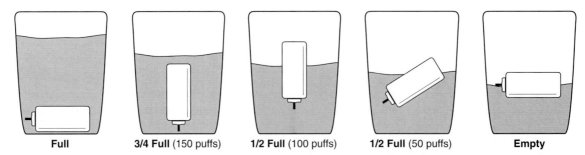

| Full | 3/4 Full (150 puffs) | 1/2 Full (100 puffs) | 1/2 Full (50 puffs) | Empty |

Figure 17-11-5. Method of estimating the amount of medication in an inhaler canister. (*From Dantzker et al, 1995; Pagliaro and Pagliaro, 1986.*)

estimate how much medication is in the canister by putting it in a glass of water. When it is empty, it floats (Figure 17-11-5). Patients should be seen in the office at least every 6 months for follow-up, even if they are feeling well. It should be discussed in advance what patients should do in case of an acute exacerbation in terms of additional (rescue) medications or if they should go to the office or emergency department for treatment.

REFERRAL TO A PULMONARY SPECIALIST

There are no hard and fast rules about referring patients to a pulmonary specialist. The history, physical examination, and initial studies of chest x-ray and PFTs should be obtained. It is recommended that patients be referred to a pulmonologist whenever a provider becomes uncomfortable with the treatment regimen. Evaluation of patients for α_1-antitrypsin deficiency, CT, lung transplant, or reduction pneumoplasty falls into the purview of the specialist.

BIBLIOGRAPHY

Berkow R, ed: *The Merck Manual of Diagnosis and Therapy,* 15th ed. Rahway, NJ, Merck Sharp & Dohme, 1987.

Braunwald E, Isselbacher KJ, Petersdorf RG, et al (eds): *Harrison's Principles of Internal Medicine,* 11th ed. Companion Handbook. New York, McGraw-Hill, 1988.

Briffa NP, Dennis C, Higenbottam T, et al: Single lung transplantation for end stage emphysema. *Thorax* 50(5):562–564, 1995.

Calverley PMA, Pride NB (eds): *Chronic Obstructive Pulmonary Disease.* London, Chapman & Hall, 1995.

Christensen L, (ed): *Identification and Treatment of COPD: Detecting and Treating COPD.* AAPA 1995 Annual Meeting Symposium Highlights. Yardley, PA, Medical Association Communications, 1995.

COMBIVENT Inhalation Aerosol Study Group: Chronic obstructive pulmonary disease: A combination of ipratropium and albuterol is more effective than either agent alone: An 85-day multicenter trial. *Chest* 105(5):1411–1419, 1994.

Dantzker DR, MacIntyre NR, Bakow ED: *Comprehensive Respiratory Care.* Philadelphia, Saunders, 1995.

De Jong JW, Postma DS, van der Mark TW, Koëter GH: Effects of nedocromil sodium in the treatment of non-allergic subjects with chronic obstructive pulmonary disease. *Thorax* 49(10):1022–1024, 1994.

Dompeling E, van Schayck CP, van Grunsven PM, et al: Slowing the deterioration of asthma and chronic obstructive pulmonary disease observed during bronchodilator therapy by adding inhaled corticosteroids. *Ann Intern Med* 118(10):770–778, 1993.

Emerman CL, Cydulka RK: Use of peak expiratory flow rate in emergency department evaluation of acute exacerbation of chronic obstructive pulmonary disease. *Ann Emerg Med* 27(2):159–163, 1996.

Fei RL, Murata GH: Contemporary management of the patient with chronic obstructive pulmonary disease. *Compr Ther* 20(5):277–281, 1994.

Fishman MC, Hoffman AR, Klausner RD, Thaler MS: *Medicine,* 2d ed. Philadelphia, Lippincott, 1985.

George RB, Light RW, Matthay MA, et al (eds): *Chest Medicine: Essentials of Pulmonary and Critical Care Medicine,* 3d ed. Baltimore, Williams & Wilkins, 1995.

Gift AG, McCrone SH. Depression in patients with COPD. *Heart Lung* 22(4):289–297, 1993.

Griffith HW, Dambro MR, Griffith J: *The 5 Minute Clinical Consult.* Philadelphia, Lea & Febiger, 1994.

Hahn MS: Chronic obstructive pulmonary disease: Understanding this progressive illness. *AdPA,* April 1996, pp 15–19.

Health after 50: Advances in the treatment of emphysema. *Johns Hopkins Med Let* 8(7):5–6, 1996.

Ikeda A, Nishimura K, Koyama H, Izumi T: Bronchodilating effects of combined therapy with clinical dosages of ipratropium bromide and salbutamol for stable COPD: Comparison with ipratropium bromide alone. *Chest* 108(6):1773–1774, 1995.

Johannsen JM: Chronic obstructive pulmonary disease: Current comprehensive care for emphysema and bronchitis. *Nurs Practi* 19(1):59–67, 1994.

Karpel JP, Kotch A, Zinny M, et al: Comparison of inhaled ipratropium, oral theophylline plus inhaled β-agonist, and the combination of all three in patients with COPD. *Chest* 105(4):1089–1094, 1994.

Kelley WN, (ed): *Essentials of Internal Medicine.* Philadelphia, Lippincott, 1994.

Kerstjens HAM, Overbeek SE, Schouten JP, et al: Airways hyperresponsiveness, bronchodilator response, allergy and smoking predict improvement in FEV_1 during long-term inhaled corticosteroid treatment. *Eur Respir J* 6:868–876, 1993.

Labus JB: *The Physician Assistant Medical Handbook.* Philadelphia, Saunders, 1995.

Little AG, Swain JA, Nino JJ, et al: Reduction pneumonoplasty for emphysema. *Ann Surg* 222(3):365–371, 1995.

McGregor CGA, Daly RC, Peters SG, et al: Evolving strategies in lung transplantation for emphysema. *Ann Thorac Surg* 57(6):1513–1520, 1994.

Miller A (ed): *Pulmonary Function Tests: A Guide for the Student and House Officer.* Orlando, FL, Grune & Stratton, 1987.

Moayyedi P, Congleton J, Page RL, et al: Comparison of nebulised salbutamol and ipratropium bromide with salbutamol alone in the treatment of chronic obstructive pulmonary disease. *Thorax* 50(8):834–837, 1995.

Nishimura K, Koyama H, Ikeda A, Izumi T: Is Oral theophylline effective in combination with both inhaled anticholinergic agent and inhaled β_2-agonist in the treatment of stable COPD? *Chest* 104(1):179–184, 1993.

O'Donnell DE, Webb KA, McGuire MA: Older patients with COPD: Benefits of exercise training. *Geriatrics* 48(1):59–66, 1993.

O'Hara MM: Understanding asthma: Why it happens and how to assess your adult patient. *J Am Acad Physician Assist* 8(3):20–35, 1995a.

O'Hara MM: Understanding asthma: New priorities in treatment. *J Am Acad Physician Assist* 8(7):60–78, 1995b.

Pagliaro AM, Pagliaro LA: *Pharmacologic Aspects of Nursing.* St. Louis, Mosby, 1986.

Peterson M, Rahr R, Blessing D, Ayachi S: Chronic obstructive pulmonary disease: Improving the outcome. *Physician Assist* 19(11):39–53, 1995.

Physicians' Desk Reference, 49th ed. Montvale, NJ, Medical Economics, 1995.

Rebuck DA, Hanania NA, D'Urzo AD, Chapman KR: The accuracy of a handheld portable spirometer. *Chest* 109(1):152–157, 1996.

Sanford JP, Gilbert DN, Sande MA: *The Sanford Guide to Antimicrobial Therapy.* Dallas, Antimicrobial Therapy, 1995.

Scientific American Medicine. SAM-CD, Jan. 1996. Online Computer Services. *Chronic Obstructive Diseases of the Lung.* New York, Scientific American, 1995.

Tardif C, Bonmarchand G, Gibon J-F, et al: Respiratory response to CO_2 in patients with chronic obstructive pulmonary disease in acute respiratory failure. *Eur Respir J* 6(5):619–624, 1993.

Ulrik CS: Efficacy of inhaled sameterol in the management of smokers with chronic obstructive pulmonary disease: A single centre randomised, double blind, placebo controlled, crossover study. *Thorax* 50(7):750–754, 1995.

Weiner P, Weiner M, Azgad Y, Zamir D: Inhaled budesonide therapy for patients with stable COPD. *Chest* 108(6):1568–1571, 1995.

West JB: *Pulmonary Pathophysiology: The Essentials,* 3d ed. Baltimore, Williams & Wilkins, 1987.

Wilson AF (ed): *Pulmonary Function Testing Indications and Interpretations: A Project of the California Thoracic Society.* Orlando, FL, Grune & Stratton, 1985.

Wyngaarden JB, Smith LH, Bennett JC (eds): *Cecil Textbook of Medicine,* 19th ed. Philadelphia, Saunders, 1992.

Chapter 18–1
ACUTE RENAL FAILURE
Donald J. Sefcik

DISCUSSION

Normally, the kidneys filter approximately 1700 L of blood per day and produce 1200 mL of urine as they remove metabolic nitrogenous by-products and regulate the volume and composition of body fluids. When an abrupt decline in renal function occurs, the body fluid milieu is disrupted and various clinical changes ensue.

Acute renal failure (ARF), a clinical condition characterized by an abrupt increase in plasma nitrogenous compounds [blood urea nitrogen (BUN) and creatinine], may manifest as a nonspecific entity or a complex array of signs and symptoms. The clinical picture tends to manifest as alterations in body fluid volume and solute composition. Early recognition and intervention have a profound impact on the long-term prognosis.

Asymptomatic elevations of BUN and creatinine (azotemia) and symptomatic renal failure (uremia) may evolve during oliguria (less than 400 mL of urine output/24 h) or with a normal urine output.

For diagnostic purposes, renal failure traditionally is discussed from a physiologic perspective. The three major classes of renal failure are categorized as

- *Prerenal:* affecting perfusion to the kidney
- *Postrenal:* affecting urine outflow distal to the kidney
- *Renal:* an intrinsic, pathophysiologic alteration within the kidney

PATHOGENESIS

The insults to the kidney that elicit renal failure are diverse. The common factor is an alteration in the ability of the kidney to remove nitrogenous compounds from plasma. Renal impairment usually is defined as a glomerular filtration rate (GFR) approximately 40 to 50 percent of normal, renal insufficiency occurs when GFR is approximately 20 to 40 percent of normal, and renal failure develops at GFRs less than 10 percent of normal. As GFR declines, BUN and creatinine accumulate and electrolyte alterations (hyperkalemia, hyperphosphatemia, and hypocalcemia), body fluid shifts (third spacing of fluids), hypertension, and an acid-base imbalance (acidosis) tend to develop.

Prerenal renal failure, the most common type (55 percent of all cases of renal failure), occurs secondary to a reduction in renal perfusion. This may be caused by volume depletion, vasodilation, and reduced cardiac output (Table 18-1-1).

Intrinsic renal failure (40 percent of all cases of ARF) results from processes that cause injury to the kidney or nephron. The term *acute tubular necrosis* (ATN) often is used in reference to intrinsic renal failure. However, many cases of ARF, regardless of etiology, are not associated with necrosis of the tubule, and this description should be reserved for histologic diagnosis. The causes include ischemia, nephrotoxins, interstitial nephritis, and miscellaneous systemic disorders (Table 18-1-1).

Postrenal renal failure (5 percent of all cases of ARF) generally results from an obstructive process. Common sites of obstruction include the bladder outlet, the ureter, and the urethra (Table 18-1-1).

SYMPTOMS

Generally, the degree of symptomatology reflects the severity of renal impairment. The inability of the kidney to regulate body fluid volume, electrolytes, and acid-base balance produces the clinical picture of ARF. Early symptoms noted by these patients may include fatigue, dizziness, swelling, anorexia, shortness of breath, and a reduction in urine output.

The early presentation of ARF is nonspecific. In addition to the general symptoms noted above, patients may have complaints that can help one determine the cause of renal failure. For example, abdominal discomfort may be a result of bladder distention in patients with bladder outflow obstruction. Flank pain may be noted in patients with hydronephrosis secondary to ureteral obstruction. Fever and rashes may be seen in some immunologic disorders associated with intrinsic renal diseases.

The diagnosis of renal failure is not generally difficult once serum chemistries have been obtained. Eliciting the type of ARF—prerenal, postrenal, or renal—poses a more difficult diagnostic challenge to a clinician (Table 18-1-1).

OBJECTIVE FINDINGS

ARF may progress through a series of phases. Commonly, an oliguric phase occurs during which GFR is reduced, BUN and creatinine rise, and problems of fluid overload and electrolyte imbalance develop. This may be followed by a diuretic phase that can last from days to weeks. Early in this phase, the urine output begins to increase, followed by a reduction in BUN and creatinine. Before the advent of dialysis, urine output could exceed 3 or 4 L per day during the recovery phase. A major emphasis in the treatment of ARF is preventing the complications that may develop.

BUN and creatinine tend to increase more than 10 mg/dL and 0.5 mg/dL daily, respectively. Simultaneously, these patients tend to develop hyperkalemia, hyperphosphatemia, hypocalcemia, fluid overload, and acidosis. As the ARF syndrome progresses, pulmonary edema, cardiac dysrhythmias, vomiting, and hypertension may develop.

If the condition becomes protracted, additional clinical manifestations including dermatologic (pruritus and uremic frost), cardiac (pericarditis and congestive heart failure), neurologic (headaches and neuropathies), osteodystrophic (osteoporosis and osteomalacia), and hematopoietic abnormalities (anemia and bleeding tendencies), may develop.

Physical findings on examination may include orthostatic hypotension, tachycardia, tachypnea, rales, jugular venous distention, peripheral edema, rashes, hypertension, flank tenderness, bladder distention, and prostatic hypertrophy, depending on the underlying pathology that initiated the ARF.

Anuria (<100 mL of urine output per 24 h) is often a sign of an obstructive (postrenal) type of ARF.

DIAGNOSTIC CONSIDERATIONS

The first problem facing a clinician is distinguishing a patient with ARF from a patient with chronic renal failure (CRF). Generally, patients with azotemia and anemia (commonly normocytic, nor-

Table 18-1-1. Major Classes of Acute Renal Failure

I. Prenal types (perceived as hypoperfusion)
  A. Hypovolemia
    1. Hemorrhage (acute blood loss)
    2. Inadequate intake
    3. Excessive output (vomiting, diarrhea, perspiration, etc.)
    4. Third spacing of bodily fluids
  B. Reduced cardiac output
    1. Myocardial disease and/or injury (intrinsic heart problem)
    2. Obstruction to cardiac filling (pericardial tamponade, etc.)
    3. Obstruction to cardiac outflow (valvular defects, etc.)
  C. Loss of vascular tone
    1. Pharmacologic drug use (vasodilators)
    2. Sepsis
    3. Anaphylaxis
II. Renal types (intrinsic renal disorders)
  A. Ischemia
    1. Renal arterial obstruction and/or stenosis
    2. Hypoperfusional states
  B. Glomerular disorders and/or injuries
    1. Glomerulonephritis
    2. Vasculitis
  C. Acute tubular disorders and/or injuries
    1. Toxins (drugs, especially aminoglycosides, contrast agents, etc.)
    2. Ischemia
  D. Interstitial nephritis
    1. Immune-mediated (drugs, especially β-lactam antibiotics)
    2. Infectious
    3. Idiopathic
III. Postrenal types (obstructive processes)
  A. Ureteral
    1. Bilateral (uncommon: tumor, stones, etc.)
    2. Unilateral (if only one functional kidney)
  B. Bladder
    1. Prostate enlargement (benign hypertrophy, tumor, etc.)
    2. Miscellaneous outlet obstruction
      a. Tumor
      b. Stone
  C. Urethral
    1. Stenosis (stricture, etc.)
    2. Extraurethral (fibrosis, etc.)

mochromic) have a more protracted type of renal failure (CRF). When prior laboratory tests are available for comparison, the knowledge that the azotemia is of recent onset is invaluable in making the determination that a patient has ARF.

LABORATORY TESTING

When one is confronted with a patient in ARF, the ultimate diagnostic challenge is to determine the underlying process that initiated the azotemia. Initially, a thorough history and physical examination (H&P) are performed to begin the search. With azotemia, the first goal is to separate patients who have a chronic form of renal failure from those with true ARF. A recent baseline laboratory is invaluable in this endeavor. Generally, during ARF, creatinine rises at a rate of 0.5 to 2.5 mg/dL per day. Once an ARF syndrome is established, the following guidelines may offer direction in delineating the cause.

Although often considered paramount in the management of ARF, quantification of the urine volume provides minimal information about the etiology. This is the case because ARF may demonstrate oliguria, polyuria, or normal urine output during various phases of its evolution. Of greater value in determining the etiology of the ARF process are an examination of the urine, especially the sediment, and selected serum chemistries.

Although it is not definitive, certain implications may be drawn from some findings on urinalysis. Sediment devoid of cellular elements is characteristically seen in both prenal and postrenal ARF. In some lower genitourinary and prostatic disorders, however, hematuria and pyuria may be seen. Typically, cellular casts tend to be more commonly associated with intrinsic renal disorders. Proteinuria, depending on quantity, may be a manifestation of glomerular filtration abnormalities or may be seen in tubular injury as a result of an ischemic or nephrotoxic insult.

During the initial assessment (H&P), one should search for clues to assist in determining the cause of renal failure. If the bladder is distended, a Foley catheter may demonstrate a urinary bladder outflow obstructive process. Renal ultrasound or CT may show signs of ureteral distention or obstruction. Renal failure indices, a combination of urine and serum chemistries, may be valuable in differentiating prenal from renal causes of azotemia and should be reviewed next (Table 18-1-2). The combination of an elevated BUN:creatinine (<20), a low fractional excretion of sodium (FENa < 1 percent), low urinary sodium (<20 meq/L), and an elevated urinary osmolality (>500 mosmol/kg) suggests a prenal ARF situation. Often, however, the distinction is not as well demarcated, and overlap exists between prenal and renal ARF indices.

Attention must be directed to the electrolytes, since hyperkalemia, hypocalcemia, hyperphosphatemia, and hypermagnesemia tend to occur. The serum pH also should be monitored, as metabolic acidosis is a common occurrence.

TREATMENT

The goals of therapy are to (1) remove any possible causes, (2) minimize additional renal injury, and (3) prevent and/or treat complications. Hospitalization of patients with ARF must be considered.

One should begin with the removal of any drugs that may be nephrotoxic or may reduce renal perfusion. If necessary, volume expansion with isotonic saline may be employed; however, it is necessary to avoid volume overload. Doses of a diuretic such as furosemide may convert oliguric to nonoliguric renal failure, which in some situations carries a better prognosis. One must avoid potentially harmful contrast agents, such as intravenous pyelography dyes. Drug levels are monitored as warranted, and drug doses are adjusted as necessary.

In all patients, meticulous attention to fluid status is critical. Serial monitoring of daily weights, fluid intake and urine output, blood pressure measurement, electrolytes, BUN, creatinine, and hemoglobin should guide management. Dialysis is indicated in some cases of ARF (see Table 18-1-3).

Table 18-1-2. Commonly Used Renal Failure Indices that Assist in Differentiating Prenal from Intrinsic (Renal) Azotemia

Index	Prerenal (Intrinsic)	Renal
Urinary sodium (mmol/L)	<10	>20
Urinary specific gravity	>1.020	<1.010
Plasma BUN/plasma creatinine	>20	<10
Urine osmolality (mosmol/kg H_2O)	>500	<300
FENa* (fractional excretion of sodium)	<1	>1

$$FENa = \frac{(\text{urinary sodium} \times (\text{plasma creatinine}) \times 100}{(\text{plasma sodium}) \times (\text{urinary creatinine})}$$

* Many consider FENa to be an extremely sensitive indicator in determining whether ARF is prenal or renal.

Table 18-1-3. Indications for Dialysis in Acute Renal
Failure Patients

Significant symptomatic pulmonary edema (secondary to volume
  overload)
Hyperkalemia (not responsive to more conservative approaches)
Toxic drug levels (amenable to correction by dialysis)
Uremia (BUN > 100 and/or creatinine > 10)
Pericarditis
Altered mental status (confusion, coma)
Significant acid-base disturbances
Bleeding (suggestive of platelet dysfunction)
Fluid overload

The management of hyperkalemia, hypocalcemia, pulmonary edema, cardiac dysrhythmias, and other miscellaneous complications should be anticipated, prevented when possible, and treated if they occur.

COMPLICATIONS AND RED FLAGS

During the treatment of renal failure, one should monitor the patient for signs of volume overload. Daily weights and attention to the patient's fluid intake and output (I&O) are important parameters. As ARF resolves, hypokalemia must be anticipated, especially if the patient demonstrates significant diuresis during recovery. Gastrointestinal bleeding may occur.

A dreaded complication is infection, which may occur in up to 75 percent of these patients. When infection occurs, it is the cause of death in as many as 75 percent of the patients who die during the course of renal failure.

PROGNOSIS

Since the development of renal dialysis, fewer patients have died from ARF. The underlying event that caused the ARF syndrome may, however, be a cause of death. Death may occur in up to 50 percent of patients in ARF, with infection being the most common cause.

The typical patient with ARF begins to show signs of improvement after about 10 days. Most cases tend to resolve over a 3- to 4-week course. Resolution often manifests as a daily increase in urine output, as renal function returns toward baseline.

Of the three broad classifications of ARF, intrinsic renal failure tends to have the most variable outcome. The majority of patients who survive a course of ARF recover enough renal function to live a normal life.

NOTES AND PEARLS

The nutritional support of the patient should be monitored. Limiting dietary proteins reduces the magnitude of the azotemia. Sodium and daily fluid intake should be monitored to avoid fluid overload. Drugs that are cleared renally often require dose adjustments, and their plasma levels should be observed closely.

BIBLIOGRAPHY

Brady HR, Brenner BM: Acute renal failure, in Fauci AS, Braunwald E, Isselbacher KJ, et al (eds): *Harrison's Principles of Internal Medicine,* 14th ed. New York, McGraw-Hill, 1998, pp 1504–1513.
Grantham JJ: Acute renal failure, in Gaarden W, Smith JB, Bennett LH Jr, Claude J: *Cecil Textbook of Medicine,* 19th ed. Philadelphia, Saunders, 1992, pp 528–532.

Chapter 18–2
BENIGN PROSTATIC HYPERPLASIA
William A. Mosier

DISCUSSION

The term *benign prostatic hyperplasia* (BPH) refers to a noncancerous abnormal enlargement of the prostate gland. The prostate gland begins to undergo hyperplastic changes during the third decade of life. Most men begin to experience some symptoms of prostate gland enlargement by age 50. However, significant problems are not common before age 60. As many as 90 percent of men between ages 70 and 90 have symptoms of BPH. The normal prostate is soft and pliable and is about the size of a walnut. When the prostate becomes hypertrophic, it often becomes rigid. This can constrict or even totally occlude the urethra. The result can be urinary retention, which eventually can lead to azotemia and irreversible bladder dysfunction. Fortunately, the condition does not progress to the severe form in most patients. It is estimated that only about 5 percent of men who undergo consideration for treatment present with severe manifestations of BPH. An estimated one in four men will require treatment for BPH symptoms by age eighty.

PATHOGENESIS

The etiology is not totally understood. However, it is thought to be related to the impact of the aging process on the hormone testosterone. An estrogen-dominant environment also plays a significant role in the development of BPH.

BPH is potentially dependent on estrogen for its development. Studies have confirmed that the ratios of estradiol (E2) to total testosterone (total T) and E2 to free testosterone (free T) are significantly correlated with prostate size. Blocking of the aromatization of testosterone to estrogen in the prostate stroma hypothetically can reverse or at least halt the progression of the disease. Studies have demonstrated that circulating autoantibodies to prostate specific antigen (PSA) exist in the serum of patients with BPH but not in the serum of patients without BPH. A possibly related factor that is considered controversial is that BPH may be associated with a diminished sex life with few or no ejaculations. This observation is based on studies that have indicated that the occurrence of BPH is higher among groups that average fewer ejaculations per month than are reported by control groups.

PATHOPHYSIOLOGY

Possibly originating within the periurethral glands, fibroadenomatosis nodules form around the periurethral region of the prostate. The hyperplastic process may form along the lateral walls of the prostate or may include tissue at the inferior margin of the vesical neck. The tissue tends to be glandular with varying amounts of fibrous stroma.

SYMPTOMS

The symptoms of BPH begin when the enlarged gland interferes with the draining of the bladder through the urethra by blocking the passage of urine. This is caused by tensing of the enlarged muscle of the prostate gland around the urethra. Common complaints include a progressive urinary frequency, urgency, nocturia, hesitancy, a feeling of a full bladder without being able to urinate, impotence, blood in the semen or hematuria, dripping or drib-

Table 18-2-1. Commonly Occurring Symptoms of BPH

Starting and stopping of the stream during urination
Sensation of incomplete emptying
Weak and diminished stream
Straining to urinate
Bladder distention
Intermittency
Impotence
Frequency
Hematuria
Hesitancy
Dribbling
Nocturia
Urgency
Dysuria

bling, and intermittency with a low-pressure flow that results in decreased force and size of the urinary stream (Table 18-2-1).

OBJECTIVE FINDINGS

Enlargement of the prostate, which can be verified on digital rectal examination, is not a prerequisite for the development of BPH symptoms. Clinically significant BPH may present with minimal or no detectable prostatic enlargement. However, when prostatic enlargement is detectable, it often presents with a rubbery consistency and a loss of the median furrow.

DIAGNOSTIC CONSIDERATIONS

When an enlarged prostate is encountered in men under age 40, venereal disease must be considered. Another important differential to screen for is cancer of the prostate. An indurated and tender prostate encountered on digital rectal examination is suggestive of prostatitis. A hard, nodular prostate usually is indicative of carcinoma or, rarely, prostatic calculi.

SPECIAL CONSIDERATIONS

It is important to avoid all instrumentation until after a patient has committed himself to definitive treatment, since any manipulation may provoke increased trauma, obstruction, and infection. The risk of obstruction caused by an enlarged prostate constricting or totally closing off the flow of urine through the urethra at the bladder neck is of major concern. The risk is increased by alcohol consumption, cold moist weather, smoking, emotional stress, and the use of drugs such as antihistamines, atropine, beta-adrenergic blockers, calcium channel blockers, and muscle relaxants.

OTHER DIAGNOSTIC TOOLS

When a patient is committed to treatment for the relief of symptoms, the following diagnostic tools may be useful in disclosing the severity of BPH. Maximum urinary flow rate and residual volume may help provide a urodynamic analysis of the severity of the symptoms. An intravenous urogram (IVU) may be useful in determining whether the terminal portions of the ureters are displaced upward or whether there is a defect at the base of the bladder. IVU is also useful in ruling out hydronephrosis or dilated ureters. A postvoiding cystogram can indicate the amount of residual urine. If the BPH is severe, catheterization after voiding can measure the residual urine and also drain it. This can be necessary for stabilizing renal function and managing a urinary

track infection. Cystoscopy is useful in estimating gland size and differentiating an obstruction that might be present, such as vesical neck contracture or prostatitis. PSA is not sufficiently accurate to distinguish between BPH and cancer of the prostate.

TREATMENT

An asymptomatic, moderately enlarged prostate does not require treatment. When treatment is initiated, it is usually at the request of a patient who is experiencing problems with urination. When the complaints are minimal, medication may be the first line of therapy to alleviate the symptoms. There are safe, effective medications currently available to treat BPH.

When a urinary tract infection or bladder outlet obstruction complicates BPH, the initial treatment must be directed toward the eradication of infection and the stabilization of renal function.

Some of the more common intervention strategies for treating BPH are

1. Pharmacologic therapy (antiandrogens or alpha$_1$-adrenergic inhibitors)
2. Prostatic incision (transurethral incision of the prostate)
3. Prostatectomy (open and transurethral)
4. Prostatic stents
5. Thermotherapy
6. Balloon dilation

Medications

Two classes of medications have proved useful in treating uncomplicated cases of BPH: antiandrogens and alpha$_1$-adrenergic inhibitors.

Antiandrogens

Because the nodular changes in the prostatic epithelium and stroma that manifest as BPH are androgen-dependent, one treatment approach is to attempt to regulate the amount of androgen available to the prostate. The 5α-reductase inhibitor agent finasteride (Proscar) is used to interfere with the conversion of testosterone to dihydrotestosterone. The goal is to decrease androgen bioavailability to the prostate tissue. It may require 6 months or more for the benefits of finasteride to become observable. A significant percentage of patients may not respond. Studies suggest that the most favorable response occurs in men with larger prostates.

Alpha-$_1$-Adrenergic Inhibitors

Hyperplasia of the prostate is primarily a phenomenon of the stroma, as opposed to the epithelial tissue, in the majority of males. The smooth muscle of the stroma receives adrenergic innervation. For this reason, the antihypertensives that function as selective alpha$_1$-adrenergic inhibitors may be useful for relaxing the smooth muscle of the prostate and the bladder neck. The mechanism by which this occurs is directly related to the fact that alpha$_1$-adrenoceptors are densely distributed in the prostate and bladder neck but only sparsely distributed in the body of the bladder. Therefore, selective alpha$_1$-adrenoceptor blocking agents such as doxazosin (Cardura), tramsulosin (Flomax), and terazosin (Hytrin) can relax the smooth muscle of the prostate and the bladder neck without interfering with bladder contractility. The usual onset of action using graduated dosing is at least 2 weeks. Many patients can maintain the benefits of treatment over time. However, some patients develop a tolerance to the treatment after as little as 6 months of therapy.

Surgery

It can take as long as 20 years after diagnosis before BPH becomes sufficiently troublesome to warrant surgical intervention. The indications for surgery include urinary retention, chronic urinary tract infections, recurrent prostate infections, persistent bleeding from the prostate, swelling or destruction of the kidney caused by urinary obstruction (revealed on x-ray), and kidney failure. The surgical procedures utilized are relatively simple. The two most widely used prostatectomies are

- *Open surgical procedure.* This approach involves removing the entire prostate through a lower abdominal incision.
- *Transurethral resection of the prostate (TURP).* TURP is considered the mainstay of urologic treatment for BPH. As the name implies, a resectoscope is passed through the urethra via the penis until it reaches the bladder neck. An electric cutting loop then is used to resect the enlarged tissue. The procedure is also done using a modified electrovaporizing loop.

Alternative procedures with flowery or fishy names such as TULIP and TUNA hold promise for simpler, safer, and more efficacious treatment for BPH. Some of these procedures are as follows:

- *Transurethral incision of the prostate (TUIP).* This procedure is similar to TURP except that rather than removing any tissue, small incisions are made in the prostate to relieve pressure on the urethra.
- *Transurethral needle ablation of the prostate (TUNA).* This procedure usually is performed using only topical urethral anesthesia, has half the cost of a TURP, and promises to be the treatment of choice in the near future.
- *Transurethral ultrasound-guided laser-induced prostatectomy (TULIP).* This is one of the first laser systems designed to treat BPH. Although it has many advantages over TURP, its two biggest disadvantages are as follows:
  1. Prolonged catheterization during the postoperative phase is required.
  2. Since no tissue is obtained, no histology sample is available to rule out prostate cancer.
- *Transurethral laser ablation of the prostate (TULAP).* This is a commonly practiced form of transurethral laser surgery.
- *Visual laser ablation of the prostate* (VLAP). Although VLAP may not always result in as complete a removal of prostatic tissue as is achieved with TURP, it is associated with a lower morbidity rate, shorter procedure time, and shorter hospitalization.
- *Endoscopic laser ablation of the prostate (ELAP).* The side effects of urinary tract infections and dysuria may be more common with this procedure; however, the need for blood transfusions appears to be less common than with TURP.
- *Transurethral microwave thermotherapy (TUMT).* This procedure can be implemented using either a high-energy or a low-energy thermotherapy protocol. It is both outpatient-based and anesthesia-free. The low-energy protocol is most beneficial in patients with a relatively small prostate.
- *Endoscopic roller ball electrovaporization of the prostate (EREV).* This is experimentally considered a safe, effective, and economic alternative to the standard TURP. It is performed using a modified TURP.

These techniques have been developed in an attempt to overcome some of the drawbacks of TURP (see "Complications and Red Flags," below). The approaches using laser energy direct a fiber, via cystoscopy, into the prostate, using heat to shrink the gland. The procedure is quicker to perform than a TURP and causes virtually no bleeding.

SUPPORTIVE MEASURES

Hot sitz baths can help relieve discomfort. It is important for the patient to drink at least eight glasses of fluid a day to promote urine production and bladder flushing. The patient also should be reminded to avoid alcohol, coffee, smoking, and spicy foods that tend to irritate the bladder.

PATIENT EDUCATION

Patient education should include a reminder of the importance of a yearly rectal examination for all male patients over age 40. If BPH has been diagnosed, a rectal examination may be indicated semiannually. The patient also should be cautioned about taking cold and allergy medications that may contain anticholinergic or sympathomimetic agents that can aggravate BPH and cause further urinary retention. Patients should be encouraged to continue an active sex life or masturbate into their advanced years. Patients should be discouraged from engaging in sexual stimulation and arousal without ejaculation. Maintaining physical fitness should be emphasized.

DISPOSITION

Since BPH develops over a protracted period, any diagnosed case of BPH should be monitored with semiannual examinations. When in doubt, a urology consult should be requested.

COMPLICATIONS AND RED FLAGS

The complications of severe untreated BPH include hydronephrosis, profuse hematuria, urinary retention, and urinary tract infections. A complaint of a burning sensation on urination with chills and fever should be assumed to be a urinary tract infection until proved otherwise. Prolonged urinary retention may lead to progressive renal failure and azotemia. Although it is well known that the open surgical procedure can result in significant sexual dysfunction, outcome studies have identified a much higher mortality and morbidity rate after TURP than was previously recognized. Studies now indicate that two-thirds of all men undergoing a TURP will experience diminished or absent ejaculation and that 5 percent will become impotent.

OTHER NOTES AND PEARLS

The availability of a self-administered questionnaire concerning BPH symptoms that a patient could complete on his own would be a valuable adjunct to standard diagnostic procedures. The International Continence Society (ICS) has developed such a tool, the ICS male questionnaire. It is considered to have a high level of validity and reliability as well as being easy for patients to complete.

An emerging treatment for BPH is transurethral microwave thermotherapy. This is a technology that not only is less costly and less invasive but also causes no identifiable adverse effects on sexual function. Various other strategies for managing BPH are being studied, such as lasers, electrocautery, and ultrasonics. However, their ability to maximize efficacy and minimize side effects has not yet been clearly established. A medication called Cernilton is being considered for the treatment of BPH.

BIBLIOGRAPHY

Andersen JT: Alpha 1 blockers vs 5-alpha reductase inhibitors in benign prostatic hyperplasia: A comparative review. *Drugs Aging* 6(5):388–396, 1995.

Barry M: Epidemiology and natural history of benign prostatic hyperplasia. *Urol Clin North Am* 17(3):495–507, 1990.

Blute ML, Tomera KM, Hellerstein DK, et al: Transurethral microwave thermotherapy for prostatism: Early Mayo Foundation experience. *Mayo Clin Proc* 67:417–421, 1992.

Boyle P, Gould AL, Roehrborn CG: Prostate volume predicts outcome of treatment of benign prostatic hyperplasia with finasteride: Meta-analysis of randomized clinical trials. *Urology* 48(3):398–405, 1996.

Bruskewitz R, Riehmann M: New Therapies for benign prostatic hyperplasia. *Mayo Clin Proc* 67:493–495, 1992.

de Wildt MJ, Debruyne FM, de la Rosette JJ, et al: High-energy transurethral microwave thermotherapy: A thermoablative treatment for benign prostatic obstruction. *Urology* 48(3):416–423, 1996.

Donovan JL, Abrams P, Peters TJ, et al: The ICS-BPH study: The psychometric validity and reliability of the ICS male questionnaire. *Br J Urol* 77(4):554–562, 1996.

Elhilali MM, Ramsey EW, Barkin J, et al: A multi center, randomized, double-blind, placebo-controlled study to evaluate the safety and efficacy of terazosin in the treatment of benign prostatic hyperplasia. *Urology* 47(3):335–342, 1996.

Eri LM, Tveter KJ: Alpha-blockade in the treatment of symptomatic benign prostatic hyperplasia. *J Urol* 154(3):923–934, 1995.

Girman CJ, Kolman C, Liss CL, et al: Effects of finasteride on health-related quality of life in men with symptomatic benign prostatic hyperplasia: Finasteride Study Group. *Prostate* 29(2):83–90, 1996.

Hill M, Hampl R, Petřík, Stárka L: Concentration of the endogenous antiandrogen epitestosterone and androgenic C19-steroids in hyperplastic prostatic tissue. *Prostate* 28(6):347–351, 1996.

Issa MM: Transurethral needle ablation of the prostate: Report of initial United States clinical trial. *J Urol* 156:426–427, 1996.

Lepor H, Shapiro E, Wang B, Liang YC: Comparison of the cellular composition of benign prostatic hyperplasia in Chinese and Caucasian-American men. *Urology* 47(1):38–42, 1996.

Lepor H, Williford WO, Barry MJ, et al: The efficacy of terazosin, finasteride, or both in benign prostatic hyperplasia: Veterans Affairs Cooperative Studies Benign Prostatic Hyperplasia Study Group. *New Engl J Med* 335(8):533–539, 1996.

Matzkin H, Cytron S, Simon D: Is there an association between cigarette smoking and gland size in benign prostatic hyperplasia? *Prostate* 29(1):42–45, 1996.

Meade WM, McLoughlin MG: Endoscopic roller ball electrovaporization of the prostate—the sandwich technique: Evaluation of the initial efficacy and morbidity in the treatment of benign prostatic obstruction. *Br J Urol* 77(5):696–700, 1996.

Roehrborn CG, Siegel RL: Safety and efficacy of doxazosin in benign prostatic hyperplasia: A pooled analysis of three double-blind, placebo-controlled studies. *Urology* 48(3):406–415, 1996.

Simpson RJ, Fisher W, Lee AJ, et al: Benign prostatic hyperplasia in an unselected community-based population: A survey of urinary symptoms, bothersomeness and prostatic enlargement. *Br J Urol* 77(2):186–191, 1996.

Span PN, Benraad ThJ, Sweep CG, Smals AG: Kinetic analysis of steroid 5-alpha-reductase activity at neutral pH in benign prostatic hyperplastic tissue: Evidence for type I isozyme activity in the human prostate. *J Steroid Biochem Mol Biol* 57(1–2):103–108, 1996.

Suzuki K, Ito K, Ichinose Y, et al: Endocrine environment of benign prostatic hyperplasia: Prostate size and volume are correlated with serum estrogen concentration. *Scand J Urol Nephrol* 29(1):65–68, 1995.

Wolff JM, Boeckmann W, Effert PJ, et al: Evaluation of patients with diseases of the prostate using prostate-specific antigen density. *Br J Urol* 76(1):41–46, 1995.

Zippe CD: Benign prostatic hyperplasia: An approach for the internist. *Cleve Clin J Med* 63(4):226–236, 1996.

Zisman A, Zisman E, Lindner A, et al: Auto antibodies to prostate specific antigen in patients with benign prostatic hyperplasia. *J Urol* 154(3):1052–1055, 1995.

Zlotta AR, Peny MO, Matos C, et al: Transurethral needle ablation of the prostate: Clinical experience in patients in urinary acute retention. *Br J Urol* 77(3):391–397, 1996.

Chapter 18–3
PROSTATITIS
Richard Dehn

DISCUSSION

Prostatitis is a broad diagnostic term that encompasses four different entities: acute bacterial prostatitis, chronic bacterial prostatitis, chronic nonbacterial prostatitis, and prostatodynia. These four diagnostic entities require different therapeutic responses, making a correct initial diagnosis important.

Acute bacterial prostatitis presents with fever and dysuria. Pain often is reported in the suprapubic, perineal, or sacral region. Symptoms of obstruction may develop as prostatic edema increases. On physical examination the patient is often febrile, and the prostate is extremely tender, enlarged, and indurated. Urinalysis shows pyuria, and microscopic examination of expressed prostatic secretions, if obtainable, shows increased leukocytes [>10 per high-power field (hpf)].

Chronic prostatitis is a chronic inflammation of the prostate. In chronic bacterial prostatitis the cause of the inflammation is bacterial. In chronic nonbacterial prostatitis the cause of the inflammation can be a nonbacterial infectious agent, but it has been hypothesized that in some cases an autoimmune mechanism may be responsible. With chronic prostatitis the patient experiences some of the symptoms of acute prostatitis without the fever and septic characteristics. The symptoms can vary from minimal to incapacitating and can include irritative voiding discomfort, perineal pain, and obstructive symptoms. Occasionally the patient will report hematuria or hematospermia. Physical examination of the prostate is generally normal. The organisms most commonly found to cause chronic bacterial prostatitis are aerobic gram-negative enteric bacteria, but occasionally enterococcus is involved. Chronic nonbacterial prostatitis can be caused by the organisms *Chlamydia trachomatis* and *Ureaplasma urealyticum* but also can be caused by a noninfectious inflammatory process. It is thought that in some cases external urinary sphincter dysfunction can produce a chronic chemical irritation that causes inflammation. The ratio of bacterial to nonbacterial cases of chronic prostatitis is 1 : 14. Most nonbacterial cases occur in younger men, and most bacterial cases involve older patients.

Prostatodynia is a syndrome of chronic prostatitis symptoms without objective evidence of prostatic inflammation. Approximately one-third of patients who present with symptoms of chronic prostatitis have no objective evidence of prostatic inflammation, and it is thought that these cases are caused by a nonprostatic organ system pathology that produces referred symptoms.

The gold standard for determining prostatic inflammation is a microscopic analysis of expressed prostatic secretions. Inflammation is suspected if more than 10 leukocytes per high-power field are observed.

PATHOGENESIS

Bacterial processes are thought to enter through the urinary tract. Recurrent chronic bacterial infections probably are related to problems with sphincter function. Chronic nonbacterial prostatitis and prostatodynia can be caused by a wide variety of pathologies, including processes outside the genitourinary system.

LABORATORY TESTING

With acute bacterial prostatitis, the urinalysis shows pyuria and the microscopic examination of expressed prostatic secretions, if obtainable, shows increased leukocytes (>10/hpf). Care should be taken in massaging the prostate, since an overly vigorous examination may cause septicemia. A complete blood count (CBC) usually will show elevated white blood cells with a shift to the left, and the urine culture usually will be positive. A culture of the prostatic secretions also will be positive.

In chronic bacterial prostatitis, the urinalysis is usually negative, although the microscopic examination of expressed prostatic secretions will show increased leukocytes (>10/hpf). A culture of the prostatic secretions usually will be positive. CBC will be normal unless it is confounded by another systemic illness.

In chronic nonbacterial prostatitis, the urinalysis is usually negative, although the microscopic examination of expressed prostatic secretions will show increased leukocytes (>10/hpf). A culture of the prostatic secretions will be negative. CBC will be normal unless it is confounded by another systemic illness.

In prostatodynia, the urinalysis is usually negative and the microscopic examination of expressed prostatic secretions will show less than 10 leukocytes per high-power field. A culture of the prostatic secretions will be negative. CBC will be normal unless it is confounded by another systemic illness.

Prostate specific antigen (PSA) is significantly elevated in acute bacterial prostatitis, but after resolution of the infection, levels return to baseline. Levels should be normal in patients with chronic prostatitis or prostatodynia. Elevations in the absence of acute prostatitis should be investigated.

Transrectal prostatic sonography may be of some value in differentiating chronic prostatitis from prostatodynia. It is sometimes possible to visualize evidence of inflammation; however, such evidence should be considered persuasive and not necessarily diagnostic.

A difference in the pH of the expressed prostatic secretions depending on the diagnosis has been observed in patients with prostatitis. In a study of 40 men with clinical prostatitis, the mean pH was found to be 7.6 for those with chronic bacterial prostatitis, 7.1 for those with chronic nonbacterial prostatitis, and 6.5 for those with prostatodynia.

DIAGNOSTIC CONSIDERATIONS

Acute and chronic infections in the genitourinary system should always be considered, such as cystitis, pyelonephritis, epididymitis, and urethritis. Anal disease and diverticulitis can present with prostatic symptoms. Prostatic cancer and bladder cancer should be ruled out in older patients with negative cultures who complain of chronic voiding symptoms.

TREATMENT

An acute bacterial prostatitis patient is usually septic enough to warrant hospitalization. After the collection of culture specimens, antibiotics should be started. Fluoroquinolones are the drugs of choice, either ciprofloxacin (Cipro) 200 mg intravenously every 12 h or ofloxacin (Floxin) 200 mg intravenously every 12 h. A less expensive alternative to this regimen is ampicillin 1 g intravenously every 6 hours and gentamicin 1.0 to 1.5 mg/kg of body weight intramuscularly every 12 h. Rapid improvement usually results from these therapies, and after the patient has been afebrile for 24 to 48 h, he should be switched to an oral antibiotic and the treatment should be continued for at least 1 month to prevent chronic prostatitis. At the end of the treatment regimen, the urine should be cultured and the prostatic secretions examined to confirm a successful outcome.

The treatment of chronic bacterial prostatitis involves a long course of antibiotic therapy. Trimethoprim-sulfamethoxazole (Bactrim DS, Septra DS) bid, ciprofloxacin (Cipro) 250 mg tid, and ofloxacin (Floxin) 200 mg bid are all acceptable regimens. Antibiotics should be continued for at least 6 weeks and possibly up to 12 weeks. If symptoms persist, suppressive therapy is helpful for the control of symptoms but is not curative.

Patients with chronic nonbacterial prostatitis should be placed on a course of doxycycline (Vibramycin) 100 mg bid or erythromycin 500 mg qid for 14 days. If the patient fails to respond to this regimen, urodynamic testing should be considered. Sphincter spasticity can be improved with terazosin (Hytrin), starting with 1 mg daily and increasing up to 10 mg. Terazosin can produce postural hypotension, and so the patient should be cautioned and advised to take the drug at bedtime. Continued symptomatology requires further consideration of pathology in other nearby structures, especially those of the genitourinary system. Occasionally improvement is attained with nonsteroidal anti-inflammatory drugs. The use of transurethral microwave thermotherapy has been investigated and has shown promise in chronic nonbacterial prostatitis patients who are resistant to other therapies. Prostatodynia treatment is similar to the treatment of chronic nonbacterial prostatitis that is nonresponsive to antibiotics.

BIBLIOGRAPHY

Chandiok S: Prostatitis—clinical and bacterial studies. *Int J STD AIDS* 3(3):180–190, 1992.

Jackson E, Fouler JE (ed): *Conn's Current Therapy, 1995.* Philadelphia, Saunders, 1995.

Presti JC, Stoller ML, Carroll PR (eds): *Current Medical Diagnosis and Treatment* 35th revision. Appleton, WI, Appleton & Lange, 1996.

Neal DE Jr: Use of terazosin in prostatodynia and validation of a symptom score questionnaire. *Urology* 43(4):460–465, 1994.

Nickel JC: Transurethral microwave thermotherapy for nonbacterial prostatitis. *J Urol* 155(6):1950–1954, 1996.

Chapter 18–4
EPIDIDYMITIS/ORCHITIS
Allan R. Riggs

Epididymitis
DISCUSSION

Although epididymitis and orchitis can occur simultaneously, they are usually separate infections and are discussed separately in this chapter.

Acute epididymitis is an inflammation of the epididymis, a tubelike structure on the posterior surface of the testis. This condition, which usually is seen in adult men, is the most common emergency involving the scrotum.[1] Epididymitis causes more than 20 percent of urologic hospital admissions.[2] Most cases of epididymitis result from retrograde infection from the urethra. The infecting organism transits the reverse pathway of the sperm. That is, the organism travels from the urethra to the prostatic urethra, to the ejaculatory duct, to the vas deferens, to the tail of the epididymis, and finally to the body and head of the epididymis. Occasionally the infection may spread to the testis (epididymoorchitis) or the spermatic cord. Most cases of epididymitis are caused by bacteria, but other etiologies can include viruses (e.g., mumps), chemical agents (e.g., urine), nonspecific causes,[3] and trauma.

The cause of epididymitis usually varies with the patient's age. In infants and children younger than 5 years old, epididymitis usually results from an anatomic abnormality such as a posterior urethral valve or an ectopic ureter or from a neurologic or functional abnormality. The inflammatory agent is usually a coliform or pseudomonad bacterium or a chemical agent such as urine.[2,3] *Haemophilus influenzae* type B bacteria can be a cause of epididymitis in prepubertal boys, and dysfunctional voiding problems can be an etiology in boys 10 to 15 yeas of age.[3]

In sexually active males under age 35, epididymitis usually is caused by a sexually transmitted organism and is associated with urethritis. In males over age 35, epididymitis usually is caused by coliform bacteria and is associated with prostatitis, urinary tract infections, and urinary tract instrumentation.[1]

Microbiology

The microbiology of epididymitis in infants and young and prepubertal boys was discussed above. In heterosexual males under age 35, epididymitis usually results from urethritis caused most frequently by *Chlamydia trachomatis* (up to 70 percent of cases) and less commonly by *Neisseria gonorrhoeae*. Some patients may be infected by both organisms. Since 30 to 50 percent of urethritis cases have no specific etiology, it is possible that an unknown pathogen that causes nonchlamydial, non-*Ureaplasma* urethritis also causes nonspecific epididymitis.[2]

Homosexual males who participate in unprotected anogenital intercourse have developed epididymitis, usually from coliforms, with one case resulting from *H. influenzae* infection.[2] In males over age 35, the causative agents are usually gram-negative urinary tract pathogens such as *Escherichia coli* and *Pseudomonas aeruginosa*.[1]

Less common infectious etiologies for epididymitis include *Streptococcus faecalis*, *Ureaplasma urealyticum*, viruses, and spirochetes.[4] Chronic epididymitis can be caused by *Treponema pallidum* and *Mycobacterium tuberculosis*.

SYMPTOMS

The presenting symptoms include a dull aching pain and swelling in the epididymis. The pain may radiate into the spermatic cord and the lower abdomen and flank. The pain of epididymitis may start slowly and increase over hours to days, in contrast to the pain of testicular torsion, which has an abrupt onset. A patient with epididymitis may report that lying down decreases the pain, whereas the pain of testicular torsion persists regardless of position.[1] The patient also may complain of urethral discharge, dysuria, and pain at the tip of the penis. Fever may be present. The symptoms may result from a physical strain such as heavy lifting or trauma or from sexual activity with a full bladder.[5]

OBJECTIVE FINDINGS

Physical examination of the testes and scrotum is best performed with the patient standing. Early in the disease, the epididymis may be firm, swollen, tender, and discrete from the testis, but as the infection persists, both the epididymis and the testicle become one swollen, tender mass. Elevation of the testis usually relieves the pain (a positive Prehn's sign), whereas this maneuver usually increases the pain of testicular torsion. Transillumination with a penlight helps differentiate hydroceles, which present as a reddish glow. Rectal examination may reveal a tender prostate, and the patient may have a fever.

If the diagnosis is uncertain on physical examination, other studies (e.g., ultrasound) should be performed.

DIAGNOSTIC CONSIDERATIONS

The most common differential diagnosis that needs to be ruled out quickly to save the testicle is testicular torsion. Although usually seen in prepubertal males, torsion occasionally is seen in young adults. It is suggested by a sudden, severe onset along with a negative urinalysis and increased pain with testicle elevation.

Torsion of the epididymal appendages, which also is usually seen in prepubertal males, is another consideration. Other differential diagnoses within the scrotum include orchitis, testicular tumor, hematocele, spermatocele, varicocele, congenital hydrocele, and incarcerated inguinal hernia.

Diagnostic considerations involving the scrotal wall include gangrene of the scrotal skin, Fournier's gangrene, abscess of the scrotal wall, fungal infection, trauma, urinary extravasation, and edema from cardiac, hepatic, or renal failure.[1,6]

SPECIAL CONSIDERATIONS

Patients undergoing immunosuppressive therapy and patients with AIDS are at risk for developing tuberculosis. Therefore, when these patients present with epididymitis, the clinician should consider *M. tuberculosis* as a possible etiology.[6]

A drug-induced epididymitis has been reported in patients on the antiarrhythmic drug amiodarone (Cordarone).[2]

LABORATORY STUDIES

In the sexually acquired form of epididymitis, Gram staining of the urethral smear may show gram-negative intracellular diplococci that are consistent with gonorrhea. The patient should not urinate for at least 2 h before the urethral swab is obtained. A urethral smear with white blood cells and no bacteria usually indicates a chlamydial infection. A urinalysis with pyuria only also may indicate chlamydial infection. It is best to get a first void urine specimen (the first 50 mL of voided urine after 2 h of continence) to identify pyuria caused by urethritis. Culture or nonculture tests for *N. gonorrhoeae* and *C. trachomatis* should be obtained.

In epididymitis that is not sexually acquired, the urinalysis usually shows bacteriuria, pyuria, and varying amounts of hematuria. Urine culture will show the causative bacterium.

The complete blood count in epididymitis shows increased white blood cells with a shift to the left. If there are suspicions of epididymitis from syphilis or tuberculosis (e.g., chronic epididymitis), a VDRL and/or a microhemagglutination assay for antibodies to *Treponema pallidum* (MHA-TP) test and a tuberculin skin test will be helpful.

RADIOLOGIC STUDIES AND OTHER IMAGING STUDIES

In selected cases where urinary tract abnormalities may be a factor, for example, in young boys and elderly men, an intravenous pyelogram (IVP) and a voiding cystourethrogram (VCUG) should be obtained. Scrotal ultrasound may help differentiate epididymitis from testicular torsion. Doppler ultrasound evaluates testicular blood flow and thus may be helpful in differentiating early testicular torsion from epididymitis. This procedure can be difficult, and the accuracy is dependent on the operator.[7] One must use caution in the interpretation because if the problem is a late torsion, there will be falsely increased blood flow because of inflamed scrotal vessels.[2]

In patients with epididymitis, technetium 99m (^{99m}Tc) pertechnetate testicular scanning shows increased perfusion through the spermatic cord vessels and increased uptake in the region of the epididymis. In contrast, there is decreased uptake of ^{99m}Tc with early torsion. Several hours after the torsion, a halo of increased uptake may surround the torsed testicle, indicating attempted collateral circulation.[8]

One must bear in mind that both technetium testicular scanning

Table 18-4-1. Antibiotics for Acute Epididymitis

Antibiotic	Dose	Bacterium	Comments
Ceftriaxone (Rocephin)	250 mg IM in a single dose	*N. gonorrhoeae*	Caution: Accompanying renal and hepatic impairment. PCN allergy
Doxycycline (Doryx)	100 mg PO bid for 10–14 days	*C. trachomatis*	Photosensitivity
Ofloxacin (Floxin)	300 mg PO bid for 10 days	*N. gonorrhoeae* *C. trachomatis*	Alternative regimen per CDC.[11] Ofloxacin contraindicated for persons ≤17 years of age
Sulfamethoxazole 800 mg-trimethoprim 160 mg (Bactrim DS)	1 DS tablet PO bid × 10 days (pediatric dose as calculated)	Coliform (e.g., *E. coli*)	For young boys and older men with pyuria and bacteriuria. Treat for 4 weeks if bacterial prostatitis is suspected
Cipofloxacin (Cipro)	250 mg PO bid × 10 days	Coliform (e.g., *E. coli*)	For older men with pyuria and bacteriuria. Treat for 4 weeks if prostatitis is suspected. Contraindicated for persons ≤17 years of age
Aminoglycoside [e.g., gentamicin (Garamycin)]	1.5 mg/kg q 8 h IV for at least 5 days, then switch to an oral antibiotic	Coliform (e.g., *E. coli*)	For systematically ill patients who require hospitalization. Reduce dose for renal impairment. Watch for nephrotoxicity and neurotoxicity

NOTE: DS = double strength; PCN = penicillin; CDC = Centers for Disease Control and Prevention.

and Doppler ultrasound can have false-positive and false-negative results.[2]

OTHER DIAGNOSTICS

A Doppler stethoscope may be a helpful adjunct to physical examination in a primary care office.

If the diagnosis of epididymitis is in doubt, a prompt urologic consultation should be made for surgical exploration of the scrotum. In young boys and elderly men with bacteriuria, cystoscopy should be performed after treatment to rule out an obstructive etiology of the epididymitis.[2]

TREATMENT

Pharmacologic Management

Since most cases of epididymitis have an infectious etiology, antibiotics should always be used (Table 18-4-1). One should start the initial antibiotics on the basis of clinical clues (e.g., sexually transmitted disease–acquired) and Gram staining of the patient's urethral smear and/or urine.

A patient with epididymitis secondary to sexually transmitted urethritis should be treated with ceftriaxone 250 mg intramuscularly and doxycycline 100 mg orally bid for 10 to 14 days to cover *N. gonorrhoeae* and *C. trachomatis,* respectively.

One should treat young boys and elderly men with bacteriuria for coliform infection as well as treating homosexuals with epididymitis resulting from anogenital intercourse. Outpatient therapy should be started with a broad-spectrum antibiotic such as trimethoprim-sulfamethoxazole or a quinolone, although quinolones are contraindicated in patients 17 years of age and younger. The appropriate length of treatment for coliform epididymitis is unknown and may need to be protracted, since relapse after 7 to 10 days can occur. If the patient is systematically ill, he should be admitted for intravenous aminoglycoside therapy.[2]

One should consider antibiotics that cover tuberculous and fungal organisms in patients with concurrent epididymitis and HIV infection.

Nonsteroidal anti-inflammatory drugs may be helpful, but steroids have not been found to be useful.[2] Antipyretics such as acetaminophen are helpful. In patients with severe pain, an anesthetic block of the spermatic cord with 1% lidocaine can be performed.[6]

Supportive Measures

Symptomatic treatment includes intermittent ice applications, sitz baths, bed rest, and scrotal elevation with a towel. The latter two treatments help with maximal lymphatic drainage. Athletic supporters may constrict and should be avoided.[2]

Patient Education

With sexually acquired epididymitis, patient education should emphasize safe sex practices such as using condoms and limiting the number of partners. The patient should be tested for and educated about other sexually transmitted diseases. He should notify his partners about receiving therapy. With epididymitis that is not sexually acquired, the patient should be advised to avoid activities that might bring on epididymitis (e.g., heavy lifting) and to seek medical care at the first symptoms of prostatitis and/or urinary tract infection. In treating epididymitis, a clinician has a golden opportunity to educate patients about testicular self-examination.

Disposition

The patient should be reevaluated if there is no improvement in 48 h. It is necessary to advise the patient that swelling and discomfort may linger for weeks or months even though the infectious agent has been eliminated. If fever persists after adequate antibiotics, an abscess may be present. This is evaluated with ultrasound and then treated with surgical drainage and/or epididymoorchiectomy.[6]

Uncomplicated epididymitis usually requires 10 to 14 days of treatment, but if there is concurrent bacterial prostatitis, antibiotics should be continued for 4 weeks. The follow-up for epididymitis is at 1 month.[6]

COMPLICATIONS AND RED FLAGS

The complications of epididymitis include testicular necrosis, testicular atrophy, abscess, and infarction. Some amount of atrophy occurs in approximately two-thirds of cases of acute epididymitis, whereas abscess and infarction are relatively rare, with a 5 percent incidence of each.[2] Infertility may occur in up to 50 percent of patients with bilateral epididymitis. Some patients may experience treatment failure or recurrence of epididymitis.

The two red flags are testicular torsion and testicular cancer. One should think torsion if a patient presents with a sudden onset of acute testicular pain, especially if the patient is age 15 or younger and epididymitis cannot be confirmed by physical examination and laboratory testing. A urologic consultation is indicated, since surgical exploration is needed within 4 to 6 h after the onset of the torsion to save the testicle.

A testicular tumor is another indication for a urologic consultation. Testicular cancer usually presents with asymptomatic swelling, but pain is a presenting symptom in approximately 20 percent of these patients.[8] Since swelling and pain are classic symptoms of epididymitis and epididymoorchitis, a follow-up evaluation to rule out a hidden malignancy should be performed after the resolution of these infections.

Other reasons for a urologic consultation include a suspected abscess, lack of response to treatment, and an unsure diagnosis of the problem. When in doubt, it is best to consult.

Orchitis

DISCUSSION

Orchitis is an inflammation of the testis that usually results from hematogenous spread during a systemic bacterial or viral illness.[8] Orchitis may be a complication of epididymitis (epididymoorchitis). Additional etiologies include syphilis (gumma of the testis), tuberculosis, and granuloma, which is thought to result from an autoimmune process directed against spermatozoa.[8] Many viruses can cause orchitis, and viruses are the most common etiology of acquired testicular failure in adults.[9] Orchitis results from the virus actually infecting testicular tissue, not from secondary inflammation. In mumps infection, orchitis is the most common complication, occurring in up to 25 percent of adult men[9] (see Chap. 9-17). Among these men, approximately 66 percent develop unilateral orchitis and the other 33 percent have bilateral orchitis. Orchitis usually follows parotitis by 3 to 4 days, but it may precede or start on the same day as parotitis.[8] After mumps, the testes may return to normal size and function or may atrophy secondary to the effect of the virus on the seminiferous tubules along with ischemia caused by pressure and edema against the inelastic tunica albuginea. Atrophy, which is usually detectable 1 to 6 months after the acute infection resolves, does not always correlate with the severity of orchitis or the development of infertility.[9]

Microbiology

The bacterial causes of orchitis are the same organisms that cause epididymitis. In sexually active males under age 35, one should treat for chlamydia and gonorrhea. In young boys, older men, and homosexuals, coliform bacteria are the likely cause of orchitis. Although rare, syphilis and tuberculosis, especially in immunocompromised patients and chronic cases, must be considered.

The viral etiologies include mumps virus, echovirus, lymphocytic choriomeningitis virus, and group B arboviruses.[9]

SYMPTOMS

Orchitis presents with testicular pain and swelling, high fever, chills, headache, nausea, and vomiting. Fever may be between 103 and 106°F (39.4 and 41.1°C) with shaking chills.[10]

OBJECTIVE FINDINGS

On physical examination the patient may have fever. The scrotum is usually erythematous, swollen, and edematous. Occasionally, epididymitis is present without orchitis and is palpable as a swollen, tender cord.[10] A hydrocele may be seen with transillumination. If the patient has orchitis caused by mumps, the parotid glands may be swollen.

DIAGNOSTIC CONSIDERATIONS

The differential diagnoses are the same as those for epididymitis and within the scrotum include testicular torsion, testicular cancer, hematocele, spermatocele, varicocele, congenital hydrocele, and incarcerated inguinal hernia. Diagnostic considerations involving the scrotal wall include gangrene of the scrotal skin, Fournier's gangrene, abscess of the scrotal wall, fungal infection, trauma, urinary extravasation, and edema. Testicular inflammation also can occur with pleurodynia, leptospirosis, melioidosis, relapsing fever, chickenpox, brucellosis, and lymphocytic choriomeningitis.[10]

SPECIAL CONSIDERATIONS

As with epididymitis, patients undergoing immunosuppressive therapy and patients with AIDS are at risk of developing orchitis from *M. tuberculosis.*

For unknown reasons, prepubertal males with parotitis do not seem to get orchitis.[8]

LABORATORY STUDIES

For a patient with a suspected bacterial orchitis, the clinician should follow the same laboratory protocols used with epididymitis: Gram stains, cultures, immunologic tests, etc., for *N. gonorrhoeae, C. trachomatis,* coliforms, *M. tuberculosis* and *T. pallidum* (see "Laboratory Studies" under "Epididymitis," above).

In viral orchitis, one should attempt a definitive diagnosis by culturing the virus from blood, urine, throat swab, CSF, and/or secretions from Stensen's duct. A rapid diagnosis of mumps can be made by immunofluorescent testing to detect viral antigen in the oropharyngeal cells.[10] Serologic tests such as enzyme-linked immunosorbent assay (ELISA) can be used to determine acute infection. Acute and convalescent sera should be obtained 2 to 3 weeks apart. A fourfold increase in titer confirms a recent infection.

With mumps orchitis, the complete blood count (CBC) may show a leukocytosis with a shift to the left. In contrast, mumps without orchitis may show a normal CBC or a mild leukopenia with a lymphocytosis. The erythrocyte sedimentation rate may rise with mumps orchitis. Serum amylase also is elevated. Plasma testosterone is low during acute orchitis but returns to normal after the illness.[10]

RADIOLOGIC STUDIES AND OTHER IMAGING

Radiologic studies usually are not indicated unless urologic abnormalities are thought to be a causative factor in orchitis. If that is the case, one should obtain an IVP and a VCUG. Scrotal ultrasound may help differentiate orchitis from epididymitis and testicular torsion. Doppler ultrasound, which evaluates testicular blood flow, may help differentiate orchitis from testicular torsion, as would ^{99m}Tc pertechnetate testicular scanning.

OTHER DIAGNOSTICS

As in epididymitis, a Doppler stethoscope may be useful for physical examination in a primary care office.

TREATMENT

Pharmacologic Management

If the orchitis is thought to be of bacterial etiology, one should start antibiotics on the basis of clinical clues (e.g., sexually transmitted disease—acquired) and on Gram staining of the patient's urethral smear and/or urine. Orchitis secondary to a sexually transmitted infection should be treated with ceftriaxone 250 mg intramuscularly and doxycycline 100 mg orally bid for 10 to 14 days. Orchitis secondary to a urologic abnormality should be treated with a broad-spectrum antibiotic such as trimethoprim-sulfamethoxazole or a quinolone. If the patient is sick enough for hospitalization, an intravenous aminoglycoside should be used until cultures and sensitivities come back.

In the rare case of symphilitic orchitis, one should use penicillin or erythromycin. In tuberculous orchitis, four antituberculous drugs may be needed, especially if multiple-drug-resistant *M. tuberculosis* is a possibility (see Chap. 9-31).

The treatment of viral orchitis is mainly palliative. Although this has not been proved in controlled studies, glucocorticoids seem to be of some benefit in decreasing fever and testicular pain and swelling. One should start with 60 mg of prednisone and taper the dose over the next 7 to 10 days.[10] When 1% lidocaine is injected into the spermatic cord, it provides quick pain relief and may decrease testicular damage by improving the local blood supply.[8] Acetaminophen and nonsteroidal anti-inflammatory drugs (e.g., ibuprofen) help with the pain and fever.

Supportive Measures

Symptomatic treatment includes bed rest, scrotal elevation, ice compresses, and sitz baths.[1]

Patient Education

If orchitis is secondary to a sexually acquired infection, the patient should be educated about safe sex practices and advised to have his partners get treatment. Testicular self-examination should be taught. If a patient presents with orchitis secondary to mumps, he should be reassured that physical activity did not bring on the orchitis. Although it is too late for a patient with mumps orchitis, other patients should be educated about prevention with the mumps vaccine.

DISPOSITION

A patient should be reevaluated in 24 to 48 h if the symptoms are worsening. A patient with mumps orchitis should be advised that the swelling, pain, and tenderness will persist for 3 to 7 days and then gradually decrease, especially when the fever breaks. A reasonable follow-up is 1 month.

COMPLICATIONS AND RED FLAGS

The complications of orchitis include atrophy and subnormal sperm counts and/or sterility. Unilateral atrophy occurs in a third of cases of mumps orchitis, and bilateral atrophy occurs in a tenth of cases.[9] If no significant atrophy has occurred, sterility is uncommon. However, if there is bilateral atrophy after mumps, below-normal sperm counts and/or sterility are very common.[10] Another complication includes pulmonary infarction that is thought to be due to thrombosis of the veins in the prostatic and pelvic plexuses, which occurs with the testicular inflammation. Priapism can be an uncommon complication.[10]

As in epididimitis, the red flags are for testicular torsion and cancer.[11] One should always consult a urologist if these diagnoses are suspected or if there are other complications or concerns that are beyond one's skills, knowledge, and experience.

REFERENCES

1. Blank BH, Schneider RE: Acute scrotal problems. *Patient Care* 24(11):154, 1990.
2. Berger RE: Acute epididimitis: Etiology and therapy. *Semin Urol* IX(1):28, 1991.
3. Bukowski TP, Lewis AG, Reeves D, et al: Epididimitis in older boys: Dysfunctional voiding as an etiology. *J Urol* 154(2):762, 1995.
4. Slanetz PA, Whitman GJ, Chew FS: Epididymal abscess. *Am J Radiol* 165(2):376, 1995.
5. Presti JC Jr, Stoller ML, Carrol PR: Urology, in Tierney LM, McPhee SJ, Papadakis MA (eds): *Current Medical Diagnosis and Treatment,* 34th ed. Norwalk, CT, Appleton & Lange, 1995, p 802.
6. Cendron M, Sant GR: Testicular disorders and disorders of the scrotal contents, in Nobel J (ed): *Textbook of Primary Care Medicine,* 2d ed. St. Louis, Mosby-Yearbook, 1996, p 1805.
7. Mettler FA: *Essentials of Radiology.* Philadelphia, Saunders, 1996, p 246.
8. Siroky MB, Krane RJ: *Manual of Urology: Diagnosis and Therapy.* Boston, Little, Brown, 1990, pp 37–38.
9. Griffin JE, Wilson JD: Disorders of the testes, in Isselbacher KJ, Braunwald E, Wilson JD, et al (eds): *Harrison's Principles of Internal Medicine,* 13th ed. New York, McGraw-Hill, 1994, p 2013.
10. Ray CG: Mumps, in Isselbacher KJ, Braunwald E, Wilson JD, et al (eds): *Harrison's Principles of Internal Medicine,* 13th ed. New York, McGraw-Hill, 1994, p 830.
11. Centers for Disease Control and Prevention: 1993 Sexually transmitted diseases treatment guidelines. *MMWR* 42(No. RR-14):88, 1993.

Chapter 18–5
RENAL LITHIASIS AND PYELONEPHRITIS
Michaela O'Brien-Norton

Renal Lithiasis
DISCUSSION

Renal colic caused by renal lithiasis (renal calculi, kidney stones) has been called the worst of all acute pains. Stones form because of the concentration of crystals in the urine, frequently as a result of some metabolic derangement caused by diet, an internal disorder, or even the environment (Table 18-5-1).

Geography, weather, and the mineral content of the local drinking water are also factors. Certain areas of the United States (the south, southwest, and west) have higher numbers of cases, but even in cold areas such as the northeast, drinking water can cause local patterns of higher incidences that vary from town to town. The stones generally are formed of calcium oxalate, calcium phosphate, cystine, and uric acid. When associated with infection, struvite (staghorn) stones form and can be quite large, encompassing the whole renal pelvis.

Kidney stones are rare in children and adolescents. The incidence of renal stones peaks between ages 30 and 50 and is somewhat higher in men.

Stones less than 5 mm usually can be passed without difficulty. Stones between 5 and 10 mm can pass approximately 50 percent of the time. Stones larger than that cause many complications, including partial or complete obstruction of the ureter and ureter

Table 18-5-1. Dietary Habits and Conditions Associated with Renal Stones

Diet
  Calcium intake
    Dairy products
    Calcium supplements
  Purine-containing foods (protein-rich food; metabolite is uric acid)
    Meat (especially red meat)
    Fish
    Poultry
  Oxalate
    Cola
    Chocolate
    Cranberries
    Tea
    Vitamin C (more than 1000 mg daily)
Diseases and conditions
  Urinary tract infection
  Gout
  Inflammatory bowel disease
  Pregnancy

lacerations. Larger stones require some type of intervention, which may include percutaneous ultrasonic lithotripsy, extracorporeal shock-wave lithotripsy, an ultrasonic transducer passed into the ureter during cystoscopy, a basket passed through a cystoscope, and nephrolithotomy. Lithotripsy is much less invasive and is replacing surgery.

SIGNS AND SYMPTOMS

Typically, there is sudden onset of flank pain that is unrelated to any activity. It often wakes the patient from a sound sleep. Usually the pain radiates to the groin, specifically the scrotum or vulva. This can be an indicator that the stone has passed to the lower third of the ureter. Once the stone passes into the bladder, frequency, urgency, and dysuria often occur, which mimic a urinary tract infection (see Chap. 18-6). Hematuria is variable, but often visible blood is present in the urine. Nausea and vomiting accompany the pain. However, these patients can present atypically.

The patient may appear agitated, apprehensive, and unable to sit or lie still. There may be costovertebral angle (CVA) tenderness. Usually the patient is afebrile. The abdomen is soft, with no rebound or guarding.

DIAGNOSTIC CONSIDERATIONS

The following diseases and conditions can mimic renal stones:

- Aneurysm of the abdominal aorta
- Acute pyelonephritis
- Biliary colic
- Appendicitis
- Pancreatitis
- Bowel obstruction
- Pelvic inflammatory disease
- Diverticulitis
- Gastroenteritis
- Perforated ulcer

SPECIAL CONSIDERATIONS

Pregnant patients should be referred to a hospital for evaluation and observation.

LABORATORY STUDIES

Urinalysis will show hematuria, either microscopic or frank blood. It also may show leukocytes when a stone is associated with a urinary tract infection (UTI). A urine culture can identify urea-splitting organisms commonly associated with struvite stones, such as *Proteus* spp. Serum electrolytes may show abnormalities reflecting the composition of the kidney stone, such as hypercalcemia and elevated uric acid.

The stone, if passed, should be retained and sent to the laboratory for analysis.

RADIOLOGIC AND IMAGING STUDIES

A KUB (kidneys, ureters, and bladder) film shows the presence of stones 90 percent of the time. Ultrasound can show the location and size of the stone as well as the condition of the kidneys. Ultrasound is the preferred choice when a patient is allergic to contrast dye. Intravenous pyelography (IVP) is the diagnostic imaging study of choice. It can determine stone location and the degree of obstruction and evaluate renal function.

TREATMENT
Pharmacologic Management

Pain Control

Ketorolac (Toradol) 60 mg intramuscularly is an effective analgesic for renal stones. It acts on the smooth muscle of the ureter, diminishing the spasms. If it fails, narcotics are indicated for pain control of renal colic. Meperidine (Demerol) 50 to 100 mg intramuscularly or morphine 10 to 15 mg intramuscularly can be used for this purpose. Even before imaging studies are performed, nausea and vomiting may need to be controlled with promethazine rectal suppositories or intramuscular promethazine. This will also help relax the patient.

Most patients can be managed on an outpatient basis. With adequate pain control, rest, sufficient oral (6 to 8 oz of water per hour) or intravenous (normal saline) hydration, and straining of the urine, 90 percent of stones can be passed. Patients should be cautioned not to overhydrate, as this can damage the kidney.

Patient Education

Appropriate diet modifications, if indicated, should be discussed. These modifications include decreased animal protein, increased fruits and vegetables, decreased dairy products, and decreased sodium.

Disposition

A referral should be made to a urologist for follow-up. The stone, if obtained, should be analyzed for its composition, and a more thorough workup can be done if warranted.

COMPLICATIONS AND RED FLAGS

Hospitalization may be required when a patient has persistent nausea and vomiting that prevents oral hydration and the use of oral analgesics, fever or other indications of sepsis, evidence of deteriorating renal function, stones larger than 5 to 7 mm, and extravasation of contrast dye from the ureter.

Drug Seekers

In the outpatient setting, providers should be aware of the "well-dressed patient from out of town who presents with classic renal colic" and is requesting a narcotic only "until the stone passes." Often this patient will have an allergy to nonsteroidal anti-inflammatory drugs (NSAIDs) (thus, eliminating the Toradol), and only Demerol will work. The patient also will request a written prescription for certain narcotics. This is the classic presentation of a drug-seeking patient. These clever patients always have gross or microscopic hematuria, which usually is added to the urine by pricking their own fingers.

Pyelonephritis

DISCUSSION

Infection of the kidneys is an acute disorder and can vary from mild symptoms to sepsis. In young, previously healthy adults, pyelonephritis frequently follows a urinary tract infection, especially when there is a delay in seeking care (see Chap. 18-6).

The predominant pathogens are gram-negative, including *Escherichia coli, Proteus* spp., *Klebsiella* spp., *Enterobacter* spp., and *Pseudomonas* spp. Bacteria ascend the ureter from the bladder and then invade the kidney.

Pyelonephritis is usually unilateral. It can rapidly progress to sepsis.

SIGNS AND SYMPTOMS

Fever, chills, flank or back pain, dysuria, nausea, vomiting, diarrhea, and tachycardia may be seen. On examination, the patient will have costovertebral tenderness, fever, and a corresponding rapid pulse and may appear sick or "toxic-looking."

DIAGNOSTIC CONSIDERATIONS

Pyelonephritis can mimic many abdominal diseases and conditions:

- Renal calculi
- Appendicitis
- Diverticulitis
- Pancreatitis
- Cholecystitis
- Obstructive uropathy (stricture, etc.)
- Pelvic inflammatory disease (especially from *Chlamydia*)

SPECIAL CONSIDERATIONS

Infants and children should always be screened for pyelonephritis and urosepsis when they present with fever, vomiting, or lethargy. The elderly may present with a vaguely altered mental status or an abdominal complaint. Immunocompromised patients presenting with fever should have a urinalysis as part of the workup. Pregnant women with fever or vomiting should always be screened.

LABORATORY STUDIES

The following studies are indicated:

- *Urinalysis with culture and sensitivity.* A catheterization specimen should be obtained if the patient is unable to void or if the patient is menstrual. Culture results take 1 or 2 days.
- *Blood culture.* Infants and young children, the elderly, and the immunocompromised if they appear toxic should have blood cultures.
- *Complete blood count with differential.* This is especially indicated if a patient is very ill-appearing.

RADIOLOGIC STUDIES

Radiologic studies usually are not indicated. If the patient is quite ill, an ultrasound may be done and can detect swelling of the kidney.

TREATMENT

Antibiotic regimens vary from 3 days to 3 weeks. A 10- to 14-day course of treatment is recommended. In outpatient settings, a single antibiotic frequently is used for mild cases. The choices include

- Trimethoprim-sulfamethoxazole 160 and 800 mg bid (Bactrim DS or Septra DS)
- Ciprofloxacin 500 mg bid (Cipro)
- Norfloxacin (Noroxin) 400 mg bid
- Clavulanic acid (Augmentin) 500 mg tid

If a patient is very ill, intravenous antibiotics are usually initiated and given until the fever is gone. Then the patient can switch to an oral antibiotic regimen consisting of

- Ceftriaxone (Rocefin) up to 2 g daily
- Ampicillin 1 g qd and gentamycin 1.5 mg/kg every 8 h

Pain medications can include acetaminophen or acetaminophen with codeine.

Supportive Measures

Supportive measures include rest and adequate fluid intake.

Patient Education

When treated in the outpatient setting, these patients need to understand the importance of taking medication as directed.

DISPOSITION

At least one follow-up visit is recommended 1 or 2 weeks after antibiotics are finished for a repeat urine culture.

COMPLICATIONS AND RED FLAGS

Hospitalization is required if a patient appears septic, has a chronic underlying disease such as diabetes, has intractable nausea and vomiting, or is very young or very old. Important considerations for others include being pregnant, male gender (young adult), and immunocompromised or immunosuppressed patients (HIV, transplants, cancer, etc.). If a patient does not improve in 48 to 72 h, renal calculi, abscess, and necrosis need to be considered.

BIBLIOGRAPHY

Coe FL, Favus MJ: Nephrolithiasis, in Fauci AS, Braunwald E, Isselbacher KJ, et al: *Harrison's Principles and Practice of Internal Medicine,* 14th ed. New York, McGraw-Hill, 1998.

Howes DS: Urinary tract infections, in Tintinalli JE, Ruiz E, Krome RL: *Emergency Medicine.* New York, McGraw-Hill, 1996, pp 527–532.

Krupp MA (ed): Urinary tract infections, in *Current Medical Diagnosis and Treatment.* Stamford, CT, Appleton & Lange, 1994.

Peacock WF: Urologic stone disease, in Tintinalli JE, Ruiz E, Krone RL: *Emergency Medicine.* New York, McGraw-Hill, 1996, pp 549–553.

Stamm WE, Hooten TM: Management of urinary tract infections in adults. *New Engl J Med* 329:1328–1334, 1993.

Stamm WE: Urinary tract infections and pyelonephritis, in Fauci AS, Braunwald E, Isselbacher KJ, et al: *Harrison's Principles and Practices of Internal Medicine,* 14th ed. New York, McGraw-Hill, 1998, pp 817–824.

Chapter 18–6
URINARY TRACT INFECTIONS
Rodney L. Moser

DISCUSSION

Urinary tract infections (UTIs) are among the most common bacterial infections in a primary care practice, especially in females of all ages. There are between 6 million and 7 million office visits annually in the United States for acute, uncomplicated UTIs, with an annual health cost that exceeds $1 billion.

There is a 50-fold increase in UTIs in adult women after they become sexually active. UTIs frequently occur in children, especially girls over age 1. Before age 1, UTIs are actually twice as common in boys. This is due to obstructive anomalies such as urethral stenosis. UTIs in healthy adult males are relatively uncommon compared to women and are predominantly related to prostate infections, although elderly men often have UTIs that result from urinary tract obstructive syndromes.

UTIs are subdivided into upper and lower tract infections. Upper tract infections include pyelonephritis (see Chap. 18-5), and lower tract infections include cystitis, urethritis, and prostatitis (see Chap. 18-3). Urethritis is an infection of the urethral opening that is seen primarily in adolescence and is associated with sexually transmitted diseases such as chlamydia (see Chap. 9-6). Cystitis is an infection of the bladder. Pyelonephritis is an infection of the renal parenchyma with systemic involvement. Infection in any part of the urinary tract may spread to another part (e.g., cystitis can spread in an ascending fashion and lead to pyelonephritis). Most infections are of the ascending type. The only anatomic defenses against ascending infections are an acidic urine, large and dilute volume, complete bladder emptying, and a tract free of any obstruction.

The commonality here is that all UTIs have a pathologic number of microorganisms causing infection and symptoms. Urine is sterile until it is contaminated with pathogens at the distal urethra. Bacteriuria is detected in over 1 percent of all females. Virtually any organism introduced into the urinary tract can cause infection. The majority of these infections are caused by fecal flora (Table 18-6-1).

Acute UTIs can cause inflammation of any part of the urinary tract, resulting in intense hyperemia and often bleeding.

SIGNS AND SYMPTOMS

In lower tract infections in women and older children, a sudden or gradual onset of dysuria (burning), frequency, and urgency is considered classic. Patients also complain of lower abdominal (suprapubic and/or bladder) discomfort and foul-smelling turbid urine. A particularly annoying symptom is strangury, or the voiding of tiny drops of urine, accompanied by urethral spasm.

Table 18-6-1. Common Microorganisms That Cause Urinary Tract Infections

Organism	Percentage of Cases
Escherichia coli	75–90
Enterobacter	2–5
Klebsiella	2–5
Proteus	1–2
Miscellaneous*	3–4

* *Pseudomonas, Staphylococcus epidermidis, Chlamydia, Ureaplasma/ Mycoplasma,* and others.

Gross hematuria is not an unusual presenting sign. Fever and other constitutional symptoms are variable. There is no true costovertebral angle (CVA) tenderness in lower tract infections, although referred low back discomfort is possible.

The symptoms of upper tract involvement are more systemic and include CVA pain and tenderness, abdominal pain, fever and chills, headache, malaise, and vomiting.

UTIs may be asymptomatic in the elderly and in diabetic patients. In children, the signs and symptoms appear to be age-related. Infants may present with irritability, fever, poor feeding, and even failure to thrive. All infants with a fever of undetermined origin should have a urinalysis. In children over age 3 or 4, the symptoms are more classic.

A large number of dysuric patients do not have a UTI, and this may explain the many negative cultures seen in "classic" patients. Urethritis secondary to sexual trauma and vaginitis, particularly monilial, are likely diagnostic considerations. In little girls, dysuria can be caused by a variety of local irritants, such as soaps (bubble baths), detergents, fabric softeners (especially the drier sheet type), poor hygiene, masturbation, and pinworms. Children who are sexually abused often present with UTIs.

DIAGNOSTIC CONSIDERATIONS

In adult women, vaginitis (particularly monilial) is the most common comorbid finding. Vaginal yeast infections can cause profound urethral irritation and dysuria. Other vaginal infections, such as bacterial vaginosis and trichomoniasis can present with dysuria (see Chaps. 12-2, 12-3, and 12-11). Sexually transmitted diseases such as chlamydia, gonorrhea, and herpes simplex infections should be considered, especially in heterosexually active women with negative or borderline bacteriuria or negative urine cultures.

Since UTIs correlate with sexual activity, urethral microtrauma during coitus can be responsible for UTI-type symptoms. Since many women with classic UTI symptoms avoid a careful examination, these findings are often missed. Colposcopy, if available, may reveal tiny periurethral fissures.

SPECIAL CONSIDERATIONS

In the pediatric population, a standard urologic recommendation is that all boys regardless of age and all girls under age 6 have a thorough workup after just one confirmed UTI. In girls over age 6, a workup is usually done after a second UTI (see "Radiologic and Imaging Studies," below).

UTIs are more common in sexually active women who use diaphragms and/or spermaticides for contraception (see Chap. 12-14). They are also more common in diabetics, immunocompromised patients, the elderly (especially those who are bedridden), and spinal cord patients (especially those who use intermittent self-catheterization or indwelling catheters).

Pregnant females may have asymptomatic bacteriuria up to 15 percent of the time. If untreated, a simple UTI has a 20 to 40 percent chance of developing into pyelonephritis, which can lead to a premature birth or other perinatal complications.

LABORATORY STUDIES

A complete urinalysis (chemical dipstick and microscopy) is a quick and cost-effective study that frequently can be done in the office. The specimen must be a fresh, clean midstream catch. One should avoid accepting specimens brought in from home in plastic containers and baby food jars. Urine is a good culture medium for bacteria, even at room temperature. The urinalysis should be done within an hour, or the specimen should be refrigerated and done within 18 h. Specimens obtained by straight catheterization or percutaneous suprapubic aspiration are also appropriate. Pediatric specimens obtained in sterile bags with an adhesive back applied over the genitalia (Tin-Kol bag) are easily contaminated with skin flora and fecal material.

Since many patients with a history of UTIs tend to medicate themselves with old antibiotics or phenazopyridine hydrochloride (Pyridium), a careful medication history is essential. Chemical dipsticks test a variety of items from pH to nitrites. Increased nitrites in the urine are a suggestive marker for a UTI.

Microscopy of fresh spun or unspun urine will quickly reveal pyuria or bacteriuria. More than 10 white blood cells (WBCs) per high-power field is considered abnormal; however, many active UTIs have "packed fields" of WBCs and red blood cells (RBCs). The presence of leukocyte casts indicates parenchymal involvement. If the urinalysis is normal, the patient should be examined carefully for other diagnostic possibilities.

Urine cultures, including sensitivity assessments, are needed in chronic or recurrent infections but need not be done routinely for cost containment.

RADIOLOGIC AND IMAGING STUDIES

Uncomplicated, infrequent UTIs do not require radiologic or imaging studies in most cases. If warranted, renal imaging studies, including a voiding cystoureterogram (VCUG) and renal ultrasonography, are the standard workup. CT may also be useful in selected patients. Intravenous pyelography is infrequently used in the evaluation of UTIs in children unless there is a strong possibility of structural anomalies. The routine use of a 99m-DMSA renal scan is useful only in acute infections.

Cystoscopy often is done to detect abnormalities of the urethra or bladder.

TREATMENT OF UNCOMPLICATED INFECTIONS

Pharmacologic Management

Although 1-day and 3-day regimens are often touted as being more cost-effective, having fewer side effects, and leading to better patient compliance, they should be limited to very select, uncomplicated patients with initial UTIs.

A variety of antibiotic choices are available to treat UTIs, including but not limited to the following 7- to 10-day regimens:

Standard Oral Regimen for Adult, Nonpregnant Women

This regimen consists of the following:

- Trimethoprim-sulfamethoxazole (Septra DS, Bactrim DS) bid for 7 to 10 days
- Nitrofurantoin monohydrate macrocrystals (Macrobid) 100 mg bid for 7 days
- Cephalexin 500 mg qid for 7 to 10 days

Treatment of Pregnant Females

Pregnant females are given nitrofurantoin monohydrate macrocrystals (Macrobid) 100 mg bid for 7 days. Penicillin and cephalosporins are also safe and effective. Aminoglycosides, tetracyclines, and quinolones should be avoided. Sulfonamides should not be used in the last 6 weeks of pregnancy.

Treatment of Children

For children older than 2 months of age who are not vomiting, oral sulfisoxazole (Gantrisin) or trimethoprim-sulfamethoxazole (Bactrim, Septra) suspension in doses based on weight can be given.

For children under 2 months, parenteral antibiotics starting with ampicillin and gentamycin or cefotaxime should be used, depending on the urine culture. Any child, regardless of age, who appears toxic should be admitted and placed on parenteral antibiotics pending clinical improvement.

Older children can be treated with antibiotic therapy similar to that used for adults, with the dose adjusted for weight.

NOTES AND PEARLS

Tired of waiting all day for an infant or toddler to urinate into a bag? Try a few minutes of rhythmic "tapping" (like percussion) over a full bladder, about once a second. This may stimulate urination in a minute or so. Have the parent hold a sterile urine cup to catch the flow. Give it a try.

BIBLIOGRAPHY

Hanno PM, Wein AJ: *Clinical Manual of Urology,* 2d ed. New York, McGraw-Hill, 1994.

Lim PB, Peterson JC: Urinary tract infection, in Tisher CC, Wilcox SG (eds): *Nephrology for the House Officer.* Baltimore, Williams & Wilkins, 1989.

Wasson J: *The Common Symptom Guide,* 3d ed. New York, McGraw-Hill, 1992.

INDEX

Page numbers followed by the letters *f* and *t* indicate figures and tables, respectively.